Imaging of Diseases
of the Chest

PETER ARMSTRONG, M.B., B.S., F.R.C.R.
Professor and Vice Chairman
Department of Radiology
University of Virginia Health Sciences Center
Charlottesville, Virginia

ALAN G. WILSON, F.R.C.P., F.R.C.R.
Consultant Radiologist
St. George's Hospital
London, England

PAUL DEE, M.B., B.S., F.R.C.R.
Professor of Radiology
University of Virginia Health Sciences Center
Charlottesville, Virginia

YEAR BOOK MEDICAL PUBLISHERS, INC.
CHICAGO • LONDON • BOCA RATON • LITTLETON, MASS.

1 2 3 4 5 6 7 8 9 0 YC 94 93 92 91 90

Library of Congress Cataloging-in-Publication Data

Armstrong, Peter, 1940–
 Imaging of diseases of the chest / Peter Armstrong, Alan G. Wilson, Paul M. Dee
   p.   cm.
 Includes bibliographies and index.
 ISBN 0-8151-0350-6
 1. Chest—Imaging. 2. Chest—Diseases—Diagnosis. I. Wilson, Alan G. II. Dee, Paul. III. Title.
[DNLM: 1. Diagnostic Imaging. 2 Lung Diseases—diagnosis. WF 600 A737i]
RC941.A75   1990
617.5′40757—dc20   89-8881
DNLM/DLC   CIP
for Library of Congress

Sponsoring Editor: James D. Ryan
Associate Managing Editor, Manuscript Services: Deborah Thorp
Production Project Coordinator: Carol A. Reynolds
Proofroom Supervisor: Barbara M. Kelly

To our families

CONTRIBUTORS

PETER ARMSTRONG, M.B., B.S., F.R.C.R.

Professor and Vice Chairman
Department of Radiology
University of Virginia Health Sciences Center
Charlottesville, Virginia

WILLIAM C. BLACK, M.D.

Assistant Professor of Radiology
National Institutes of Health
Bethesda, Maryland

VALERIE A. BROOKEMAN, PH.D., M.D.

Assistant Professor of Radiology
University of Virginia Health Sciences Center
Charlottesville, Virginia

BARBARA Y. CROFT, PH.D.

Associate Professor of Radiology
University of Virginia Health Sciences Center
Charlottesville, Virginia

PAUL DEE, M.B., B.S., F.R.C.R.

Professor of Radiology
University of Virginia Health Sciences Center
Charlottesville, Virginia

THEODORE E. KEATS, M.D.

Professor and Chairman
Department of Radiology
University of Virginia Health Sciences Center
Charlottesville, Virginia

THOMAS L. POPE, JR., M.D.

Associate Professor of Radiology
Department of Radiology
University of Virginia Health Sciences Center
Charlottesville, Virginia

ALAN G. WILSON, F.R.C.P., F.R.C.R.

Consultant Radiologist
St. George's Hospital
London, England

PREFACE

This book has been written to provide radiologists, chest physicians, and thoracic surgeons with a one-volume account of chest imaging, primarily in the adult patient. An attempt has been made to present an integrated review of the appearances encountered in diseases of the lungs, pleura, and mediastinum using the various imaging modalities available in a modern radiology department. Clearly, the plain chest radiograph remains the most frequently used modality in patients with chest disease, and its interpretation continues to be a great challenge. Therefore, the chest radiograph has been accorded the preeminence it deserves, but at the same time, attention has been directed to ultrasound, magnetic resonance imaging, radionuclide imaging, and, above all, computed tomography.

The clinical and pathological aspects of conditions such as bronchial carcinoma, pulmonary embolism, and chest trauma are widely known, and detailed discussion of these aspects has been deliberately avoided. On the other hand, in less commonly encountered conditions, such as the immunological disorders and drug- or radiation-induced disease, we have chosen to deal with the clinicopathologic aspects in more detail. Our aim has been to provide answers to the many questions that, in our experience, arise in the day-to-day practice of chest radiology.

Peter Armstrong, M.B., B.S., F.R.C.R.

—ACKNOWLEDGMENTS

So many individuals contribute to a medical text book that it is impossible to acknowledge all their help individually. We have had the help of many superb secretaries. In particular, Pat West, Shirley Yowell, Geneva Shifflett, Diana Bowman, and Kelly Powell of the University of Virginia (UVa) and Pat Vecchi of St. George's Hospital, London, have all helped with typing manuscripts and making photocopies. Sherry Deane, the best personal secretary anyone could ever hope to have, typed and retyped the many drafts of chapters, prepared reference lists, and generally assisted with the preparation of manuscripts and photographs. To her go my heartfelt thanks. Carol Chowdhry, our editorial assistant, was completely invaluable both for the many hours spent educating and re-educating us on points of style and grammar and for checking and numbering the numerous references in this book. Ursula Bunch of the UVa Department of Biomedical Communications, was equally obsessional in preparing the photographs to an extremely high standard. Without good images, a book such as this is of little value. We are, therefore, pleased to express our sincere gratitude to them both for all their efforts. The mammoth task of sorting photographs fell to my daughter Natasha who from age 13 to 15 spent many hours correlating photographs with original radiographs/scans—all by pattern recognition. Her contribution to this book is gratefully acknowledged. My great friend and collaborator on so many projects, Dr. Martin Wastie of Nottingham, England, gave generously of his time and considerable expertise in suggesting revisions for the chapter on pulmonary embolism and contributed many of the pictures. Dr. William C. Black contributed several of the magnetic resonance images in this book.

Chest radiology is a team effort between radiologists, chest surgeons, and pulmonary internists. It has been my great fortune to have always worked with thoracic surgeons and physicians who were friendly, cooperative colleagues with a great interest in radiology. First, Mr. Angus MacArthur of King's College Hospital, London, inspired me with his clear-thinking, intelligent approach to thoracic surgery and his insights into the radiology of the chest. He, together with that great teacher of chest radiology, Dr. George Simon, were my early mentors. On arriving in Charlottesville, I found Dr. George Minor to be a fine and knowledgeable surgeon. He was succeeded by another remarkable surgeon, Dr. Tom Daniel. They will recognize in these pages many of the cases that they have operated or consulted upon. Equally, Dr. Philip Hugh-Jones of King's College Hospital and Dr. Dudley Rochester of UVa, together with all physicians in their respective departments, have contributed, not only to this book but to my education. Thanks also to Year Book Medical Publishers, notably Jim Ryan, Carol Reynolds, and Deborah Thorp. I would also like to thank Dr. Norman J. Knorr and Dr. Robert M. Carey, both of whom were Dean of the University of Virginia Medical School during the period this book was being written. Without the support and resources of the medical school this book would not have been possible. Finally, I would like to thank Dr. Theodore E. Keats, Chairman of the Department of Radiology, for his continued support and friendship. His unfailing sense of humor and his wide knowledge of radiology have been an inspiration to all who have worked and trained at UVa.

Peter Armstrong, M.B., B.S., F.R.C.R.

CONTENTS

Technical Considerations

PLAIN CHEST RADIOGRAPHS

The standard views of the chest are the erect posteroanterior (PA) and lateral projections, both of which are exposed at total lung capacity. In a properly positioned PA examination, the medial ends of the clavicles are seen equidistant from the edges of the relevant thoracic vertebrae. (Clearly, in patients with scoliosis or chest wall deformity this assessment is more difficult.) The scapulae should be held as far to the side of the chest as possible. This position is best achieved by rotating the patient's shoulders forward and placing the backs of his or her wrists on the iliac crests. In a correctly exposed film, the entire lung should be visible, including the portions behind the heart, as well as the complex interfaces of the lung with the mediastinum. Just how much lung is visible depends on the technical factors, notably the kilovoltage used for the examination and the film-screen combination chosen.

The trend over the past 10 to 15 years has been to convert from low kilovoltage (60 to 80 kV) to high kilovoltage (above 125 kV) examinations. (At one time 350-kV examinations were used, but as no diagnostic advantages over 140-kV examinations were demonstrated,[6] the technique has been abandoned.) Low-kV films do, however, have some advantages. They are excellent for demonstrating those portions of the lung not "hidden" by the heart, mediastinum, ribs, and breast shadows, and the contrast between the lung vessels and surrounding air in the lung is the best that can be achieved with conventional filming. Similarly, lung nodules,[7] particularly miliary nodulation of the lungs, stand out more clearly with low kV images and calcifications are seen to advantage.

High-kV films have several advantages over the low-kV films.[9] The better penetration of the mediastinum, heart, and breast tissues allows one to see lung and airway details through these structures. Also, because the coefficients of x-ray absorption of bone and soft tissue approach one another with higher kilovoltage, the skeletal structures no longer hide the lungs to the same degree. It is sometimes a surprise to realize how much of the lung is overlaid by ribs and clavicles. The high-kV images thus demonstrate much more of the lung. High-kV images are preferable for routine examinations of the lungs and mediastinum because most information about the mediastinum on plain chest radiographs depends on distortions of the lung interfaces with the mediastinum and on seeing the major airways. Also, because the exposure times are shorter and less scattered radiation strikes the intensifying screen with high-kV technique, structures within the lung have a sharper outline. (Scattered radiation is greater with higher kilovoltage, but the use of a grid or an air gap means that there is a net reduction of scattered radiation degrading the image compared with low-kV, nongrid techniques.)

At high kilovoltage, an air gap can be used to disperse scattered radiation. Such air gaps are typically 6 inches in depth. The image produced is comparable to that obtained with a grid, and radiation exposure to the patient is also comparable.[14] The potential disadvantage of an unsharp image and unwanted magnification that results from increasing the distance between the object and film is compensated for by increasing the focus-film (source-to-image) distance. This increased distance is technically possible with high-kV techniques, and focus-film distances of 10 to 12 feet are commonly employed.

Films Made With Portable Equipment

The use of portable x-ray machines to obtain chest radiographs has the obvious and very real advantage that the examination can be done without moving the patient from his or her bed. There are, however, many disadvantages to using portable equipment. The shorter focus-film distance results in undesirable magnification, and high-kV techniques cannot be used because of the impracticability of aligning the x-ray beam with a grid. The maximum milliamperage available is also severely limited, necessitating longer exposure times to obtain adequate film blackening. Longer exposure times risk significant blurring of the image because of patient movement. Portable lateral studies, though technically possible, are not used routinely because they so often require long exposure times which lead to blurred images. Also, the radiation exposure to adjacent patients and to staff is inevitably higher than in frontal films. Not only is the machinery limited, but the fact that the patient is in bed imposes certain restrictions. They may have to be examined while supine or half upright and are often rotated. Even if the patient sits up, the chest is rarely as vertical as it is in a standing patient. More important, the patient cannot take as deep a breath if he or she is sitting in bed. This restriction is particularly true of obese subjects. Therefore, radiographs should be acquired with portable equipment only if the limitations of the technique are outweighed by the advantages of not having to move a patient.

Film-Screen Combinations

The recording medium is as important as the exposure factors. Film-screen combinations have changed dramatically over the past 10 to 15 years. Two major advances have occurred: (1) the introduction of "faster" screens without loss of resolution, through the use of rare earth phosphors, and (2) the introduction of wide-latitude film.

All conventional chest radiographs are produced by exposing cassettes containing a film sandwiched between intensifying screens. The film is exposed directly by the x-rays, but most of the film blackening comes from light emitted from the intensifying screens. The introduction of a variety of rare earth crystals has improved light emission over that of the calcium tungstate crystal screens previously in universal use. This advance reduced the exposure necessary to cause film blackening and permitted shorter exposure times with resulting sharper images, a particular advantage for films being exposed with portable equipment.

Not only did the intensifying screens improve, but new film emulsions were introduced. Wide-latitude film is of particular interest to the chest radiologist. Compared with conventional film, wide-latitude film provides the ability to display minor differences in x-ray absorption (similar to widening the window width at computed tomography [CT].

Extra Views

The frontal and lateral projections suffice for most radiographic purposes. Other useful views include the lateral decubitus, lordotic, and oblique views.

1. *Lateral decubitus view.* This view is not, as its name would imply, a lateral view. It is a frontal view taken with a horizontal beam while the patient is lying on his or her left or right side. Its major purpose is to demonstrate movement of fluid, usually pleural fluid. If a pleural effusion is not loculated, it will gravitate, to some extent, into the dependent portions of the pleural cavity. If the patient is lying on his or her side, the fluid will layer between the chest wall and lung edge. Because the ribs, unlike the diaphragm, are always identifiable, the comparison of standard frontal views with lateral decubitus views provides a reliable way of diagnosing free pleural fluid (see Chapter 14). Similarly, air-fluid levels can be confirmed by proving their constant horizontal orientation regardless of the position of the patient. Lateral decubitus views have also been recommended to show shifts in pulmonary edema with change in position, but few centers have adopted this practice.

2. *Lordotic view.* A lordotic view is a form of oblique view in which the beam is angled 15° to 20° craniad. This angulation is achieved either by positioning the patient upright and angling the beam or by leaving the beam horizontal and leaning the patient backward. The lordotic view is intended to demonstrate the lung apices free from the superimposed shadows of the clavicle and first rib. It is particularly

useful in distinguishing pulmonary shadows, which could be significant, from incidental osteochondromas or bony irregularities of the costochondral junctions. If a pulmonary lesion is clearly present but further details are needed, then investigation with tomography, either computed or conventional, is usually preferable to the lordotic view.

3. *Oblique view.* Oblique views are the standard extra views for demonstrating rib lesions. They are rarely used in cases of pulmonary disease except, on occasion, to localize a pulmonary nodule.

Conventional Tomograms

In conventional tomography, the x-ray tube is linked to the film cassette holder by a bar, so that the tube and cassette move in opposite directions around an axis. The concept exploits the fact that blurring of an object is least when it is on the same level as the axis of rotation of the x-ray tube and cassette.

Conventional tomography in chest disease has been superseded by CT. Where CT is not available, the indications for conventional tomography are

1. To show the edge of an intrathoracic mass (e.g., a pulmonary nodule) and to detect any calcification or cavitation within it.
2. To accurately localize an opacity.
3. To clarify the presence of rib destruction.
4. To analyze hilar shadows.
5. To clarify an indefinite pulmonary lesion. It should, however, be realized that conventional tomography, unlike CT, will rarely demonstrate an abnormality in areas that are clearly normal on conventional radiographs.

NEWER IMAGING MODALITIES

The technology available for chest examinations in a modern x-ray department is very complex. In this chapter we will explain the principles of producing images with the newer modalities of digital radiography, CT, and magnetic resonance imaging (MRI) (radionuclide studies are discussed in Chapter 8) using language that is as nontechnical as possible. Before the modalities are discussed individually, two basic components of all imaging techniques, including conventional radiology—namely, contrast and spatial resolution—are worth considering.

Contrast resolution is the comparison of degrees of blackness of particular areas on the image. It re-

flects the number of shades of gray that can be demonstrated. To be useful, this contrast must be appreciable by the human eye on the image being examined. Spatial resolution refers to the minimum size (area) that can be resolved. Spatial resolution is usually expressed as line pairs per millimeter, a unit which refers to the greatest number of lines that can be separately identified on an image. Line pairs refer to alternating black and white lines of equal thickness, adjacent black and white lines constituting a line pair, so that one line pair per millimeter would be a black and white line of ½ mm each, and four line pairs per millimeter would be four alternating black and white lines, each line being ⅛ mm thick.

Both contrast and spatial resolution are important in interpreting an image. Unless one can distinguish some difference in contrast between two areas on a radiograph, it is not possible to see the edge between them, however good the spatial resolution. Engineers designing imaging systems strive for excellence in both spatial and contrast resolution. Certain examinations have inherently good contrast: for example, CT, MRI, radionuclide imaging, and ultrasound. However, spatial resolution with these systems is not as good as with conventional radiography, the system that has the best spatial resolution, but also has significant limitations of contrast resolution. Digital radiography is being developed to improve the contrast resolution of conventional filming while trying to preserve the same spatial resolution.

The best images are seen when both spatial and contrast resolution are excellent, but considerable information is obtainable from images that are excellent in just one or the other of these parameters. For instance, radionuclide images have poor spatial resolution, but contrast differences between normal and pathologic tissues are often so great that valuable information is still obtained.

Contrast resolution with CT and MRI is excellent. The range of densities is in excess of 2,000, and these can, if desired, all be displayed. The spatial resolution of CT and MRI is poor compared with that of conventional film. Thus, CT scanning is useful when excellent contrast resolution is valuable, whereas plain films retain their utility when spatial resolution is the key. For example, plain films may demonstrate the edge of a pulmonary shadow to advantage, whereas CT demonstrates the range of densities within that shadow. One point about contrast resolution may at first glance appear confusing. CT, despite its poor spatial resolution, can demonstrate smaller pulmonary nodules than can be seen with conventional techniques. But the pulmonary nodule is seen because enough picture elements show soft tissue density contrasted against the low density of the adjacent lung.

Digital Chest Radiography

Digital imaging is used in many ways in the modern radiology department; CT and MRI are exclusively digital techniques. The term digital radiograph refers to a digitized image with the same basic characteristics as a conventional radiograph, but formed from digital information.[5] Such an image can be viewed or photographed from a TV monitor, or it can be "written" onto a film by a laser device.

All conventional radiographic images, whether on film or on TV monitors from a fluoroscope, are analog pictures. In other words, the image is made up of a continuous range of densities. A digital image is composed of a preset number of discrete densities with a small, but definite, "jump" between each. The specific density is represented by a number that can be manipulated by a computer. Digital computers cannot process analog data without conversion to digital form.

The advantage of creating digital chest radiographs are

1. A greater range of contrast in the image. Digital systems generally provide 2^{10} (1,024) or more discrete contrast levels. The blackening of conventional film is nonlinear, so that contrast differences at the extremes are less than in the midrange. Digitization allows all contrast levels to be displayed equally.

2. The ability to use a computer to manipulate contrast levels and windows and to process the image. This allows the radiologist to see on just one image such low-contrast interfaces as the mediastinal boundaries, intrathoracic catheters and tubes, nodules behind the heart or the domes of the diaphragm, and subtle calcification within pulmonary nodules.

3. With digital imaging, the image density can be controlled, and acceptable images can, therefore, be generated at radiation doses that would result in severely overexposed or underexposed conventional radiographs. Also, in some of the systems, x-ray dose reduction can be achieved.

4. The ability to store the information in high-density form on digital archiving devices allows rapid and easy retrieval. Digital images will be required if picture archiving and communications systems (PACS) are to become a reality. Currently, images derived from CT, MRI, nuclear medicine, ultrasound, and angiography comprise approximately 25% of the images in a large modern radiology department. The eventual aim of digital radiography is to be the final step on the road to an all-digital imaging department. Such a department could eliminate the problems of film storage, lost films, and unavailability of images when more than one physician wishes to view them simultaneously.

There are four basic methods of producing a digital radiograph of the chest:

1. The conventional chest radiograph can be digitized.[10] The major application is to create a digitized image for transmission to another site (teleradiology).

2. The image from a fluorescent screen can be digitized. This is usually done using a digital TV camera placed at a port on the image intensifier. This method has been widely used for digital subtraction angiography. For chest radiography, it requires an image intensifier with a diameter of at least 40 cm. With such a system, a chest radiograph is exposed in the conventional way, and the whole chest is imaged with a single broad-area x-ray beam using a very short exposure time.[4, 13] The spatial resolution of such systems depends on the matrix, which currently is in the order of 1,024 × 1,024.

3. A fan-shaped or pencil-shaped (flying spot) x-ray beam that progressively scans the chest can be directed through the patient on to an array of digital detectors.[1, 3, 8] A major advantage of narrow beams and detectors aligned to those beams is reduction in scatter. (Scattered radiation is a major cause of reduced contrast and spatial resolution in broad-area beam systems.) These systems take several seconds to complete an image, and any movement of the patient causes the image to be disjointed. Again, the spatial resolution depends on the matrix, which currently is 1,024 × 1,024.

4. The fourth type of system uses standard radiologic equipment but employs a reusable photostimulable phosphor plate (europium-doped barium fluorohalide) instead of an x-ray film or screen.[11] The plate fits into standard film cassettes. A latent image is formed on the plate that can be converted into a digital code by a laser scanning device. The plate can be reused once the latent image has been erased. The digital information can then be manipulated and displayed in whatever fashion is desired. A major advantage is that the plates can be exposed with standard x-ray equipment and can therefore be

used for portable x-ray examinations. Other advantages include the short exposure time, the excellent exposure latitude of the system (overexposure or underexposure of films becomes virtually impossible), and the relatively high spatial resolution (2.5 to 4 line pairs/mm for an adult chest). The disadvantages are predominantly related to the high cost of processing the image.

It was hoped that the greater contrast resolution inherent in digital imaging would provide diagnostically useful information. So far, this extra information has been limited and has not justified widespread use of the equipment.[5] The competition from the conventional chest radiograph is substantial. Despite its poor contrast range, the conventional radiograph with appropriate exposure factors reveals almost all interfaces that can be seen with digital radiography. The plain chest radiograph offers excellent spatial resolution—on the order of 5 line pairs/mm. The spatial resolution of a digital system depends on the matrix size and on the size of the field of view. Modern digital systems use matrices of up to 1,024 × 1,024, and high-resolution TV monitors can display such a matrix without loss. If the whole chest is to be viewed at once on a TV monitor, this translates to a spatial resolution of somewhat less than 2 line pairs/mm. An approximate comparison between conventional and digital systems would be that the equivalent resolution of a 14 × 14-in. plain chest radiograph requires a matrix of the order of 7,000 × 7,000.[2] Zooming into a limited area using a 1,024 × 1,024 display matrix (say fourfold magnification) can come reasonably close to the spatial resolution of a plain chest radiograph.

The limiting factor in matrix size is cost. For each doubling of the matrix, the amount of digital information increases fourfold. The increase from 512 × 512 to 1,024 × 1,024 requires a fourfold increase in processing and storage power, and the increase to 2,048 × 2,048 will require yet another fourfold increase in capacity. This increase in data is of little use unless it can be rapidly transmitted along cables and displayed on TV monitors with an appropriate matrix.

Computed Tomography

CT scanning depends on the same basic physical principles as conventional radiography: namely, the absorption of x-rays by the atoms of the tissues. The difference is that by using multiple projections and computer calculations of radiographic density, it is possible to record finer differences in absorption than can be achieved with conventional films. Also, these differences can be displayed in sectional format without blurring.

The basic components of a CT machine are:

1. The x-ray tube, which is similar to the x-ray tube of a conventional machine.

2. An array of electronic x-ray detectors, placed opposite the tube, is housed in a scanning gantry. In stationary-rotate systems, there are up to 2,400 stationary detectors arranged in a ring around the patient, and the x-ray tube rotates within this ring, emitting a fan-shaped beam that always covers the whole width of the body part to be examined. In the rotate-rotate system, both the tube and x-ray detector array rotate synchronously around the patient, the number of detectors being enough to cover the fan-shaped beam, but no more.

3. Control devices to rotate the tube (and the detectors where appropriate) around the patient in a short enough time to ensure an image in one breath hold. With all modern machines, CT scanning of the chest can be performed with a total exposure time of 2 to 3 seconds per section. Ultrafast exposure of 50 msec can be achieved with specialized equipment.

4. A computer to reconstruct the image from x-rays received by the detectors.

5. Display devices.

The image is composed of a matrix of picture elements (pixels), the diameter of which determines the resolution of the image. Most machines operate with a fixed number of pixels in the matrix. Thus, the size of each pixel varies according to the diameter of the circle to be scanned. The narrower the scan circle, the smaller the area represented by the pixel and the higher the resolution. Pixel size on modern machines varies between 0.25 mm and 1 mm. By the selection of specific areas (so-called "targeting"), the optimal resolution of the image can be displayed, making available to the operator information that is in the raw data but not displayed when the whole-body section is viewed at one time.

The height of the pixel is determined by the thickness of the section and is chosen by the operator. In chest work, sections are usually 8–10 mm thick. Thus, each pixel has a definite volume. For this reason, it is frequently referred to as a volume element (voxel). The average radiographic density of each voxel is calculated by the computer, and the resulting image consists of a representation of the average density of each of the voxels in the section.

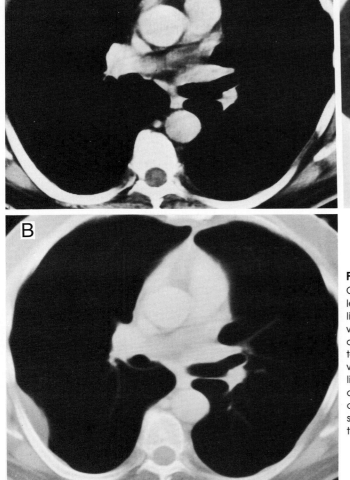

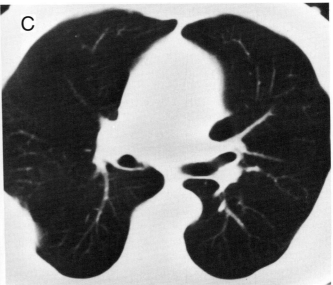

FIG 1–1.
CT scans of the chest illustrating the effects of varying window levels and window widths. The section shows an extrapleural lipoma lying against the right chest wall. **A,** window center 30 HU, window width 350 HU shows mediastinal soft tissue differences to advantage but does not show lung detail, nor is the lipoma easy to see. **B,** window center 30 HU, window width 1,500 HU shows the whole range of densities so that bone detail is well seen, the lipoma is recognizable as a soft tissue mass, and the mediastinal and the lung structures are visible but subtle distinctions of contrast are invisible. **C,** window center −600 HU, window width 1,000 HU shows lung detail to advantage but provides no information about the mediastinum other than outline.

The units have been arbitrarily chosen so that zero is water density and −1,000 is air density. These units have been named Hounsfield units (HUs) to commemorate Godfrey Hounsfield, the English engineer who developed the early CT machines. The image is displayed on video monitors, which are viewed directly by the operator and from which a photographic record can be made. The range of densities to be viewed is selected by the operator. This is necessary because neither the display systems nor the human eye can appreciate more than approximately 22 shades of gray, so no one image can reveal all the available information. Two variables are employed: (1) window width and (2) window center.

The window width is the number of Hounsfield units to be displayed. Any densities greater than the upper limit of the window are displayed as white, and any below the limit of the window are displayed as black. Between these two limits, the densities are displayed in shades of gray. The median density of the window chosen is the "center" or "level," and this center can be moved higher or lower at will, thus moving the window up or down through the range (Fig 1–1). The narrower the window width, the greater the contrast discrimination within the window. For individual problems, the operator can inspect the TV monitor while varying the window and center to select the image that best demonstrates the findings. In routine work, the window widths and centers selected vary from institution to institution.

The settings used by the author for hard copy images are:

1. For the mediastinum and chest wall: a window of 300 to 500 HU and a center of +30 HU.

2. For the lungs: a very wide window of 1,000 HU or more and a center of −400 to −600 HU.

3. For skeletal structures: the widest possible window and a center of 30 HU.

Advantages of Computed Tomography

1. The superior contrast resolution of CT allows the demonstration of structures within the mediastinum, and is far superior to the plain chest radiograph in demonstrating calcification in the pulmonary nodule.

2. The transaxial sectional display is a particular advantage in demonstrating the position of lesions seen in only one view on plain chest radiographs and in showing areas overlaid by other structures; for example, in the subpleural regions, the costophrenic sulci, and the perimediastinal areas.

3. The sectional image without superimposition from overlying structures may reveal details not available in nonsectional images. This advantage is exploited particularly in high-resolution, thin-section CT scans of the lung parenchyma.

Indications for Computed Tomography

1. CT scanning is used to elucidate abnormalities identified or suspected on plain chest radiographs, particularly mediastinal abnormalities. Outside the mediastinum, the major use of CT is to define the size, shape, and position of a shadow that cannot be satisfactorily evaluated from plain films alone.

2. More rarely, CT is used in patients with normal plain chest radiographs. To be cost effective, a definite indication must exist. In general, the indications are:

- Myasthenia gravis, to search for possible thymoma.
- Endocrinologic evidence of a possible mediastinal tumor (e.g., corticotropin-producing carcinoid tumors of the thymus, or hyperparathyroidism with no evidence of neck tumor).
- Malignant neoplasm known to involve or metastasize to mediastinal lymph nodes (e.g., bronchial carcinoma and lymphoma).
- Malignant neoplasm with a propensity to metastasize to the lung, provided the detection of pulmonary nodules would influence management.
- Lung carcinoma suspected because of repeated hemoptysis or positive sputum cytologic evidence in the face of negative findings at bronchoscopy.

Technique

When the whole chest is to be examined, the usual routine is to place the patient supine and obtain contiguous 8–10 mm-thick sections from the extreme lung bases to the apices. Thinner sections may be chosen if the lesion being investigated is very small or if partial volume artifacts may be influencing the interpretation of the image. If thinner sections are chosen, higher exposures and, therefore, greater radiation doses, are needed to maintain an adequate signal-to-noise ratio.

Selected patients are given intravenous contrast-enhancement, primarily to opacify the mediastinal and hilar blood vessels and the cardiac chambers. To achieve maximum opacification at desired levels, 50 to 100 cc of a standard water-soluble, iodine-containing contrast solution is given, either as a continuous infusion diluted in 200 to 300 cc of saline or as one or more boluses. Contrast enhancement is rarely needed for the interpretation of lung abnormalities. The degree to which contrast enhancement is used for hilar and mediastinal disorders varies greatly from center to center. In patients with average or greater than average mediastinal fat, the mediastinal vessels are easily identified from their known anatomy. Similarly, hilar anatomy is sufficiently constant to make contrast opacification optional. An opposing view, to which we subscribe, is that, since the risk from intravenous contrast material is low and the extra information obtainable is unpredictable, intravenous contrast material should be used whenever hilar or mediastinal disease is a serious consideration unless there are specific contraindications.

When giving intravenous contrast material it is necessary to remember that the agent rapidly diffuses out of the vascular space into the tissues and that the best contrast differentiation between blood and soft tissues is seen on the first pass through the vessels. This principle is particularly exploited in dynamic scanning, where scans are obtained to coincide with various phases of opacification of a vessel or a lesion. Often, multiple scans are obtained at the same level as rapidly as possible in order to demonstrate the passage of a bolus of contrast agent. To do this effectively, one has to cover the expected transit time of the bolus. Following injection of the contrast agent into the patient's arm, the superior vena cava is best opacified on average at 6 seconds after injection, the pulmonary artery at 8 seconds, the ascending aorta at 13 seconds, and the descending aorta at 14 seconds. Technically, one usually has to choose one level to analyze at a time, because it is rarely practicable to cover multiple levels in the available time. The heat loading on the x-ray tube and the relatively slow table movement combine to make rapid multilevel scanning impossible with the standard machines. The primary indications for dynamic scanning are demonstrating aortic dissection and proving whether a particular density is or is not a blood vessel.

Each examination should be tailored to the clinical problem. The examination can be limited in scope when the aim is to elucidate a localized abnormality discovered on plain chest radiograph. Also, the protocol for suspected aortic dissection (see Chapter 15) and for the evaluation of a solitary pulmonary nodule (see Chapter 5) differs significantly from the standard examination.

Magnetic Resonance Imaging

The physical principles governing MRI are quite different from those of CT and are more complex. The major advantages are that sectional images may be obtained with equal ease in the axial, coronal, sagittal, or even oblique planes, and that no ionizing radiation is employed. So far, MRI appears harmless at current imaging field strengths. MR images are primarily dependent on three intrinsic tissue parameters: proton density and the tissue relaxation times, T1 and T2. Chemical characteristics such as fat content and the hydration state at the cellular level also contribute to the intensity of the signal.

Physical Phenomena

MRI provides a map of the distribution of those nuclei that precess when placed in a magnetic field. Precession is similar to the movement of a gyroscope in a gravitational field. The frequency of precession (ω_0) for a particular atomic nucleus is directly proportional to the magnetic field (B_0) (Fig 1–2). It can be expressed by the Larmor equation

$$\omega_0 = \gamma\, B_0$$

where ω_0 is the frequency of precession, B_0 is the imposed magnetic field, and γ is a constant for a particular nucleus—the gyromagnetic ratio.

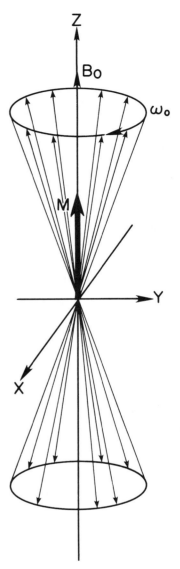

FIG 1–2.
Hydrogen nuclei precessing with random phase and frequency ω_0 in applied magnetic field B_0. Net magnetization M is parallel to B_0.

Precession in a magnetic field occurs only with those nuclei that have a magnetic moment or intrinsic "spin." Intrinsic spin is a concept in quantum physics that is observed only in nuclei with an odd number of protons or neutrons. Although many nuclei, such as hydrogen, carbon 13, fluorine 19, sodium 23, and phosphorous 31 have this property, the only one with sufficient abundance in the body for imaging with current MRI techniques is the hydrogen nucleus. The signal intensity in a hydrogen MR image reflects the hydrogen nuclei (protons) in mobile water and lipids within the body. Water is the most common source of hydrogen nuclei in the body.

The precessional frequency of the hydrogen nucleus at 1 tesla is 42.25 MHz. The tesla is a unit of magnetic field strength, and 1 tesla equals 10,000 gauss. By comparison, the earth's magnetic field is approximately 0.5 gauss. Currently, the magnetic fields used in clinical MRI range in strength from 0.02 to 2 tesla.

It is necessary to consider both the behavior of the individual hydrogen protons and also their net effect, for it is the net effect that is detected and imaged. The magnetic moment of each hydrogen nucleus can be thought of as a tiny magnet. In the absence of an applied magnetic field, the magnetic moments of the hydrogen nuclei are randomly oriented, pointing in all directions. When an external magnetic field, B_0, is applied, they line up either parallel (low energy state) or antiparallel (high energy state) to the magnetic field with a slight excess (1.4 in 1 million) in the parallel configuration at equilibrium. It is this excess of protons that results in a net magnetization M in the direction of the applied magnetic field B_0 (see Fig 1–2).

MRI is based on the phenomenon of resonance. In a uniform magnetic field the hydrogen nuclei precess with a constant frequency ω_0 about the axis of the applied magnetic field B_0. Normally, these nuclei precess with randomly different phases (i.e., they are all "out of step," and no radio signal can be detected from them with a receiving antenna). However, with the application of a precisely calculated pulse of radiofrequency, ω_0, the hydrogen nuclei absorb energy, resulting in transitions between the parallel and antiparallel states and causing the individual nuclear dipoles to precess in-phase (synchronously). As a consequence, their net magnetization M now has a component M_{XY} precessing in a plane perpendicular to B_0 (Fig 1–3). This in-phase rotating magnetization induces an oscillating voltage in a pick-up coil, which corresponds to the net magnetization M_{XY} perpendicular to the magnetic field B_0. From the frequency characteristics of this oscillating voltage, information can be obtained about the location of the hydrogen nucleus and its environment.

Once the radiofrequency pulse is turned off, the protons begin to dephase and to realign with the stationary magnetic field B_0, and the net magnetization M begins to return to equilibrium, namely parallel to B_0. This realignment and dephasing is known as relaxation and has two basic components: T1 and T2.

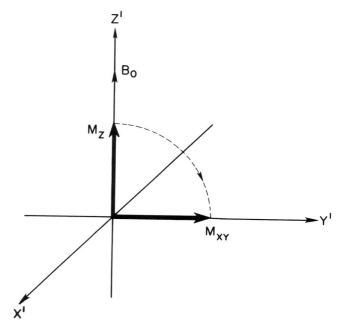

FIG 1–3.
Application of a 90° pulse of radiofrequency energy results in the net magnetization having a component M_{XY} precessing at frequency ω_0 in a plane perpendicular to B_0. This component appears stationary in the reference frame X'Y'Z' rotating at ω_0.

T1 and T2 Relaxation Times

There are two processes involved in relaxation, both of which are exponential in time, somewhat analogous to radioactive decay, and are characterized by the time constants T1 and T2. The net magnetization M returns to its equilibrium, parallel to the applied magnetic field B_0, with time constant T1, the time for the net magnetization to recover to 63% of its maximum equilibrium value (Fig 1–4). T1 depends on how fast energy can be exchanged from the precessing nuclei to the surrounding lattice of atoms by random thermal molecular collisions.

Immediately following application of the radiofrequency pulse, the hydrogen nuclei precess synchronously in phase. After removal of the pulse, however, they become increasingly out of phase as local magnetic fields affect each individual proton differently. This dephasing of the precessing nuclei occurs with a relaxation time T2, which is also called the spin-spin relaxation time because it refers to the effects of the interactions between the precessing nuclear spins (Fig 1–5). In solid tissues, the local magnetic fields that contribute to dephasing are significant because the molecules, and hence their local magnetic fields, are relatively fixed in space. T2 for solid materials is very short (in the order of microseconds). By comparison, in a liquid, the molecules

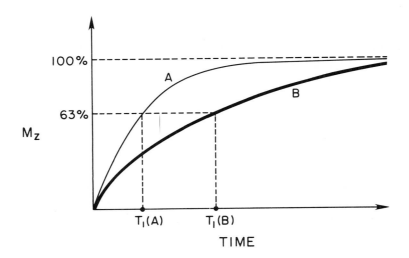

FIG 1–4.

Spin-lattice relaxation: recovery of magnetization M_Z in the Z direction with time constant T1. Tissue A has shorter time constant T1(A) and therefore faster recovery than tissue B, T1(B). The 100%

fluctuate rapidly, and the resultant local magnetic fields average to nearly zero and contribute little to the dephasing of neighboring precessing protons. Thus, T2 for liquids is longer (in the order of seconds) than for solids. T2 is always shorter than T1; and as liquids become solids, the value of T2 approaches that of T1.

Thus, after a radiofrequency pulse, one component of the magnetization is recovering (owing to spin-lattice relaxation with time constant T1) (see Fig 1–4), while the other is decaying (owing to proton dephasing or spin-spin relaxation with time constant T2) (see Fig 1–5). The net magnetization

equilibrium value depends on the density of protons in the tissue. If tissues A and B have different proton densities, their equilibrium values will be different.

M rises because M is returning to the equilibrium state parallel to B_0.

Spatial Localization

Paul Lauterbur, in 1973, devised a method of obtaining spatial information from magnetic resonance. Lauterbur's work was a major breakthrough that allowed the well-established technique of nuclear magnetic resonance for chemical assay to be used for imaging purposes. The principle derives from the Larmor equation. The value of the applied stationary magnetic field B_0 determines the particular resonant frequency ω_0 for a particular nucleus.

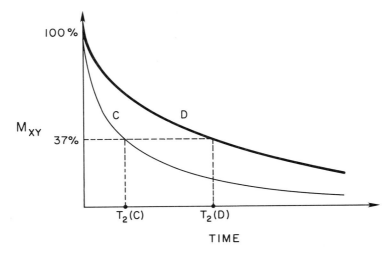

FIG 1–5.

Spin-spin relaxation: dephasing protons result in M_{XY} decreasing with time constant T2. Tissue C has shorter time constant, T2(C), and therefore dephases faster than tissue D, T2(D). If tissues C and D have different proton densities, their 100% starting values will be different.

However, if another magnetic field is applied so that there is a gradient of magnetic field in one direction, then each plane perpendicular to the direction of the gradient will experience a slightly different net magnetic field. Thus, the hydrogen nuclei within each plane will resonate at proportionately different frequencies according to the Larmor equation. Therefore, spatial information in one direction may be obtained. The superimposed gradient magnetic field is applied using a "gradient coil."

By applying magnetic field gradients to two or all three directions, the magnetic field can be defined, not only for a particular plane but also for a line or a point within the object being imaged. The received resonant signal can be analyzed by computer using the Fourier transformation technique into its composite frequencies. Planar images can be generated with equal ease in sagittal, coronal, or axial directions.

In MRI, there are many possible sequences for applying the radiofrequency pulse; the most common is the spin-echo sequence.

Spin-Echo Technique

First, a 90° radiofrequency pulse is applied to flip the net magnetization (M) 90° from the Z direction (parallel to B_0) to the XY plane (perpendicular to B_0). The net magnetization then precesses in the XY plane once the radiofrequency pulse is removed. As previously described, the individual precessing nuclei, originally in phase, will begin to dephase as a result of the different local magnetic fields they ex-

perience (Fig 1–6). However, if after a time t another pulse is applied to flip the precessing nuclei 180° about the Y axis (but still in the XY plane), they will continue to precess in the same direction, but after time t will be back in phase again, and generate a coherent echo signal. The analogy of horses running around a race track may be helpful. After the race begins, the horses running around the track spread out, or dephase. If after a certain time t they could be stopped and their progress exactly reversed, then, after an additional time t the horses would arrive synchronously back at the starting gate.

The echo signal, representing the net magnetization after time $2t$ will be less intense than the original resonant signal for the following reason: the different local magnetic fields experienced by the hydrogen nuclei, and causing them to dephase as they precess, arise from two sources—inhomogeneities in the external applied field B_0 and also time-dependent random variations in the local magnetic fields. The former are cancelled out by the 180° reversing pulse of the spin-echo technique; but the latter, because of their time dependence, are irreversible and represent T2 decay owing to spin-spin relaxation as described previously.

TR and TE

As already discussed, T1 and T2 are intrinsic relaxation times of the nuclei being imaged and depend on their local chemical environment and the field strength produced by the magnet. They are independent of the operator. Two parameters that can

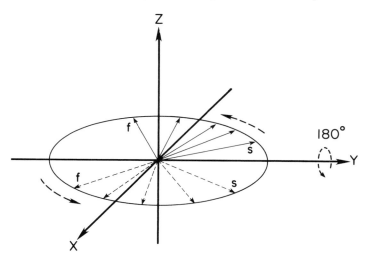

FIG 1–6.
In the spin-echo sequence, at time t after the 90° pulse the dephasing precessing protons are flipped 180° about the Y axis in the XY plane and generate an echo signal after time $2t$. Fast "f" and slow "s" protons arrive back synchronously to create the coherent echo signal.

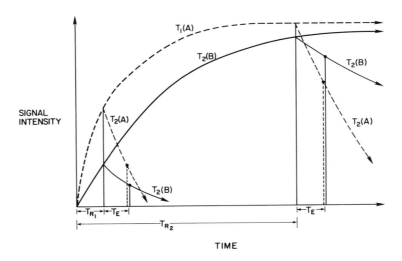

FIG 1–7.
Composite graph of the recovery and decay of the signal intensity with relaxation times T1 and T2, respectively. The relative signal intensities represented in the MR image for two tissues A and B will vary, depending on the values chosen for repetition time TR and echo time TE. TR₁ gives a T1-weighted image (tissue A, with shorter T1, is hyperintense relative to tissue B). TR₂ gives a T2-weighted image (tissue B, with longer T2, is hyperintense relative to tissue A).

be selected by the operator to generate images at different time points in the relaxation processes are TR, the repetition time of the pulsing sequence, and TE, the echo time. The radiofrequency pulsing sequence is repeated many times during the MR imaging process. The time between successive repetitions is called TR, the repetition time. TR determines how far the net magnetization M has been allowed to recover back to its equilibrium value before the next series of pulses (Fig 1–7). Therefore, TR is associated with the spin-lattice relaxation time T1. TE is the echo time $2t$, the time between the initial 90° pulse and the resonant echo signal in a spin-echo sequence, as outlined in the previous section. Therefore, TE is associated with the spin-spin relaxation time T2.

Typical TR values are 0.1 to 3 seconds. If the TR value is too short, there is not enough time for the net magnetization M to recover before the pulse sequence is repeated. Therefore, the initial signal intensity is not strong enough. Very long TR values are unnecessary, as the net magnetization of most tissues being imaged will have fully recovered in less than 3 seconds. TE values selected for imaging range from 15 to 300 msec.

The TR and TE values selected for a series of MR images determine the extent of T1 recovery and T2 decay in the tissues being imaged and, therefore, the intensity of the recorded signals (see Fig 1–7). Typically, more than one combination of TR and TE is selected, so that different sets of images with different relative signal intensities from different tissues are recorded. Some degree of tissue characterization can thus be obtained.

Images recorded using short TR and short TE values are "T1-weighted." The short TE value allows for little T2 decay, and the short TR value maximizes the differences in the T1 relaxation times of different tissues. Images recorded using long TR and long TE values are "T2-weighted." The long TR value allows for almost full recovery of the net magnetization of most tissues being imaged, and therefore the T1 relaxation time is no longer of consequence, whereas the long TE value emphasizes the different T2 relaxation times of different tissues. A combination of long TR and short TE values results in minimal T1 and T2 dependence, but reflects differences in proton density of the tissues.

Table 1–1 provides a summary of the relative relaxation times, T1 and T2, and relative signal intensities of various tissues in the body for T1-weighted (short TR/TE) and T2-weighted (long TR/TE) spin-echo pulse sequences.

Machine Components

The MR imaging machine includes a large magnet that imposes the external applied magnetic field, a set of gradient coils for spatial localization, and a radiofrequency transmitter antenna to induce resonance of the hydrogen nuclei. An antenna also receives the resonant signal which is amplified, filtered, and digitized. A computer system performs the control, data acquisition, processing, analysis, and display.

TABLE 1–1.
Relative Relaxation Times and Signal Intensities of Various Body Tissue Types

Tissue	Relaxation Time		Signal Intensity	
	T1	T2	Short TR/TE	Long TR/TE
Fluid	Very long	Very long	Very dark	Very bright
Fat	Short	Long	Very bright	Bright
Fibrous tissue	Long	Short	Dark	Dark
Solid organs	Moderate	Short	Intermediate	Dark
Tumors	Long	Long	Dark	Bright
Fresh hemorrhage	Long	Very short	Dark	Dark
Air	—	—	Very dark	Very dark
Calcification	—	—	Very dark	Very dark

The magnetic field may be generated either by a permanent magnet or by electrical current, whereby a magnetic field is generated around conducting wire. The current-carrying conducting wire can be resistive, which requires a continuous driving voltage from a power supply, or superconducting, which means that there is no electrical resistance in the conducting wire and therefore no power loss. Currently, superconducting wires in MR imager magnets must be cooled to $4.2°$ K ($-453.8°F$) by liquid helium. The advantages of superconducting magnets include the higher maximum magnetic field that can be obtained, the negligible power required, and excellent stability.

The two-dimensional section image is usually 256×256 pixels (picture elements). The voxel (volume element) size is the product of the pixel size and the slice thickness. The slice thickness is comparable to that used in CT: namely, about 0.5 cm. The number of slices that can be recorded during one pulsing sequence is determined by TR. Display and photography of the sectional MR images are very similar to those of CT.

Motion Artifacts

MR images are degraded by periodic motion of respiratory and cardiovascular origin, resulting in both image blurring and the superposition of ghost images. The higher the magnetic field, the greater the degradation of MR image quality by motion artifacts. The ghost images are more intense at higher magnetic fields because of the higher signal-to-noise ratio.

Cardiovascular motion artifacts can be reduced most simply by cardiac triggering. However, the period of the cardiac cycle determines the TR value, which must equal the R-R interval or multiples thereof.

The greatest source of motion degradation of MR images is the periodic motion of the patient's lungs, chest wall, diaphragm, and abdomen during breathing. Various methods have been attempted to reduce the effect of respiratory motion on MR images. These include physical restraint, breathholding, respiratory gating, and several data acquisition and processing techniques including averaging, rephasing, pseudogating, STIR (short inversion recovery), and reordering of phase encoding (ROPE, COPE, and EXORCIST being particular manufacturers' methods). It is beyond the scope of this general introduction to go into details of these methods, which have been reviewed elsewhere.[12]

For the patient to hold his or her breath during MR imaging, specialized fast imaging techniques, such as gradient echo sequences with a TR as short as 30 msec, can be employed. However, they result in reduced signal-to-noise ratio. Respiratory gating, whereby data are acquired during only a part of the respiratory cycle, requires a complex respiratory monitor, which is inconvenient for routine imaging and prolongs the imaging time.

No one method is routinely used, and combinations of two or more methods may be employed.

REFERENCES

1. Barnes GT, Sones RA, Tesic MM: Digital chest radiography: Performance evaluation of a prototype unit. *Radiology* 1985; 154:801–806.
2. Barrett HH, Swindell WH: *Radiologic Imaging: The Theory of Image Formation, Detection and Processing.* New York, Academic Press, 1981; vol 1, pp 55–59.
3. Fraser RG, Breatnach E, Barnes GT: Digital radiography of the chest: Clinical experience with a prototype unit. *Radiology* 1983; 148:1–5.
4. Fujita H, Doi K, McMahon H, et al: Basic imaging properties of a large image intensifier–TV digital chest radiographic system. *Invest Radiol* 1987; 22:328–335.
5. Goodman LR, Wilson CR, Foley WD: Digital radiog-

raphy of the chest: Promises and problems. *AJR* 1988; 150:1241–1252.

6. Herman PG, Drummey J, Swensson RG, et al: 350 kV chest radiography has no diagnostic advantage: A comparison with 140 kV technique. *AJR* 1982; 138:485–489.

7. Kelsey CA, Moseley RD, Mettler FA, et al: Comparison of nodule detection with 70-kVp and 120-kVp chest radiographs. *Radiology* 1982; 143:609–611.

8. Kushner DC, Cleveland RH, Herman TE, et al: Low-dose flying spot digital radiography of the chest: Sensitivity studies. *Radiology* 1987; 163:685–688.

9. Revesz G, Shea FJ, Kundel HL: The effects of kilovoltage on diagnostic accuracy in chest radiography. *Radiology* 1982; 142:615–618.

10. Sommer FG, Smathers RL, Wheat RL, et al: Digital processing of film radiographs. *AJR* 1985; 144:191–196.

11. Sonoda M, Takano M, Miyahara J, et al: Computed radiography utilizing scanning laser stimulated luminescence. *Radiology* 1983; 148:833–838.

12. Stark DD, Bradley WG Jr: *Magnetic Resonance Imaging.* St Louis, CV Mosby Co, 1988.

13. Templeton AW, Dwyer SJ, Cox GG, et al: A digital radiology imaging system: Description and clinical evaluation. *AJR* 1987; 149:847–851.

14. Trout ED, Kelley JP, Larson VL: A comparison of an air gap and a grid in roentgenography of the chest. *AJR* 1975; 124:404–411.

Principles of Diagnostic Testing

The technology of diagnostic imaging has developed rapidly in recent years. In many instances, the newer imaging modalities such as ultrasound, computed tomography (CT), and magnetic resonance imaging (MRI) have helped clinicians diagnose disease more accurately, quickly, and safely than was possible in the past. In other instances, however, the bewildering array of testing options has caused confusion, waste, and harm to patients. To ensure the appropriate use of such a large diagnostic armamentarium, it is vital that clinicians be familiar with the basic principles of diagnostic testing. Although the principles apply to the broad field of medicine, the illustrative examples will be confined to the subject of chest disease.

SENSITIVITY AND SPECIFICITY

When selecting a diagnostic test, one of the most important considerations is the accuracy, or efficacy, of the test. Diagnostic efficacy is best described in terms of sensitivity and specificity.[15, 21] Stated simply, sensitivity is the ability of a test to recognize disease, and specificity is the ability of a test to recognize normality. These concepts can be illustrated with the help of a binary table that depicts the correlation between test interpretation and the presence or absence of disease in the population under study (Fig 2–1). The binary table categorizes patients into four mutually exclusive outcomes: positive test result and disease present, true positive (TP); positive test result and disease absent, false positive (FP); negative test result and disease present, false negative (FN); and negative test result and disease absent, true negative (TN).

The sensitivity of a test is the proportion of patients with disease who have positive test results. In other words, it is the ability of the test to recognize disease.

$$\text{Sensitivity} = \frac{TP}{TP + FN} \qquad (2-1)$$

The specificity of a test is the proportion of patients without disease who have negative test results. In other words, it is the ability of the test to recognize normality, or the absence of a particular disease.

$$\text{Specificity} = \frac{TN}{TN + FP} \qquad (2-2)$$

Example 1

In a recent study,[7] CT scanning was used to evaluate the mediastinum in patients with known lung carcinoma. CT scans showing mediastinal lymph nodes with a short-axis diameter of at least 1.0 cm were considered positive for metastasis, while CT scans revealing no nodes larger than 1.0 cm were considered negative for mediastinal involvement. Following surgery, the patients were categorized according to their CT scan results and pathologic findings (Fig 2–2). Surgical pathology was presumed to be infallible and was thus the "gold stan-

		\multicolumn{2}{c}{DISEASE}
		PRESENT	ABSENT
T E S T	POSITIVE	TRUE POSITIVE	FALSE POSITIVE
	NEGATIVE	FALSE NEGATIVE	TRUE NEGATIVE

FIG 2–1.
Binary table correlating test results *(left)* with presence or absence of disease in the patient. For explanation, see text.

dard" against which the CT scan was compared. In this series,

$$\text{Sensitivity} = 20/21$$
$$= 0.95;$$
$$\text{Specificity} = 18/28$$
$$= 0.64$$

PRETEST AND POST-TEST PROBABILITIES

Before requesting a diagnostic test, the clinician usually has some idea of the probability of a particular disease in his patient. This prior, or pretest, probability can be thought of as the prevalence of the disease in a population of patients similar to the one under consideration. If the patient is representative of a well-defined population, a very precise estimate of prevalence may be available. For example, suppose a pulmonologist wants an estimate of the pretest probability of lung cancer in a 50-year-old

		\multicolumn{2}{c}{SURG-PATH}
		MALIGNANT	BENIGN
C T	POSITIVE*	20	10
	NEGATIVE	1	18

*Short-axis diameter ≥ 1.0 cm

FIG 2–2.
Correlation of CT diagnosis with mediastinal node biopsy findings in patients with lung cancer. (Data from Glazer GM, Orringer MB, Gross BH, et al: The mediastinum in non-small cell lung cancer: CT-surgical correlation. *AJR* 1984; 142:1101–1105.

man who smokes more than one pack of cigarettes per day. Such an estimate is available from a reference population of male smokers over 45 years of age, who have a prevalence of lung cancer of 0.6%.[10] When the patient does not conform so neatly to a reference population, the pretest probability of disease is a more subjective clinical estimate.

In example 1, the pretest probability of mediastinal involvement in patients with newly diagnosed lung cancer is:

$$\text{Pretest probability} = 21/49$$
$$= 0.43$$

Knowing the sensitivity and specificity of a test is helpful when deciding whether to request a test; however, once the result has been obtained, this knowledge is not sufficient to answer the question "what is the probability of disease now that the test result is known?" This answer is provided by the post-test probability of disease, a figure that incorporates not only the sensitivity and specificity of the test, but also the pretest probability of the disease in question. (Post-test probabilities are often expressed as positive or negative predictive value [PPV or NPV]. The PPV is equal to the post-test probability of disease. The NPV, however, is equal to one minus the post-test probability.)

In example 1, the post-test probability of mediastinal involvement when the CT scan is positive is the ratio of patients with true positive test results over all patients with positive results.

$$\text{Post-test probability} (+) \quad \begin{aligned} &= \frac{\text{TP}}{\text{TP} + \text{FP}} &&(2\text{–}3)\\ &= 20/30 \\ &= 0.67 \ (67\% \ \text{PPV}) \end{aligned}$$

With a negative CT result, the post-test probability is the ratio of patients with false negative results over all patients with negative results.

$$\text{Post-test probability} (-) \quad \begin{aligned} &= \frac{\text{FN}}{\text{TN} + \text{FN}} &&(2\text{–}4)\\ &= 1/19 \\ &= 0.05 \ (95\% \ \text{NPV}) \end{aligned}$$

The term "accuracy" refers to the ratio of patients with either true positive or true negative results over all patients in the study. This term is of limited value, because it lumps together positive and negative results. In example 1:

$$Accuracy = 38/49$$
$$= 0.78$$

It is extremely important to understand that post-test probability and accuracy are strongly dependent on the pretest probability of disease. Suppose a study similar to that quoted in example 1 is performed on patients who have primary lung cancers that are all smaller than 2 cm in diameter (Fig 2–3). Because smaller primary tumors are less likely to have distant spread, the proportion of patients with mediastinal involvement would be expected to be smaller (say 0.10). Although the sensitivity and specificity of the CT scan might remain the same (sensitivity = 20/21 = 0.95, specificity = 121/189 = 0.64), the post-test probabilities and overall accuracy would change significantly:

$$Post\text{-}test\ probability\ (+) = 20/88$$
$$= 0.23$$
$$Post\text{-}test\ probability\ (-) = 1/121$$
$$= 0.01$$
$$Accuracy = 144/210$$
$$= 0.68$$

These differences are explained by the lower pretest probability in the second study (0.10 vs. 0.43). The example demonstrates certain principles. The sensitivity and specificity of a test are generally independent of disease prevalence and are, therefore, often called the intrinsic operating characteristics of the test. On the other hand, the post-test probabilities and accuracy are highly dependent on the prevalence of disease and thus cannot be generalized over settings where the prevalence varies. For this reason, reports of sensitivity and specificity are

		SURG-PATH	
		MALIGNANT	**BENIGN**
C	**POSITIVE***	20	68
T	**NEGATIVE**	1	121

*Short-axis diameter ≥ 1.0 cm

FIG 2–3.
CT/surgical-pathologic correlation of mediastinal lymph nodes in early-stage cancer of the lung (lesions < 2 cm in diameter).

more reliable than reports of post-test probabilities and accuracy, which are greatly influenced by regional variation of disease prevalence.

BAYES THEOREM

It is not necessary to construct a binary table each time the post-test probability is determined. Using simple algebra, equations (2–3) and (2–4) can be written in terms of sensitivity (S), specificity (Sp), and pretest probability (P).[1]

$$\begin{array}{ll} Post\text{-}test \\ probability\ (+) \end{array} = \frac{P \times S}{P \times S + (1 - P) \times (1 - Sp)} \quad (2\text{-}5)$$

$$\begin{array}{ll} Post\text{-}test \\ probability\ (-) \end{array} = \frac{P \times (1 - S)}{P \times (1 - S) + (1 - P) \times Sp} \quad (2\text{-}6)$$

With negative test results, the post-test probability is influenced more by sensitivity than specificity. For positive test results the opposite is true. Looking at equation (2–5), if the specificity of a test is 1.0, then the post-test probability of a positive test result is 1.0. With equation (2–6), if the sensitivity of a test is 1.0, then the post-test probability of a negative test is zero.

RECEIVER-OPERATOR-CHARACTERISTICS ANALYSIS

The sensitivity and specificity of a test depend on the criteria chosen for interpretation.[9, 11] As the criteria for calling a test result positive are made more stringent, specificity improves at the expense of sensitivity. Conversely, as the criteria are relaxed, sensitivity improves while specificity diminishes.

When the investigators in the original CT study[7] chose a lymph node diameter of 2.0 cm instead of 1.0 cm as the criterion for CT positivity, the sensitivity and specificity differed (Fig 2–4):

$$Sensitivity = 14/21$$
$$= 0.67$$
$$Specificity = 27/28$$
$$= 0.97$$

The specificity of mediastinal CT scanning increased, but its sensitivity declined. As the criteria for positivity varied from 0.5 cm to 3.0 cm, the sensitivity and specificity varied. This relationship can be demonstrated on a receiver-operator-charac-

		SURG-PATH	
		POSITIVE	**NEGATIVE**
C	**POSITIVE***	14	1
T	**NEGATIVE**	7	27

*Short-axis diameter ≥ 2.0 cm

FIG 2–4.
Changes in sensitivity and specificity from Figures 2–2 and 2–3 with lymph node diameters of 2.0 cm.

teristics (ROC) curve (Fig 2–5). This curve is generated by plotting the sensitivity (true positive rate) verses one minus the specificity (false positive rate) for the different interpretation criteria. The fundamental principle illustrated by the ROC curve is that there is an inherent limit to the diagnostic efficacy of a test. Once this limit has been reached, the interpreter can only improve sensitivity at the expense of specificity, and vice versa.

The ROC curve can be used to select the "best" cutoff criteria for positivity, taking the pretest probability and the relative costs (in terms of patient out-

MALIGNANT MEDIASTINAL METASTASIS IN LUNG CANCER

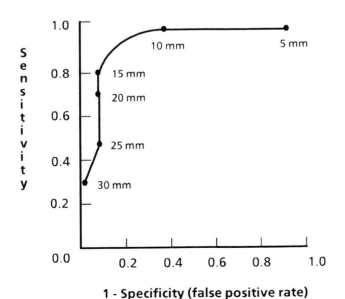

FIG 2–5.
ROC curve for chest CT in the evaluation of lung cancer patients for mediastinal lymph node metastasis.

come) of false positive and false negative test results into account.[9] Using principles of decision theory, it can be shown that the best cutoff point on the ROC curve is where

$$\text{Slope} = \frac{1 - P}{P} \times \frac{C_{FP}}{C_{FN},}$$

where C_{FP} and C_{FN} are the costs of the false positive and negative test results, respectively.

When the pretest probability is intermediate and the relative costs of false positive and false negative results are similar, the best cutoff point is where the slope is near one (the middle of the curve). When the pretest probability of disease is either very high or very low, or when the costs of false positive and false negative results are very different, then the cutoff point would be at the extremes of the ROC curve.

For example, consider the role of CT of the chest in the evaluation of potentially operable lung cancer patients. Most surgeons will not attempt surgical cure on patients with mediastinal lymph node metastases. Where mediastinoscopy is readily available, the cost of a false positive CT result (unnecessary mediastinoscopy) is small in comparison to the cost of a false negative result (inappropriate attempt at curative resection). Therefore, the best cutoff point would lie on the shallow (upper right) portion of the ROC curve, where the sensitivity of CT is high. On the other hand, if mediastinoscopy were not available, then the cost of a false positive CT result (denial of potentially curative resection) would be greater than the cost of a false negative result (unnecessary surgery). In this situation, the appropriate cutoff point would be on a steeper (lower left) section of the ROC curve, where the specificity of CT is high.

Additionally, ROC curves are useful in comparing the performance of different tests because they allow for a wide range of different (positivity) criteria. The area under the ROC curve of a perfect test is 1.0, while the area under the curve of a test with no predictive value is 0.5.

LIKELIHOOD RATIO

Describing test efficacy in terms of the ROC curve and calculating post-test probabilities from equations 2–5 and 2–6 can be arduous and impractical tasks for the busy clinician. Fortunately, the likelihood ratio (LR) offers an easier method of communicating the significance of test results. This concept has recently been illustrated in the literatures of internal medicine,[18] radiology,[2] and pathology.[16]

The LR is the probability of a particular test result given disease, divided by the probability of the same test result given no disease. LR can be derived from the sensitivity (S) and specificity (Sp) of the test. For a positive test result,

$$LR = \frac{S}{1 - Sp}$$

and for a negative result

$$LR = \frac{1 - S}{Sp}$$

The LR varies in value from zero to infinity, depending on the degree of positivity or negativity of the test result. A test result that is strongly positive has a LR much greater than 1.0, whereas a test result that is strongly negative has a LR close to zero. A test result that is neither strongly positive nor negative has a LR near 1.0.

For example, in the CT study where 1.0 cm is the cutoff for mediastinal lymph node diameter, the LR for a "positive" result is

$$LR (+) = \frac{20/21}{20/28}$$
$$= 2.7$$

For a "negative" result,

$$LR (-) = \frac{1/21}{18/28}$$
$$= 0.07$$

Most diagnostic tests are capable of generating a spectrum of possible results for which the designations "positive" and "negative" are too simplistic. A major advantage of LR is that it can be applied to a range of test results. The LR for each different test result is determined by dividing the probability of a particular test result in a patient with disease by the probability of the same test result in a patient without disease. For example, in the series of patients with lung cancer described earlier, the LR associated with a lymph node measuring between 15 and 20 mm is the probability of a lymph node measuring between 15 and 20 mm in a patient with mediastinal involvement divided by the probability of a lymph node measuring between 15 and 20 mm in a patient

without mediastinal involvement: 3.3. Similarly, the LRs for mediastinal lymph nodes of different sizes can be determined (Table 2–1). Note that the LR can be applied to several different categories of lymph node size, while the terms sensitivity and specificity impose a positivity criterion that places all lymph nodes into only one of two broad categories.

Not only is the LR useful as a means of concisely communicating the degree of positivity or negativity of a test result, it also facilitates the integration of the test result and the clinical setting. The complex form of Bayes theorem, equations (2–5) and (2–6), can be reduced to a more intuitive linear equation when LR is substituted for sensitivity and specificity, and probabilities are converted to odds:

$$\text{Post-test odds} = \text{Pretest odds} \times \text{LR}$$

Odds and probabilities are related as follows:

$$\text{Odds} = \frac{P}{1 + P}$$

$$P = \frac{\text{odds}}{1 + \text{odds}}$$

This multiplicative form of Bayes theorem allows the significance of a test result to be easily understood. Consider a typical lung cancer patient with a pretest probability of mediastinal involvement of 0.25 or pretest odds of 1:3 (0.25/0.75 = 1:3). If chest CT reveals a mediastinal lymph node measuring between 15 and 20 mm, then post-test odds of mediastinal involvement

$$= 1:3 \times 3.3$$
$$= 1.1:1$$

With roughly even odds of mediastinal involvement, mediastinoscopy might be advised prior to an attempt at curative surgery.

Furthermore, the linearity of the multiplicative form provides for the easy integration of other test

TABLE 2–1.

Likelihood Ratios of Mediastinal Lymph Nodes in Lung Cancer Patients

Short-Axis Diameter (mm)	Likelihood Ratios
0–9	0.08
10–14	0.50
15–19	3.3
20–29	13.3
30–infinity	Infinity

results. For any number of conditionally independent tests, post-test odds can be determined as a linear function of the pretest odds and LRs of the tests performed:

Post-test odds =
   Pretest odds $\times$ LR$_1$ $\times$ LR$_2$ $\times$ . . . $\times$ LR$_N$

This equation is useful for evaluating a patient with multiple test results, particularly when some of them conflict.

Unfortunately, the subject of test independence is complex, and a rigorous analysis of this subject is beyond the scope of this chapter. In simple terms, however, tests that detect disease in a similar fashion are more interdependent than those that detect disease by different means. For example, plain chest radiographs and chest CT scans both enable detection of mediastinal lymph node metastases when these nodes become enlarged. Because the results of these two tests are dependent on lymph node size, the tests are somewhat interdependent, and the sequential application of Bayes theorem does not apply.

The likelihood ratio has other limitations. Its practical application is limited by the same restrictions that govern the use of sensitivity and specificity. The disease must be regarded as either present or absent, and only one disease process can be considered at a time. Bayes theorem can be applied to a disease of varying severity and to differential diagnosis,[19] but the analysis is too complicated to be included in this brief introduction to principles of diagnostic testing.

METHODOLOGICAL CONSIDERATIONS

There are numerous diagnostic efficacy studies appearing in the medical literature. Unfortunately, virtually all of these studies are compromised to some degree by methodological and statistical limitations and, not surprisingly, produce conflicting results.[14, 17] Sorting out those results that are valid and relevant to patient management is facilitated by some understanding of study design and biostatistics. We briefly discuss some important methodological and statistical considerations, using hypothetical examples for illustration.

Methodology

Patient Selection

The method of patient selection should be clearly defined so that the study results are repro-

ducible and applicable to other patients prospectively. Retrospective studies are generally flawed because they consider patients who are not necessarily representative of those for whom the test is being advocated. Patient selection can be best controlled with a prospective study.

For example, an article states that the sensitivity and specificity of chest CT are 0.90 for the diagnosis of pulmonary metastasis in children. The diagnosis is based on the finding of one or more pulmonary nodules measuring greater than 5 mm in diameter. Can these results be applied to the evaluation of an otherwise healthy middle-aged man from Southwestern Virginia, a region where histoplasmosis is endemic? Probably not. If one were to study such a population, CT scanning would probably detect nodules over 5 mm in diameter in a large proportion of patients without pulmonary metastases, and the specificity of CT would be far lower than 0.90. The point is that in studies demonstrating a high sensitivity or specificity of a diagnostic test usually a highly select group of patients have been examined. Results from such studies are not necessarily applicable to patients of a different description, particularly when these patients are likely to have normal variants or other disease processes that mimic the disease in the diagnostic efficacy study.

Disease Severity

The disease entity under investigation should be clearly defined in terms of its stage or severity. A test will generally be more sensitive and specific in the detection of advanced disease.

For example, consider the sensitivity and specificity of the plain chest radiograph in the detection of lung cancer. Not infrequently, stage I lung cancer (primary tumor $\leq$ 3 cm, no hilar or mediastinal lymph node metastases) is overlooked on the plain chest radiograph. In fact, it has been reported in a prospective study that nearly 90% of small lung cancers were initially overlooked on earlier chest radiographs. For this reason, the sensitivity of the chest radiograph in the detection of stage I lung cancer would be relatively low, perhaps only 50%. The specificity of plain chest radiographs would also be expected to be rather low, considering all the nonspecific benign parenchymal diseases and spurious shadows that can produce an irregular density. On the other hand, the sensitivity and specificity of plain chest radiographs are virtually 100% for patients with stage IV lung carcinoma (large masses with mediastinal invasion).

Test Review Bias

The interpretation of the test being evaluated should not be influenced by knowledge of the ultimate diagnosis. The criteria for test positivity should be objective, clearly defined, and consistently applied. Ideally, the interpreter should be "blinded" from the diagnosis and also from the results of other tests. "Blinding" is optimal when the study is prospective.

For example, in a study of plain chest radiographs in patients with chronic obstructive pulmonary disease (COPD), the investigator finds increased anteroposterior diameter, low flat diaphragm, or inhomogeneous pulmonary vascular pattern in virtually all patients with known COPD, and considers these chest radiographs positive. On the other hand, in patients known to be healthy, he or she finds at least one normal feature on the radiograph. By varying the test criteria for each case, consciously or unconsciously, the investigator can achieve a spuriously high sensitivity and specificity for the diagnosis of COPD. Such a high degree of accuracy would not be duplicated if the radiologist were blinded from the diagnosis of COPD and if the criteria were more consistently applied.

Diagnostic Review Bias

The ultimate diagnosis should not be influenced by the interpretation of the test being evaluated.

A radiologist claims he or she can reliably make a specific diagnosis of benignancy with percutaneous needle biopsy. He or she then performs a prospective study of patients with coin lesions in which both the biopsy specimen and all pertinent clinical information are given to the pathologist for review. The pathologist may be strongly, albeit unconsciously, influenced by the patient's history. The pathologist may be more inclined to report "consistent with inflammation" when he sees nonspecific inflammatory cells in a young, nonsmoking patient. But seeing the identical slide in an older patient who smokes, the pathologist might report "insufficient material for diagnosis," fearing that the sample is not representative and that the patient has lung cancer. Not surprisingly, this diagnostic strategy produces very few false diagnoses of benign disease, but not because needle biopsy is highly accurate. Instead, it is the strong predictive value of the clinical information that prevents the pathologist from making a false negative diagnosis.

Like test review bias, diagnostic review bias falsely increases the correlation between test results and diagnosis, thereby leading to spuriously elevated sensitivity and specificity. Unlike test review bias, diagnostic review bias can occur even in a prospective study.

Work-up Bias

Work-up bias can be subtle and difficult to eliminate, even with prospective study design. It occurs when the interpretation of the test under scrutiny influences the further evaluation of the patient. Patients with positive test results are usually investigated more thoroughly than those whose tests are negative, and the latter are often lost to follow-up. In these circumstances, sensitivity is usually overestimated. Specificity may be either overestimated or underestimated, depending on how patients with negative test results are counted in the study.

When negative test results are assumed to be true negatives, even though the absence of disease has not been proved, both the sensitivity and specificity of the test are overestimated. This phenomenon is easiest to explain with a binary table. Patients who actually have false negative test results are misplaced into the true negative cell, so that sensitivity is calculated with a spuriously low denominator (TP + FN) and specificity with a spuriously high numerator (TN) (Fig 2–6). Consequently, both sensitivity and specificity are overestimated. This methodologic flaw might be expected, for example, in a study of the diagnostic efficacy of the chest radiograph for early lung cancer, in which many patients with false negative studies would be lost to follow-up.

When patients with negative test results are excluded from a diagnostic efficacy study, the specificity is underestimated. This occurs because both the true negative and false negative patients are underrepresented in the binary table. The specificity is

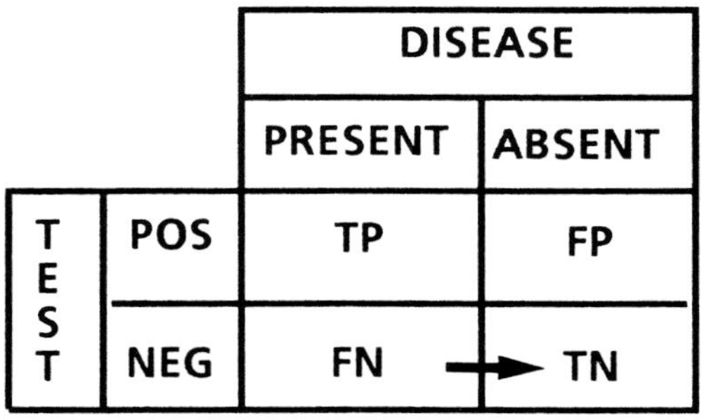

FIG 2–6.
Effect on sensitivity of assuming negative test results to be true negatives; numeric values for FN (false negatives) in the binary table will be too low and TN (true negative) too high in resulting calculations (see text).

then calculated using a spuriously low numerator (Fig 2–7). An example might be a study evaluating the diagnostic efficacy of the ventilation/perfusion (V/Q) lung scan in pulmonary embolism, where the diagnosis is established by pulmonary angiography. Because it would be unethical to perform pulmonary angiography on all patients with completely normal V/Q scans, many patients with either true negative or false negative V/Q scans would be excluded from the study. The exclusion of the true negative cases would lead to an underestimate of the specificity of the V/Q scan. (The sensitivity of the V/Q scan would be overestimated.)

Modality Bias

Modality bias plays a major role in comparing the efficacy of competing modalities if there is no neutral "gold standard" or if the investigator favors one modality over its competitor.[6] Obviously, if one modality is considered the ultimate standard then the competing modality can never achieve a higher sensitivity or specificity. Any difference in the test results will be considered either a false positive or false negative result for the comparison modality. Even if a neutral gold standard can be found, the investigator cannot usually be "blinded" from the knowledge of which modality he or she is reading (e.g., MRI vs. CT). Having a vested interest in the modality he or she chooses to write about, the investigator will usually apply this modality more skillfully or thoroughly than the other. This bias is most pronounced in comparison studies of newer modalities versus older ones. Even if test review, diagnostic review, and work-up biases are carefully eliminated by "blinding" and prospective guidelines are followed for patient entry, evaluation, and follow-up, modality bias may be impossible to eliminate completely. In contrast to other forms of bias, modality bias may actually be less of a problem in retrospective studies, in which the readings are less likely to have been made by a biased investigator.[6]

Diagnostic efficacy studies that do not adhere to the above methodologic guidelines produce results which may not represent reality. Generally, the sensitivity and specificity of diagnostic imaging have been overestimated, particularly those of the newer modalities, because investigators have been biased toward producing results which promote their technical expertise. However, the same methodologic flaws can allow an underestimate of diagnostic efficacy when the investigator wants to demonstrate a lack of efficacy, a phenomenon that is becoming more prevalent with the growing desire for containing costs.

Sample Size

In addition to methodologic design, the size of the study population from which efficacy results are derived is an important factor for critical review. The precision of an experimentally derived estimate, such as sensitivity, specificity, or LR, is dependent on the sample size. Precision is best represented with a confidence interval, the range of which is inversely related to sample size.

For a simple proportion, p, the confidence interval can be calculated as follows:

$$CI = [p + A/2 \pm Z \sqrt{p(1-p)/n + A/4n}]/(1+A)$$
$$(2-11)$$

where $Z = 1.96$ for a 95% confidence interval,[20] $A = Z^2/n$, and n = sample size. In Figure 2–2, for example, the 95% confidence interval for the specificity of CT is:

$$CI = 0.41 - 0.82$$

In other words, there is a 95% probability that the specificity of CT is between 0.41 and 0.82 based on the sample size of 28 patients. If the specificity were based on a sample size of 2,800 patients instead of 28, then the 95% confidence interval for specificity would be 0.62 to 0.66.

DECISION ANALYSIS

As stated previously, diagnostic efficacy is an important consideration for appropriate test selection. However, knowledge of a test's efficacy is not always sufficient for determining the test's clinical usefulness. Other factors, such as the pretest probability of disease, the natural history of disease, the benefits

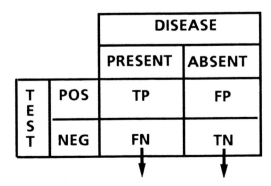

		DISEASE	
		PRESENT	**ABSENT**
TEST	**POS**	TP	FP
	NEG	FN	TN

FIG 2–7.
Effect on specificity of excluding negative test results from the study. (For key to abbreviations, see Figure 2–6.)

and risks of treatment, the risk of the test, and financial constraints must also be considered.[12, 13, 23] Although decisions regarding the use of diagnostic tests are usually made intuitively, the need for a more precise and consistent decision-making process is mounting. The growth of information pertaining to diagnostic and therapeutic modalities is increasing the complexity of medical decisions. Furthermore, these decisions are being heavily influenced by medicolegal and economic concerns. Concomitant with the increasing need for a quantitative decision-making process is the increasing availability of personal computers and decision support software, which are beginning to make the application of decision analysis to clinical medicine practicable.

The first, and perhaps most important, step in performing decision analysis is to design a decision tree, which illustrates the downstream effects of a choice. By convention, a square box designates a "choice" node, from which various strategy options emanate (Fig 2–8). For example, a surgeon may be trying to decide between two different management strategies for a patient with known lung cancer. One strategy is to proceed directly to an attempt at curative surgery (Fig 2–9). The other strategy is to perform chest CT and operate only if the CT is negative for mediastinal involvement (Fig 2–10).

Under the strategy NO CT, there is a risk of perioperative death. If the patient survives surgery, there are two possible outcomes, both of which are beyond the control of the surgeon: (1) the patient does not have mediastinal involvement and is surgically cured; (2) the patient has mediastinal metastasis and has undergone unnecessary surgery. The chance occurrence of events is indicated by the presence of circular "chance" nodes. Each outcome in the strategy is assigned a numeric value, usually in terms of quality-adjusted-life-years (QALYS). QALYS represent life expectancy modified by a factor which takes into account morbidity the patient may suffer because of testing and/or treatment used in the strategy. In this example, the value of the early disease outcome might be 9.9 QALYS (10 years being the average life expectancy from curative surgery, with 0.1 years deducted for the morbidity of surgery). Calculated in a similar fashion, the value of the outcome in advanced disease might be 0.9 QALYS. Death outcomes are generally assigned a value of zero QALYS. The probability of the death outcome in the NO CT strategy is simply the mortality rate (MT) for surgical resection of lung cancer. The probability of the advanced disease outcome is one minus surgical mortality times the pretest prob-

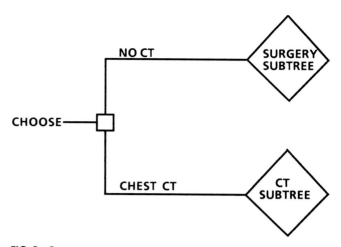

FIG 2–8.
Decision tree for management of lung cancer indicating choices of chest CT and no CT.

ability of mediastinal metastasis. Similarly the probability of the early disease outcome is one minus the mortality of surgery times one minus P. The expected clinical utility of the NO CT strategy is determined by adding together the product of each outcome's value and probability.

Expected Utility NO CT = $0 \times MT$ +
$0.9 \times P \times (1 - MT)$ +
$9.9 \times (1 - P) \times (1 - MT)$

The number of possible outcomes in the second strategy (see Fig 2–10) is five if CT is interpreted as either positive or negative. The first chance node in

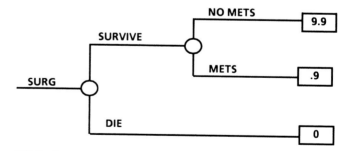

FIG 2–9.
NO CT subtree depicting events following decision to perform surgery. Numbers in rectangular boxes—terminal nodes—represent estimates of quality-adjusted patient life expectancy, in years, associated with outcome. From top to bottom, the probabilities of the five different outcomes are

$(1 - MT) \times (1 - P)$
$(1 - MT) \times P$
MT

P = prevalence; MT = mortality of surgery.

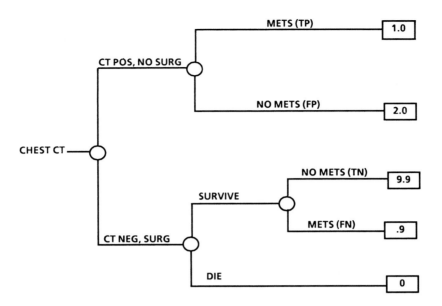

FIG 2–10.
CT subtree depicting events following decision to perform chest CT. Numbers in rectangular boxes—terminal nodes—represent estimates of quality-adjusted patient life expectancy, in years, associated with outcome. The probability of each outcome is determined by Bayes theorem. From top to bottom, the probabilities of the five different outcomes are:

$(P \times S)$
$(1 - P) \times (1 - Sp)$
$(1 - MT) \times (1 - P) \times Sp$
$(1 - MT) \times P \times (1 - S)$
$MT \times [(1 - P) \times Sp + P \times (1 - S)]$

S = sensitivity of CT; Sp = specificity of CT; P = prevalence; MT = mortality of surgery.

the strategy indicates that CT may be either positive or negative. With a positive result, another chance node indicates that the positive result may either be correct or incorrect. Similarly, a negative result may or may not be correct. Thus, there are five possible outcomes of the CT strategy. The first two outcomes are a true positive CT result with surgery appropriately withheld and a false positive CT result with surgery inappropriately withheld. The false positive CT outcome might be associated with a value of 2.0 QALYS. The other three outcomes parallel those of the NO CT strategy: a true negative CT result with curative surgery, a false negative CT result with unnecessary surgery, and perioperative death. For simplicity, we have assumed that the morbidity and mortality of chest CT are zero.

The probabilities of the five different outcomes in the CT strategy from top to bottom are calculated using Bayes theorem. Just as with NO CT, the expected clinical utility of CT is calculated by summing the products of the outcome values and probabilities.

If the sensitivity and specificity of CT are 0.95 and 0.65, the pretest probability of mediastinal metastasis, 0.50, and the surgical mortality, 0.05, then the expected clinical utility of the NO CT strategy is

greater than that of the CT strategy: 5.1 QALYS versus 3.9 QALYS. In other words, a patient undergoing chest CT would be expected to live, on the average, 1.2 years less than the patient going directly to surgery. This difference in outcome can be attributed largely to the relatively low specificity of chest CT and the high cost (in terms of patient outcome) of a false positive test result. In fact, if the other variables are held constant, the specificity of CT must exceed 0.98 for the CT strategy to be beneficial. Alternatively, if all the variables are held constant except for the pretest probability of mediastinal metastasis, it can be shown that this latter variable must exceed 0.95 for the CT strategy to increase patient life expectancy. In like fashion, breakeven points or thresholds can be identified for key variables where the expected utilities of competing strategies are the same. By varying the input data, decision analysis can be tailored to a particular patient or medical environment without necessarily changing the structure of the decision tree. This ability to play out "what if" scenarios is a major advantage of decision analysis over the traditional intuitive decision process.

In addition to varying the input data, the structure of the decision tree can be modified to allow for refinements in a diagnostic or treatment strategy. In the earlier example, an additional branch might be grafted onto the decision tree indicating that positive CT scans are confirmed with mediastinoscopy, so that patients with false positive CT studies are not denied potentially curative surgery. This CT/mediastinoscopy strategy would actually provide a slightly greater patient life expectancy than the NO CT strategy and also reduce overall dollar costs of medical management.[3]

Sometimes the result of a decision analysis is a "close call"[8] in which no particular strategy is favored. However, such a "close call" result may still be useful in that it reassures the decision maker and patient that relevant information has been explicitly and impartially taken into account.

Cost-Effectiveness Analysis

In addition to estimating expected clinical utility, decision analysis can also estimate expected cost of a medical strategy. In those situations where one strategy has both a greater clinical utility and lower cost than another, the former strategy is clearly preferable. However, when one strategy has a greater clinical utility and greater cost, then the trade-off must be considered within a particular context. This trade-off is conventionally represented as a cost-effectiveness ratio (CER): the ratio of marginal cost (dollars of medical expenditure) to marginal benefit (QALYS).[4, 22]

$$\text{Marginal CER} = \frac{\text{Cost}_1 - \text{Cost}_2}{\text{QALYS}_1 - \text{QALYS}_2}$$

The higher the ratio, the less cost-effective is the one strategy relative to the other. The ultimate goal of cost-effectiveness analysis is not necessarily to choose the strategy with the lowest CER. Such an approach would largely eliminate medical intervention, even that which is highly beneficial. Instead, cost-effectiveness analysis should be used to maximize the benefit of diagnostic testing given a CER constraint. The concept of CER helps put the relative usefulness of various medical and other public health measures into perspective so that they can be more consistently applied (Table 2–2). Ultimately, society as a whole will have to define what maximum CER is acceptable.

More sophisticated techniques of decision analysis are beginning to take into account the dynamic nature of disease processes. Diseases fluctuate in their severity and are frequently fatal. With Markov models, the transition rates between levels of severity

TABLE 2–2.

Costs Per Year of Life Saved for Some Health Investments

Mandatory air bags [22]	$ 540
Coronary artery bypass (three-vessel) [22]	7,200
Screening mammography [24]	18,000
Hemodialysis [22]	25,000
Liver transplant—1-year survival [22]	250,000

(including death) can be used to estimate the QALYS associated with decision tree outcomes.[1] Sometimes the question is not if the test should be done, but when. Considering the problem of patient follow-up, it has been shown that the optimal scheduling of tests is a function of the rate of disease recurrence (hazard rate), the time delay between when a disease is detectable by the examination and when it presents clinically (lead time), and cost-benefit constraints.[5] These and other developing techniques are increasing the applicability of the relatively new discipline—medical decision making—to clinical practice.

REFERENCES

1. Beck JR, Pauker SG: The Markov process in medical prognosis. *Med Decis Making* 1983; 3:419–458.
2. Black WC, Armstrong P: Communicating the significance of radiologic test results: The likelihood ratio. *AJR* 1986; 147:1313–1318.
3. Black WC, Armstrong PA, Daniel TM: Cost-effectiveness of chest CT in T1NOMO lung cancer. *Radiology* 1988; 167:373–378.
4. Doubilet PM: Cost effective: A trendy, often misused term. *AJR* 1987;148:827–828.
5. Dwyer AJ, Prewitt JMS, Ecker JG, et al: Use of the hazard rate to schedule follow-up exams efficiently. An optimization approach to patient management. *Med Decis Making* 1983; 3:229–244.
6. Gelfan DW, Ott DJ: Methodologic considerations in comparing imaging modalities. *AJR* 1985; 144:1117–1121.
7. Glazer GM, Orringer MB, Gross BH, et al: The mediastinum in non-small cell lung cancer: CT-surgical correlation. *AJR* 1984; 142:1101–1105.
8. Kassirer JP, Pauker SG: The toss-up. *N Engl J Med* 1981; 305:1467–1469.
9. McNeil BJ, Keeler E, Adelstein SJ: Primer on certain elements of medical decision making. *N Engl J Med* 1975; 293:211–215.
10. Melamed MR, Flehinger BJ, Zaman MB, et al: Screening for early lung cancer. Results of the Memorial Sloan-Kettering study in New York. *Chest* 1984; 86:44–53.

11. Metz CE: Basic principles of ROC analysis. *Semin Nucl Med* 1978; 8:283–298.

12. Pauker SG, Kassirer JP: Decision analysis. *N Engl J Med* 1987; 316:250–260.

13. Pauker SG, et al: The threshold approach to clinical decision making. *N Engl J Med* 1980; 302:1109–1116.

14. Philbrick JT, Horwitz RI, Feinstein AR: Methodologic problems of exercise testing for coronary artery disease: Groups, analysis and bias. *Am J Cardiol* 1980; 46:807–812.

15. Philips WC, Scott JA, Blaszcynski GI: How sensitive is "sensitivity"; how specific is "specificity"? *AJR* 1983; 140:1265–1270.

16. Radack KL, et al. The likelihood ratio. *Arch Pathol Lab Med* 1986; 110:689–693.

17. Ransohoff DF, Feinstein AR: Problems of spectrum and bias in evaluating the efficacy of diagnostic tests. *N Engl J Med* 1978; 299:926–930.

18. Sackett DL: Interpretation of diagnostic data. 5. How to do it with simple math. *Can Med Assoc J* 1983; 129:947–954.

19. Schwartz WB, Wolfe JH, Pauker SG: Pathology and probabilities: A new approach to interpreting and reporting biopsies. *N Engl J Med* 1981; 305:917–923.

20. Simon R: Confidence intervals for reporting results of clinical trials. *Ann Intern Med* 1986; 105:429–435.

21. Sox HC: Probability theory in the use of diagnostic tests. *Ann Intern Med* 1986; 104:60–66.

22. Weinstein MC: Challenges for cost-effectiveness research. *Med Decis Making* 1986; 6:194–198.

23. Weinstein MC, et al: *Clinical Decision Analysis*. Philadelphia, WB Saunders, 1980.

3

The Normal Chest

In this chapter we will consider the normal anatomy of the lungs, mediastinum, and diaphragm as demonstrated on the plain chest radiograph (Fig 3–1), conventional contrast examinations, computed tomography (CT), and magnetic resonance imaging (MRI).

THE LUNGS AND AIRWAYS

The Central Airways

The trachea is a straight tube which, in children and young adults, passes downward and backward in the midline. With unfolding and ectasia of the aorta, the trachea deviates to the right as it descends into the chest. It may also bow forward. In cross section, it is round, oval, or oval with a flattened posterior margin. The upper limit of normal for its coronal and sagittal diameters in adults is 25 and 27 mm respectively for men and 21 and 23 mm for women.[5]

The trachea divides into the two main-stem bronchi at the carina. In children the angles are symmetrical, but in adults the right main-stem bronchus has a steeper angle than the left. The range of angles is wide, and alterations in angle can only be diagnosed by right-left comparisons, not by absolute measurement.

The lobar and segmental branching pattern is shown in Figure 3–2. There are many variations. These are of greater interest to the bronchoscopist and surgeon than to the radiologist now that bronchography is almost never performed.

The Hili

Understanding the appearances of the normal pulmonary hili requires an appreciation of the anatomy of the major bronchi (see Fig 3–2) and hilar blood vessels (Figs 3–3 and 3–4)[21, 38, 55, 57] because it is these structures that are demonstrated with imaging (Figs 3–5, 3–6, 3–7, and 3–8). The normal lymph nodes, nerves, and connective tissue do not contribute significantly to the bulk of the hili, and the small amounts of fat between the vessels is, for practical purposes, visible only at MRI.

The following points of anatomy should be remembered:

1. The right main bronchus has a more vertical course than the left main bronchus. Also, the right upper lobe bronchus arises more proximally than the left upper lobe bronchus.

2. The right main-stem bronchus and its divisions into the right upper lobe bronchus and bronchus intermedius are outlined posteriorly by lung so that the posterior wall of these portions of the bronchial tree is seen as a thin stripe (Figs 3–7 and 3–9). This region is, therefore, a sensitive area in which to look for masses, such as lymphadenopathy. On the left side, the lower lobe artery intervenes between the lung and the bronchial tree, and only a small tongue of lung can invaginate between the left lower lobe artery and the descending aorta to contact the posterior wall of the left main-stem bronchus (see Fig 3–7).[56]

3. The right pulmonary artery passes anterior to the major bronchi to reach the lateral aspect of the

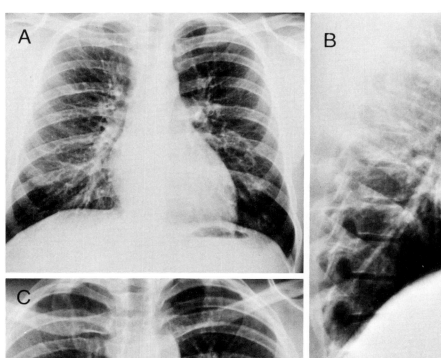

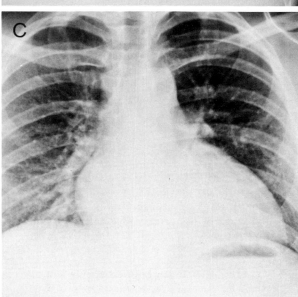

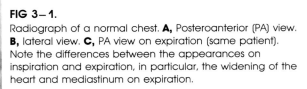

FIG 3–1.
Radiograph of a normal chest. **A,** Posteroanterior (PA) view.
B, lateral view. **C,** PA view on expiration (same patient).
Note the differences between the appearances on
inspiration and expiration, in particular, the widening of the
heart and mediastinum on expiration.

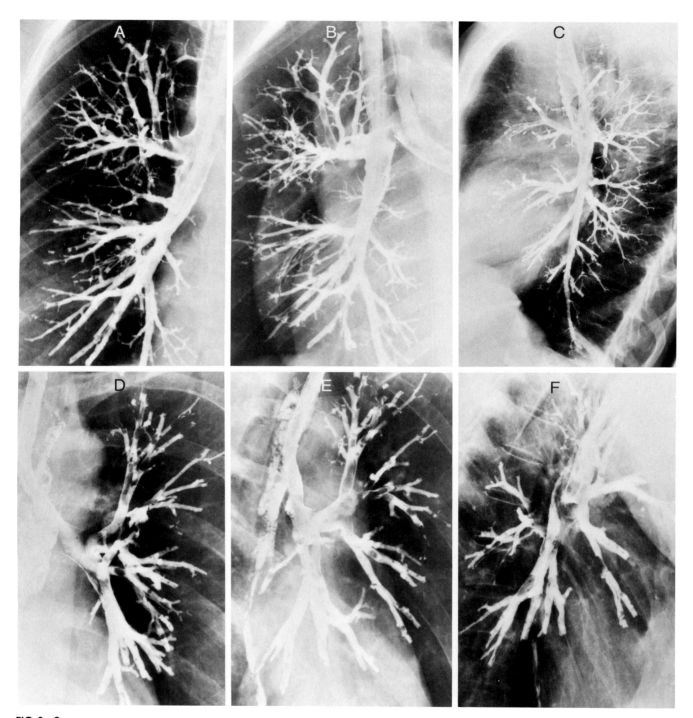

FIG 3–2.
The divisions of the bronchial tree shown by bronchography. **A,** right bronchial tree—anteroposterior (AP) view. **B,** right bronchial tree—right posterior oblique view. **C,** right bronchial tree—lateral view. **D,** left bronchial tree—AP view. **E,** left bronchial tree—left posterior oblique view. **F,** left bronchial tree—lateral view.

(Continued.)

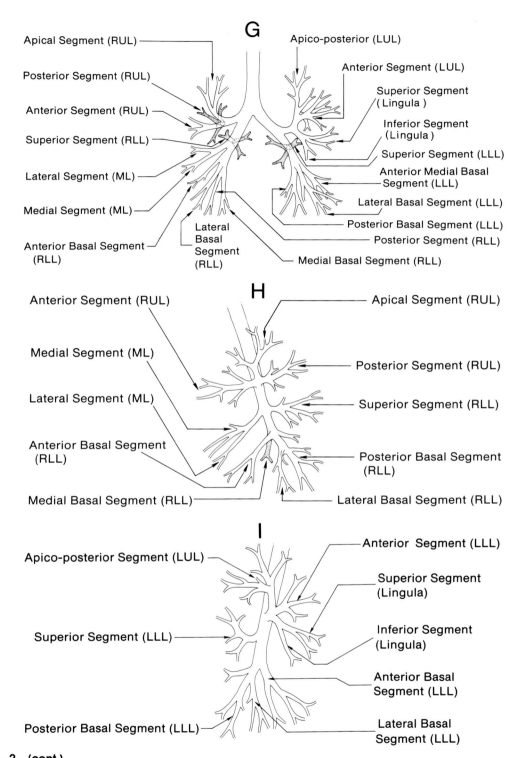

FIG 3–2   (cont.).
G, diagram of AP view. **H,** diagram of lateral view of right bronchial tree. **I,** diagram of lateral view of left bronchial tree.

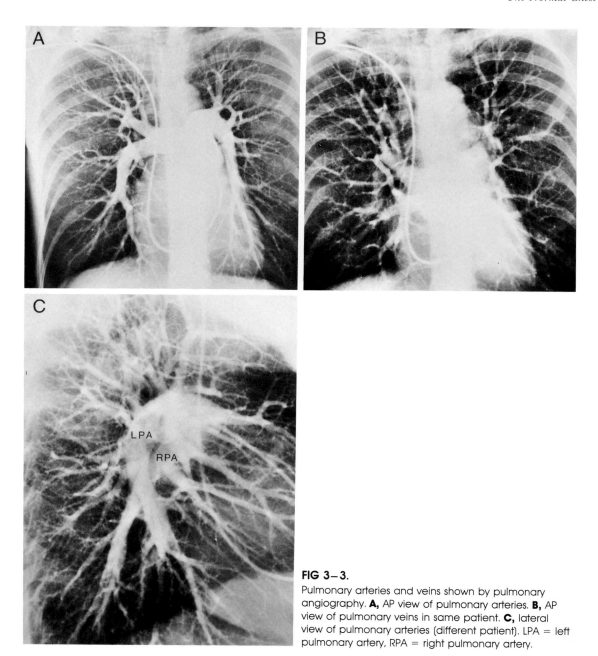

FIG 3–3.
Pulmonary arteries and veins shown by pulmonary angiography. **A,** AP view of pulmonary arteries. **B,** AP view of pulmonary veins in same patient. **C,** lateral view of pulmonary arteries (different patient). LPA = left pulmonary artery, RPA = right pulmonary artery.

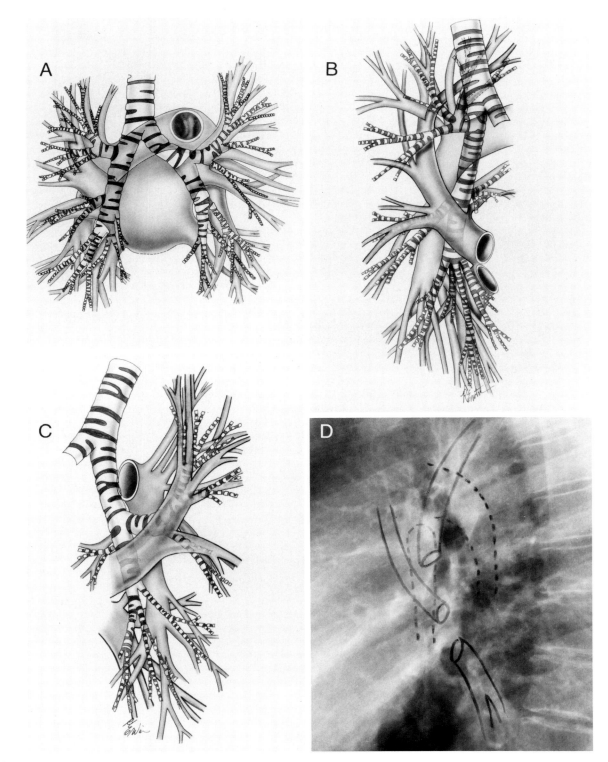

FIG 3-4.

Diagram of hilar structures. **A,** frontal view. **B,** right hilus: oblique view. **C,** left hilus: oblique view. **D,** lateral radiograph with position of central pulmonary arteries and veins drawn in. The left and right pulmonary arteries are indicated by *dotted lines* (the left lies pos- terior to the right). The inferior pulmonary veins are similar on the two sides and are superimposed (only one is drawn in). The right superior pulmonary vein is on a more anterior plane than the left superior pulmonary vein.

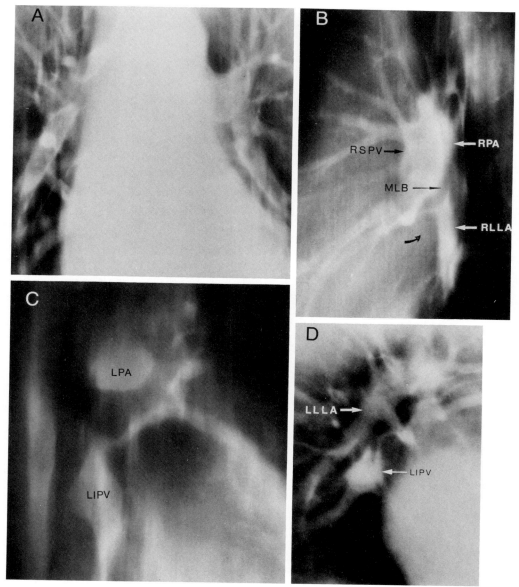

FIG 3—5.
Conventional tomograms of hilar structures. **A,** AP view. **B,** lateral view of right hilus. **C,** oblique view of left hilus. **D,** lateral view of left hilus. LIPV = left inferior pulmonary vein, LLLA = left lower lobe artery, LPA = left pulmonary artery, MLB = middle lobe bronchus, RPA = right pulmonary artery, RLLA = right lower lobe artery, RSPV = right superior pulmonary vein. The *curved black arrow* points to the angle between the middle and lower lobe bronchi, which is devoid of a normal rounded shadow.

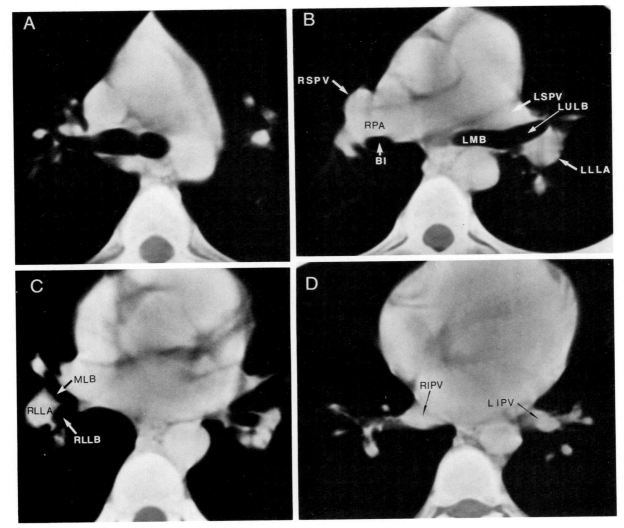

FIG 3–6.
CT scans of pulmonary hili. **A,** at level of tracheal carina. The hilar vessels at this level are segmental divisions. **B,** at level of bronchus intermedius. Note the lack of major vessels behind the bronchus intermedius and the conglomerate density formed by the right pulmonary artery and the right superior pulmonary vein. **C,** at the level of the inferior (right) middle lobe bronchus. **D,** at the level of the inferior pulmonary veins. BI = bronchus intermedius, LIPV = left inferior pulmonary vein, LLLA = left lower lobe artery, LMB = left main bronchus, LSPV = left superior pulmonary vein, LULB = left upper lobe bronchus, MLB = middle lobe bronchus, RIPV = right inferior pulmonary vein, RLLB = right lower lobe bronchus, RPA = right pulmonary artery, RSPV = right superior pulmonary vein.

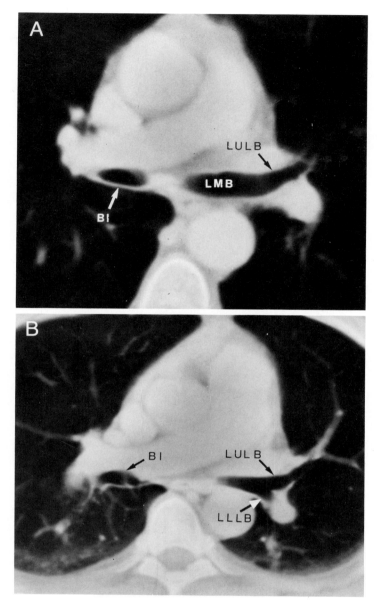

FIG 3–7.
A and **B,** CT scans illustrating posterior relationships of left and right bronchial tree. BI = bronchus intermedius, LLLB = left lower lobe bronchus, LMB = left main bronchus, LULB = left upper lobe bronchus. Section **A** is 1 cm higher than section **B.**

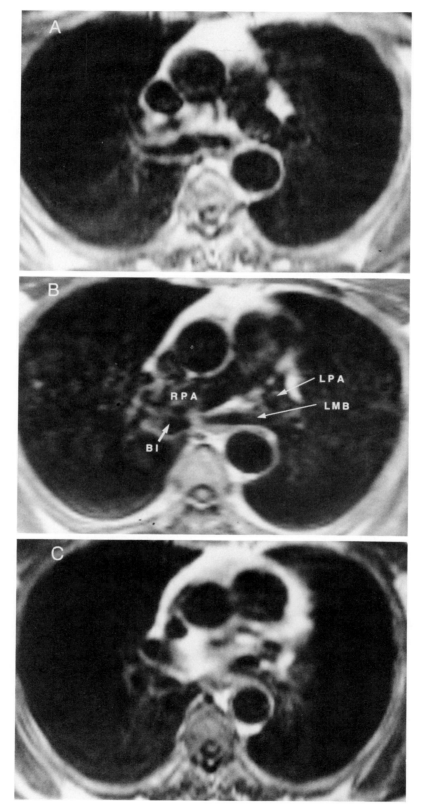

FIG 3–8.
A–C, MR images of pulmonary hili: three adjacent sections. Note the relative lack of signal in the hilar regions. BI = bronchus inter-medius, LMB = left main bronchus, LPA = left pulmonary artery, RPA = right pulmonary artery.

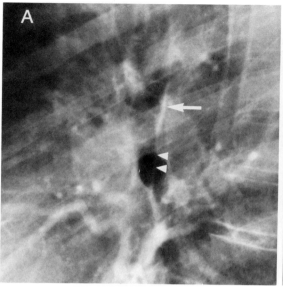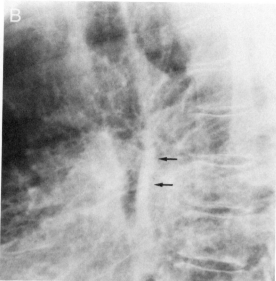

FIG 3—9.

A, lateral radiograph of normal pulmonary hili. The *arrow* points to the posterior wall of the right main bronchus and the *arrowheads* point to the posterior wall of the bronchus intermedius. **B,** lateral view in a patient with lymphangitis carcinomatosa shows thickening of the tissues posterior to the bronchus intermedius *(arrows).*

bronchus intermedius and right lower lobe bronchus, whereas the left pulmonary artery arches over the left main bronchus and left upper lobe bronchus to descend posterolateral to the left lower lobe bronchus.

4. The pulmonary veins are similar on the two sides. The superior pulmonary veins are the anterior structures in the upper and midhilus on both sides, and the inferior pulmonary veins run obliquely forward beneath the divisions of each lower lobe artery to enter the left atrium. Because the central portions of the pulmonary arteries are so differently organized on the two sides, the relationship of the major veins to the arteries differs. On the right, the superior pulmonary vein is separated from the central bronchi by the lower division of the right pulmonary artery, whereas on the left, the superior pulmonary vein is separated from the lower division of the left pulmonary artery by the bronchial tree.

5. On the plain chest radiograph, the transverse diameter of the lower lobe arteries prior to their segmental divisions can be measured with reasonable accuracy. The arteries should normally be 9 to 16 mm in diameter (Fig 3—10). The large round shadow seen on the lateral and oblique views of the right hilus, both on plain films and conventional tomography, is a combination of the right pulmonary artery and the superior pulmonary vein (see Fig 3—5, B). The combined shadows of these two vessels may be sufficiently large to be confused with a mass.

6. Another feature of note with conventional radiographs, particularly tomograms, is that normally there are no large vessels traversing the angle between the middle and the lower lobe bronchi on the right or the angle between the upper and lower lobe bronchi on the left (see Fig 3—5). Therefore, a rounded shadow larger than 1 cm in either of these angles is unlikely to be a normal vessel. Caution is needed, however, because the superior pulmonary vein may, on occasion, appear in sharp focus on a tomogram in the same section as the middle lobe or left upper lobe bronchus. In these circumstances it is usually possible to trace the shadow out into the lungs and confirm that it is indeed the superior pulmonary vein.

The Lungs Beyond the Hili

The *segmental bronchi* divide into progressively smaller airways until, after six to 20 divisions, they no longer contain cartilage in their walls and become bronchioles. The bronchioles divide, and the last of the purely conducting airways is known as the terminal bronchiole. Beyond the terminal bronchioles lie the gas-exchange units of the lung, the acini. The walls of the segmental bronchi are invisible on chest radiograph except when seen end-on as ring shadows. The entire airway down to the terminal bronchiole can, however, be identified on a well-filled bronchogram (Fig 3—11). The acinus, which is 5 to 6

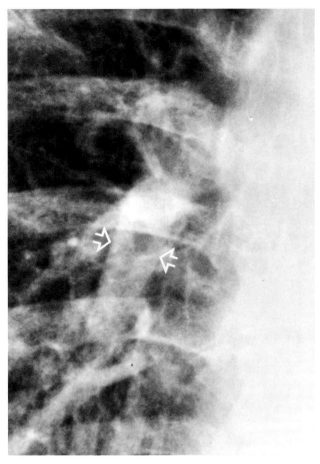

FIG 3–10.
Right lower lobe artery. The diameter indicated by the *arrows* should be between 9 and 16 mm.

The *pulmonary blood vessels* (see Fig 3–3) are responsible for the branching linear markings within the lungs both on conventional films and at CT scanning. It is not possible to distinguish arteries from veins in the outer two-thirds of the lungs except by angiography. More centrally, the orientation of the arteries and veins differs: the inferior pulmonary veins draining the lower lobes run more horizontally; the lower lobe arteries, more vertically. In the upper lobes, the arteries and veins show a similar gently curving vertical orientation, but the upper lobe veins (when not superimposed on the arteries) lie lateral to the arteries and can sometimes be traced to the main venous trunk—the superior pulmonary vein. These anatomic differences are best demonstrated at tomography.

The diameter of the blood vessels beyond the hilus varies according to the position of the patient. On chest films taken with the patient in the upright position, there is a gradual increase in the diameter of both the arteries and the veins from apex to base. For such comparisons to be valid, the measurements must be made equidistant from the hilus. These changes in vessel size correlate with physiologic studies of perfusion which show that, with the patient erect, there is a gradation of blood flow increasing from apex to base, a difference that is less marked in the supine subject. Although general statements re-

mm in diameter, comprises respiratory bronchioles, alveolar ducts, and alveoli. Three to five acini are grouped together in lobules which, in the lung periphery, are separated by septa. When thickened by disease, these septa form the so-called septal lines or Kerley B lines.

The bronchopulmonary segments are based on the divisions of the bronchi (see Fig 3–2). The boundaries between segments are complex in shape, and the segments have been likened to the pieces of a three-dimensional jigsaw puzzle. With the rare exception of accessory fissures, there is no septation between them. Although processes such as atelectasis or pneumonia may predominate in one segment or another, these processes never conform precisely to the whole of just one segment, since collateral air drift occurs across segmental boundaries and intrapulmonary fluid may also spread from segment to segment without any visible sign of the segmental boundary.

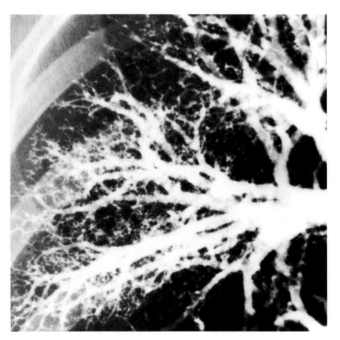

FIG 3–11.
Terminal bronchiolar filling by bronchography.

garding differences in regional blood vessel size can be made, it is difficult to make meaningful measurements of individual peripheral pulmonary vessels, since it is not known whether the vessel being measured is an artery or a vein, nor can one know the degree of magnification. Certain measurements have been suggested for upright chest films:[31]

- The artery and bronchus of the anterior segment of either or both upper lobes are frequently seen end-on. The diameter of the artery is usually much the same as the diameter of the bronchus (4 to 5 mm).
- Vessels in the first anterior interspace should not exceed 3 mm in diameter.

A rich network of *lymphatics* drains the lung and pleura. The subpleural lymphatic vessels are found just beneath the pleura, at the junction of the interlobular septa and pleura, where they interconnect with each other as well as with the lymphatic vessels in the interlobular septa. The lymph then flows to the hilus by way of lymphatic channels that run peribronchially and in the deep septa. Under normal circumstances the lymphatic network is radiographically invisible, but in certain conditions, for example if the lung is edematous or if the lymphatic channels are occluded by tumor, the enlarged septa containing the dilated lymphatics may become visible (see Chapter 5).

There are a few intrapulmonary lymph nodes which are small and are not identified on plain chest radiographs. Very occasionally they may be seen at CT as small, peripherally located nodules.

The Fissures

The lobes of the lungs are separated by fissures that, in the majority of people, are incomplete. In other words, lung tissue passes from one lobe to another through holes in the fissures.[59] These defects are important because they allow collateral air drift between lobes and also limit the accumulation of pleural fluid in the interlobar portions of the pleural cavity.[11]

The anatomy of the fissures is dealt with in detail in Chapter 14; only an outline is given here. The *major fissures* on each side are similar. The left major (oblique) fissure divides the left lung into an upper and lower lobe. The right lung has an additional fissure, the minor (horizontal) fissure, which separates

the middle from the right upper lobe. The major fissures run obliquely forward and downward, passing through the hilus, commencing at approximately the fifth thoracic vertebra to contact the diaphragm 0 to 3 cm behind the anterior chest wall. Portions of one or both major fissures are frequently seen on the lateral chest radiograph. It is, however, very unusual to be able to trace both fissures in their entirety. Each major fissure follows a gently curving plane somewhat similar to that of a propeller blade, with the upper portion facing forward and laterally and the lower portion facing forward and medially. Below the hili, the lateral portions of the major fissures lie further forward than do the medial portions, whereas above the hili, this relationship reverses. Because of these undulations, it is sometimes possible to identify the lateral aspect of the upper portion of either major fissure in the frontal view.[41, 42] Though these undulations can be identified at CT,[42] they cannot, in general, be traced on the plain chest radiograph. On a lateral view, therefore, one cannot be certain which portion of the fissure is being profiled, and it is easy to misinterpret a fissure as displaced when it is in fact in normal position. The inferior few centimeters of either or both major fissures are often wide, as a result of fat or pleural thickening between the leaves of the pleura. This thickening may lead to loss of silhouette where the fissure contacts the diaphragm.

The *minor fissure* fans out forward and laterally in a horizontal direction from the right hilus. On a standard upright frontal chest radiograph, the minor fissure contacts the lateral chest wall at, or close to, the axillary portion of the right sixth rib. The fissure curves gently, the anterior and lateral portion usually curving downward. Because of the undulations of the major fissure, the minor fissure may be projected posterior to the right major fissure on a normal lateral view.

On standard CT examination (Fig 3–12), the normal fissures are less frequently visible as a line. Their position can, however, usually be predicted from the position of the relatively avascular zone that forms the outer cortex of the lobe.[36, 42] The region of the major fissures is seen as a band of avascularity, or a zone with much smaller vessels, traversing the lung. The minor fissure appears as an oval deficiency of vessels on one or more sections at the level of the bronchus intermedius.[27] Because the major fissures run obliquely through the section, the fissure is usually either invisible or is

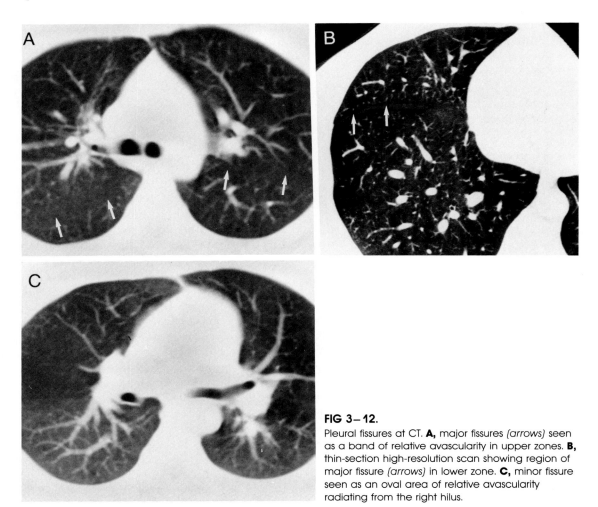

FIG 3—12.
Pleural fissures at CT. **A,** major fissures *(arrows)* seen as a band of relative avascularity in upper zones. **B,** thin-section high-resolution scan showing region of major fissure *(arrows)* in lower zone. **C,** minor fissure seen as an oval area of relative avascularity radiating from the right hilus.

a poorly defined band of density. On very thin sections, the fissure will more frequently be seen as a line.

Occasionally, other fissures are present. The most common, seen in up to 1% of the population, is the "azygos lobe fissure" (Fig 3–13), so called because it contains the azygos vein within its lower margin. The fissure results from failure of normal migration of the azygos vein from the chest wall to its usual position in the tracheobronchial angle, so that the invaginated visceral and parietal pleurae persist to form a fissure. The altered course of the azygos vein together with the fissure is readily seen at CT.[52] Since there is no corresponding alteration in the segmental architecture of the lung, the term "lobe" is a misnomer. It is supplied by branches of the apical segment bronchus with or without a contribution from the posterior segmental airway.[4] It is not unduly susceptible to disease.

Fissures may, very rarely, be seen at the bound-

aries between bronchopulmonary segments.[26] A minor fissure, similar to the minor fissure on the right, can occur on the left separating the lingular segments from the remainder of the upper lobe. A horizontally oriented fissure—the superior accessory fissure—may be seen separating the superior segment from the basal segments in either lower lobe. An inferior accessory fissure is common in one or the other lower lobe, particularly on the right, separating the medial basal segment from the remaining segments.[54] This accessory fissure is usually not deep enough to be seen on plain chest radiographs but, when visible, runs obliquely upward and medially toward the hilus from the diaphragm.

The inferior pulmonary ligaments are pleural reflections, analogous in shape to the peritoneal reflections which form the broad ligaments of the uterus. These ligaments invest the hili and connect the mediastinal surface of each lower lobe to the mediastinum. They are discussed further in Chapter 14.

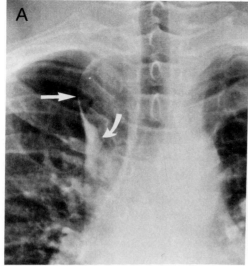

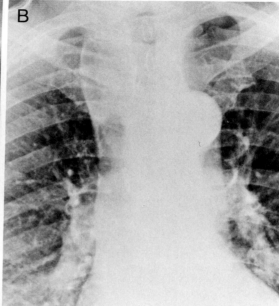

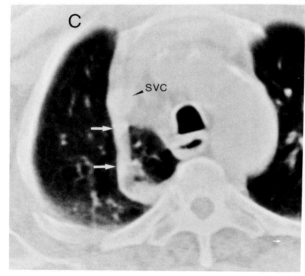

FIG 3–13.
Azygos lobe fissure. **A,** typical example. The *horizontal arrow* points to the fissure. The *curved arrow* points to the azygos vein running in the lower margin of the fissure. Note that the azygos vein is not in its usual position in the tracheobronchial angle. **B,** an example in which the lung lying medial to the azygos fissure appears opaque. This opacity can be normal and does not represent disease—as is shown in **C,** a CT scan through the azygos lobe in the same patient. The band of the azygos vein *(arrows)* crossing through the lung to join the superior vena cava *(SVC)* is well seen.

THE MEDIASTINUM

The mediastinum is divided by anatomists into superior, anterior, middle, and posterior divisions.* The exact anatomic boundaries between these divisions are unimportant to the radiologist because they do not provide a clear-cut guide to disease, nor do these boundaries form barriers to the spread of disease. Moreover, almost every writer on the subject seems to have a different definition.[16, 18, 30, 60] We will start by describing the mediastinal structures and spaces as seen at CT and MRI and then move on to a description of their appearance on plain film, because the complex interfaces between the mediastinum and the lungs are best understood by careful correlation with cross-sectional images.

The Normal Mediastinum

The normal mediastinal structures that are always identified at CT and MRI (Fig 3–14) can be divided into the heart and blood vessels that make up the bulk of the mediastinum, the major airways, and

---

*According to *Gray's Anatomy,*[12] the mediastinum is divided into superior and inferior compartments by an imaginary line from the manubriosternal angle to the fourth intervertebral disk. The inferior compartment is divided into anterior, middle, and posterior. The anterior mediastinum lies anterior to the pericardium and the ascending aorta. The posterior mediastinum is bounded in front by the trachea, the pulmonary vessels, and the pericardium, and behind by the vertebral column. Its contents include the descending aorta, the esophagus, the azygos and hemiazygos veins, and the thoracic duct.

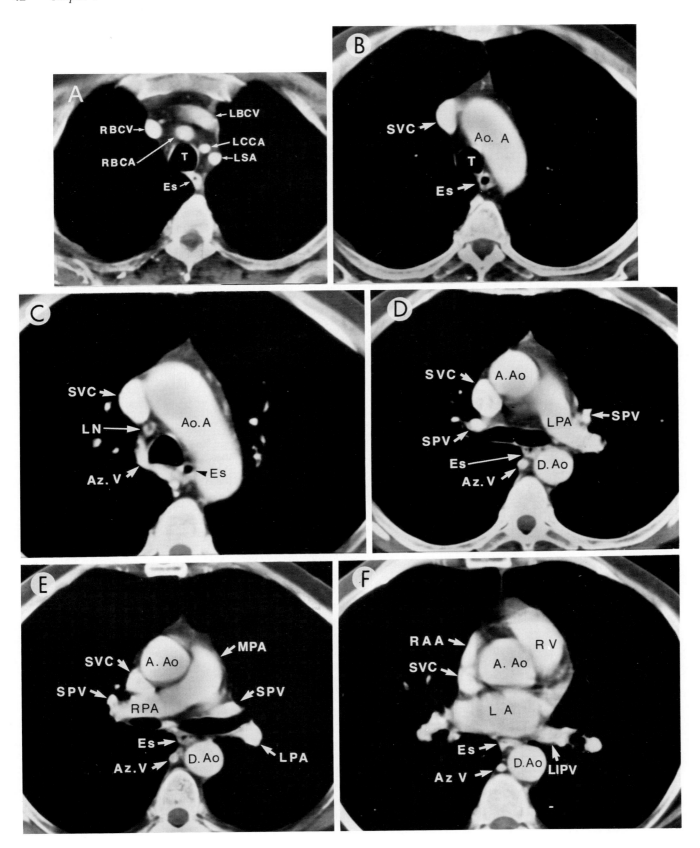

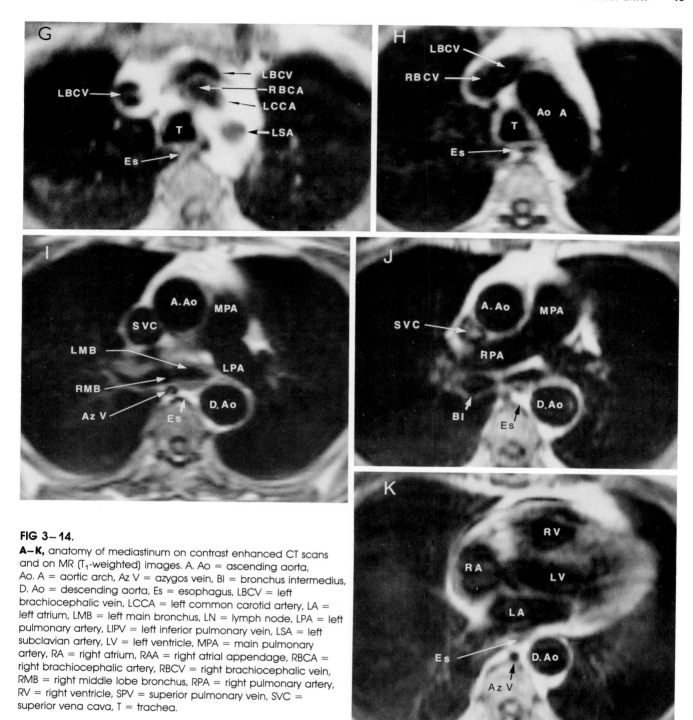

FIG 3–14.
A–K, anatomy of mediastinum on contrast enhanced CT scans
and on MR (T$_1$-weighted) images. A. Ao = ascending aorta,
Ao. A = aortic arch, Az V = azygos vein, BI = bronchus intermedius,
D. Ao = descending aorta, Es = esophagus, LBCV = left
brachiocephalic vein, LCCA = left common carotid artery, LA =
left atrium, LMB = left main bronchus, LN = lymph node, LPA = left
pulmonary artery, LIPV = left inferior pulmonary vein, LSA = left
subclavian artery, LV = left ventricle, MPA = main pulmonary
artery, RA = right atrium, RAA = right atrial appendage, RBCA =
right brachiocephalic artery, RBCV = right brachiocephalic vein,
RMB = right middle lobe bronchus, RPA = right pulmonary artery,
RV = right ventricle, SPV = superior pulmonary vein, SVC =
superior vena cava, T = trachea.

the esophagus. These structures are surrounded by a variable amount of connective tissue, largely fat, within which lie lymph nodes, the thymus, the thoracic duct, and the phrenic and laryngeal nerves.

Mediastinal Blood Vessels

On transaxial images, the vertically oriented ascending and descending portions of the aorta appear round, whereas the arch is seen as a tapering oval that becomes narrower as it gives rise to the arteries to the upper body. The average diameter of the ascending aorta is 3.5 cm; that of the descending aorta is 2.5 cm.[28] Sections above the aortic arch show the three major aortic branches arranged in a curve lying anterior and to the left of the trachea, their order, from right to left, being the brachiocephalic (innominate), left common carotid, and left subclavian arteries. The brachiocephalic artery is appreciably larger than the other two vessels. It varies slightly in position. In about half the population it is directly anterior to the trachea; in the remainder, while still anterior to the trachea, it is either slightly to the right or left of the midline.[20] The left common carotid artery lies to the left of the trachea; the left subclavian artery also lies either to the left of the trachea or posterior to it. It is the most lateral vessel of the three and often contacts the left lung.

In 0.5% of the population, the right subclavian artery arises as a fourth major branch of the aorta, instead of arising from the brachiocephalic artery. Known as an aberrant right subclavian artery, it runs behind the esophagus from left to right, at or just above the level of the aortic arch, to lie against the right side of the vertebral bodies before entering the neck. In individuals with an aberrant right subclavian artery, the brachiocephalic artery (really the right common carotid artery) is smaller than usual, being similar in diameter to the left common carotid artery.

As the descending aorta travels through the chest it gradually moves from a position to the left of the vertebral bodies to an almost midline position before exiting from the chest through the aortic hiatus in the diaphragm. The diameter should remain nearly constant, but with increasing age dilatation and tortuosity may develop.

The mediastinal venous anatomy[25] is illustrated in Figure 3–15. The superior vena cava (SVC) has an oval or round configuration on transaxial section. Its diameter is usually one-third to two-thirds the diameter of the ascending aorta.[28] It can, however, be considerably smaller and may be much flattened in shape.

On occasion (in 0.3% to 0.5% of the healthy population, but in 4.4% to 12.9% of those with congenital heart disease[6, 8]), there may be a left SVC (Fig 3–16). This anomaly results from failure of obliteration of the left common cardinal vein during fetal development. A right SVC and an interconnecting brachiocephalic vein are also present in most cases. A left SVC arises from the junction of the left jugular and subclavian veins and travels vertically through the left mediastinum, passing anterior to the left main bronchus before joining the coronary sinus on the back of the heart. From this point the blood flows through the coronary sinus into the right atrium, the coronary sinus being significantly larger than normal because of the increased blood flow. A left SVC may be confused with lymphadenopathy if the full course of the vessel is not appreciated.

The left brachiocephalic vein forms a curved band anterior to the arteries arising from the arch of the aorta. Since it takes an oblique, downward course to joint the SVC, its image on axial sections may be oval rather than tubular in shape. The right brachiocephalic vein, which travels vertically, lies anterolateral to the trachea in line with the three major arteries. This vein is identifiable as the farthest right of the vessels; it is larger than the arteries, and is oval in shape. The junction of the right and left brachiocephalic veins is frequently identifiable.

The azygos vein travels anterior to the spine, either behind or to the right of the esophagus, until at some variable point it arches forward to join the posterior wall of the SVC. Usually it remains within the mediastinum and occupies the right tracheobronchial angle. In the 1% of the population who have an azygos lobe, the azygos vein traverses the lung before entering the SVC, in which case the SVC may appear distorted.

The hemiazygos and accessory hemiazygos veins also lie against the vertebral bodies, but in a more posterior plane, usually just behind the descending aorta. The accessory hemiazygos vein drains into the left superior intercostal vein, which arches around the aorta more or less at the junction of the arch and the descending portion, and joins the left brachiocephalic vein. The left superior intercostal vein is much smaller than the azygos vein and is only rarely identified on CT scans.

Occasionally, the inferior vena cava (IVC) does not develop in the usual fashion, and the azygos vein forms the venous conduit draining inferior vena caval blood back to the heart. The hepatic veins in these cases drain into the right atrium, not into the IVC. The azygos vein will, therefore, be a very large

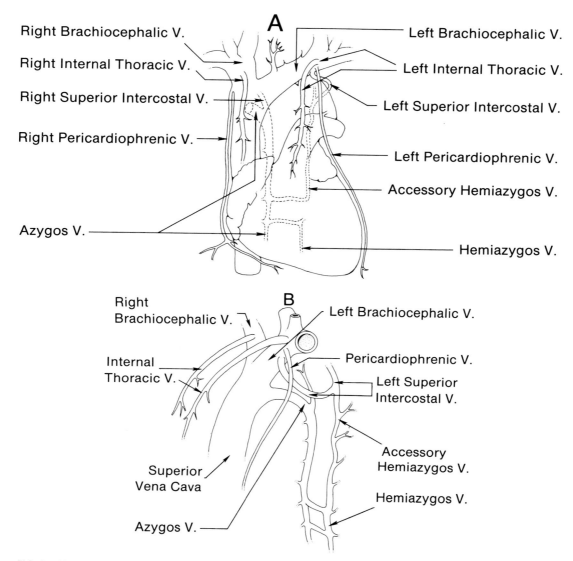

Right Brachiocephalic V.
Right Internal Thoracic V.
Right Superior Intercostal V.
Right Pericardiophrenic V.
Azygos V.

A

Left Brachiocephalic V.
Left Internal Thoracic V.
Left Superior Intercostal V.
Left Pericardiophrenic V.
Accessory Hemiazygos V.
Hemiazygos V.

B

Right Brachiocephalic V.
Internal Thoracic V.
Superior Vena Cava
Azygos V.

Left Brachiocephalic V.
Pericardiophrenic V.
Left Superior Intercostal V.
Accessory Hemiazygos V.
Hemiazygos V.

FIG 3–15.
A and **B,** diagram illustrating mediastinal venous anatomy. Redrawn from Godwin JD, Chen JTT. Thoracic venous anatomy. *AJR* 1986; 147:674–684.

structure, only slightly smaller than the IVC. Its anatomy is otherwise unaltered. Azygos continuation of the IVC may resemble a mediastinal mass or lymphadenopathy.

The main pulmonary artery runs obliquely backward and upward to the left of the ascending aorta. It divides into right and left branches. The right branch travels more or less horizontally through the mediastinum, between the ascending aorta and SVC anteriorly and the major bronchi posteriorly. The left pulmonary artery arches higher than the right pulmonary artery and passes over the left main bronchus to descend posterior to it. This configuration leads to two important observations: the left

pulmonary artery is often seen on a higher section than the right pulmonary artery; and the lung abuts the posterior wall of the right airway, but is partly or totally excluded from contact with the left airway by the descending limb of the left pulmonary artery. The external diameter of the main pulmonary artery is slightly smaller than that of the ascending aorta, averaging 2.8 cm in the series by Guthaner et al.[28] The right pulmonary artery is two-thirds the diameter of the main pulmonary artery.

The Esophagus

The esophagus is visible on all axial sections from the root of the neck down to the esophageal hi-

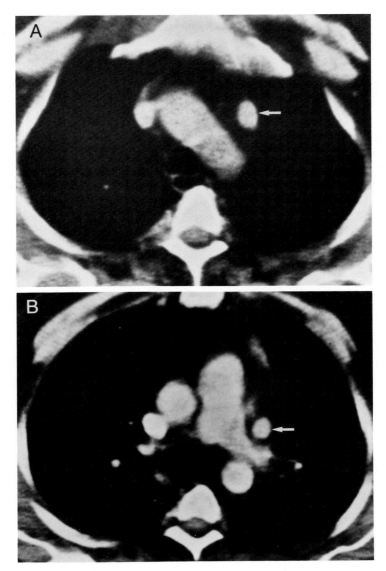

FIG 3–16.
Persistent left superior vena cava *(arrow).* **A,** section at level of aortic arch. **B,** section 3 cm lower.

atus through the diaphragm. In approximately 80% of normal persons, the esophagus contains air, sometimes just a small amount. If there is sufficient mediastinal fat, the entire circumference of the esophagus can be identified. If air is present in the lumen, the uniform thickness of the wall can be appreciated. Without air, the collapsed esophagus appears either circular or oval and is usually approximately 1 cm in its narrowest diameter. At MRI the signal intensity on T1-weighted images is similar to that of muscle, but on T2-weighted images the esophagus often shows a much higher signal intensity than muscle (Fig 3–17).

The Thymus

The thymus is situated anterior to the aorta and the right ventricular outflow tract or pulmonary artery. At CT scanning it is usually found inferior to the left brachiocephalic vein and superior to the level of the horizontal portion of the right pulmonary artery; it is often best appreciated on a section through the aortic arch (Fig 3–18).[37]

In childhood prior to puberty,[29] the thymus fills in most of the mediastinum in front of the great vessels (see Fig 3–18). In this period the gland varies so greatly in size that measurement is of little value in deciding normality. Shape is a more useful criterion.

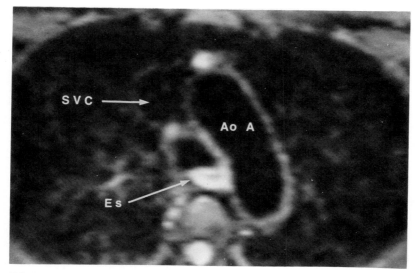

FIG 3–17.
MR image (T$_2$-weighted) of mediastinum showing the high signal intensity of the esophagus. Ao A = ascending aorta, Es = esophagus, SVC = superior vena cava.

The thymus is soft and fills in the spaces between the great vessels and the anterior chest wall as if moulded by these structures. The lateral margins may be convex, straight, or bulged outward, and approximate symmetry is the rule. A sharp angular border equivalent to the sail sign on plain films is occasionally visible at CT.[29] In young children, the thymus may extend all the way into the posterior mediastinum[10, 17] and may, very occasionally, be confused with a posterior mediastinal mass.[50]

The gland consists of two lobes, each enclosed in its own fibrous sheath[47]; up to 30% of the population have a fat cleft visible by CT at the junction of the two lobes. Of the two lobes, the left is usually larger[13] and is situated slightly higher than the right.[48] But these asymmetries are moderate, and it is not always possible to clearly define the two lobes.[37] A large lobe on one side with little or no thymic tissue visible on the other suggests a mass. At CT, the thymus is bilobed, triangular, or shaped like an arrowhead. The maximum width and thickness of each lobe decrease with advancing age. Between ages 20 and 50, the average thickness measured by CT decreases from 8 or 9 mm to 5 or 6 mm, the maximum

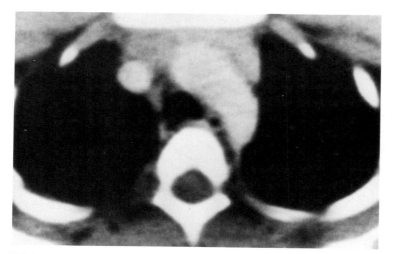

FIG 3–18.
Normal thymus in a 12-year-old boy. The thymus fills in most of the mediastinum and moulds to the aorta and superior vena cava.

thickness of one lobe being up to 1.5 cm.[3, 17] These diameters are greater at MRI, presumably because MRI demonstrates the thymic tissue even when it is partially replaced by fat.[13] At MRI sagittal images demonstrate that the gland is 5 to 7 cm in craniocaudad dimension.[13] It is impractical to measure the craniocaudad dimension at CT scanning, but the gland may be visible over a similar distance.[3, 17]

In younger patients the CT density of the thymus is homogeneous and close to that of other soft tissues. The gland often enhances appreciably with intravenous contrast material, but to a lesser extent than the great vessels.[29] After puberty, the density gradually decreases owing to fatty replacement.[51] In patients older than age 40, the thymus may have an attenuation value identical to that of fat.[3] In some patients, the whole gland shows fat density[3, 14] and is therefore indistinguishable from mediastinal fat. In others, residual thymic parenchyma is visible as a streaky or nodular density (Fig 3–19).[14, 37]

Early reports of the MRI appearances of the normal thymus suggest that the gland is always visible.[13] On T1-weighted images, the intensity is appreciably lower than that of mediastinal fat though, as would be expected, this difference decreases with age. On T2-weighted images, the intensity is similar to fat and does not vary with age. Proton density images show significantly less signal than the surrounding fat.

The "Mediastinal Spaces"

The nomenclature of the connective tissue spaces within the mediastinum is not standard, and there are no exact definitions for the boundaries between them. Nevertheless, the terms in common use need to be understood by radiologists. There are five named spaces surrounding the central airways (Fig 3–20): (1) the pretracheal space, (2) the aortopulmonary window, (3) the subcarinal space, (4) the right paratracheal space, and (5) the posterior tracheal space. All five contain lymph nodes that drain the lung and are therefore likely to be involved by bronchial carcinoma. In addition to these central spaces, there are the junction areas, so-called because in these areas the two lungs approximate each other. One lies anterior to the aorta and pulmonary artery and is variously known as the anterior junction[44] or the prevascular space[20]; the other lies posterior to the esophagus and is known as the posterior junction.[43] Finally, there are the paraspinal lines on either side of the spine and the junctional area between mediastinum and retroperitoneum known as the retrocrural space.

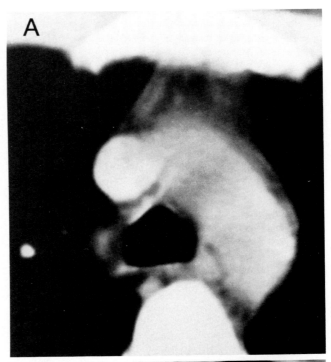

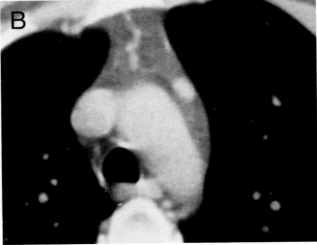

FIG 3–19.
Normal thymic remnants. **A,** streaky linear remnants in a 21-year-old woman. **B,** nodular remnants in a 36-year-old man.

Pretracheal Space

The pretracheal space[49] has no boundary with the lung and is therefore not imaged on plain chest radiographs. It is well known to surgeons, because it is the space explored by transcervical mediastinoscopy. The space is triangular in cross section—the three boundaries being the trachea or carina posteriorly, either the superior vena cava or the right innominate vein anteriorly and to the right, and the ascending aorta with its enveloping superior pericardial si-

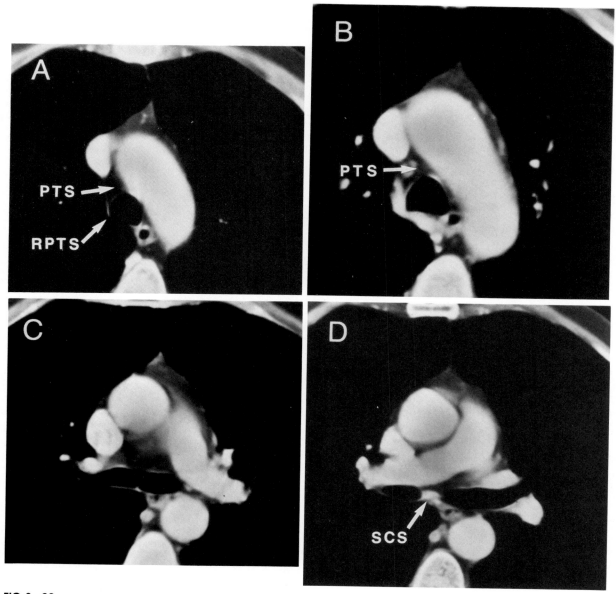

FIG 3–20.
A–D, the mediastinal spaces. PTS = pretracheal space, RPTS = right paratracheal space, SCS = subcarinal space. The four sections **(A–D)** are adjacent sections.

nus anteriorly and to the left.[1] Being centrally located, it is continuous with the right paratracheal space, the aortopulmonary window, and the subcarinal space. Consequently, lymph nodes or other masses arising in any of these spaces may grow large enough to encroach on the pretracheal space and vice versa.

The Aortopulmonary Window

The aortopulmonary window is situated under the aortic arch above the left pulmonary artery. It is bounded medially by the trachea and esophagus and laterally by the lung. Its fatty density is not always appreciated at CT scanning because so often the sections include either the aortic arch or the left pulmonary artery, and volume averaging results in higher than fat density.

The ligamentum arteriosum and the recurrent laryngeal nerve traverse this space. How often they can be identified is not clear, but in any event, they are not likely to be confused with lymphadenopathy or other masses.

The Subcarinal Space

The subcarinal space, lying beneath the tracheal carina, is bounded on either side by the major bronchi. The azygoesophageal recess of the right lung lies behind the subcarinal space, and distortions of the azygoesophageal recess are a sensitive method of detecting masses, usually lymphadenopathy, in this region. The posterior boundary is partly formed by the esophagus; hence, the use of the barium swallow examination to assess subcarinal swellings.

The Right Paratracheal Space and Posterior Tracheal Space

These two adjacent spaces (they should more properly be called stripes) are best considered together. Normally, the right lung is separated from the trachea only by a thin layer of fat (the only exception being at the tracheobronchial angle where the azygos vein lies between the lung and the airway). The degree to which the lung envelops the posterior wall of the trachea is variable. In up to half the population, a substantial portion of the posterior tracheal wall is outlined by lung as it interposes between the spine and the trachea to contact the esophagus.

The Anterior Junction

The *anterior junction*[44] (prevascular space) lies anterior to the pulmonary artery, the ascending aorta, and the three major branches of the aortic arch. This space lies between the two lungs and is bounded anteriorly by the chest wall. If the two lungs approximate each other closely enough, the intervening mediastinum may consist of little more than four layers of pleura and is then sometimes known as the anterior junction line (see Fig 3–24). Coursing through the prevascular space superiorly is the left brachiocephalic vein. The internal mammary vascular bundles are to be found laterally and are only visible at CT if intravenous contrast material is administered. Embedded within the prevascular space are lymph nodes, the thymus, and the phrenic nerve. Otherwise there is only a variable amount of fat and other connective tissue, which can be so small in amount that the two lungs abut one another or so great that the separation is several centimeters.

The Posterior Junction and Paraspinal Areas

The term *posterior junction* describes the mediastinal region posterior to the trachea and the heart, where the two lungs lie close to each other.[43] The right lung always invaginates behind the right hilar structures and the heart to contact the pleura overlying the azygos vein and the esophagus. This tongue of lung is therefore known as the azygoesophageal recess. Displacement of the lung from the azygoesophageal recess is an important sign of a subcarinal mediastinal mass, particularly adenopathy. Above the level of the azygos arch, contact is with the esophagus alone.

On the left, the lung interface is with the aortic arch and descending aorta rather than with the esophagus, but in some individuals the left lung below the aortic arch invaginates anterior to the descending aorta to almost reach the midline.

The paraspinal areas are contiguous with the posterior junction. Normally there is little or no discernible connective tissue between the lateral margins of the spine and the lungs. The only structures contained in these areas are intercostal vessels and small lymph nodes.

The Retrocrural Space

The aorta exits the chest by passing through the aortic hiatus, which is bounded by the diaphragmatic crura and the spine (Fig 3–21). The diaphragmatic crura are ligaments that blend with the anterior longitudinal ligament of the spine. Apart from the aorta, the structures that pass through the aortic hiatus are the azygos and hemiazygos veins, intercostal arteries, and splanchnic nerves. All these structures are small, too small to be mistaken for lymphadenopathy.[7]

Mediastinal Lymph Nodes

Lymph nodes are widely distributed in the mediastinum. The nomenclature for these nodes is not

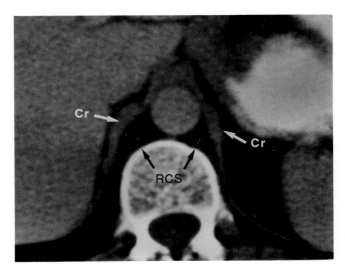

FIG 3–21.
Retrocrural spaces (RCS). Cr = diaphragmatic crura.

standardized nor, unfortunately, does it correspond exactly with the terms used for the mediastinal spaces. The following description uses terms in keeping with the nomenclature of the American Thoracic Society (ATS) designed for the staging of carcinoma of the bronchus (Table 3–1)[23, 24, 53] (Fig 3-22).

Anterior mediastinal nodes lie anterior or anterolateral to the aorta and the innominate artery (Station 6 in the ATS definitions).

TABLE 3–1.

American Thoracic Society Definitions of Regional Nodal Stations*

X	Supraclavicular nodes
2R	Right upper paratracheal nodes: nodes to the right of the midline of the trachea, between the intersection of the caudal margin of the innominate artery with the trachea and the apex of the lung
2L	Left upper paratracheal nodes: nodes to the left of the midline of the trachea, between the top of the aortic arch and the apex of the lung
4R	Right lower paratracheal nodes: nodes to the right of the midline of the trachea, between the cephalic border of the azygos vein and the intersection of the caudal margin of the brachiocephalic artery with the right side of the trachea
4L	Left lower paratracheal nodes: nodes to the left of the midline of the trachea, between the top of the aortic arch and the level of the carina, medial to the ligamentum arteriosum
5	Aortopulmonary nodes: subaortic and paraaortic nodes, lateral to the ligamentum arteriosum or the aorta or left pulmonary artery, proximal to the first branch of the left pulmonary artery
6	Anterior mediastinal nodes: nodes anterior to the ascending aorta or the innominate artery
7	Subcarinal nodes: nodes arising caudal to the carina of the trachea but not associated with the lower lobe bronchi or arteries within the lung
8	Paraesophageal nodes: nodes dorsal to the posterior wall of the trachea and to the right or left of the midline of the esophagus
9	Right or left pulmonary ligament nodes: nodes within the right or left pulmonary ligament
10R	Right tracheobronchial nodes: nodes to the right of the midline of the trachea, from the level of the cephalic border of the azygos vein to the origin of the right upper lobe bronchus
10L	Left peribronchial nodes: nodes to the left of the midline of the trachea, between the carina and the left upper lobe bronchus, medial to the ligamentum arteriosum
11	Intrapulmonary nodes: nodes removed in the right or left lung specimen, plus those distal to the main-stem bronchi or secondary carina

*From Glazer GM, Gross BH, Quint LE, et al: Normal mediastinal lymph nodes: Number and size according to American Thoracic Society mapping. *AJR* 1985; 144:261–265. Used with permission.

Tracheobronchial nodes encircle the trachea and main bronchi except where the aorta, pulmonary artery, and esophagus are in direct contact with the airway. There is no clear division between the various nodes in this group, but they can be divided according to site:

1. Right and left paratracheal nodes, which can be further subdivided into upper and lower groups, depending on whether they lie above or below the level of the top of the aortic arch (Stations 2R, 4R, 2L, and 4L). In the ATS-approved nomenclature this group includes the pretracheal nodes.

2. Aortopulmonary window nodes, which include nodes along the lateral surfaces of the aorta and left or main pulmonary arteries (Station 5).

3. Subcarinal nodes, a group that comprises all the nodes found beneath the carina and main bronchi (Station 7).

4. Tracheobronchial and hilar nodes. Tracheobronchial nodes (Stations 10R and 10L) lie adjacent to right and left main stem bronchi and are, therefore, mediastinal in location. The lower tracheobronchial nodes may, however, be removed at standard pneumonectomy. The hilar nodes (Stations 11R and 11L) are defined as nodes distal to the main stem bronchi, and these are always part of standard pneumonectomy.

The *posterior mediastinal nodes* are divided into paraesophageal (Station 8) and pulmonary ligament nodes (Station 9). Glazer et al.[24] include nodes around the descending aorta with Station 8 nodes. Nodes are also present in the retrocrural areas and in the anterior cardiophrenic angles.

Normal Lymph Node Size

There are three CT series to date in which normal lymph node size in the mediastinum has been measured, and these are in general agreement.[22, 23, 49] In these studies, 95% of normal mediastinal lymph nodes are less than 10 mm in diameter, and the remainder are, with very few exceptions, less than 15 mm in diameter. There is a significant variation in the number and size of lymph nodes seen in the different locations within the mediastinum. Nodes in the region of the brachiocephalic veins are generally smaller, over 90% being 5 mm or less, whereas nodes in the aortopulmonary window, the pretracheal and lower paratracheal spaces, and the subcarinal compartment are often 6 to 10 mm in diameter.

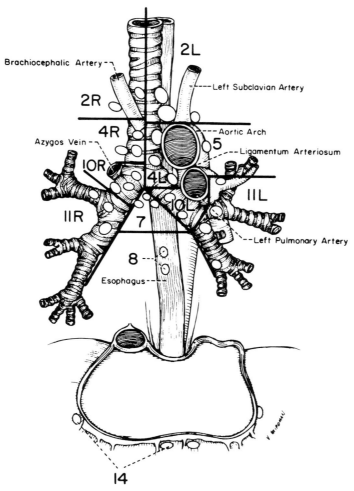

Brachiocephalic Artery

2L

2R

Left Subclavian Artery

4R

Aortic Arch

Azygos Vein

5

Ligamentum Arteriosum

IOR

4L

IIL

IIR

7

Left Pulmonary Artery

8

Esophagus

I4

FIG 3–22.
American Thoracic Society lymph node mapping scheme. Reprinted with permission from Glazer HS, Aronberg DJ, Sagel SS, et al: CT demonstration of calcified mediastinal lymph nodes: A guide to the new ATS classification. *AJR* 1986; 147:17–25. See Table 3–1 for definitions.

Normal Mediastinal Contours on Plain Chest Radiographs

Plain chest radiographs provide limited information regarding mediastinal anatomy, since only the interfaces between the lung and the mediastinum are visualized. For descriptive convenience we will treat the frontal and lateral projections separately, although in practice the information from these two views should be integrated. For further details of the normal appearances in the lateral projection, the reader is referred to the excellent accounts by Proto and Speckman.[45, 46]

Frontal Projection

The Left Mediastinal Border.—Above the aortic arch, the mediastinal shadow to the left of the trachea is of low density and is due to the left carotid and left subclavian arteries and the jugular veins. The usual appearance in the frontal projection is a gently curving border formed by the left subclavian artery, which fades out where the artery enters the neck. A separate interface may occasionally be discernible for the left carotid artery. The outer margin of the left tracheal wall is almost never outlined because the lung is separated from the trachea by the aorta and great vessels.

Below the aortic arch, the left mediastinal border is formed by the aortic-pulmonary pleural stripe,[32] the main pulmonary artery, and the heart. A small "nipple" may occasionally be seen projecting laterally from the aortic knob. This "nipple" is caused by the left superior intercostal vein arching forward around the aorta just beyond the origin of

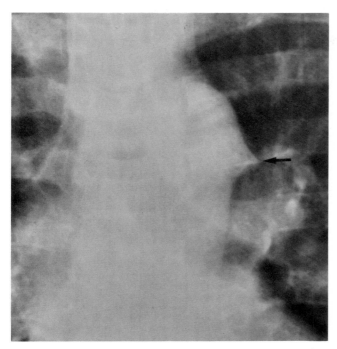

FIG 3–23.
The left superior intercostal vein *(arrow)* seen as the so-called "aortic nipple."

the left subclavian artery before entering the left brachiocephalic vein (Fig 3–23). This vein should not be misinterpreted as adenopathy projecting from the aortopulmonary window. Fat can sometimes be identified in the aortopulmonary window beneath the aortic arch.

The Right Mediastinal Border.—The right mediastinal border is normally formed by the right brachiocephalic (innominate) vein, the SVC, and the right atrium. The right paratracheal stripe can be seen through the right brachiocephalic vein and SVC because the lung contacts the right tracheal wall from the clavicles down to the arch of the azygos vein (Fig 3–24). This stripe, which should be of uniform thickness and no greater than 3 mm in width, is visible in approximately two-thirds of healthy subjects. It consists of the wall of the trachea and adjacent mediastinal fat, but there should be no focal bulges due to individual paratracheal lymph nodes. The diagnostic value of this stripe is that it excludes space-occupying processes in the area where the stripe is visible and appears normal. The azygos vein is outlined by air in the lung at the lower end of this stripe. The diameter of the azygos vein in the tracheobronchial angle is variable; it may be considered normal when 10 mm or less. The nodes immediately beneath the azygos vein, which are sometimes known as azygos nodes, are not recognizable on normal chest radiographs.

The Anterior Junction.—The two lungs approximate each other above the level of the heart and below the manubrium; therefore, the term "anterior junction" has been applied to this area of the mediastinum[44]. When the two lungs are separated only by pleura, the anterior junction forms a visible line (see Fig 3–24). This line, known as the anterior junction line, is usually straight and diverges to fade

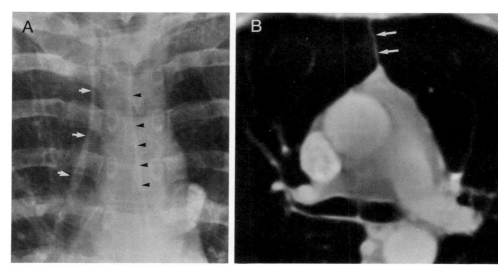

FIG 3–24.
A, anterior junction line *(black arrowheads)* and right paratracheal stripe *(white arrows)*. The lowest white arrow points to the azygos vein. **B,** CT scan in another patient shows anterior junction line *(arrows)*.

out superiorly as it reaches the clavicles. It descends for a variable distance, usually deviating to the left. Sometimes it follows a vertical course or, very rarely, it may deviate to the right. It cannot extend below the point where the two lungs separate to envelop the right ventricle. Since the line is only occasionally seen, failure to identify it is of no significance. More often the two lungs are separated by fat and thymus, with the result that the borders of the anterior junction are invisible on plain film, or only one or other border can be identified. Bulging of one or both borders indicates the presence of a mass. In young children, the thymus can be a prominent structure; the sail shape is characteristic (Fig 3–25).

Proto et al.[44] used the terms superior and inferior recesses to describe the lung interfaces above and below the anterior junction region. The interfaces of the superior recesses are concave laterally. They are formed by mediastinal fat anterior to the arteries that supply the head and neck. (The left and right brachiocephalic veins course through this fat but do not form visible borders on the frontal view.) The inferior recesses[44] are due to divergence of the lungs around fat in the lower mediastinum anterior to the heart.

The Posterior Junction.— In some patients, the lungs almost touch each other behind the esophagus to form the posterior junction line—a structure which can be thought of as an esophageal mesentery (Fig 3–26).[30] This line, unlike the anterior junction line, diverges to envelop the aortic and azygos arches. Above the aortic arch, the posterior junction line extends to the lung apices, where it diverges and disappears at the root of the neck, well above the level of the clavicles. The differences in the superior extent of the anterior and posterior junction lines are related to the sloping boundary between the thorax and the neck. Once again the width of the line depends on the amount of mediastinal fat. Whether both sides of the line are seen on plain chest radiograph depends on the tangent formed with the adjacent lung. Bulging of the borders of any portion of the posterior junction line or its superior recesses suggests a mass or other space-occupying process. The only normal convexities are those attributable to the azygos vein or aortic arch.

Whether or not there is a visible posterior junction line above the aortic arch, the interface between the lung and the right wall of the esophagus can often be seen as a very shallow S extending from the lung apex down to the azygos arch. If there is air in the esophagus, which there frequently is, the right wall of the esophagus will be seen as a stripe, usually 3 to 5 mm thick.[9] This interface is known as the pleuroesophageal line or stripe (Fig 3–27).

Below the aortic arch, the right lower lobe makes contact with the right wall of the esophagus and the azygos vein as it ascends next to the esophagus. This portion of lung is known as the azygoesophageal recess, and the interface is known as the azygoesophageal line (Fig 3–28). The shape of the azygos arch

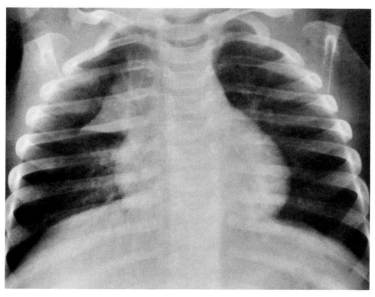

FIG 3–25.
Normal thymus in a 3-year-old child. The sail shape projecting to the right of the mediastinum is characteristic.

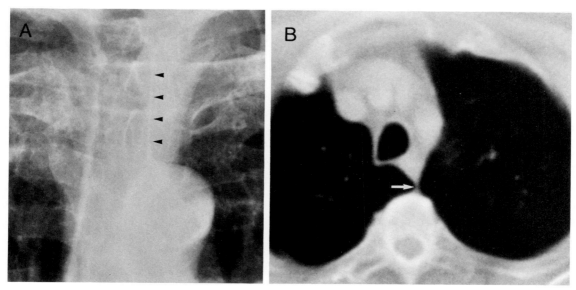

FIG 3–26.
A, posterior junction line *(arrowheads).* **B,** CT scan shows origin of the line *(arrow)* in the same patient.

varies considerably in different subjects and, therefore, the shape of the upper portion of the azygoesophageal line varies accordingly. The upper few centimeters of the azygoesophageal line are, however, always straight or concave toward the lung. A convex shape suggests a subcarinal mass. The azygoesophageal line can be traced down into the posterior costophrenic angle in subjects with normal anatomy.

The left wall of the esophagus (Fig 3–29) is rarely visible; the near vertical border seen through the heart represents the left wall of the descending aorta. This border can be traced, with virtually no loss of continuity, upward to the aortic arch and downward to the diaphragm. In a few subjects, a small segment of aortic outline may be invisible because of contact between the aorta and the descending division of the left pulmonary artery behind the left main bronchus.

Occasionally, the lung contacts the left wall of the esophagus, and then the esophagus will be outlined both from the right and the left. Because air is frequently present in the esophagus, it may even be possible to identify separately the thickness of the right and left walls. The usual site for air to be trapped is just beneath the aortic arch (see Fig 3–29).

The Paraspinal Lines.—The term "paraspinal line" refers to a stripe of soft tissue density parallel to the left and right margins of the thoracic spine. Although lymph nodes and intercostal veins share this space with mediastinal fat and pleura, these structures cannot normally be recognized individu-

ally. With little fat, the interface may closely follow the undulations of the lateral spinal ligaments. With larger quantities of fat, these undulations are smoothed out. The thickness of the left paravertebral space is usually greater than that of the right. The paravertebral stripes are usually less than 1 cm in width, though they can be wider in obese subjects. Aortic unfolding contributes to the thickness of the left paraspinal line; as the aorta moves posteriorly it strips the pleura from its otherwise close contact with the profiled portions of the spine.

Lateral View

The Mediastinum Above the Aortic Arch.—A variable portion of the aortic arch and the head and neck vessels are visible in the lateral view, depending on the degree of aortic unfolding. The brachiocephalic artery is the only artery recognized with any frequency. It arises anterior to the tracheal air column. Unless involved by atheromatous calcification, the origin is usually invisible, but after a variable distance, its posterior wall can be seen as a gentle S-shaped interface crossing the tracheal air column. The left and right brachiocephalic veins are also visible in the lateral view. The left brachiocephalic vein often forms an extrapleural bulge behind the manubrium. The posterior border of the right brachiocephalic vein and the SVC can occasionally be identified curving downward in much the same position and direction as the brachiocephalic artery, but are sometimes traceable below the upper margin of the aortic arch.

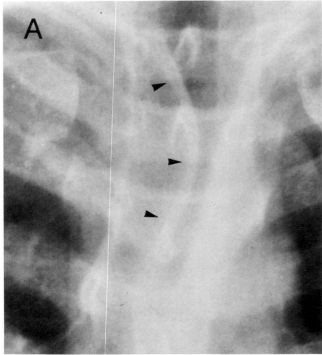

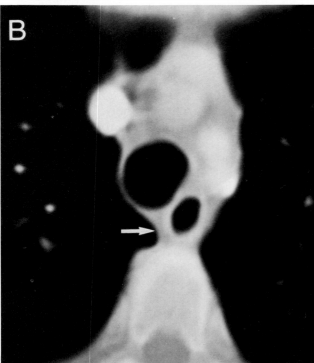

FIG 3–27.
A, pleuroesophageal line *(arrowheads).* **B,** CT scan shows the origin of the line *(arrow)* in the same patient.

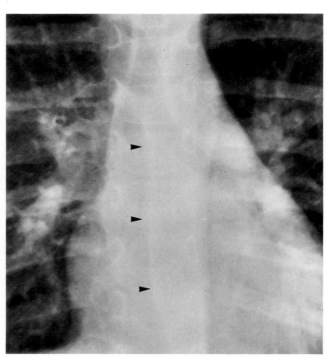

FIG 3–28.
Azygoesophageal line *(arrowheads).*

The Trachea and Retrotracheal Area.—The air column in the trachea can be seen throughout its length as it descends obliquely downward and posteriorly. The course of the trachea in the lateral view of adult subjects is straight, or bowed forward in patients with aortic unfolding, with no visible indentation by adjacent vessels. The carina is not visible on the lateral view. The anterior wall of the trachea is visible only in a minority of patients, but its posterior wall is usually visible because lung often passes behind the trachea, thereby allowing one to see the "posterior tracheal stripe or band" (Fig 3–30).[2] This stripe is seen in 50% to 90% of healthy adults.[2, 39] It is uniform in width and measures up to 3 mm (rarely, 4 mm). There is, however, a problem in applying this measurement. Because air is frequently present in the esophagus, the anterior wall of the esophagus may contribute to the thickness of the stripe in healthy subjects.[39] Alternatively, the lung may be separated from the trachea by the full width of a collapsed esophagus, leading to a band of density 1 cm or more in thickness (Fig 3–31). Thus, caution is needed if abnormalities are to be diagnosed on the basis of an increase in thickness of the posterior tracheal stripe. CT study has shown that the visibility of the posterior tracheal stripe is dependent on the degree to which the lung passes behind the trachea.[34] Sometimes there is little space between the

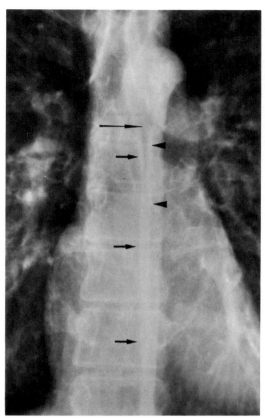

FIG 3–29.
The right and left walls of the esophagus. The *arrowheads* point to the left wall. The *arrows* point to the right wall (azygoesophageal line). The *uppermost arrow* points to air in the lumen of the esophagus trapped beneath the aortic arch.

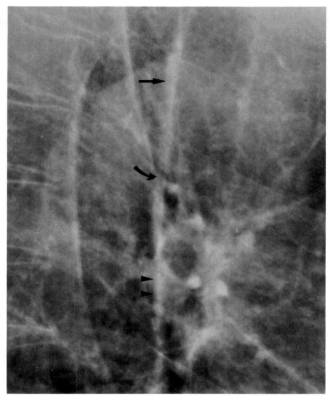

FIG 3–30.
Posterior tracheal band *(straight arrow)*. Note that the posterior walls of the trachea, right main bronchus *(curved arrow)*, and bronchus intermedius *(arrowheads)* are seen as a continuous thin band.

airway and the spine and, what little there is, is occupied by the esophagus and connective tissue. Clearly, the quantity of mediastinal fat is an important factor in determining how much lung invaginates behind the trachea.

The Retrosternal Line.—A bandlike opacity simulating pleural or extrapleural disease is often seen in healthy individuals along the lower half or third of the anterior chest wall on the lateral view (Fig 3–32).[58] This density is due to the differing anterior extent of the left and right lungs. The left lung does not contact the most anterior portion of the left thoracic cavity at these levels because the heart and its epicardial fat occupies the space.

The Inferior Vena Cava.—In most healthy subjects the posterior wall of the inferior vena cava is visible just before it enters the right atrium. Even patients with azygos continuation of the inferior vena cava may show a similar vessel formed by the contin-

uation of the hepatic veins as they drain into the right atrium. In approximately 5% of healthy people the posterior wall of the inferior vena cava is not visible on the lateral chest radiograph.

THE DIAPHRAGM

The diaphragm consists of a large, dome-shaped central tendon with a sheet of striated muscle radiating from the central tendon to attach to ribs 7 through 12 and to the xiphisternum.[19, 33, 40] The two crura arise from the upper three lumbar vertebrae and arch upward and forward to form the margins of the aortic and esophageal hiati. The median arcuate ligament connecting the two crura forms the anterior margin of the aortic hiatus, and the crura themselves form the lateral boundary of the aortic hiatus. Accompanying the aorta through this opening are the azygos and hemiazygos veins and the thoracic duct. Anterior to the aortic hiatus lies the esophageal hiatus, through which run the espoha-

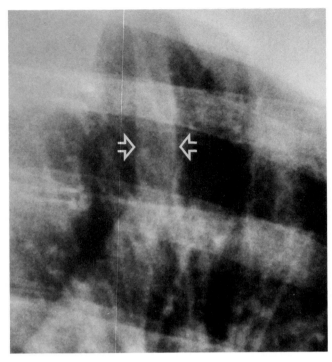

FIG 3—31.
Normal collapsed esophagus appearing as a band shadow *(arrows)* posterior to the trachea.

gus, the vagus nerve, and the esophageal arteries. The most anterior of the three diaphragmatic hiati is the hiatus for the IVC, which is situated within the central tendon immediately beneath the right atrium. The diaphragm has a smooth dome shape in most individuals, but a scalloped outline is also common.

The position of the diaphragm in healthy subjects on upright plain chest radiographs taken at full inspiration was investigated by Lennon and Simon.[35] They used the anterior ribs to describe the position of each hemidiaphragm, because the dome is closer to the anterior chest wall, and both the domes and the anterior ribs are closer to the film in the PA projection. The normal right hemidiaphragm is found at about the level of the anterior sixth rib, being slightly higher in women and in individuals over 40 years of age. The range is approximately one interspace above or below this level. In most people, the right hemidiaphragm is 1½ to 2½ cm higher than the left, but the two hemidiaphragms are at the same level in some 9% of the population. In a few, 3% in the series by Felson,[15] the left hemidiaphragm is higher than the right, but by less than 1 cm. The normal excursion of the diaphragm is usually between 1.5 and 2.5 cm, though greater degrees of movement are not uncommon.

Incomplete muscularization, known as eventration, is also very common. An eventration is composed of a thin membranous sheet replacing what should be muscle. Usually it is partial, involving one-half to one-third of the hemidiaphragm, frequently the anteromedial portion of the right hemidiaphragm. The lack of muscle manifests itself radiographically as elevation of the affected portion of the diaphragm, and the usual pattern is a smooth hump on the contour of the diaphragm. When the entire hemidiaphragm is involved, it will be elevated and, on fluoroscopy, there will be poor, absent, or paradoxical movement. In severe cases it is impossi-

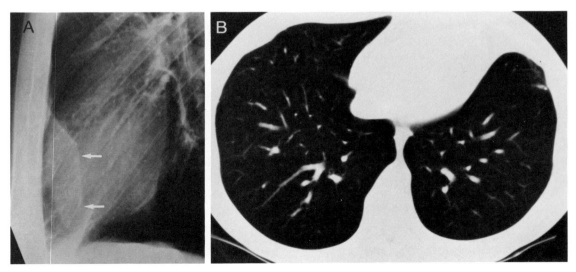

FIG 3—32.
A, the retrosternal line *(arrows).* **B,** CT scan in the same patient shows that the anterior margin of the left lung lies more posterior than the anterior margin of the right lung, in part because of the heart and in part because of epicardial fat.

ble to distinguish congenital eventration from acquired paralysis of the phrenic nerve.

REFERENCES

1. Aronberg DJ, Peterson RR, Glazer HS, et al: The superior sinus of the pericardium: CT appearance. *Radiology* 1984; 153:489–492.
2. Bachman AL, Teixidor HS: The posterior tracheal band: A reflector of local mediastinal abnormality. *Br J Radiol* 1975; 48:352–359.
3. Baron RL, Lee JKT, Sagel SS, et al: Computed tomography of the normal thymus. *Radiology* 1982; 142:121–125.
4. Boyden EA: The distribution of bronchi in gross anomalies of the right upper lobe, particularly lobes subdivided by the azygos vein and those containing pre-eparterial bronchi. *Radiology* 1952; 58:797–807.
5. Breatnach E, Abbott GC, Fraser RE: Dimensions of the normal human trachea. *AJR* 1984; 142:903–906.
6. Buirski G, Jordan SC, Joffe HS, et al: Superior vena caval abnormalities: Their occurrence rate, associated cardiac abnormalities and angiographic classification in a paediatric population with congenital heart disease. *Clin Radiol* 1986; 37:131–138.
7. Callen PW, Korobkin M, Isherwood I: Computed tomographic evaluation of retrocrural prevertebral space. *AJR* 1977; 129:907–910.
8. Cha EM, Khoury GH: Persistent left superior vena cava: Radiologic and clinical significance. *Radiology* 1972; 103:375–381.
9. Cimmino CV: The esophageal-pleural stripe: An update. *Radiology* 1981; 140:607–613.
10. Cohen MD, Weber TR, Sequeira FW, et al: The diagnostic dilemma of the posterior mediastinal thymus. CT manifestations. *Radiology* 1983; 146:691–693.
11. Dandy WE: Incomplete pulmonary interlobar fissure sign. *Radiology* 1978; 128:21–25.
12. Davies DV, Coupland RE (eds): *Gray's Anatomy*, ed 34. London, Longmans, Green and Co, 1967.
13. deGeer G, Webb WR, Gamsu G: Normal thymus: Assessment with MR and CT. *Radiology* 1986; 158:313–317.
14. Dixon AK, Hilton CJ, Williams CT: Computed tomography and histological correlation of the thymic remnant. *Clin Radiol* 1981; 32:255–257.
15. Felson B: *Chest Roentgenology*. Philadelphia, WB Saunders, 1973.
16. Felson B: The mediastinum. *Semin Roentgenol* 1969; 4:41–58.
17. Francis IR, Glazer GM, Bookstein FL, et al: The thymus: Re-examination of age-related changes in size and shape. *AJR* 1985; 145:249–254.
18. Fraser RG, Pare JAP, Pare PD, et al: *Diagnosis of Diseases of the Chest*, ed 3. Vol 1. Philadelphia, WB Saunders, 1988.
19. Gale ME: Anterior diaphragm: Variations in the CT appearance. *Radiology* 1986; 161:635–639.
20. Gamsu G: Computed tomography of the mediastinum, in Moss AA, Gamsu G, Genant HK (eds): *Computed Tomography of the Body*. Philadelphia, WB Saunders, 1983.
21. Genereux GP: Conventional tomographic hilar anatomy emphasizing the pulmonary veins. *AJR* 1983; 141:1241–1257.
22. Genereux GP, Howie JL: Normal mediastinal lymph node size and number: CT and anatomic study. *AJR* 1984; 142:1095–1100.
23. Glazer GM, Gross BH, Quint LE, et al: Normal mediastinal lymph nodes: Number and size according to American Thoracic Society mapping. *AJR* 1985; 144:261–265.
24. Glazer HS, Aronberg DJ, Sagel SS, et al: CT demonstration of calcified mediastinal lymph nodes: A guide to the new ATS classification. *AJR* 1986; 147:17–20.
25. Godwin JD, Chen JTT: Thoracic venous anatomy. *AJR* 1986; 147:674–684.
26. Godwin JD, Tarver RD: Accessory fissures of the lung: Pictorial essay. *AJR* 1985; 144:39–47.
27. Goodman LR, Golkow RS, Steiner RM, et al: The right mid-lung window. *Radiology* 1982; 143:135–138.
28. Guthaner DF, Wexler L, Harell G: CT demonstration of cardiac structures. *AJR* 1979; 133:75–81.
29. Heiberg E, Wolverson MK, Sundaram M, et al: Normal thymus: CT characteristics in subjects under age 20. *AJR* 1982; 138:491–494.
30. Heitzman ER: *The Mediastinum: Radiologic Correlations With Anatomy and Pathology*, ed 2. Berlin, Springer-Verlag, 1988.
31. Jefferson K, Rees S: *Clinical Cardiac Radiology*. London, Butterworths, 1973.
32. Keats TE: The aortic-pulmonary mediastinal stripe. *AJR* 1972; 116:107–109.
33. Kleinman PK, Raptopoulos V: The anterior diaphragmatic attachments: An anatomic and radiologic study with clinical correlations. *Radiology* 1985; 155:289–293.
34. Kormano M, Yrjana J: The posterior tracheal band: Correlation between computed tomography and chest radiography. *Radiology* 1980; 136:689–694.
35. Lennon EA, Simon G: The height of the diaphragm in the chest radiograph of normal adults. *Br J Radiol* 1965; 38:937–943.
36. Marks BW, Kuhns LR: Identification of the pleural fissures with computed tomography. *Radiology* 1982; 143:139–141.
37. Moore AV, Korobkin M, Olanow W, et al: Age-related changes in the thymus gland: CT-pathologic correlation. *AJR* 1983; 141:241–246.
38. Naidich DP, Khouri NF, Scott WW, et al: Computed tomography of the pulmonary hila: Normal anatomy. *J Comput Assist Tomogr* 1981; 5:459–467.

39. Palajew MJ: The tracheo-esophageal stripe and the posterior tracheal band. *Radiology* 1979; 132:11–13.

40. Panicek DM, Benson CB, Gottlieb RH, et al: The diaphragm: Anatomic, pathologic, and radiologic considerations. *RadioGraphics* 1988; 8:385–425.

41. Proto AV, Ball JB: The superolateral major fissures. *AJR* 1983; 140:431–437.

42. Proto AV, Ball JB: Computed tomography of the major and minor fissures. *AJR* 1983; 140:439–448.

43. Proto AV, Simmons JD, Zylak CJ: The posterior junction anatomy. *Crit Rev Diagn Imaging* 1983; 20:121–173.

44. Proto AV, Simmons JD, Zylak CT: The anterior junction anatomy. Crit Rev Diagn Imaging 1983; 19:111–173.

45. Proto AV, Speckman JM: The left lateral radiograph of the chest. Part one. *Med Radiogr Photogr* 1979; 55:30–74.

46. Proto AV, Speckman JM: The left lateral radiograph of the chest. Part two. *Med Radiogr Photogr* 1980; 56:36–64.

47. Rosai J, Levine GD: Normal thymus, in *Atlas of Tumor Pathology*, 2nd series Fascicle 13, Armed Forces Institute of Pathology, 1976.

48. Sagel SS, Aronberg DJ: Thoracic anatomy and mediastinum, in Lee JKT, Sagel SS, Stanley RJ (eds): *Computed Body Tomography*. New York, Raven Press, 1982.

49. Schnyder PA, Gamsu G: CT of the pretracheal retrocaval space. *AJR* 1981; 136:303–308.

50. Shackleford G, McAlister W: The aberrantly positioned thymus. *AJR* 1974; 120:291–296.

51. Siegelman SS, Scott WW, Baker RR, et al: CT of the Thymus, in Siegelman SS (ed): *Computed Tomography of the Chest*. New York, Churchill Livingstone, 1984.

52. Speckman JM, Gamsu G, Webb WR: Alterations in CT mediastinal anatomy produced by an azygos lobe. *AJR* 1980; 137:47–50.

53. Tisi GM, Friedman PJ, Peters RM, et al: Clinical staging of primary lung cancer. American Thoracic Society recommendations. *Am Rev Respir Dis* 1983; 127:659–663.

54. Trapnell DH: The differential diagnosis of linear shadows in chest radiographs. *Radiol Clin North Am* 1973; 11:77–92.

55. Vix VA, Klatte EC: The lateral chest radiograph in the diagnosis of hilar and mediastinal masses. *Radiology* 1970; 96:307–316.

56. Webb WR, Gamsu G: Computed tomography of the left retrobronchial stripe. *J Comput Assist Tomogr* 1983; 7:65–69.

57. Webb WR, Glazer G, Gamsu G: Computed tomography of the normal pulmonary hilum *J Comput Assist Tomogr* 1981; 5:485–490.

58. Whalen JP, Meyers MA, Oliphant M, et al: The retrosternal line. *AJR* 1973; 117:861–872.

59. Yamashita H: *Roentgenologic Anatomy of the Lung*. Tokyo, Igaku-Shoin, 1978.

60. Zylak CJ, Pallie W, Jackson R: Correlative anatomy and computed tomography: A module on the mediastinum. *RadioGraphics* 1982; 2:255–592.

Normal Variants That May Simulate Disease

Proper interpretation of chest films involves not only the detection of disease but also the avoidance of misinterpretations of normal anatomic variations or variations in appearance produced by operator technique. Errors of commission of this type may be an even greater error than the error of omission, for we may then subject a healthy patient to unwarranted investigation and treatment, with all its concomitant anxiety.

The illustrations that follow (Figs 4–1 through 4–38) demonstrate some of the normal entities which may confuse the oberver if he or she is not familiar with them. Appropriate references are appended for those who wish to explore this subject further. The interested reader may also wish to consult a larger work on the same subject (Keats TE: *Atlas of Normal Roentgen Variants That May Simulate Disease,* ed 4. Chicago, Year Book Medical Publishers, 1988).

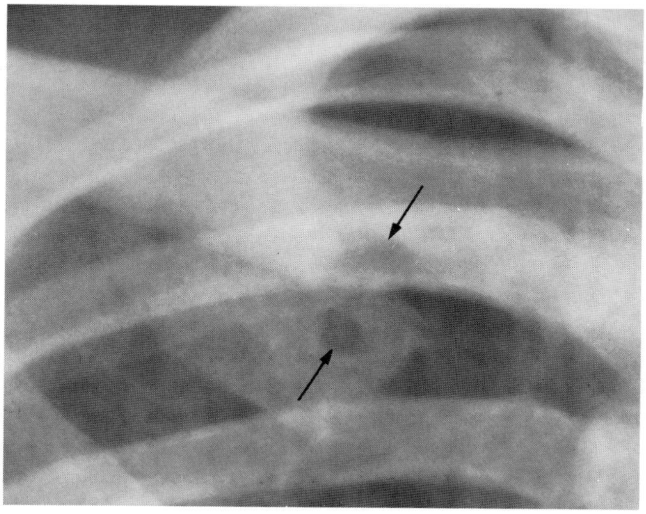

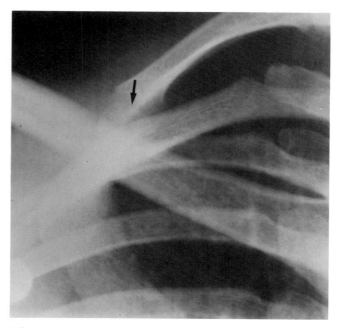

FIG 4–1.
Two possibly confusing anatomic variants are shown in this illustration. The defect in the clavicle *(upper arrow)* is the rhomboid fossa; the *lower arrow* points to a fossa in the anterior end of the first rib.

FIG 4–2.
An anomalous articulartion in the first rib *(arrow)* which should not be mistaken for fracture or destructive lesion. This entity is seen most commonly in the first rib, particularly on the right side.

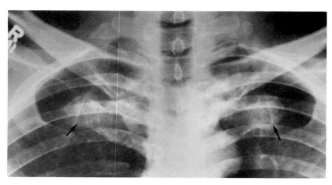

FIG 4–3.
Developmental hypoplasia of the first ribs bilaterally, but with presence of the costal cartilage, which are calcified *(arrows)*.

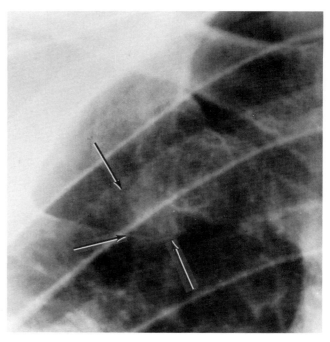

FIG 4–4.
Hypertrophic calcified costal cartilage at the anterior end of the first rib *(arrows)* may simulate a lesion in the lung.

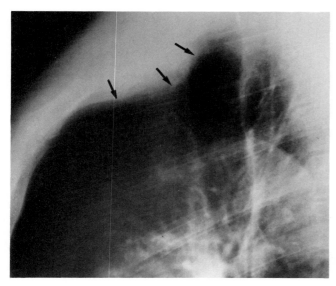

FIG 4–5.
The anterior extrapleural line *(arrows)* represents a deviation of the pleura produced by the innominate artery and vein and the costal cartilage of the first ribs. It should not be mistaken for a lesion of the sternum or a mediastinal mass. (Reference: Whalen JP, et al: Anterior extrapleural line: Superior extension. *Radiology* 1975; 115:525.)

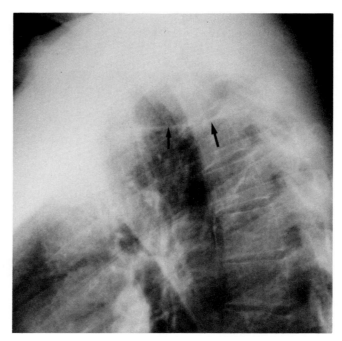

FIG 4–6.
In an improperly positioned chest study, the spine of the scapula may overlap the lung and produce a shadow *(arrows)* that may be mistaken for a pneumothorax. (Reference: Harbin WP, Cimmino CV: The radiographic innominate lines of the scapular spine. *Va Med* 1974; 101:1050.)

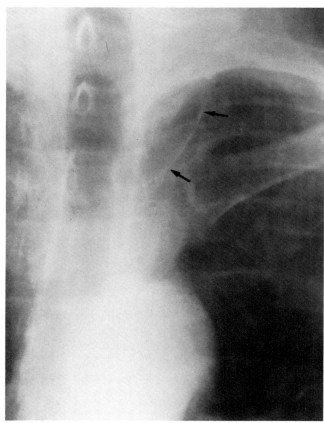

FIG 4–7.
The accessory fissure of the left upper lobe *(arrows)*, also known as the left azygous lobe. (Reference: Schmitz-Cliever E: On the occurrence of left-sided venous azygous lobe. *Fortschr Geb Roentgenstr* 1965; 72:728.)

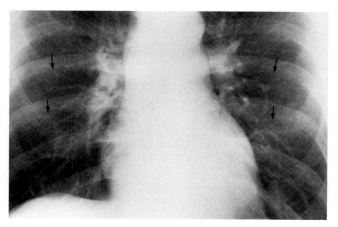

FIG 4–8.
Lack of definition of the inferior aspects of the posterior portions of the middle ribs *(arrows)* is due to the thin flange of bone at the lower margins of these ribs. This entity may be confused with a destructive process.

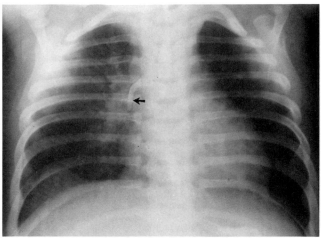

FIG 4–9.
An intrathoracic rib *(arrow)*—an anomaly of no clinical significance. (Reference: Weinstein AS, Mueller CF: Intrathoracic rib. *AJR* 1965; 94:587.)

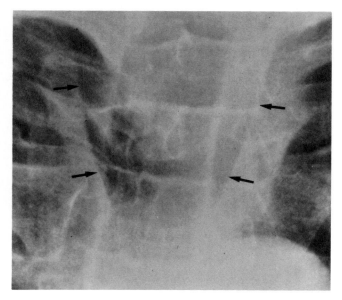

FIG 4–10.
The suprasternal fossa *(arrows)* may be quite deep and cast a radiolucency that might be mistaken for an abnormal accumulation of air, such as an esophageal diverticulum. (Reference: Ominsky S, Berinson HS: The suprasternal fossa. *Radiology* 122:311.)

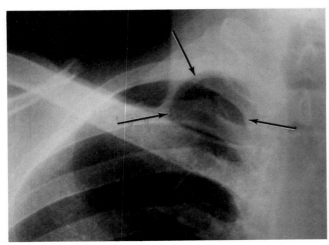

FIG 4–11.
The confluence *(arrows)* of the shadows of the sternocleidomastoid muscle, the first ribs, and the clavicle may simulate a bulla or cavity in the apex of the lung.

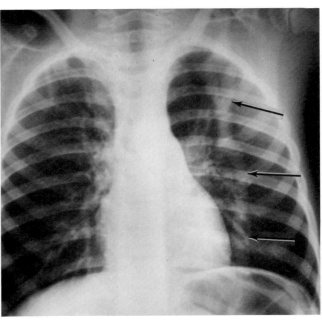

FIG 4–12.
Hair braids *(arrows)* produced this unusual appearance of the left lung.

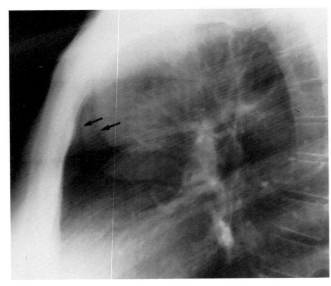

FIG 4–13.
Redundant soft tissues of the axilla produce rounded densities *(arrows)* projected into the mediastinum.

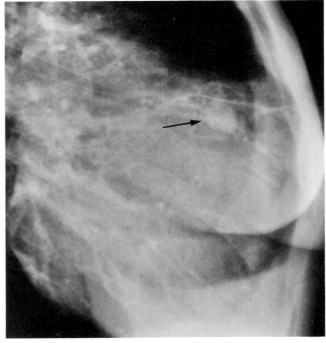

FIG 4–14.
Nipple shadows *(arrow)* may cause confusing images in the lateral projection in poorly positioned patients, in this case simulating a nodular lesion in the lung.

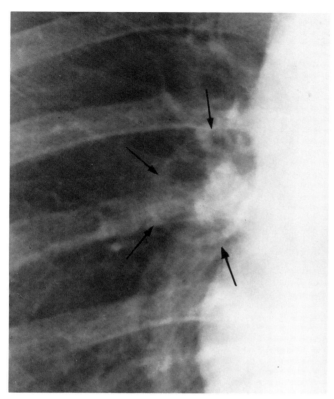

FIG 4–15.
Superimposed shadows of vessels *(arrows)* may simulate a cavitary lesion.

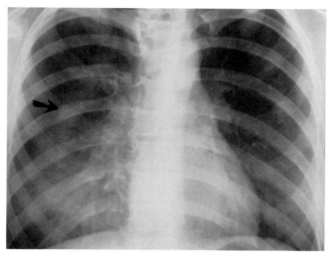

FIG 4–16.
The opacity in the right base in this 13-year-old patient is due to the dense juvenile breast, accentuated by slight rotation of the patient to the left at the time of filming. The linear shadow above *(arrow)* is due to a hair braid.

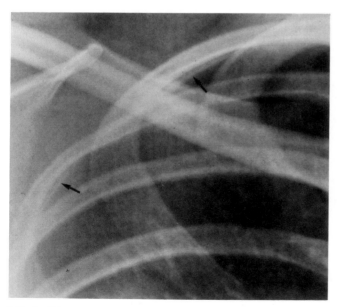

FIG 4–17.
The companion soft tissue shadows of the upper ribs and the radiolucency laterally *(arrows)* should not be mistaken for a pneumothorax.

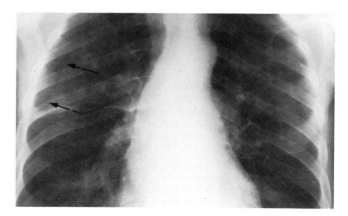

FIG 4–18.
Skin folds in the elderly *(arrows)* may simulate a pneumothorax. Note that the edge of the fold has a fading margin in contrast to the sharp pleural line seen with a true pneumothorax. (Reference: Fisher JK: Skin folds versus pneumothorax. *AJR* 1978; 130:791.)

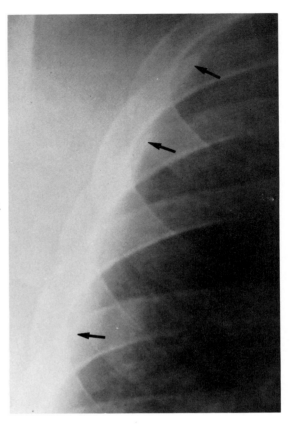

FIG 4–19.
In obese individuals, extrapleural fat *(arrows)* may simulate pleural thickening. The absence of blunting of the costophrenic angles is a useful differential clue. (Reference: Vix VA: Extrapleural costal fat. *Radiology* 1974; 112:563.)

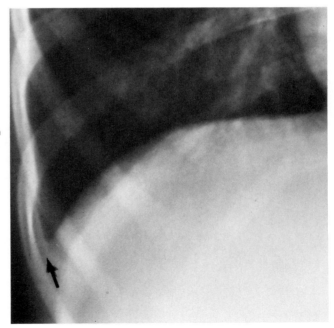

FIG 4–20.
Blunted costophrenic angles *(arrow)* in young adults are often seen as an apparently normal finding. This is apt to be misinterpreted as evidence of pleural effusion. It is possibly related to redundancy of the pleura or possibly as a reflection of the presence of the small amount of pleural fluid which is normally present in the pleural space. (Reference: Ecklof O, Torngren A: Pleural fluid in healthy children. *Acta Radiol* [Diagn] (Stockh) 1971; 11:346.)

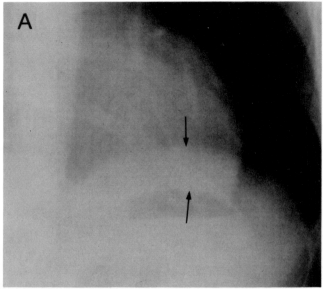

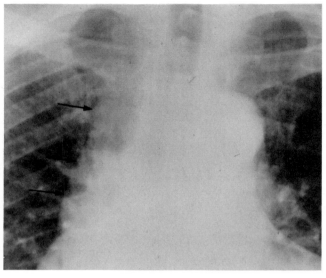

FIG 4–22.
Mediastinal fat will produce widening of the mediastinal silhouette *(arrows)*. This may be seen in simple obesity, in Cushing's disease, and in patients receiving steroids. (Reference: Price JF, Rigler LG: Widening of the mediastinum resulting from fat accumulation. *Radiology* 1970; 96:497.)

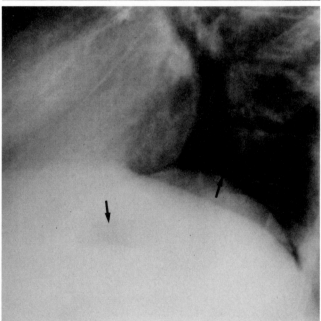

FIG 4–21.
A, the increased distance between the stomach gas bubble and the diaphragm *(arrows)* suggests a subpulmonic effusion. **B,** the lateral projection indicates that this appearance is due to the fact that the posterior portion of the left diaphragm, seen posteriorly *(right arrow),* is higher than the anterior portion, which is adjacent to the gas bubble *(left arrow).*

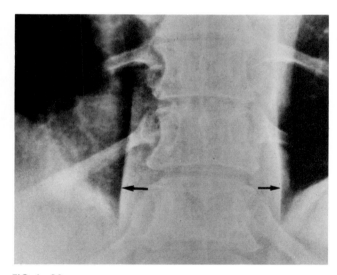

FIG 4–23.
Paraspinous fat deposition *(arrows)* will displace the paravertebral pleural reflections and may simulate a disease process. (Reference: Streiter ML, et al: Steroid induced thoracic lipomatosis: Paraspinal involvement. *AJR* 1982; 139:679.)

FIG 4–24.
The manubrium presents laterally because of slight rotation and scoliosis and may simulate a mediastinal mass *(top arrow)*. The azygous arch is seen below *(lower arrows)*.

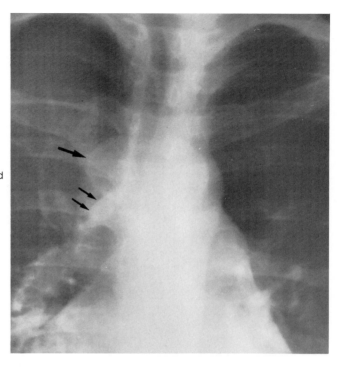

FIG 4–25.
The retrosternal line. This mass-like density is produced by the interface between the two lungs and the mediastinal fat. (Reference: Whalen JP, et al: The retrosternal line. A new sign of an anterior mediastinal mass. *AJR* 1973; 117:861.) (See also Fig 3–32.)

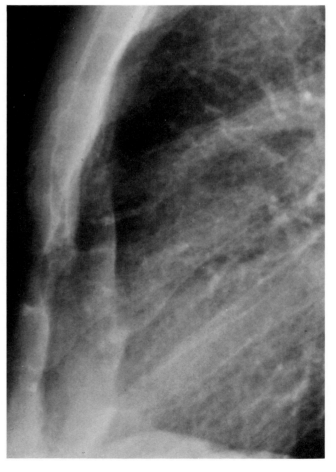

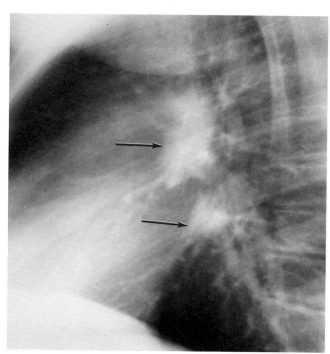

FIG 4–26.
This normal lateral projection demonstrates the pulmonary artery *(upper arrow)* and a confluence of the pulmonary veins *(lower arrow)*. The latter is sometimes mistaken for a nodular lesion in the lung.

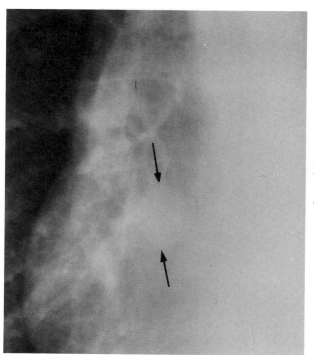

FIG 4–27.
The confluence of the pulmonary veins at the left atrium may present as a nodular density *(arrows)*, which should not be confused with a mass lesion.

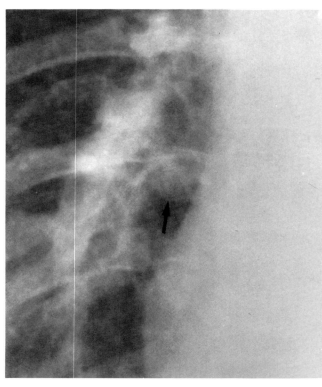

FIG 4−28.
A large transverse process *(arrow)* may simulate a nodular pulmonary lesion.

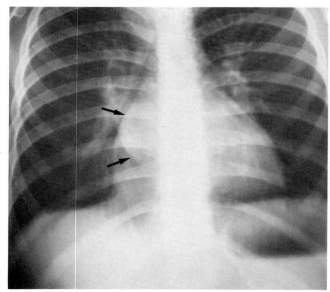

FIG 4−29.
The right border of the left atrium *(arrows)* may be seen in healthy individuals and should not be mistaken for chamber enlargement or mediastinal mass.

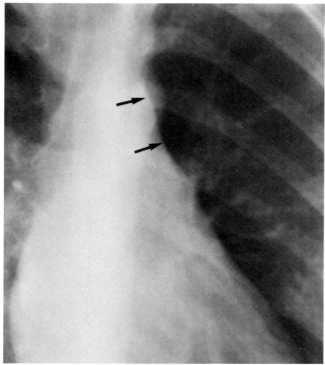

FIG 4–30.
The aortic-pulmonary stripe is a reflection of the mediastinal pleura from the aorta to the pulmonary artery *(arrows)*. This should not be confused with displacement of the mediastinal pleura resulting from adenopathy. (Reference: Keats TE: The aortic-pulmonary mediastinal stripe. *AJR* 1972; 116:107.)

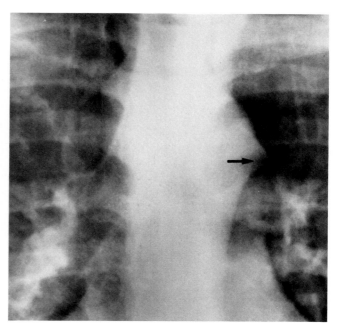

FIG 4–31.
The aortic nipple *(arrow)*. This normal shadow is produced by the highest intercostal vein and should not be mistaken for an aortic or mediastinal lesion. (Reference: Ball JB, Proto AV: The variable appearance of the left superior intercostal vein. *Radiology* 1982; 144:445.)

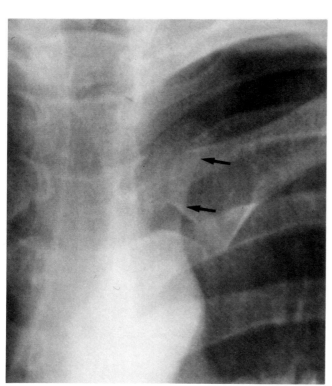

FIG 4–32.
The shadow of the left subclavian artery *(arrows)* may simulate a pleural or parenchymal density.

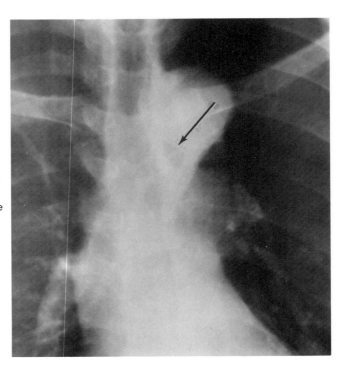

FIG 4–33.
Air in the esophagus may be confused with free air in the mediastinum. In elderly people, the esophagus follows the ectatic descending aorta, and air is trapped in the knuckle of the esophagus below the arch *(arrow)*. (Reference: Proto AV: Air in the esophagus: A frequent radiologic finding. *AJR* 1977; 129:433.)

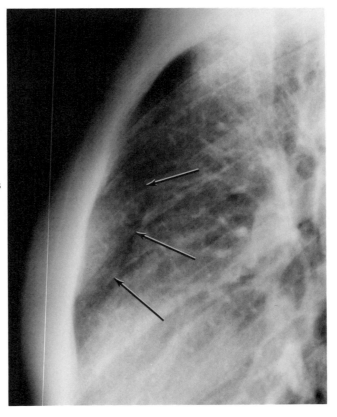

FIG 4–34.
The mammary anterior mediastinal pseudotumor. The lateral aspects of dense, small breasts of young women *(arrows)* may project into the anterior mediastinum in the lateral projection and simulate a mediastinal mass. (Reference: Keats TE: Mammary anterior mediastinal pseudotumor. *J Can Assoc Radiol* 1976; 27:262.)

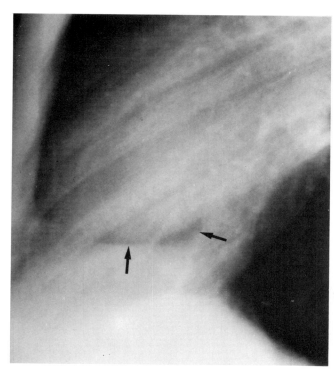

FIG 4–35.
Confusing radiolucencies may be produced by the inferior vena cava. With full inspiration, it is possible to clear a portion of the diaphragmatic surface of the heart and expose the anterior wall of the inferior vena cava *(right arrow)*. This results in a triangular area of radiolucency *(arrows)*. (Reference: Tonkin IL, et al: Radiographic isolation of the inferior vena cava. *AJR* 1977; 129:657.)

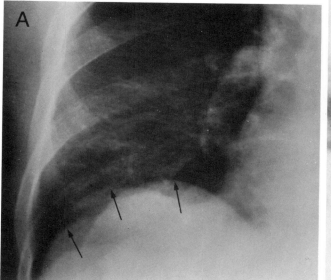

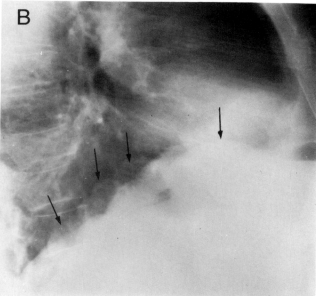

FIG 4–36.
"Scalloping" of the diaphragm *(arrows)* is a normal variation in the muscular architecture of the diaphragm. **A,** posteroanterior radiograph. **B,** lateral radiograph.

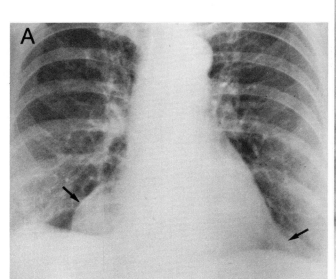

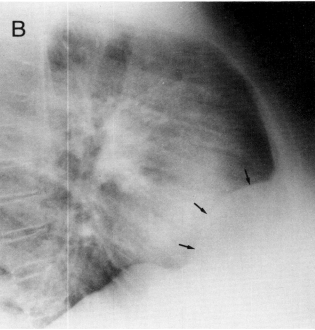

FIG 4–37.
Epipericardial fat pads *(arrows)*. Note their relative lucency in the frontal film **(A)** and the anterior position of the fat pad in the lateral projection **(B).** These fat collections may be confused with cysts and neoplasms. They vary in size with the weight of the patient. (Reference: Holt JF: Epipericardial fat shadows in differential diagnosis. *Radiology* 1947; 48:472.)

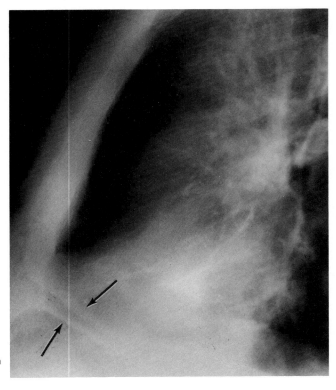

FIG 4–38.
The sternal insertions of the diaphragm *(arrows)* can be seen occasionally in healthy individuals.

5

Radiologic Signs of Diseases of the Lungs

Imaging studies are performed for two basic reasons: to diagnose disease and to assess the extent or progress of a known disorder. The role of the radiologist is to define the size and shape of any abnormalities that may be present, to determine their location as accurately as possible, and, in those cases where the diagnosis is not yet known, to suggest the diagnosis and differential diagnosis. The diagnostic considerations for any particular radiographic pattern are narrowed by reviewing the appearances on serial images and by correlating the pattern with the clinical and laboratory data.

One of the most crucial diagnostic decisions is establishing the location of any lesion, in particular whether the process is primarily in the lung, the hilus, the mediastinum, the pleura, the chest wall, or the diaphragm. Indeed these distinctions are so important that most textbooks, including this one, are organized according to anatomic divisions. In this chapter we will confine our discussion to the signs of pulmonary abnormalities, the other sites being considered in their relevant chapters. Plain chest radiographs should be viewed with optimal lighting, including a bright light facility. Low-contrast shadows may be "brought out" by viewing the tilted radiograph, a simple technique which is really the antithesis of bright lighting. Although search patterns among experienced viewers are far from orderly it seems wise, particularly for the inexperienced, to adopt some sort of systematic scanning pattern to try to ensure that the search is complete. The apices, the hili, the retrocardiac regions, the lung below the

domes of the diaphragm, and the strip just inside the chest wall should be specifically examined, because experience has shown that opacities in these areas are easily overlooked. As discussed later, some subtle opacities may be detected not so much by their density as by the obliteration of a normal contour. Two interrelated signs will be considered first—the silhouette sign and the air bronchogram sign—because these two signs have widespread applicability in the diagnosis of a variety of chest disorders.

The Silhouette Sign

Felson popularized the term "silhouette sign" to indicate an obliteration of the borders of the heart, mediastinum, or diaphragm by an adjacent opacity (Fig 5–1). In his original description, Felson assumed that the mechanism of the sign was dependent on direct contact.[18] He wrote, "an intrathoracic lesion touching a border of the heart, aorta, or diaphragm will obliterate that border on the roentgenogram. An intrathoracic lesion not anatomically contiguous with a border of one of the structures will not obliterate that border. We have applied the term silhouette sign to indicate the obliteration of a portion of these borders by adjacent disease." The lesion responsible for obliterating a silhouette does not have to be large; a small pulmonary opacity will do so just as effectively as a large mass (Fig 5–2). Nor does the opacity have to originate within the lung; pleural fluid, extrapleural fat, chest wall deformity, and medi-

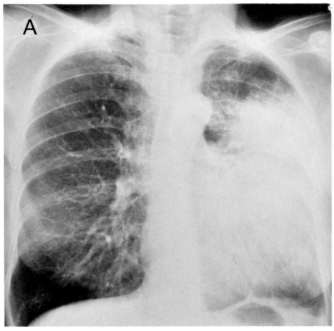

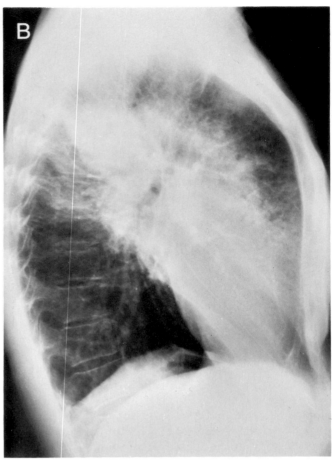

FIG 5–1.
The silhouette sign. The left heart border is invisible because of consolidation in the adjacent left upper lobe. **A,** posteroanterior (PA) view. **B,** lateral view.

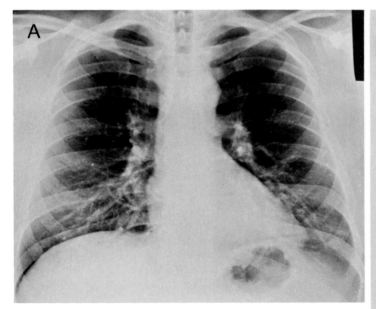

FIG 5–2.
The silhouette sign. **A,** a small patch of pneumonia in the anterior segment of the left lower lobe has resulted in lack of visibility of the outer half of the left hemidiaphragm. (The lateral view in this patient is shown in Figure 5–15.) **B,** normal diaphragm outline after the pneumonia has resolved.

astinal masses all may cause a loss of silhouette.

The mechanism responsible for the sign is debated. According to Felson,[18] the sign depends on direct contact, but another possible explanation is that the sign may simply be due to absorption of x-rays by whatever lies in the path of the beam, and the reason the border is lost only in cases of direct contact is that precise anatomic conformity of shape occurs only when intimate contact is present.

Regardless of mechanism, the silhouette sign can be used in two ways: (1) to localize a radiographic density (Figs 5–3 and 5–4) and (2) to detect lesions of low radiopacity when the shadow is less obvious than the loss of silhouette (see Fig 5–2). Since either direct contact or precise anatomic conformity of shape is required to efface a silhouette, the lesion must lie immediately adjacent to the structure in question. With a process that is remote from the interface and merely overlaps it on the radiograph, the radiographic boundary will still be visible through the opacity, though it may be more difficult to appreciate. Thus, opacities in the right middle lobe or lingula may obliterate the right and left bor-

ders of the heart, respectively (Figs 5–1 and 5–5), whereas opacities in the lower lobes may partially obliterate the outline of the descending aorta and diaphragm, but leave the cardiac outline clearly visible (Figs 5–6 and 5–7). Similarly, the aortic knob will be rendered invisible if there is no air in the apicoposterior segment of the left upper lobe. The best example of detecting lesions of low radiopacity is collapse of the right middle lobe (see Fig 5–5).

Felson and Felson[18] warned that mistakes will be made in identification of the sign unless the following points are borne in mind:

1. The technical quality of the roentgenogram must be such that the diseased area is adequately penetrated. Underpenetration may result in loss of visibility of a normal border.

2. The outline of a portion of the cardiovascular structure in question must be clearly visible beyond the shadow of the spine. In many healthy individuals, the right border of the heart and ascending aorta do not project into the right thorax. In these

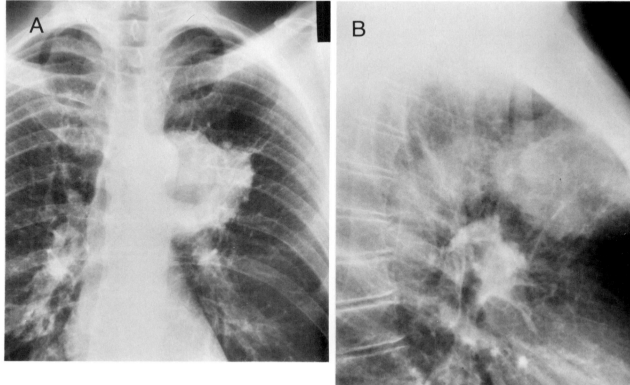

FIG 5–3.
A, preservation of the silhouette of the aortic knob and descending aorta in the PA view is good evidence that the pulmonary mass does not lie in the superior segment of the left lower lobe. **B,** the lateral view shows that the mass, in fact, lies well anteriorly. (It proved to be a squamous cell carcinoma.)

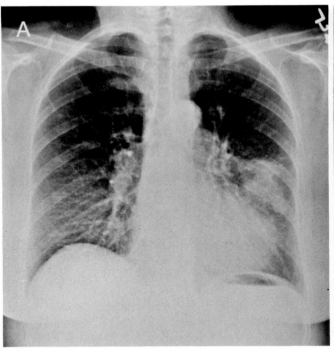

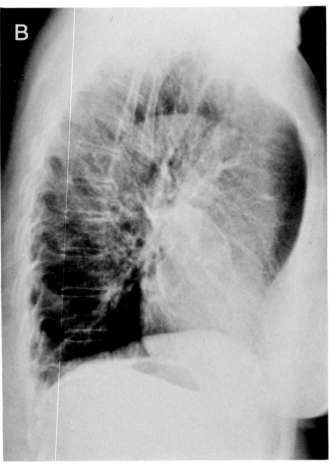

FIG 5–4.
A, the loss of silhouette of the left cardiac border in the frontal view localizes the pulmonary consolidation to the lingula. **B,** the lateral view confirms the interpretation: it proved to be postobstructive pneumonia beyond a carcinoma in the lingular bronchus.

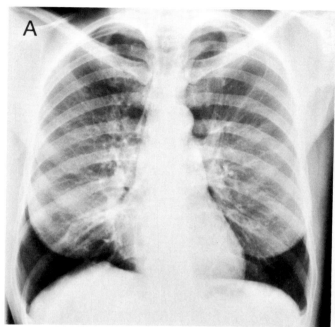

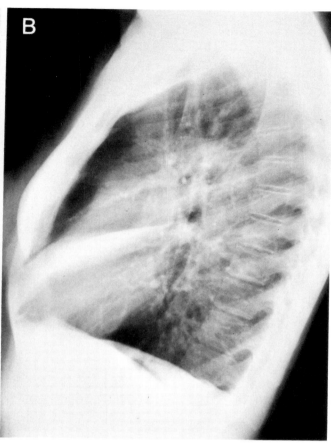

FIG 5–5.
Right middle lobe collapse/consolidation obliterating the right
heart border. **A,** PA view. **B,** lateral view.

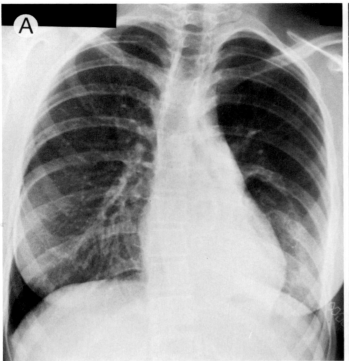

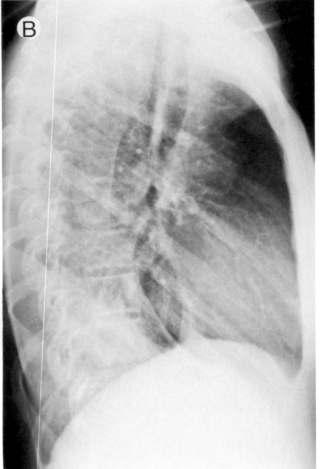

FIG 5–6.
Left lower lobe collapse/consolidation obliterating the outline of the adjacent descending aorta and medial left hemidiaphragm.

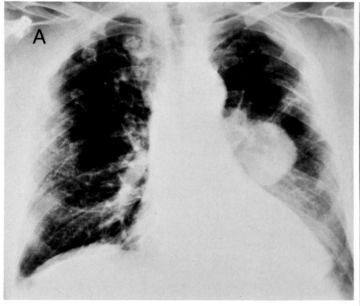

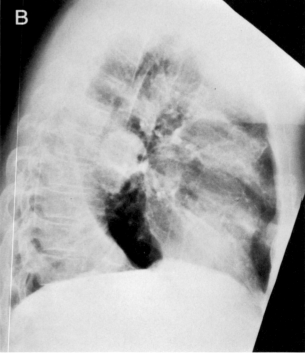

FIG 5–7.
Left lower lobe collapse/consolidation obliterating the outline of the left hemidiaphragm but leaving the outline of the left heart border clearly defined. The lobar collapse was due to a large carcinoma of the bronchus. (Widespread pleural calcification resulting from previous exposure to asbestos is present.) **A,** PA view. **B,** lateral view.

patients the silhouette sign cannot be applied on the right side.

3. In patients with pectus excavatum, the right border of the heart is commonly obliterated because the depressed thoracic wall replaces aerated lung alongside the cardiac silhouette (Fig 5–8).

It should also be pointed out, as Felson himself warned, that there are patients in whom no disease and no satisfactory explanation will be found for the loss of the right heart border.[18] These cases are, however, few and far between and do little to reduce the value of the sign.

The Air Bronchogram

Normal intrapulmonary airways are invisible unless end-on to the x-ray beam, but air within bronchi or bronchioles passing through airless parenchyma may be visible as branching linear lucencies (Fig 5–9). An air bronchogram within an opacity is a reliable sign which indicates that the opacity must be

TABLE 5–1.

Causes of an Air Bronchogram

Normal expiratory radiograph
Consolidation
Pulmonary edema
Non-obstructuve pulmonary atelectasis
    Hyaline membrane disease
    Compression atelectasis (e.g., pleural effusion, pneumothorax)
    Fibrotic scarring, for example
        Radiation fibrosis
        Bronchiectatic lobe
Severe interstitial disease
    Sarcoidosis
    Fibrosing alveolitis
Certain neoplasms, notably
    Bronchioloalveolar carcinoma
    Lymphoma
    Pseudolymphoma

intrapulmonary, not pleural or mediastinal, in location. The sign is particularly well demonstrated with computed tomography (CT) (Fig 5–10).

The most common causes of an air bronchogram (Table 5–1) are pneumonia and the various

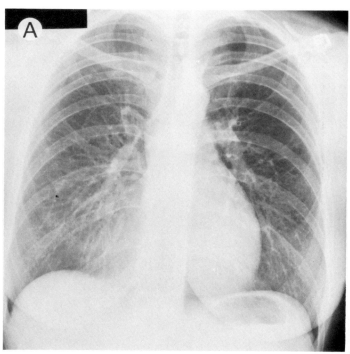

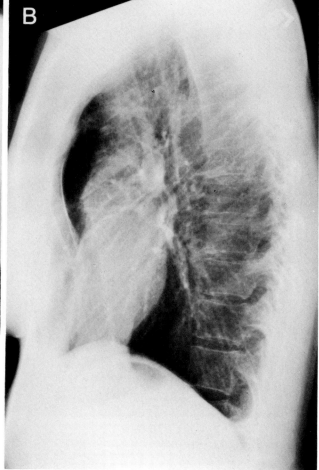

FIG 5–8.
Pectus excavatum causing obliteration of the right border of the heart. **A,** PA view. **B,** lateral view.

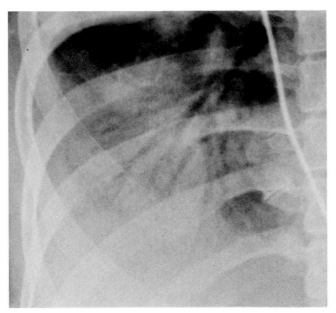

FIG 5–9.
Air bronchogram. The branching linear lucencies within the consolidation in the right lower lobe are particularly well demonstrated in this example of staphylococcal pneumonia.

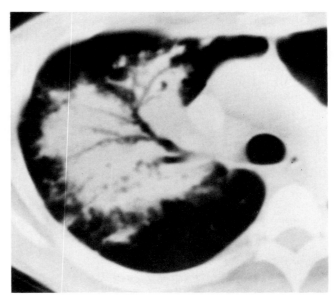

FIG 5–10.
Air bronchogram shown by CT in a patient with pneumonia.

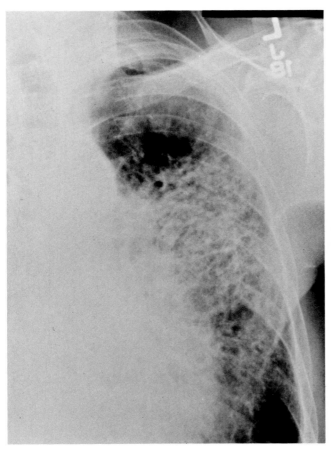

FIG 5–11.
Air bronchogram in bronchioloalveloar cell carcinoma.

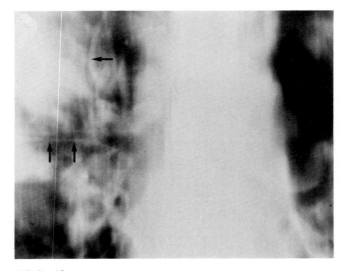

FIG 5–12.
Sarcoidosis of the lung showing an air bronchogram *(arrows)* in an area of severe pulmonary involvement.

forms of pulmonary edema. Air bronchograms are also seen in atelectatic lobes provided the airway is patent as, for example, in collapse due to pleural effusion or pneumothorax or in collapse associated with bronchiectasis. Similarly, widespread air bronchograms are also seen with hyaline membrane disease.

There are four less predictable situations in which air bronchograms may be seen.[75]

1. Some tumors, such as alveolar cell carcinoma (Fig 5–11), lymphoma, and pseudolymphoma, grow around the airways without compressing them.

2. Interstitial fibrosis may be so intense that it renders the lung parenchyma airless, producing an air bronchogram because the bronchi remain patent. Thus, the nodular and consolidative lesions of sarcoidosis (Fig 5–12) may show an air bronchogram as may advanced fibrosing alveolitis and radiation fibrosis (Fig 5–13).[74]

3. Air bronchograms can sometimes be seen in postobstructive pneumonia, even though one might have expected replacement of air by secretions beyond the obstruction.

4. Air bronchograms can be normal at low lung volumes and also, in children, in segmental bronchi behind the heart.

PULMONARY OPACITY

Focal pulmonary opacity is detected in the frontal view by comparing one lung with the other. In the lateral view, such right/left comparisons are not possible. A reliable rule for the lateral view in the normal patient is that as the eye travels down the spine, each thoracic vertebral body appears blacker than the one above it, until the diaphragm is reached. Pulmonary opacity projected over the spine will interrupt this continuum and permit recognition of a shadow that might otherwise be overlooked (Fig 5–14). Another helpful point to bear in mind is that in the radiograph of a healthy subject there is no abrupt change in density across the heart shadow in the lateral projection (Fig 5–15). The rib shadows are, of course, an exception and they have to be mentally subtracted from the image. Also, but less reliably, the high retrosternal area is usually more transradiant than all other areas on the lateral chest radiograph except the region immediately behind the heart.

The *characteristics* of a shadow on a radiograph depend on the absorptive capacity and geometry of

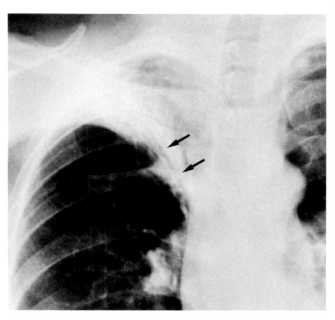

FIG 5–13.
Air bronchogram *(arrows)* in radiation fibrosis of right upper lobe following treatment of carcinoma of the breast.

the object. In order of increasing absorptive capacity, the major components of the chest are air, fat, fluid and soft tissues, and bone. For practical purposes, fluid and soft tissues, apart from fat, are isodense. The following geometric features are worth noting (Fig 5–16).

1. Interfaces tangential to the x-ray beam are sharp and distinct, whereas interfaces oblique to the beam are not seen because the thin end of the wedge just fades off and cannot be identified (Fig 5–16, *a*).

2. Hollow cylinders and hollow spheres are most absorptive at their edges because, at the edge, the beam has a longer path within the object and is therefore more attenuated. Also, marginal interfaces inside and out are sharp and distinct (Fig 5–16, *b*).

3. A thin sheet perpendicular to an x-ray beam will probably cause no detectable opacity (Fig 5–16, *c*). A thin sheet that is oriented along the beam (tangential) becomes much more absorptive and casts a definite shadow (Fig 5–16, *d*).

There are innumerable patterns of pulmonary opacity, with no clear-cut divisions between them. Despite the imperfections, it is worth the effort to categorize these patterns. The more certain one is of the categorization of an individual case, the shorter the differential diagnostic list will be. The following classification of pulmonary shadows is suggested

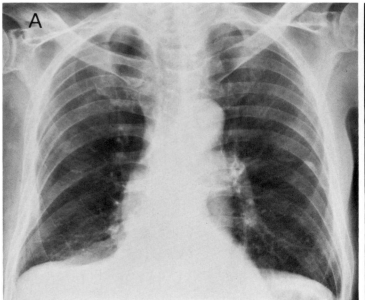

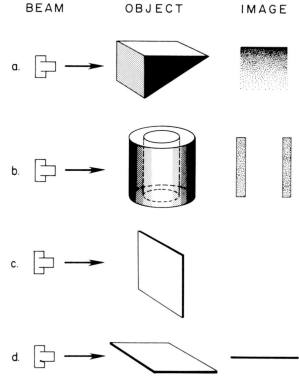

FIG 5–14.
Alteration in opacity of thoracic vertebrae on the lateral projection as a sign of lower lobe density. In this case the increasing opacity of the vertebral bodies as the eye travels down the spine is one of the most obvious signs indicating the presence of right lower lobe collapse. **A,** PA view. **B,** lateral view.

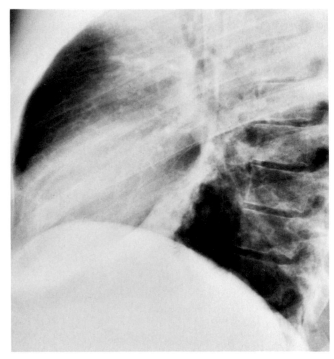

FIG 5–15.
Abrupt change in density overlying cardiac shadow. Lateral view in a patient with pneumonia in the anterior segment of the left lower lobe. (PA view of this patient is shown in Fig 5–2).

FIG 5–16.
Density characteristics of pulmonary shadows. See text for explanation.

(pleural shadows are considered separately in Chapter 14):

1. Air-space filling,
2. Collapse (atelectasis),
3. Pulmonary mass (nodule),
4. Line shadows,
5. Ring shadows, cysts, and bullae,
6. Widespread nodular, reticulonodular, and honeycomb shadowing.

More than one pattern may be present. Calcification and cavitation should be looked for as they will further limit the number of diagnostic possibilities.

AIR-SPACE FILLING

There is considerable confusion over the terminology that should be used to describe one or more discrete, ill-defined pulmonary densities. Infiltrate, consolidation, and air-space filling are the most popular descriptive terms. Certain purists believe that all three are unjustifiable because they imply histologic knowledge.

The expressions "air-space filling" or "air-space shadows" seem to be the best because they imply a radiographic appearance.[20] The word "consolidation" can be confusing because pathologists use it synonymously with exudate, whereas its use by radiologists is more catholic. The word "infiltrate" is also used differently by radiologists and pathologists. Radiologists use the term liberally to describe almost any pulmonary shadow, whereas pathologists mean the specific histologic features of infiltration. We will use the phrase "air-space filling/shadowing" for a radiographic appearance that implies replacement of air in the distal airways and alveoli by fluid or, very occasionally, by other material such as tumor or alveolar proteinosis, with no destruction or displacement of the gross morphology of the lung. The fluid can be a transudate, an exudate, or blood. Where it is possible to be certain that the shadow is caused by edema, the expression pulmonary edema will be used instead. The term consolidation will be restricted to those shadows thought to be due to exudate, blood, or tumor. Thus, edema and consolidation are subdivisions of the term air-space filling.

The radiologic features of air-space filling are one or more shadows with ill-defined margins, except where the shadow abuts the pleura. When multiple, the shadows typically coalesce. An air bronchogram may be visible, often as scattered branches or small twigs. The normal vascular markings within the shadow are invisible, because of the silhouette sign. The lack of clarity of the edge of the shadows results, in part, from the piecemeal spread of the process through the bronchi and alveoli, the poorly defined margin being analogous to the edge of a three-dimensional jigsaw puzzle. Once the process abuts a fissure, the edge appears sharp. The ease with which it is possible to appreciate this edge on plain chest radiographs depends on how much of the fissure is tangential to the x-ray beam.

The distribution of air-space filling is often characteristic, being lobar, sublobar, or showing the so-called bat's wing or butterfly pattern. Many sublobar processes are vaguely conical in configuration, sometimes resembling the shape of a segment. Precise conformity to a segment almost never occurs because, with the rare exception of accessory fissures, there are no anatomic barriers to prevent the spread of fluid or other processes across segmental boundaries. Air-space filling is often peripheral in location, crossing segmental boundaries with impunity. Spherical consolidations are also seen, but are rare.

Ill-defined nodular shadows between 0.5 and 1 cm are sometimes seen in, and adjacent to, the larger opacities of air-space filling, particularly with pulmonary edema and infection. They are a notable feature in varicella and tuberculous infection (Fig 5–17). These shadows have been called "acinar shadows" since they are believed to be opaque acini contrasted against aerated lung.[103] They are most often seen at the edge of large opacities and coalesce

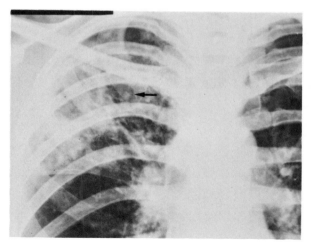

FIG 5–17.
Acinar shadows in pulmonary tuberculosis (arrow). In the lateral portion of the right upper lobe, the acinar shadows have become confluent.

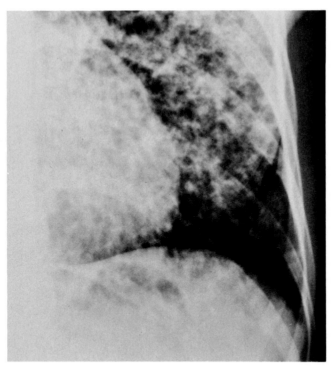

FIG 5–18.
Air alveologram in bronchogenic spread of tuberculosis.

as the disease progresses. The converse of the acinar shadow is the "air alveologram" (Fig 5–18), a pattern of small rounded lucencies due to aerated acini surrounded by fluid-filled lung.

The term "ground glass" is sometimes applied to a homogeneous veiling opacity. Such opacity is seen in a large number of conditions including air-space filling disorders and interstitial pulmonary diseases.

Cavitation may occur within areas of air-space filling. The term "cavitation" implies necrosis and liquefaction of lung tissue. If the necrotic center communicates with the bronchial tree, air will enter the cavity (Fig 5–19) and will be seen as a translucency within the shadow, often accompanied by an air-fluid level (Fig 5–19).

Computed tomographic (CT) scanning may, on occasion, provide additional information about air-space filling.[64] It will show acinar filling to advantage (Fig 5–20). The excellent contrast discrimination of CT allows pneumonia, in the immunocompromised host, for example, to be diagnosed when the plain chest radiographs still have a normal appearance. It can also demonstrate the size, shape, and precise position of any cavities (Fig 5–21).[37] Because of its greater contrast sensitivity and three-

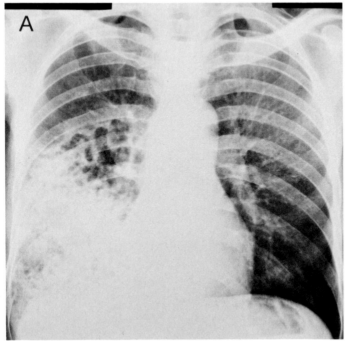

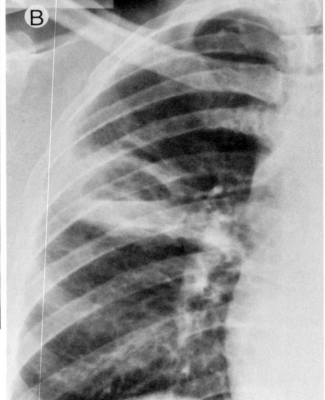

FIG 5–19.
Cavitation. **A,** in this example of staphylococcal pneumonia, there are multiple transradiant areas within the consolidation but no air-fluid levels. **B,** another patient, illustrating an air-fluid level in a cavity within an area of pneumonia.

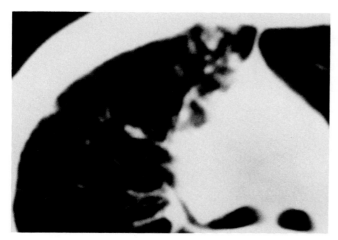

FIG 5–20.
Post primary tuberculosis. CT scan shows acinar shadows.

dimensional imaging capability, CT may show more cavities than plain films. Better definition of a cavity or the demonstration of multiple cavities may improve diagnostic accuracy but, if a cavity is clearly demonstrated on plain films, then CT usually has little additional information to offer. Other morphologic features of air-space filling that are particularly well demonstrated by CT are air bronchograms (see Fig 5–10), the satellite lesions of infectious granulomatous inflammation, and the conformity of radiation fibrosis to the radiation port (Fig 5–22).

Genereux[25] has suggested that measuring CT numbers can, on occasion, be helpful in diagnosing the nature of air-space shadowing. The CT density may be high in pulmonary hemorrhage, progressive massive fibrosis, and pulmonary calcinosis, and be low in lipoid pneumonia.[46] Great care must be taken in accepting a low CT number, however, because part of the volume being measured could be air in aerated alveoli or bronchi.

Differential Diagnosis of Air-Space Filling

The differential diagnosis of air-space shadows is long and covers diseases that require quite different forms of management. Creating smaller categories according to the radiographic features is difficult. It is helpful, however, to divide these opacities into those that are single and those that are multiple. (The differential diagnosis of nodular and reticulonodular shadowing is discussed separately in the section "Widespread Nodular, Reticulonodular, and Honeycomb Shadowing," later in this chapter.)

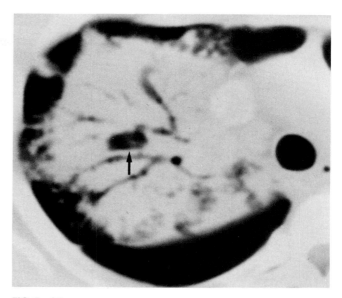

FIG 5–21.
CT scan showing cavitation *(arrow)* in area of pneumonia.

Solitary Air-Space Shadows

Solitary air-space shadowing (Fig 5–23) is usually the result of pneumonia, atelectasis, infarction, or hemorrhage (Fig 5–24). Neoplasms, particularly bronchioloalveolar carcinoma (see Fig 5–11), malignant lymphoma (Fig 5–25) and pseudolymphoma, may occasionally appear ill-defined enough to be called consolidation. The full list of causes of solitary air-space shadows is given in Table 5–2.

Multiple Air-Space Shadows

Air-space filling is often multifocal and tends to coalesce as it progresses (Fig 5–26). The list of con-

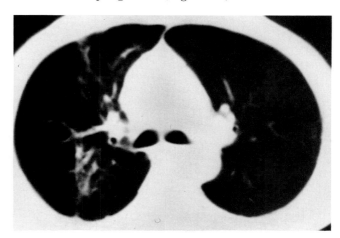

FIG 5–22.
CT scan showing conformity of radiation fibrosis to the radiation port.

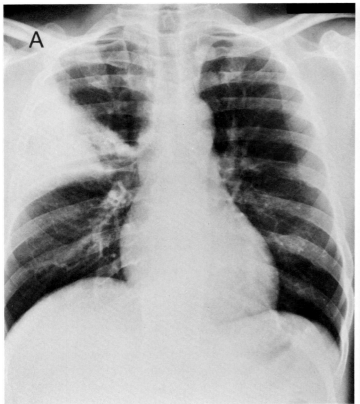

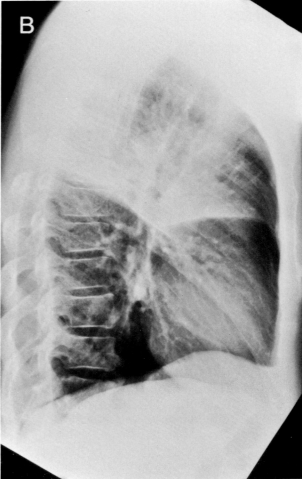

FIG 5—23.
Solitary air space shadow, in this case resulting from bacterial pneumonia. **A,** PA view. **B,** lateral view.

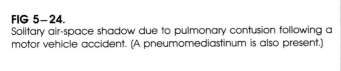

FIG 5—24.
Solitary air-space shadow due to pulmonary contusion following a motor vehicle accident. (A pneumomediastinum is also present.)

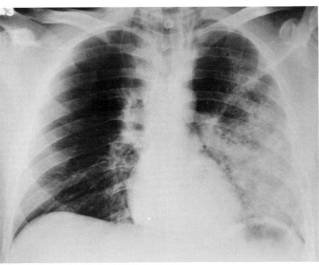

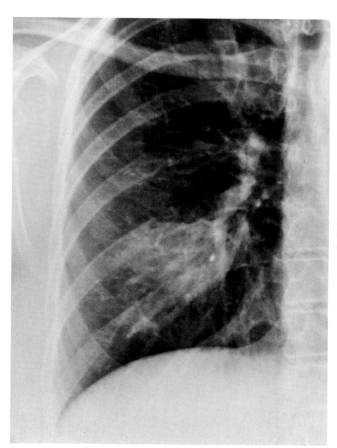

FIG 5–25.
Solitary air-space shadow in Hodgkin's disease of the lung parenchyma.

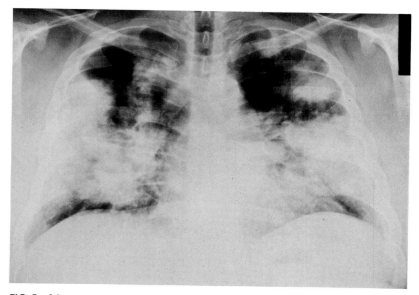

FIG 5–26.
Multiple air-space shadows resulting from bacterial pneumonia.

TABLE 5–2.

Differential Diagnosis of a Solitary Air-Space Shadow

Diagnosis	Comment
Pneumonia	Pneumonia (bacterial, including tuberculous, viral, fungal, and parasitic) is the most common cause of solitary air-space filling. The opacity may be almost any shape from segmental/lobar to round or irregular. Cavitation and accompanying pleural effusion are both distinct features. In adults, an associated hilar mass suggests a centrally located neoplasm causing post-obstructive pneumonia, whereas in children, an associated hilar mass suggests primary tuberculosis.
Atelectasis	The diagnosis of atelectasis is based on its characteristic shape. The appearances and causes are discussed in the section "Atelectasis/Collapse" later in this chapter. Discoid atelectasis results in a characteristic bandlike shape coursing through the lung, often in a horizontal orientation. Large areas of atelectasis that do not conform to either of these patterns may be indistinguishable from the other causes of air-space shadowing listed in this table.
Infarction/hemorrhage associated with pulmonary embolism	Infarcts are usually segmental in size, rarely larger. One surface is invariably in contact with the pleura. The rounded hump pointing toward the hilus known as Hampton's hump (see Chapter 8) is a well known but infrequent sign suggestive, but not diagnostic, of the condition. Septic infarcts cavitate frequently, whereas bland infarcts rarely cavitate.
Pulmonary contusion	Contusions appear within hours of injury and clear within a few days. They are usually maximal in the general area of injury, though contrecoup damage may be seen at a distance. Pneumatocele formation is a distinct feature. Pulmonary contusion may surround a pulmonary hematoma. Hematomas resemble masses, may liquefy and cavitate, and take much longer to clear than contusions.
Collagen vascular disease/vasculitis	These conditions are infrequent causes of solitary air-space shadowing. They need to be considered in patients with appropriate clinical features. The opacity is usually sublobar in size and nonspecific in shape. Cavitation may be seen. Most solitary shadows in patients with collagen vascular disease/vasculitis will be pneumonia or infarction.
Drug reactions and allergic reactions	Air-space shadows in these conditions are rarely solitary. They may be almost any shape except lobar.
Hemorrhage	Solitary air-space shadows due to hemorrhage are usually due to pulmonary emboli or to pulmonary contusion. When due to systemic disease, pulmonary hemorrhage is usually multifocal. When single, the opacity can be any shape even including lobar.
Neoplasm	Post-obstructive pneumonia is a common cause of solitary air-space shadowing. Some neoplasms, particularly bronchioloalveolar carcinoma, malignant lymphoma, and pseudolymphoma, can closely resemble focal pneumonia and may even contain air bronchograms. The absence of clinical features of pneumonia and the lack of change of the shadow over many weeks point to one of these neoplasms. The longer the opacity persists, particularly if it grows slowly, the more likely it is to be a neoplasm.
Radiation pneumonitis/fibrosis	Air-space shadowing due to radiation therapy conforms fairly precisely to the shape of the radiation port, a feature that is particularly evident in CT scans. The shape and the fact that radiation therapy was given usually permits a specific diagnosis to be made.
Eosinophilic pneumonia	Air-space shadowing in this condition is almost invariably multifocal; it is very rarely solitary. The opacity is likely to be noticeably peripheral in location.
Amyloidosis	Amyloidosis is an extremely rare cause of a solitary air-space shadow. When encountered, the opacity is nonspecific in appearance.

ditions to be included in the differential diagnosis (Table 5–3) is even longer than that for solitary air-space shadows.

It is useful to separate out those cases that conform to the so-called butterfly or bat's wing pattern, because the presence of the pattern modifies the probability of the various conditions that can cause multiple air-space shadows. These fanciful terms are an attempt to describe bilateral shadowing that is perihilar in distribution (Fig 5–27). The shadowing consists of coalescent densities with ill-defined borders, and there may be acinar shadows at the periphery. Bat's wing shadowing may be symmetric, but more often it is worse on one side than the other. The outer portion of each lobe is less involved than the perihilar area, and often the outer portion is normal. Air bronchograms and air alveolograms may be prominent features.

Multiple air-space shadows that are clearly lobar or segmental in shape constitute another potentially useful subgroup (Fig 5–28) (Table 5–4).

Certain generalizations may be helpful when considering air-space shadows:

1. Clinical correlation is essential in virtually every case and is often decisive. A few examples will suffice to emphasize this point: (a) In patients with noncardiogenic pulmonary edema, the chest film may only become abnormal several hours after the onset of symptoms, whereas with cardiogenic pulmonary edema, the pulmonary shadowing is almost always evident early on. (b) Widespread pneumonia is almost invariably accompanied by cough and fever. (c) Aspiration should be suspected as the cause of air-space shadowing in patients who have known predisposing factors such as alcoholism, a recent sei-

TABLE 5–3.

Multiple Coalescent Air-space Shadows

Cause	Likelihood of Bat's Wing Pattern*
Exudates/Transudates	
Pneumonia	+ +
Pulmonary emboli causing infarction (bland or septic)	+
Eosinophilic pneumonia	0
Collagen vascular disease/vasculitis	+
Pulmonary edema, both circulatory and non-circulatory (ARDS)†	+ + +
Inhalation of noxious gases/liquids	+ + +
Hydrocarbon ingestion	+
Drug reactions	+
Allergic reactions	+
Alveolar proteinosis	+ + +
Amyloidosis	+
Hemorrhage	
Pulmonary contusion/hematoma	+
Hemorrhage due to pulmonary embolus	+
Aspiration of blood	+ +
Spontaneous hemorrhage, Goodpasture's syndrome, anticoagulant therapy, bleeding tendency	+ + +
Neoplasm	
Bronchioloalveolar carcinoma	+ +
Lymphangitis carcinomatosa	+ +
Nonlymphangitic metastases	0
Malignant lymphoma	+
Pseudolymphoma	0
Miscellaneous	
Sarcoidosis	0
Silicosis/coal workers pneumoconiosis	0
Alveolar microlithiasis	+ +
Diffuse pulmonary calcification	+ +

*+ + + = common pattern for particular disease, + + = occasional pattern for particular disease, + = rare pattern for particular disease, and 0 = extremely rare or nonexistent pattern for particular disease.
†ARDS = adult respiratory distress syndrome.

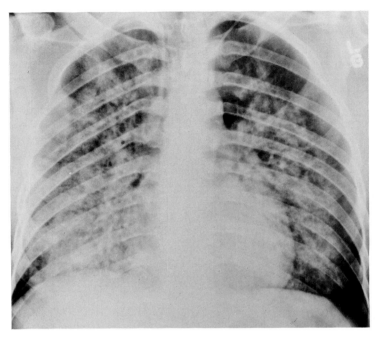

FIG 5–27.
"Bat's wing" pattern due to pulmonary edema. This example is typical in that it is bilateral, but asymmetric. The shadowing is maximal in the central (perihilar) portions of the lung, and the outer portion of the lungs are relatively clear.

zure, or a period of unconsciousness. (d) Immunocompromised patients are a special and complicated group. Pulmonary shadows in such patients are usually indicative of infection, often from opportunistic organisms. (e) Pulmonary hemorrhage associated with widespread pulmonary consolidation has a variety of causes including Goodpasture's syndrome, idiopathic pulmonary hemorrhage (also known as primary pulmonary hemosiderosis), pulmonary hemorrhage associated with glomerulonephritis, Wegener's granulomatosis, hematologic malignancy, bleeding disorders such as hemophilia or anticoagulant therapy, and trauma. (f) In a leukemic patient, the diagnosis for widespread air-space filling regardless of distribution will usually be pneumonia. The important differential diagnostic possibilities are diffuse pulmonary hemorrhage (which will usually, but not always, be accompanied by hemoptysis); leukemic infiltration, particularly if the peripheral white blood cell count is very high; drug reaction; or pulmonary edema, particularly if there is a circulatory cause for the edema.

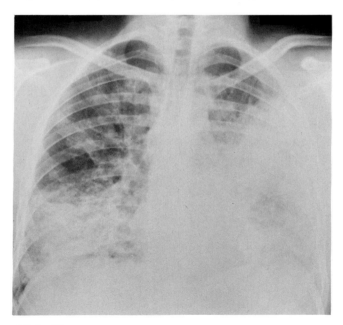

FIG 5–28.
Multiple air-space shadows with a lobar/segmental distribution, in this case of bacterial pneumonia.

TABLE 5–4.

Differential Diagnosis of Multiple Air-space Shadows When Their Shape Is Clearly Lobar or Segmental

Pneumonia
Infarction/hemorrhage due to pulmonary emboli
Pulmonary edema*
Neoplasm (bronchioloalveolar carcinoma,
　　lymphangitis carcinomatosa,* malignant
　　lymphoma)

*Segmental or lobar shapes are a rare manifestation of the entity.

2. Opacity of the whole of a lobe with no loss of volume is virtually diagnostic of pneumonia: this remains true even if a small portion of the lobe is spared (Fig 5–29). The common causes of lobar consolidation without atelectasis are pneumococcal or mycoplasma pneumonia, and pneumonia distal to a bronchial neoplasm. Obstruction of a lobar bronchus by a tumor usually causes some degree of atelectasis, but true consolidation without loss of volume is not uncommon. In these cases, the tumor obstructs the drainage of secretions, and bacterial pneumonia supervenes. Clinically, the condition of these patients may closely resemble simple pneumonia, but the consolidation, though it may improve with appropriate treatment, does not clear completely if it is secondary to an underlying tumor. Because the tumor in such cases involves a lobar bronchus, it is always readily visible at bronchoscopy.

Bronchioloalveolar carcinoma (see Fig 5–11) and malignant lymphoma may, on occasion, mimic lobar pneumonia radiologically. The lobar consolidation in these cases is due to the tumor itself spreading through the alveolar spaces without necessarily occluding the central bronchi.

3. Lobar consolidation with expansion of the lobe strongly suggests bacterial pneumonia (particularly *Streptococcus pneumoniae*, *Klebsiella pneumoniae*, *Pseudomonas aeruginosa*, and *Staphylococcus aureus* pneumonia) or obstructive pneumonia due to a centrally positioned carcinoma of the bronchus.

4. A consolidative process that is spherical in shape is likely to be due to pneumonia (Fig 5–30). The organisms most likely to cause round (spherical/nodular) pneumonia are *S. pneumoniae*, *S. aureus*, *K. pneumoniae*, *P. aeruginosa*, *Legionella pneumophila* or *L. mcdadii*, *M. tuberculosis*, and several of the fungi. Clearly, the major differential diagnosis is from neoplasm.

5. Air lucencies within consolidated lung may be due to (a) resolution of the process with interven-

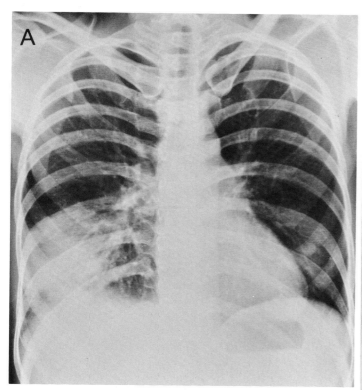

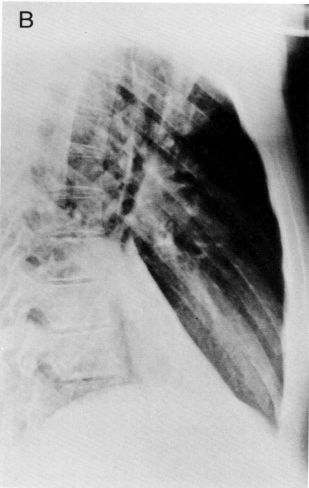

FIG 5–29.
Lobar consolidation resulting from bacterial pneumonia. In this case, the superior segment of the right lower lobe is spared. **A,** PA view. **B,** lateral view.

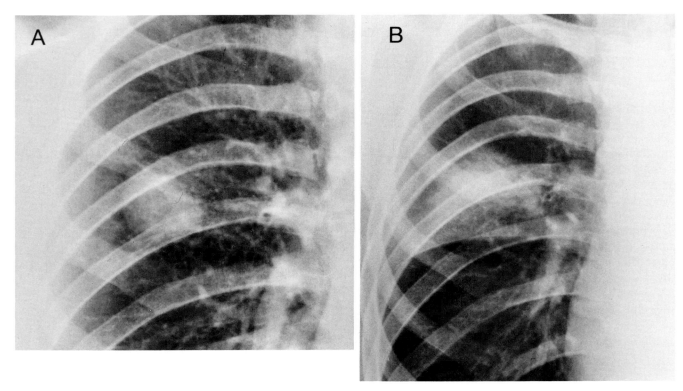

FIG 5–30.
Round (spherical) pneumonia, in a case of bacterial pneumonia. **A,** radiograph on admission to hospital. **B,** one day later the pneumonia has spread through the adjacent lung.

ing normal lung, (b) necrosis of tissue with cavitation, and (c) pneumatoceles.[73] The development of air-fluid levels in an area of consolidation that is known or presumed to be pneumonia strongly suggests necrotizing pneumonia (true abscess formation). Bacteria are the likely pathogens, notably *Staph. aureus,* gram-negative bacteria (especially *Klebsiella, Proteus,* and *Pseudomonas*), anaerobic bacteria, and tuberculosis. A meniscus or halo of air within an area of segmental or lobar consolidation is an almost specific appearance for invasive aspergillosis or invasive mucormycosis. Those few cases of segmental or lobar consolidation with cavitation not due to infection will be due to a vasculitis or, rarely, to lymphoma. (Cavitation in pulmonary masses is a separate subject and is dealt with later in this chapter.)

6. Nonsegmental air-space shadows which are widespread, yet clearly peripheral in location (sometimes called "the photographic negative of pulmonary edema"), are highly indicative of chronic eosinophilic pneumonia (Figs 5–31 and 5–32).[23]

7. By far the most common cause of the bat's wing pattern is pulmonary edema (see Fig 5–27), particularly if air bronchograms, air alveolograms, or acinar shadows are present. The coexistence of Kerley B lines removes all differential diagnoses other than lymphangitis carcinomatosa. Those cases of bat's wing shadowing not due to pulmonary edema are likely to be due to pneumonia, inhalation of noxious gases or liquids (including aspiration of gastric contents), multifocal pulmonary hemorrhage (Fig 5–33), or neoplasm. Multifocal pneumonia can be due to a vast array of organisms, but the bat's wing pattern in the immune-competent patient should particularly suggest aspiration pneumonia, gram-negative bacterial pneumonia, and nonbacterial pneumonias such as mycoplasma, viral, and rickettsial pneumonia. Pneumonia in the immunocompromised host often results in the bat's wing pattern, most notably in infections with opportunistic organisms such as *Pneumocystis carinii* and various fungi.

Bat's wing shadowing that remains unchanged over several weeks and is associated with nonspecific chronic symptoms suggests alveolar proteinosis (Fig 5–34) or a neoplasm, notably lymphangitis carcinomatosa (Fig 5–35), bronchioloalveolar carcinoma, and malignant lymphoma. Amyloidosis, sarcoidosis,

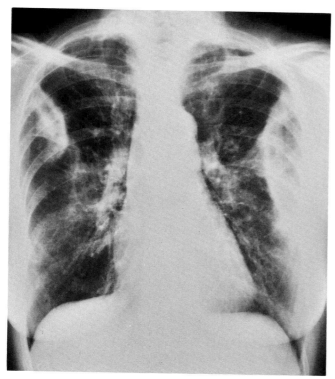

FIG 5—31.
Chronic eosinophilic pneumonia showing a nonsegmental strikingly peripheral distribution of the air-space shadowing.

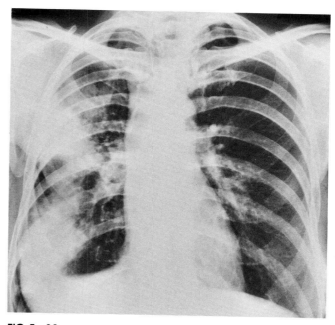

FIG 5—32.
Chronic eosinophilic pneumonia with unilateral, nonsegmental, peripherally located air-space shadowing.

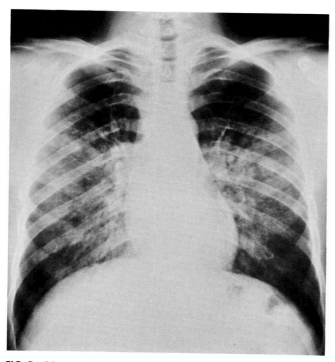

FIG 5—33.
"Bat's wing" shadowing resulting from idiopathic pulmonary hemorrhage.

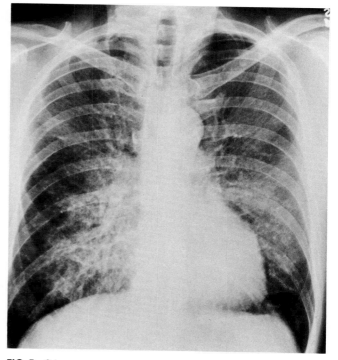

FIG 5—34.
"Bat's wing" shadowing in alveolar proteinosis.

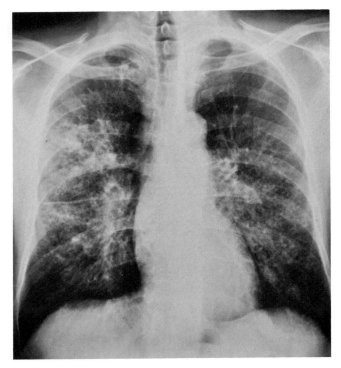

FIG 5–35.
"Bat's wing" shadowing in lymphangitis carcinomatosa.

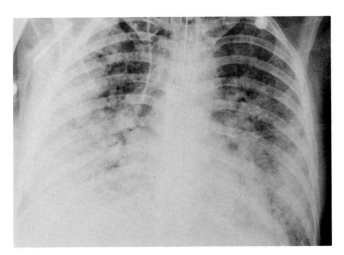

FIG 5–36.
Widespread, uniform air-space shadowing in adult respiratory distress syndrome.

and Wegener's granulomatosis are extremely rare possibilities for such shadowing.

8. Many of the causes of multiple air-space shadows appear rapidly, but pulmonary edema is the only one that can clear within hours.

9. Air-space shadowing that resolves only to reappear either in the same area or in some other part of either lung suggests pulmonary edema; eosinophilic pneumonia, either acute or chronic; or asthma, particularly when associated with bronchopulmonary aspergillosis.

10. Adult respiratory distress syndrome (ARDS) is the most likely diagnosis for uniform opacity of the whole of both lungs without pleural effusion (Fig 5–36). Air bronchograms are a noteworthy feature in these patients. The presence of associated pneumothorax or pneumomediastinum increases the likelihood of ARDS.

11. Sarcoidosis occasionally causes patchy shadows in the lungs which tend to be spherical in shape, to contain air bronchograms, and to be associated with obvious hilar and mediastinal lymph node enlargement. Sometimes these opacities dominate the picture and, when irregular in shape, are radiologically indistinguishable from pneumonia (Fig 5–37 and 5–38).

12. Progressive massive fibrosis may resemble

air-space shadowing (Fig 5–39). It is rarely misdiagnosed, however, because the lesions are so characteristic in shape and position and because the other findings of pneumoconiosis are almost invariably visible.

ATELECTASIS/COLLAPSE

The terms atelectasis, collapse, and loss of volume are used synonymously. They imply reduced inflation of the lung. There are several mechanisms for loss of volume, the most frequent being bronchial obstruction.

In adults, bronchial obstruction is usually the result of bronchial neoplasm, foreign body, or mucus. On occasion, it is due to inflammatory or post-traumatic bronchostenosis, a broncholith, or extrinsic compression by such phenomena as enlarged lymph nodes, aortic aneurysm, or left atrial enlargement. Because bronchial tumors are uncommon in children, the probable causes of lobar atelectasis differ significantly from those in adults. In young children the airways are smaller and more vulnerable to mucus obstruction. Thus, pneumonia is the most common cause of atelectasis in children, the inflammatory exudate and mucus causing significant airway obstruction. Other than pneumonia, the most likely causes of lobar collapse in children are inhaled foreign body or mucus plug obstruction in conditions such as asthma or cystic fibrosis. Less frequent causes of bronchial obstruction in children include inflammatory or post-traumatic bronchostenosis and compression of the bronchial tree by anomalous vessels.

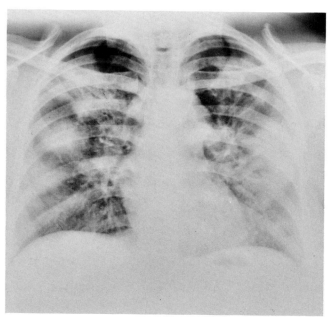

FIG 5–37.
Sarcoidosis showing multiple, rounded, ill-defined areas of pulmonary shadowing. Note also the bilateral hilar and mediastinal adenopathy.

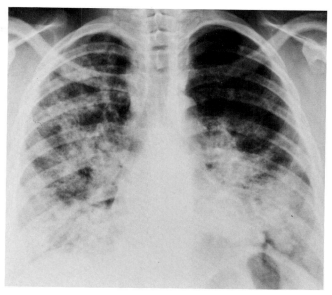

FIG 5–38.
Sarcoidosis showing widespread nonspecific pulmonary shadowing closely resembling pneumonia.

The position of an obstructing lesion can be predicted by recognizing which lobes are collapsed. Obliteration or narrowing of the bronchial air column at the site of obstruction is often visible, particularly at CT scanning.[62] Opaque foreign bodies or calcified broncholiths may be directly visible. All these findings are helpful in determining the need for bronchoscopy and in directing the procedure.

Another useful sign is the *Golden S sign,* which allows one to recognize that a lobe has collapsed around a large central mass (Figs 5–40 and 5–51). The mass may prevent the central portion of the lobe from losing volume. Because the peripheral lung collapses and the central portion does not, the relevant fissures are convex centrally and concave peripherally; the shape of the fissure, therefore, resembles an S or a reverse S—hence the name Golden S sign, after Golden's description of cases of lobar collapse caused by carcinoma of the lung.[32]

Apart from bronchial obstruction, the major mechanisms for atelectasis are (1) compression by adjacent masses or overinflated lung, (2) retraction of the lung associated with large pneumothorax or pleural effusion, (3) cicatrization of the lung, and (4) so called "adhesive atelectasis," which occurs when the surfaces of the alveoli adhere to each other as, for example, in hyaline membrane disease of the newborn and in discoid atelectasis.

The middle lobe and lingula are particularly vulnerable to collapse, possibly because their "lobar" bronchi arise at a relatively acute angle, and there are many lymph nodes surrounding these bronchi. In addition, in patients with complete minor and major fissures, the opportunity for collateral drift to the middle lobe is limited. In one series of 129 pa-

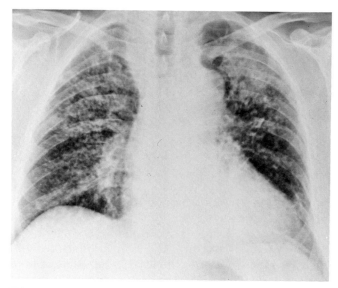

FIG 5–39.
Progressive massive fibrosis (PMF) in a coal miner. The conglomerate PMF shadow in the left upper lobe is ill-defined enough to resemble air-space shadowing, but the typical location and the presence of widespread small nodules in the lungs are characteristic of a mineral dust pneumoconiosis.

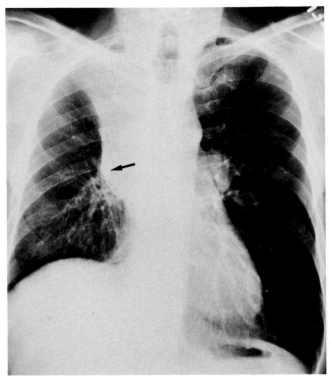

FIG 5–40.
Right upper lobe collapse with Golden "S" sign. The outward bulge *(arrow)* of the displaced minor fissure indicates an underlying mass, which proved to be a bronchial carcinoma.

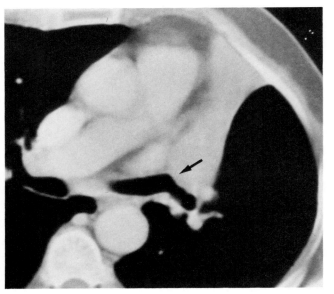

FIG 5–41.
Carcinoma of the bronchus obstructing the left upper lobe bronchus and causing left upper lobe collapse. The bronchial occlusion by the tumor *(arrow)* is well shown by CT.

tients with chronic disease in the right middle lobe and/or lingula, 58 had no evidence of central obstruction, either by endobronchial or exobronchial masses.[78] These patients, most of whom were middle-aged women, were labeled as having "the middle lobe syndrome" (see Fig 5–54). The condition was originally thought to be due to tuberculous lymphadenopathy pressing on the lobar bronchus, but recent reports suggest that the entity is due to chronic inflammatory disease, presumably pneumonia, which clears very slowly because of lack of collateral drift.[11]

Even though the signs of pulmonary collapse are most obvious at CT scanning, that modality is only occasionally needed. Plain films are usually sufficient to diagnose the presence of a collapsed lobe, but CT can be useful when the plain film findings are ambiguous. This occurs particularly when pleural fluid and pulmonary disease processes are both present. In these circumstances it can be very difficult to quantitate the relative contribution of the two processes from plain films alone. CT is also accurate in demonstrating the site and size of an obstructing lesion in lobar collapse[62] (Figs 5–41 and 5–42), but

is rarely used for this purpose because bronchoscopy is usually more informative.

The Signs of Lobar Collapse

The fundamental signs of lobar collapse[71] are opacity of the lobe and evidence of loss of volume of the lobe. The signs can be divided into (1) direct signs, such as displacement of fissures, pulmonary

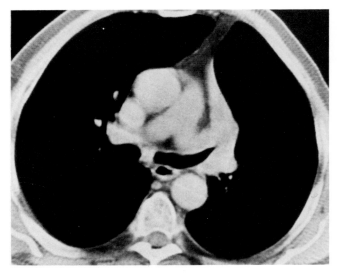

FIG 5–42.
Carcinoma of the bronchus causing "rat tail" narrowing of the left upper lobe bronchus and collapse of the left upper lobe.

blood vessels, and major bronchi, and (2) shift of other structures to compensate for the loss of volume. The compensatory shifts will be discussed first, to be followed by a detailed description of the appearances of collapse of individual lobes.

Compensatory overexpansion of the adjacent lobe results in spreading out of the vessels within that lobe. The concept here is that there will be fewer vessels per unit volume when a lobe undergoes compensatory expansion. Though this is a well-known sign, it can be difficult to evaluate and should not be relied upon if it is an isolated finding since previous lung damage, from infection for example, can lead to a similar appearance. Also, the sign may be difficult to recognize, even in cases of severe compensatory overexpansion.

Another sign of compensatory expansion is the shifting granuloma. Displacement of adjacent lung can be difficult to identify, but displacement of a granuloma, particularly when calcified, is often easy to recognize (Fig 5–43).

The amount of *mediastinal shift* accompanying lobar collapse is variable. In general, it is greatest with lower lobe collapse and with chronic fibrotic upper lobe collapse, relatively mild with acute upper lobe collapse, and virtually nonexistent with collapse of the middle lobe. Its recognition depends on noting displacement of the trachea and mediastinum. Displacement of the trachea is much the more reliable

sign. Normally, on a correctly centered frontal view, the trachea lies midway, or slightly to the right of the midpoint, between the medial ends of the clavicles. Minor obliquity of the chest radiograph does not make much difference because the trachea is only just behind the plane of the medial ends of the clavicles. Aortic unfolding, however, may move the trachea to the right.

The normal size and position of the mediastinum varies so greatly that displacement of the mediastinal shadow is an insensitive sign of pulmonary collapse. Normally one-fifth to half of the cardiac shadow lies to the right of the midline. More or less than this suggests mediastinal shift.

Hemidiaphragm elevation is another form of compensatory shift. It is usually unrecognizable in right middle lobe collapse and subtle in right upper lobe collapse. Collapse of either lower lobe or of the left upper lobe may lead to obvious elevation of the ipsilateral hemidiaphragm. The sign is, however, of limited value because the position of the normal diaphragm is highly variable, particularly in a hospital population. It depends on many factors, including the amount of gas in the stomach, and can vary from day to day in the same individual. Therefore, great care must be taken when using this sign to support the diagnosis of lobar collapse.

Inward movement of the chest wall causes narrowing of the spaces between the affected ribs. This sign,

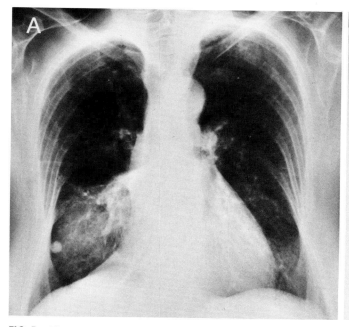
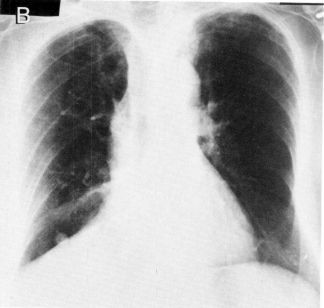

FIG 5–43.
Displacement of a calcified granuloma secondary to right lower lobe collapse. **A,** at a time when mild right lower lobe collapse is present. **B,** when complete collapse of the right lower lobe is present.

which is only seen with a severely collapsed lobe, can be difficult to evaluate on chest films. It is much easier to recognize with CT where the volume of each hemithorax can be readily compared. Clearly, confusion with preexisting chest wall deformity, particularly when consequent to scoliosis, may cloud the issue.

Right Upper Lobe Collapse

Right upper lobe collapse (Figs 5–40 and 5–44), is the easiest lobar collapse to recognize on plain chest radiographs. The major and minor fissures move upward toward each other rather like a half-closed book, the spine of which is represented by the hilus. At the same time, these fissures rotate toward the mediastinum, with the result that the right upper lobe packs against the mediastinum and lung apex. The more the collapse, the greater the concavity of the minor fissure. Eventually, with extreme collapse, the minor fissure parallels the mediastinum and thoracic apex and resembles pleural thickening or mediastinal widening. The lobe is attached to the

hilus by a conical wedge of collapsed lung and, therefore, the curving inferior margin of the lobe always connects to the hilus. The intrinsic bulk of the central vessels and bronchi means that there is a limit to the loss of volume possible at the hilus; hence, an outward bulge will be discernible at the hilus in examples of extreme collapse even when no hilar mass is present. Because the collapsed right upper lobe has extensive contact with the mediastinum, the normal superior vena caval border is "silhouetted" out on the frontal chest film, as is the ascending aorta on the lateral view.

The middle and lower lobes expand to occupy the vacated space, leading to outward and upward displacement of the lower lobe artery. Because this displacement is easy to see on frontal radiographs, it is a good sign to look for. The corresponding upward angulation of the right main stem and lower lobe bronchi is more difficult to recognize. Overexpansion of the opposite upper lobe is usually minor. For practical purposes it is visible only at CT scanning.

On the lateral view, the upward displacement of

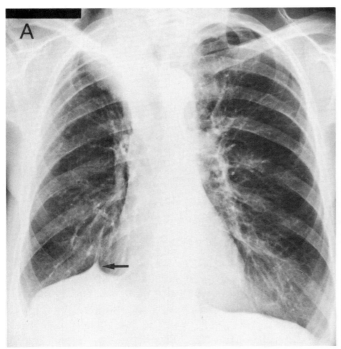

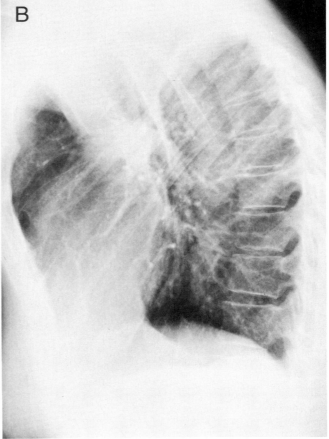

FIG 5–44.
Right upper lobe collapse. Typical example. Also note the juxtaphrenic peak *(arrow)*. **A,** PA view. **B,** lateral view.

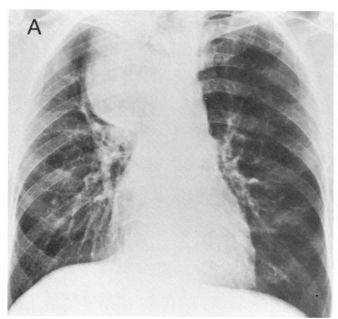

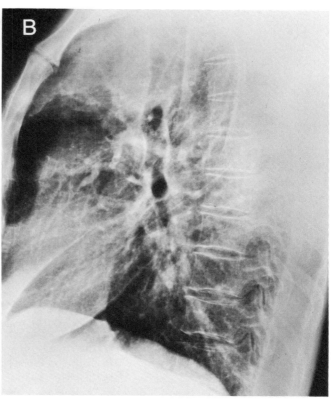

FIG 5–45.
Right upper lobe collapse around a large, centrally obstructing bronchial carcinoma (Golden "S" sign) resembling a mediastinal mass. The best clue to the correct interpretation is the elevation of the right lower lobe artery. **A,** PA view. **B,** lateral view.

the major and minor fissures is usually obvious. Often, the wedge of collapsed lung radiating out from the hilus is no more than an indistinct density on lateral views, since no portion is tangential to the x-ray beam. The elevation of the right pulmonary trunk

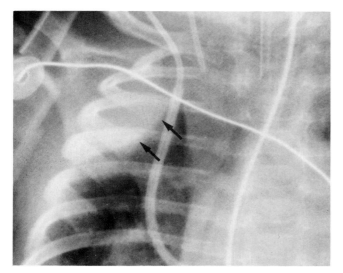

FIG 5–46.
"Peripheral atelectasis" of right upper lobe *(arrows)* in an infant following cardiac surgery. The lobe has collapsed against the chest wall.

and the anterior displacement of the right bronchial tree can be identified on the lateral projection,[97] but only with great difficulty.

Occasionally, collapse of the right upper lobe around a large obstructing bronchial tumor can closely mimic a mediastinal mass (Fig 5–45). An error in interpretation can be avoided by carefully analyzing the film for compensatory shift of other intrathoracic structures.

On rare occasions, the normal chest wall contact is maintained even in severe collapse. This appearance (Fig 5–46), which is almost always confined to young children, has been termed "peripheral atelectasis"[21] because the collapsed lobe lies against the chest wall and the overexpanded lower lobe lies centrally.

A recently popularized sign is the so-called *juxtaphrenic peak*.[48] The term refers to a small triangular shadow based on the apex of the dome of the right hemidiaphragm with loss of silhouette of the hemidiaphragm at the point of contact in both frontal and lateral projections (see Fig 5–44). The sign is probably due to traction on either the lower end of the major fissure, the inferior accessory fissure or the inferior pulmonary ligament.[29]

At CT scanning,[28, 61–63] the collapsed right up-

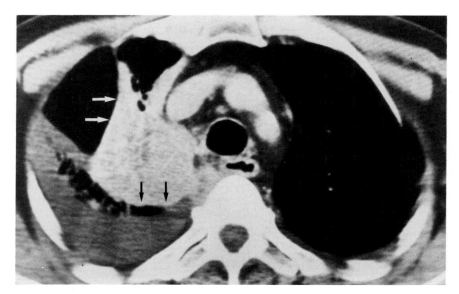

FIG 5—47.
CT scan showing right upper lobe collapse. The *black arrows* point to the major fissure. The *white arrows* point to the minor fissure. (There is also a right pleural effusion.)

per lobe appears as a triangular soft tissue density lying against the mediastinum and the anterior chest wall. The border formed by the major fissure posteriorly and the minor fissure laterally is sharp. (Fig 5—47). In the absence of large intrapulmonary masses, each fissural boundary should be uniformly concave or convex, not a combination of the two. A severely collapsed right upper lobe assumes a band-like configuration plastered against the mediastinum, an appearance that can be confused with me-

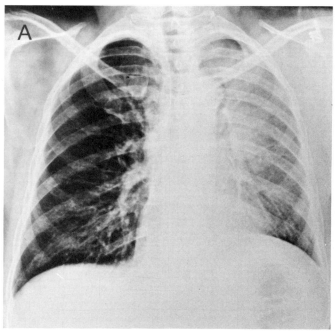

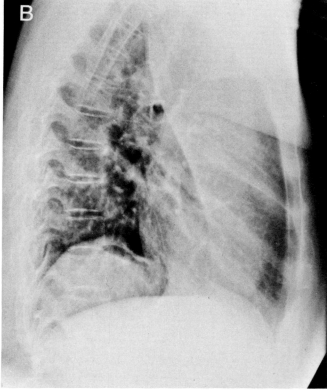

FIG 5—48.
Left upper lobe collapse in a patient with bronchial carcinoma. **A,** PA view. **B,** lateral view.

diastinal disease. Sometimes the hyperexpanded superior segment of the lower lobe may insinuate itself between the mediastinum and the medial border of the collapsed lobe. Elevation of the right upper lobe bronchus may cause the bronchus intermedius to move laterally,[28] and the right middle lobe bronchus may be displaced anteriorly and reoriented in a more horizontal position.

Left Upper Lobe Collapse

Because there is no minor fissure on the left, the appearance of collapse of the left upper lobe is significantly different from collapse of the right upper lobe (Fig 5–48). The collapse is predominantly forward, pulling the expanding lower lobe behind it. Except at the edges, the lobe in its collapsed state retains much of its original contact with the anterior chest wall and mediastinum. Since the lobe thins as the fissure is pulled forward, the usual appearance on a frontal radiograph is a hazy density extending out from the left hilus, often reaching the lung apex, and fading laterally and inferiorly.

The loss of the left cardiac and mediastinal silhouette is a striking feature on the frontal view. With mild loss of volume—provided the lobe is opaque—the entire cardiac and upper mediastinal border, together with the diaphragm outline adjacent to the cardiac apex, becomes invisible. With increasing loss of volume, the upper margin of the aortic knob will once again become visible because the superior segment of the lower lobe takes the place of the posterior segment of the upper lobe. With further loss of volume the upper border of the pulmonary opacity becomes hazy and its medial border becomes sharp because the apex is now occupied by the greatly overexpanded superior segment of lower lobe (Fig 5–49). The superior mediastinal and left hemidiaphragm contours will then reappear but, with very few exceptions (Fig 5–50), the left border of the heart remains effaced even in the most severe cases of complete left upper lobe collapse.

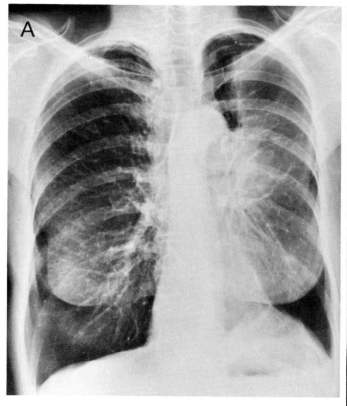

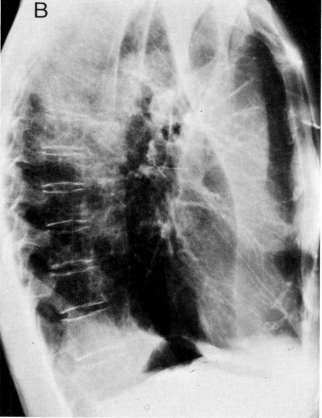

FIG 5–49.
Left upper lobe collapse. In this example, the greatly expanded superior segment of the left lower lobe occupies the apex and consequently the upper surface of the aortic arch is visible. **A,** PA view. **B,** lateral view.

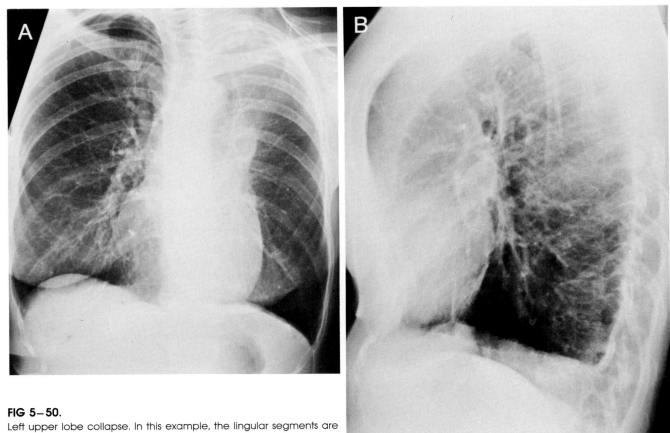

FIG 5–50.
Left upper lobe collapse. In this example, the lingular segments are so reduced in volume that there is no detectable loss of silhouette of the left border of the heart. (There is also a pectus excavatum which is responsible for the loss of the right border of the heart.) **A,** PA view. **B,** lateral view.

The overexpansion of the left lower lobe results in elevation of the left hilus and outward angulation of the left lower lobe artery. The left bronchial tree assumes an **S**-shaped configuration, the left main bronchus assuming a near horizontal course and the lower lobe bronchus running more vertically than usual (Fig 5–51).

On the lateral view, the lateral portion of the major fissure is usually seen as a clearly defined concave margin running approximately parallel to the anterior chest wall. The inevitable wedge of tissue radiating from the hilus is indistinct on the lateral projection unless there is a hilar mass to alter the tangents. The lingula segment, being thinner to start with, often appears to be no more than a sliver. The whole fissure may be so far forward that a collapsed upper lobe can be overlooked or misinterpreted as an anterior mediastinal density. Sometimes the fissure rotates, so that no part of it is tangential to the x-ray beam and, in these cases, the edge of the shadow is ill-defined in the lateral view also.

A striking feature of left upper lobe collapse is herniation of the opposite lung into the left hemithorax in front of the aorta (see Fig 5–41), which leads to increased visibility of the ascending aorta on the lateral chest radiograph (Figs 5–48 and 5–49), a feature which should not be misinterpreted as the anterior edge of the collapsed lobe, and certainly not as a mediastinal mass. In rare instances, the edge of the herniated lung can be seen projected over the aortic knob on a frontal film. The more usual cause of aerated lung lying medial to the opacity of a collapsed left upper lobe is overexpansion of the left lower lobe invaginating between the collapsed lung and the mediastinum (see Fig 5–49).

A juxtaphrenic peak on the hemidiaphragm (Figs 5–42 and 5–52) and the phenomenon of "peripheral" atelectasis may be seen on the left just as they may with collapse of the right upper lobe.

At CT (see Figs 5–41, 5–42, 5–47, and 5–53)[28, 61–63] collapsed left and right upper lobes appear similar, but with left upper lobe collapse, the airless lingular segments are identified on sections below the carina as a narrow triangular density

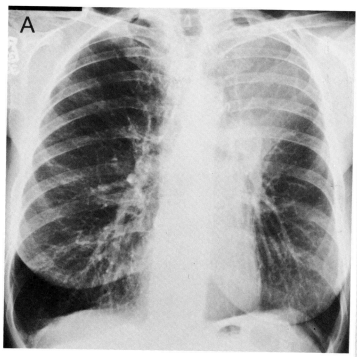

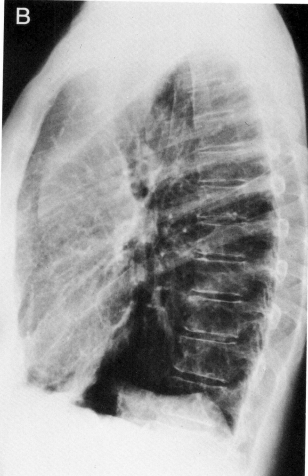

FIG 5–51.
Left upper lobe collapse showing reorientation of the left main-stem bronchus and the left lower lobe bronchus. Note the near horizontal alignment of the main-stem bronchus and a near vertical alignment of the lower lobe bronchus. **A,** PA view. **B,** lateral view.

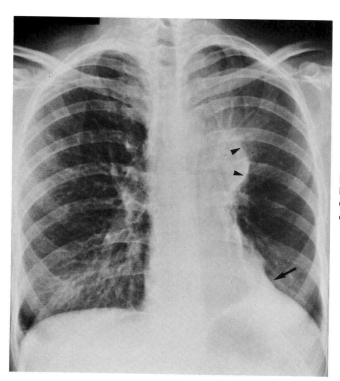

FIG 5–52.
Left upper lobe collapse showing juxtaphrenic peak *(arrow)* and Golden "S" sign *(arrowheads)*. The collapse was due to a centrally obstructing bronchial carcinoma.

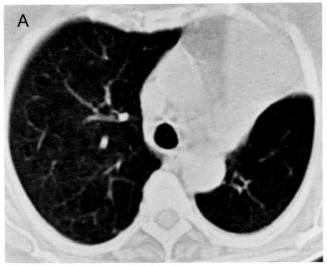

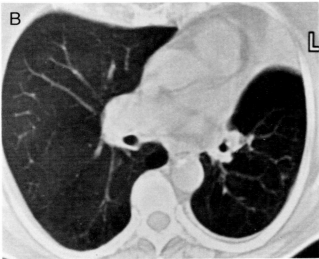

FIG 5–53.
CT scans showing left upper lobe collapse. Note the forward displacement of the major fissure and the mediastinal shift to the left. **A,** section above the level of the left main-stem bronchus showing collapsed anterior, posterior, and apical segments. **B,** section through the collapsed lingular segments.

based on the heart and anterior chest wall extending almost to the diaphragm. The herniation of the right lung anterior to the aorta is particularly well demonstrated at CT scanning.

Right Middle Lobe Collapse

The opacity of a collapsed middle lobe on the frontal chest radiograph may, in severe cases, be so minimal that middle lobe atelectasis is easy to overlook, because its depth in the plane of the beam may be no more than a few millimeters (Fig 5–54). Loss

of silhouette of the right border of the heart is almost always a feature. The bronchial and vascular realignments in right middle lobe collapse are so slight that there is no recognizable alteration in the appearance of the right hilus. The collapsed lobe is, however, easily and reliably recognized on the lateral chest radiograph. The major and minor fissures approximate one another and, if the collapse is pronounced, the lobe diminishes in volume and resembles a curved, elongated wedge. The wedge tapers in two directions: medial to lateral, and anterior to posterior. Because the wedge can be relatively thin, much of it is end-on to the beam in the lateral projection. The image on the lateral chest radiograph is, therefore, a well-defined, curved triangular band of density, lying between the major and minor fissures, extending downward and forward from the hilus. The collapsed lobe may be so thin that it may be misinterpreted as a thickened fissure. Clearly, since the fissures form the boundary of the collapsed lobe, they should not be separately visible in their normal positions—an important point in the differential diagnosis from fluid, fibrosis, or tumors lying within the fissures.

At CT (Fig 5–55),[28, 61–63] right middle lobe collapse appears as a triangular density bounded posteriorly by the major fissure, medially by the mediastinum at the level of the right atrium, and anteriorly by the minor fissure. The posterior boundary should be well defined. Unless the minor fissure is pulled well down, the anterior margin will be poorly defined on the CT images. The right middle lobe bronchus enters the posteromedial corner of the opacity, an important point in the differential diagnosis from loculated pleural fluid. Because the collapsed middle lobe is effectively a sheet of tissue running obliquely through the chest, the axial sections of CT are not aligned with the lobe, and only small portions of the collapsed lobe are seen on any one section.

Right and Left Lower Lobe Collapse

The appearances seen with collapse of the lower lobes are sufficiently similar on the two sides that it is convenient to consider them together. Collapse may affect the whole lobe, but the superior segment is frequently spared.

With collapse of either lower lobe (Figs 5–56 and 5–57), the major fissure rotates backward and medially, and the upper half of the fissure swings downward. Thus, collapsed lower lobes lie posteromedially in the lower thoracic cavity. The resulting

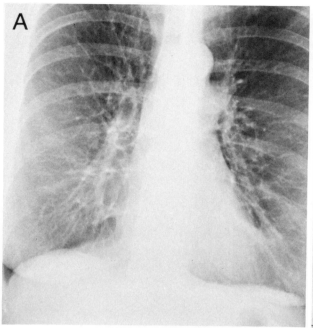

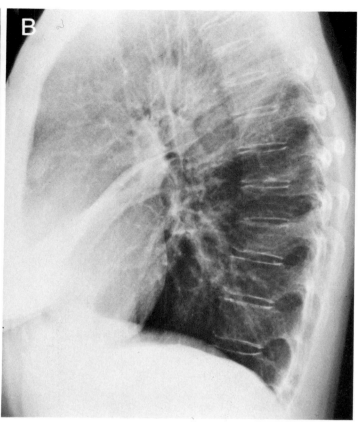

FIG 5–54.
Right middle lobe collapse. **A,** the lobe is so severely atelectatic that the opacity in the frontal view is difficult to see. There is, however, loss of the right heart border owing to the silhouette sign. **B,** the lateral view shows the collapsed lobe to advantage. In this case, the collapse was chronic and the result of "middle lobe syndrome."

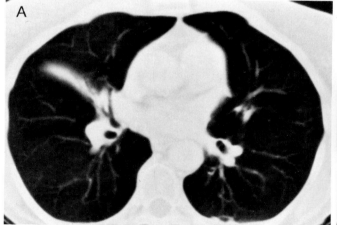

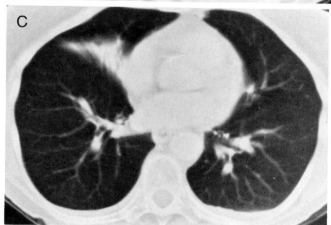

FIG 5–55.
CT scans of right middle lobe collapse in the same patient shown in Figure 5–54. Note the patent middle lobe bronchus and the air bronchogram. Three adjacent sections are shown: **A,** the most superior section at the level of the right middle lobe bronchus; **B,** one section lower; **C,** the lowest section.

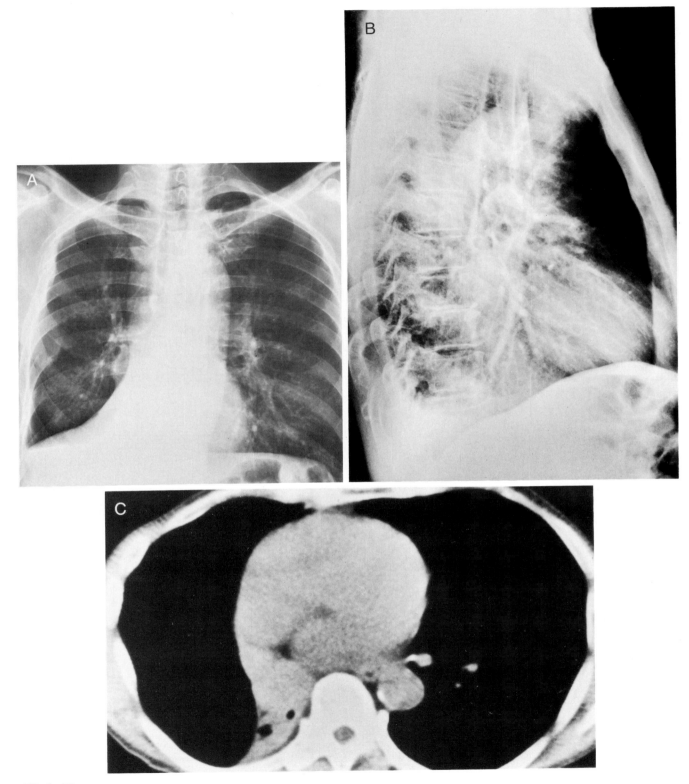

FIG 5–56.
Right lower lobe collapse resulting from bronchial carcinoma. (A metastasis is present in the right eighth rib, and there are multiple old fractures of the right ribs). **A,** PA radiograph. **B,** lateral radiograph. **C,** CT scan.

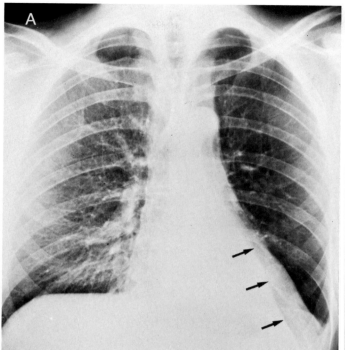

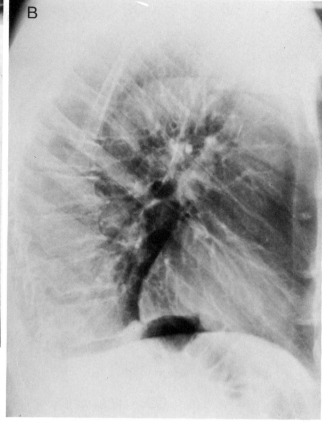

FIG 5–57.

Left lower lobe collapse resulting from bronchial carcinoma. (The *arrows* point to the displaced major fissure.) In this example, the displacement of the left hilar vessels is particularly well demonstrated. The left lower lobe artery is invisible because it is within the collapsed lobe. Note also the splaying of blood vessels in the over expanded left upper lobe. The flat waist sign is also present. **A,** PA view. **B,** lateral view.

triangular opacity is based on the diaphragm and mediastinum, with the fissure running obliquely through the thorax. On frontal projection, the opacity of a collapsed lower lobe is easier to recognize on the right than on the left because on the left it is often hidden by the heart, especially if the film is underpenetrated. With severe loss of volume the lobe becomes notably thin and appears as a sliver lying against the mediastinum (Fig 5–58). Sometimes, presumably because the inferior pulmonary ligament does not attach to the diaphragm, the lobe plasters against the mediastinum, but has little if any contact with the diaphragm. In these cases, the collapsed lobe assumes a rounded configuration and resembles a mediastinal mass (see Fig 14–19).

If the superior segment remains aerated, the upper half of the major fissure will often be identified on the frontal view as a line that may run horizontally to contact the spine (Fig 5–59). In these cases, the major fissure may be confused with the minor fissure, a misinterpretation that can be avoided by remembering that the minor fissure does not cross medial to the hilus.

Lower lobe collapse is sometimes most obvious in the lateral view. With mild loss of volume, the opaque lobe and the displaced major fissure are readily recognizable, but with more severe loss of volume the fissure rotates, and the triangular opacity in the lower posterior quadrant of the chest has an ill-defined anterior margin. Unless the collapse is severe, the outline of the posterior half of the right or left hemidiaphragm shadow will be lost. With very severe collapse, the outline of the ipsilateral hemidiaphragm once again becomes visible because compensatory expansion of the upper and/or middle lobes brings them into contact with the previously effaced diaphragm (see Fig 5–58). The opacity of the collapsed lobe may be difficult to recognize unless one is careful to observe the density of the vertebrae. Normally, on lateral projection each vertebra should appear blacker as one descends through the thorax to the diaphragm. In lower lobe collapse, the lower

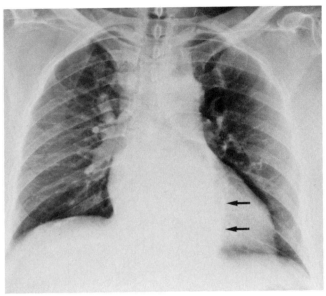

FIG 5–58.
Very severe collapse of the left lower lobe. The collapsed lobe *(arrows)* is no more than a sliver against the mediastinum. The altered configuration of the left hilus is perhaps the most striking sign in this example.

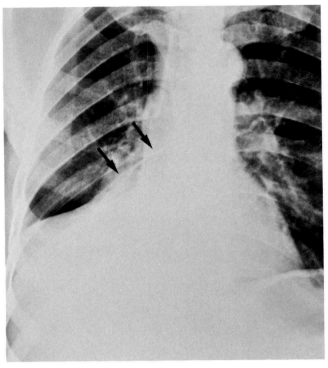

FIG 5–59.
Right lower and right middle lobe collapse with partial aeration of the superior segment of the right lower lobe. *Arrows* point to the displaced major fissure.

vertebrae appear whiter than those higher up (see Figs 5–56 and 5–57).

The major vascular trunks supplying the lobes are displaced but, more importantly, they are invisible because they are coursing through an opaque lobe. Therefore, with complete lower lobe collapse, the lobar and segmental divisions of the pulmonary artery will be displaced and invisible. Careful analysis of the hilus may, however, be needed to recognize this difference because displaced middle or upper lobe trunks may resemble the lower lobe arteries. A similar analysis of the bronchi may be even more revealing. The lower lobe bronchus will enter the collapsed lobe, and in most cases, the air within the bronchus can be identified as it enters the triangular density.

Bronchial displacement can also be recognized on lateral chest films, but the signs are more subtle and demand confident knowledge of the normal.[97] Normally, the central bronchi run in the same direction as the trachea and course obliquely backward as they descend, so that the right and left major airways are virtually superimposed on one another in a true lateral projection. The only difference is the higher origin of the right upper lobe bronchus and the differences inherent in the right lung having a middle lobe. Lower lobe collapse leads to backward displacement of the relevant airways. This displacement is of particular practical use when there is

doubt as to whether an opacity is due primarily to pleural fluid or to lower lobe collapse. With collapse, the bronchi are pulled back, whereas with pleural fluid the bronchi may be pushed forward.[68]

The appearance of the upper mediastinal contours may occasionally be helpful in drawing attention to, or confirming, the possibility of lower lobe collapse. Kattan[47] has emphasized three signs:

1. The upper triangle sign[49] refers to a low-density, clearly margined triangular shadow on frontal chest radiographs that resembles right-sided mediastinal widening. It is seen in right lower lobe collapse and is caused by rightward displacement of the anterior junctional tissues of the mediastinum (Fig 5–60). The appearance superficially resembles right upper lobe collapse but should not be confused with it, because the fissural, vascular, and bronchial realignments all point to overexpansion of the right upper lobe rather than to collapse.

2. The flat waist sign[50] refers to flattening of the contours of the aortic knob and adjacent main pulmonary artery (see Fig 5–57). It is seen in severe collapse of the left lower lobe and is due to leftward displacement and rotation of the heart. The appear-

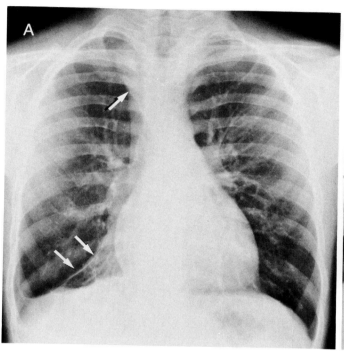

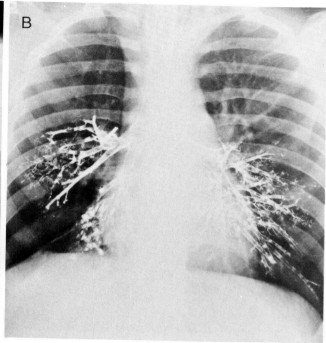

FIG 5–60.

Right lower lobe collapse due to bronchiectasis showing the upper triangle sign *(upward pointing arrow)*. The displaced major fissure *(downward pointing arrows)* and the right lower lobe artery

entering the collapsed lobe are well demonstrated. **A,** PA radiograph. **B,** bronchogram showing the arrangement of the bronchi.

ance, therefore, resembles a shallow right anterior oblique view of the normal mediastinum.

3. The outline of the top of the aortic knob may be obliterated in severe left lower lobe collapse.[47]

At CT scanning,[28, 61–63] a collapsed lower lobe produces a triangular opacity of soft tissue density in the posterior chest against the spine (Figs 5–56 and 5–61). The major fissure rotates to lie obliquely across the thoracic cavity. The lobe is fixed at the hilus, and the medial basal segment cannot move further back than the attachment of the inferior pulmonary ligament to the mediastinum. In cases where the inferior pulmonary ligament is incomplete, collapse of the basal segments may simulate a mass on CT just as it may on the plain chest radiograph.[27]

Whole Lung Collapse

Whole lung collapse on either side leads to opacity of the whole hemithorax. The signs of compensatory shift are usually obvious. Mediastinal shift is invariably present, and herniation of the opposite lung is usually a striking feature (Fig 5–62).

Combined Right Upper and Middle Lobe Collapse

Because there is no single bronchus to the right upper and middle lobes that does not also supply the right lower lobe, collapse of these two lobes with normal aeration of the lower lobe is unusual. The appearances are virtually identical to those seen with left upper lobe collapse (Fig 5–63).

Combined Right Lower and Middle Lobe Collapse

The combination of right lower and middle lobe collapse is seen with obstruction to the bronchus intermedius. The appearances are very similar to collapse of the right lower lobe alone in both the PA and lateral projections except that, as Proto and Tocino have noted,[71] if the abnormal density extends all the way to the lateral costophrenic angle, combined middle and lower lobe collapse should be suspected (Fig 5–64). Similarly, on the lateral view, the opacity extends from the front to the back of the thorax.

Diagnosing combined middle and lower lobe collapse is much easier at CT, where the three-dimensional anatomy is clearly displayed. Because the bronchi can be individually identified, it is possible

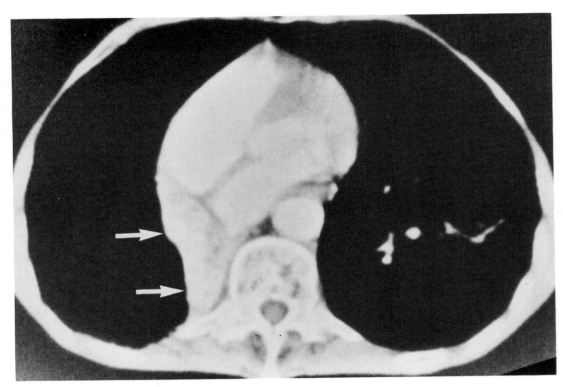

FIG 5–61.
CT scan of collapsed right lower lobe. *Arrows* point to the displaced major fissure.

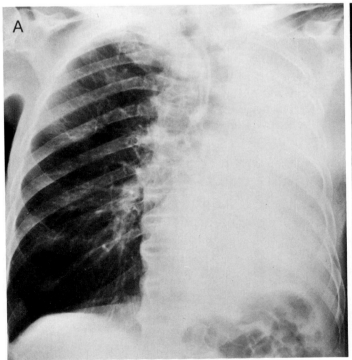

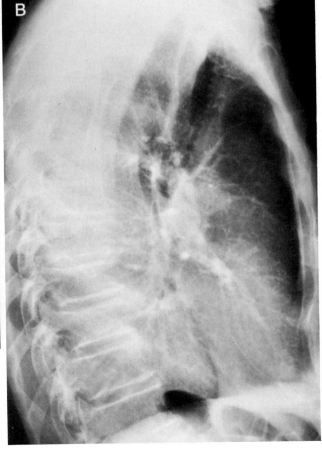

FIG 5–62.
Collapse of the left lung. The left lung is opaque, and there is striking shift of the mediastinum. **A,** PA view. **B,** lateral view.

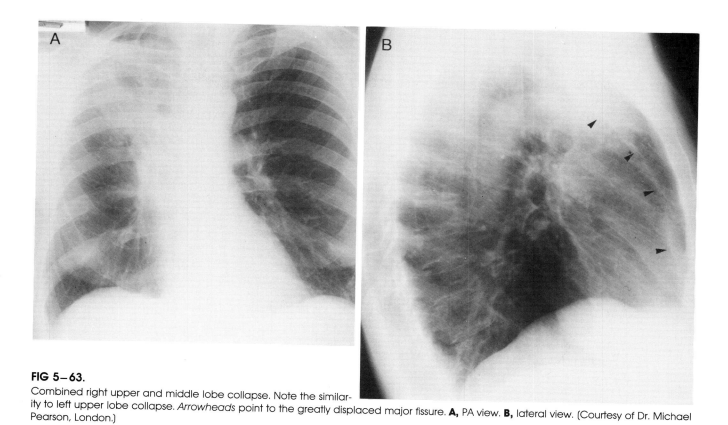

FIG 5–63.
Combined right upper and middle lobe collapse. Note the similarity to left upper lobe collapse. *Arrowheads* point to the greatly displaced major fissure. **A,** PA view. **B,** lateral view. (Courtesy of Dr. Michael Pearson, London.)

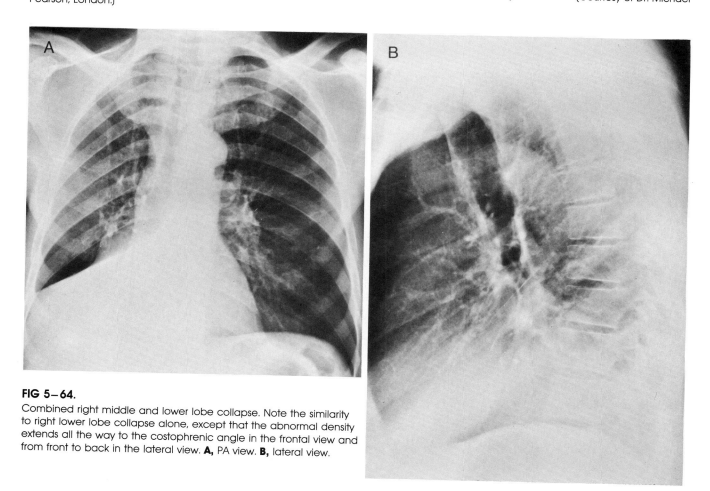

FIG 5–64.
Combined right middle and lower lobe collapse. Note the similarity to right lower lobe collapse alone, except that the abnormal density extends all the way to the costophrenic angle in the frontal view and from front to back in the lateral view. **A,** PA view. **B,** lateral view.

to identify the middle lobe specifically and so diagnose or exclude the presence of combined middle and lower lobe collapse.

Distinguishing Lower Lobe Collapse From Pleural Fluid

Lower lobe collapse can be difficult, and sometimes impossible, to distinguish from pleural effusion on conventional PA and lateral radiographs. This diagnostic dilemma is most frequent in postoperative or acutely ill patients and is compounded by the fact that these patients are frequently examined with portable equipment in frontal projection only.

The diagnosis of lobar collapse depends on recognizing shift of structures, particularly the fissures, the hilar blood vessels, and the major bronchi. If the position of the fissures can be confidently established, then the diagnosis is easy. If not, attention should be turned to the hili, particularly the position of the lower lobe arteries and bronchi, because these structures are large and can often be identified with confidence. Two questions should be addressed. First, do these structures enter the opacity in question and, second, are they displaced in a direction that suggests collapse? For example, in a patient with basal opacity, if the lower lobe artery is obscured and the lower lobe bronchus runs vertically through the opacity, then lower lobe collapse should be diagnosed. If, on the other hand, the lower lobe artery is clearly seen lateral to the opacity and the bronchus is not surrounded by the density, then the opacity is not the result of lower lobe collapse.

Lateral decubitus views may be necessary to distinguish between lower lobe collapse and pleural fluid. Provided fluid is free in the pleural cavity, it will layer against the lateral chest wall, whereas in lobar collapse there is little change in the shape or position of the density in question. If the pleural fluid is loculated, the decubitus view may not be helpful.

Distinguishing between pleural effusion and lobar collapse is easy at CT (Fig 5–65), but CT is only occasionally needed because the lateral decubitus view is a simpler means of diagnosis. At CT, the density of the collapsed lobe is usually appreciably greater than that of the pleural effusion, even more so if intravenous contrast enhancement is used.[62, 63] Also, blood vessels and bronchi can be traced into the compressed lung.

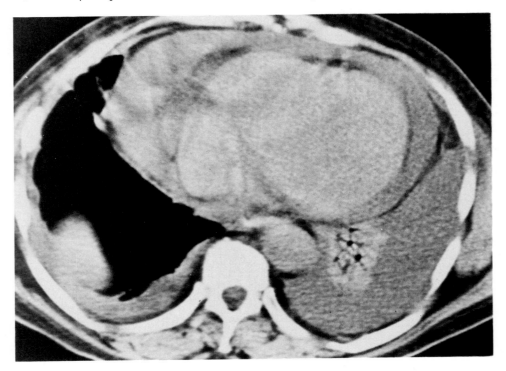

FIG 5–65.
CT scan of combined pleural effusion and left lower lobe collapse. The collapsed lobe with its air bronchogram is clearly distinguishable from the adjacent left pleural effusion. (The patient, who suffered from small cell carcinoma of the lung, also has extensive mediastinal adenopathy, a pericardial effusion, and a right pleural effusion.)

Cicatrization Atelectasis

Pulmonary fibrosis leads to loss of lung volume owing to a combination of lung destruction and loss of compliance. There are many different patterns; the precise radiographic features depend on the distribution of the primary disease.

Following infection, a lobe may lose volume because of destruction and fibrosis (Figs 5–62 and 5–66). Bronchial occlusion and dilatation may accompany the fibrosis and, if the disease affects the dependent portions of the lung, the patients may have the clinical features of bronchiectasis. Naidich et al.[63] have pointed out the following features, all of which are best seen at CT, but which may be inferred from plain chest radiographs: no endobronchial mass; dilated, thick-walled bronchi within the atelectatic lobe; and associated extensive pleural thickening. The loss of volume can be very severe and may be greater than is generally observed in lobar collapse caused by endobronchial obstruction.

Widespread interstitial pulmonary fibrosis causes generalized loss of lung volume. Reticulonodular shadowing of the lung is then the dominant radiographic feature (see the section "Widespread Nodular, Reticulonodular, and Honeycomb Shadowing" later in this chapter).

Round Atelectasis

Round atelectasis, also known as folded lung, is a unique form of chronic atelectasis that resembles a mass.[4, 9, 67, 80] The process is frequently associated with asbestosis.[59, 94]

The mechanism that leads to the formation of round atelectasis is uncertain. One suggestion[38] is that a pleural effusion occurs initially and causes elevation and compression atelectasis of the adjacent lower lobe. The atelectatic lung may adhere to the parietal pleura and to the major fissure. As the pleural effusion clears, the atelectatic lung folds in on itself, leading to the condition of round atelectasis.

The major feature on plain films and CT scans is the peripheral location, usually in one or other lower lobe in contact with the pleura, which is thickened both over the lesion and sometimes in other parts of the pleural cavity as well (Figs 5–67 and 5–68). Plaques of thickened or calcified pleura resulting from asbestosis exposure may be seen in both thoracic cavities. Round atelectasis is never completely surrounded by aerated lung, but there is often aerated lung between the lesion and the diaphragm. The opacity is usually in direct contact with the posterior chest wall (see Fig 5–66), but may be seen in contact with the diaphragm (see Fig 5–68). The top, bottom, and lateral edges are usually smooth, but the anterior edge is often irregular and blends with curved bronchi and blood vessels that lead into the atelectatic mass. Round atelectasis is usually oval in configuration and angled with respect to the pleural surface (see Fig 5–67). Air bronchograms may be seen within the opacity, and the volume of the affected lobe is usually reduced. The condition is most often unilateral, but may be bilateral. Though usually static, round atelectasis may occasionally shrink.[38]

CT (Figs 5–67 and Fig 5–68) shows all the features to advantage[13, 26, 94] and may show that the pleural disease is more extensive than was previously appreciated. The CT findings may be definitive so that further investigation to exclude carcinoma as the cause of the mass is unnecessary.

Discoid Atelectasis

Discoid atelectasis (also known as plate or linear atelectasis) is a form of peripheral pulmonary collapse that is not secondary to bronchial obstruction.

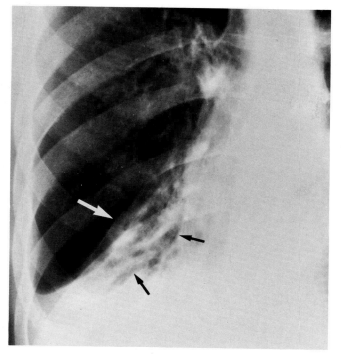

FIG 5–66.
Right lower lobe collapse due to bronchiectasis. The air in dilated bronchi *(black arrows)* is an important clue to the cause of the collapsed lobe. The *white arrow* points to the displaced major fissure.

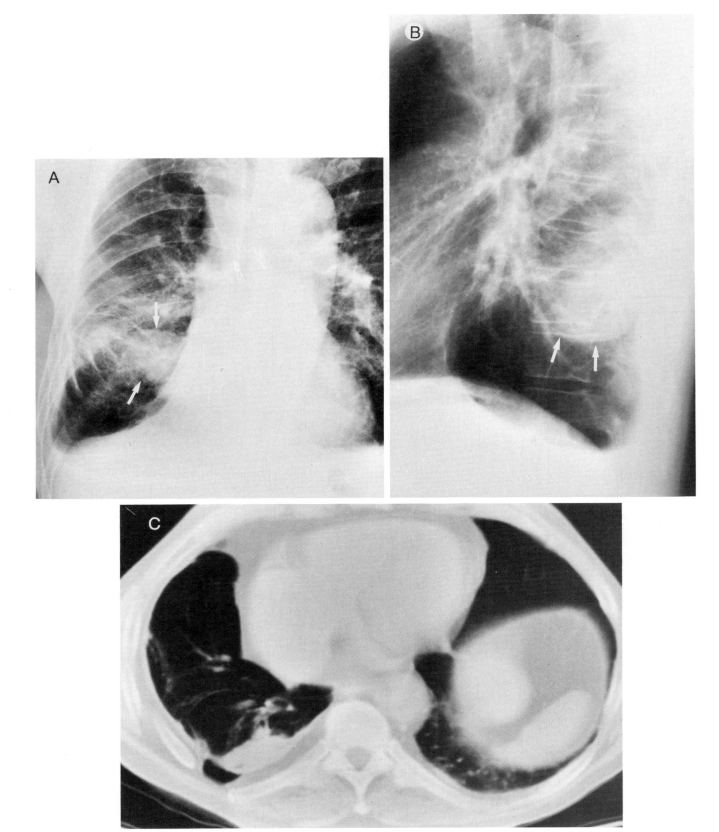

FIG 5–67.
Round atelectasis *(arrows)*. These examples show the typical features of an oval mass aligned obliquely in contact with pleural thickening along the posterior chest wall. **A,** PA radiograph. **B,** lateral radiograph. **C,** CT scan.

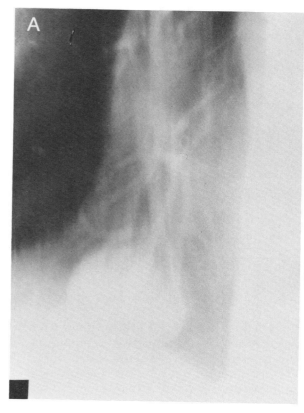

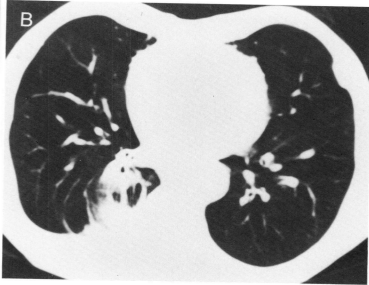

FIG 5—68.
Round atelectasis showing distortion of blood vessels entering the lesion.
A, lateral tomogram. **B,** CT scan.

First described by Fleischner,[19] and therefore sometimes known as Fleischner lines, the atelectasis takes the form of a disk (Fig 5—69). Sometimes the disk is so wide that it crosses the whole lobe. Discoid atelectasis may be single or multiple. It usually abuts the pleura and is perpendicular to the pleural surface[96] with no predisposition to point toward the hilus. The thickness ranges from a few millimeters to a centimeter or more, and the lesions are, therefore, usually seen as line or band shadows.

Westcott and Cole[96] have recently reviewed in great detail the mechanisms that lead to discoid atelectasis. The subject is complex but, put simply, discoid atelectasis is due to hypoventilation, which leads to alveolar collapse. Alveoli lying at the lung bases and those lying posteriorly are most likely to collapse, not only because they have the lowest volume but also because the physiologic mechanisms responsible for keeping the small airways and alveoli open are at their most vulnerable in these sites.

Discoid atelectasis is common, particularly in hospitalized patients. Since it reflects hypoventilation, it is seen in a large variety of conditions, including painful breathing (e.g., pleurisy following surgery, general anesthesia, trauma), pneumonia, pulmonary edema, pulmonary embolism, neoplasms, masses or fluid in the abdomen, or shallow breathing from any other cause. Discoid atelectasis by itself is usually of little clinical importance though the conditions it is associated with may be of great significance. Occasionally, discoid atelectasis is of such magnitude and so widespread that it may be a cause of hypoxemia. Here it should be remembered that plain films may substantially underestimate the extent of the condition. Following general anesthesia, for example, widespread discoid atelectasis can be clinically significant, even in cases which show few signs on plain chest radiograph.

Compressive and Passive Atelectasis

The distinction between compressive and passive atelectasis is not clear-cut. The lung is inherently elastic and, therefore, any process that requires increased space within the thorax will either compress the lung or allow it to retract. For example, pleural effusion or pneumothorax allows retraction of the adjacent lung. With large pleural effusions the lobes surrounded by fluid may collapse completely. Large masses in any intrathoracic location frequently press on the lung and therefore acquire an ill-defined margin because of adjacent atelectatic lung. Simi-

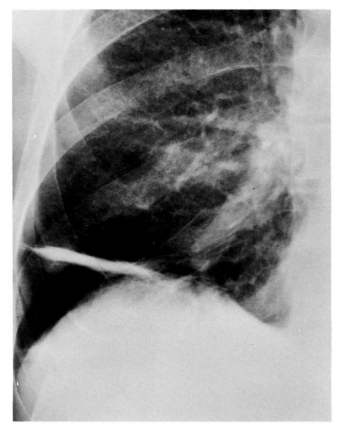

FIG 5–69.
Discoid atelectasis showing typical bandlike shadow.

larly, emphysematous bullae are often surrounded by atelectatic lung. The shape of the collapsed lung in these cases reflects the cause.

THE PULMONARY MASS (NODULE)

The term pulmonary mass refers to an essentially spherical opacity with a well-defined edge. Although the Fleischner Society[20] and others use the word "nodule" for a lesion of up to 3 cm in diameter and "mass" for lesions greater than 3 cm in diameter, we will use the two terms interchangeably. The differential diagnosis is given in Table 5–5.

Masses may be single or multiple and range in size from a few millimeters to many centimeters in diameter. The 2- to 5-mm nodules seen with widespread nodular or miliary shadowing are a separate category and are discussed in the section "Widespread Nodular, Reticulonodular, and Honeycomb Shadowing" later in this chapter. There will, of course, be times when it is impossible to distinguish

between air-space shadowing and a mass. In these circumstances, fortunately not frequent, the differential diagnosis will include many, if not all, of the diagnoses listed previously in Tables 5–2 and 5–5.

Solitary Pulmonary Nodule

The solitary pulmonary nodule (SPN) is one of the most common diagnostic problems in pulmonary radiology. The possible diagnoses are numerous and are given in Table 5–5 (Fig 5–70), but it is worth remembering that over 95% fall into one of three groups:

1. Malignant neoplasm, either primary or metastatic
2. Infectious granulomas, either tuberculous or fungal
3. Benign tumors, notably hamartomas.

Nonradiologic factors are clearly vital when considering differential diagnosis. For example, bronchogenic carcinoma is very rare in patients under 35 years of age and is relatively rare in nonsmokers. Also of importance is whether the patient has an extrathoracic tumor of a type known to metastasize to the lungs. The chances of a solitary pulmonary nodule being a metastasis is very low if the patient does not have a known primary tumor and there are no clinical features to indicate the presence of such a tumor at the time of presentation. In the large multicenter series reported by Steele, only three of 877 resected SPNs were the result of metastasis.[87] In the study of 705 patients without a known tumor reported by Good and Wilson, only one nodule was due to a metastasis.*[35]

Patients with SPN are generally divided into two groups: those in whom malignant neoplasm is either unlikely or impossible; and those in whom malignancy remains a serious consideration. If there is no known extrathoracic primary tumor, the problem usually centers on deciding whether or not the patient has a primary malignant neoplasm of the lung, notably bronchial carcinoma.

Morphologic features such as size, shape and cavitation, which can be of help in making the distinction, will be discussed later, but it must be em-

---

*There is an important practical point here. Imaging tests that search for an occult extrathoracic primary tumor to help in deciding whether an SPN is or is not a metastasis will inevitably be counterproductive. With such low probability of an extrathoracic primary tumor, the false positive results of the various imaging procedures would swamp the true positive findings, even with tests of high specificity.

TABLE 5–5.

Differential Diagnosis of a Solitary Pulmonary Nodule or Mass

Neoplastic
    Bronchial carcinoma*
    Metastasis*
    Lymphoma*
    Adenoma
    Hamartoma
    Benign connective tissue and neural tumors, e.g., lipoma,
        fibroma, neurofibroma, mesothelioma

Inflammatory
    Infective
        Granuloma* e.g., tuberculosis, histoplasmosis, cryptococcosis, blastomycosis,
            coccidioidomycosis, nocardia, dirofilariasis
        Round pneumonia, acute or chronic*
        Lung abscess*
        Hydatid cyst*
    Noninfective
        Rheumatoid arthritis*
        Wegener's granulomatosis*
        Lymphomatoid granulomatosis*
        Necrotizing sarcoidal angiitis
        Lipoid pneumonia
        Behçet's disease*

Congenital
    Arteriovenous malformation
    Sequestration*
    Lung cyst*
    Bronchial atresia with mucoid impaction

Miscellaneous
    Pulmonary infarct*
    Round atelectasis
    Intrapulmonary lymph node
    Progressive massive fibrosis*
    Mucoid impaction*
    Hematoma*
    Amyloidosis*

*May cavitate.

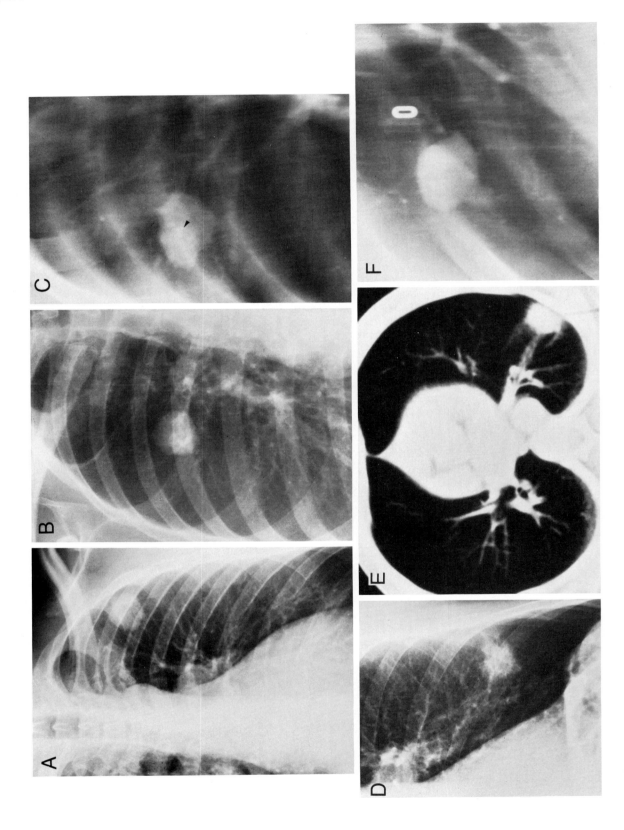

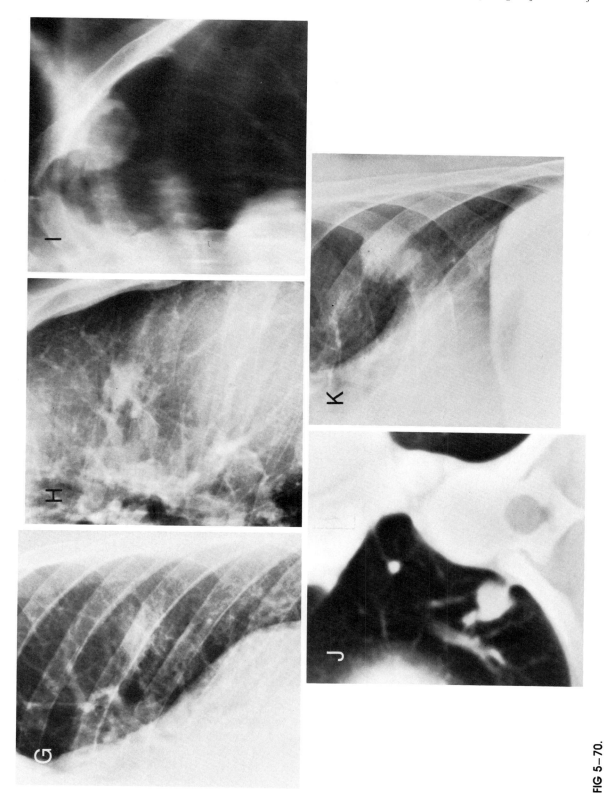

FIG 5–70.

Examples of various causes of solitary pulmonary nodules. **A,** bronchial carcinoma (adenocarcinoma). **B,** hamartoma. **C,** tuberculous granuloma. Note the punctate calcification *(arrowhead)*. **D** and **E,** organizing pneumonia. **F,** hydatid cyst. **G** and **H,** Wegener's granulomatosis. **I,** rheumatoid nodule in a patient with rheumatoid arthritis. **J,** hematoma 6 weeks after motor vehicle accident. **K,** pulmonary infarct.

phasized that there are no radiologic features that are entirely specific for lung carcinoma (or other primary malignant tumors). There are, however, three observations that exclude the diagnosis with reasonable certainty, namely: (1) specific types of calcification; (2) a rate of growth that is either too slow or too fast for the nodule to be primary lung cancer; (3) clear-cut identification of enlarged feeding and draining vessels, indicating that the nodule is an arteriovenous malformation.

Calcification

1. Concentric (laminated) calcification is virtually specific to tuberculous or fungal granulomas (Fig 5−71).

2. Popcorn calcifications—namely, randomly distributed, often overlapping, small rings of calcification—are only seen when there is cartilage in the nodule, a feature specific to hamartoma and cartilage tumors (Fig 5−72).

3. Punctate calcification occurs in a variety of benign and malignant lesions: granuloma; hamartoma; amyloidoma; and metastases, particularly osteosarcoma and chondrosarcoma. Punctate calcification is almost never seen in bronchial carcinoma unless the

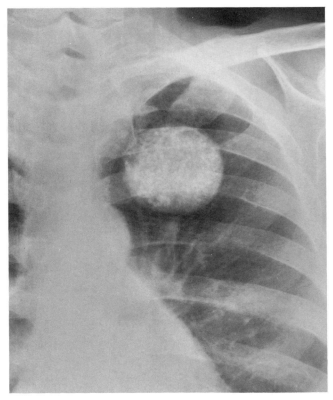

FIG 5−72.
Popcorn calcification in a pulmonary hamartoma.

tumor engulfs a preexisting calcified granuloma (Fig 5−73) in which case the calcification is virtually never at the center of the nodule or randomly distributed throughout the nodule. It should be remembered, therefore, that the presence of one or more focal calcifications arranged in an eccentric group, though reducing the probability of lung cancer, does not eliminate the possibility of carcinoma.

4. Widespread or uniform calcification of a nodule virtually excludes the diagnosis of bronchial carcinoma. Such calcification may be visible on plain chest radiograph. It is better seen with low-kVp examinations than on films taken with high-kVp technique. Many radiologists exploit fluoroscopic equipment to maneuver the patient so as to project the nodule clear of overlying ribs or other structures and to take advantage of the fact that fluoroscopic equipment often has x-ray tubes with fine focal spot sizes and can operate at low kVp. Fluoroscopy can be used to locate a nodule prior to tomography when the position of the nodule is not certain from standard radiographs. The depth of the nodule can be estimated by observing its position in various oblique projections.

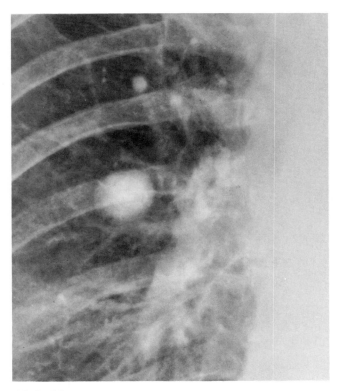

FIG 5−71.
Concentric laminated calcification in a histoplasmosis granuloma.

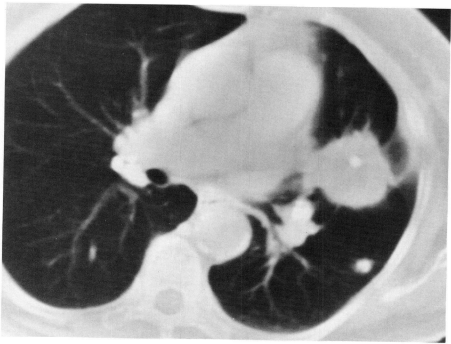

FIG 5—73.

Bronchial adenocarcinoma. CT scan shows focal calcification in a granuloma engulfed by the tumor. Note the completely separate similar granuloma in the lung behind the tumor and the widespread calcification in hilar lymph nodes.

Conventional tomography provides better visualization of calcification within a nodule than plain chest radiography,[42] but has largely been superseded by CT for this purpose. Linear rather than pluridirectional movement appears preferable for detecting calcification, probably because of the differences in blur characteristics between the two movements.[8]

Digitizing the conventional chest film and measuring the variation in optical density within the nodule improves the sensitivity of detecting calcification.[82] The principle here is to compare the optical density of the pixels within the nodule to each other. It remains to be seen how sensitive and specific this method proves to be.

CT, because of its superb density discrimination, is the most sensitive technique for the detection of calcification in an SPN (Fig 5—74). (Techniques using dual-energy CT data which should provide more accurate density measurements are being developed, but have not yet been adequately evaluated.) Siegelman et al. used CT to identify nodules as benign by determining the CT density of the nodule.[84] They measured the CT density of 91 nodules classed as uncalcified on conventional tomography and derived the "representative CT (RCT) number," a number representing the CT density of the 32 most dense contiguous voxels. On a Pfizer American Scientific Engineering scanner, the average RCT number for bronchogenic carcinomas was 92 Hounsfield units (HU); no carcinoma had an RCT number higher than 147 HU. Twenty of the thirty-three benign lesions examined had a RCT number higher than 164 HU (164 HU was derived by adding four standard deviations to 92 HU). They concluded that CT densitometry of pulmonary nodules would be a clinically useful technique for determining that an SPN was benign, if it had an appropriately high RCT number. Proto and Thomas, using an Omni Medical 600 scanner, confirmed these results but recommended a RCT number of 200 HU for the cutoff point above which the diagnosis of a benign lesion could be made.[69]

It has become clear that the RCT number has to be evaluated carefully because the technical factors involved in measuring the attenuation values of intrathoracic nodules are complex.[101, 102] The density measurements, which can differ by as many as 250 HU, vary according to the scanner being used and can even vary from one examination to another with the same machine. Density measurements are also affected by the anatomy and size of the patient, by the diameter and position of the nodule within the lung, by the kilovoltage chosen for the examina-

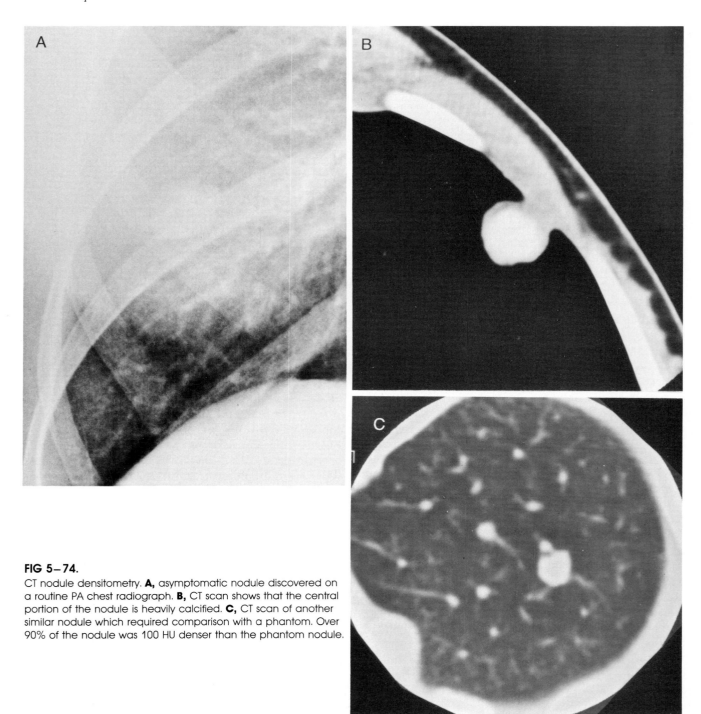

FIG 5–74.
CT nodule densitometry. **A,** asymptomatic nodule discovered on a routine PA chest radiograph. **B,** CT scan shows that the central portion of the nodule is heavily calcified. **C,** CT scan of another similar nodule which required comparison with a phantom. Over 90% of the nodule was 100 HU denser than the phantom nodule.

tion, and by the reconstruction algorithm being used.[43, 102, 103] The density of the nodule measured by CT is inversely related to the kilovoltage, a phenomenon that is more pronounced at high concentrations of calcium.[43] To overcome these problems, Zerhouni et al.[99] designed a reference phantom that can simulate the shape, dimensions, and density of the thorax at multiple levels. Cylinders of various diameters made of resins containing radiopaque materials can be placed within the phantom. The CT density of these cylinders corresponds to 180 HU on the scanner originally used by Siegelman and coworkers. The aim is to simulate the conditions under which an SPN is measured, so as to provide a meaningful measure of the density of the patient nodule regardless of equipment-related or patient-related variations. The technique involves taking 1.5- to 2-mm sections of the patient's nodule. A reference cylinder with a diameter close to that of the patient's nodule is then placed within the phantom in a position that corresponds to the position of the nodule in the thorax. The chest wall thickness of the phantom is adjusted to correspond to the patient's body habitus, and the phantom is then scanned using the same table position and identical technical factors used for the patient examination. The images of the patient's nodule and the simulated nodules are then compared. If more than 10% of the voxels in the patient nodule are higher in density than the density of the reference cylinder, the nodule is considered to be above the critical density level. If the high density is either uniformly distributed or clearly lies centrally within the nodule, then the nodule is almost certainly not a bronchial carcinoma. But, as with plain film and conventional tomographic evaluation, CT scans may show eccentric calcification within a bronchial carcinoma if the tumor engulfs a preexisting calcified granulomatous lesion.[69, 83] There are, however, a few well-documented reports of clear-cut diffuse calcification in bronchial carcinoma [33, 54, 88, 102] (Fig 5–75). To avoid misdiagnosing a benign lesion in the very few cases of carcinoma that show calcification, it is recommended that a high-density lesion be considered benign only if the edge of the nodule is smooth.[83, 102] Also, evaluation of a nodule by CT scanning rarely yields a confident diagnosis of benign disease if the nodule is larger than 3 cm. CT densitometry is therefore not recommended for lesions greater than 3 cm in diameter or for nodules with irregular or spiculated borders.[102]

The phantom is a useful aid in nodule densitometry, but just how necessary it is with the newest scanners has been questioned.[12, 80] The number of patients who benefit from CT densitometry of an SPN is relatively small.[30, 79] In most patients, the decision to perform surgery is still based on plain film characteristics, particularly the rate of growth of the nodule.

Rate of Growth

Bronchial carcinomas usually take between 1 month and 18 months to double their volume, the average time being 4.2 to 7.3 months, depending on cell type.[24] A few take as long as 24 months, and a few double their volume in under a month.[7, 24, 58, 85, 89, 95] Therefore, doubling times faster than 1 month or slower than 18 months make

bronchial carcinoma unlikely, but do not exclude the diagnosis completely (Fig 5–76).

Doubling times faster than 1 month suggest infection,[66] infarction,[66] histiocytic lymphoma,[14] or a fast-growing metastasis from tumors such as germ cell tumor and certain sarcomas.[10] Doubling times slower than 18 months suggest processes such as granuloma, hamartoma, bronchial carcinoid, and round atelectasis. One point to bear in mind is that since primary lung tumors close to 1 cm are usually invisible on plain chest radiograph, it is not possible to calculate an accurate growth rate for small nodules developing in areas that were previously normal.

Those patients with a solitary pulmonary nodule with a rate of growth that is either indeterminate or is in keeping with bronchial carcinoma, who do not have an extrathoracic primary tumor, and who do not have a benign pattern of calcification in the nodule, form a discrete group. The proportion of solitary pulmonary nodules that fall into this category varies greatly according to geography and the type of patients being seen. In the series reported by Good[34, 35] this group formed 40% of patients with an SPN. In Europe the proportion will be higher than in the United States because of the virtual absence of fungal granulomas. Figures from the large series of Steele,[87] Good and Wilson,[35] Bateson,[2] Toomes et al.,[91] and Huston and Muhm[42] suggest that between 25% and 50% of such cases in patients above 35 years of age will prove to be bronchial carcinoma, with the remainder composed of the various lesions listed previously in Table 5–5. Analyzing the size and shape of an SPN and noting the presence or absence of cavitation may provide useful information.

Size

An SPN resulting from lung cancer can be any size, but those less than 9 mm in diameter are virtually never visible on plain chest radiograph. Hence, a well-defined nodule of smaller size which is clearly seen is likely to be calcified and, therefore, likely to be benign. When the nodule is between 1 and 4 cm in diameter, there are no diagnoses in Table 5–5 that can be excluded on the basis of size alone. Above 4 cm, however, the probabilities begin to change dramatically. Most nodules larger than 4 cm in diameter are bronchial carcinoma. With few exceptions, SPNs above this size that are not primary or metastatic carcinoma will prove to be lung abscess, Wegener's granulomatosis, lymphomatoid granulomatosis, round pneumonia, round atelecta-

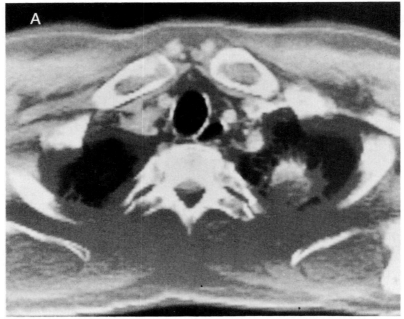

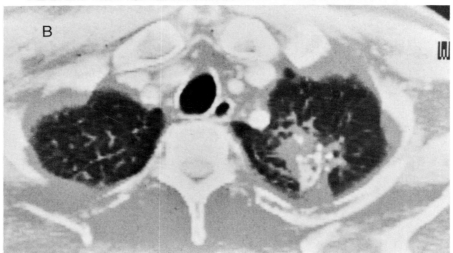

FIG 5–75.
A and **B,** adjacent CT sections showing a primary adenocarcinoma of the lung with widespread punctate, conglomerate calcification . On histologic examination, the calcification proved to be necrotic foci of tumor. (Courtesy of Dr. John Pitman, Williamsburg, Va.).

sis, or hydatid cyst. The first three resemble each other and may be indistinguishable from bronchial carcinoma. The latter three, however, may show characteristics that permit a specific diagnosis to be made.

Shape

There is substantial disagreement in the literature over how much attention should be paid to the shape of a nodule when trying to determine the nature of an SPN. Good[34] believed that calcification and lack of growth were the only important factors, and many subsequent authors have agreed. However, certain shapes do provide important diagnostic information and, in practice, shape is often used to make management decisions.[42]

A very irregular edge makes bronchial carcinoma highly probable, and a corona radiata, the appearance of numerous strands radiating into the surrounding lung, is almost specific for bronchial carcinoma.[42] Exceptions do exist, however. For example, chronic inflammatory lesions may, on occasion, have a very irregular edge (see Fig 5–70 and Fig 5–77) and may even show a corona radiata.

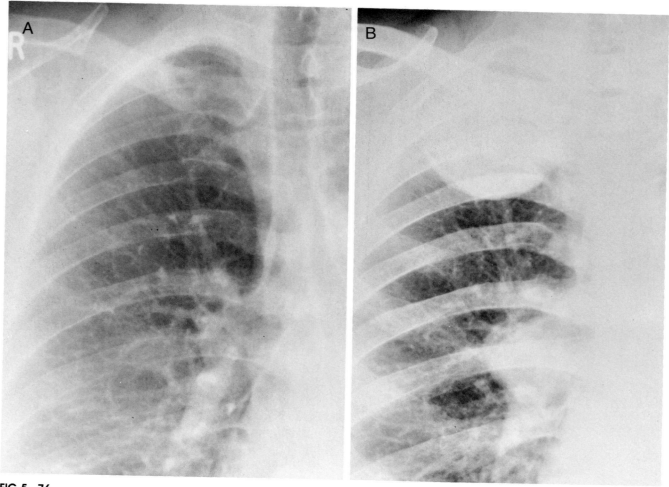

FIG 5–76.
Unusually rapid growth of a primary large cell carcinoma of the lung. The two views (**A** and **B**) were taken 2 months apart.

Lobulation and notching are seen with almost all the diagnostic possibilities, but the more pronounced these signs are, the more likely it is that the lesion is a bronchogenic carcinoma. A well-defined, smooth, nonlobulated edge is most compatible with hamartoma, granuloma, and metastasis. It is rarely seen in patients with bronchial carcinoma.

If, on high-quality tomography, the opacity is seen to be composed of one or more narrow linear shadows without focal nodularity, then the chances of bronchial carcinoma are so low that benignancy can be assumed and follow-up need be the only recommendation.[42]

The presence of a *pleuropulmonary tail* in peripherally located nodules is not helpful in the differential diagnosis of an SPN. Much has been written about the "tail" sign because at one time it was believed to be of potential diagnostic value. However, it turns out that the sign is seen with a variety of lesions, both malignant and benign, particularly granulomas.[5,41,81]

Cavitation

A cavity is defined by the Fleischner Society[20] as a gas-filled space within a zone of pulmonary consolidation, a mass, or a nodule. There may or may not be an accompanying fluid level. The features that have the most discriminative value in diagnosing the nature of masses that show cavitation are size, number, wall thickness, regularity and smoothness of outline, and position.

As can be seen from Table 5–5, many of the causes of SPN may result in cavitation, so the presence or absence of cavitation is of limited diagnostic value. The morphology of the cavity may, however, be helpful. Lung abscess and benign lesions in general have a thinner, smoother wall than cavitating malignant neoplasms. Woodring and Fried[98] com-

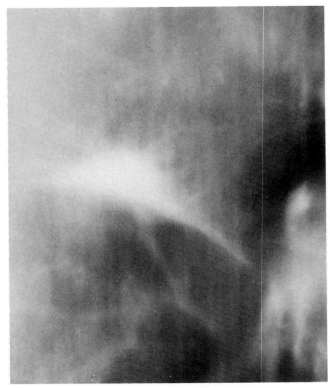

FIG 5–77.
Organizing pneumonia with very irregular edges. The lesion was resected because it was thought to be a bronchial carcinoma.

pared 126 patients with solitary cavities and found that when maximum wall thickness was 16 mm or above only 4 cases were benign, whereas 35 cases were due to malignant neoplasm. Conversely, with maximum wall thickness of 4 mm or less, only 2 cases were malignant neoplasm and 30 were benign. Between 4 and 16 mm, the cases were almost equally divided, with 33 cases being benign and 22 being malignant.

In practice the diagnosis of most acute lung abscesses usually depends on the clinical features together with the appearance of a cavity evolving in an area of undoubted pneumonia. The more difficult problem is distinguishing between cavitating neoplasm and chronic inflammatory processes. Fungal pneumonia, particularly cryptococcus and blastomycosis, and various collagen vascular diseases, particularly Wegener's granulomatosis and rheumatoid arthritis nodules, can appear identical to carcinoma of the lung and may even be indistinguishable clinically.

A cavity may contain a mass within it, the air within the cavity forming a peripheral halo or crescent of air between the intracavitary mass and the cavity wall, giving rise to the so-called "air-crescent" or "air-meniscus" sign. Intracavitary masses are most often due to fungal mycetomas. Other causes include complicated hydatid disease, blood clot (as a result of tuberculosis, laceration with hematoma, or infarct), abscess and necrotizing pneumonias (particularly due to *Klebsiella* or *Aspergillus fumigatus*), and necrotic neoplasm.

CT is a good modality for diagnosing the presence of a cavity within the lung, but it has little or no advantage over plain films in diagnosing the nature of the cavity because it rarely limits the differential diagnosis. CT can, however, distinguish with great reliability between lung abscess and empyema where this is a problem on plain chest radiograph (see Chapter 6).[1, 86]

RING SHADOWS/CYSTS

Ring shadows are characterized by an annular shadow with a central transradiancy. There is no clear distinction between cavitating consolidation, cavitary masses, and ring shadows, but the term ring shadow is usually restricted to discrete round or oval spaces within the lung, surrounded by a thin wall of up to 2 mm.[31] Such ring shadows can be of any size and may be single or multiple, unilocular or multilocular. They may contain fluid, manifest as an air-fluid level. The term "cyst" is often reserved for cavitary lesions that are more than 1 cm in diameter and are evenly thin-walled (less than 4 mm in diameter). By common use, the word *pneumatocele* is confined to air cysts that develop after lung trauma (Fig 5–78), infection (Fig 5–79), and hydrocarbon ingestion. CT may be useful in selected cases to define more accurately the shape, position, and contents of a ring shadow. CT is particularly helpful in distinguishing between loculated pneumothorax and an intrapulmonary cyst or bleb and in demonstrating any related pulmonary disease.[72]

The causes of ring shadows/cysts are listed in Table 5–6.

MULTIPLE PULMONARY NODULES

The differential diagnosis for multiple pulmonary nodules is given in Table 5–7. Once again the list is long, but well over 95% of multiple pulmonary nodules are the result of either metastases or tuberculous/fungal granulomas. The great majority of pa-

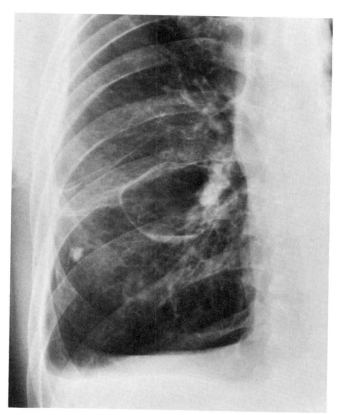

FIG 5–78.
Pulmonary pneumatocele due to previous trauma. A small amount of fluid is present in the pneumatocele.

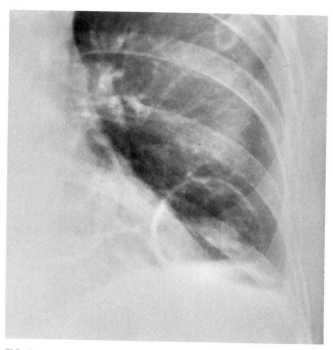

FIG 5–79.
Pneumatocele at the left lung base resulting from staphylococcal pneumonia. A second smaller pneumatocele is seen in the left mid zone.

tients who have multiple noncalcified nodules on plain chest radiographs will have metastases, and the presence of an extrathoracic primary tumor will usually be known or at least suspected clinically. The larger and more variable in size the nodules, the more likely they are to be neoplastic. The same statistic does not apply to nodules found only by CT; here the probability of multiple metastases is much lower and the chance of multiple granulomas is higher because much smaller nodules can be detected.

The following points may help in limiting the diagnostic possibilities listed in Table 5–7.

1. Metastases (Fig 5–80) are usually spherical and have well-defined outlines, though metastases with irregular margins and poorly defined edges are occasionally encountered. Metastases usually vary considerably in size.

2. Nodules containing calcification are usually infectious granulomas, notably tuberculous or histoplasma granulomas (Fig 5–81). On rare occasions, they will be multiple hamartomas or even amyloido-

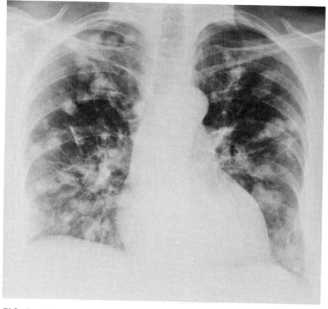

FIG 5–80.
Multiple pulmonary nodules owing to metastases from squamous cell carcinoma of the salivary gland.

TABLE 5–6.
Pulmonary Ring Shadows/Cysts of More Than 1 cm

Congenital	Sequestered segment Bronchogenic cyst Cystic adenomatoid malformation
Infection	Bacterial abscess, notably: anaerobic bacteria, *Staphylococci,* tuberculosis Fungal abscess, notably coccidioidomycosis Echinococcus cyst

Collagen
  vascular
  disease
	Rheumatoid necrobiotic nodule
	Wegener's granulomatosis

Neoplasm	Bronchial carcinoma, notably squamous cell Metastases, notably squamous cell Laryngeal papillomatosis with pulmonary spread Malignant lymphoma
Thromboembolism	Infarct, notably septic infarcts
Airway disease	Blebs/bullae Bronchiectasis (individual ring shadows due to dilated bronchi)
Pneumatoceles	Pulmonary laceration Pulmonary infection, notably staphylococcal Hydrocarbon ingestion
Mimics	Bowel herniation Empyema Lucite plumbage

mas. Thus, nodules that are extensively calcified can, with one important exception, be assumed to be benign. The one exception is in patients with osteosarcoma or chondrosarcoma, because metastases from these tumors frequently calcify (Fig 5–82). In the case of metastases from chondrosarcoma, the calcification may be the typical popcorn calcification of cartilage tumors. If both calcified and noncalcified nodules coexist, the presence of the calcified nodules cannot be taken as proof that the noncalcified nodules are also benign.

3. Growth rate can be a useful discriminator between granuloma and metastasis. Strauss,[89] reviewing the literature on the doubling times of pulmonary metastases, found a very wide range, much wider than for primary lung carcinoma: 11 to 745 days for breast carcinoma; 11 to 150 days for colorectal carcinomas; 10 to 205 days for testicular tumors; 17 to 253 days for soft tissue and bone sarcomas. Thus, to exclude the diagnosis of metastasis in the case of tumors with slow growth rates requires that the nodule in question must have remained the

same size or grown very slowly indeed over several years. Some tumors, for example choriocarcinoma and osteosarcoma, may show explosive growth, doubling their volumes in less than a month.[44] Others, for example thyroid carcinoma, can remain the same size for a very long time.[56]

4. Small pulmonary granulomas are common in the U.S. histoplasmosis belt. Elsewhere in the United States granulomas are less common. In parts of the world where fungal disease is uncommon, pulmonary granulomas are also uncommon and are usually caused by tuberculosis. Thus, the likelihood of pulmonary nodules being granulomas is strongly influenced by where the patient has lived.

5. Multiple arteriovenous malformations can usually be diagnosed with certainty by noting large feeding arteries and draining veins. They are very rare and are usually part of the Osler-Weber-Rendu syndrome.

6. Cavitation is seen in many of the disorders listed in Table 5–7. The major diagnostic value

TABLE 5–7.

Differential Diagnosis of Multiple Pulmonary Nodules/Masses

Neoplastic
  Malignant
    Metastatic*
    Malignant lymphoma*/lymphomatoid granulomatosis*
  Benign
    Hamartomas
    Laryngeal papillomatosis*

Inflammatory
  Infective
    Granulomas,* e.g., tuberculosis, histoplasmosis,
      cryptococcosis, coccidioidomycosis, nocardia
    Round pneumonias*
    Lung abscesses* especially septicemic
    Atypical measles
    Hydatid cysts*
    Paragonimiasis*
  Noninfective
    Rheumatoid arthritis*/Caplan's syndrome*
    Wegener's granulomatosis*
    Sarcoidosis
    Drug-induced

Congenital
  Arteriovenous malformations
Miscellaneous
  Progressive massive fibrosis*
  Hematomata*
  Amyloidosis*
  Pulmonary infarcts*
  Mucoid impactions*

*May cavitate.

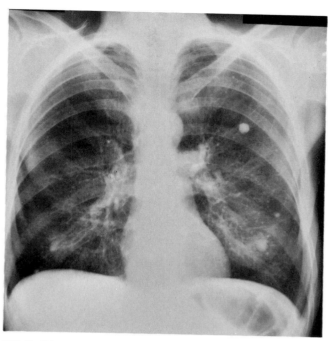

FIG 5–81.
Multiple calcified pulmonary nodules due to histoplasmosis granulomas.

of cavitation is that it indicates an active disease process. It is not a feature of incidental lesions such as inactive granulomas or multiple hamartomas.

7. Sarcoidosis can produce multiple nodular shadows in the lung that may resemble metastases or lymphoma. The uniform size, the slightly ill-defined edge, and the accompanying hilar/mediastinal adenopathy are important indicators of the diagnosis of sarcoidosis (Fig 5–83). Also, the age of the patient and the frequent lack of signs and symptoms of malignant neoplastic disease often help resolve the diagnostic difficulty.

8. Multiple nodules are a feature of coal worker's pneumoconiosis and chronic silicosis. When greater than 1 cm in diameter, they are known as progressive massive fibrosis. The presence of widespread nodulation in the rest of the lung and the characteristic shape and location of progressive massive fibrosis lead to a specific diagnosis in virtually every case (Fig 5–84). (The nodules of Caplan's syndrome may be more difficult to distinguish from me-

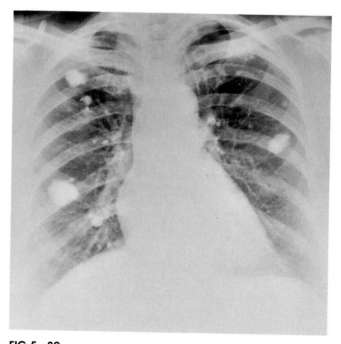

FIG 5–82.
Multiple calcified pulmonary nodules due to metastases from an extrathoracic osteosarcoma.

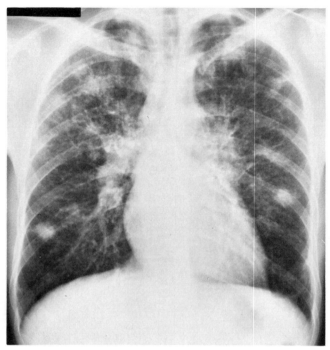

FIG 5–83.
Multiple pulmonary nodules due to sarcoidosis. Note that there is also hilar and mediastinal adenopathy. As is so often the case in sarcoidosis, the nodules are ill-defined in outline and much the same size.

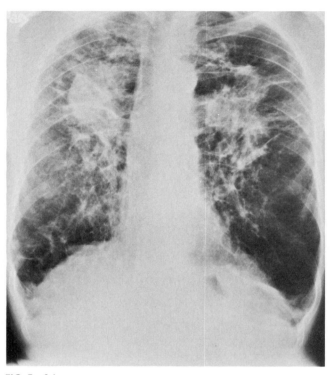

FIG 5–84.
Multiple pulmonary nodules due to progressive massive fibrosis *(PMF)*. The diagnosis here is easy because of the characteristic location, the shape of the PMF shadows, the background nodulation of the lungs, and the generalized emphysema.

tastases, because the other signs of coal worker's pneumoconiosis are often absent). The patient's work history is of great importance in diagnosing progressive massive fibrosis because, on rare occasions, neoplasms (Fig 5–85) or inflammatory conditions such as Wegener's granulomatosis can cause a similar appearance (Fig 5–86).

LINE/BAND SHADOWS

The term "band shadow" is usually reserved for linear opacities that are more than 5 mm wide, whereas linear densities less than 5 mm wide are simply referred to as line shadows. The causes of abnormal line/band shadows are given in Table 5–8. A feature that may help in limiting the differential diagnosis is branching, a phenomenon that is seen only with vascular malformations and bronchiectatic or obstructed, secretion-filled airways (bronchoceles/mucoid impaction).

Of the items listed in Table 5–8, only septal lines, mucoid impaction, and bronchial wall thickening will be discussed further in this section. The other entities are described elsewhere in this book.

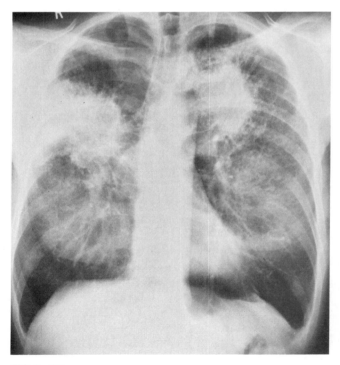

FIG 5–85.
Bilateral primary bronchial carcinoma mimicking progressive massive fibrosis.

TABLE 5–8.

Causes of Line/Band Shadows

Skin fold
Clothing, tubes, etc.
Wall of a bleb or pneumatocele
Bronchial/peribronchial thickening, the causes of which
    are:
    Pulmonary edema
    Lymphangitis carcinomatosa
    Asthma
    Bronchiolitis
    Cystic fibrosis
    Bronchiectasis
Bronchocele (mucoid impaction)
Pleuroparenchymal scar
Discoid atelectasis
Anomalous blood vessels or feeding and draining vessels
    to arteriovenous malformation
Thickening of pleural fissures
Pleural tail associated with pleural nodule
Septal lines (Kerley lines), the causes of which are given in
    Table 5–9.

Mucoid Impaction

With mucoid impaction (bronchocele, mucocele), a bandlike opacity is seen pointing to the hilus. The lesion is often very broad (1 cm or more) and is sharply marginated with branches which have been likened to fingers—the so-called "gloved finger shadow." The presence of such shadows always implies segmental bronchial obstruction.[16] Mucoid im-

pactions are found typically in allergic bronchopulmonary aspergillosis (Fig 5–87), but may be seen with a variety of obstructing lesions provided collateral air drift maintains aeration to the affected segment (Fig 5–88). Felson,[16] in his review of the subject, found that radiologically visible mucoid impaction had also been reported in primary and metastatic carcinoma of the lung, bronchial carcinoid, tuberculous bronchostenosis, broncholithiasis, bronchial atresia (Fig 5–89), sequestration, pulmonary bronchogenic cyst, and foreign body aspiration.[16] If the surrounding lung collapses or consolidates, the shadow of the mucoid impaction becomes invisible because of the silhouette effect.

Septal Lines

The interstitial septa of normal lungs are not visible by current methods of imaging except in a small minority of thin patients and then only on very high

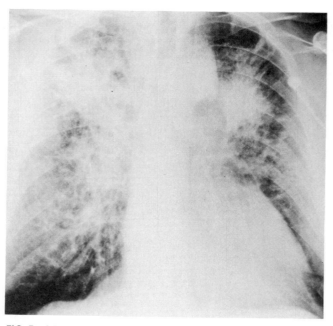

FIG 5–86.
Wegener's granulomatosis of the lung mimicking progressive massive fibrosis.

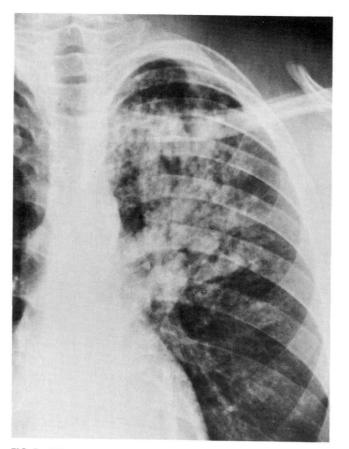

FIG 5–87.
Mucoid impaction (mucocele) of bronchi in the left upper lobe in a patient with allergic bronchopulmonary aspergillosis. Branching tubular shadows, such as those illustrated, have been likened to a "gloved finger."

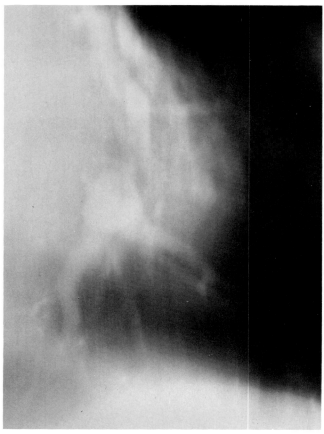

FIG 5–88.
Bronchocele in the left lower lobe presumed to be secondary to congenital bronchial atresia. The branching pattern is typical of a bronchocele.

quality plain chest radiographs. For practical purposes it is only when the septa are thickened that they become radiographically visible (Fig 5–90).[40, 92]

Septal lines were first described by Kerley in patients with pulmonary edema.[51] He named them A, B, and C lines because he was not certain of their anatomic basis. "Septal lines" is a more descriptive and, therefore, better term because the lines represent thickening of connective tissue septa within the lung.[40, 93]

The septa are anatomically divided into deep septa and peripheral interlobular septa.[77] Deep septal lines (Kerley A lines) are up to 4 cm in length, radiate from the hili into the central portions of the lungs, do not reach the pleura, and are most obvious in the mid and upper zones. Interlobular septal lines (Kerley B lines) are usually less than a centimeter in length and parallel one another at right angles to the pleura. They may be very thin and sharply defined or may be a few millimeters in width and fairly ill-defined. They are located peripherally in contact with the pleura but are generally absent along fissural surfaces.[77] They may be seen in any zone, but are most frequently observed at the lung bases.

The term "C lines" should be dropped altogether from the radiologist's vocabulary, because the crisscrossing lines that Kerley designated as C lines are, in fact, due to superimposition of many B lines.[40] Kreel et al.[53] described thick septal lines due to pulmonary edema that resemble discoid atelectasis.

Septal lines need to be distinguished from blood vessels. Blood vessels are not seen in the outer centimeter of the lung, whereas interlobular septa, even though narrower in diameter, may be visible by virtue of having substantial depth along the trajectory of the x-ray beam. Similarly, the deep septa are seen as narrow, dense lines because they are thin sheets of tissue seen end-on. Blood vessels of such a narrow diameter would be either invisible or of extremely low density. Another helpful feature is that deep septal lines, though they may interconnect or superimpose, do not branch in as uniform a manner as blood vessels.

The identification of septal lines is an extremely useful diagnostic feature, since thickened septal lines occur in few conditions (Table 5–9). If transient or rapid in development, they are virtually diagnostic of interstitial pulmonary edema.

Bronchial Wall (Peribronchial) Thickening

In normal chest radiographs, the walls of the bronchi beyond the hili are invisible unless they are end-on to the x-ray beam. The few that are seen end-on have a thin, well-defined, ringlike wall. Portions of the walls of the lobar bronchi within the hili are also routinely visible in the healthy patient. The posterior wall of the bronchus intermedius should measure less than 3 mm.[70] Since this particular portion of the bronchial tree is clearly seen in lateral

TABLE 5–9.
Causes of Septal Lines (Kerley Lines)

Pulmonary edema
Lymphangitis carcinomatosa/malignant lymphoma
Congenital lymphangiectasia
Viral and mycoplasma pneumonia
Interstitial pulmonary fibrosis from any cause
Pneumoconiosis
Sarcoidosis
Lymphocytic giant cell interstitial pneumonitis
Late-stage hemosiderosis
Lymphangiomyomatosis (tuberous sclerosis)

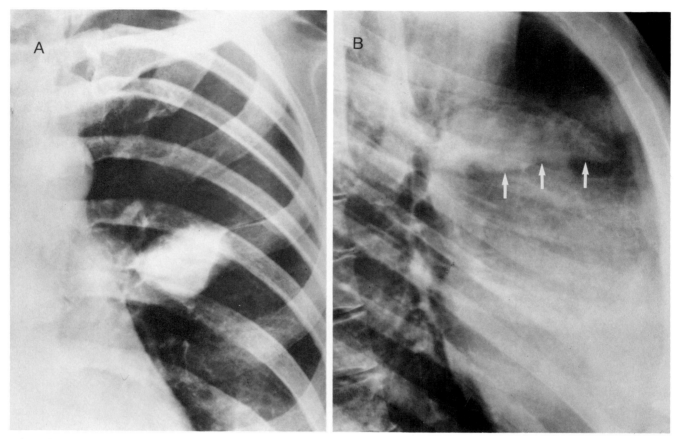

FIG 5–89.
Bronchocele *(arrows)* in the left upper lobe showing a nonbranching, mucus-filled, dilated bronchus resulting from bronchial atresia. **A,** PA view. **B,** Lateral view.

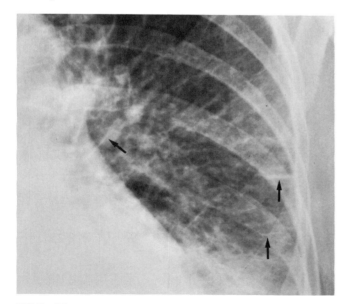

FIG 5–90.
Septal lines due to pulmonary edema. The B lines are the short horizontal lines at the lung periphery *(vertical arrows).* The A lines are the lines radiating from the hili *(oblique arrow).*

chest radiographs and is even easier to identify on CT scans, it is a useful site at which to assess central bronchial wall thickening.

Intraparenchymal bronchial wall thickening (Fig 5–91, A and B) is seen in disorders of the bronchial wall such as recurrent asthma, allergic aspergillosis, bronchiolitis, cystic fibrosis, and bronchiectasis. It is also seen with edema or neoplastic infiltration (lymphangitis carcinomatosa) of the peribronchial tissues. It is useful to note whether the bronchial wall thickening is associated with bronchial dilatation, a combination that would establish the diagnosis of bronchiectasis as the cause of the bronchial wall thickening.

If edema or inflammatory/neoplastic cells infiltrate the peribronchial interstitial space, the combination of the bronchial wall and the widened interstitium produces visible bronchial/peribronchial thickening. Not only do the bronchial walls appear thick, they are also usually less well-defined. Though bronchial wall thickening may resemble two adjacent blood vessels, the distinction can be made by identi-

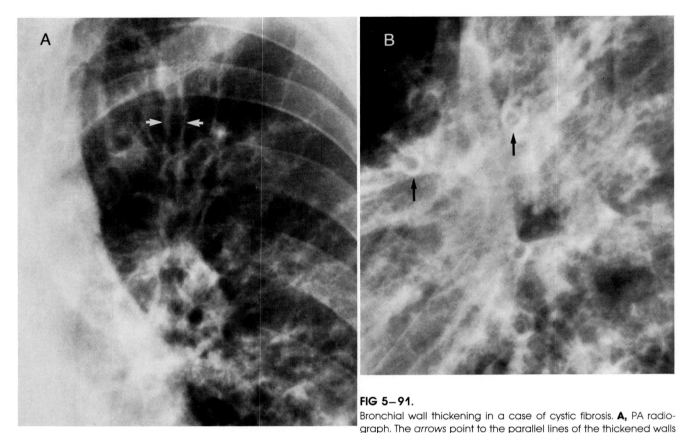

FIG 5–91.
Bronchial wall thickening in a case of cystic fibrosis. **A,** PA radiograph. The *arrows* point to the parallel lines of the thickened walls of a representative moderately dilated bronchus. **B,** lateral radiograph. The *arrows* point to two examples of ring shadows due to thickened bronchial walls seen end on.

fying the parallelism of the walls and by observing Y-shaped branching parallel walls where the bronchi divide.

WIDESPREAD NODULAR, RETICULONODULAR, AND HONEYCOMB SHADOWING

A large number of diseases cause widespread small pulmonary opacities. Occasionally, the chest radiograph provides enough information for the diagnosis, but usually it is just one piece of information in a complex of clinical features and laboratory tests.

The numerous small opacities seen on chest radiographs probably do not represent the individual lesions seen by the pathologist; rather, the pattern appears to be produced by summation. Carstairs[6] showed that when multiple superimposed sheets of small nodules are radiographed, the resulting image is a reticulonodular pattern. This observation is important because it suggests that the size and shape of the nodules and lines on the chest radiograph are not a precise reflection of the responsible lesion.

Some authors have advocated two classes of diffuse lung disease—alveolar and interstitial—based on plain radiographic findings.[22, 36] Alveolar disease is said to be manifest by opacities which are lobar, segmental, or "butterfly" in distribution.[15, 39] The individual shadows have ill-defined margins (except when they contact a fissure), tend to coalesce, and may contain air bronchograms or air alveolograms. "Acinar" shadows, it is claimed, are distinctive enough to narrow the differential diagnosis of pulmonary opacities to those diseases which cause filling of the alveolar air-spaces. "Acinar" shadows are ill-defined coalescent nodular opacities, approximately the size of an acinus, which may initially appear as rosettes of small densities.[103] Interstitial disease, on the other hand, is manifest by relatively well-defined linear, nodular, irregular, or honeycomb shadows together with septal lines, subpleural thickening, perivascular haze, or peribronchial cuffing.

The problem with this division is that it is often difficult to categorize widespread small shadows into one or the other group. Indeed, one would not expect it to be easy because, on pathologic examination, few diseases are purely alveolar or purely interstitial. Many diseases that are regarded pathologically as alveolar show radiographic features of interstitial disease and, conversely, there is an appreciable list of so-called interstitial diseases that show the radiographic signs ascribed to alveolar disease.[76] Even "acinar" shadows have been shown to correspond to interstitial processes.[45] Nevertheless, the division of diffuse lung disease into alveolar and interstitial patterns does have its merits, always provided that these divisions are carefully applied and used as a conclusion, not as a starting point, for the description. The recent and developing use of high-resolution, thin-section CT will probably refine the radiologist's ability to more accurately categorize diffuse lung disease into alveolar and interstitial categories.

It is equally possible[17] and probably preferable to generate the differential diagnostic list according to the combination of radiographic signs without regard to an intermediate decision as to whether the process is predominantly alveolar or interstitial (see Table 5–12).

Many descriptive terms have been proposed for widespread small lung shadows on the plain chest radiograph; only a few are widely accepted. For diagnostic purposes, the following are recommended[52]:

1. *Reticular or linear pattern.* This pattern consists of fine linear shadows, usually in an irregular netlike arrangement forming rings with thin walls and surrounding spaces of air density (Fig 5–92). Kerley A and B lines (septal lines) are a specific form of linear shadowing of great diagnostic importance because their presence is reliable evidence of interstitial thickening.

2. *Nodular pattern.* This pattern consists of clearly defined round or irregular opacities, ranging from a diameter of 1 to 2 mm (Fig 5–93) up to 1 cm. Such lesions may be partially or completely calcified. Above this size, the nodules represent individual lesions, and the differential diagnosis is discussed on p. 129.

3. *Reticulonodular pattern.* This pattern represents a mixture of nodular and reticular patterns. The nodules are usually irregular in shape. A reticulonodular appearance is much more common than a purely reticular or purely nodular pattern.

4. *Honeycomb pattern.* This term should be used to describe a coarse reticular or reticulonodular pattern in which the crisscrossing linear elements surround small cystic air-spaces. This appearance corresponds to what the pathologist calls honeycomb lung when viewing the surface of a cut section of lung (Fig 5–94).

5. *Cystic pattern.* Widespread ring shadows of 1 cm or more are diagnostic of cystic bronchiectasis (Fig 5–95).

6. *Haze or ground-glass pattern.* These terms refer to a diffuse increase in density and loss of clarity of the pulmonary vessels and, to a variable extent, the diaphragmatic outlines. The abnormality may be subtle, and the sign can be highly subjective. In severe, advanced, diffuse lung disease, the disease process, even if interstitial in origin, may replace virtu-

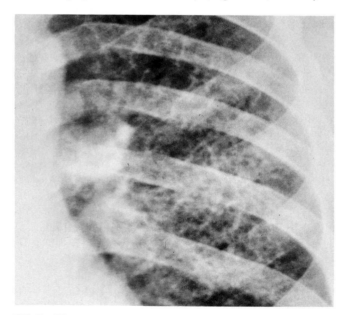

FIG 5–92.
Reticular pattern in a patient with histiocytosis X.

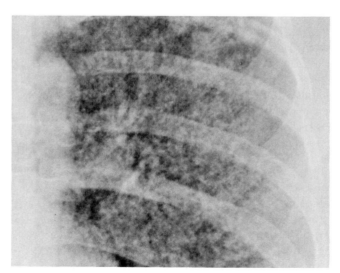

FIG 5–93.
Nodular pattern in a patient with miliary tuberculosis.

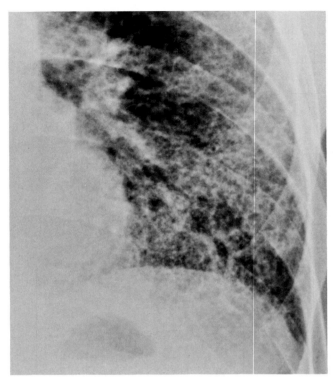

FIG 5-94.
Reticulonodular pattern in a patient with interstitial pulmonary fibrosis due to scleroderma.

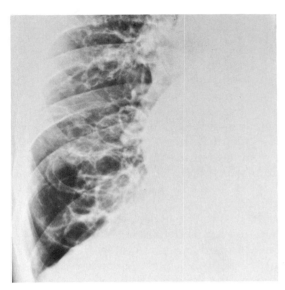

FIG 5-95.
Cystic pattern in a patient with cystic bronchiectasis.

ally all the air in the alveoli, and the affected lung then becomes uniformly opaque except possibly for air bronchograms.

These six terms usually provide a reasonably accurate description of diffuse lung disease. They do not imply a specific disease process but are used to generate a differential diagnostic list. In some situations, notably industrial lung disease, the problem is not diagnosis but quantification of the severity of disease. The International Labor Office and other groups have drawn up a classification based on reference radiographs to provide standardized descriptions (see Chapter 9).

Other factors to note when deciding on differential diagnostic possibilities are zonal predominance, if any, and such signs as a reduction in lung volume, bronchial wall thickening, presence of air-space shadowing, masses, adenopathy, and pleural effusions.

All the plain radiographic signs have their counterparts on CT (Fig 5-96, A and B). Spatial resolution is best seen with thin sections which avoid partial volume artifact and high-resolution (non-smoothed) reconstruction algorithms targeted to

small fields of view.[3, 55, 65, 100] (An appropriate technique is to sample at centimeter intervals through the region of interest with sections of 1.5- to 2-mm thickness). An important point to remember when reviewing CT scans for diffuse lung disease is that the degree of inflation of the dependent lung is relatively poor.[90] Thus, with the patient in the supine position, the posterior lung shows vessel crowding that is easily confused with lung disease. Images should, therefore, be taken when the patient is at deep inspiration and, in cases of diagnostic difficulty, additional images can be taken with the patient prone. The areas of suspicion will then appear normal if no disease is present. The window centers and levels are of considerable importance because the apparent size of very small objects changes quite significantly with different parameters. A good rule is to set the center midway between the CT density of the object being imaged and the CT density of the surrounding tissue. In the case of diffuse lung disease, the midpoint between soft tissue and air is approximately −400 HU. The window width should be very wide: 1,000 HU or more. Thin sections require higher than usual milliamperage values to increase signal-to-noise ratio.

Zerhouni et al.[100] identified four categories of signs in interstitial lung disease.

1. Thickened and irregular interfaces (see Fig 5-96). The interface between the pleura and the extreme lung edge appears finely irregular and thickened. Similarly, the pleural fissures appear irregular

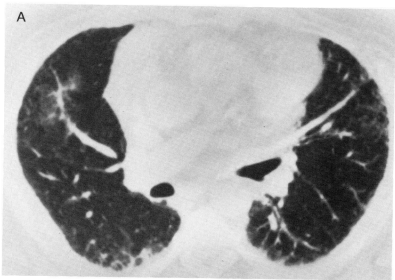

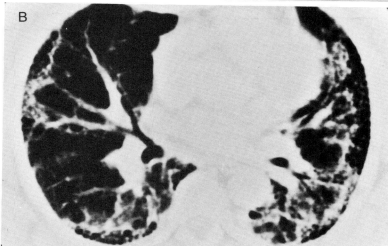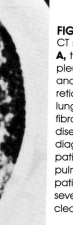

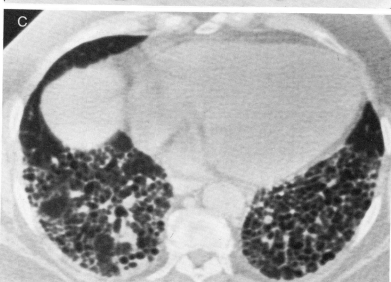

FIG 5–96.
CT scans of fibrosing alveolitis (interstitial fibrosis).
A, there are thickened and irregular interfaces at the pleural boundary, along the intrapulmonary vessels, and adjacent to the bronchi. There is also a fine reticular pattern maximal in the outer third of the lung. The patient had symptomatic idiopathic fibrosing alveolitis with clinical and CT features of the disease but a normal chest radiograph. The diagnosis was proved by open lung biopsy. **B,** a patient with rheumatoid arthritis showing advanced pulmonary fibrosis. The plain chest radiograph in this patient is shown in Figure 5–99. **C,** a patient with severe idiopathic fibrosing alveolitis showing clear-cut honeycomb pattern.

instead of smooth, and the intrapulmonary blood vessels and bronchial walls also show irregular interfaces with adjacent lung. The bronchial wall thickening makes the airways visible beyond the medial half of the lungs.

2. Short linear densities, which can be divided into three distinct groups. (a) A 1- to 2-cm polyhedral grouping of lines corresponding to the septa between the secondary pulmonary lobules. These lines are the CT equivalent of Kerley A and B lines. (b) A reticular pattern with crisscrossing lines enclosing spaces of perhaps a quarter or less of the area of the secondary pulmonary lobule. (c) A fine reticular pattern, which can represent interstitial disease but which also may be seen in poorly inflated portions of dependent normal lung.

3. Nodular densities of about 1 mm in diameter. These nodules need to be distinguished from normal vessels running vertically through the section. Most often, the nodular densities are associated with linear elements; they are maximal where the lines cross each other.

4. Increased background density of the lung appearing as a featureless hazy or ground-glass appearance. Unlike air-space filling, the vessels and bronchi can still be identified through the hazy density.

Tables 5–10 through 5–12 provide a general guide to the differential diagnosis of widespread nodular and reticulonodular shadowing. The tables are a simplified approach, and it is important to re-

TABLE 5–10.

Diffuse Bilateral Small Nodular Opacities of the Lungs (Miliary Pattern)

Miliary tuberculosis
Nontuberculous infection, notably:
Histoplasmosis
Blastomycosis
Coccidioidomycosis
Cryptococcosis
Nocardiosis
Viral infection
Bronchiolitis obliterans
Pneumoconiosis, notably:
Coal worker's
Silicosis
Siderosis
Berylliosis
Stannosis
Sarcoidosis
Metastases
Histiocytosis X
Amyloidosis
Alveolar microlithiasis

TABLE 5–11.

Causes of Diffuse Bilateral Reticulonodular Opacities of the Lungs

Idiopathic interstitial pulmonary fibrosis
Rheumatoid lung disease (interstitial fibrosis)
Scleroderma/dermatomyositis/systemic lupus erythematosus
Drug reaction/noxious gases (acute or fibrotic stages)
Extrinsic allergic alveolitis (acute or fibrotic stages)
Pneumoconiosis, notably:
Coal worker's
Silicosis
Asbestosis
Berylliosis
Extrinsic allergic alveolitis:
Acute stage
Fibrotic stage
Sarcoidosis
Histiocytosis X
Interstitial pneumonia, notably:
Fungi, particularly histoplasmosis
Mycoplasma pneumoniae
Viruses
Chronic aspiration
Bronchiolitis obliterans
Pulmonary edema
Lymphangitic spread of carcinoma/lymphoma
Lymphangiomyomatosis (tuberous sclerosis)
Lymphocytic interstitial pneumonitis/Waldenstrom's macroglobulinemia
Amyloidosis
Hemosiderosis:
Idiopathic/Goodpasture's syndrome
Secondary to mitral valve disease
Talc granulomatosis
Alveolar microlithiasis
Gaucher's disease
Alveolar proteinosis
Neurofibromatosis

alize that there are many exceptions. Certain generalizations can be applied with caution:

1. Acute conditions should be considered separately. If multiple linear markings appear acutely—that is, within hours or days—the most likely diagnosis is pulmonary edema, particularly cardiogenic edema, or pneumonia. In the immune-competent patient with fever, viral or mycoplasma pneumonia should be the major consideration. The line shadows indicate thickening of the interstitial septa of the lung, which may produce clear-cut septal (Kerley) lines or, if numerous, may appear as a reticular pattern owing to the superimposition of many thickened septa. In the case of cardiogenic edema, the other signs of circulatory overload will often be present.

TABLE 5–12.

Signs That Limit the Differential Diagnosis of Diffuse Bilateral Reticulonodular Opacities of the Lungs

Acute appearance of shadows suggests:
   Pulmonary edema (both cardiac and noncardiac)
   Pneumonia, notably mycoplasma, viral, or opportunistic
Lower zone predominance of the opacities together with decrease in lung volume suggests:
   Idiopathic interstitial pulmonary fibrosis
   Rheumatoid lung disease (interstitial fibrosis)
   Scleroderma/dermatomyositis/systemic lupus erythematosus (interstitial fibrosis)
   Drug reaction/noxious gases (fibrotic stage)
   Extrinsic allergic alveolitis (fibrotic stage)
   Asbestosis
   Chronic aspiration
Mid/upper zone predominance of the opacities suggests:
   Chronic tuberculous and fungal disease
   Pneumoconiosis (coal worker's, silicosis, berylliosis)
   Sarcoidosis
   Histiocytosis X
   Extrinsic allergic alveolitis (fibrotic stage)
   Ankylosing spondylitis (fibrosis)
Associated increase in lung volume or bullae suggests:
   Underlying emphysema
   Cystic fibrosis
   Histiocytosis X
   Lymphangiomyomatosis (tuberous sclerosis)
   Neurofibromatosis
Associated septal (Kerley) lines suggest:
   Pulmonary edema
   Lymphangitic spread of carcinoma/lymphoma
   Viral/mycoplasmal pneumonia
   Sarcoidosis
   Extrinsic allergic alveolitis
   Interstitial pulmonary fibrosis (idiopathic, collagen vascular disease, etc.)
   Pneumoconiosis (notably silicosis)
Associated hilar lymphadenopathy suggests:
   Sarcoidosis
   Lymphangitis carcinomatosa
   Lymphoma
   Infections, notably:
      Tuberculosis
      Viral
   Pneumoconiosis, notably:
      Silicosis
      Berylliosis
Associated hilar node calcification suggests:
   Sarcoidosis
   Silicosis
   Chronic tuberculosis or histoplasmosis
   Treated lymphoma
Associated pleural effusion suggests:
   Pulmonary edema
   Lymphangitic spread of carcinoma/lymphoma
   Collagen vascular disease
   Lymphangiomyomatosis (particularly if effusion is chylous)
   NB: Pleural effusions are notably absent in idiopathic interstitial pulmonary fibrosis
Associated pleural thickening suggests:
   Asbestosis, particularly if pleural calcification is present.

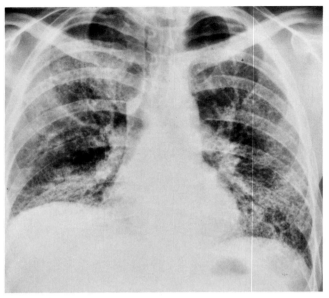

FIG 5–97.
Interstitial pulmonary fibrosis in a patient with scleroderma. The peripheral and basal predominance of the shadowing, combined with the small lung volumes, is typical of diffuse interstitial pulmonary fibrosis.

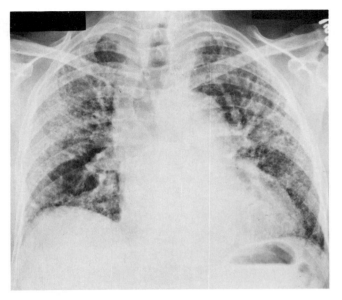

FIG 5–98.
Idiopathic fibrosing alveolitis (interstitial fibrosis). This case demonstrates a peripheral predominance to the shadowing. Note the small volume of the lungs.

2. The distribution of the shadows can be of help in differential diagnosis:
   a. Reticulonodular shadows maximal at the bases and/or at the lung periphery, together with loss of lung volume but without pleural effusion or hilar adenopathy, are almost invariably due to one of the forms of interstitial pulmonary fibrosis (fibrosing alveolitis) (Figs 5–97 through 5–99). The major causes are idiopathic pulmonary fibrosis, asbestosis, rheumatoid lung disease, scleroderma, and dermatomyositis. Extrinsic allergic alveolitis and drug toxicity may also show this pattern. With chronic bilateral aspiration, bronchopneumonia may convert from consolidation to interstitial fibrosis and bronchiectasis, causing reticulonodular shadowing that may closely resemble late-stage idiopathic fibrosing alveolitis.
   Bergin and Muller divided the lungs as seen on axial CT scans into central (which they called axial), middle, and peripheral thirds.[3] Fibrosing alveolitis, rheumatoid lung, and scleroderma showed a definite peripheral predominance of reticulonodular shadowing (see Figs 5–96 and 5–99); in lymphoma, the abnormal densities tended to be central; in silicosis, the small nodular shadows were seen predominantly in the middle third. The pulmonary shadowing in lymphangitis carcinomatosa involved all three compartments.
   b. Unilateral reticulonodular shadowing without zonal or lobar predominance, particularly if septal lines are obvious and pleural effusions are present, is virtually diagnostic of lymphangitis carcinomatosa

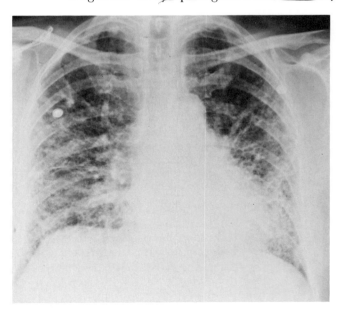

FIG 5–99.
Diffuse interstitial pulmonary fibrosis in a patient with rheumatoid arthritis. This example shows mid-zone and lower-zone predominance with only mild loss of volume.

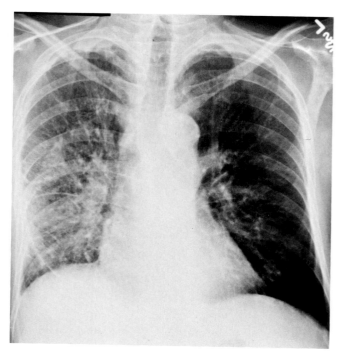

FIG 5–100.
Lymphangitis carcinomatosa showing unilateral reticulonodular shadowing. Note the fissural thickening and the septal lines.

(Fig 5–100). Aspiration pneumonia may occasionally give this appearance, and sarcoidosis may, rarely, cause unilateral reticulonodular shadowing.

c. Coarse reticulonodular shadowing maximal in the upper zones, particularly when associated with fibrotic contraction of the upper lobes, is seen particularly in chronic tuberculous (Fig 5–101, A) or fungal disease, notably histoplasmosis (Fig 5–101, B), the fibrotic end-stage of extrinsic allergic alveolitis (Fig 5–101, C), sarcoidosis (Fig 5–101, D), ankylosing spondylitis, and radiation fibrosis.

d. Clear-cut reticular shadowing with pronounced upper zone predominance strongly suggests histiocytosis X, particularly if air spaces greater than 1 cm are seen.

e. Coarse shadowing radiating from the hili into the mid and upper zones, but sparing the extreme apices, is highly suggestive of sarcoidosis (Fig 5–102). The presence of hilar lymphadenopathy makes the diagnosis virtually certain.

f. Uniformly distributed, very small miliary nodules are virtually confined to miliary tuberculosis, sarcoidosis (Fig 5–103), or pneumoconiosis from coal, silica, or other inorganic dusts. The presence of bilateral

lymphadenopathy makes sarcoidosis much the most likely, but does not exclude the other possibilities. Signs of mitral valve disease will suggest the diagnosis of secondary hemosiderosis (Fig 5–104)

g. Miliary nodules maximal in the upper zones are strongly suggestive of coal worker's pneumoconiosis, silicosis, or other mineral dust pneumoconioses. The denser the nodules, the more likely is pneumoconiosis.

3. The components of the pattern itself may also be of help:

a. Obvious septal lines are seen only in those conditions listed in Table 5–9. The most common cause by far is pulmonary edema, the next most frequent causes are lymphangitis carcinomatosa and interstitial pneumonia. Usually the other signs on the films, taken together with the knowledge of the patient's symptoms, permit one of the alternatives to be chosen, particularly if the chronicity or acuteness of the disease is known. For example, rapid appearance or disappearance of septal lines occurs only in pulmonary edema. Viral and mycoplasma pneumonia are associated with acute febrile illness, whereas relentless progression over weeks is virtually diagnostic of lymphangitis carcinomatosa. The CT equivalent of septal lines is a polyhedral linear pattern, the lines being 1 to 2 cm in length. In lymphangitis carcinomatosa this large reticular meshwork shows lines of variable thickness and associated nodularity, giving a pattern that may prove to be specific to the condition.[60, 100]

b. True honeycomb pattern is virtually diagnostic of end-stage interstitial pulmonary fibrosis (fibrosing alveolitis) of many causes, histiocytosis X, or lymphangiomyomatosis. The honeycomb pattern is particularly well demonstrated at thin-section high-resolution CT.

c. Multiple, partially, or totally calcified small nodular shadows are seen in only a few conditions. Most of the cases encountered will be the result of calcification of widespread patchy pneumonia due to either disseminated histoplasmosis, tuberculosis, or varicella infection (Fig 5–105). Occasionally, pneumonia due to coccidiomycosis or blastomycosis may calcify. In each instance, the responsible pneumonia will have occurred several years before. The presence of calci

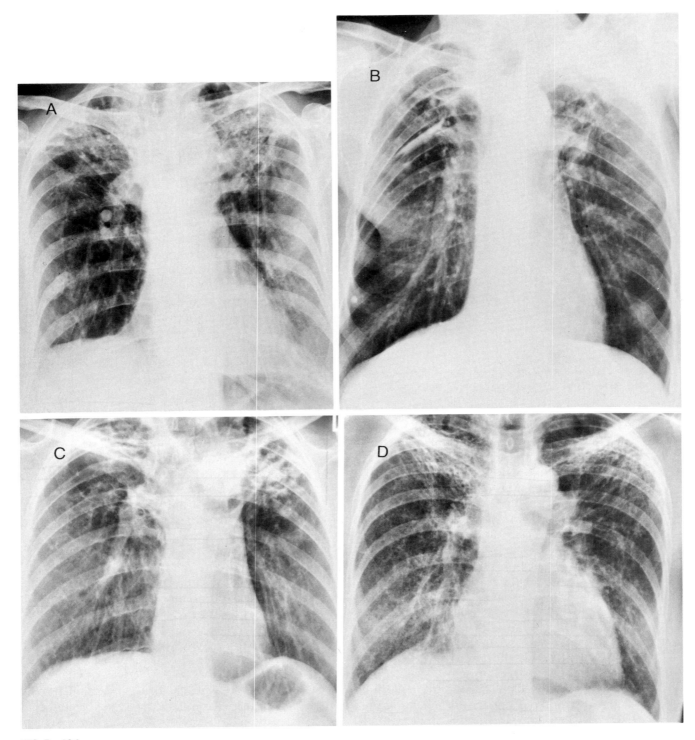

FIG 5–101.
Coarse upper zone reticulonodular shadowing with fibrotic contraction of the upper lobes. **A,** tuberculosis. Note the patchy small calcifications within the fibrotic upper lobes. **B,** histoplasmosis. **C,** extrinsic allergic alveolitis: a case of bird fancier's disease. **D,** sarcoidosis.

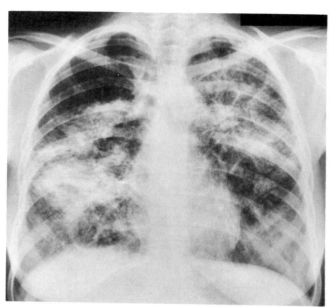

FIG 5–102.
Pulmonary fibrosis due to sarcoidosis. The mid-zone predominance radiating from the hili with relative sparing of the extreme apices and bases is typical of sarcoidosis.

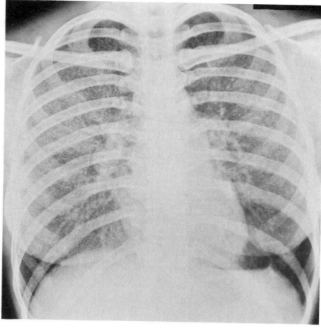

FIG 5–103.
Uniformly distributed fine nodular shadowing in a patient with sarcoidosis. Note also the bilateral hilar adenopathy.

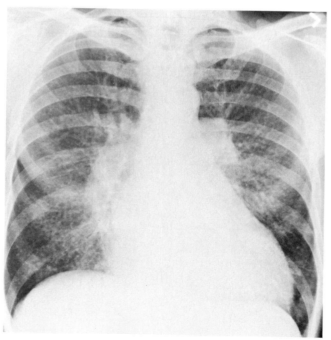

FIG 5–104.
Uniformly distributed fine nodular shadowing due to hemosiderosis in a patient with mitral valve disease. Note the other signs of mitral valve disease.

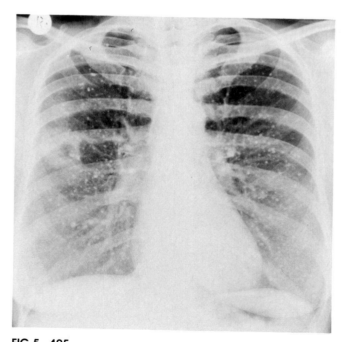

FIG 5–105.
Multiple small calcifications in the lungs due to old healed varicella pneumonia. (The patient also has a carcinoma of the right upper lobe.)

fication indicates healing but, in the case of tuberculous and fungal infections, does not necessarily mean the disease is inactive.

Radiologically visible calcification in metastases is very uncommon and, for practical purposes, is seen only with osteogenic sarcoma and chondrosarcoma.

d. High-density miliary nodulation may be seen with silicosis, stannosis, baritosis, or microlithiasis. The opacity of the nodules in baritosis may be even greater than calcific density.

e. Multifocal pulmonary ossification is occasionally seen in long-standing mitral valve disease (Fig 5–106). If the resulting small nodules clearly contain bony trabeculae, the diagnosis is easy. In most cases, however, only amorphous calcification can be recognized radiographically, and the distinction from postinfective calcification becomes impossible. Nowadays the entity is rare.

f. Cloudlike punctate calcification of the lung is seen only in alveolar microlithiasis (Fig 5–107) and hypercalcemia due to conditions such as hyperparathyroidism, particularly secondary hyperparathyroidism due to renal failure[57] (Fig 5–108, A and B). In each instance the calcifications may be so minute that it is not possible to appreciate that the cloudlike shadows are, in fact, due to a myriad of calcifications. The appearance may then be confused with the other causes of multiple air-space shadows.

4. Certain combinations may make one diagnosis or a group of diagnoses more likely:

a. The combination of overinflation of the lung, widespread or basally predominant reticulonodular shadowing, and pleural effusion in a middle-aged woman is virtually diagnostic of the rare entity lymphangiomyomatosis (Fig 5–109).

b. The combination of small irregular shadows, maximal in the upper zone, with bronchial wall thickening and overinflation of the lungs in a younger patient is virtually diagnostic of cystic fibrosis (Fig 5–110).

c. The presence of bilateral conglomerate shadows greater than 1 cm in diameter in the upper zones together with widespread or upper zone predominant small nodules in the lungs makes pneumoconiosis virtually certain.

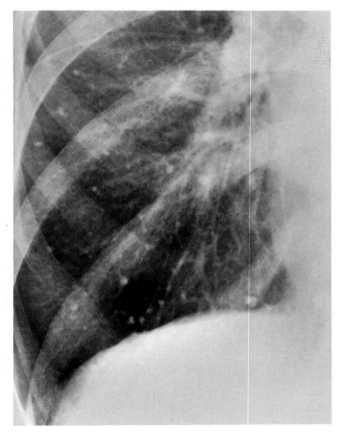

FIG 5–106.
Multifocal ossification in the lungs due to long-standing mitral valve disease.

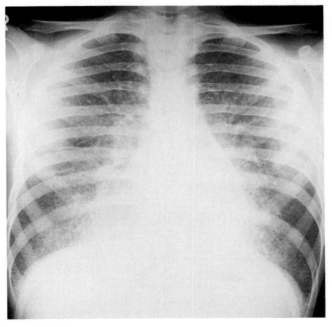

FIG 5–107.
Alveolar microlithiasis. The innumerable fine pulmonary calcifications are so small that they appear cloudlike. (Courtesy of Dr. Michael C. Pearson, London.)

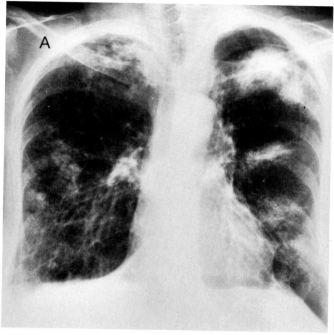

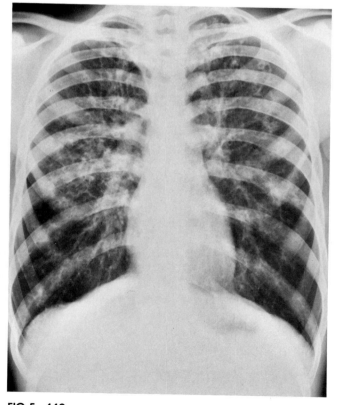

FIG 5–108.
Pulmonary calcification due to hyperparathyroidism. The fine calcifications are deposited in the lung in a patchy fashion and produce coalescent cloudlike shadows. The patient died despite parathyroidectomy. **A,** PA radiograph. **B,** xerograph taken at autopsy shows the pulmonary calcifications.

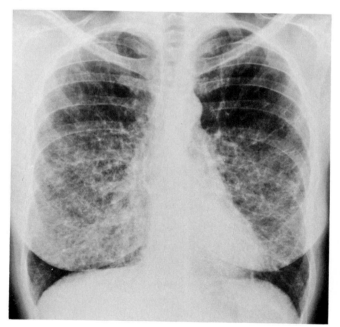

FIG 5–109.
Lymphangiomyomatosis of the lung. Typical example in a middle-aged woman showing lower zone predominant reticulonodular shadowing and low, flat hemidiaphragms.

FIG 5–110.
Cystic fibrosis. Note the combination of small irregular shadows in the upper lobe, bronchial wall thickening, and overinflation of the lung in a 20-year-old man.

INCREASED TRANSRADIANCY OF THE LUNG

True increase in transradiancy of the lungs (i.e., not due to technical factors) can be divided according to distribution into widespread, affecting both lungs; unilateral, affecting all or the majority of one lung; and focal, affecting a portion of one lobe only. (Increased transradiancy within a pulmonary opacity or contained within a cyst/cavity are separate topics discussed earlier in this chapter).

Widespread increase in transradiancy of both lungs is seen in two basic conditions: airway disease, notably emphysema, bronchiolitis and asthma; and obstruction to blood flow from the right side of the heart, usually associated with right to left cardiac shunting, e.g., Fallot's tetralogy, Eisenmenger's physiology, or severe widespread peripheral pulmonary arterial stenoses. Massive pulmonary embolism is a theoretical possibility for widespread pulmonary oligemia, but in practice, is virtually never seen.

Focal increase in transradiancy is seen with emphysema and bullous disease, and in some patients with pulmonary emboli.

Increased transradiancy of one lung (also known as unilateral hyperlucent lung) is a fairly commonly encountered radiographic finding. Basically, the causes may be subdivided as follows:

1. Radiographic artifact. Output of x-rays from the x-ray tube may not be uniform across the radiographic field. This so-called heel-toe effect is normally adjusted vertically so that output increases from the apices to the bases. If the heel-toe effect operates across the thorax, one hemithorax may appear more penetrated (i.e., more transradiant) than the other. A similar appearance may result from slight rotation of the patient; the side to which the patient is rotated is the more penetrated, regardless of whether the film has been taken PA or anteroposterior. In both situations, one should compare the relative exposures of the soft tissues, especially around the shoulder girdles. A clear-cut difference in penetration of these structures may then explain why one lung appears more lucent.

2. Thoracic wall and soft tissue abnormalities. These are the most common cause of a unilateral hyperlucent lung (notably, a mastectomy on the ipsilateral side). Other causes include a congenital defect of the pectoral muscles (Poland syndrome).

3. Diminished vascular perfusion of the lung. A substantial reduction in vascular perfusion of one lung may cause that lung to be abnormally lucent. Causes may be either congenital (e.g., aplasia of a

pulmonary artery or hypoplasia of the lung) or acquired (e.g., thromboembolic disease, fibrosing mediastinitis, tumor infiltration, or Swyer-James syndrome) (Fig 5–111).

4. Overexpansion of the lung. The lung as a whole may be relatively hyperexpanded when compared with the opposite lung. This state may result, for example, from foreign body impaction with obstructive emphysema. On occasion, emphysema, especially with bulla formation, may be asymmetric. Lobar collapse on one side with compensatory emphysema in the rest of the lung can appear superficially as a transradiant thorax, particularly if the collapse is chronic and extreme, since the collapsed lobe may be a relatively inconspicuous sliver of tissue wedged against the upper mediastinum or the lower paravertebral regions. Careful study of the hilar airway and vascular anatomy should resolve this confusion. On occasion, a lobar resection may have been performed leaving remarkably little radiographic evidence of previous surgical intervention.

5. Sometimes mild, generalized, increased opacity of one lung is misinterpreted as increased transradiancy of the opposite normal lung. Examples are the filtering effect of a large pleural effusion layering out posteriorly in a supine patient and the occasional case of uniform loss of volume of a lung. The

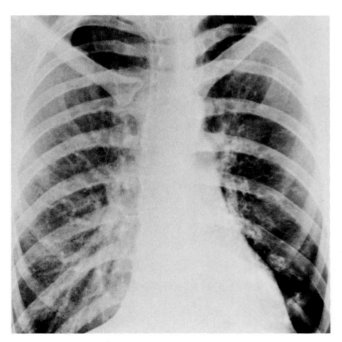

FIG 5–111.
Swyer-James (McLeod's) syndrome. Note the relative transradiancy of the left hemithorax, the reduction in size of the hilar vessels, and the small intrapulmonary vessels in the left lung.

latter applies particularly to intensive care patients with mucus plugging. Some patchy pulmonary parenchymal density is likely to be present, but it may not be as obvious as an isolated lobar collapse. One may, however, appreciate that the projected area of the involved lung is smaller than the other lung. The unobstructed lung, however, in these cases may appear relatively hyperlucent.

REFERENCES

1. Baber CE, Hedlund LW, Oddson TA, et al: Differentiating empyemas and peripheral pulmonary abscesses. The value of computed tomography. *Radiology* 1980; 135:755–758.
2. Bateson EM: An analysis of 155 solitary lung lesions illustrating the differential diagnosis of mixed tumors of the lung. *Clin Radiol* 1965; 16:51–65.
3. Bergin CJ, Muller NL: CT of interstitial lung disease: A diagnostic approach. *AJR* 1987; 148:8–15.
4. Blesovsky A: The folded lung. *Br J Dis Chest* 1966; 60:19–22.
5. Bryk D: Participating tail: New roentgenographic sign of pulmonary granuloma. *Am Rev Respir Dis* 1969; 100:406–408.
6. Carstairs LS: The interpretation of shadows in a restricted area of the lung field on a chest radiograph. *Proc R Soc Med* 1961; 54:978–980.
7. Chahinian P: Relationship between tumor doubling time and anatomoclinical features in 50 measurable pulmonary cancers. *Chest* 1972; 61:340–345.
8. Chasen MH, McCarthy MJ: Pulmonary nodules: Detection of calcification by linear and pluridirectional involvement in tomographic study. *Radiology* 1985; 156:589–592.
9. Cho SR, Henry DA, Beachley MC, et al: Round (helical) atelectasis. *Br J Radiol* 1981; 54:643–650.
10. Collins VP, Loeffler RK, Tivey H: Observations on growth rates in human tumors. *AJR* 1956; 76:988–1000.
11. Culiner MM: The right middle lobe syndrome, a non-obstructive complex. *Dis Chest* 1966; 50:57–66.
12. de Geer G, Gamsu G, Cann C, et al: Evaluation of a chest phantom for CT nodule densitometry. *AJR* 1986; 147:21–25.
13. Doyle TC, Lawler GA: CT features of rounded atelectasis of the lung. *AJR* 1984; 143:225–228.
14. Dunnick NR, Parker BR, Castellino RA: Rapid onset of pulmonary infiltration due to histiocytic lymphoma. *Radiology* 1976; 118:281–285.
15. Felson B: The roentgen diagnosis of disseminated pulmonary alveolar diseases. *Semin Roentgenol* 1967; 2:3–21.
16. Felson B: Mucoid impaction (insipissated secretions) in segmental bronchial obstruction. *Radiology* 1979; 133:9–16.
17. Felson B: A new look at pattern recognition of diffuse pulmonary disease. *AJR* 1979; 133:183–189.
18. Felson B, Felson H: Localization of intrathoracic lesions by means of the postero-anterior roentgenogram: The silhouette sign. *Radiology* 1950; 55:363–374.
19. Fleischner F: Uber das Wesen der basalen horizontalen Schattenstreifen im Lungenfeld. *Wien Arch Intern Med* 1936; 28:461.
20. Fleischner Society: Glossary of terms for thoracic radiology: Recommendation of the nomenclature committee of the Fleischner Society. *AJR* 1984; 143:509–517.
21. Franken EA, Klatte EC: Atypical (peripheral) upper lobe collapse. *Ann Radiol* 1977; 20:87–93.
22. Fraser RG, Pare JAP, Pare PD, et al: *Diagnosis of Diseases of the Chest.* ed 3. Philadelphia, WB Saunders Co, 1988.
23. Gaensler EA, Carrington CB: Peripheral opacities in chronic eosinophilic pneumonia: The photographic negative of pulmonary edema. *AJR* 1977; 128:1–13.
24. Garland LH, Coulson W, Wollin E: The rate of growth and apparent duration of untreated primary bronchial carcinoma. *Cancer* 1963; 16:694–707.
25. Genereux GP: CT of acute and chronic distal air space (alveolar) disease. *Semin Roentgenol* 1984; 19:211–221.
26. Glass TA, Armstrong P, Dyer RB, et al: Computed tomographic features of rounded atelectasis. *J Comput Tomogr* 1980; 7:183–185.
27. Glay J, Palayew MJ: Unusual patterns of left lower lobe atelectasis. *Radiology* 1981; 141:331–333.
28. Glazer HS, Aronberg DJ, Van Dyke JA, et al: CT manifestations of pulmonary collapse, in Siegelman SS (ed): *Computed Tomography of the Chest.* New York, Churchill Livingstone Inc, 1984.
29. Godwin JD, Tarver RD: Accessory fissures of the lung. *AJR* 1985; 144:39–47.
30. Godwin JD, Speckman JM, Fram EK, et al: Distinguishing benign from malignant pulmonary nodules by computed tomography. *Radiology* 1982; 144:349–351.
31. Godwin JD, Webb WR, Savoca CJ, et al: Multiple, thin walled cystic lesions of the lung. *AJR* 1980; 135:593–604.
32. Golden R: The effect of bronchostenosis upon the roentgen-ray shadows in carcinoma of the bronchus. *AJR* 1925; 13:21–30.
33. Goldstein MS, Rush M, Johnson P, et al: A calcified adenocarcinoma of the lung with very high CT numbers. *Radiology* 1984; 150:785–786.
34. Good CA: The solitary pulmonary nodule: A problem of management. *Radiol Clin North Am* 1963; 1:429–438.
35. Good CA, Wilson TW: The solitary circumscribed pulmonary nodule: Study of seven hundred five

cases encountered roentgenologically in a period of three and one half years. *JAMA* 1958; 166:210–215.

36. Gould DM, Dalrymple GV: A radiological analysis of disseminated lung disease. *Am J Med Sci* 1959; 238:621–637.

37. Gross BH, Glazer GM, Wimbish KJ: CT of solitary cavitary infiltrates. *Semin Roentgenol* 1984; 19:236–242.

38. Hanke R, Kretzschmar R: Round atelectasis. *Semin Roentgenol* 1980; 15:174–182.

39. Heitzman ER: *The Lung—Radiologic-Pathologic Correlations*, 2 ed. St Louis, CV Mosby Co, 1984.

40. Heitzman ER, Ziter FM, Markarian B, et al: Kerley's interlobular septal lines: Roentgen-pathologic correlation. *AJR* 1967; 100:578–582.

41. Hill CA: "Tail" signs associated with pulmonary lesions: Critical reappraisal. *AJR* 1982; 139:311–316.

42. Huston J, Muhm JR: Solitary pulmonary opacities on plain tomography. *Radiology* 1987; 163:481–485.

43. Im JG, Gamsu G, Gordon D, et al: CT densitometry of pulmonary nodules in a frozen human thorax. *AJR* 1988; 150:61–66.

44. Ishihara T, Kikuchi K, Ikeda T, et al: Metastatic pulmonary diseases: Biologic factors and modes of treatment. *Chest* 1973; 63:227–232.

45. Itoh H, Tokunaga S, Asamoto H, et al: Radiologic-pathologic correlations of small lung nodules with special reference to peribronchiolar nodules. *AJR* 1978; 130:223–231.

46. Joshi RR, Cholankeril JV: Computed tomography in lipoid pneumonia. *J Comput Assist Tomogr* 1985; 9:211–213.

47. Kattan KR: Upper mediastinal changes in lower lobe collapse. *Semin Roentgenol* 1980; 15:183–186.

48. Kattan KR, Eyler WR, Felson B: The juxtaphrenic peak in upper lobe collapse. *Semin Roentgenol* 1980; 15:187–193.

49. Kattan KR, Felson B, Holder LE, et al: Superior mediastinal shift in right lower lobe collapse. The "upper triangle sign." *Radiology* 1975; 116:305–309.

50. Kattan KR, Wiot JF: Cardiac rotation in left lower lobe collapse "the flat waist sign." *Radiology* 1976; 118:275–279.

51. Kerley P: Radiology in heart disease. *Br Med J* 1933; 2:594–597.

52. Kerr IH: Interstitial lung disease: The role of the radiologist. *Clin Radiol* 1984; 35:1–7.

53. Kreel L, Slavin G, Herbert A, et al: Intralobar septal oedema: D lines. *Clin Radiol* 1975; 26:209–221.

54. Mallens WMS, Nijhuis-Heddes JMA, Bakker W: Calcified lymph node metastases in bronchioloalveolar carcinoma. *Radiology* 1986; 161:103–104.

55. Mayo JR, Webb WR, Gould R, et al: High-resolution CT of the lungs: An optimal approach. *Radiology* 1987; 163:507–510.

56. McGee AR, Warren R: Carcinoma metastatic from the thyroid to the lungs: A twenty-four year follow up. *Radiology* 1966; 87:516–517.

57. McLachlan MSF, Wallace DM, Seneriratne C: Pulmonary calcification in renal failure. Report of three cases. *Br J Radiol* 1968; 41:99–106.

58. Meyer JA: Growth rate versus prognosis in resected primary bronchogenic carcinomas. *Cancer* 1973; 31:1468–1472.

59. Mintzer RA, Gore RM, Vogelzang RL, et al: Rounded atelectasis and its association with asbestosis–induced pleural disease. *Radiology* 1981; 139:567–570.

60. Munk PL, Muller NL, Miller RR, et al: Pulmonary lymphangitic carcinomatosis: CT and pathologic findings. *Radiology* 1988; 166:705–709.

61. Naidich DP, Ettinger N, Leitman BS, et al: CT of lobar collapse. *Semin Roentgenol* 1984; 19:222–235.

62. Naidich DP, McCauley DI, Khouri NF, et al: Computed tomography of lobar collapse: 1. Endobronchial obstruction. *J Comput Assist Tomogr* 1983; 7:745–757.

63. Naidich DP, McCauley DI, Khouri NF, et al: Computed tomography of lobar collapse: 2. Collapse in the absence of endobronchial obstruction. *J Comput Assist Tomogr* 1983; 7:758–767.

64. Naidich DP, Zerhouni EA, Hutchins GM, et al: Computed tomography of the pulmonary parenchyma: Part 1: Distal air space disease. *J Thorac Imaging* 1985; 1:39–53.

65. Nakata H, Kimoto T, Nakayama T, et al: Diffuse peripheral lung disease: Evaluation by high-resolution computed tomography. *Radiology* 1985; 157:181–185.

66. Nathan MH, Collins VP, Adams RA: Differentiation of benign and malignant pulmonary nodules by growth rate. *Radiology* 1962; 79:221–232.

67. Payne CR, Jacques PF, Kerr IH: Lung folding simulating peripheral pulmonary neoplasm (Blesovky's syndrome). *Thorax* 1980; 35:936–940.

68. Proto AV, Merhar GL: Central bronchial displacement with large posterior pleural collections. Findings on the lateral chest radiograph and CT scans. *J Can Assoc Radiol* 1984; 35:128–132.

69. Proto AV, Thomas SR: Pulmonary nodules studied by computed tomography. *Radiology* 1985; 156:149–153.

70. Proto AV, Speckman JM: The left lateral radiograph of the chest. *Med Radiogr Photogr* 1979; 55:30–74.

71. Proto AV, Tocino I: Radiographic manifestations of lobar collapse. *Semin Roentgenol* 1980; 15:117–173.

72. Putman CE, Godwin JD, Silverman PM, et al: CT of localized lucent lung lesions. *Semin Roentgenol* 1984; 19:173–188.

73. Reed JC: *Chest Radiology: Plain Film Patterns and Differential Diagnosis*, ed 2. Chicago, Year Book Medical Publishers, 1987.

74. Reed JC, Madewell JE: The air bronchogram in interstitial disease of the lungs. *Radiology* 1975; 116:1–9.

75. Reed JC: Pathologic correlations of the air bronchogram: A reliable sign in chest radiology. *Crit Rev Diagn Imag* 1977; 10:235–255.

76. Reeder MM, Felson B: *Gamuts in Radiology: Comprehensive Lists of Roentgen Differential Diagnosis.* Cincinnati, Audiovisual Radiology of Cincinnati, 1975.

77. Ried L: The connective tissue septa in the adult human lung. *Thorax* 1959; 14:138–145.

78. Rosenbloom SA, Ravin CE, Putman CE, et al: Peripheral middle lobe syndrome. *Radiology* 1983; 149:17–21.

79. Sagel SS: The solitary pulmonary nodule: Role of CT, commentary. *AJR* 1986; 147:26–27.

80. Schneider JH, Felson B, Gonzales LL: Rounded atelectasis. *AJR* 1980; 134:225–232.

81. Shapiro R, Wilson GL, Yesner R, et al: A useful roentgen sign in the diagnosis of localized bronchioloalveolar carcinoma. *AJR* 1972; 114:516–524.

82. Sherrier RH, Chiles C, Johnston GA, et al: Differentiation of benign from malignant pulmonary nodules with digitized chest radiographs. *Radiology* 1987; 162:645–649.

83. Siegelman SS, Khouri NF, Leo FP, et al: Solitary pulmonary nodules: CT assessment. *Radiology* 1986; 160:307–312.

84. Siegelman SS, Zerhouni EA, Leo FP, et al: CT of the solitary pulmonary nodule. *AJR* 1980; 135:1–13.

85. Spratt JS, Spjut HJ, Roper CI: The frequency distribution of the rates of growth and the estimated duration of primary pulmonary carcinomas. *Cancer* 1963; 16:687–693.

86. Stark DD, Federle MP, Goodman PC, et al: Differentiating lung abscess and empyema: radiography and computed tomography. *AJR* 1983, 141:163–167.

87. Steele JD: The solitary pulmonary nodule—report of a cooperative study of resected asymptomatic solitary pulmonary nodules in males. *J Thorac Cardiovasc Surg* 1963; 46:21–39.

88. Stewart JG, MacMahon H, Vyborny CJ, et al: Dystrophic calcification in carcinoma of the lung: Demonstration by CT. *AJR* 1987; 148:29–30.

89. Strauss MJ: The growth characteristic of lung cancer and its application to treatment design. *Semin Oncol* 1974; 1:167–174.

90. Strickland B, Brennan J, Denison DM: Computed tomography in diffuse lung disease: Improving the image. *Clin Radiol* 1986; 37:335–338.

91. Toomes H, Delphendahl A, Marike HG, et al: The coin lesion of the lung: A review of 955 resected coin lesions. *Cancer* 1983; 51:534–537.

92. Trapnell DH: The peripheral lymphatics of the lung. *Br J Radiol* 1963; 36:660–672.

93. Trapnell DH: The differential diagnosis of linear shadows in chest radiographs. *Radiol Clin North Am* 1973; 11:77–92.

94. Tylen V, Nilsson V: Computed tomography in pulmonary pseudotumors and their relation to asbestos exposure. *J Comput Assist Tomogr* 1982; 6:229–237.

95. Weiss W: Tumor doubling time and survival of men with bronchogenic carcinoma. *Chest* 1974; 65:3–8.

96. Westcott JL, Cole S: Plate atelectasis. *Radiology* 1985; 155:1–9.

97. Whalen JP, Lane EJ: Bronchial rearrangements in pulmonary collapse as seen on the lateral radiograph. *Radiology* 1969; 93:285–288.

98. Woodring JH, Fried AM: Significance of wall thickness in solitary cavities of the lung: A follow-up study. *AJR* 1983; 140:473–474.

99. Zerhouni EA, Boukadoum M, Siddiky MA, et al: A standard phantom for quantitative CT analysis of pulmonary nodules. *Radiology* 1983; 149:767–773.

100. Zerhouni EA, Naidich DP, Stitick FP, et al: Computed tomography of the pulmonary parenchyma: Part 2. Interstitial disease. *J Thorac Imaging* 1985; 1(1):54–64.

101. Zerhouni EA, Spivey JF, Morgan RH, et al: Factors influencing quantitative CT measurements of solitary pulmonary nodules. *J Comput Assist Tomogr* 1982; 6:1075–1087.

102. Zerhouni EA, Stitik FP, Siegelman SS, et al: CT of the pulmonary nodule: A cooperative study. *Radiology* 1986; 160:319–327.

103. Ziskind MM, Weill H, Rayzant AR: The recognition and significance of acinus-filling processes of the lung. *Am Rev Respir Dis* 1963; 87:551–559.

6

Infections of the Lungs and Pleura

PNEUMONIA

Pneumonias are most usefully classified according to the responsible infecting organism because the organism dictates the treatment. Unfortunately, radiologic techniques are poor at predicting even the broad category of infectious agent let alone the specific organism.[315] Radiology does, nevertheless, have many important roles in patients with suspected pulmonary infection. The plain chest radiograph remains the best available method of establishing the presence of a pneumonia and of determining its location and extent. Predisposing conditions, notably bronchial carcinoma, may be visible, and complications, such as pleural effusion, empyema, and abscess formation are readily demonstrated. Once pneumonia and its complications have been diagnosed, chest radiographs become an excellent method for following the patient's response to treatment.

The essential radiographic feature of pneumonia is pulmonary consolidation, which may show cavitation and may be accompanied by pleural effusion. The appearance of individual areas of pulmonary consolidation varies almost infinitely from one or more small, ill-defined shadows to large air-space shadows involving the whole of one or more lobes, the pattern depending not only on the infecting organism but also on the integrity of the host's defenses.

Pneumonias are sometimes divided according to their chest radiographic appearances into bronchopneumonia, lobar pneumonia, spherical (round or nodular) pneumonia, and interstitial pneumonia. Though widely used, these terms are in reality of limited value, as several patterns may be produced by the same organism and because there is often overlap of patterns in the individual patient. Also, the pathologist and radiologist do not always agree in their use of these descriptive phrases.

Bronchopneumonia is the most common of the three patterns. In bronchopneumonia the inflammatory exudate is multifocal and centered on large inflamed airways. It is therefore distributed in a way that reflects the course of the bronchial tree. In other words, it is roughly segmental in shape. Both pathologically and radiologically, the consolidations are patchy, involving some acini and sparing others. Thus, on radiologic examination, bronchopneumonia is characterized by patchy consolidation, loss of volume, and the absence of air bronchograms (Fig 6–1). Later on, as affected areas coalesce, the shadowing may become more uniform and resemble lobar pneumonia. Though the term "segmental consolidation" is in common use, consolidation conforming precisely to the segmental anatomy is rarely seen, because there are no physical barriers to prevent the spread of infection from one segment to another within the same lobe.

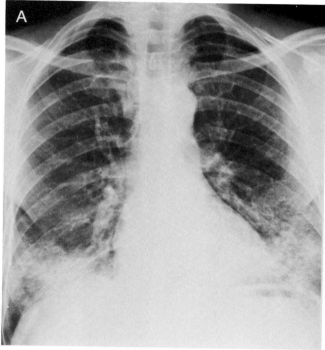

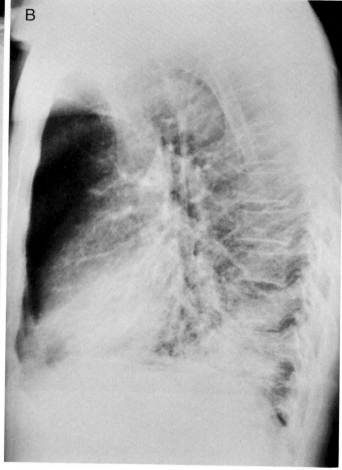

FIG 6—1.
Bronchopneumonia. Bilateral lower-zone predominant aspiration pneumonia in an alcoholic patient. **A,** PA view. **B,** lateral view.

In lobar pneumonia (Fig 6–2), the inflammatory exudate begins in the distal air spaces and spreads by way of the pores of Kohn across segmental boundaries, giving rise to uniform nonsegmental consolidation. Eventually, the pneumonia may involve a whole lobe, but usually the process stops well before the entire lobe is consolidated. The consolidation is usually confined to one lobe, though multilobar involvement is not uncommon. As the airways are not primarily affected, there is little or no volume loss, and visible air bronchograms are common.

Some pneumonias present as spherical or nodular-shaped consolidations (Fig 6–3). Usually, the nodules are fairly ill-defined and may contain air bronchograms. They may cavitate, in which case they are referred to as abscesses.

Interstitial pneumonia refers to a radiographic pattern comprising peribronchial thickening and ill-defined reticulonodular shadowing of the lungs (Fig 6–4). Patchy subsegmental or discoid atelectasis is common. This pattern, though it may show a lobar or segmental distribution, is frequently independent of the lobar architecture of the lung. The usual causes of interstitial pneumonia are viral and mycoplasmal infections.

Diagnosing the Cause of Pneumonia

Pneumonias caused by viruses or *Mycoplasma pneumoniae* are usually self-limiting and resolve without treatment, in marked contrast to bacterial pneumonias, which require accurate diagnosis and therapy if serious complications, and even death, are to be avoided. It is bacterial pneumonia, therefore, that forms the bulk of cases seen in hospital. The choice of which antibiotic to use may have to rest upon an informed guess, based on the combination of clinical and radiographic features, because the results of

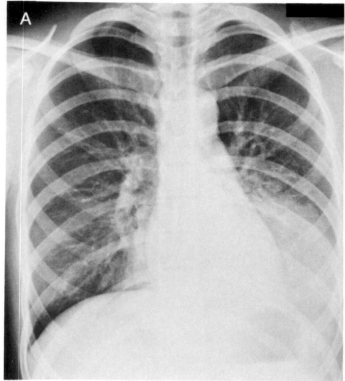

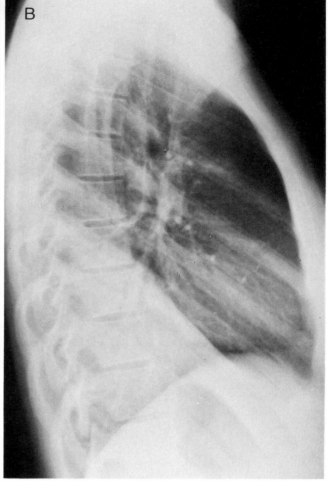

FIG 6–2.
Lobar pneumonia. Pneumococcal pneumonia involving the whole of the left lower lobe. **A,** PA view. **B,** lateral view.

bacteriologic tests are often delayed. Once the results of cultures or other bacteriologic tests are known, the initial antibiotic regimen can then be revised. Such guesses are based on many factors:

1. The *age* of the patient and any history of specific exposure.

2. The *source of the infection,* particularly whether it was acquired in hospital or in the community. Pneumococcal, mycoplasmal, and viral pneumonias are the common community-acquired pneumonias,[140] with *Staphylococcus aureus, Streptococcus pyogenes, Klebsiella, Chlamydia, Rickettsia* and *Legionella pneumophila* as alternative agents, whereas gram-negative bacilli, *S. aureus,* anaerobic organisms, and pneumococci are the particularly prevalent causes in hospital-acquired infections.[22] Nearly half the cases have more than one potential pathogen.[22]

3. The *character of the illness.* Bacterial pneumonia typically presents as an acute illness with chest

pain, chills, high fever, and cough productive of purulent sputum. Neutrophilia is common. Mycoplasmal and viral pneumonias, on the other hand, usually have prodromal symptoms, mild pyrexia, and less sputum. Neutrophilia is absent, and the total white blood cell count is usually only slightly elevated.

4. *Predisposing conditions.* The list of predisposing conditions for pneumonia is long and complex. An important example is aspiration pneumonia due to anaerobic organisms or gram-negative bacteria, which is particularly likely in patients who are alcoholics or who have had recent general anesthesia or a bout of unconsciousness, and those with disturbances of swallowing.[120] Other examples include pneumococcal pneumonia, which is particularly likely in sickle cell disease and following splenectomy, whereas *Pseudomonas aeruginosa* or *S. aureus* are the likely pathogens responsible for pneumonia in patients with cystic fibrosis.[77, 180] Patients who are

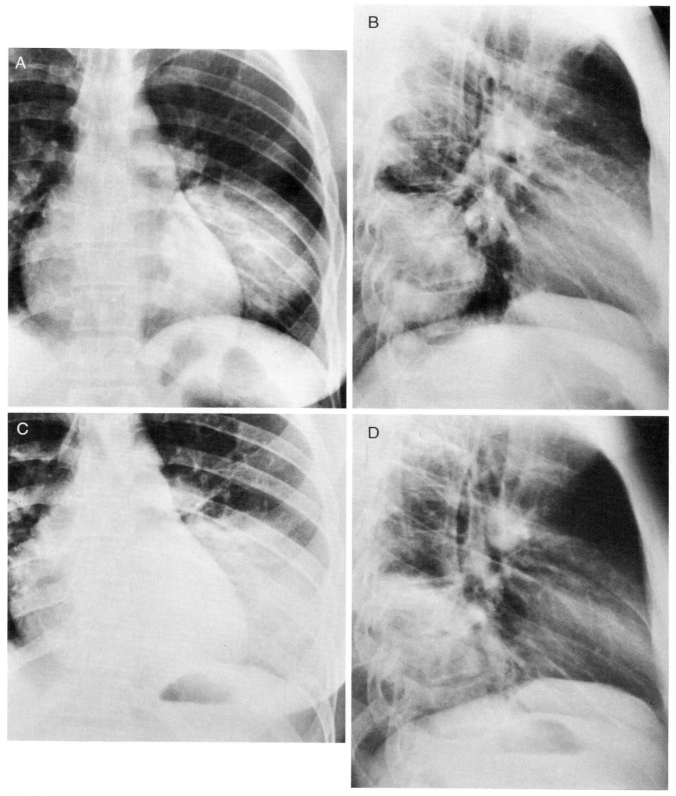

FIG 6–3.
Round pneumonia in the left lower lobe due to pneumococcal pneumonia. **A** and **B,** PA and lateral radiographs on patient's ad- mission to hospital. **C** and **D,** 12 hours later the round pneumonia has progressed to become more lobar in shape.

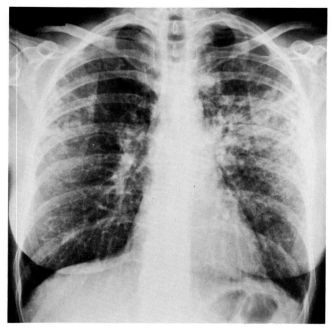

FIG 6–4.
Interstitial viral pneumonia; note the bilateral streaky shadowing radiating from the hili.

immunocompromised present a special category and are discussed in the section "Pulmonary Infection in the Immunocompromised Patient" later in this chapter.

Much has been written about the chest radiograph in the individual pneumonias. The information is difficult to remember, because there is so little that is specific to a particular organism. We will provide a detailed review for the interested reader, but will start with some generalizations, which we hope will be of value:

1. Consolidation of the whole or most of a lobe is usually bacterial in origin (see Fig 6–2). Post-obstructive pneumonia should also be strongly considered. When lobar consolidation results from a primary bacterial infection, the usual organism will be *S. pneumoniae* (pneumococcus); occasionally the infection will be due to *Klebsiella, S. aureus, Mycobacterium tuberculosis, L. pneumophila,* or aspiration of anaerobic or gram-negative bacteria from the upper respiratory tract or pharynx. Expansion of the lobe due to intense exudate is virtually diagnostic of *Klebsiella* or pneumococcal pneumonia.

2. Aspiration pneumonia frequently causes patchy consolidation in the dependent portions of the lungs (see Fig 6–1). The consolidations are usually multilobar and bilateral in distribution.

3. Consolidation with cavitation (Fig 6–5) suggests bacterial or fungal disease rather than viral or mycoplasmal infection. The bacteria that commonly cause cavitation are *S. aureus,* gram-negative bacteria (especially *Klebsiella, Proteus,* and *Pseudomonas*), anaerobic bacteria, and *M. tuberculosis.* A solitary large abscess in a patient without underlying lung disease, the so-called primary lung abscess, is usually attributable to anaerobic bacteria.

Pneumatocele formation (see p. 128) can be difficult to distinguish from cavitation (Fig 6–6). When the result of pneumonia, the responsible organism is likely to be *S. aureus,* though pneumatoceles have also been described in infants with pneumonia due to *S. pneumoniae.*[8]

Pulmonary gangrene is a rare but interesting form of cavitation which produces sloughed lung within a large cavity (Fig 6–7). It is secondary to thrombosis of the pulmonary vessels as they pass through the pneumonia. The two agents most frequently reported as responsible are *S. pneumoniae* and *Klebsiella* sp.[68, 229] The condition is unusual with the other gram-negative pneumonias.[136] Pulmonary

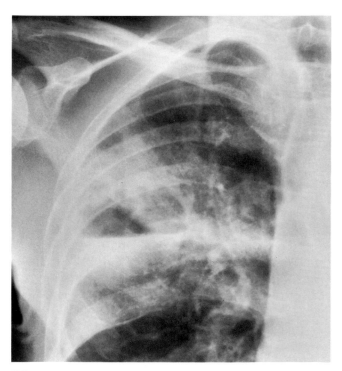

FIG 6–5.
Consolidation with cavitation, due to gram-negative bacterial pneumonia.

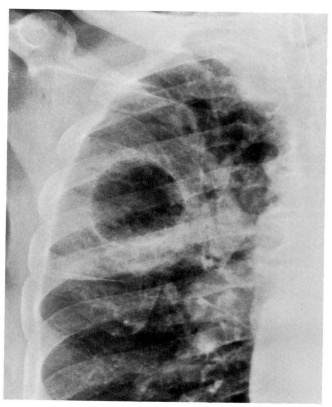

FIG 6—6.
Pneumatocele formation in staphylococcal pneumonia.

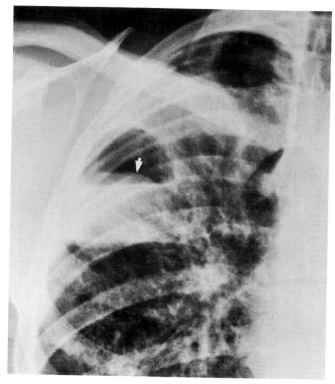

FIG 6—7.
Pulmonary gangrene. The sloughed lung *(arrow)* can be seen projecting above the air-fluid level in the cavity. The organism in this case was *Pseudomonas aeruginosa*.

gangrene has also been described with *M. tuberculosis,*[172] with aspergillosis and mucormycosis in the immunocompromised host,[347] and possibly also with anaerobic bacteria.[229]

4. Nodular (spherical) pneumonia (see Fig 6—3) is usually the result of pneumococcal infection,[272] *L. pneumophila,*[76] *L. micdadei,*[245] Q-fever,[215] or fungal disease. It may also result from the hematogenous spread of bacteria, *S. aureus* infection being the common bacterial pneumonia to spread by way of septic emboli. Though spherical pneumonia can be confused with lung carcinoma, the distinction is relatively straightforward when the pneumonia is bacterial in origin, as spherical pneumonia usually has a less well defined edge, may contain air bronchograms, expands to involve the adjacent lung over the next few hours or days, and is associated with obvious clinical features of acute bacterial infection (see Fig 6—3). Also, spherical pneumonia is most common in children, an age at which lung carcinoma does not occur. Spherical pneumonias resulting from fungal infections, however, are often chronic and may closely resemble carcinoma of the lung both clinically and radiographically.

5. Pneumonia which presents with widespread, small, ill-defined reticulonodular shadows (Fig 6—8), whether or not lobar or segmental opacities are also present, is likely to be due to viral or mycoplasmal infection.[62] In exceptional cases, fungal and streptococcal infection give rise to this pattern.

6. Miliary nodulation in the lungs has many causes. When due to infection, the likely organisms are *M. tuberculosis* (Fig 6—9) and various fungi. The nodules are even in size, usually 2 to 4 mm in diameter, are well-defined, and are uniformly distributed.

7. Patchy upper lobe consolidations (Fig 6—10) are very suggestive of tuberculous or fungal infection, notably histoplasmosis, but occasionally North American blastomycosis, cryptococcosis, and coccidioidomycosis. Patchy lower lobe consolidations together with loss of volume suggest one of the aspiration pneumonias (*S. aureus*, anaerobic or gram-negative bacterial pneumonia).

8. Pleural effusions which are seen early, are large, or change rapidly are most commonly due to

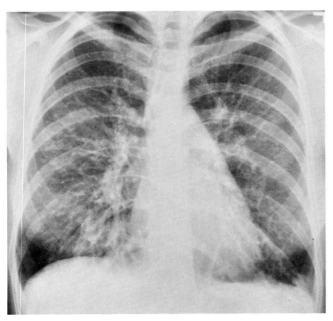

FIG 6—8.
Mycoplasma pneumonia showing widespread reticulonodular shadowing in the lung.

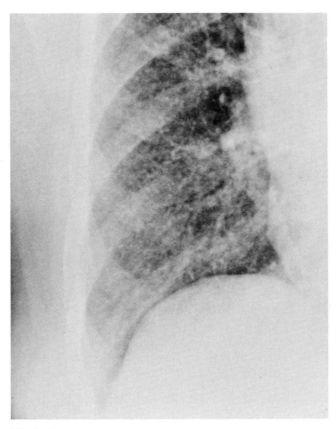

FIG 6—9.
Miliary tuberculosis.

anaerobic bacteria, gram-negative bacteria, *S. aureus*, and *S. pyogenes*. Empyemas are radiologically indistinguishable from pleural effusions but should be considered if the effusion is large, delayed in appearance, or loculates rapidly—particularly if the effusion accompanies a pneumonia in which empyema is known to be common.

9. Most pneumonias resolve radiologically within a month, often within 10 to 21 days, and most of the remainder by 2 months. The most indolent shadowing is seen with tuberculosis, anaerobes, *Coxiella burnetii*, *L. pneumophila*, *C. psittaci* and some cases of *M. pneumoniae*. Consolidation persisting beyond 2 months represents delayed resolution, and an explanation should be sought. The most likely reasons are that the patient is old or has some systemic disease. Alternatively, the pneumonia may have been extensive or have been complicated by atelectasis, cavitation, or empyema. If none of these explanations appears satisfactory, a predisposing local cause such as obstructing neoplasm or bronchiectasis should be carefully looked for.

BACTERIAL PNEUMONIA

Streptococcus pneumoniae Pneumonia

Streptococcus pneumoniae (pneumococcal) pneumonia occurs in patients of any age, is the most common community-acquired bacterial pneumonia,[299] and is also a leading cause of hospital-acquired infection. Chronic illness, alcoholism, and splenectomy are all predisposing factors. Clinically, pneumococcal pneumonia typically presents with sudden onset of high fever, shaking chills, pleuritic pain, and cough productive of sputum that is sometimes streaked with blood.

A variety of radiographic patterns are described. Pneumococcal pneumonia is the prototype of lobar consolidation (Fig 6—11). Bacteria are inhaled into the periphery of a lobe, where they incite an intense inflammatory reaction, which is seen radiographically as an area of homogeneous shadowing (Fig 6—12). Air bronchograms may be evident. The exudate spreads rapidly across the interalveolar connections rather than by way of the bronchial tree. It crosses segmental boundaries and, therefore, does not show a true segmental pattern. If untreated, the pneumonia may involve the whole of the lobe, which may be expanded by the intense exudate. Frequently, the gravitationally dependent portions of the lobes are the most densely opacified. Sometimes

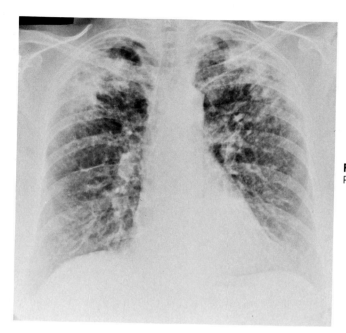

FIG 6–10.
Patchy upper zone consolidations due to histoplasmosis.

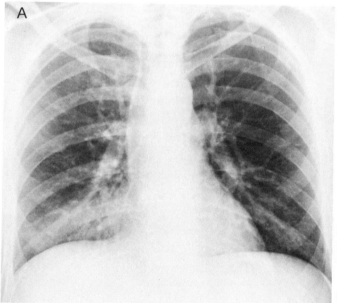

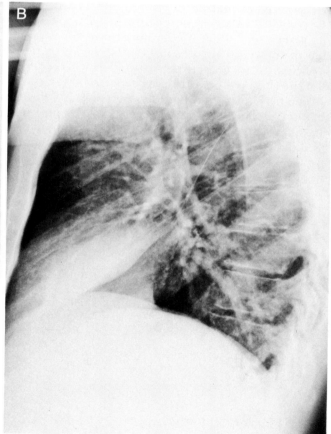

FIG 6–11.
Pneumococcal pneumonia presenting as lobar pneumonia of the middle lobe. **A,** PA view. **B,** lateral view.

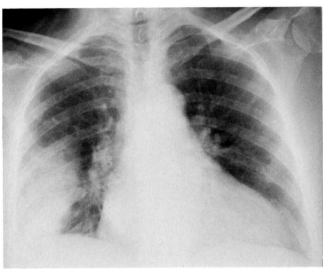

FIG 6–12.
Pneumococcal pneumonia presenting as a large peripheral consolidation in the right lower lobe.

more than one lobe is involved. If seen early in its course, before any pleural boundaries have been reached, the pneumonia may be spherical in shape, particularly in children.

Nowadays this classic picture of lobar pneumonia is seen less often. Two reports have emphasized that the more usual pattern is that of patchy or peribronchial consolidation (Fig 6–13), which occurred in 57 (61%) of the 94 patients reported by Ort and colleagues[230] and in 28 of 40 patients (70%) in Kantor's series.[165] A widespread small nodular and linear pattern resembling interstitial disease was seen in 22% of Kantor's patients; others do not emphasize this pattern, presumably regarding it as one of the bronchopneumonic varieties.

With appropriate treatment the pneumonia usu-ally clears within 10 to 14 days. Pleural effusion is seen in up to 57% of patients,[195, 312] and occasionally, particularly if appropriate treatment has been delayed, the effusion turns into an empyema. The presence of parapneumonic effusions correlates with the duration of symptoms before admission, with bacteremia and with prolonged fever after commencement of therapy.[312]

Cavitation is distinctly unusual (Fig 6–14). A very rare complication is pulmonary gangrene.[68, 229]

Streptococcus pyogenes Pneumonia

Streptococcus pyogenes pneumonia is now much less common than pneumococcal pneumonia. In the early part of this century, it was a major cause of

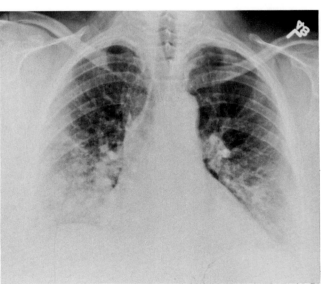

FIG 6–13.
Pneumococcal pneumonia presenting as bilateral mid- and lower-zone patchy consolidations.

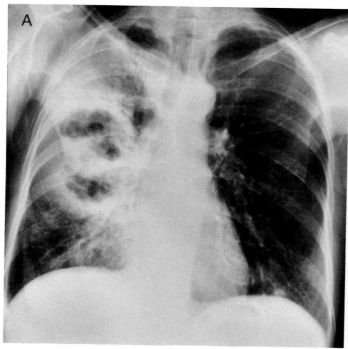

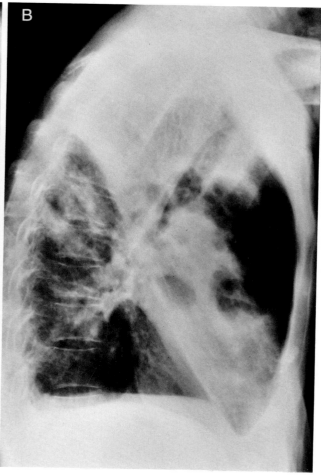

FIG 6–14.
Pneumococcal pneumonia showing extensive cavitation in lobar consolidation of the right upper and middle lobes. **A,** PA view. **B,** lateral view.

pneumonia in both adults and children. It may complicate viral infections or may follow streptococcal upper respiratory tract infections. Radiographically (Fig 6–15), *S. pyogenes* pneumonia causes confluent or patchy consolidation, with lower lobe predominance. Large pleural effusions and empyema are common.[23]

Staphylococcal Pneumonia

Pneumonia due to *S. aureus* usually follows aspiration of organisms from the upper respiratory tract, occurring particularly in debilitated hospitalized patients. It may also be a community-acquired disease, particularly in infants and elderly individuals, often complicating influenza. Pneumonia from hematogenous spread may result from endocarditis, thrombophlebitis, or staphylococcal infection of indwelling catheters. Septicemic infection is also seen in drug addicts and immunocompromised patients.

Typically, the plain chest radiograph[335] (Fig

6–16) shows patchy segmental consolidation, often with loss of volume. Air bronchograms are rare. The consolidation may spread rapidly and become confluent, resembling that of lobar pneumonia (Fig 6–17). Several lobes are frequently involved and the disease may be bilateral. Abscess cavities may form within the pneumonia and are common at any age (see Fig 6–17). Pneumatoceles (Fig 6–18) are much more frequent in childhood than adult infection and they may lead to pneumothorax. Pleural effusions, which may develop rapidly, are common. In one large series of adults they were seen in just under 40% of cases.[335] Empyema formation is a common and serious complication, particularly in children. Septicemic infection, in contrast to that following aspiration, causes multiple spherical (round) consolidations, which may cavitate (Fig 6–19).[224]

Anthrax

Anthrax, a major scourge prior to the introduction of vaccines originated by Louis Pasteur, is due

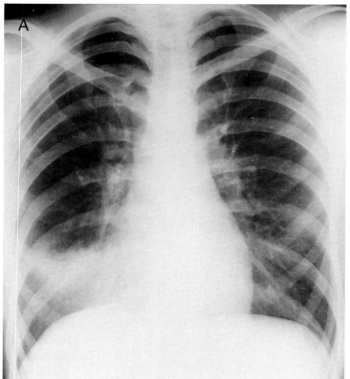

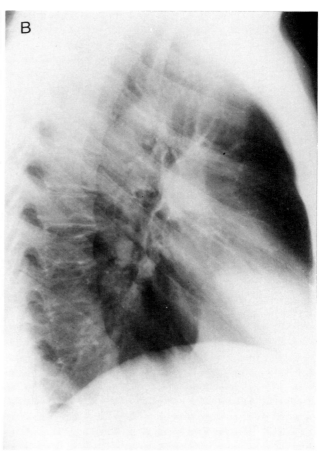

FIG 6–15.
β-Hemolytic streptococcal pneumonia showing homogeneous area
of consolidation in the right middle lobe. **A,** PA view. **B,** lateral view.
(Courtesy of Dr. Michael C. Pearson, London.)

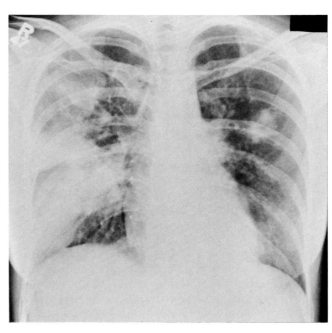

FIG 6–16.
Staphylococcal pneumonia showing bilateral multifocal
consolidation.

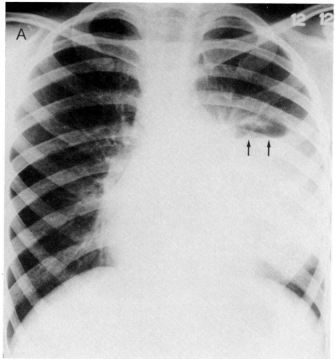

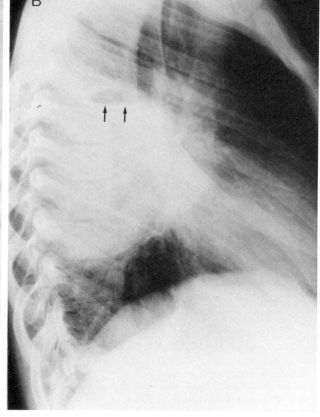

FIG 6–17.
Staphylococcal pneumonia showing confluent lobar-type consolidations with cavitation *(arrows* point to air-fluid level in the superior segment of the left lower lobe). **A,** PA view. **B,** lateral view. (Courtesy of Dr. Michael C. Pearson, London.)

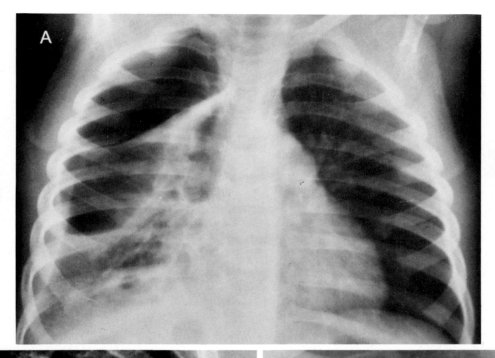

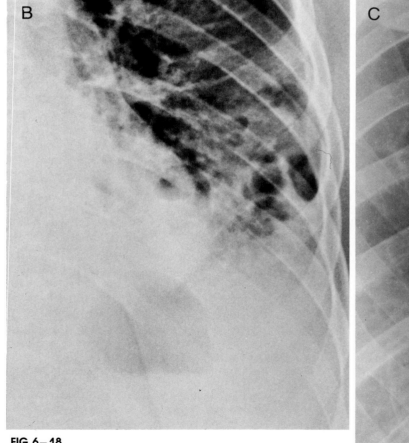

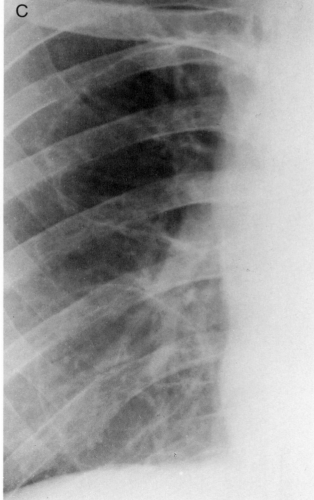

FIG 6–18.
Pneumatocele formation in staphylococcal pneumonia. **A,** young child with large pneumatoceles in pneumonia in right lung. **B,** young adult with multiple small pneumatoceles in left lower lobe pneumonia. **C,** thin-walled residual pneumatoceles following staphylococcal pneumonia in another young adult.

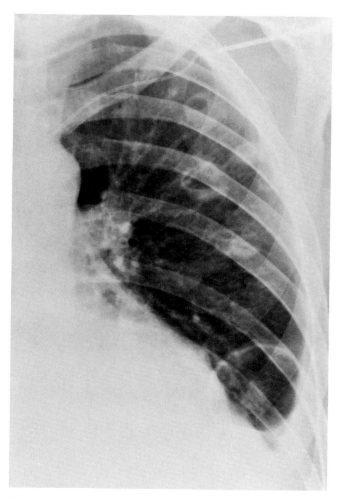

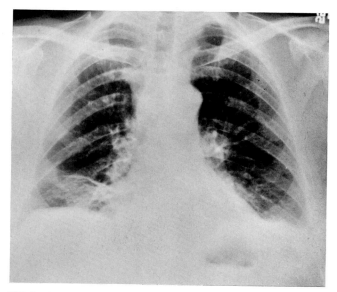

FIG 6–20.
Anthrax pneumonia in a carpet cleaner who developed pneumonia with severe fever, shaking chills, and hypotension. There are bilateral basal consolidations, and there is mediastinal and hilar lymphadenopathy.

Gram-Negative Bacterial Pneumonia

Many aerobic gram-negative bacteria cause pneumonia.[243] The most important are the *Enterobacteriaceae* (notably, *Klebsiella, Enterobacter, Serratia marcescens, Escherichia coli,* and *P. mirabilis*), *P. aeruginosa, Acinetobacter, Hemophilus influenzae,* and *L. pneumophila.* Together with *S. aureus* these organisms are much the most frequent cause of hospital-acquired pneumonia and are a major cause of morbidity and mortality. They contaminate hospital equipment such as ventilators and the soaps, liquids, or jellies used to care for wounds and catheters. (*Klebsiella* and *Legionella* pneumonias have features that differentiate them from other gram-negative bacterial pneumonias and are discussed in the following section.)

Affected patients usually have a known predisposing factor, such as chronic obstructive pulmonary disease or a major medical condition, or have recently had surgery. The bacterial flora of the upper respiratory tract changes in such patients, and when aspiration occurs, they are in great danger of developing a gram-negative bacterial pneumonia. Aspiration is believed to be the common method by which the disease enters the lungs, but pneumonia following inhalation of organisms or spread by way of the bloodstream is also occasionally seen.

The radiologic pattern of the gram-negative bac-

FIG 6–19.
Septic emboli resulting from staphylococcal septicemia in a patient on renal dialysis with an infected dialysis shunt site. Note the multiple, round pulmonary cavities with thin walls.

to *Bacillus anthracis,* a gram-positive aerobic bacillus. Anthrax is now an extremely rare cause of pneumonia in the United States and the United Kingdom. It is usually acquired from contact with infected goats or their products, particularly unfinished hides and wools imported from endemic areas in Asia, the Middle East, or Africa (Fig 6–20). The spores may be inhaled directly into the lungs, but cutaneous anthrax is the usual clinical presentation, the spores being carried to regional lymph nodes, from which they may disseminate to the lungs, causing hemorrhagic pneumonia. Mediastinal widening due to lymphadenopathy appears to be a common radiographic feature.[323] The lungs may also show patchy consolidation, particularly at the bases, and pleural effusions may be seen.

FIG 6–21.
Hemophilus influenzae pneumonia causing bilateral basal patchy consolidations, predominantly in the right lower lobe.

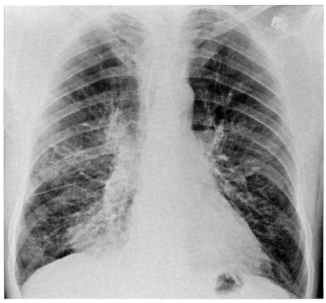

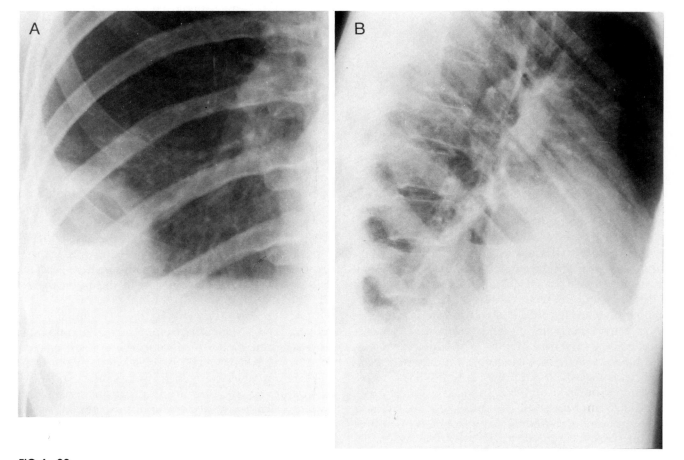

FIG 6–22.
Right lower lobe abscess due to *E. coli* infection. **A,** PA view. **B,** lateral view. (Courtesy of Dr. Michael C. Pearson, London.)

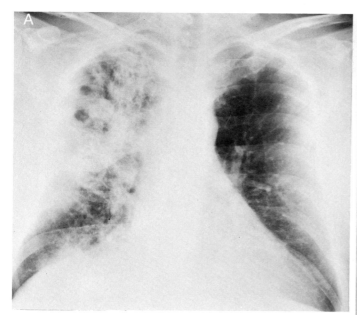

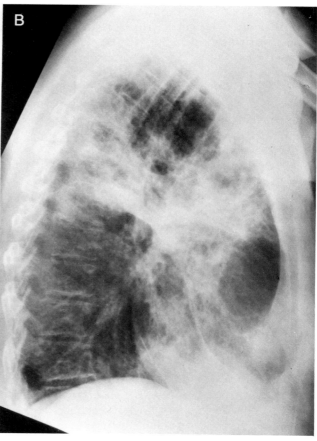

FIG 6–23.
Klebsiella pneumonia of the right upper lobe showing numerous cavities. **A,** PA view. **B,** lateral view.

terial pneumonias closely resembles that already described for staphylococcal pneumonia.* The appearances vary from small ill-defined nodules to patchy consolidation (Fig 6–21), which may sometimes be confluent and resemble lobar pneumonia or pulmonary edema.[151] Usually the consolidations are multifocal, with the lower lobes nearly always affected, usually bilaterally. About half the time the upper and middle lobes are involved as well.[322] Cavitation is common (Figs 6–5 and 6–22),[206] but it should be realized that radiographic lucencies in areas of consolidation, though often due to abscess formation, are sometimes due to spared normal acini surrounded by pneumonia.[263] Renner et al.[263] also point out that the microabscesses seen at pathologic study are not identified on the plain chest radiograph; it is only once they coalesce to form cavities of 2 cm or more and communicate with an airway that they become visible.

Parapneumonic pleural effusions are common in

*Those readers interested in the articles which describe the appearances for each individual organism should consult references 15, 241, 263, 316–318, and 322.

most gram-negative pneumonia, with empyema an important and fairly frequent complication.[317, 318]

Klebsiella *Pneumonia*

Pneumonia due to *K. pneumoniae* (Friedlander's pneumonia), like the other gram-negative pneumonias, usually affects people with chronic debilitating illnesses or alcoholism. The pneumonia presents clinically with high fever and toxemia and resembles severe pneumococcal pneumonia. Radiologically,[93, 148] the consolidation is also similar to that seen with *S. pneumoniae*—the disease often being confined to one lobe, with homogeneous nonsegmental consolidation that spreads rapidly to become a lobar pneumonia[106] (Fig 6–23, A and B). Multilobar and bilateral consolidations may occur.[148] The advancing edge of the pneumonia is sharp and distinct. In one series, there was a striking predilection for the upper lobes,[148] a finding not supported by Frommhold's cases.[106] Also, lobar expansion was a noteworthy feature in the early series,[93, 148] but it is our impression that in the modern antibiotic era both these features are unusual.

Cavitation, which may occur early and progress

very quickly, is seen in 30% to 50% of cases, a feature that distinguishes it from pneumococcal pneumonia, in which cavitation is rare. The cavities are frequently multiple and may attain great size. Solitary large chronic abscesses are occasionally encountered.[260] Massive necrosis, so-called pulmonary gangrene, is a rare phenomenon. Pleural effusion and empyema are relatively uncommon.[148, 243]

Legionella pneumophila *Pneumonia*

Legionnaires' disease, which results in a severe pneumonia with a high mortality, is due to *L. pneumophila,* an aerobic gram-negative bacillus found in water and humidifier systems. (*L. micdadei* pneumonia is considered separately in the section on immunocompromised patients later in this chapter.) Infection is believed to come from these sources rather than by person-to-person contact. The disease may be sporadic or occur in epidemics, as in the 1976 outbreak at the American Legion Convention, where 29 of 182 affected delegates died, from which the name Legionnaires' disease is derived. The infection is characterized by malaise, myalgias, headaches, abdominal and chest pain, nausea, vomiting and diarrhea, high fevers, and rigors, with cough and dyspnea. Predisposing chronic diseases are common and may be either pulmonary, such as chronic bronchitis and emphysema, or systemic, such as malignant disease or renal failure. The organism is difficult to culture, so the diagnosis is usually established serologically and is therefore delayed.

The appearances on the chest radiograph have been reviewed in detail by Meenhorst and Mulder[211] and by Kroboth et al.[177] The initial finding is peripherally situated patchy consolidation (Fig 6–24) that spreads rapidly, often involving more than one lobe and becoming bilateral in half the cases (Fig 6–25). There may be a slight predilection for the lower lobes, but this has not been seen in all series.[211] The consolidations may coalesce to resemble those of lobar pneumonia[76, 87] or they may assume a spherical configuration.[76] Cavitation, though reported, is unusual[177] (see Fig 6–25); it appears to be most frequent in immunocompromised patients.[2] Pleural effusions, which are usually small but may on occasion be massive, are documented in up to two thirds of cases,[177, 211] and frank empyema formation may occur.[256] The radiographic resolution is slow, particularly in immunocompromised patients, and lags behind the clinical improvement. The changes usually persist for at least 3 to 8 weeks after the acute illness.

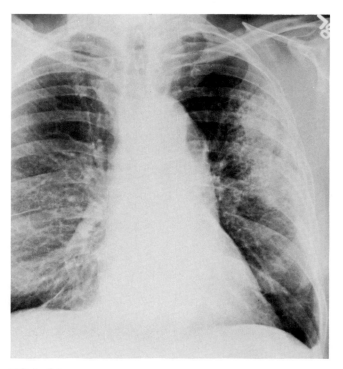

FIG 6–24.
Legionella pneumophila pneumonia showing a rounded peripheral area of consolidation in the left upper lobe.

Pertussis (Whooping Cough)

Whooping cough is caused by the aerobic gram-negative coccobacillus *Bordetella (Hemophilus) pertussis.* Pneumonia due to this organism is less common now that immunization is available.

Radiographically,[19, 32, 90] the striking feature is extensive streaky peribronchial consolidation in one or more lobes. A recently reported large series comprising 238 patients ill enough to require admission to hospital provides a good indication of the chest radiographic findings in the modern era.[32] Sixty-three patients (26%) had abnormal findings on the chest radiograph. Pulmonary consolidation, which was predominantly peribronchial in distribution, was present in 50 patients, pulmonary collapse in 9 and visible lymphadenopathy in 22. The pulmonary changes showed a tendency to involve the right lung, particularly the lower and middle lobes. The peribronchial consolidation may be maximal close to the mediastinum (Fig 6–26), giving rise to an appearance that has been dubbed the "shaggy heart" sign.[19]

Melioidosis

Melioidosis[88] is due to the gram-negative bacillus *Pseudomonas pseudomallei,* an organism that resides in

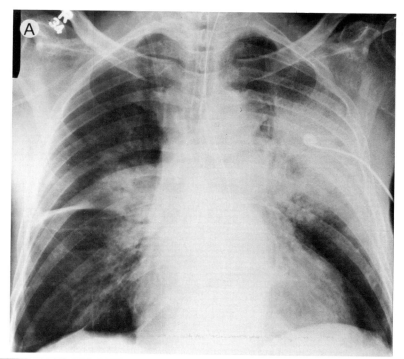

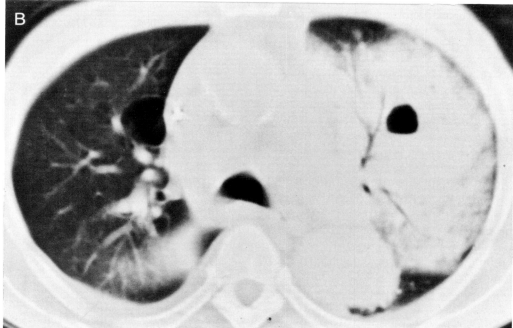

FIG 6–25.
Legionella pneumophila pneumonia showing multilobar confluent consolidation. The cavitation that can be seen in the plain film **(A)** is better demonstrated in the computed tomographic scan **(B)**.

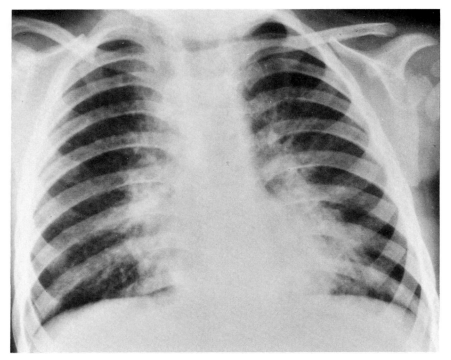

FIG 6–26.
Pertussis pneumonia showing peribronchial consolidation adjacent to the heart, giving rise to the "shaggy heart" sign.

dust and soil. Pneumonia due to this organism is rare except in the flooded fields and marshes of Southeast Asia. The pneumonia may be acute or subacute. The acute form is characterized by fulminating septicemia and acute prostration and it can be rapidly fatal. The subacute form consists of chest pain, occasional hemoptysis, low-grade fever, and weight loss. Some patients have few symptoms and are diagnosed only because pulmonary disease is found on chest radiography.

Radiographically,[156, 311] the acute pneumonia shows widespread bilateral small round ill-defined areas of consolidation, which may coalesce to form segmental or lobar opacities (Fig 6–27), and which have an affinity for the upper lobes. Cavitation is frequent, and the cavities may be thin-walled. Pleural effusion and empyema, though reported, are rare, as is hilar adenopathy.

In the subacute form, the plain chest radiograph shows segmental or lobar consolidation which often cavitates[311] and may be accompanied by empyema. In the subclinical form, the chest radiograph closely resembles post-primary tuberculosis with patchy upper lobe consolidation and cavitation.

Plague

Plague is due to *Yersinia (Pasteurella) pestis*, a gram-negative coccobacillus, which is still found in some areas of Asia, Africa, South America, and the Southwestern portions of the United States.[3, 261] Pneumonia may be primary, due to inhalation of infected droplets, or it may be spread hematogenously from infected swollen axillary or femoral lymph nodes, sometimes known as buboes. The resulting pneumonia is severe, with high fever and, in fatal cases, numerous petechiae and ecchymoses, the appearance of which gave rise to the name "Black Death" in the fearful epidemic which swept Europe in the 14th century.

Radiographically,[3] the pneumonia causes rapidly progressive dense patchy consolidations that may be nodular, segmental or lobar in shape. Eventually multiple lobes are involved, and mediastinal adenopathy and pleural effusions may be present. In some cases of bubonic plague the mediastinal/hilar adenopathy may be the only radiographic finding.

Tularemia

Tularemia, named after Tulare County in California, is due to *Francisella tularensis*, an aerobic

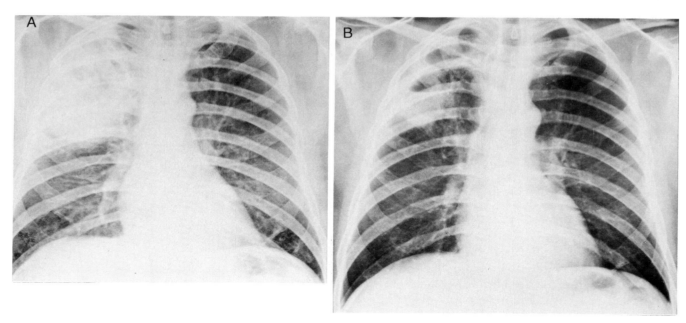

FIG 6–27.
Melioidosis pneumonia showing a large area of consolidation in right upper lobe **(A).** Six weeks later **(B)** the pneumonia has partially resolved, leaving a thin-walled abscess.

gram-negative coccobacillus. The disease is endemic in many parts of the world, including Europe, Asia, and North America. Though relatively uncommon, it is widely distributed in the United States.[276] Human infection is acquired in a variety of ways: through the skin in individuals who handle infected animals (rabbits, squirrels, skunks, dogs, game birds, and many others) or their skins; by bites from infected insect vectors, notably ticks and fleas; by bites from the infected animals themselves; or by inhalation of organisms from infected carcasses, dust, or following laboratory accidents. Pneumonia is a common finding in patients with tularemia.

The radiographic signs of tularemia pneumonia[9, 75, 216, 233, 276] are lobar, segmental, rounded, oval, or patchy pulmonary consolidations, which may be unilateral or bilateral in distribution (Fig 6–28). The most common pattern is unilateral patchy consolidation. Cavitation may occur but is unusual, and a pattern resembling pulmonary edema may also be encountered. Miliary nodulation was seen in one case in a large series.[276] The pulmonary changes may be accompanied by cardiomegaly owing to pericarditis with pericardial effusion. Hilar adenopathy is frequent, as are pleural effusions, both of which may be unilateral or bilateral. Empyema and bronchopleural fistula may supervene. The consolidations may, on rare occasions, heal with

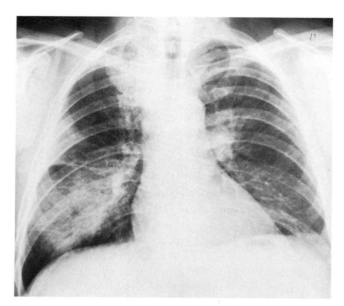

FIG 6–28.
Tularemia pneumonia showing multiple areas of consolidation in the right lung. Two weeks before this film was taken, the patient had run over a rabbit while mowing the lawn.

fibrosis and calcification and thus resemble tuberculosis and histoplasmosis.

Anaerobic Lung Infection

Most anaerobic lung infections result from aspiration of infected oral contents, and overt periodontal disease is seen in the majority of patients.[21] Predisposing factors such as a recent episode of altered consciousness, dysphagia, or alcoholism are almost always present.[21] Underlying bronchial carcinoma was found in 9% of patients in one large series.[21]

The infection is usually indolent or subacute,[181] though an acute febrile illness, closely resembling pneumococcal pneumonia but without shaking chills, may be seen.[20, 21] Often the sputum is putrid, a feature not encountered in pneumonia due to aerobic bacteria. In about half the cases, anaerobic organisms alone are responsible (the common ones are *Bacteroides, Fusobacterium, Peptococcus* and *Peptostreptococcus*, microaerophilic *Streptococcus*, and *Propionibacterium*); in the other half, mixed anaerobic and aerobic bacteria are found on culture. A pitfall here is that the anaerobic bacteria may not be appreciated unless especially cultured, and it may therefore be assumed that aerobic organisms are wholly responsible for the pneumonia.

The radiographic findings have been described in two large series of 69[181] and 143[21] patients. The appearances can be conveniently divided into pulmonary parenchymal infection, pneumonia with cavitation, and discrete lung abscess, each of which may be associated with empyema.

Anaerobic pneumonia has a strong predilection for the lower lobes (Figs 6–1 and 6–29), the right lung being more commonly affected than the left. These sites are entirely compatible with the belief that the pneumonia follows aspiration from the upper respiratory tract. There is usually one predominant focus of disease, but multilobe involvement is also common.

Cavitation within consolidation is seen in 30% to 40% of cases and it may develop while the patient is in the hospital on appropriate antibiotic therapy. One third of cases will have a discrete lung abscess (Fig 6–30). Discrete lung abscesses occur chiefly in the posterior portions of the lungs, usually in the posterior segments of the upper lobes or in the superior segments of the lower lobes. Those cases that develop cavitation or lung abscess take longer to resolve, with resolution sometimes taking 6 weeks or more. Hilar and mediastinal adenopathy may accompany lung abscess,[269] and such cases

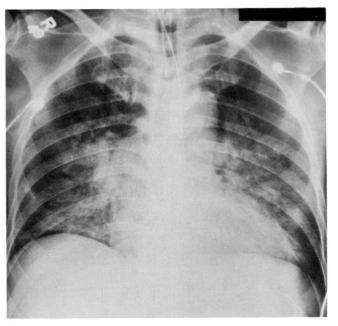

FIG 6–29.
Anaerobic aspiration pneumonia showing bilateral mid and lower zone consolidation.

may, therefore, closely resemble carcinoma of the lung.

One-third to one-half of cases will have an empyema.[21, 181] Both anaerobic and aerobic organisms are frequently grown from the pleural fluid. Over half the patients in one series of anaerobic bacterial empyema had no apparent parenchymal disease.[181] If pleural effusion is seen in association with anaerobic lung infection, it is virtually certain to be an empyema.[181] The infected fluid can be mobile, but is frequently loculated. Very large empyemas may be seen, and bronchopleural fistula is a recognized complication.

Leptospirosis

Leptospirosis, due to the spirochete *Leptospira*, is common in the tropics where it is the cause of Weil's disease, a syndrome comprising fever, jaundice, hemorrhage, nephritis, and meningitis.

Pneumonia occurs in one-fifth to two-thirds of patients with leptospirosis. The pulmonary consolidations are due to hemorrhagic pneumonitis and usually appear as poorly defined patchy areas of consolidation without loss of volume,[184] which in severe cases may be extensive and confluent.[184] Patchy discoid atelectasis and pleural effusions are common. Hilar/mediastinal adenopathy does not appear to be a feature.

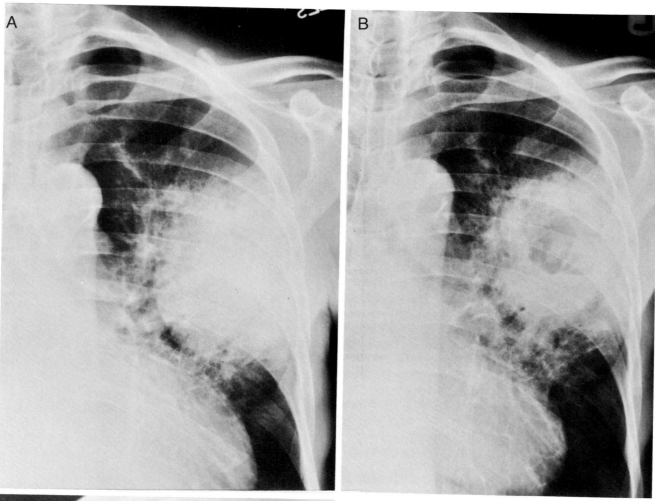

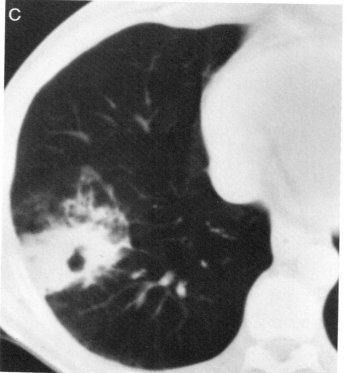

FIG 6–30.
Anaerobic bacterial lung abscess in an alcoholic patient with bad teeth. **A,** early in the course of the disease, there is a rounded area of pneumonia. **B,** two days later there is a discrete lung abscess. **C,** CT scan in another patient shows anaerobic bacterial pneumonia with cavitation.

Rickettsial Infections

Pneumonia due to rickettsial organisms is rare. The commonest is Q-fever, caused by *Coxiella burnetti*. Rocky Mountain spotted fever, caused by *Rickettsia rickettsii*, is occasionally encountered in the United States, mostly in the southeastern states, where it is transmitted through tick bites.

Q-fever occurs worldwide and is acquired from cattle or sheep products, infected dust, or occasionally from the bite of infected ticks or mites. The disease occurs sporadically and in epidemics. The symptoms are sudden in onset comprising a flulike illness with fever, dry cough, myalgias, arthralgias, and headache. Less than half those infected develop pneumonia. The usual radiographic appearance of Q-fever pneumonia[127, 215] (Fig 6–31) is subsegmental, segmental, or lobar consolidation, frequently accompanied by patchy atelectasis that is often discoid in shape. Spherical (round) pneumonia is common, particularly in epidemic cases. Pleural effusions are seen in some patients, particularly in sporadic infection. The disease is self-limiting, but resolution of pulmonary consolidation may be slow—up to 70 days, with the average time being 30 days.[215]

Small vessel inflammation is the basic pathologic process in Rocky Mountain spotted fever. The resulting pulmonary vasculitis leads to a variety of radiographic patterns of pulmonary infection, varying from unifocal or multifocal consolidations resembling bacterial pneumonia, to widespread pulmonary infection resembling pulmonary edema, combined in some cases with pleural effusions.[185, 204] The pulmonary edema pattern is probably caused by pulmonary capillary endothelial damage combined with the effect of increased hydrostatic forces due to left-sided heart failure.[78] The pathological end result is interstitial and alveolar edema and hemorrhage, together with a mononuclear and lymphocytic interstitial infiltrate.[204] Bacterial superinfection appears to be rare.[78] The clinical diagnosis depends on recognizing a multiorgan vasculitis, notably of the skin and meninges, in an acutely febrile patient during the tick season in endemic areas.

Chlamydia Infections

Chlamydia psittaci infection, so-called ornithosis or psittacosis, is usually acquired from infected birds. Infection with the psittacosis agent may result in disease of wide clinical spectrum, ranging from completely asymptomatic infections recognized only by serologic means to overwhelming illness involving multiple organ systems.[292] Usually the patient complains of fever, malaise, headache, and a nonproductive cough, and the clinical picture may be indistinguishable from acute bacterial pneumonia with pleuritic chest pain, productive cough, hemoptysis, shortness of breath, and shaking chills. The chest radiograph reveals patchy pulmonary consolidation (Fig 6–32), which can be very extensive. Another described pattern is patchy reticular shadowing with lower zone predominance which appears more severe than would be expected from the clinical features. Pleural effusions are rare.

Chlamydia trachomatis is a recently recognized cause of pneumonia in neonates and infants, where it may cause widespread streaky consolidations and air trapping similar to that seen with acute bronchiolitis of viral origin.[253] In the few reported cases in adults, the chest radiographs showed focal streaky consolidation without evidence of air trapping. Pleural effusion, though reported, is not a striking feature.[84, 309]

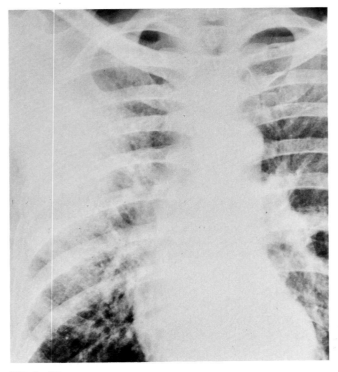

FIG 6–31.
Q-fever. There is a large focal consolidation in the right upper lobe.

PULMONARY TUBERCULOSIS

In economically developed countries tuberculosis is no longer the scourge it was at the turn of the

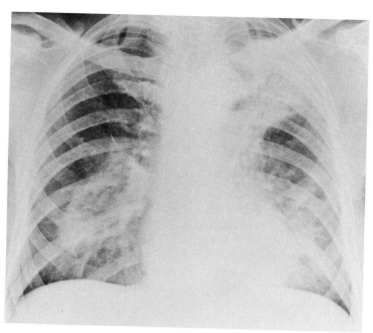

FIG 6–32.
Psittacosis pneumonia. Multifocal bilateral consolidations are seen.

century. Nevertheless, some 22,000 new cases were reported in the United States in 1985.[49] Many cases represent reactivation of tuberculosis acquired when the disease was more prevalent. Social deprivation or substance abuse plays a role in many of the new cases of tuberculosis, and the increasing prevalence of acquired immune deficiency syndrome (AIDS) raises the specter of a rising incidence of complicating tuberculosis with additional risks to health workers and other persons.[244] Almost all cases are caused by infection with the human strain of *M. tuberculosis* and the remainder by the so-called atypical mycobacteria, notably *M. kansasii* and *M. avium-intracellulare*.

The inflammatory response to tuberculous infection differs from the usual inflammatory response to infecting microorganisms in that it is modified substantially by a hypersensitivity reaction to components of the tubercle bacillus. It is uncertain to what extent the hypersensitivity reaction is advantageous or deleterious in resisting and controlling infection.

The initial response to primary tuberculous infection[246] is a polymorphonuclear leukocyte infiltration akin to the usual inflammatory reaction to bacterial infection. The response, however, devolves to a greater extent upon macrophages and lymphocytes, resulting in a more indolent inflammatory reaction. The macrophages become compacted and modified to form epithelioid cells, and multinucleated giant cells and lymphocytes infiltrate the pe-

riphery of the tubercles. Delayed hypersensitivity becomes manifest some 4 to 10 weeks after the initial infection, a positive tuberculin reaction being evidence of this development. The hallmark of hypersensitivity is the development of caseous necrosis in the pulmonary focus or in the involved lymph nodes. The periphery of the tubercle shows fibrocyte proliferation, with the laying down of a capsule of collagen. Inflammatory involvement of the regional lymph nodes in the hilus and in the mediastinum is a dominant feature, particularly in the younger individual. In primary tuberculous infections, the pulmonary focus and the adenopathy may resolve without trace, or may leave a focus of caseous necrosis, scarring, or calcification.

Various terms are applied to the form of tuberculosis which develops and progresses under the influence of established hypersensitivity. These terms include post-primary, secondary, or reactivation tuberculosis. The term reactivation tuberculosis, though not ideal because the disease may on occasion evolve from primary tuberculosis without a latent interval, does serve to emphasize that most cases represent reactivation of endogenous infection rather than reinfection with *M. tuberculosis*.[304] Reactivation tuberculosis develops under the immediate influence of hypersensitivity, which accelerates the changes described above. In particular, caseous necrosis occurs at an early stage in the process. Involvement of the regional lymph nodes is not a feature of reactivation tuberculosis; whether this is by virtue of the hypersensitivity reaction or acquired immunity is uncertain. Factors that predispose to reactivation of tuberculosis include aging, malnutrition, uremia, diabetes mellitus, alcoholism, silicosis, cancer, familial and acquired immune deficiency diseases, and drug-induced immunosuppression.[186, 244]

The gross morphologic features of reactivation tuberculosis[246] can be subdivided into:

1. The foci of acute tuberculous infiltration in the pulmonary parenchyma.

2. Cavity formation. Air spaces in a tuberculous process may represent excavated foci of caseous necrosis or, alternatively, pneumatoceles or bullae which follow fibrous contraction or endobronchial disease.

3. Fibrosis and distortion of lung architecture.

The extent of the fibrosis and damage to the lung will depend on such factors as the amount of caseous necrosis and the severity of associated endobronchial and pleural disease. Fibrous tissue contracts as it matures, and even quiescent lesions may show increased contraction and distortion over an extended period of observation.

4. Calcification. Dystrophic calcification may occur in foci of caseous necrosis. Such calcification takes a considerable time to become radiographically visible and is, therefore, often associated with pulmonary fibrosis or tuberculoma formation.

5. Tuberculoma formation: namely, a focus of tuberculosis in which the processes of activity and containment are finely balanced. The result is a fairly discrete nodule or mass in which repeated extensions of infection have created a core of caseous necrosis surrounded by a mantle of epithe-

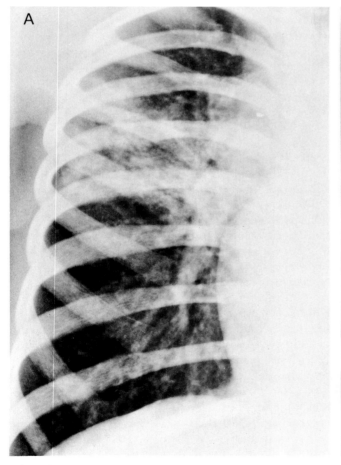

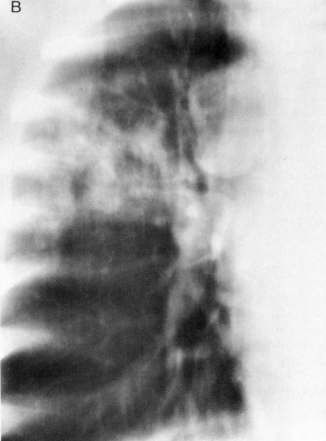

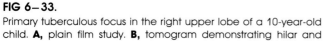

FIG 6–33.
Primary tuberculous focus in the right upper lobe of a 10-year-old child. **A,** plain film study. **B,** tomogram demonstrating hilar and mediastinal adenopathy to better advantage. Note the slight constriction of the right upper lobe bronchus.

lioid cells and collagen with peripheral round-cell infiltration.

Both primary and reactivation tuberculosis may extend to extrathoracic sites such as the gastrointestinal tract, larynx, kidneys, bones and joints, and the central nervous system. In these cases it is generally thought that the primary portal of entry is the lungs, even though in many instances there is no radiographic evidence of pulmonary tuberculosis. Tuberculosis of the larynx and gastrointestinal tract both have a high association with visible active pulmonary tuberculosis.[13, 302]

The Radiographic Appearances of Pulmonary and Pleural Tuberculosis

Tuberculosis may involve the lungs in patterns of disease which reflect a number of factors: the host's immune status, the existence of hypersensitivity from previous infection, the method of spread of disease, and an incompletely understood tendency of the disease to affect certain portions of the lungs. The radiographic appearances can be considered under the broad headings of primary tuberculosis and reactivation tuberculosis. These very broad patterns of disease may overlap or undergo transformation from one pattern to another.

Primary Tuberculosis

Formerly, the initial infection with *M. tuberculosis* usually occurred in childhood; however, primary tuberculosis has been increasingly encountered in an adult population. In a recent series,[341] over half the cases of primary tuberculosis occurred in individuals 18 years of age or older, and one-quarter of all adult cases were deemed to represent the primary form of the disease. The division between primary tuberculosis and post-primary or reactivation tuberculosis is by no means clear-cut, and some 10% of all cases of primary tuberculosis may evolve without any interval into a chronic progressive form of the disease indistinguishable from reactivation tuberculosis.[118]

Classically, the tubercle bacillus causes a nonspecific focal pneumonitis (Fig 6–33). In approximately one-half of cases, the primary pulmonary foci are never identified or documented. Indeed the chest radiograph may remain entirely normal despite definite conversion of tuberculin sensitivity or the presence of positive sputum cultures. The predominant radiographic feature of primary tuberculosis is the presence of adenopathy in the appropriate lymph drainage pathways (Figs 6–33 and 6–34). The resultant hilar adenopathy is usually unilateral, and any mediastinal adenopathy is contiguous to the affected hilus. In some patients, hilar adenopathy may

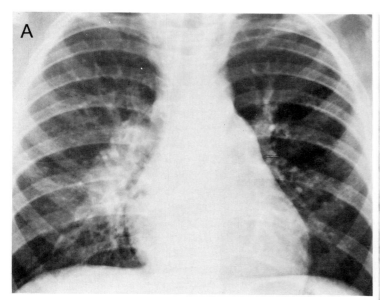

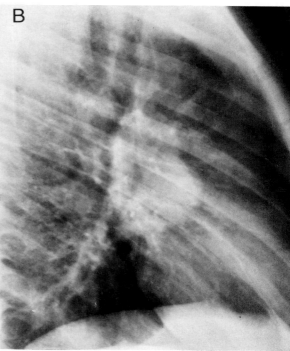

FIG 6–34.
Primary tuberculosis in a 5-year-old child with right hilar adenopathy but no pulmonary consolidation. **A,** PA view. **B,** lateral view.

be bilateral, or mediastinal adenopathy may occur alone. The adenopathy may be strikingly severe and extensive, particularly in African and Asian individuals (Fig 6–35), and may closely resemble lymphoma, metastatic disease, or sarcoidosis. In the middle-aged or elderly patient lymph node enlargement is, in general, far less common and less apparent than it is in the child.[35]

The pulmonary foci of primary tuberculosis are randomly distributed and range from small, ill-defined parenchymal shadows to segmental or lobar consolidation. Slight expansion of consolidated lobes may be noted (Fig 6–36). In the absence of cavitation, consolidation of segments or lobes produces a radiographic picture indistinguishable from that of the bacterial pneumonias. The time course is, however, different, with tuberculous pneumonia being much more indolent, often taking weeks or months to clear. Primary tuberculosis may be masslike and, in an adult, the disease may be confused with conditions such as Wegener's granulomatosis or pulmonary neoplasia (Fig 6–37). A single pulmonary focus occurs in most instances, but multiple foci may be encountered. The incidence of cavitation varies, having been found in 10%[55] to 30% of cases.[341] The pulmonary focus frequently resolves without trace or, alternatively, it may evolve into a small nodule or

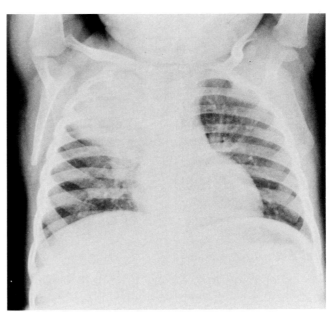

FIG 6–36.
Primary tuberculosis, with a large area of consolidation in the right upper lobe causing expansion of the lobe.

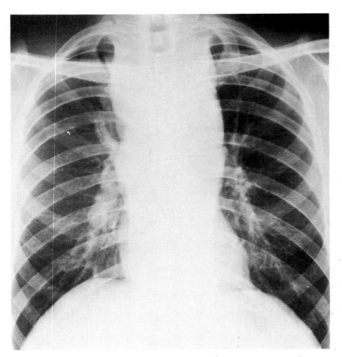

FIG 6–35.
Massive mediastinal adenopathy and slight right hilar adenopathy in a young black man with primary tuberculosis.

scar which may then calcify. Such calcifications may be observed following primary tuberculosis in up to 20% of patients. Hilar or mediastinal lymph node calcification is observed more frequently, being seen in some 35% of cases[329] (Fig 6–38). Single or multiple tuberculomas may develop in primary tuberculosis, but they are seen much less frequently than in reactivation tuberculosis.

Pleural effusions are fairly common, at least in those cases which have been studied in major hospitals, occurring in approximately one-quarter of patients. The effusions are generally unilateral and are usually associated with some identifiable pulmonary parenchymal abnormality.

Segmental or lobar airway narrowing is frequent and may be caused by endobronchial tuberculosis or by extrinsic pressure from enlarged lymph nodes (Fig 6–39). The result is usually segmental or lobar atelectasis, but air-trapping may occur occasionally (Fig 6–40).

Pulmonary tuberculosis associated with AIDS has many of the clinical and radiographic features of primary tuberculosis, even when there is strong evidence that the disease represents reactivation of previously acquired infection.[244] The hypersensitivity reaction appears to be in abeyance, and cavitation does not usually occur. The consolidations may be noted in any part of the lungs and hilar and mediastinal adenopathy are usual. Extrathoracic dissemina-

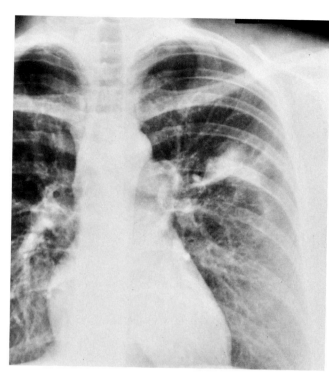

FIG 6–37.
Primary tuberculosis in a young adult resembling neoplasm. There is an area of rounded consolidation in the left upper zone together with left hilar adenopathy.

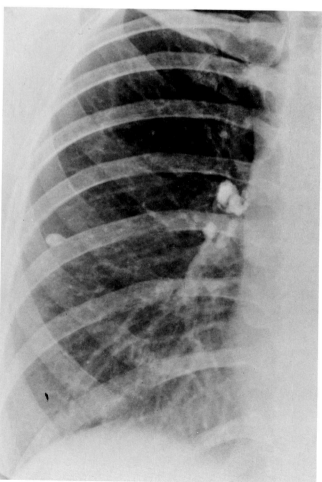

FIG 6–38.
A calcified tuberculous focus with calcification in the corresponding hilar lymph nodes.

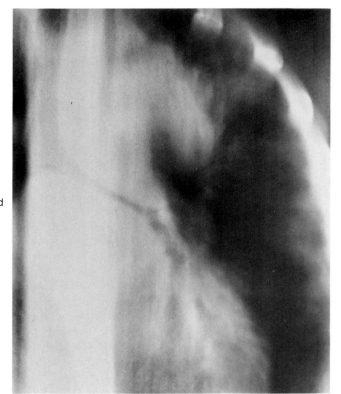

FIG 6–39.
Primary tuberculosis in the left upper lobe with elongation and narrowing of the left main stem bronchus.

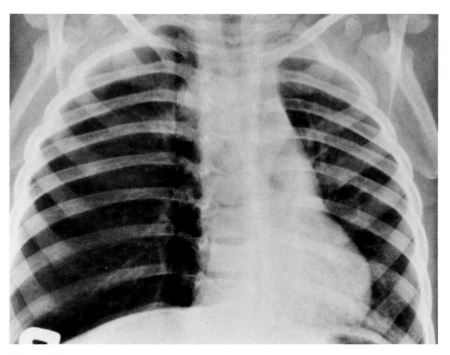

FIG 6–40.
Radiograph of a child with bronchoscopically proved primary endobronchial tuberculosis. There is right paratracheal adenopathy and marked hyperexpansion of the entire right lung.

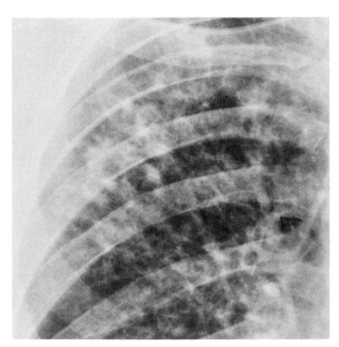

FIG 6–41.
Early reactivation tuberculosis showing patchy small shadows with
ill-defined margins.

tion, miliary tuberculosis, and endobronchial spread
are definite risks in patients with AIDS, and there is
a much higher than normal incidence of positive
sputum cultures for *M. tuberculosis*. Concomitant infections, for example with *Pneumocystis carinii*, are
common and may result in diagnostic confusion.

Reactivation Tuberculosis

Focal Pulmonary Tuberculosis

In the earlier phases, reactivation tuberculosis
gives rise to patchy subsegmental consolidations with
ill-defined margins (Fig 6–41) and a tendency to coalesce so that there may be small satellite foci in the
adjacent lung. There is a predilection for the posterior aspects of the upper lobes and the superior segments of the lower lobes, although no portion of the
lungs is immune (Fig 6–42). Bilateral and multilobar
involvement is fairly frequent. The consolidations
are usually peripheral in location and, therefore, air
bronchograms are not present. Some focal pleural
thickening may be present in the early stages, even
in the absence of pleural effusions (Fig 6–43).

Cavitation is a distinct feature of reactivation tuberculosis and is a finding of considerable diagnostic
significance since it indicates a high likelihood of activity (Fig 6–44). Even quite small pulmonary foci
may cavitate, and multiple cavities of varying size
may be present. Fluid levels may be present (see Fig
6–44) and may aid in the recognition of cavities, the

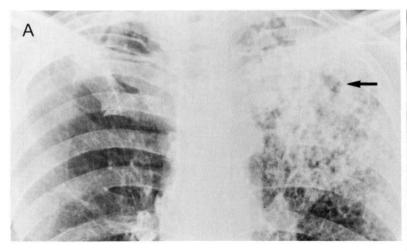
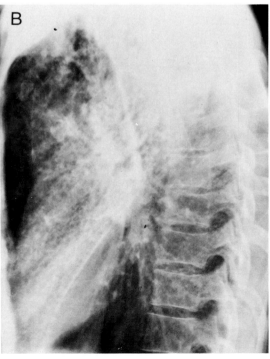

FIG 6–42.
Reactivation tuberculosis involving the left upper lobe with at least one area of
cavitation *(arrow)*. **A,** frontal view. **B,** the lateral radiograph indicates
predominant involvement of the apical and posterior segments of the left
upper lobe.

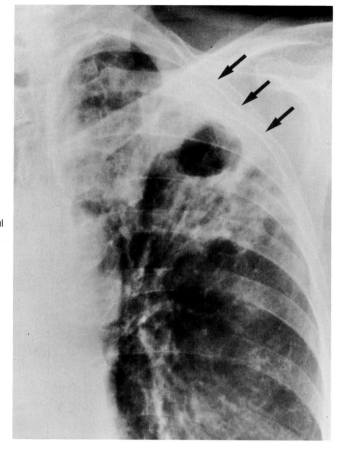

FIG 6–43.
Cavitary reactivation tuberculosis showing localized pleural thickening *(arrows)*.

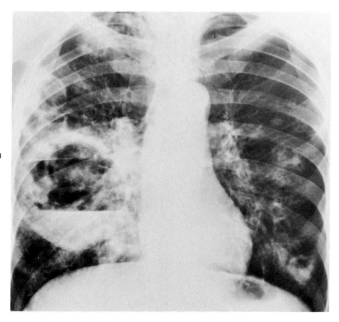

FIG 6–44.
Reactivation tuberculosis with a large cavitary lesion containing an air-fluid level in the right lower lobe. Other smaller cavitary lesions are seen in other lobes.

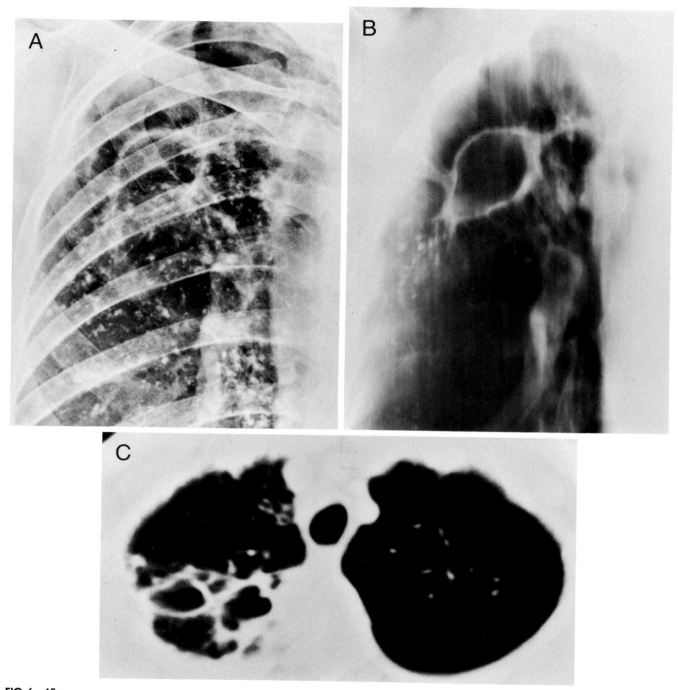

FIG 6–45.
Fibrocalcific reactivation tuberculosis with cavitation. **A,** plain film. **B,** conventional tomogram in the same patient showing the cavity clearly. **C,** CT examination in a different patient showing cavitation in reactivation tuberculosis of the posterior segment of the right upper lobe.

walls of which may be indistinct or obscured by overlying densities.[203] Frequently, however, fluid levels are not present. Apical bullae, if present, may be misinterpreted as cavitation, a mistake that can often be avoided if it is borne in mind that cavities are centered within areas of consolidation and do not merely overlap them. Additional views such as apical lordotic views, conventional tomography, or CT may be employed if there is doubt about the presence of possible cavitation (Fig 6–45). Patients with cavitary disease represent an actual or potential threat to those who come into contact with them and, therefore, it may be entirely appropriate to institute immediate infective precautions on the basis of the radiographic findings alone.

Even in the absence of specific therapy there is a tendency for the lesions to become contained by the granulomatous and fibrous response of the adjacent lung. In the preantibiotic era the response was, of course, a fairly prolonged process that was often measured in years. Specific antituberculous therapy has radically shortened the time required for healing, and the healing process is usually more complete. Radiographically, containment is suggested by increasing definition of the tuberculous foci and the development of fibrosis in the surrounding lung. Gradual fibrous contraction of the affected segment or lobe is shown by fissural displacement or distortion of the vascular structures in the hilus. Bronchiectasis develops in the affected lung and is often much more severe than can be appreciated from plain films (Fig 6–46). Calcification is often seen in areas of caseous necrosis coincident with the increasing fibrosis. Fluid levels in cavities, when present,

disappear. The cavities themselves either disappear or remain as chronic cavities, often with a relatively smooth inner wall.

Tuberculous Lobar Pneumonia and Bronchopneumonia

An entire lobe can become consolidated (Fig 6–47), and cavitation often occurs within the affected lobe. Heavy seeding of the bronchial tree is likely, particularly in the presence of cavitation, and smaller foci of disease may be found in other parts of the lungs. Although overshadowed by the lobar pneumonia, these foci may be extremely important in indicating the true nature of the process. Sequential films will show that tuberculous lobar pneumonia is more chronic and indolent than the usual cavitary pneumonias.

Widespread bronchopneumonia presumably results from a breakdown in host defenses with spread of disease by way of the airways. It is usually patchy and bilateral (Fig 6–48) and may involve portions of lung less commonly affected by tuberculosis such as the middle lobe or the anterior segments of the upper lobes. Fibrocalcific changes may be seen else-

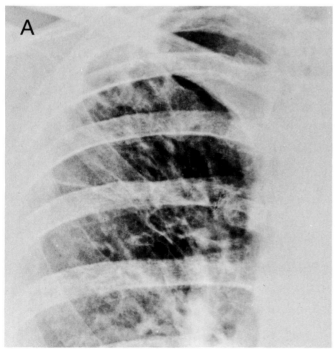

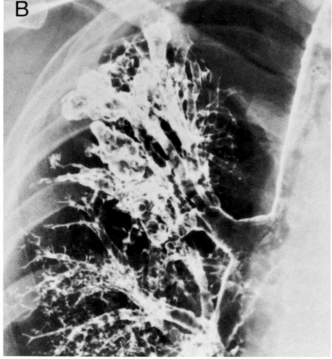

FIG 6–46.
Fibrous contraction of the right upper lobe. **A,** plain film showing possible small peripheral cavities. **B,** bronchogram in the same patient revealing the full extent and the severity of the underlying bronchial changes.

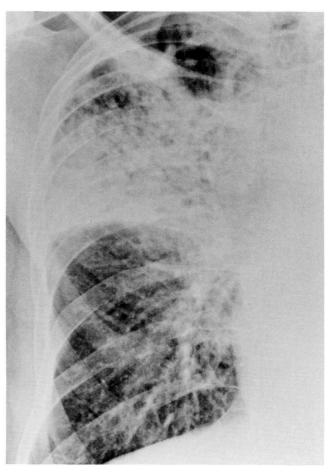

FIG 6–47.
Tuberculous pneumonia showing lobar consolidation of the right upper lobe.

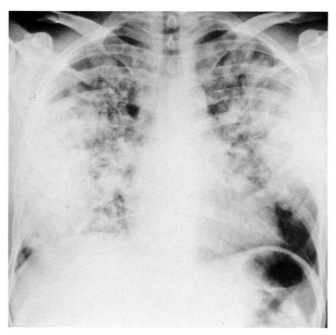

FIG 6–48.
Tuberculous bronchopneumonia without evidence of cavitation or any identifiable originating focus.

where in the lungs if the bronchopneumonia stems from breakdown of preexisting chronic fibrocaseous tuberculosis.

In immunocompromised hosts, tuberculous bronchopneumonia may become very extensive and may be rapidly fatal. Cavitation need not be present in the early phases even when extensive patchy confluent perihilar consolidation is present.

Endobronchial Tuberculosis

On occasion, a tuberculous focus may arise in or extend into a major bronchus. Tuberculous granulations and granulomatous cicatrization may then cause a bronchial stricture, which in turn can cause obstructive emphysema or atelectasis. The associated pulmonary parenchymal lesions may be obscured by the atelectasis, and it may be difficult or impossible to ascertain the underlying cause of the atelectasis from the chest radiographs (Fig 6–49).

Broncholiths represent an interesting late complication of pulmonary tuberculosis (Fig 6–50).[325] A calcified lymph node may erode into an adjacent airway and be associated with hemoptysis or pneumonia. The peripheral lung may show evidence of atelectasis resulting from bronchial obstruction or areas of consolidation related to aspiration of blood or post-obstructive pneumonia. On occasion, air trapping may occur if the broncholith causes ball valve obstruction. A broncholith in one of the segmental bronchi is easy to overlook because calcifications at hilar level are assumed to be in lymph nodes outside the bronchial lumen. Broncholiths in the lobar or main bronchi may be more clearly centered within the airway, a finding that is readily confirmed by using tomography, particularly CT.[293] Bronchoscopic removal of broncholiths may be attended by severe hemoptysis caused by coincident erosion of the broncholith into the accompanying branch of the pulmonary artery. Hence establishing the diagnosis noninvasively has practical significance. Broncholithiasis may also be diagnosed retrospectively if a previously documented calcification disappears.

Tuberculoma Formation

Tuberculomas are discrete tumor-like foci of tuberculosis in which there is a fine balance between activity and repair. The margins of a tuberculoma

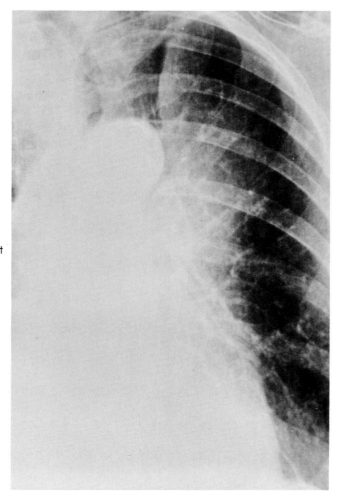

FIG 6–49.
Endobronchial tuberculosis producing complete collapse of the left upper lobe.

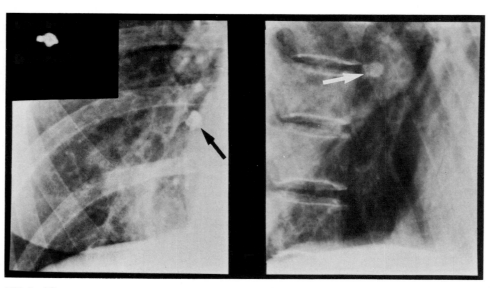

FIG 6–50.
A peripheral broncholith in the right lower lobe *(arrows)* with a wedge of peripheral consolidation. The insert *(top left)* shows the broncholith removed at bronchoscopy.

are usually well circumscribed, although there may be some irregularity or focal loss of definition because of adjacent fibrous changes (Fig 6–51). Tuberculomas may be multiple and on occasion may become large, up to 5 cm in diameter. Some growth may be perceptible over an extended period of observation. Calcification develops in the central caseous core with time, and it is often detectable radiographically. It may be amorphous, and if the core is large in relation to the cellular mantle, a nodule of uniform increased density will result, whereas with a more confined central core of calcification a line of demarcation may be apparent (Fig 6–52). Calcifications that are more laminar, flecklike, or punctate also occur and are then easier to appreciate because variable density is noted within the nodule. Tuberculomas show little tendency to break down, and cavitation is rare. Cavitation strongly suggests reactivation.

Miliary Tuberculosis

Miliary tuberculosis, which results from hematogenous dissemination of the disease, is an infrequent but feared complication of both primary and

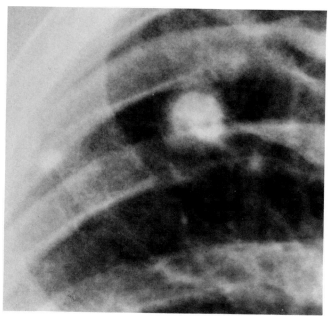

FIG 6–52.
Two apical tuberculomas. The smaller, lateral tuberculoma is uniformly dense. Contrast its density with that of the adjacent ribs. The larger tuberculoma has a low-density mantle around a large calcified core.

reactivation tuberculosis. The lungs are beset by myriads of 2- to 3-mm granulomata, likened in size and appearance to millet seeds. Radiographically, the result is widespread fine nodules, which are uniformly distributed and equal in size (Fig 6–53). Because there is a threshold below which the nodules are invisible, miliary tuberculosis can be present in patients whose chest radiographs show no abnormalities. Then, when the nodules reach a critical threshold in size or number they may suddenly become visible. Similarly, on or about this threshold the nodules may disappear and reappear on serial radiographs. Miliary tuberculosis does not leave residual calcifications. Miliary nodulation of the lung has numerous causes other than tuberculosis but tuberculosis is the preeminent consideration because prompt diagnosis and treatment are vital.

Miliary tuberculosis is a rare cause of the adult respiratory distress syndrome and, in such cases, the diagnosis can be extraordinarily difficult because the miliary nodules are superimposed on a more diffuse, less structured background of pulmonary density.[70] Equally problematic are the rare cases in which miliary tuberculosis complicates preexisting interstitial lung disease. In the illustrated case of miliary tuberculosis complicating silicosis, the diagnosis was only established at autopsy (Fig 6–54). Even

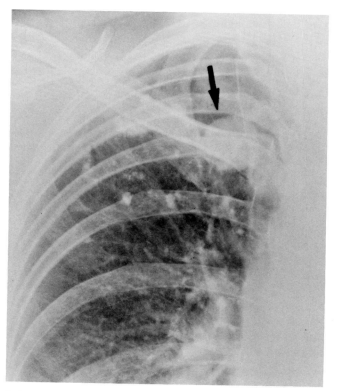

FIG 6–51.
Tuberculoma. Note the well-defined pulmonary nodule *(arrow)* as well as the associated fibrocalcific scarring in the adjacent lung.

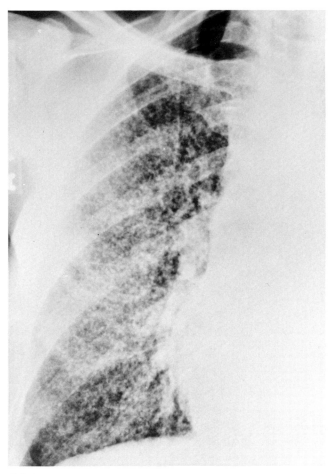

FIG 6–53.
Miliary tuberculosis showing widespread uniformly distributed fine nodulation of the lungs.

with successful therapy the miliary nodulation may take weeks or months to clear.

Tuberculous Pleuritis

Any tuberculous focus may involve the adjacent pleura, and some degree of focal pleural thickening and scarring is relatively common. Pleural effusions are not infrequent in patients with widespread tuberculosis. Tuberculous pleuritis, which may occur in the absence of a visible pulmonary focus, must be considered in the differential diagnosis of any large unilateral pleural effusion for which no adequate cause can be established radiographically, clinically, or by pleural fluid analysis. CT scans may demonstrate a pulmonary focus that is not visible on the plain chest radiograph.[149] On occasion, pleural biopsy may be necessary to establish the diagnosis of tuberculous pleuritis.

The response of tuberculous pleurisy to appropriate treatment is varied. All traces of pleural reaction may clear, but it is common to have some residual pleural scarring with obliteration of the costophrenic sulcus and distortion of the diaphragm. Residual thickening may be quite severe, and it is in these cases particularly that the lung can become restricted by the encompassing fibrous tissue and calcification.

Tuberculous pleurisy may become localized and form a tuberculous empyema. The empyema may break through the parietal pleura to form a subcutaneous abscess, the so-called empyema necessitans. The empyema cavity may also be connected to the bronchial tree by a fistulous track (Figs 6–55 and 6–56). Drainage of such lesions may result in a chronic bronchopleural fistula that can be extremely resistant to treatment. CT scanning is extremely useful in delineating foci of activity in pleural tuberculosis evidenced by fluid collections within the rind of pleural thickening. Even bronchopleural fistulae may be delineated by these axial images.[149] Tuberculosis was at one time a fairly common cause of spontaneous pneumothorax, although today this complication is rare.

Assessment of Activity

Chest radiography clearly plays a vital role in the detection and control of pulmonary tuberculosis. Serial radiography is important in gauging the activity of lesions and their response to treatment. It is hazardous to gauge activity on the basis of a single radiographic examination; even though fibrous infiltration and calcification may be prominent features, active foci may nonetheless be present. Tuberculous foci which appear inactive over an extended period of observation may contain viable organisms with the potential to break down under adverse circumstances. Miliary nodulation definitely indicates activity, and cavitation is a strong indication of active disease. In actual practice, one is often obliged to base certain judgments on the findings in a single radiographic examination. For example, isolation and aggressive investigation may be urged for one patient, whereas another may be allowed to proceed to routine surgery in the face of some seemingly "inactive" fibrocalcific apical scarring. Nevertheless, one cannot afford to be too cavalier about the latter type of case and some minimum additional study is advisable— for example, comparison with any previous radiographic studies or a follow-up examination.

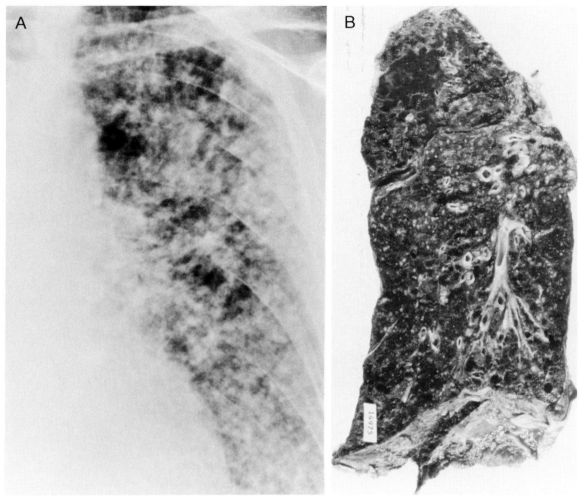

FIG 6–54.
Studies of an 85-year-old male with silicosis. **A,** plain chest radiograph. **B,** autopsy specimen showing miliary tuberculosis *(white dots)* set on a background of extensive anthracotic nodulation.

Hemoptysis in Pulmonary Tuberculosis

Hemoptysis is an important feature of active pulmonary tuberculosis. It may also be seen in patients whose disease is inactive, but who have developed a complication. For instance, bronchial carcinoma may have developed in an area damaged by tuberculous disease[266] or, alternatively, the tuberculous lesion may have become reactivated because of an alteration in the cancer patient's immune system.[166] A mycetoma may have developed in a tuberculous cavity (see the discussion of pulmonary aspergillosis in the section "Fungal Disease" later in this chapter), or the bleeding may be from bronchiectasis that resulted from the tuberculous infec-tion. The bronchial arteries supplying the bronchiectatic lung can be enormous (Fig 6–57). Finally, and very rarely, a mycotic aneurysm, the so-called Rasmussen aneurysm, may have developed[257] (see p. 384).

Effects of Pulmonary Collapse Therapy

Some of the most remarkable radiographs result from various forms of collapse therapy dating from the preantibiotic era. The thoracoplasty involved resecting a varied number of ribs to collapse the chest wall onto the underlying lung (Fig 6–58). In many instances, only a small portion of the lung at the base remained aerated, and the majority of the lung was

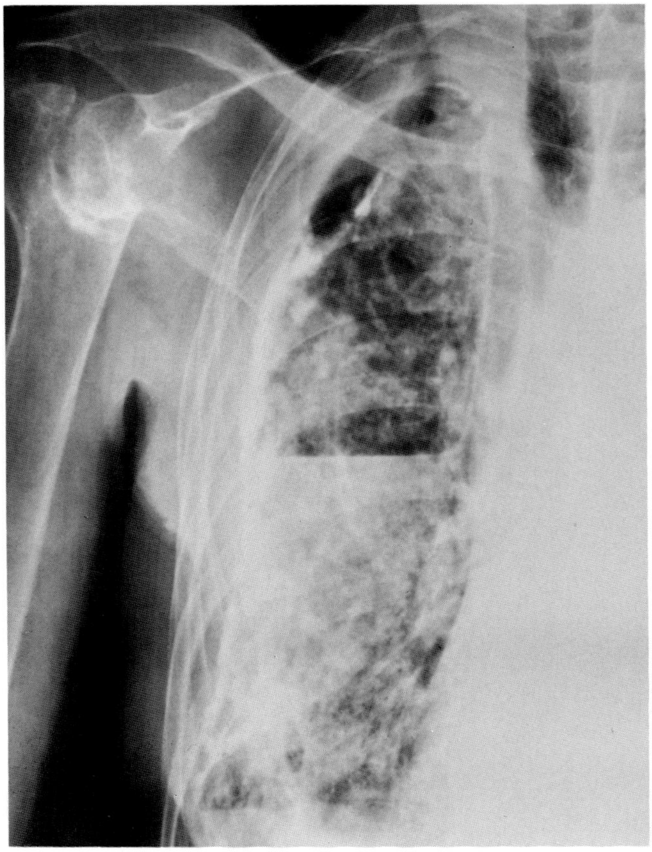

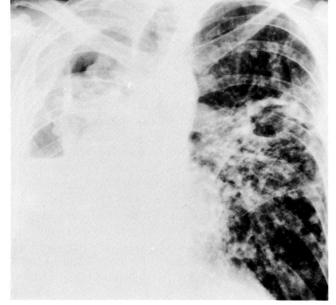

FIG 6–55.
Radiograph of an elderly man with long-standing tuberculosis. There is extensive partially calcified pleural thickening, a bronchopleural fistula resulting in a hydropneumothorax, and tuberculous arthritis of the shoulder.

FIG 6–56.
A middle-aged alcoholic patient with widespread reactivation tuberculosis. The right lung is almost destroyed and a bronchopleural fistula has resulted in a hydropneumothorax.

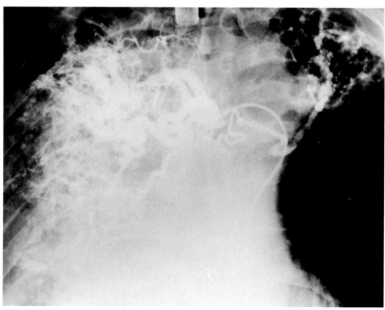

FIG 6–57.
A selective bronchial arteriogram in a patient with chronic fibrocavitary tuberculosis and hemoptysis. The bronchial artery has dimensions comparable to those of a normal femoral artery.

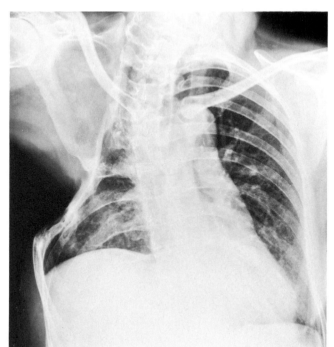

FIG 6–58.
View of a right thoracoplasty involving the upper eight ribs with partial collapse of the underlying lung. There was no evidence of active disease for many years.

obliterated. There was, of course, at least some residual fibrocalcific thickening underlying the thoracoplasty. Various other materials or objects were inserted extrapleurally to compress the underlying lung. These included paraffin, mineral oil, and lucite balls (Fig 6–59, A and B). Collapse therapy with pneumothoraces produced pleural thickening.

THE ATYPICAL MYCOBACTERIA

A number of mycobacteria other than *M. tuberculosis* have been identified as causes of pulmonary infection. These include *M. kansasii, M. avium-intracellulare, M. fortuitum,* and *M. gordonae.* It appears that *M. kansasii* is the most common cause of atypical mycobacterial infection.

One of the problems in the study of the clinical and radiographic manifestations of atypical mycobacterial infections has been that these organisms may occur as incidental contaminants. A further problem is that atypical mycobacterial infections have a predilection for individuals with preexisting chronic obstructive pulmonary disease, and it may be difficult to determine the clinical significance of a positive culture for one of the atypical mycobacteria in such patients.

The classic features of atypical mycobacterial infections of the lung are, in essence, those of a chronic indolent fibrocavitary process usually involving one or both apical regions of the lungs in a middle-aged or older individual with underlying chronic obstructive pulmonary disease. In many instances the radiographic features are indistinguishable from those of reactivation tuberculosis (Fig 6–60). The response to antituberculous therapy may be poor, and a seemingly inexorable progression of the disease over a period of years is frequent. This applies especially to infections with *M. avium-intracellulare.* Localized pleural reactions occur, but pleural effusions are uncommon. Adenopathy is distinctly unusual, as

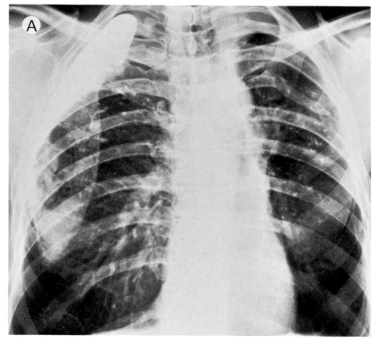

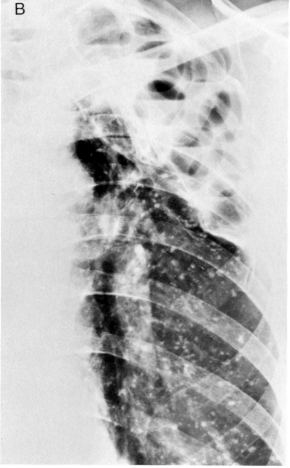

FIG 6–59.
A, collapse therapy by mineral oil injection (oleothorax). **B,** collapse therapy using lucite balls.

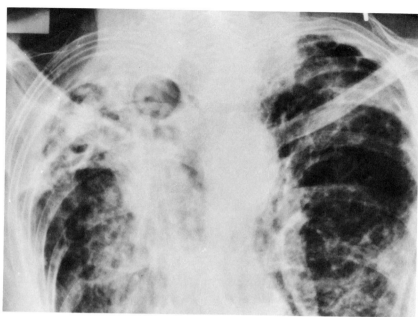

FIG 6–60.
Study of elderly male with long-standing obstructive pulmonary disease. Indolent fibro-cavitary disease in both lungs is caused by *M. avium-intracellulare*.

is miliary spread of disease. The lesions have the same predilection for the posterior aspects of the upper lobes or the superior segments of the lower lobe as reactivation tuberculosis.

Cavitation is a distinct feature of atypical mycobacterial infection and occurs in up to 96% of patients.[56] Some emphasis has been placed on a tendency for the cavity or cavities to be thin walled (Fig 6–61), but this was found in only one-third of Christensen's cases.[56]

In their series, Albelda et al.[1] placed greater reliance on the tissue diagnosis of the atypical mycobacterioses and in doing so were able to identify a separate group of patients who did not match the classic radiologic description. They found a subgroup in whom patchy nodular infiltrates were observed in a peribronchial distribution. Upper lobe prevalence was not present. In one-half of the group, cavities were noted in the nodules, and this feature—combined with the distribution of the lesions—gave a superficial resemblance to bronchiectasis. The radiographic findings in individual cases were, on the whole, fairly nonspecific and unlikely to suggest more than chronic diffuse lower airway disease. Ordinarily such cases may not be subjected to the aggressive investigation seemingly required for their identification. In practice, it is the group with the classic features of indolent inexorably progressive apical fibrocavitary disease resistant to antituberculous therapy that is likely to be

aggressively investigated. Hence, the radiographic descriptions may have concentrated on this group of patients to the exclusion of cases with more diffuse and less obvious radiographic manifestations. Nevertheless, it seems intuitively likely that

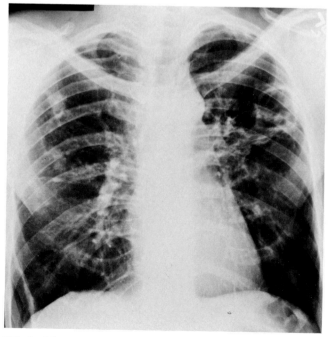

FIG 6–61.
Atypical mycobacterial infection in an alcoholic patient showing thin-walled cavities bilaterally, particularly in the left upper lobe.

the cases with obvious progressive lung destruction are clinically the most significant.

NOCARDIOSIS

Most cases of pulmonary nocardiosis are due to *Nocardia asteroides*, though other *Nocardia* species are occasionally implicated, notably *N. brasiliensis*. *Nocardia* is a filamentous, gram-positive, weakly acid-fast bacillus. It is related to *Actinomyces israelii* and to the *Mycobacteria*[326] and may be confused with either of these organisms. Infections by the *Nocardia* species occur worldwide. The organism is both very slow growing and difficult to culture, and there is no effective serologic test. It is often stated that nocardiosis is seen in patients on steroid therapy or in individuals with chronic illness, notably underlying immunologic deficiency or alveolar proteinosis (Fig 6–62).[50, 238, 275, 326] But in several reviews,[29, 65, 92] a substantial proportion, almost half in one large series,[336] had no recognizable underlying condition. Dissemination from the lungs to other organs, notably the brain, may occur.

In the lung, *Nocardia* typically causes single or

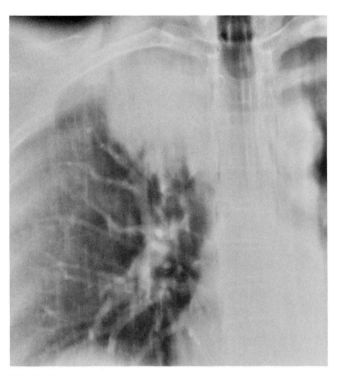

FIG 6–63.
Nocardia brasiliensis pneumonia in the right upper lobe.

multiple chronic abscesses similar to the lesions caused by pyogenic bacteria. Fibrosis is a late development, and pleural involvement is frequent, usually either fibrous thickening or empyema.

The chest radiographic findings are variable.* Pulmonary consolidation is the most frequent. The consolidations are usually large and frequently cavitate (Figs 6–63 and 6–64). They may be unifocal or multifocal, and can be patchy, segmental or occasionally lobar. Expansion of a lobe is recorded.[135] Some patients show either single or multiple round pneumonias (Fig 6–65), which can be irregular and may break down, giving rise to a thick-walled cavity. When solitary, the distinction from bronchial carcinoma may be difficult.[43] Similarly, the very rare endobronchial mass due to nocardiosis may exactly mimic a tumor radiologically and bronchoscopically.[143] Occasionally, diffuse consolidations or widespread reticulonodular shadows are encountered. Pleural effusion, which may be empyema, and hilar/mediastinal adenopathy are all reported features of the disease. Rarely, *Nocardia* may form a fungus ball similar to an aspergilloma.[222]

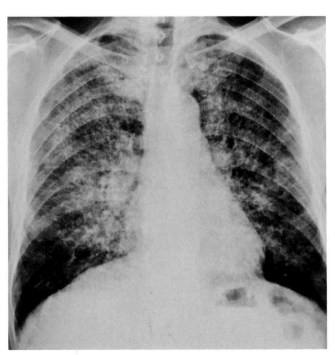

FIG 6–62.
Nocardial infection complicating pulmonary alveolar proteinosis. The pulmonary shadowing is largely, if not totally, due to the alveolar proteinosis. The complicating nocardial infection cannot be diagnosed radiologically.

*References 16, 92, 103, 135, 222, 225, 288, and 336.

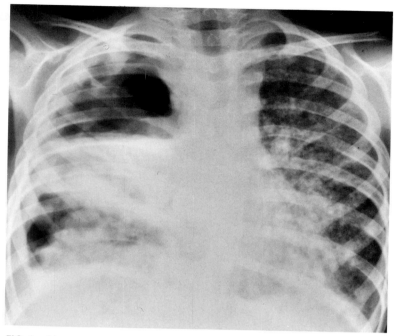

FIG 6–64.
Nocardia asteroides pneumonia in a child. These multifocal consolidations and large right lung abscess developed within 1 week.

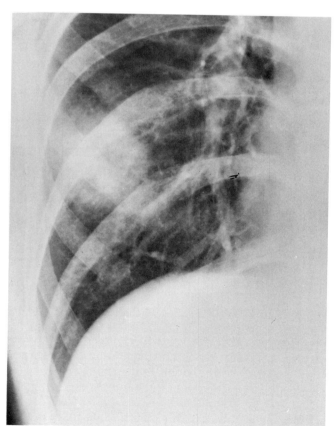

FIG 6–65.
Round pneumonia due to *N. asteroides*. Note the resemblance of this area of pneumonia to bronchial carcinoma.

ACTINOMYCOSIS

Actinomycosis is caused by *Actinomyces israelii,* an anaerobic gram-positive filamentous bacterium, which was at one time erroneously classified as a fungus. Unlike the related nocardiosis, actinomycosis is not an opportunistic infection.[326] The disease occurs when local conditions favor growth, namely when organisms that reside as commensals in the mouth and oropharynx gain access to devitalized or infected tissues. Once *A. israelii* is able to proliferate within the tissues, it causes a chronic inflammatory reaction characterized by abscesses which typically contain tiny sulfur granules in thick pus.[44]

The disease is most common in the cervicofacial region and abdomen.[326] The lungs, which are involved in less than one-quarter of cases,[44] are infected either because of aspiration of oral debris containing the organism, or because of direct spread from abdominal or cervicofacial disease.[44] Because actinomycosis tends to cross fascial planes, the pneu-

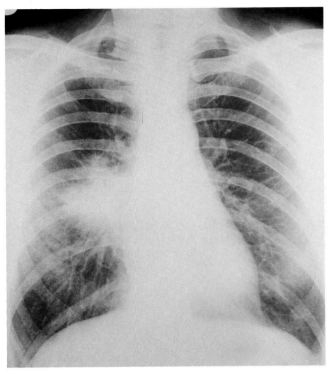

FIG 6–67.
Round pneumonia due to actinomycosis resembling bronchial carcinoma. (Courtesy of Dr. Michael C. Pearson, London.)

monia readily spreads to the pleura, producing empyema, and may spread extrapleurally to give rise to abscesses and sinus tracks in the chest wall, the bones of the thorax, and the pericardium.[24] Hematogenous dissemination is rare.

The chest radiograph[14, 24, 98, 102, 285] usually reveals an area of persistent consolidation (Fig 6–66) or a mass (Fig 6–67), either of which may cavitate. The similarity to bronchogenic carcinoma frequently leads to diagnostic confusion.[218] Focal fibrosis and contraction may be striking. Widespread small nodular shadowing has been reported.[24, 97] The infection readily transgresses the pleura and will therefore cross fissures and extend into the chest wall. Chest wall invasion may be less common now that effective antibiotic therapy is available.[102]

Pleural involvement is manifest by pleural effusion, pleural thickening, or empyema formation, but is seldom associated with large accumulations of fluid. Rib involvement leads to lysis and visible periostitis (Fig 6–68), which may be demonstrated to advantage by CT (Fig 6–69). Similarly, if the spine is involved, there may be a lytic lesion in the spine adjacent to the pulmonary or pleural shadowing.[345] CT has the advantage over plain radiography in that it can demonstrate chest wall and paraspinal inva-

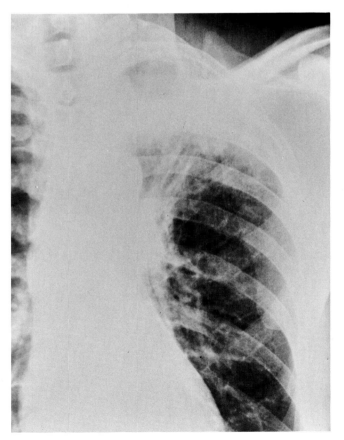

FIG 6–66.
Pneumonia due to actinomycosis. There is extensive consolidation in the apical portion of the left upper lobe. The patient complained of shoulder pain, suggesting chest wall invasion.

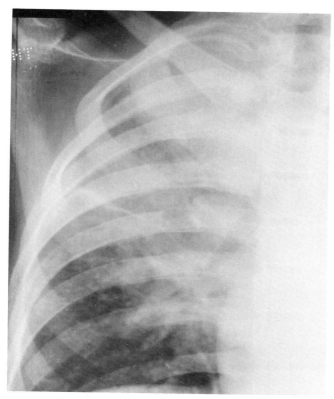

FIG 6—68.
Actinomycosis pneumonia invading the chest wall and causing periostitis of the upper six ribs. (Courtesy of Dr. Michael C. Pearson, London.)

sion even if no bone destruction is visible on the chest radiograph.[328]

FUNGAL DISEASE

Fungi are defined as mushrooms, molds, and yeasts.[137] A mold is a microscopic, multibranched tubular structure that grows at its expanding margin by the elongation of hyphal tips and by the production of new branches, known as hyphae. The yeast shape is another morphological form taken by some fungi. Yeasts are single, ovoid to spherical cells with rigid walls, in which multiplication occurs by the development of buds, the cytoplasm and at least one nucleus moving into the bud. The distinction between certain bacteria and fungi is not clear-cut, and some pathogenic organisms such as *Nocardia* and *Actinoymyces*, often thought of as fungi, are now considered to be bacteria (see the previous two sections). In the following section we will discuss those fungal agents that are responsible for most fungal pulmonary disease, namely histoplasmosis, cryptococcosis,

coccidioidomycosis, and North American blastomycosis, and then briefly describe sporotrichosis and geotrichosis. Fungal pneumonias in the immunocompromised host due to *Candida*, *Aspergillus*, and mucormycosis are discussed separately in the section "Pulmonary Infection in the Immunocompromised Patient" later in this chapter.

It is a popular myth that fungal disease of the lung shows the same radiographic features as tuberculosis. Though this is largely true of histoplasmosis, it is a serious misstatement for cryptococcosis, coccidioidomycosis, and blastomycosis. Although the diseases caused by these fungi may resemble tuberculosis in some of their manifestations, it must be emphasized that they show a variety of patterns and may be seriously confused with bronchial carcinoma.

Pulmonary Histoplasmosis

Histoplasmosis is due to the fungus *Histoplasma capsulatum*, which grows as a septate mycelium in the soil in many temperate zones of the world. Birds such as chickens, starlings, and pigeons may contain the fungus in their excreta and feathers. The mixture of droppings and soil produces an enriched growth medium for the fungus, the droppings providing inorganic nitrogen. Bats are a particularly potent source of infection. Unlike birds, bats are infected and pass the yeast form in their excreta. Thus many reported cases of histoplasmosis occur after the patients have been cleaning chicken houses or exploring bat-infested caves. Infection with the organism is particularly prevalent in the central and eastern United States, in the Mississippi and Ohio Valleys, Texas, Virginia, Delaware, and Maryland.

Human infection results from inhalation of airborne spores, which germinate and convert to the yeast form. Other routes of infection are possible, but apparently infrequent. Dissemination occurs by way of the blood and lymphatics, and organisms are removed from the blood by the cells of the reticuloendothelial system in the liver, spleen, and bone marrow. In immune competent individuals, the fungus multiplies intracellularly until cell-mediated immunity has developed. The macrophages can then kill the fungus and produce intense inflammation. Caseous necrosis occurs, and calcification will follow. In infants, as well as in patients on steroids or immunosuppressive drugs, and in those with AIDS, cellular immunity is overwhelmed or fails to develop, and progressive dissemination occurs.[162] Acute infection in the normal host, though very common, is usually asymptomatic. Goodwin et al.[123] suggest that most

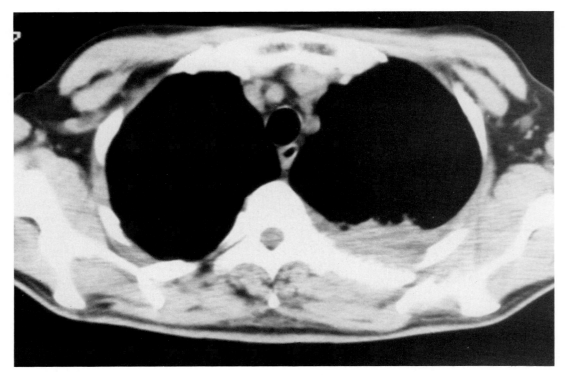

FIG 6–69.
Actinomycosis invading the chest wall. CT scan demonstrates periostitis and soft-tissue mass.

cases of symptomatic histoplasmosis occur in patients with either a structural defect in the lungs, such as emphysema, or in patients with some immunologic defect which may or may not be definable.

The definitive diagnosis of histoplasmosis depends on either growing the organism from infected sites or on demonstrating it histologically in biopsy material. Culturing *H. capsulatum* is difficult, but more importantly such cultures take time. Therefore, in acutely ill patients the diagnosis has to be made on the basis of histologic evidence. In disseminated disease the bone marrow is the best source; in one relatively recent series, the bone marrow examination yielded the organism in 15 of 19 cases.[69]

There are several tests that depend on the immune response to histoplasmosis. All suffer from sometimes being negative in disseminated disease, and all may be positive in the absence of active disease, previous exposure presumably being responsible for the positive result. Skin testing is now recommended only for epidemiologic studies, not for the diagnosis of active disease. The complement fixation test, the immunodiffusion test, the radioimmunoassay, and the enzyme immunoassay will give more quantitative results. The first two are insensitive but specific, whereas the latter two are very sensitive, but nonspecific.[162] A new radioimmunoassay of antigen (rather than antibody) in urine and serum has been introduced that may prove to be particularly useful in diagnosing disseminated histoplasmosis in immunocompromised patients.[333]

A classification of pulmonary histoplasmosis is given in Table 6–1.

Asymptomatic Infection

The widespread development of skin hypersensitivity to histoplasmin is taken as evidence that millions of people in endemic areas become infected with the fungus. More than 80% of individuals from

TABLE 6–1
Classification of Pulmonary Histoplasmosis*

Histoplasmosis in normal hosts
   Asymptomatic infection
   Symptomatic infection
Opportunistic infections
   Disseminated histoplasmosis (immune defect)
   Chronic pulmonary histoplasmosis (structural defect)
Histoplasmoma
Excessive fibrosis (mediastinal fibrosis)

*Modified from Goodwin RA, Lloyd JE, Des Prez RM: Histoplasmosis in normal hosts. *Medicine* 1981; 60:231–266.

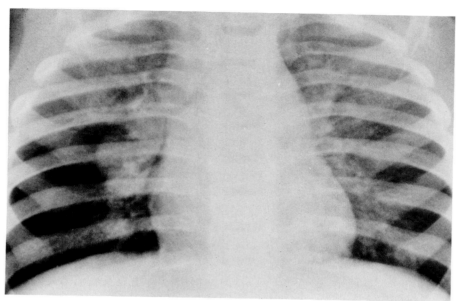

FIG 6—70.
Asymptomatic histoplasmosis, with enlargement of the right hilar lymph nodes.

highly endemic areas demonstrate skin test reactivity by age 20.[86] There is usually no definable clinical illness, but many adults in endemic areas show radiographic evidence of infection, usually calcified foci of healed disease.[205]

The chest film findings (Fig 6—70) of asymptomatic infection include*:

1. One or more patches of pneumonia, which often cluster together, and may be in any lobe. The consolidations, particularly the larger ones, often leave a calcified remnant, though they may disappear totally.[237] In young children the calcification takes just months to occur, but in adults it occurs more slowly.[237]

2. Regional lymph node enlargement and/or calcification, both of which can be striking. The calcifications are in areas of necrosis, and since the necrosis is focal, the result is tiny nodular calcifications which, when multiple, are sometimes called mulberry calcification.

3. One or more histoplasmomas.

Each of these phenomena may occur alone or in combination.[334] It is generally held that cavitation is not a feature of the asymptomatic form of the disease,[265] but this assumption has been questioned,[25, 53] and there are reported cases of cavitation in asymptomatic patients.[61]

*References 61, 123, 237, 265, 290, and 334.

Symptomatic Infection in the Normal Host

The symptoms of pulmonary histoplasmosis range from brief, mild malaise to severe, protracted illness. The illness resembles influenza, the chief features being fever and headache. There may also be substernal discomfort, loss of appetite, and nonproductive cough. The liver and spleen may be enlarged, and erythema nodosum and erythema multiforme may be encountered.

The important factors in determining whether symptomatic infection will occur are the quantity of the airborne inoculum and, to a lesser extent, the host hypersensitivity prior to exposure. Thus, individuals from endemic areas are likely to suffer either a mild illness or no illness at all. Symptomatic histoplasmosis usually resolves without therapy.

The chest radiograph often has a normal appearance in patients with mild symptoms. When abnormalities are seen, they usually consist of one or more small patchy consolidations involving the lower lobes, with or without hilar adenopathy[162] (Fig 6—71).

Exceptionally heavy exposure can occur in epidemics, often from a single source. The clinical manifestations are then more severe with higher fever. Respiratory failure and death will occur on rare occasions.[162] The radiographs may show[10, 123, 223, 290, 327]:

1. Multiple small nodules or irregular shadows (Fig 6—72) (less than 1 cm in diameter), which may

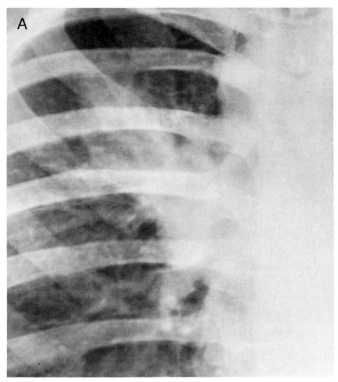
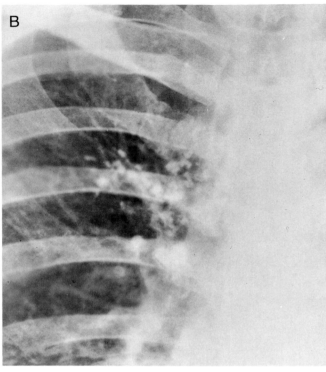

FIG 6–71.

Symptomatic histoplasmosis in an otherwise healthy patient. **A,** focal area of pulmonary consolidation, plus right hilar lymphadenopathy. **B,** many years later there is coarse calcification in the region of the previous pneumonia and in the affected hilar and mediastinal lymph nodes.

disappear or may leave small calcifications (Fig 6–73).

2. Widespread fine nodular shadows 2 to 3 mm in size (miliary nodulation).

Disseminated Histoplasmosis

Disseminated histoplasmosis is rare; approximately one-third of cases develop during the patient's first year of life.[265] The rest occur in adults, notably in their 6th and 7th decades of life. There is a striking male predominance of approximately 4 to 1.[125]

Dissemination usually indicates a failure of immune response either known or, as conjectured by Goodwin,[122, 125] "a consequence of transient defects in the immunological apparatus such as are known to complicate certain viral infections." Disseminated histoplasmosis may be the presenting feature in patients with AIDS. Dissemination may involve all organs, but it has a predilection for the reticuloendothelial system. Oropharyngeal ulcers are a particular feature of low-grade chronic disease in adults.[170]

The chest film may be normal, but usually shows widespread pulmonary shadowing. The pattern varies. Widespread miliary nodules identical to miliary tuberculosis (Fig 6–74), interstitial shadowing, nodular shadowing, and patchy consolidations with or without cavities are all reported.[61, 99, 125, 170, 237] In babies the chest film may remain normal despite overwhelming disease.[265]

Chronic Pulmonary Histoplasmosis

Chronic pulmonary histoplasmosis is now regarded as an opportunistic infection in the sense that persistent infection only occurs in the abnormal pulmonary air spaces of emphysema.[124] Such infection may then spread by way of the bronchi to produce chronic patchy pneumonitis. The colonization of large bullous spaces may produce infected cavities which at first are thin-walled, but later develop thick fibrous walls. The cavities may enlarge slowly and destroy lung, thus exacerbating the symptoms of underlying chronic obstructive lung disease. The majority will eventually heal without treatment. In those few cases that become progressive, there is a relentlessly downhill course. In one large study of 50 patients who relapsed following treatment, 15 died.[239]

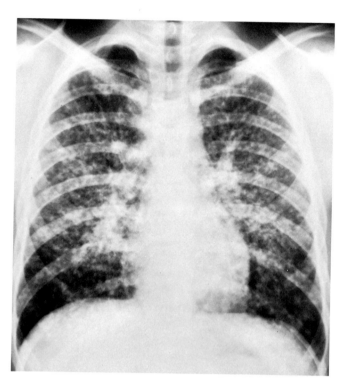

FIG 6–72.
Acute inhalational histoplasmosis in an otherwise healthy patient. This young man developed fever and cough after tearing down an old barn. The study shows bilateral hilar adenopathy.

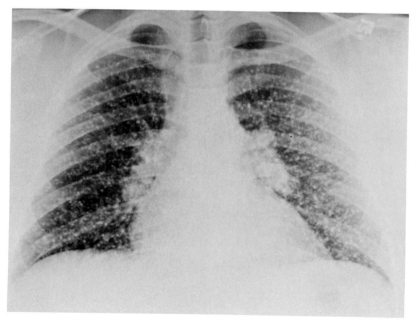

FIG 6–73.
Innumerable small calcifications in the lungs resulting from previous acute inhalational histoplasmosis. There is residual hilar adenopathy.

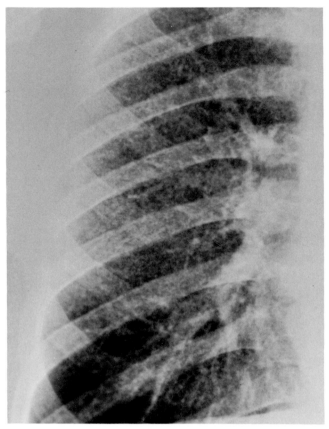

FIG 6–74.
Disseminated miliary histoplasmosis in an immunocompromised patient. Note the similarity to miliary tuberculosis.

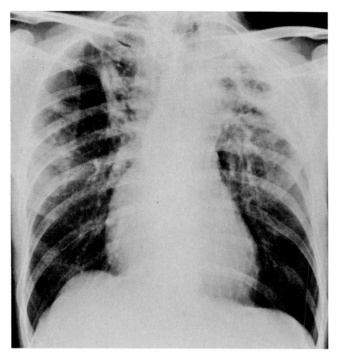

FIG 6–75.
Chronic histoplasmosis showing upper lobe consolidation, contraction, and cavitation. Note the similarity to post-primary tuberculosis.

The symptoms of chronic pulmonary histoplasmosis are similar to those of pulmonary tuberculosis, with mild to moderate malaise, fever, weight loss, and productive cough. Hemoptysis occurs in more than one-third of patients with cavitary disease, and chest pain can be a distinct feature.[122]

The radiographic appearances closely resemble postprimary tuberculosis. The multiple, small, patchy consolidations show a striking predilection for the upper lobes (Fig 6–75). Though the lower lobes may show evidence of infection in severe cases, they are rarely, if ever, involved in isolation. The consolidations, though they may be unilateral, are frequently bilateral. It is now realized that cavitation, previously thought to be a common feature,[26, 198] in fact occurs in a minority of patients (Fig 6–76). The original published studies dealt only with the most severe examples, and it is now appreciated that a milder, self-limiting form of the disease constitutes about 80% of the cases.[124] The infected cavities involve the upper lobes particularly and are frequently bilateral.[26, 198] The cavities may resolve, but fre-

quently they persist or progress, particularly those with a thick wall.[124] As with tuberculosis, the upper lobes contract due to scarring and destruction by the infection. Pleural effusion may occur but is rare, and lymphadenopathy is unusual.[61, 290]

Histoplasmoma

Histologically, the histoplasmoma is a small necrotic focus of infection surrounded by a relatively massive fibrous capsule.[126] Radiologically, the typical histoplasmoma is a well-defined spherical nodule (Fig 6–77). It may be of soft tissue density or contain discrete calcifications. Calcification in the necrotic center is an early feature and may be seen 3 months after the lesion is first identified. As the fibrous capsule grows, calcification is laid down in laminations that may cause a general increase in density or may, on occasions, appear as concentric rings on radiologic examination. Histoplasmomas may be single or multiple (Fig 6–78,A and B). The detection of increased density due to the presence of this calcification (Fig 6–79) is the basis of the CT diagnosis of benignity in the assessment of pulmonary nodules (see p. 123).

Usually the edge of the histoplasmoma is smooth or slightly lobular. There are, however, many cases

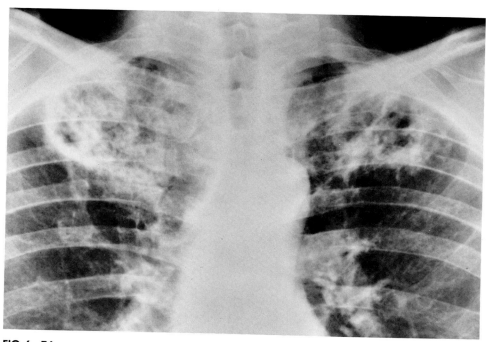

FIG 6–76.
Chronic cavitary histoplasmosis. Note the striking upper zone predominance of the shadows. Multiple large cavities are present in this case.

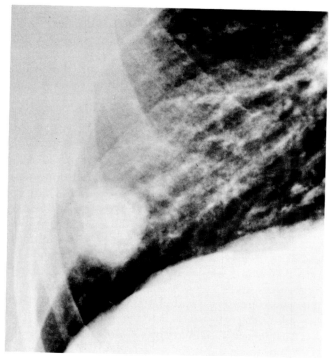

FIG 6–77.
Histoplasmoma, showing a well-defined spherical nodule. The central portion of the nodule shows calcification.

on record in which the edge is irregular, sometimes markedly so. Indeed, the edge may be so shaggy that on rare occasions it is indistinguishable from the corona radiata seen with bronchial carcinoma. Occasionally histoplasmomas, both single and multiple,[236] will be seen to enlarge over the years. The enlarging histoplasmoma, even if it is cavitary or multiple, does not appear to pose a problem of dissemination of disease.[237, 290] In one series,[126] the increase in diameter averaged approximately 2 mm/year. This increase in size has at times led to confusion with carcinoma of the lung, particularly in those cases in which the characteristic calcifications were not present. In general, however, the growth is far slower than that observed with malignant lesions.

Broncholithiasis

The term broncholith refers to a portion of calcified lymph node lying within a major airway. The phenomenon is seen in both histoplasmosis and tuberculosis and the radiographic features are identical in the two diseases.[325] The subject is discussed and illustrated in the section on tuberculosis earlier in this chapter (see p. 185).

Mediastinal Fibrosis

The subject of mediastinal fibrosis due to histoplasmosis is discussed in Chapter 15.

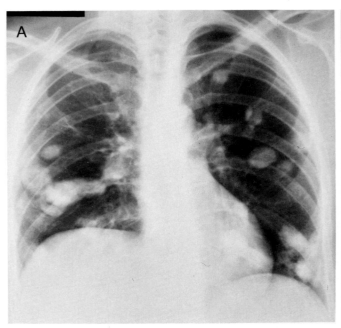

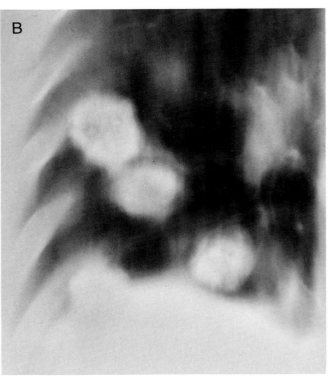

FIG 6–78.
Multiple calcified histoplasmomas. **A,** plain film. **B,** conventional tomogram showing concentric organization of the calcification.

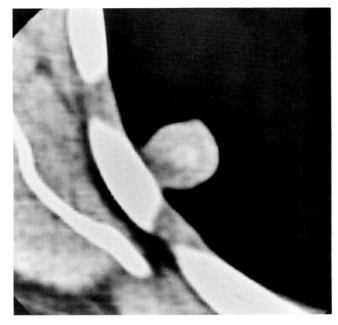

FIG 6–79.
CT scan of histoplasmoma showing the central ringlike calcification.

Cryptococcosis

Cryptococcosis, also known as torulosis *(Torula histolytica)* or European blastomycosis, is an infection caused by inhaling spores that contain *Cryptococcus neoformans.* The organism is a nonmycelial budding yeast found in the soil and in bird droppings, particularly from pigeons.

The lung, being the portal of entry, is a common site of this disease. From here it may spread to many organs, meningitis and meningoencephalitis being the most serious consequences.[189] The disease may occur in persons of any age, but is most common in adults. The prevalence is difficult to determine as there is no good skin test or serum antibody assay for cryptococcosis, and the question of saprophytic colonization as opposed to invasive disease cannot be assessed from either culture of sputum or the currently available serologic tests.[45, 139] An antigen latex agglutination test can be used for diagnosis of individual cases, since it is reasonably specific; its sensitivity is, however, poor.[45]

Fever, chest pain, cough, and mucoid sputum production are the usual symptoms,[171] but many patients with cryptococcal pneumonia have no symptoms, and the pulmonary lesions seen radiographi-

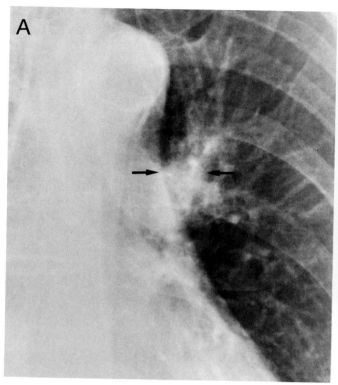

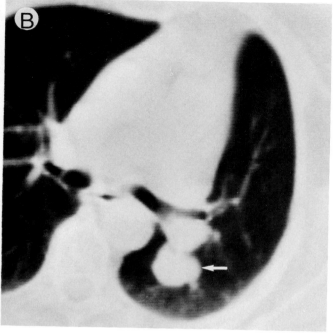

FIG 6-80.
Cryptococcus nodule. **A,** plain film (the *arrows* point to the lesion). **B,** CT scan showing uniform soft-tissue density of the nodule. The nodule *(arrow)* is indistinguishable from a bronchial carcinoma.

cally heal spontaneously. Approximately one-half to two-thirds of the cases of symptomatic infection are associated with immunodeficiency from conditions such as AIDS,[176] lymphoma, leukemia, diabetes mellitus, and particularly drugs; and in these patients, extrapulmonary dissemination is common.[171]

Cryptococcal pneumonia may be the presenting feature of AIDS.[176] Patients with underlying disease tend to develop cryptococcal meningitis with a greater frequency than those without a predisposing condition.[18] Meningeal spread is extremely common in immunocompromised patients[171]; it was seen in one series in 18 of 27 AIDS patients.[176]

A large variety of appearances may be seen on chest radiographs. The descriptions and classifications vary considerably, as do the incidence of the various findings.* This variation may be due to the relative frequency of immunodeficiency in the patient populations being described. As expected, patients who are immunocompromised have more extensive findings.[173] In general three patterns are en-

*References 42, 91, 128, 155, 171, 173, and 340.

countered, the first two of which are the most common and approximately equal in frequency:

1. One or more spherical nodules/masses
2. One or more areas of patchy consolidations
3. Multiple small nodules or irregular shadows.

Nodules/Masses

The size of these mass lesions varies from barely visible to huge. They are usually single (Fig 6–80), but may be multiple and vary in location, with no predilection for any one lobe or zone. Some are composed largely of fungus with little associated inflammatory response,[91, 128] a form of disease which produces a well-defined mass and, in the few cases reported, is not associated with lymphadenopathy, cavitation, or pleural effusion. The remainder are predominantly due to fibrous tissue with central caseation and abundant organisms.[301] These lesions are usually poorly defined and may show cavitation and associated lymphadenopathy, both phenomena being more frequent in immunocompromised patients.[173]

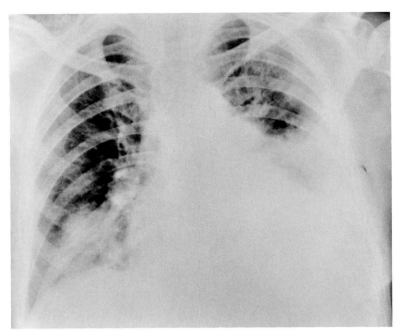

FIG 6–81.
Cryptococcal pneumonia showing extensive bilateral mid- and lower-zone consolidation.

From this description it will be clear that the distinction from bronchial carcinoma is often difficult,[212] usually requiring biopsy. Sputum cultures and bronchial washings which grow *C. neoformans* do not exclude the diagnosis of carcinoma. *Cryptococcus* colonizes the respiratory tract in a large number of chronic disorders and, therefore, will often be found in patients with bronchial carcinoma. In one series of 28 patients with roentgenographic parenchymal lung lesions and *C. neoformans* in the respiratory tract, 25% had lung cancer.[82]

Patchy Consolidation

As with the masses, the size, location, and multiplicity of consolidation varies greatly; even lobar consolidation has been reported.[199] In some series a predilection is shown for the lower zones (Fig 6–81),[197] and in some there is a predominance of upper lobe presentations.[128] Air bronchograms may be present. Cavitation (Fig 6–82) and associated lymphadenopathy both occur, but are relatively unusual. Unlike the consolidative lesions in histoplasmosis and tuberculosis, subsequent loss of volume and calcification do not appear to be prominent features.[301]

Widespread Small Nodules or Irregular Shadows

This pattern is the least frequent and is indistinguishable from that of a host of other interstitial diseases. When nodular, it resembles miliary tuberculosis and other fungal infections.

Pleural Effusions

Pleural effusions appear to be relatively rare in pulmonary cryptococcosis.[91] A 1980 review showed that the 30 cases reported in the English-language literature were divided almost equally between localized and disseminated disease.[344]

Coccidioidomycosis

Coccidioidomycosis is caused by *Coccidioides immitis*, a fungus found in the soil. The disease is limited mainly to the U.S. Southwestern states and northern Mexico, where it is endemic. Pulmonary infection is acquired by inhalation of the fungus; transmission by person-to-person contact is extremely rare. As with histoplasmosis, the incidence of infection as shown by coccidioidin skin test conversion exceeds that of clinical symptoms,[28] but the incidence of symptoms is higher than in histoplasmosis, the prev-

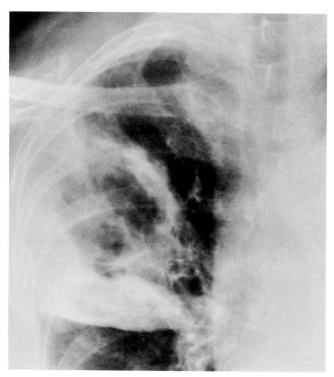

FIG 6–82.
Cryptococcal pneumonia showing extensive cavitation in the right upper lobe.

alence of symptoms being approximately 40%.[28, 287] The infection usually occurs in adults and is mild and self limiting. Occasionally, it is severe and prolonged. Dissemination is rare, but has serious consequences.

The standard diagnostic tests are precipitin and complement fixation tests. The most definitive diagnosis is made by the identification or culture of the organism in body fluids or tissues, but the success of this approach varies greatly. Organisms are almost always found in purulent drainage from skin and soft tissues, sometimes in sputum and lung or bronchial aspirates, and rarely in pleural fluid, though organisms can usually be demonstrated by biopsy of granulomas in the pleura.[188]

The disease is classified in various ways. This presentation will use the same groupings for the pulmonary manifestations as those used by Drutz and Catanzaro in their major review article.[80]

Primary Coccidioidomycosis

The illness in primary coccidioidomycosis is non-specific and resembles a mild viral infection; sometimes a severe pneumonia is seen, and very occasion-

ally the disease becomes disseminated. The usual symptoms are fatigue, cough, and chest pain, accompanied not infrequently by dyspnea, arthralgia, headache, and sore throat. A maculopapular rash and erythema nodosum are common skin manifestations. "Valley fever" is a relatively specific complex consisting of erythema nodosum, erythema multiforme, and arthritis.

Radiographically,[157, 209, 278] asymptomatic patients may have fibrous scars or small, calcified pulmonary or nodal granulomata. Alternatively, the chest film may show no abnormalities. Symptomatic patients show unifocal or multifocal segmental consolidation that may take a month or two to resolve.

Hilar/mediastinal adenopathy and pleural effusion are each seen in approximately one-quarter of patients,[38, 131] usually in combination with a pulmonary shadow (Fig 6–83,A and B). Such adenopathy can be quite pronounced[157] and, if isolated, needs to be distinguished from sarcoidosis or lymphoma.[131] Paratracheal adenopathy may, on rare occasions, be associated with granulomatous masses in the trachea or major bronchi, particularly in children.[33, 219]

Persistent Pulmonary Coccidioidomycosis

Most patients with primary coccidioidomycosis recover within 2 to 3 weeks. Those whose symptoms or radiographic abnormalities persist after 6 to 8 weeks are considered to have persistent coccidioidomycosis. The most common complaint is hemoptysis.[80] Patients with persistent and extensive pneumonia are often very sick. Fatal cases are usually, but not always, in immunocompromised patients.

Systemic dissemination is rare except in immunocompromised patients, occurring in less than 1% of cases; it is much more common in non-Caucasians than in Caucasians.[287] Dissemination occurs most frequently to skin, followed by soft tissue, synovium, bone, lymph nodes, meninges and urinary tract.[188] In general, dissemination is accompanied by anergy to coccidioidin and by high complement fixation titers.

The radiographic findings of persistent pulmonary coccidioidomycosis are coccidioidal nodules (coccidioidoma), persistent coccidioidal pneumonia, and miliary coccidioidomycosis. Coccidioidal nodules are areas of round pneumonia. On plain chest radiographs they are usually subpleural in location[267] and mostly in an upper lobe (Fig 6–84). Cavitation is a major characteristic.[150] The wall may be thick, but is often thin, in some cases strikingly so. On the whole the cavities are small, averaging 1.5 cm in diameter,[209] but

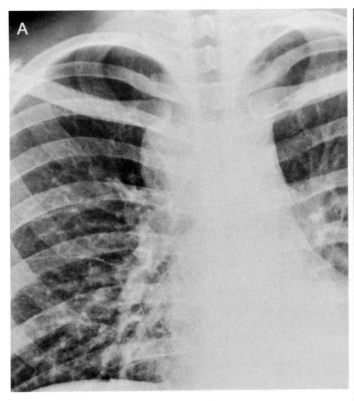

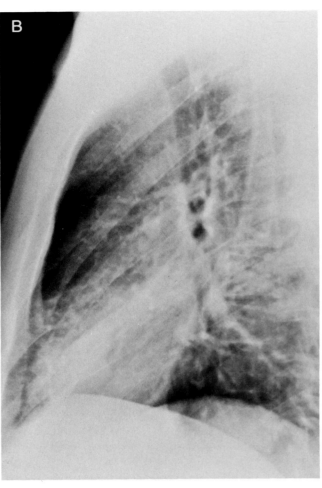

FIG 6–83.
Primary coccidioidomycosis in a patient who had visited California. There is consolidation in the right middle lobe and substantial right paratracheal adenopathy. **A,** PA view. **B,** lateral view.

they may reach 6 cm.[38] Rapid change in size is a characteristic feature of the cavities,[157] and pneumothorax or pyopneumothorax may be a complication.[80, 85] Calcification is unusual.[267, 280, 287]

Patients with *chronic progressive coccidioidal pneumonia* may have prolonged symptoms and show upper lobe fibrocavitary disease with loss of volume very similar to that seen with tuberculosis or histoplasmosis.[283] Miliary spread, a frequently fatal complication, may be an early manifestation of the disease or may complicate chronic pulmonary or extrapulmonary disease. The miliary nodulation is similar in appearance to miliary tuberculosis. Associated mediastinal lymph node enlargement is common.[287]

North American Blastomycosis

Blastomyces dermatitidis is a dimorphic fungus that grows in mycelial form at room temperature and is a yeast form at body temperature. Most cases of blastomycosis occur in the central and southeastern parts of the United States, bordering on the Mississippi and Ohio River Valleys, but documented examples have been reported from Africa,[282] the Middle East, Canada, and Central and South America.[52] The source of the fungus is difficult to prove but it is believed to be the soil,[282] possibly enhanced by decaying wood and bird droppings. Person-to-person transmission of the disease has not been demonstrated.[284] Blastomycosis may occur sporadically or as outbreaks from a common source. Sporadic cases show a predilection for middle-aged men, especially those exposed by occupation to the soil (e.g., farmers, construction workers and those involved in the timber industry). Single-source outbreaks affect both sexes and all ages equally. The common thread appears to be exposure to soil in wooded areas, whether at work or play.[48] The usual portal of entry is the lung.[286] After being inhaled, the organism converts to the yeast form at body temperature, with resulting infection of the lungs and skin and, to a lesser extent, of the bones and the male genitourinary sys-

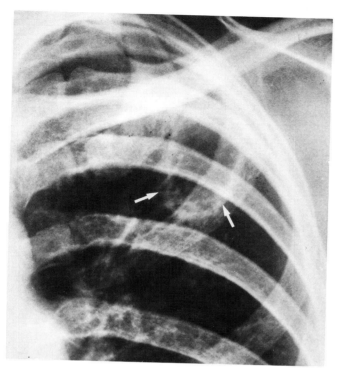

FIG 6–84.
Thin-walled cavity *(arrows)* resulting from coccidioidal pneumonia.

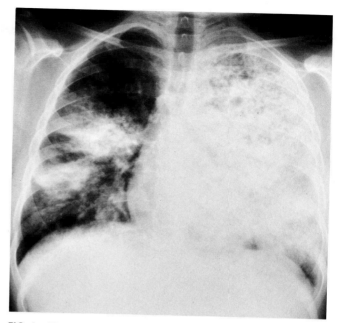

FIG 6–85.
Blastomycosis pneumonia in a 12-year-old girl. There are bilateral consolidations, predominantly in the left upper lobe.

tem.[27, 282] The central nervous system and gastrointestinal system are rarely involved. Subcutaneous abscesses, which go on to become ulcerations, are the most common clinical manifestation of the disease.[282] A small minority of affected patients are immunocompromised.[258]

Because there is no general screening test, knowledge regarding the prevalence of the disease is inadequate. The diagnosis is established by demonstrating a rising antibody titer or by culture of the organism. Skin tests are no longer used, and complement fixation tests are negative for disease in 50% or more of patients.[289] However, a new enzyme immunoassay test is under development.[174] The definitive diagnosis requires the recognition of the organism on microscopic examination of smears from infected sites or, more definitively, by culture.

The pulmonary infection is often asymptomatic. When symptoms occur, the manifestations are variable, in some cases resembling acute pneumonia. The symptoms may be similar to those of influenza—with fever, chills, headache, myalgia, arthralgia, and cough. In the more chronic cases, the disease may closely resemble carcinoma of the lung, clinically and radiologically. The skin nodules and ulcerations are an important clinical clue to the diagnosis. The outcome is also variable; most patients recover and remain well, but progressive pulmonary disease and dissemination may occur.

Pulmonary involvement is an almost constant finding at autopsy, but only 60% of patients with systemic blastomycosis demonstrate significant abnormalities on the plain chest radiograph.[7] Several series and reviews have documented the radiographic findings.* A major feature of acute infection is ill-defined consolidation in the lung that is indistinguishable from acute pneumonia. The consolidation may be unifocal or multifocal and range from subsegmental to lobar, occurring more frequently in the upper than the lower lobes (Figs 6–85 and 6–86). In a minority of cases the consolidations are widespread bilaterally. Cavitation occurs in approximately 10% to 20% of cases. A pattern closely resembling fibrocavitary tuberculosis or histoplasmosis is seen in some cases of chronic blastomycosis[141, 252, 289] (Fig 6–87). Calcification is, however, a less prominent feature. A few patients, averaging 5% to 10% in the various series, show a spherical pneumonia, usually 3 to 6 cm in diameter which, if it does not contain air bronchograms, will be radiographically indistinguishable from bronchial carcinoma.

Accompanying pleural changes are not infrequent. Usually they take the form of pleural thickening adjacent to the pulmonary process, but there

*References 7, 39, 138, 141, 183, 242, 252, 289, and 339.

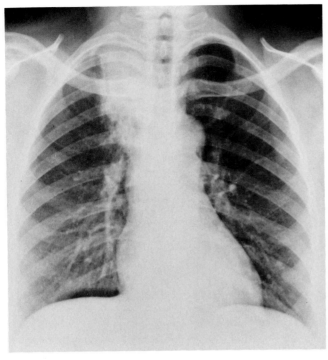

FIG 6–86.
Blastomycosis pneumonia in a middle-aged woman showing right upper lobe consolidation and loss of volume, initially thought to be post-obstructive pneumonia beyond a carcinoma.

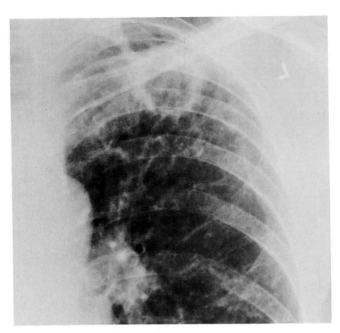

FIG 6–87.
Blastomycosis showing fibrocavitary disease in the left upper lobe.

may occasionally be a small ipsilateral pleural effusion. Direct invasion of the chest wall with the development of an extrapleural mass and rib destruction is very occasionally encountered.[141] Lytic lesions in the bones due to hematogenous spread are more frequent than direct spread,[141] the pattern being identical to that seen with metastatic malignant neoplasm.

Lymph node enlargement is infrequent and, when present, is usually hilar in location and mild in degree.

A variable proportion of cases are reported as causing miliary nodulation in the lungs (Fig 6–88), which can be indistinguishable from miliary tuberculosis. This pattern appears to be more common in patients who are immunocompromised.[305]

Pulmonary Aspergillosis

The genus *Aspergillus* is a ubiquitous dimorphic fungus present in soil and water and abundant in decaying and moldy vegetation. There are over 300 species of *Aspergillus* but *A. fumigatus* is by far the most frequent pathogen in man.[161] It is a unique fungus in that it can cause a wide spectrum of pulmonary disease, ranging from simple colonization to life-threatening invasive aspergillosis, depending on the immunologic status of the host, individual susceptibility, or preexisting lung disease. It has been suggested that pulmonary aspergillosis be considered as a spectrum instead of the conventional divisions into (1) mycetoma, (2) invasive aspergillosis, and (3) allergic bronchopulmonary aspergillosis,

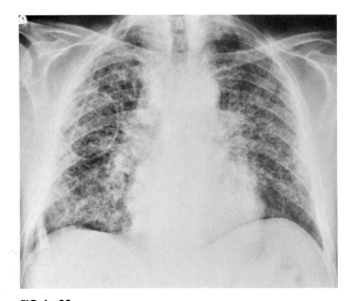

FIG 6–88.
Blastomycosis in an immunocompromised patient showing widespread miliary nodulation in the lungs.

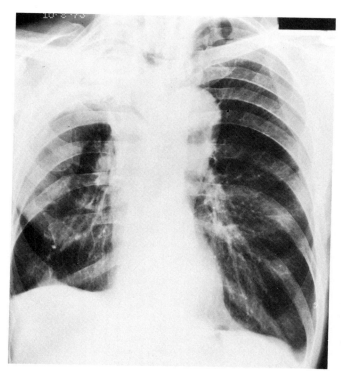

FIG 6–89.
Mycetoma in the pleural space following a right upper lobectomy.

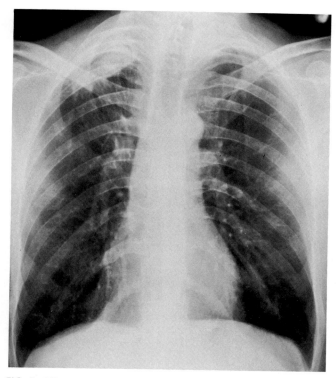

FIG 6–90.
Mycetoma in a fibrotic contracted right upper lobe resulting from long-standing ankylosing spondylitis.

particularly as these three entities may overlap with one another in an individual patient and with other *Aspergillus*-related phenomena such as mucoid impaction, eosinophilic pneumonia, bronchocentric granulomatosis, extrinsic allergic alveolitis, or asthma.[130] Also, limited invasion may occur with mycetoma in patients with mild immunosuppression or underlying lung disease.[113] The subject of colonization and mycetoma is discussed here. Invasive aspergillosis is considered later in this chapter and allergic aspergillosis is discussed in Chapter 11.

Saphrophytic colonization is seen in patients with chronic obstructive airway disease who are debilitated and who are receiving prolonged courses of multiple antibiotics or corticosteroids.[161] Aspergillus has been found in 7% of sputum cultures in patients with a wide variety of chest diseases and in 24% of sputum cultures of asthmatics. Some patients may show evidence of an immunologic response, such as increased total immunoglobulin E, positive precipitins, and immediate or late skin reactivity to *Aspergillus* antigen.[161]

The term aspergilloma (mycetoma, fungus ball) is used to describe a ball of coalescent mycelial hyphae which typically colonize preexisting chronic cavities, most of which are in the lung, although mycetomas may also form in chronic pleural cavities[63, 83, 213] (Fig 6–89). The pulmonary cavities are usually due to old healed pulmonary tuberculosis, though cavities from a variety of other causes including fungal infection, sarcoidosis, ankylosing spondylitis (Fig 6–90), interstitial pulmonary fibrosis, bronchiectasis and pulmonary infarct/lung abscess may also be colonized by the fungus.*

Pathologically,[51] an intracavitary aspergilloma is a compact, spherical conglomerate of hyphae which may be attached to the wall of the cavity but usually is not. Microscopically, the fungus ball is composed of concentric or convoluted layers of radially arranged and intertwined hyphae. Those in the center are often nonviable. Although hyphae can be found along the surface and within the fibrous wall of the cavity, invasion into the adjacent lung parenchyma does not occur unless host defense mechanisms are otherwise compromised, in which case the condition can take a locally destructive form known variously as chronic necrotizing pulmonary aspergillosis[37] or "semi-invasive" aspergillosis.[113] The underlying abnormality may be locally diseased lung—for exam-

*References 83, 89, 95, 104, 154, 167, 254, 268, and 291.

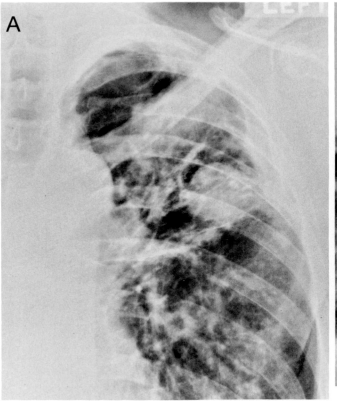

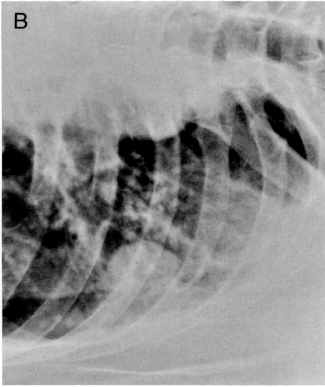

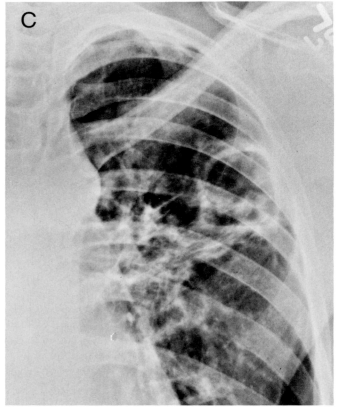

FIG 6–91.
Mycetoma showing intracavitary ball of fungus. Note the crescent of air above the mycetoma, the adjacent pleural thickening, and the movement of the fungus ball. In this case the underlying fibrocavitary disease was due to atypical mycobacterial infection. **A,** frontal view. **B,** lateral decubitus view. **C,** frontal view 1 year earlier shows preexisting cavity with an air-fluid level, but no recognizable mycetoma.

ple, chronic obstructive lung disease, prior irradiation, or pneumoconiosis. Mild systemic immunocompromise such as connective tissue disorders, poor nutrition, diabetes mellitus, or low-dose corticosteroid therapy, may also be present.

Most patients with mycetoma are over 40 years of age and more likely to be men than women.[207, 268] The mycetoma may be asymptomatic and first discovered incidentally on a chest radiograph, but hemoptysis is frequent, being seen in 50% to 80% of patients.[89, 104, 160, 167] The mechanism of bleeding is not known, but it has been attributed to friction between the fungus ball and the hypervascular cavity wall, to endotoxins liberated from the fungus, and to type III reaction in the cavity wall.[161] Occasionally, the hemoptysis is so massive as to be life-threatening.[160, 254] Other symptoms include productive cough, chest pain, fever, dyspnea, weight loss, and fatigue, due mainly to the underlying condition rather than to the mycetoma itself.[254] Precipitin tests are species-specific; therefore, the occasional negative serum precipitin test result will be seen when the responsible *Aspergillus* organism is not *A. fumigatus*.

The diagnosis is, in essence, established on radiographic grounds. Skin tests and sputum cultures for *Aspergillus* may be positive, but neither test is sensitive or specific.[207] Positive precipitating antibodies to *Aspergillus* antigens can be demonstrated in the serum in over 90% of patients,[104] but again the test is not specific for mycetoma, as it is also positive in many of the forms of pulmonary aspergillosis, including temporary colonization of the airway by fungal hyphae.[161]

The essential finding on plain film is the mycetoma itself,[104, 153, 348] a rounded mass of soft tissue density lying within a preexisting cavity (Fig 6–91). Because most of the preexisting cavities are due to old tuberculosis or histoplasmosis, mycetomas are found most often in the upper lobes or in the superior segment of the lower lobes. Usually, the mass only fills a portion of the cavity, so air is seen between the fungus ball and the wall. This air takes the shape of a meniscus and is usually referred to as the "air-meniscus sign" or the "air-crescent sign" (Fig 6–92). This sign, though not specific to mycetoma, strongly suggests the diagnosis when an intracavitary mass is seen in an area of focal pulmonary scarring. Another very useful diagnostic sign is that a fungus ball can be made to roll around the cavity, so that it changes position when comparisons are made between erect, supine, prone, and lateral decubitus views (Fig 6–93). In some cases, the mycetoma will

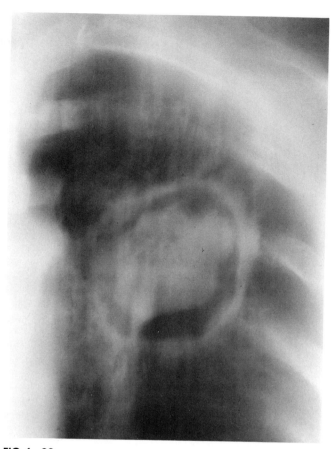

FIG 6–92.
Tomogram of mycetoma showing an air-crescent sign between the fungus ball and the preexisting cavity wall. (Courtesy of Dr. Michael C. Pearson, London.)

more or less fill the cavity, and no longer be able to roll around within it.

Because the cavity wall is lined by fungus, it may appear thick[196] (Fig 6–94), a sign that is seen most often in long-standing mycetoma with obvious intracavitary mass, but also with early colonization before the fungus ball itself is obvious. Pleural thickening of up to 2 cm adjacent to the cavity is a frequent finding of *Aspergillus* superinfection.[190] An air-fluid level may be present within the cavity.[104, 190, 196]

All the plain film findings are better seen with tomography,[104] and CT scanning demonstrates the features even better. It shows a spongelike mass that contains irregular air spaces (Fig 6–95).[268] The air-crescent sign and the wall of the preexisting cavity are well seen, and the mobility of the fungus ball can be readily demonstrated with extra views in the prone and lateral decubitus positions, if necessary. The spongelike appearance is so characteristic that, in patients with positive precipitins in the serum, the

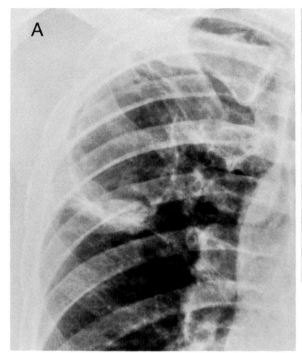

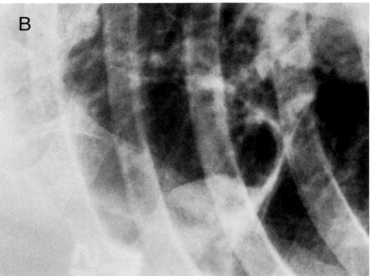

FIG 6—93.
Mycetoma in a preexisting cavity showing change in position. **A,** supine view. **B,** on the lateral decubitus view the fungus ball has rolled to the dependent portion of the cavity.

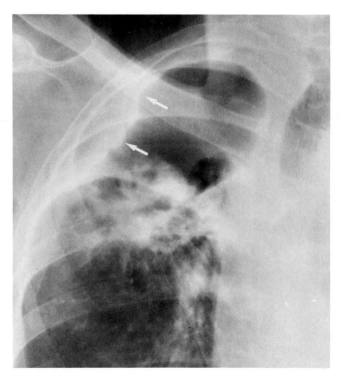

FIG 6—94.
Mycetoma in preexisting histoplasmosis cavity showing thickening of the pleura *(arrows)* constituting the cavity wall.

diagnosis is secure even in cases in which the mycetoma fills the cavity, and therefore neither the air-crescent sign nor evidence of mobility can be demonstrated. The diagnosis of mycetoma formation can be made earlier with CT by noting fungal strands either lining the cavity or within the lumen before they have formed a ball that can be recognized on a plain chest radiograph.

In the semi-invasive form,[37, 113] the fungus may produce extensive local consolidation and destruction of the lung parenchyma (Fig 6—96). There need not be a previous cavity; the appearance may simply be an area of chronic pulmonary consolidation that undergoes progressive cavitation and subsequent mycetoma formation. Once the mycetoma has formed, the appearances resemble the noninvasive form except that the cavity continues to grow slowly under observation.[113]

A stable, noncavitary, nodular or masslike form of pulmonary aspergillosis has also been described[295] in which there is no evidence of a preexisting cavity and the lesion resembles a pulmonary neoplasm on both plain film and CT scans. None of the three reported patients was immunocompromised. The authors suggested that the lesions represented a locally invasive form of infection, but the relationship of these masses to semi-invasive or chronic necrotizing pulmonary aspergillosis is not clear.

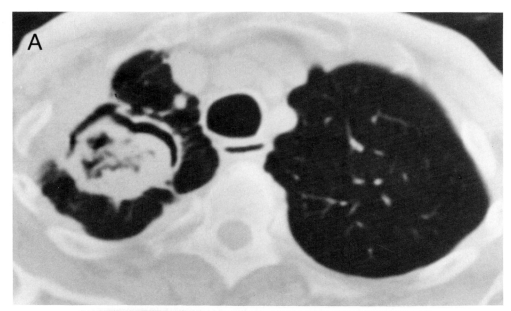

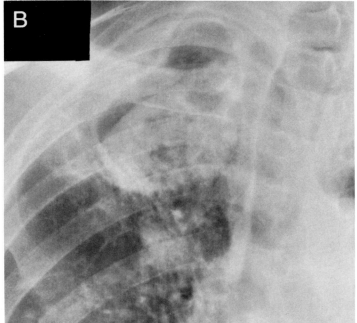

FIG 6–95.

A, CT scan of mycetoma showing the intracavitary mass with multiple linear lucencies. Note the air-crescent sign and the lateral wall formed by pleural thickening. **B,** plain film on same day for comparison.

Unusual Fungi

Sporotrichosis is usually a lymphocutaneous infection obtained by direct implantation of the fungus *Sporothrix schenckii*. The highest incidence of the common lymphocutaneous form is in agricultural workers, nurserymen, and similar occupations.[270]

Skin tests are not available, and the serologic tests are highly specialized. The best method of diagnosis is culture of the fungus from sputum specimens, bronchial brushings or washings, or pleural biopsies. Pulmonary involvement may be secondary to skin infection, but most cases of pulmonary disease are caused by inhalation of spores, and occupational ex-

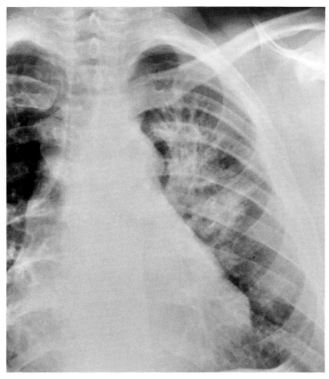

FIG 6–96.
Semi-invasive aspergillosis showing focal ill-defined consolidation in an otherwise normal appearing lung. The patient had no known immunocompromise.

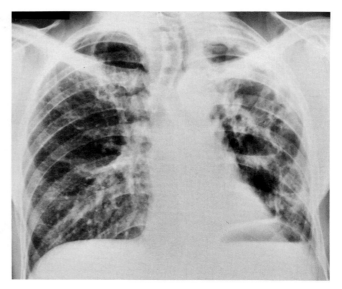

FIG 6–97.
Sporotrichosis showing multiple thin-walled cavities containing air-fluid levels and adjacent pleural thickening. Note the close resemblance to pulmonary tuberculosis.

posure does not play as great a role.[34, 217, 270] Systemic dissemination may occur. The usual symptoms of pulmonary disease are productive cough and low-grade fever. The chest radiographic findings (Fig 6–97) are variable, mostly areas of consolidation that may give rise to thin-walled cavities and fibronodular densities in the upper lobes closely resembling pulmonary tuberculosis,[34, 60] even to the extent that fungus balls may grow in sporotrichosis cavities.[270]

Geotrichosis is due to *Geotrichum candidum*, a fungus that normally inhabits the pharynx and gastrointestinal tract. It may cause bronchitis, asthma, or pneumonia. In parenchymal infection the radiograph may show upper lobe consolidation and thin-walled cavities.

MYCOPLASMA PNEUMONIA

Mycoplasma pneumoniae (Eaton agent) is the most common nonbacterial cause of pneumonia. It usually affects children and young adults between the ages of 5 and 25. It sometimes occurs in localized outbreaks in families, schools, or military groups; the disease is spread by inhalation of droplets and has a 10- to 20-day incubation period. The symptoms resemble those of a viral infection; there is usually malaise, fever, chills, headache, a nonproductive cough, and a variety of nonrespiratory manifestations.[221] The physical findings on examination of the chest are often less than might be expected from the chest radiograph. The diagnosis is usually established retrospectively by an elevated or rising cold agglutinin titer. The disease, which responds to tetracycline or erythromycin, usually runs a self-limiting course, although fatal cases are recorded[175] as is the development of interstitial fibrosis.[169]

The chest radiographic findings are variable.* The most common pattern is patchy consolidation, which may coalesce to resemble lobar pneumonia.[57] Usually the pneumonia is unilateral, often involving one lobe only (Fig 6–98,A and B). Occasionally the consolidation spreads to involve other lobes.[96, 142] There appears to be a predilection for the lower lobes (Fig 6–98,C), though solitary upper lobe involvement is well recognized.[96, 117, 129] An alternative pattern is nodular or reticular shadowing resembling an interstitial process (Fig 6–99). In most series, this pattern was relatively uncommon, but in

*References 47, 96, 101, 142, 249, and 306.

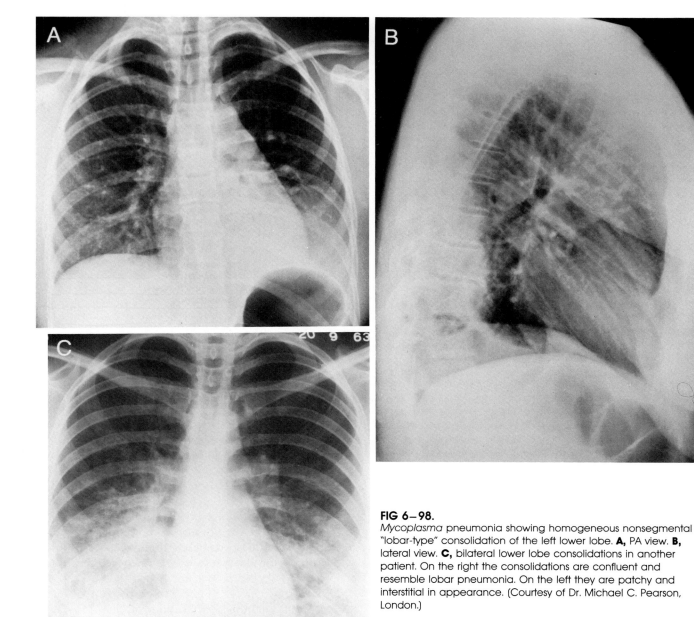

FIG 6–98.
Mycoplasma pneumonia showing homogeneous nonsegmental "lobar-type" consolidation of the left lower lobe. **A,** PA view. **B,** lateral view. **C,** bilateral lower lobe consolidations in another patient. On the right the consolidations are confluent and resemble lobar pneumonia. On the left they are patchy and interstitial in appearance. (Courtesy of Dr. Michael C. Pearson, London.)

one large series it was seen in the majority of patients.[306] In the series of Putman et al.[249] an interstitial pattern was often associated with a more indolent and longer course, without high fever or cough.

Cavitation does not appear to occur. Pleural effusion is variously reported as rare or occurring in up to 20% of cases,[94] probably reflecting the use or nonuse of lateral decubitus views. Large effusions,

which may be hemorrhagic, are seen occasionally.[249] Both adenopathy (Fig 6–100) and pleural effusion are commoner in children.[47, 74, 133, 306, 308] Pneumatoceles have been reported, but they are rare.[116]

The appearance of the chest radiograph may take several weeks to return to normal. In the series reported by Finnegan and co-workers, only 40% had cleared by 4 weeks, but almost all were clear by 8 weeks.[96]

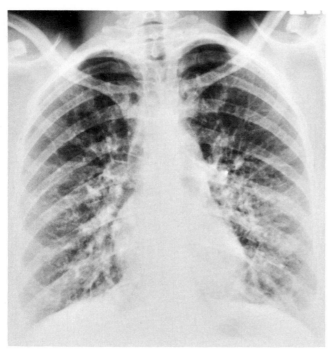

FIG 6–99.
Mycoplasma pneumonia showing widespread linear shadowing of an interstitial type.

VIRAL PNEUMONIA

Viruses are the major cause of respiratory tract infection in the community, particularly in children. Droplet transmission from human to human is the usual mode of spread. Mostly, it is the upper respiratory tract and airways that are involved. Pneumonia is relatively uncommon. In infants and young children, the most common viruses causing pneumonia are respiratory syncytial virus, parainfluenza, adenovirus, and influenza virus; in older children and adults, they are the influenza virus and adenovirus.

Pathologically,[62, 301] viral pneumonia begins with destruction and sloughing of the respiratory ciliated, goblet, and mucous cells. The bronchial and bronchiolar walls, together with the interstitial septa of the lungs, become thickened as a result of edema and inflammation, the inflammatory cells being primarily lymphocytes. This so-called interstitial pneumonitis is often patchy, affecting predominantly the peribronchial portions of the lobules. With more severe inflammation the alveoli will fill with inflammatory exudate, which may be hemorrhagic in nature, and hyaline membranes may form. Resolution is the rule, but permanent mucosal damage may occur, as may chronic interstitial fibrosis. Viral pneumonias are one of the causes of bronchiolitis obliterans.

In general, the radiologic findings in viral pneumonia[62, 158, 231] are not sufficiently different from those of bacterial or mycoplasmal pneumonia to allow a reliable distinction to be made,[315] nor are there features that allow one to diagnose a specific virus infection. The basic sign is consolidation, which is often composed of widespread small patchy shadows that may coalesce to a variable degree (Fig 6–101,A and B). Multilobar involvement is usual. Sometimes the pulmonary shadows are composed of multiple poorly defined 2- to 3-mm nodules (Fig 6–102,B). Bronchial wall thickening and peribronchial shadows are a striking and common feature. Such shadowing frequently radiates outward from the hili. Cavitation is not a feature. Flattening of the diaphragm and increased retrosternal space due to air-trapping are often present. Hilar adenopathy is very variable, being common in measles pneumonia and in infectious mononucleosis but rare with other viral pneumonias. Pleural effusions are not a prominent feature, though small ones do not negate the diagnosis.

Infections with influenza virus occur in epidemics and pandemics, and sporadically. Influenza A and B are the subtypes most commonly responsible for the severe outbreaks associated with pneumonia. The symptoms include fever, dry cough, myalgias, and headaches. Rhinitis, pharyngitis, bronchitis, and bronchiolitis may develop. When pneumonia occurs, it may be due to bacterial superinfection, *S. aureus*, *Pneumococcus*, and *H. influenza* being the common secondary invaders. The virus itself may cause pneumonia, and when it does, the infection is often very severe. Pneumonia is both more common and more serious in the elderly, in late pregnancy, and in those with underlying disorders, particularly cardiopulmonary disease.

Radiologically (see Fig 102), in one large series of over 100 patients with influenza pneumonia,[108] the findings were multifocal, 1- to 2-cm patchy consolidations that rapidly became confluent, with the majority showing bilateral consolidation and basilar predominance. Lobar and segmental consolidations were unusual. Pleural effusions, though encountered and sometimes large, were not a feature. Cavitation was notably rare. The appearance can resemble pulmonary edema, and the complicating bacterial pneumonia can be difficult to distinguish from the pneumonia due to the influenza virus itself.

Parainfluenza virus pneumonia occurs predominantly in outbreaks in winter, affecting mainly children. Usually parainfluenza infection causes upper respiratory symptoms, notably croup, and bronchi-

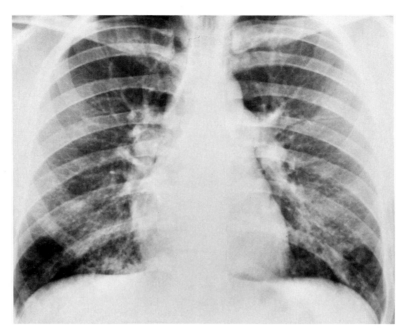

FIG 6–100.
Mycoplasma pneumonia showing bilateral hilar lymph node enlargement as well as interstitial pulmonary shadowing.

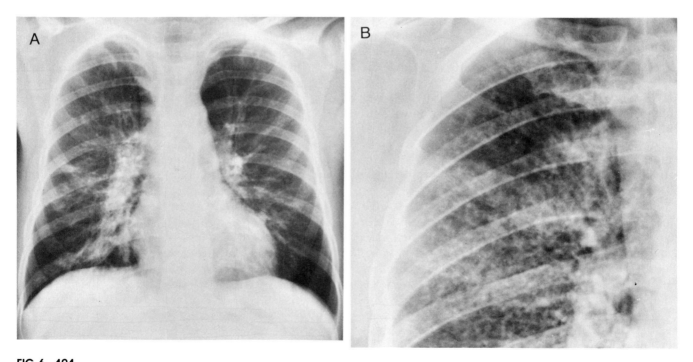

FIG 6–101.
Viral pneumonia: **(A)** in a child, showing scattered, small, ill-defined consolidations in both mid and lower zones; **(B)** an adult, showing widespread small nodular shadows.

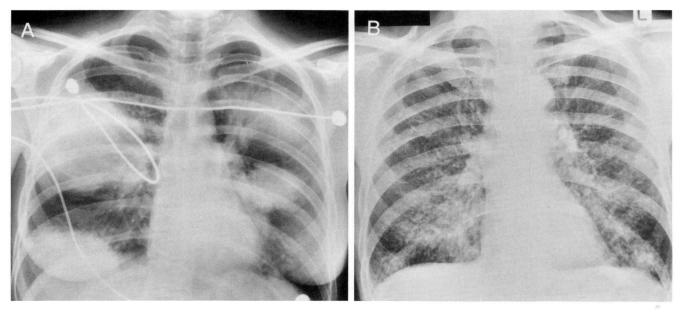

FIG 6–102.
Two examples of influenza pneumonia: **(A)**, showing multiple focal pulmonary consolidations; **(B)** showing multiple small, ill-defined nodular shadows scattered throughout the lungs, maximal at the bases.

olitis; pneumonia is relatively uncommon, particularly in adults. Pneumonia may result from bacterial superinfection. Radiologically, the appearances are those of patchy peribronchial consolidations, mainly in the lower lobes and pleural effusions may be seen.[332]

Respiratory syncytial virus is a major cause of bronchiolitis and bronchopneumonia in infants and young children. The plain chest radiograph shows streaky peribronchial opacities associated with overinflation of the lungs.[264, 298] Lobar collapse is a frequent finding,[251] and lobar consolidation is occasionally seen.[264]

Coxsackie, rhinovirus, and *ECHO (enteric cytopathic human orphan)* viruses are all related. They usually cause a flulike illness and upper respiratory tract symptoms. Very occasionally they cause pneumonia. The ECHO viruses usually affect infants; the other two may affect children and adults.[115] Radiologically,[116] the appearances are nonspecific, with reticulonodular shadowing radiating from the hilar region predominantly into the lower zones. These shadows may become confluent. Hilar adenopathy may be present.

Rubeola (measles) virus may cause pneumonia in addition to its other systemic and skin manifestations, particularly in children but also occasionally in adults.[132, 250] The pneumonia frequently contains multinucleated epithelial giant cells containing inclu-

sion bodies, a feature believed to be specific to measles and given the name giant cell pneumonia. The pneumonia usually develops before, or coincident with, the measles skin rash. Radiologically, in those with pneumonia,[90] the lungs show a widespread reticular pattern, often accompanied by hilar adenopathy. Lobar atelectasis of varying degree is common.

Superinfection with *Sta. aureus, Pneumococcus, H. influenza,* and *Str. pyogenes* may occur, in which case the pneumonia shows more focal confluent areas and sometimes also cavitation.

Usually the viral pneumonia clears with the resolution of the disease, but the radiographic changes may persist for many months.

Children who have been immunized with inactivated measles virus may develop atypical measles when exposed to the measles virus. The radiographic appearance of pneumonia in atypical measles[346] differs from that seen in the usual form, by showing more nodular (spherical) and segmental consolidations. The nodular consolidations may persist and be confused with pulmonary masses such as metastatic neoplasm, or sequestration. Hilar adenopathy frequently accompanies the pneumonia in atypical measles, as may pleural effusion.

Infectious mononucleosis due to the Epstein-Barr virus is a very common infection in the community but is a rare cause of pneumonia. The great majority of patients with infectious mononucleosis show no abnormalities on plain chest radiographs. The most frequent intrathoracic manifestation is hilar adenopathy. Pulmonary shadows are rare. When present, they are usually streaky or interstitial in appearance.[5, 182]

Adenovirus is a relatively frequent cause of mild infection of the respiratory tract. Pneumonia is uncommon and confined largely to infants and young children. The chest radiograph[119, 232, 296] shows patchy or confluent widespread consolidations, though consolidations confined to one lobe are also encountered. Bronchial wall thickening and peribronchial shadowing are striking findings. Air trapping is very common in young children. Lobar collapse is also frequent. Small pleural effusions are seen in approximately one-third of patients. The infection can be highly damaging, leaving bronchiectasis[232] or bronchiolitis obliterans, and the Swyer-James (McLeod) syndrome may result.[201]

Herpes simplex viruses are divided into two basic types, one that causes mucocutaneous vesicles and another that causes genital tract infection and is spread by means of sexual intercourse or acquired during birth.

Pneumonia is extremely uncommon except in the immunocompromised patient. Herpes simplex pneumonia is a particular problem for patients with AIDS (see the section "Pulmonary Infection in the Immunocompromised Patient" later in this chapter).

Chicken pox and *herpes zoster (shingles)* are both caused by the varicella-zoster virus. Pneumonia due to the virus is rare in children, bacterial superinfection being the likely cause if a child with chicken pox develops pneumonia. Over 90% of cases of varicella-zoster pneumonia occur in adults, in patients with lymphoma, and in those who are immunocompromised for a variety of reasons. Symptoms of pneumonia develop 1 to 6 days after the onset of the skin rash.[319] The plain chest film[281, 319] differs slightly from that seen with other viral infections in that the pneumonia causes multiple 5 to 10 mm ill-defined nodules (Fig 6–103), that may be confluent and which may come and go in different areas of the lungs. Hilar adenopathy and small pleural effusions occur during the acute phase of the disease, but are unusual. The small, round consolidations resolve quickly after the disappearance of the skin lesions, usually within a week or so, but can persist for months. In a few patients, the lesions calcify and can then be seen forever as numerous well-defined randomly scattered 2 to 3 mm dense calcifications in otherwise healthy lungs (see Fig 5–105). The appearance resembles the calcifications seen following disseminated histoplasmosis.

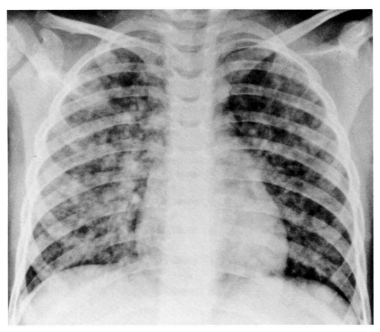

FIG 6–103.
Chickenpox pneumonia showing widespread ill-defined 5- to 10-mm nodular shadows.

PROTOZOAL INFECTIONS

Amebiasis is due to the *Entamoeba histolytica*, a protozoan that is found worldwide. The condition is usually asymptomatic. Symptomatic infections are usually confined to the gastrointestinal tract and liver. Pleural effusion and lower lobe consolidation may be present contiguous to an amebic abscess in the liver or subphrenic space, just as they may accompany any other suppurative process in these sites. An amebic liver abscess may extend through the diaphragm into the pleura giving rise to empyema, and may even extend into the lung causing pneumonia and lung abscess.[152, 307] The most common symptoms are fever and cough, which may be productive of chocolate-colored pus. Hemoptysis and chest or abdominal pain are also frequent.[307] Fistulae may form connecting the liver abscess to the airways, the pericardium, and very rarely to the skin.

The radiographic findings are empyema and adjacent pulmonary consolidation or lung abscess, which may be combined with signs of an elevated hemidiaphragm[152, 330, 338] (Fig 6–104). Signs of liver or subphrenic abscess will be visible on CT or ultrasound examination.

Hematogenous spread of amebic liver abscess to the lungs is very rare. When it occurs, it causes transient areas of pneumonia or lung abscess.

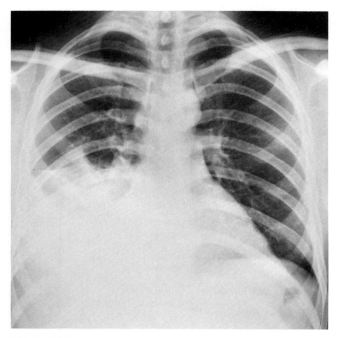

FIG 6– 104.
Intrathoracic changes secondary to amebic lung abscess. There is a large right pleural effusion with collapse/consolidation of the right lower lobe.

HELMINTHIC INFECTION

Roundworm, Hookworm, and *Strongyloides* Infections

Ascaris lumbricoides (roundworms), *Ankylostoma duodenale*, *Necator americanus* (hookworms), and *Strongyloides stercoralis* are all roundworms that, as part of their life cycle, pass through the lung. *Ascaris* eggs are ingested in food contaminated by infected feces and hatch in the small intestine to penetrate the bowel wall and enter the lymphatics and bloodstream. *Ankylostoma* and *Strongyloides* eggs hatch in human feces deposited in soil and penetrate the skin of the hands or feet of those that come into contact with infected soil or dust. In some cases, *Strongyloides* eggs may reenter the same host by way of the intestinal mucosa or perianal skin. Regardless of the route by which these organisms enter the bloodstream, they are carried to the lung, where they burrow through the alveolar walls to enter the airways and ascend in the tracheobronchial tree, eventually to be swallowed into the intestine, where they grow to their adult form. *Strongyloides* may also grow to adult form within the lung itself. The clinical features are largely related to the skin and gastrointestinal tract. Pulmonary symptoms are uncommon with all three organisms and include an unproductive cough, substernal chest pain, and, occasionally, hemoptysis and dyspnea. *Strongyloides*, if they grow to adult form in the lung, may give rise to a syndrome resembling asthma. Strongyloidiasis may also be responsible for overwhelming infection in immunocompromised patients.[248]

In most instances, there are no pulmonary complications with any of these worms but, in a few patients, an allergic reaction may occur in the lung parenchyma, which manifests itself radiographically as dense transient migratory infiltrates without recognizable segmental distribution.[30] Blood and sputum eosinophilia are often present, and the entity is therefore included as one of the causes of acute pulmonary infiltrates with eosinophilia (Löffler syndrome).[114] Cavitation does not occur, nor does hilar/mediastinal lymphadenopathy. Pleural effusions are not a feature.

Filariasis

The filarial worm that most commonly causes pulmonary manifestations is *Wuchereria bancrofti*. The major disease caused by this organism is the disfiguring condition of elephantiasis, owing to filarial obstruction of cutaneous lymphatics. This organism is also believed to be the cause of tropical eosinophilia, a syndrome consisting of cough, wheezing, and severe blood eosinophilia.[226] The chest radiograph[146, 321] may be normal but usually shows widespread fine nodular or reticulonodular shadowing. The appearances may closely resemble those of miliary tuberculosis. Occasionally, localized consolidation is seen. The pulmonary shadowing, which is due to eosinophilic and histiocytic infiltration,[321] is believed to be due to an immunologic response to microfilaria rather than to direct infection. Although pleural thickening may be demonstrated, pleural effusion does not appear to be a feature.[321] Generalized lymphadenopathy may occur, but radiographically visible mediastinal/hilar adenopathy is uncommon.[226] The radiologic changes usually resolve with treatment, but sometimes resolution takes months, and in some cases interstitial fibrosis may supervene.[321] Though *W. bancrofti* is believed to be the major inciting organism in tropical eosinophilia, other filaria, *Brugia malayi* for example, are thought to be responsible for a small proportion of cases.

Very rarely the filarial worm *Dirofilaria immitis* (dog heartworm) can cause pulmonary infection in humans. It usually infects dogs, but can be transferred to humans by mosquito bites. The larvae travel to the walls of the right-sided cardiac chambers and may dislodge and embolize into the pulmonary vascular bed, where they cause a granulomatous reaction that manifests itself as a solitary 1- to 2-cm subpleural pulmonary nodule on chest radiograph.[54] *Dirofilaria* granulomas are usually found in adults. Since the blood eosinophil count is usually normal and there are no reliable skin or serologic tests, the granulomas are usually excised in the belief that they may be bronchial carcinoma.

Other worms that may cause a localized granulomatous reaction in the lung are dog and cat *Ascaridoidea* worms, *Toxocara canis*, and *Toxocara cati* (visceral larva migrans). Symptoms include cough, wheezing, dyspnea, and a number of extrapulmonary manifestations. Infections with these organisms usually occur in children and produce patchy areas of consolidation on the plain chest radiograph associated with peripheral blood eosinophilia (Fig 6–105).

Schistosomiasis

Pulmonary disease due to schistosomiasis is rare. Of the flukes responsible for schistosomiasis (*Schistosoma mansoni*, *S. japonicum*, and *S. haematobium*), *S. mansoni* and *S. haematobium* are those most likely to be implicated in pulmonary disease. Various species of freshwater snails act as the intermediate hosts, being infected by larvae hatched from eggs that reach the water in feces or urine. Cercariae, the infective larvae, leave the snails and penetrate the skin or mucus membranes of humans as they swim or paddle in the water. The cercariae migrate to the mesenteric veins or, in the case of *S. haematobium*, to the venous

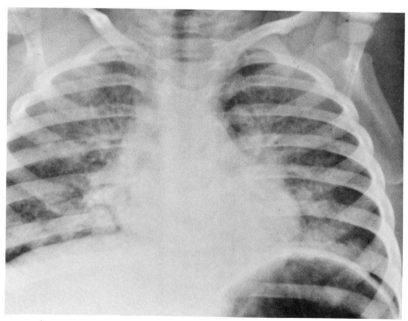

FIG 6–105.
Toxocara canis infection with widespread pulmonary consolidation.

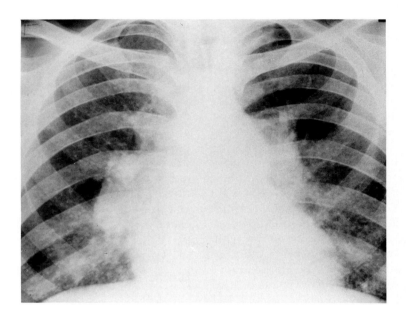

FIG 6–106.
Schistosomiasis with widespread, basally predominant, reticulo-nodular shadows in both lungs. The cardiac enlargement and large central pulmonary arteries are due to the associated pulmonary arterial hypertension. (Courtesy of Dr. Michael C. Pearson, London.)

plexuses of the bladder, prostate, or uterus. The adult flukes mate and deposit eggs in the veins, and the eggs are carried to various sites where they induce inflammation, ulceration, and fibrosis. Deposition of eggs in the small vessels of the lungs is rare, but when it occurs, the resulting granulomatous inflammation causes luminal obliteration[159] and may result in increased pulmonary vascular resistance.[110] In these cases, the major radiographic features are those of pulmonary arterial hypertension but, on occasion, a widespread fine reticular nodular shadowing representing ova with surrounding inflammatory changes or fibrosis may be seen (Fig 6–106).[73, 159]

Patchy consolidations due to Löffler's syndrome may be seen early in the course of the infection as the flukes migrate through the lungs. Very rarely a solitary nodule may be identified (Fig 6–107).[240]

Paragonimiasis

Paragonimiasis is usually the result of infection by the lung fluke *Paragonimus westermani*. The disease, which is endemic in Southeast Asia, Indonesia, West Africa, and South America, is acquired by eating crustaceans and water snails that act as the intermediate host. The immature flukes penetrate the bowel wall, travel through the peritoneal cavity, and migrate through the diaphragm to enter the lung parenchyma. Infection, as documented by positive serologic tests, may be asymptomatic and show no radiographic abnormalities. Symptoms include hemoptysis, pleuritic chest pain, and chronic cough, which may produce sputum containing the ova of the infecting organism.

The pulmonary changes result from chronic

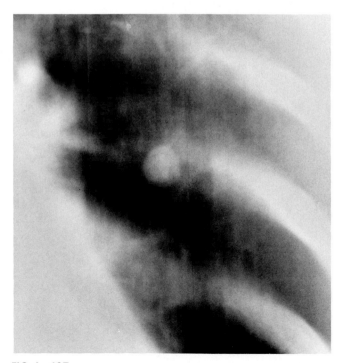

FIG 6–107.
Schistosomiasis causing a solitary pulmonary granuloma.

inflammation in areas surrounding the worm. Radiographically[163, 227, 313] (Fig 6–108), these areas are seen as multiple round, poorly defined consolidations in any lung zone, but most often in the mid zones. The consolidations may be fleeting and associated with blood eosinophilia.[12] As time goes by, the lesions become better defined, often appear nodular and may excavate, leaving cystic air spaces. Because the flukes penetrate the diaphragm and pleura, pleural effusions are common.[163]

Echinococcus Infection

Hydatid disease is caused by tapeworms: *Echinococcus granulosus* and *E. multilocularis* (alveolaris). The life cycle involves primary and intermediate mammalian hosts. Dogs are the usual primary host. The intermediate host is usually a sheep or a cow, but is sometimes man. The disease is endemic in sheep-rearing areas of South America and the Mediterranean Basin, particularly North Africa and Greece. It is even more common in Australia. Cases are, however, occasionally encountered from infections acquired in other parts of the world, including North America and Wales. The so-called Sylvatic form[67] has deer and moose as intermediate hosts and is endemic in the frozen north.

The adult worm lives in the small intestine of the primary host. Ova are passed in feces and ingested by the intermediate host. Larvae develop in the duodenum of this new host, where they enter the bloodstream and travel to the liver and lungs and occasionally even into the systemic circulation. The life cycle is completed when another primary host eats the remains of an infected intermediate host.

Disease in humans is due to the cysts that form around the parasite. Eosinophilia above 5% occurred in 40% of patients in a series reported from Lebanon.[17] The most reliable serologic test uses partially purified hydatid antigen or antigen 5. Complement fixation, hemagglutination, latex agglutination, and bentonite flocculation tests are also available. The Casoni skin test is not recommended because of its low sensitivity and specificity.[164] The structure of these cysts is important in the understanding of the radiographic findings. As they grow, hydatid cysts compress the adjacent lung into a fibrotic capsule known as the pericyst. The cyst itself has a thin, smooth wall composed of two adherent layers—the laminated ectocyst and the delicate lining endocyst from which hang the daughter cysts. The pulmonary cysts may grow rapidly, and approximately two-thirds rupture. Most rupture into the surrounding lung and bronchial tree, and secondary infection of the ruptured cyst is common. Occasionally the cyst will rupture into the pleural cavity. Rupture may result in an acute allergic reaction, sometimes accompanied by life-threatening hypotension. Cysts that

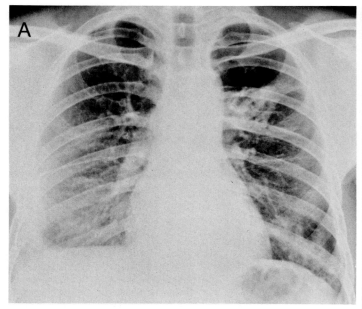

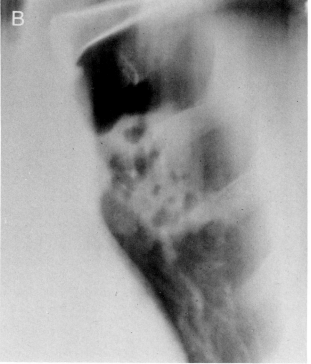

FIG 6–108.
Paragonimiasis. **A,** there is ill-defined consolidation. **B,** the tomogram shows complex central cavitation in the consolidation.
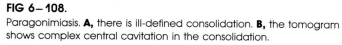

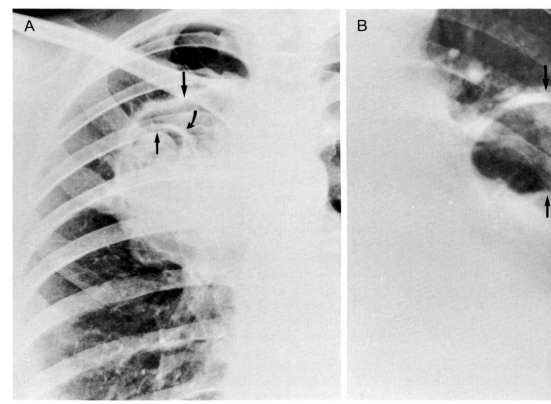

FIG 6–109.
Ruptured hydatid cyst. **(A)** showing the pericyst *(downward pointing arrow)*, the ectocyst *(curved arrow)*, and daughter cyst *(upward pointing arrow)*. There are air-crescents between the ectocyst and the pericyst and also between the daughter cyst and the ectocyst. **B,** another patient, showing the pericyst *(downward pointing arrow)* and the ectocyst *(upward pointing arrow)* with air between them.

have not ruptured usually do not give rise to symptoms, and the diagnosis is then made on the basis of a routine chest film.

The cardinal radiographic features* are one or more spherical or oval well-defined smooth masses of homogeneous density in otherwise normal lung, usually in the mid or lower zones. Multiple cysts are seen in about one-third of patients and are bilateral in 20%[31]; sometimes more than ten cysts are seen. There is a predilection for the lower lobes, the posterior segments, and the right lung.[17, 31] CT scanning[279] reveals the fluid contents of the cyst with a density close to that of water; the daughter cysts, when present, appear as curved septations. At CT scanning the cyst walls range in thickness from 2 mm up to 1 cm, the wall at CT representing the combined pericyst, ectocyst, and endocyst. The cysts may be very large; cysts of 10 cm and even 20 cm have been reported. The rate of growth

*References 17, 31, 41, 210, and 277.

may be fairly rapid, with doubling times of less than 6 months. A striking feature is that the cyst is relatively pliant and moulds to adjacent structures, resulting in indentations, lobulations, or flattenings. Surrounding inflammation may cause the edge of the lesion to be ill-defined. Calcification, which is such a common feature of hydatid cysts in the liver, is extremely rare in cysts that arise in the lungs.

If the pericyst ruptures (Fig 6–109), air dissects between the fibrotic lung forming the pericyst and the ectocyst of the parasite, leading to a visible crescent of air between the two, known as a "meniscus" or "crescent" sign. If the cyst itself ruptures, then an air-fluid level results, and daughter cysts may even be seen floating in the residual fluid. On rare occasions, air is seen on both sides of the true cyst wall; that is, a crescent of air is seen surrounding the cyst and air-fluid levels are also present. Sometimes, the cyst wall is seen crumpled up and floating in fluid, which lies within the noncollapsed pericyst—a pathognomonic appearance imaginatively described as the "water lily" sign or the "camalote" sign. All these signs are particularly well demonstrated at CT.[279] With secondary infection, the membranes may disintegrate and the walls thicken, so that the picture is indistinguishable from bacterial lung abscess.

Hydatid cysts may also be present in the pleura, in which case they may be secondary to seeding of the pleura following rupture. In some cases, the pleural location can be the primary site of disease. Mediastinal cysts are relatively rare. They form smooth round or oval masses in the mediastinum that may compress adjacent mediastinal structures such as the major airways or erode the bone of the thoracic cage.[255]

PULMONARY INFECTION IN THE IMMUNOCOMPROMISED PATIENT

The ability of an individual to combat infections may be impaired by a variety of mechanisms (Table 6–2). In summary, these mechanisms are:

1. *Granulocytopenia.* Granulocytes are an essential line of defense against microorganisms, and any deficiency of their numbers will weaken the host's defenses. Granulocytopenia may be a feature of the actual disease process or, alternatively, be a consequence of drug or radiation therapy. The incidence of pulmonary infections shows a steep rise as granulocyte counts fall below 1,000 cells/cu mm.

2. *Reduced cell-mediated immunity.* T-lymphocyte–dependent immune responses are an important line

TABLE 6–2.

Impairment of Human Immunity to Infection

Impaired Cell	Nature of Immunocompromise	Causes of Impairment	Common Infecting Organisms
Granulocyte	Altered inflammatory response	Acute and chronic myelocytic leukemia Steroids Drugs, including chemotherapeutic agents Chronic granulomatous disease Irradiation	Bacteria: E. coli, H. influenza S. aureus Serratia marcescens Pseudomonas Klebsiella Nocardia Fungi: Aspergilla, Candida
T lymphocyte	Reduced cell-mediated immunity	Lymphoma Acquired immune deficiency syndrome Steroids Chemotherapeutic agents Renal insufficiency Irradiation	Bacteria: Legionella, Listeria Nocardia, M. tuberculosis Viruses: Cytomegalovirus, varicella Fungi: Aspergillus Cryptococcus Parasites: Pneumocystis Toxoplasma
B lymphocyte	Reduced antibody formation	Lymphoma Acute and chronic lymphocytic leukemia Multiple myeloma Hypogammaglobulinemia Steroids Chemotherapeutic agents	Bacteria: E. coli, Pseudomonas Klebsiella S. pneumoniae Viruses: Cytomegalovirus Parasites: Pneumocystis
Macrophage	Impaired granulomatous response	Silica	Bacteria: M. tuberculosis Fungi: Blastomyces Histoplasma

of defense, particularly against obligate intracellular parasites as well as against nonpathogenic commensals in the respiratory tract.

3. *Reduced humoral immunity.* Impairment of B-lymphocyte function reduces the antibody response to infective agents, thereby diminishing host resistance. A reduction of circulating antibodies may also be a serious feature of hypoglobulinemic states. Similarly, thymic aplasia, asplenia, or splenectomy can result in humoral immunodeficiency, leading to marked susceptibility to infections with organisms such as *Str. pneumoniae.*

4. *Incompetence of cellular elements.* Inability of granulocytes to combat certain microorganisms is seen in patients with chronic granulomatous disease. It has been suggested that silica particles in some way damage pulmonary macrophages and thereby reduce the ability of the lungs to mount an adequate response to microorganisms such as *M. tuberculosis* or the fungi.[2, 144]

5. Nonspecific reduction in host resistance. Advanced age, alcoholism, diabetes mellitus, starvation or malnutrition, cancer, or other debilitating diseases may reduce the ability of an individual to combat infections.

A commonly encountered clinical problem is the immunocompromised patient with fever and pulmonary shadows. Before discussing the differential diagnosis in more detail, a number of generalized statements may be made in connection with pulmonary disease in the immunocompromised host.[273]

1. Seventy-five percent of pulmonary complications in these patients result from infection (in patients with severe neutropenia or in those with focal pulmonary lesions, the figure is 90%). In the remaining 25%, the complications relate to pulmonary drug reactions, pulmonary manifestations of the underlying disease, or unrelated diseases such as cardiac edema or pulmonary emboli. In up to 30% of cases, more than one pulmonary complication is present.

2. Diffuse pulmonary shadowing is associated with an overall mortality approaching 50%. Establishing the exact nature of the complication improves the outcome by no more than 10% to 20%. Even at autopsy the exact diagnosis is never established in 15% to 20% of cases.

3. The chest radiograph almost never provides an exact diagnosis; the most that can be expected is a list of differential diagnoses to be correlated with the clinical and laboratory findings.

Bacterial Pneumonia

Bacteria are the most frequent cause of pneumonia in the immunocompromised patient. In general terms, the pneumonias caused by organisms such as *Str. pneumoniae, Sta. aureus,* or *P. aeruginosa* do not differ from their counterparts in the general population. Patients with neutropenia may show a slight lag in the appearance of pulmonary consolidation and, in the group as a whole, pleural effusions and empyema are uncommon. On occasion, bacterial pneumonias may become widely disseminated in the lungs of immunocompromised patients, an occurrence that is unusual in otherwise healthy individuals (Fig 6–110).

Patients on steroids and patients with renal transplants are particularly susceptible to Legionella-like organisms. These organisms include *L. pneumophila* and *L. micdadei* (Pittsburgh agent). *Legionella pneumophila* pneumonia shows a spreading pattern of focal consolidation involving wide areas of lung, sometimes with cavitation and pleural effusion. *Legionella micdadei* pneumonia is particularly prevalent in renal transplant recipients. It has a fairly characteristic radiographic pattern[245] consisting of fairly well circumscribed nodular densities which show a distinct tendency to central cavitation in the lungs

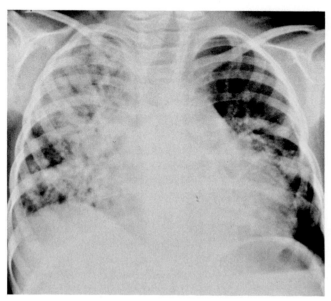

FIG 6–110.
Disseminated *E. coli* pneumonia in a child with leukemia.

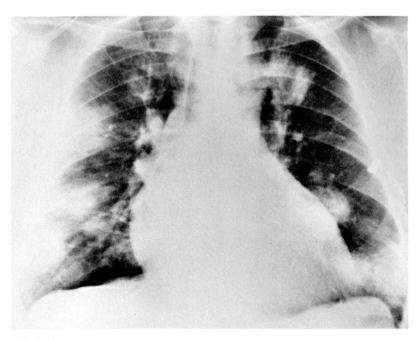

FIG 6–111.
A renal transplant patient with multiple rounded areas of *L. micdadei* pneumonia.

(Fig 6–111). The number of these densities is variable, and the distribution may be widespread and random.

Tuberculosis is always feared in the immunocompromised patient but, in practice, is rare. This presumably reflects the decline of tuberculosis in the general population. Those cases that are encountered represent reactivation of quiescent lesions and, in these patients, there is often a history of previous tuberculosis or a positive tuberculin skin test. It is feared, however, that the developing AIDS epidemic may bring with it a recrudescence of tuberculosis. In a study of patients with AIDS and complicating tuberculosis, Pitchenik and Rubinson[244] found that the radiographic features most often resembled primary tuberculosis despite strong indications that most cases, in fact, represented reactivation (see the discussion "Reactivation Tuberculosis" earlier in this chapter). Tuberculosis occurring as a result of steroid therapy is clinically and radiographically indistinguishable from reactivation tuberculosis. On rare occasions, tuberculosis may disseminate in a fulminant fashion, resulting in diffuse pulmonary consolidation (Fig 6–112).

Nocardia asteroides infection is fairly common in the immunocompromised host, particularly in patients on corticosteroids and immunosuppressive agents. The clinical presentation is subacute, and the radiographic features are slow in development. The radiographic features are discussed in the section "Nocardiosis" earlier in this chapter.

Fungal Infection

Aspergillus fumigatus, a rare cause of primary pneumonia in the general population, achieves a major role in the immunocompromised group, particularly in patients with lymphoma or leukemia.[145] The pulmonary aspergilloses are a spectrum of disease ranging from bronchopulmonary aspergillosis in the hyperimmune host, through pulmonary mycetoma formation in lung cavities of patients with normal immune status, to invasive pulmonary aspergillosis in the immunocompromised host. Overlap between these entities occurs, and "semi-invasive" pulmonary aspergillosis has been reported as a chronic cavitary disease process in patients with mild immuno-compromise and underlying lung damage.[113] The following discussion is confined to the acute invasive form of pulmonary aspergillosis, which pathologically is characterized by mycotic vascular invasion, thrombosis, and infarction leading to necrosis and cavitation. The lungs may be seeded by means of the airways (particularly in the more localized forms of disease) or the blood stream.

The diagnosis of invasive aspergillosis is not easy

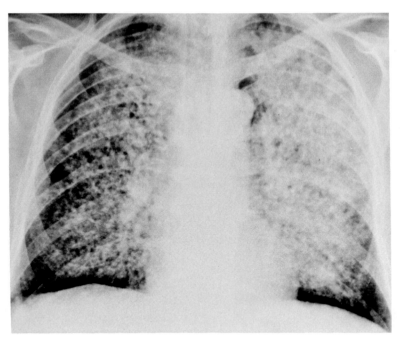

FIG 6–112.
Leukemic patient with biopsy-proved disseminated tuberculosis. A chest radiograph 1 month earlier was normal in appearance.

to make, particularly in the early phases before cavitation supervenes. Indeed, in perhaps one-third of cases the chest radiographs taken soon after the onset of symptoms may appear normal.[343] There are basically two initial radiographic patterns: single or multiple areas of rounded pneumonia, and disseminated miliary or nodular pulmonary shadows. Of these two, the rounded pneumonia pattern occurs much more frequently.[191] The regions of rounded pneumonia are randomly distributed in the lung, and the margins are indistinct (Fig 6–113). CT is particularly suited to demonstrating the rounded nature of the pneumonias and the indistinct invasive margin.[179] CT may also demonstrate very early lesions not visualized on chest radiographs. On isolated occasions, an air bronchogram may be seen within the area of consolidation.

Cavitation is not usually seen on the initial radiographs. There is evidence that cavitation occurs with recovery from neutropenia when leukocytes mobilize in the area of infiltration.[112] Thus, cavitation is paradoxically a favorable sign indicating a significant defensive response. The earliest sign of cavitation is the air-crescent sign in which a lucent crescent of air develops toward the margin of the rounded pneumonia.[66] The air-crescent is usually seen toward the upper margin of the pneumonia. The lucency enlarges and extends to form a true cavity often with

mural nodulation (see Fig 6–113).[134] An interesting precursor of the air-crescent sign, which may be seen on CT, is the development of a band of decreased attenuation around the margin of rounded pneumonia.[179] This CT halo is thought to represent a zone of tissue demarcation in which the air-crescent will develop.

The single or multiple areas of rounded pneumonia enlarge slowly over a period ranging from 7 to 28 days and may eventually become segmental or lobar consolidations. Hilar adenopathy is not a feature and pleural effusions are, in general, seen only if hemorrhagic infarction supervenes. Invasion of the chest wall or mediastinal structures is described but is exceedingly rare.[4, 200]

Disseminated pulmonary invasive aspergillosis may arise de novo or complicate the more localized form. The pulmonary shadows in these patients range from a miliary to a more coarsely nodular pattern.[40, 190] Hematogenous dissemination from a distant focus, as might be expected, involves the lungs fairly evenly (Fig 6–114), whereas a heavy airway inoculum may give a more central unevenly distributed pattern of bronchopneumonia (Fig 6–115).

Candida albicans species may cause pneumonia, either alone or in combination with other fungi, particularly *Aspergillus* species. A significant proportion of patients with *C. albicans* pneumonia have leuke-

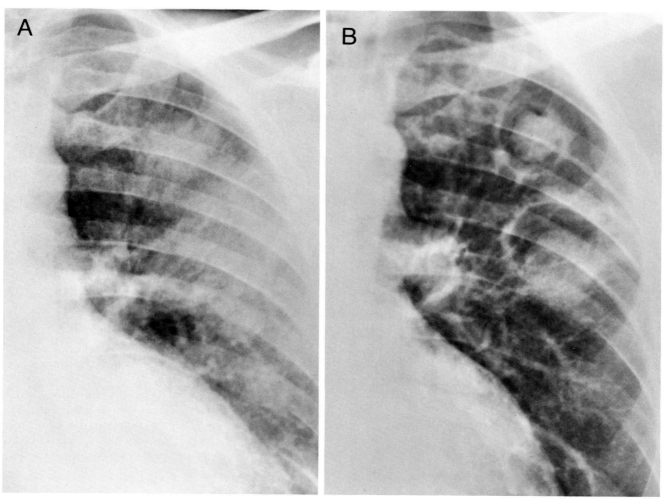

FIG 6–113.

Aspergillus pneumonia in a leukemic patient. **A,** a nondescript area of consolidation in the lung. **B,** 12 days later two rounded cavities, each with a central slough surrounded by a rim of air, have developed, while the remainder of the pneumonia has cleared.

mia or lymphoma often in the later stages of treatment.[46] The great majority have widespread systemic dissemination of the organism.[72] Aspiration *Candida* pneumonia without systemic involvement is stated to be rare.[271]

The diagnosis of *C. albicans* pneumonia is difficult, partly because pneumonia caused by other opportunistic organisms may also be present, and partly because the presence of superficial colonization by *Candida* species may be discounted. Typically, the patient with disseminated candidiasis has severe and prolonged neutropenia, persistent fever in spite of antibiotic therapy, hepatomegaly, obvious colonies of *C. albicans* on the mucous membranes, and pulmonary shadowing on chest radiograph. Buff et al.[46] have analyzed the radiographic appear-

ances in 20 histologically proved cases of "pure" pulmonary candidiasis. The great majority were identified at autopsy, and the radiographs, obtained within 48 hours of death, presumably reflected advanced disease. Nearly half the patients had radiographic changes suggesting diffuse bilateral nonsegmental patchy disease of an alveolar or mixed alveolar-interstitial character. The remaining patients had unilateral or bilateral lobar or segmental areas of pulmonary consolidation. These authors found that cavitation, adenopathy, masslike infiltrates, or miliary infiltrates were not observed. On the other hand, Pagani and Libshitz[235] described a pattern of miliary-nodular infiltration in pulmonary candidiasis more akin to the findings seen in Figure 6–116. It is possible that this pattern represents an earlier mani-

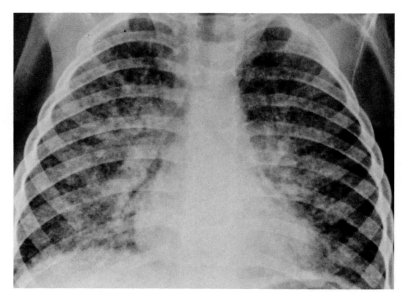

FIG 6–114.
Disseminated aspergillosis in a child with chronic granulomatous disease.

festation of pulmonary candidiasis. All the patients in the series of Buff et al. succumbed to disseminated candidiasis, whereas the patient illustrated in Figure 6–116 responded satisfactorily to treatment. Dubois et al.[81] failed to find any specific radiographic patterns in pulmonary candidiasis, partly because of the high frequency of other pulmonary infections, edema, and hemorrhage. These authors stressed the need for the early institution of antifungal therapy based primarily on clinical grounds.

The *phycomycetes (Rhizopus, Mucor, Mortierella, Absidia,* and *Basidiobolus)* may, on rare occasions, cause a pneumonia in immunocompromised patients. The commonly accepted designation for infection with these species of fungi is mucormycosis. Mucormycosis has a 100% mortality in the absence of treatment

FIG 6–115.
Disseminated *Aspergillus* pneumonia in a patient with chronic lymphatic leukemia.

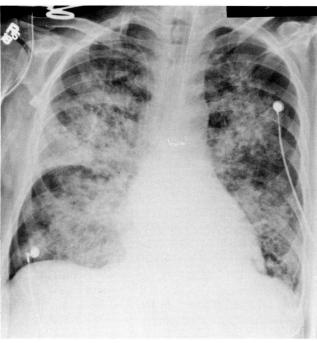

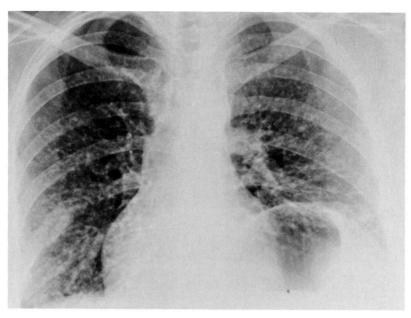

FIG 6–116.
Biopsy-proved disseminated pulmonary candidiasis in a young man with immuno-blastic leukemia.

and a very high mortality even with aggressive therapy. Approximately 75% of patients with mucormycosis have leukemia or lymphoma, and diabetes mellitus figures prominently among the remainder.[220] The most striking feature of the pathology of mucormycosis is fungal vascular invasion resulting in infarction.[214] An inexorable centrifugal pattern of spread is very common. This is characteristically seen with infection of the paranasal sinuses, with direct extension to involve the brain and the meninges being frequent. The diagnosis of pulmonary mucormycosis is difficult. A single focus of disease in the lung is common, and this may be manifest either as a pulmonary nodule or mass, or as lobar consolidation (Fig 6–117).[107, 259] Cavitation is frequently seen and is probably related to vascular invasion by the phycomycetes with consequent infarction. The cavity may contain a fungus ball or a slough.[262] Foci of consolidation may be multiple and will spread centrifugally with an ill-defined edge until the lobar boundaries are reached. Pleural effusions are recorded, but there has been no report of direct spread across fissural boundaries.

Cryptococcus neoformans pneumonia occurs in immunocompromised patients (Fig 6–118), although the majority have no demonstrable cellular or humoral immunocompromise. In immunocompromised hosts, the pneumonia is often overshadowed by cryptococcal meningitis. Cryptococcal pulmonary

infection is discussed in detail under "Cryptococcosis" in the section on fungal disease earlier in this chapter.

Widespread dissemination of blastomycosis, coccidioidomycosis, and histoplasmosis does occur in immunocompromised patients with serious consequences, but given the frequency of these diseases in certain geographic areas it is surprising that these fungi are so rarely implicated as opportunistic infective agents. Specific diagnostic features are lacking, and the clinical thrust is likely to be toward excluding infection by the more common opportunistic fungi.

Viral Infection

The most common virus to cause pneumonia in the immunocompromised patient is the *cytomegalovirus*. Infection is typically related to a defect in cell-mediated immunity and, therefore, is seen in lymphoma or transplant patients. Cytomegalovirus pneumonia may coexist with or even predispose to other pneumonias especially *P. carinii* pneumonia. The radiographic appearances are of diffuse interstitial shadows with basal predominance extending from the bases to give a diffuse, patchy, often slightly nodular pattern. The overlap with *P. carinii* pneumonia is considerable both radiologically and pathologically.

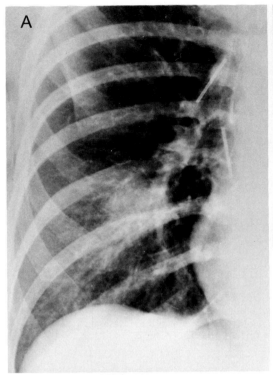

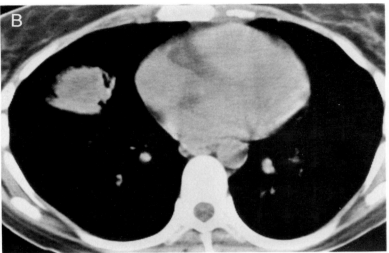

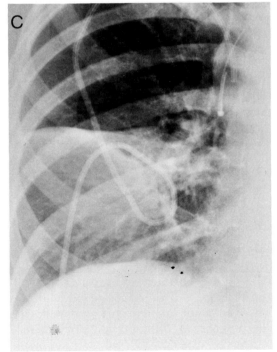

FIG 6–117.
Mucormycosis. Isolated pulmonary consolidation is seen in the middle lobe in a patient with lymphoma. **A,** PA radiograph. **B,** CT scan. **C,** PA radiograph 6 weeks later showing progression of the consolidation.

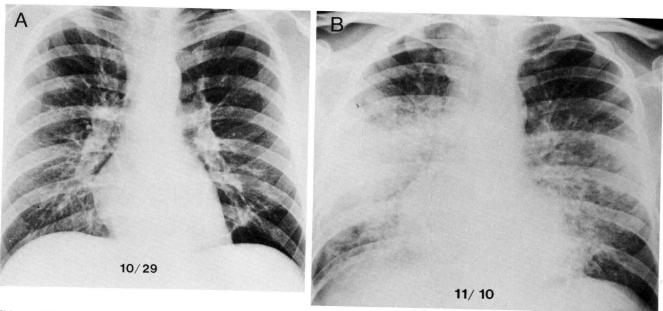

FIG 6–118.
A and **B,** cryptococcal pneumonia in a young man with lymphoma.

The other viruses capable of causing severe pneumonia especially in lymphoma patients are the zoster/varicella virus and the herpes simplex virus. Varicella/zoster pneumonia is fulminant with the development of extensive patchy areas of parenchymal consolidation which may become widely confluent (Fig 6–119). The diagnosis is rendered much more likely if the patient has coincident disseminated herpes zoster or varicella.

Parasitic Infection

The protozoan *Pneumocystis carinii* was first identified in 1909 by Chagas. This organism may be widespread in the animal kingdom as a commensal, and it was only in the 1960s and 1970s that the organism became increasingly recognized and sought as a pathogen in immunocompromised individuals. The advent of AIDS in the 1980s has brought *Pn. carinii*

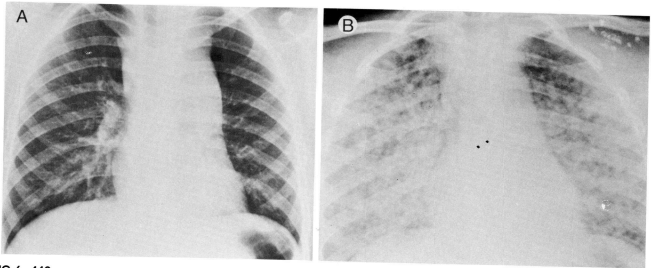

FIG 6–119.
Varicella pneumonia in a patient with lymphoma. **A,** prior to chemotherapy. **B,** after beginning chemotherapy.

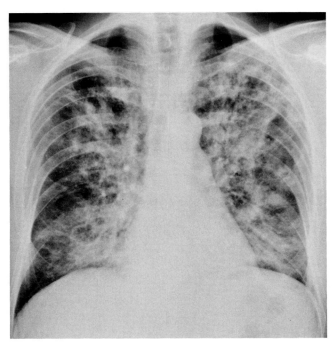

FIG 6—120.
Pneumocystis carinii pneumonia in a homosexual man with AIDS. Combined infection with cytomegalovirus.

pneumonia into public prominence, since it is the cause of up to 75% of pulmonary complications in AIDS patients and is a major cause of death in these individuals[310] (Fig 6—120).

Histologic studies show that *Pn. carinii* pneumo-nia is predominantly an alveolar filling process with only a minor interstitial inflammatory component.[71] *Pneumocystis carinii* rarely penetrates the alveolar wall, and systemic dissemination does not occur, except possibly in AIDS patients. Furthermore, *Pn. carinii* pneumonia is often associated with pneumo-nia caused by other opportunistic organisms such as cytomegalovirus or fungi. This association may in part explain the more focal patterns described in *Pn. carinii* pneumonia.[208] Nevertheless, the most usual form of *Pn. carinii* pneumonia is a diffuse synchro-nous alveolar filling process, which results in death from respiratory insufficiency rather than any sys-temic toxic effect.

It is common for patients with *Pn. carinii* pneu-monia to have entirely normal-appearing chest ra-diographs in the early phases of the disease.[111, 320] In such instances the infiltrates have not reached the threshold of radiographic visibility even though gallium-67 scans may provide unequivocal evidence of diffuse lung disease (Fig 6—121). Indeed, Ga-67 scanning is a highly sensitive method of determin-ing the presence of diffuse opportunistic infections of the lungs, with a 95% to 100% sensitivity in patients with *Pn. carinii* pneumonia.[59, 342] A normal Ga-67 scan has a predictive value of over 90% in ruling out *Pn. carinii* pneumonia.[342] On the other hand, Ga-67 scanning has a low specificity, as other opportunistic infections can equally well result in positive scans.

Correlation of the pathologic and radiologic

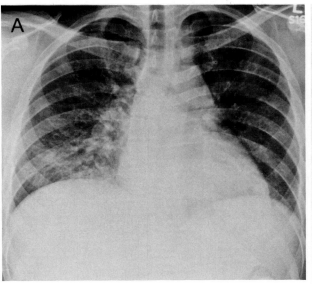
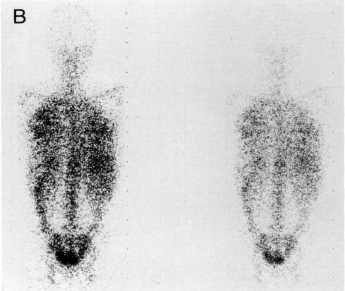

FIG 6—121.
Pneumocystis carinii pneumonia in a man with AIDS. **A,** the chest radiograph showed early diffuse pulmonary infiltration. **B,** the gallium scan shows markedly increased uptake in lungs.

findings in *Pn. carinii* pneumonia is difficult because of the relatively high frequency of associated disease processes.[109] These include other opportunistic infections, pulmonary manifestations of the underlying disease process, drug reactions, and agonal changes. Typical or classical changes will be described first, and consideration will then be given to variant appearances.

Even though *Pn. carinii* pneumonia is predominantly an alveolar filling process the earliest radiographic changes can appear "interstitial" in character (Fig 6–122). Thus, a diffuse fine nodular pattern is common, and there may be a slight reticular component. Progression of disease, however, leads to increasing confluence and density of the shadows, and an alveolar filling pattern becomes increasingly apparent (Fig 6–123). Typically, the shadows are diffuse and symmetric with a tendency to spare the periphery and the apices of the lungs (Fig 6–124). With severe involvement, however, this perihilar predominance may be lost, and the shadows may involve all parts of the lung. Certain portions of lung may be spared either because of preexisting disease such as bullous emphysema or because they lie within the field of previous irradiation.[100] Normal vascular structures become obscured, and air bronchograms may be a striking feature. This progres-

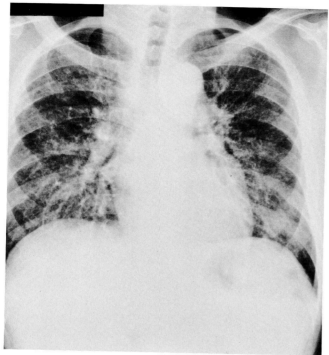

FIG 6–122.
Pneumocystis carinii pneumonia in a leukemic patient showing early diffuse infiltration, slightly "interstitial" in character.

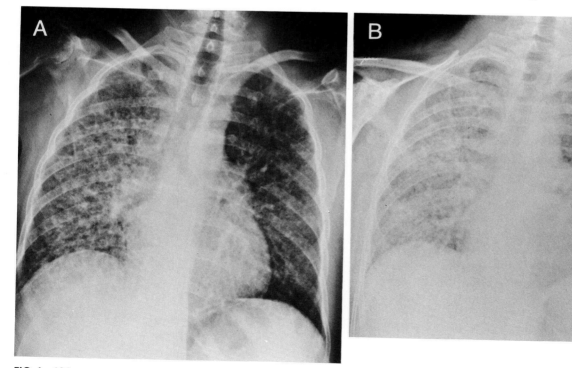

FIG 6–123.
Pneumocystis carinii pneumonia in a hemophiliac patient with AIDS shows progression to involve all parts of both lungs. **A** and **B,** the two views were obtained 5 days apart.

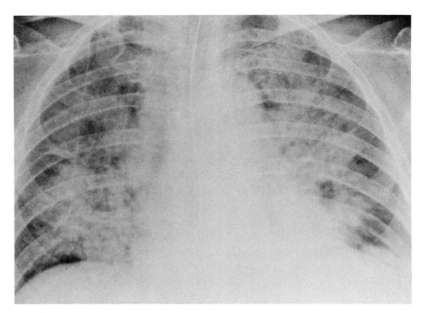

FIG 6–124.
Autopsy-proved *Pn. carinii* pneumonia in a lymphoma patient.

sion from a normal chest radiograph to severe diffuse air-space shadows occurs usually over a 3- to 5-day period.[79] With successful treatment, chest radiographs that were initially normal may remain so. Otherwise, the time for pulmonary shadowing to disappear is proportional to the initial severity, with a case of moderate severity usually clearing in some 10 to 14 days.

The most common variant is randomly distributed lobar consolidation, usually involving at least two lobes (Fig 6–125). Such cases may have coincident opportunistic infections, and the diagnosis is difficult without identifying the responsible organism.[147] Cavitation has been described in a very few cases but, in these cases, it has been difficult to positively incriminate *Pn. carinii* as the cause of the cavitation.[58] Pleural effusions are described but are certainly uncommon in "uncomplicated" *Pn. carinii* pneumonia,[79] and spontaneous pneumothorax has been described in a few patients.[121] Hilar or mediastinal adenopathy has been observed in isolated cases in some series,[79, 310] but it is difficult in such cases to exclude adenopathy caused by the patient's underlying disease or by a coincident infection such as tuberculosis. An exceptional manifestation of *Pn. carinii* pneumonia is the presence of pulmonary nodules, either single or multiple.[36, 64] Here, the potential for confusion with a malignant process such as Kaposi's sarcoma in an AIDS patient is considerable.

The Differential Diagnosis of Pulmonary Shadowing in the Immunocompromised Host

Fever and pulmonary shadows are a commonly encountered problem in the immunocompromised patient. Elucidation of such cases requires consider-

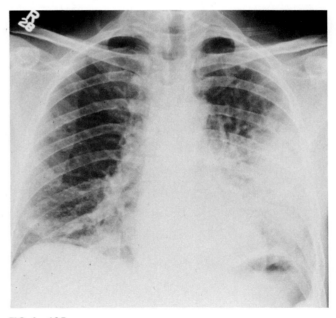

FIG 6–125.
Pneumocystis carinii pneumonia in a young man with AIDS. The pneumonia is atypical in that it is more asymmetric and focal than is usual.

ation of the nature of the immunocompromise (see Table 6–2), the results of previous tuberculin testing, whether the infection was acquired in or out of hospital, whether there is any known potential source of infection, and the results of blood or sputum cultures and of serologic testing. The possibility that the pulmonary shadowing is a noninfective complication should also be considered. In most cases, it is only by such a multipronged approach that one can reasonably expect to determine the likely diagnosis or to decide the basis for rational therapy.

In addition to the infections discussed in the preceding pages, pulmonary shadows in immunocompromised patients may be caused by one or more of the following: neoplastic involvement of the lung; pulmonary complications related to therapy; pulmonary hemorrhage; and nonspecific interstitial pneumonitis.

Neoplastic Involvement of the Lung

Patients with neoplasm, particularly those with leukemia or lymphoma, may be immunocompromised because of the treatment they are receiving or on occasion because of the primary disease. In these patients, the differential diagnosis of opportunistic pneumonia will include neoplastic involvement of the lung. Leukemic infiltrates, which may produce shadowing indistinguishable from that of opportunistic pneumonia, are discussed on p. 320. The radiographic differentiation between pneumonia and lymphomatous involvement of the lung can be ex-

tremely difficult, and often impossible, when the pulmonary shadowing is not masslike or nodular in appearance. Pleural effusions may occur in both leukemia and lymphoma and do not necessarily indicate a complicating infection.

Pulmonary Complications Related to Therapy

Included in this category are adverse drug reactions, transfusion reactions, graft-vs.-host reactions, and radiation pneumonitis. The radiographic features of adverse drug reactions and radiation pneumonitis are discussed in Chapter 10. Adverse drug reactions are sufficiently common, particularly with the cytotoxic agents, to make these a very real diagnostic possibility as a cause of focal or diffuse pulmonary infiltrates.

Transfusion reactions are usually acute, and the temporal relationship to the transfusion of blood or its fractions is clearcut. The reaction may simply be one of volume overload with pulmonary edema. More capricious are the agglutinin reactions resulting from an excess of antibodies in the donor serum directed against the recipient's cells, particularly granulocytes. The result is the abrupt onset of fever, chills, tachypnea, and tachycardia coincident with the development of varying patterns of pulmonary edema (Fig 6–126). The edema pattern may persist for 24 to 48 hours and a response to corticosteroid therapy may be appreciated.

Graft-vs.-host disease occurs in some 25% to 50% of patients following bone marrow transplantation. Transplanted immunocompetent lymphocytes

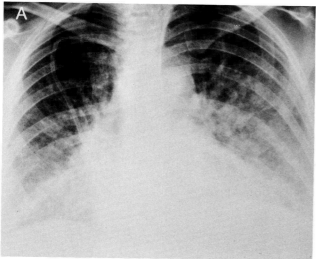
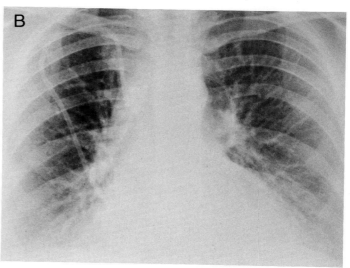

FIG 6–126.

Agglutinin reaction in a 40-year-old woman who had had a bone marrow transplant. **A,** chest radiograph at the height of the transfusion reaction. **B,** chest radiograph 12 hours later following steroid therapy.

react to the tissues of the patient and, in effect, the transplanted cells are rejecting the host.[178] Pulmonary manifestations of this condition develop some 3 to 12 months following the transplant. Clinically, the patients develop cough, bronchospasm, and an obstructive pulmonary function pattern. Pathologically, a lymphocytic bronchitis is found, and in severe cases there may be bronchiolitis obliterans. The radiographs reflect the airway distribution of disease with patchy nondescript perihilar infiltration (Fig 6–127). In severe cases, a diffuse pulmonary interstitial pattern is seen in the lungs.[234]

Pulmonary Hemorrhage

Leukemia may be associated with a profound bleeding tendency, and pulmonary hemorrhage may be one manifestation of this tendency. The clinical features may clearly indicate the bleeding tendency, and the abrupt appearance of patchy acinar densities with hemoptysis and a fall in the hematocrit may allow the diagnosis to be made.

However, it is difficult to ascertain the incidence of pulmonary hemorrhage in leukemia, particularly as the coagulopathy may preclude biopsy. Pulmonary hemorrhage varying from microscopic to massive hemorrhage is seen in some three-quarters of

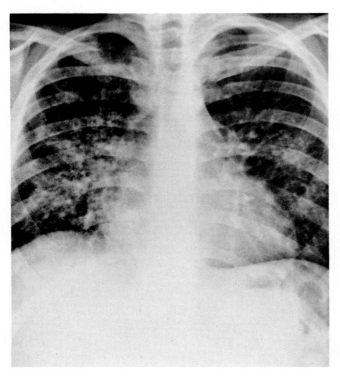

FIG 6–127.
Graft-vs.-host disease in a leukemic patient 4 months following bone marrow transplantation.

leukemic patients at autopsy.[202] The issue is complicated by the fact that pulmonary hemorrhage may be associated not only with a bleeding tendency but also with infection or diffuse alveolar damage.[202, 300] Tenholder and Hooper[314] suggest that the incidence of pulmonary hemorrhage as a sole cause of pulmonary shadowing in leukemic patients may be as high as 40%. This seems a high figure but it does serve to emphasize that pulmonary hemorrhage is probably underdiagnosed.

Nonspecific Interstitial Pneumonitis

In many cases exhaustive investigation fails to establish the cause of pulmonary densities in an immunocompromised patient. Recourse may then be made to lung biopsy, either open biopsy or by the transbronchial route. In a significant number of patients, the only result is a diagnosis of nonspecific diffuse alveolar damage and interstitial pneumonitis. Clearly the cases proceeding to biopsy tend to be the problematic ones, but in this select group nonspecific interstitial pneumonitis may be found in some 30% to 45% of cases.[168, 187, 274]

Nonspecific interstitial pneumonitis has been found to be frequent in AIDS patients with clinically evident pneumonitis. In an exhaustive study by Simmons et al.[297] it was found that although 50% of their AIDS patients proved to have *P. carinii* pneumonitis, 34% had nonspecific interstitial pneumonitis. Nonspecific interstitial pneumonitis was found to be clinically and radiologically indistinguishable from *P. carinii* pneumonitis. Nonspecific interstitial pneumonitis is, therefore, a highly significant clinical "entity." It seems likely, however, that this "entity" will ultimately prove to have more than one distinct cause.

Patients with AIDS and the AIDS-related complex may develop a lymphocytic interstitial pneumonia (LIP), which is radiographically difficult to distinguish from opportunistic infections.[228] LIP is probably much more common in the AIDS population than in the population at large. Positive identification of this lymphoproliferative disorder requires biopsy. As discussed on p. 315, LIP may evolve into a lymphoproliferative malignancy, but this conversion is rarely seen in AIDS patients, possibly because of their limited survival.

PARAPNEUMONIC PLEURAL EFFUSIONS AND EMPYEMA

There is no precise definition that distinguishes an uncomplicated parapneumonic pleural effusion from an empyema. By one definition, positive pleural fluid cultures are needed.[192] By another,[331] the pleural fluid must have a specific gravity of greater than 1.018, and a white blood cell count of greater than 500 cells/mm³ or a protein level greater than 2.5 gm/dl. Vianna[324] defined an empyema as pleural fluid with either positive cultures for the same microorganism from at least two consecutive samples or a white blood cell count greater than 15,000/mm³ and a protein level above 3.0 gm/dl.

According to the American Thoracic Society,[6] the evolution of an empyema can be divided into three stages which gradually merge together. These divisions have been amplified by Light in his recent reviews[192, 193]:

> First is the *exudative stage* characterized by the rapid outpouring of sterile pleural fluid into the pleural space in response to inflammation of the pleura. The associated pneumonic process is usually contiguous with the visceral pleura and results in increased permeability of the capillaries in the visceral pleura. The pleural fluid in this stage is characterized by a low

white blood count, a low lactic dehydrogenase (LDH) level, a normal glucose level and a normal pH.[194] If appropriate antibiotic therapy is instituted at this stage, the pleural effusion progresses no further, and the insertion of chest tubes is not necessary. If appropriate antibiotic therapy is not instituted, bacteria invade the pleural fluid from the contiguous pneumonic process, and the second, *fibropurulent,* stage evolves. This stage is characterized by the accumulation of large amounts of pleural fluid with many polymorphonuclear leukocytes, bacteria, and cellular debris. Fibrin is deposited in a continuous sheet covering both the visceral and parietal pleura in the involved area and the tendency is to loculation. These loculations prevent extension of the empyema, but make drainage of the pleural space with chest tubes increasingly difficult. As this stage progresses, the pleural fluid pH and glucose level become progressively lower and the LDH level progressively higher. The last stage is the *organization stage,* in which fibroblasts grow into the exudate from both the visceral and parietal pleural surfaces and produce an inelastic membrane called the pleural peel (Fig 6–128, A and B). This pleural peel encases the lung and renders it virtually

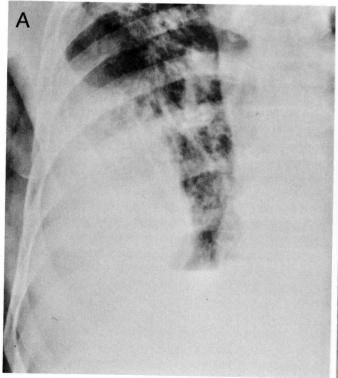 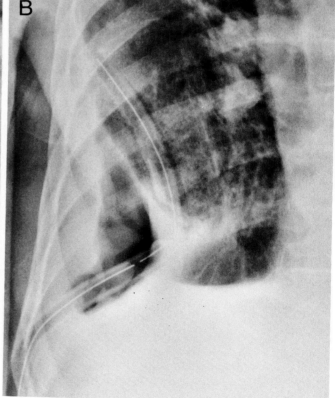

FIG 6–128.
Pleural peel in a tuberculous empyema. **A,** empyema prior to tube drainage. **B,** following tube drainage air has entered the empyema space, allowing one to recognize the greatly thickened parietal and visceral pleura.

functionless. At this stage the exudate is thick, and if the patient has remained untreated, the fluid may drain spontaneously through the chest wall (empyema necessitatis) or into the lung, to produce a bronchopleural fistula.

Most empyemas are associated with a recognizable pneumonia. The usual bacteria responsible for nontuberculous empyemas or "parapneumonic" effusions are anaerobic bacteria, *Sta. aureus, Str. pneumoniae,* other streptococcal species, and various gram-negative bacteria.

The clinical picture of patients with aerobic bacterial pneumonia and pleural effusion is quite similar to that of patients with bacterial pneumonia but no effusion. The incidence of pleuritic chest pain and the degree of leukocytosis are comparable, whether or not there is an accompanying pleural effusion.[195] Patients with anaerobic bacterial infections of the pleural space usually present with a subacute illness.[21] The majority have a history of alcoholism, an episode of unconsciousness, or another factor that predisposes to aspiration.

The diagnosis of parapneumonic effusion and empyema depends on recognizing fluid in the pleural cavity and performing thoracentesis for analyzing the fluid. Because empyemas are so protein-rich, there is a strong tendency for the pleural fluid to loculate and, therefore, ultrasound or CT may be required to appreciate the full size of the pleural fluid collection. With free fluid, lateral decubitus views will suffice to quantitate the fluid. Light et al.[195] recommend diagnostic thoracentesis in patients with pneumonia and pleural effusion if a layer of 1 cm or more of pleural fluid can be demonstrated on the lateral decubitus view. Lesser quantities of fluid will clear with antibiotic treatment and, therefore, the thoracentesis is not required.[195]

The appearance on plain chest radiographs varies with the evolution of the parapneumonic fluid collection. Uncomplicated, sterile effusions appear identical to pleural fluid collections that may accompany noninfectious consolidations such as pulmonary emboli, postpericardiotomy syndrome, and pancreatitis. Previous scarring of the pleural cavity may lead to loculation, but otherwise the fluid is mobile. Fibropurulent fluid collections have a strong tendency to loculate. Loculated fluid does not fall to the most dependent portion of the pleural cavity, so images taken in various positions will show fixed collections of fluid density.

The distinction between pulmonary consolidation/abscess and loculated pleural fluid on conventional radiographs can be difficult but has important therapeutic consequences. Empyema requires early tube drainage, whereas adequate antibiotic therapy obviates the need for drainage in most cases of lung abscess. The radiographic features that need to be analyzed are shape and the appearance of any air within the opacity. Loculated collections of pleural fluid, with the exception of interlobar fluid, are based on the parietal pleura and cause an oval, lens-shaped, or rounded expansion of the pleura (Fig 6–129). The shape is often the single most definitive feature. If an air-fluid level is present, then the comparative length in frontal and lateral projections may help distinguish lung abscess and empyema (Fig 6–130). Since empyema spaces are usually lenticular in shape, the air-fluid level will often be substantially longer in one view than it is in the other.[105] Intrapulmonary abscesses are usually spherical, and the spherical cavity will have an air-fluid level that is the same length regardless of projection. Also, in empyema the air-fluid level may reach to the chest wall, whereas a lung abscess is often surrounded by lung parenchyma and the air-fluid level is therefore less likely to reach the chest wall. Proto and Merhar[247] observed that large collections of pleural fluid could displace the hilar structures away from the lesion, whereas lung abscesses, which destroy rather than compress lung, do not displace these structures in the same fashion. This sign, which can be of great value, can also be misleading in individual cases.[337] When profiled, the inner margin of the empyema is sharply defined and shows a curved smooth interface with the adjacent lung, but very often, one or more interfaces with the lung are not tangential to the beam, and the density, therefore, fades off with an imperceptible border.

Round pneumonias do not show the very smooth, well-defined interface with the adjacent lung that is seen in empyema. Also, although they may contact the pleura, round pneumonias are rarely as broadly based on the pleura.

Interlobar loculated pleural fluid results in a unique appearance. The opacity is centered on a fissure and is lens shaped with a more pronounced bulge inferiorly than superiorly, reflecting the gravitational effect of the fluid suspended within the fissure. In the lateral projection, interlobar fluid in the major fissure appears as a well-defined lens shape, whereas in frontal projection the opacity is circular and fades off in all directions. It is, therefore, in the frontal view that confusion with pneumonia is most likely to occur.

CT scanning can be very valuable in deciding between empyema and a peripherally positioned lung

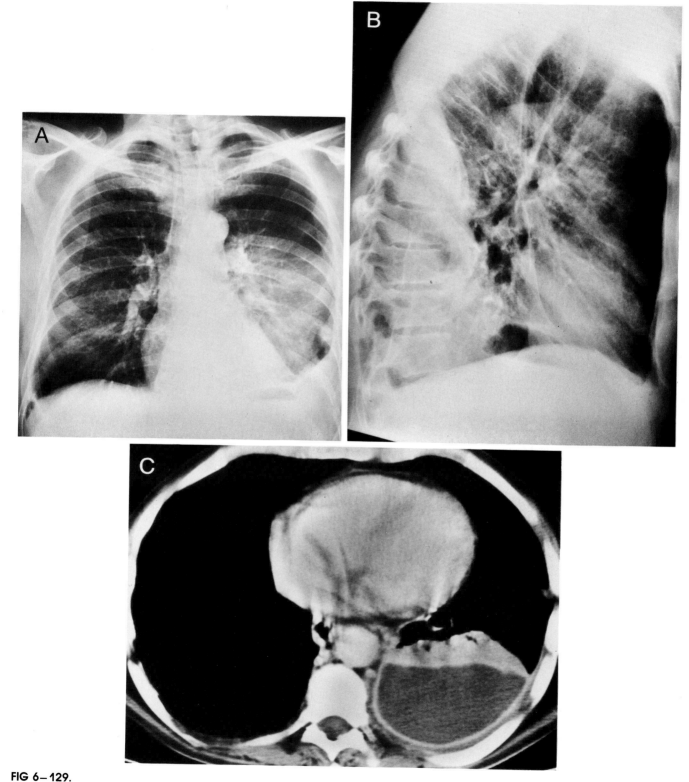

FIG 6–129.
Typical shape of empyema on plain film and CT scans. **A,** frontal view. **B,** lateral view showing lens-shaped pleural expansion. **C,** CT scan showing the pleural fluid collection displacing and compressing the adjacent left lower lobe.

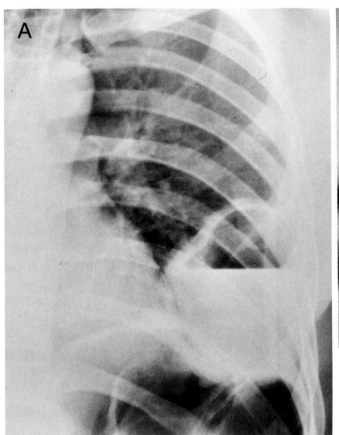

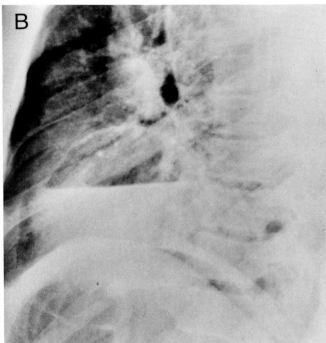

FIG 6—130.
Air-fluid level in empyema. On the frontal view, the air-fluid level reaches the chest wall. A comparison of the length of the air-fluid level in the two projections shows a disparity in length, suggesting that the true shape of the cavity is lens-shaped rather than spherical. **A,** PA view. **B,** lateral view.

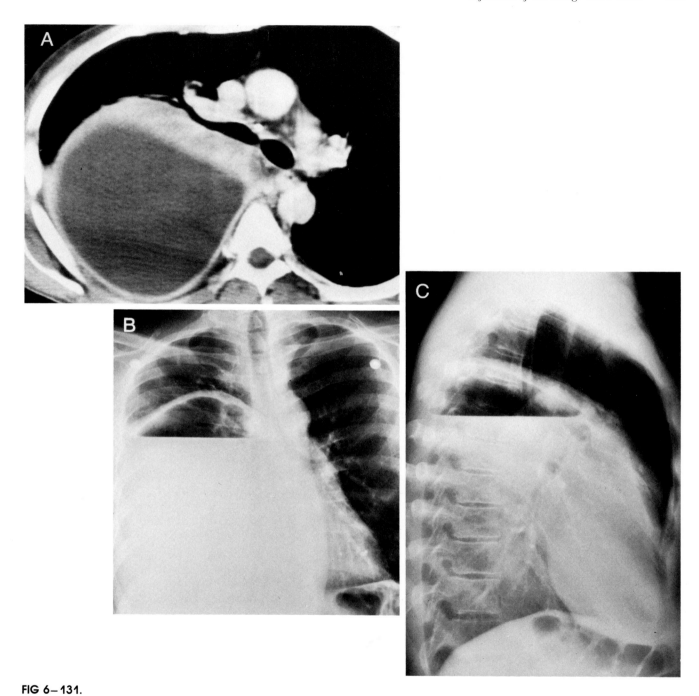

FIG 6–131.
A, CT scan of pleural empyema showing homogeneous oval fluid collection based on the chest wall with a very smooth outline and no evidence of bubbles of gas in the wall of the fluid collection. Note also the forward displacement of the ipsilateral central bronchi. PA radiograph **(B)** and lateral radiograph **(C)** for comparison with the CT scan.

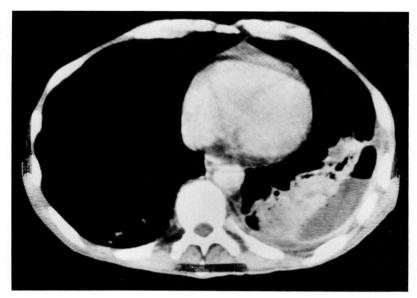

FIG 6–132.
CT scan of pleural empyema showing lens shape and short air-fluid level. There is pneumonia in the underlying lung.

abscess in those cases when the plain chest radiographic features are ambiguous. In one series of 70 patients with empyema or lung abscess, it proved possible to correctly characterize the lesion in all cases with CT.[303] The distinguishing features at CT are[11, 294, 303, 337] (Figs 6–129 through 6–135):

1. *Shape.* Empyemas, unless very large, are basically lenticular in shape. The angle formed at the interface with the chest wall is obtuse or tapering. Large collections, however, may be more spherical and may show acute angles. Lung abscesses, on the other hand, tend to be spherical and show acute angles at their margins with the chest wall. Also, fluid collections in the pleural space may change their shape as the patient changes position, whereas lung abscesses are fairly rigid and retain approximately the same shape in upright, supine, prone, or decubitus views.

2. *Wall characteristics.* The walls of an empyema are formed by thickened visceral and parietal pleura. This thickened pleura is of uniform thickness and uniform soft-tissue density, with a smooth inner and outer wall, enclosing the empyema fluid— a combination of findings to which the term "split pleura sign" has been given.[303] The thickened pleura may enhance following the administration of intravenous contrast medium.

The wall of a lung abscess is irregular in thickness and has an irregular inner and outer margin. It also tends to be thicker than that of an empyema and it may contain multiple dots of air and, on occasion, may even show distorted air bronchograms.

3. *Appearance of the adjacent lung.* The lung adjacent to an empyema may be clear, but often it is compressed. This compression may lead to distortion of the adjacent vessels, and if the collection is very large, hilar vessels and bronchi may be displaced. Because lung abscesses destroy rather than displace, the adjacent vessels and bronchi tend to remain in their normal position, or are pulled toward the atelectasis or parenchymal destruction. When consolidation is seen adjacent to the fluid collection, it is of little help in differential diagnosis, as pneumonia is the primary cause of most empyemas, and lung abscesses usually form within areas of pneumonia.

In summary, the CT features associated with empyema include lenticular shape; thin, uniform, smooth walls; compression of the adjacent lung; obtuse angles at the interface with the chest wall; and separation of pleural layers. The features associated with lung abscess include round shape; thick, nonuniform, irregular walls; acute angles at the interface of the chest wall; and absence of evidence of lung compression. Both empyemas and lung abscesses may contain one or more pockets of air and show air-fluid levels, but most empyemas do not show dots of air in their walls, whereas the wall of a lung abscess often contain bubbles of air.

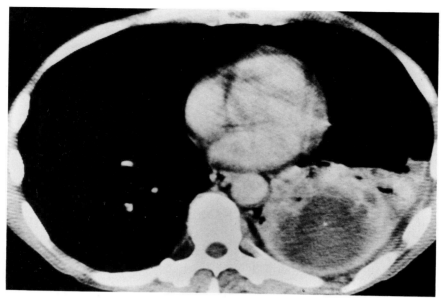

FIG 6–133.
Lung abscess at CT that resembles an empyema. The wall of the abscess is relatively thick and irregular and contains bubbles of gas. The fluid collection is spherical.

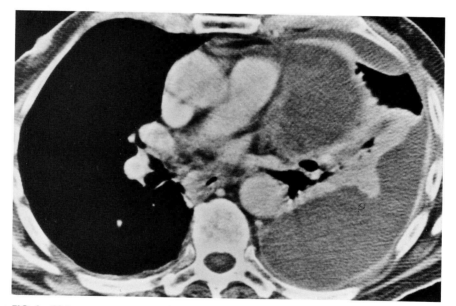

FIG 6–134.
Multilocular pleural empyema. Each empyema space shows the typical CT features of pleural empyema.

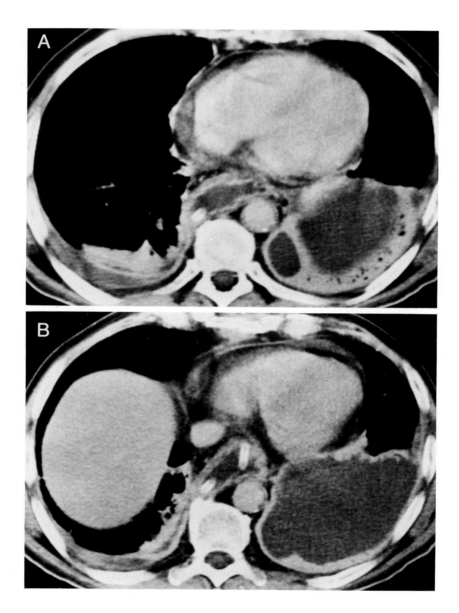

FIG 6–135.
Potential pitfall in the diagnosis of pleural empyema. The pleural empyema in this patient lies largely in a subpulmonary location; therefore, in section **(A)** the lung is draped over the fluid collection and air bronchograms in compressed lung are seen between the empyema and the chest wall. **B,** a lower section shows the more typical features of pleural empyema.

REFERENCES

1. Albelda SM, Kern JA, Marihelli DL, et al: Expanding spectrum of pulmonary disease caused by nontuberculous *Mycobacteria. Radiology* 1985; 157:289–296.
2. Alison AC, Hart PDA: Potentiation by silica of the growth of mycobacterium tuberculosis in macrophage cultures. *Br J Exp Pathol* 1968; 49:465–476.
3. Alsofrom DJ, Mettler FA, Mann JM: Radiographic manifestations of plague in New Mexico, 1975–1980: A review of 42 proved cases. *Radiology* 1981; 139:561–565.
4. Altman AR: Thoracic wall invasion secondary to pulmonary aspergillosis: A complication of chronic granulomatous disease of childhood. *AJR* 1977; 129:140–142.
5. Andiman WA, McCarthy P, Markowitz RI, et al: Clinical, virologic, and serologic evidence of Epstein-Barr virus infection in association with childhood pneumonia. *J Pediatr* 1981; 99:880–886.
6. Andrews NC, Parker EF, Shaw RR, et al: Management of nontuberculous empyema. American Tho-

racic Society: A statement of the subcommittee on surgery. *Am Rev Respir Dis* 1962; 85:935–936.

7. Armstrong JD: Common fungal diseases of the lungs: Blastomycosis. *Radiol Clin North Am* 1973; 11:169–173.

8. Asmar BI, Thirumoorthi MC, Dajani AS: Pneumococcal pneumonia with pneumatocele formation. *Am J Dis Child* 1978; 132:1091–1093.

9. Avery FW, Barnett TB: Pulmonary tularemia: A report of five cases and consideration of pathogenesis and terminology. *Am Rev Respir Dis* 1967; 95:584–591.

10. Babbit DP, Waisbren BA: Epidemic pulmonary histoplasmosis. *AJR* 1960; 83:236–250.

11. Baber EC, Hedlund LW, Oddson TA, et al: Differentiating empyemas and peripheral pulmonary abscesses: The value of computed tomography. *Radiology* 1980; 135:755–758.

12. Bahk YW: Pulmonary paragonimiasis as a cause of Loeffler's syndrome. *Radiology* 1962; 78:598–601.

13. Bailey CM, Windle-Taylor PC: Tuberculous laryngitis: A series of 37 patients. *Laryngoscope* 1981; 91:93–100.

14. Balikian JP, Cheng TH, Costello P, et al: Pulmonary actinomycosis: A report of three cases. *Radiology* 1978; 128:613–616.

15. Balikian JP, Herman PG, Godleski JS: *Serratia* pneumonia. *Radiology* 1980; 137:309–311.

16. Balikian JP, Herman PG, Kopit S: Pulmonary nocardiosis. *Radiology* 1978; 126:569–573.

17. Balikian JP, Mudarris FF: Hydatid disease of the lungs: A roentgenologic study of 50 cases. *AJR* 1974; 122:692–707.

18. Balmes JR, Hawkins JG: Pulmonary cryptococcosis. *Semin Respir Med* 1987; 9:180–186.

19. Barnhard HJ, Kniker WT: Roentgenologic findings in pertussis with particular emphasis on the "shaggy heart" sign. *AJR* 1960; 84:445–450.

20. Bartlett JG: Anaerobic bacterial pneumonitis. *Am Rev Respir Dis* 1979; 119:19–24.

21. Bartlett JG, Finegold SM: Anaerobic infections of the lung and pleural space. *Am Rev Respir Dis* 1974; 110:56–77.

22. Bartlett JG, O'Keefe P, Tally FP, et al: Bacteriology of hospital acquired pneumonia. *Arch Intern Med* 1986; 146:868–871.

23. Basiliere JL, Bistrong HW, Spence WF: Streptococcal pneumonia: Recent outbreaks in military recruit populations. *Am J Med* 1968; 44:580–589.

24. Bates M, Cruickshank G: Thoracic actinomycosis. *Thorax* 1957; 12:99–123.

25. Baum GL: Cavitation in histoplasmosis: Some further comments, letter. *Chest* 1975; 67:625–626.

26. Baum GL, Schwarz J: Chronic pulmonary histoplasmosis. *Am J Med* 1962; 33:873–879.

27. Baum GL, Schwarz J: North American blastomycosis. *Am J Med Sci* 1959; 238:661.

28. Bayer AS: Fungal pneumonias; pulmonary coccidioidal syndromes: Part 1. *Chest* 1981; 79:575–583. Part 2. *Chest* 1981; 79:686–691.

29. Beaman BL, Burnside J, Edwards B, et al: Nocardial infections in the United States, 1972–1974. *J Infect Dis* 1976; 134:286–289.

30. Bean WJ: Recognition of ascariasis by routine chest or abdomen roentgenograms. *AJR* 1965; 94:379–384.

31. Beggs I: The radiology of hydatid disease: A review. *AJR* 1985; 145:639–648.

32. Bellamy EA, Johnston IDA, Wilson AG: The chest radiograph in whooping cough. *Clin Radiol* 1987; 38:39–43.

33. Beller TA, Mitchell DM, Sobonya RE, et al: Large airway obstruction secondary to endobronchial coccidioidomycosis. *Am Rev Respir Dis* 1979; 120:939–942.

34. Bennett JE: *Sporothrix schenckii,* in Mandell GL, Douglas RG, Bennett JE (eds): *Principles and Practice of Infectious Diseases,* ed 2. New York, John Wiley & Sons, 1985.

35. Berger HW, Granada MG: Lower lung field tuberculosis. *Chest* 1974; 65:522–526.

36. Bier S, Halton K, Krivisky B, et al: *Pneumocystis carinii* pneumonia presenting as a single pulmonary nodule. *Pediatr Radiol* 1986; 16:59–60.

37. Binder RE, Faling LJ, Pugatch RD, et al: Chronic necrotizing pulmonary aspergillosis: A discrete clinical entity. *Medicine* 1982; 61:109–124.

38. Birsner JW: The roentgen aspects of five hundred cases of pulmonary coccidioidomycosis. *AJR* 1954; 72:556–573.

39. Blastomycosis cooperative study of the Veterans Administration: Blastomycosis: A review of 198 collected cases in Veterans Administration Hospitals. *Am Rev Respir Dis* 1964; 89:659–672.

40. Blum J, Reed JC, Pizzo SV, et al: Miliary aspergillosis associated with alcoholism. *AJR* 1978; 131:707–709.

41. Bonakdarpour A: Echinococcus disease: Report of 112 cases from Iran and a review of 611 cases from the United States. *AJR* 1967; 99:660–667.

42. Bonmati J, Rogers JV, Hopkins WA: Pulmonary cryptococcosis. *Radiology* 1956; 66:188–194.

43. Brown A, Geyer S, Arbitman M, et al: Pulmonary nocardiosis presenting as a bronchogenic tumor. *South Med J* 1980; 73:660–663.

44. Brown JR: Human actinomycosis: A study of 181 subjects. *Hum Pathol* 1973; 4:319–330.

45. Buechner HA, Seabury JH, Campbell CC, et al: The current status of serologic, immunologic and skin tests in the diagnosis of pulmonary mycoses. *Chest* 1973; 63:259–270.

46. Buff SJ, McLelland R, Gallis HA, et al: *Candida albicans* pneumonia: Radiographic appearance. *AJR* 1982; 138:645–648.

47. Cameron DC, Borthwick RN, Philp T: The radiographic patterns of acute *Mycoplasma* pneumonitis. *Clin Radiol* 1977; 28:173–180.

48. Campbell GD, Chapman SW: Blastomycosis. *Semin Respir Med* 1987; 9:164–169.

49. CDC tuberculosis—United States 1985. *MMWR* 1986; 35:669–703.

50. Chandler FW, Watts JC: Mycotic, actinomycotic, and algal infections, in Kissane JM (ed): *Anderson's Pathology*, ed 8. St Louis, CV Mosby Co, 1985, pp 371–400.

51. Chandler FW, Watts JC: Fungal infections, in Dail DH, Hammar SP (eds): *Pulmonary Pathology.* New York, Springer-Verlag, 1988.

52. Chick EW: Epidemiologic aspects of the pulmonary mycoses. *Semin Respir Med* 1987; 9:123–129.

53. Chick EW, Bauman DS: Acute cavitary histoplasmosis—fact or fiction, editorial. *Chest* 1974; 65:479–480.

54. Cholankeril JV, Napolitano J, Ketyer S, et al: Computed tomography in the evaluation of *Dirofiliaria immitus* granuloma of the lung. *J Comput Tomogr* 1983; 7:305–309.

55. Choyke PL, Soskman HD, Curtis AM, et al: Adult-onset pulmonary tuberculosis. *Radiology* 1983; 148:357–362.

56. Christensen EE, Dietz GW, Ahn CH, et al: Radiographic manifestations of pulmonary *Mycobacterium kansasii* infections. *AJR* 1978; 131:985–993.

57. Cockcroft DW, Stilwell GA: Lobar pneumonia caused by *Mycoplasma pneumoniae. Can Med Assoc J* 1981; 124:1463–1468.

58. Cohen BA, Pomeranz S, Rabinowitz JG, et al: Pulmonary complications of AIDS: Radiologic features. *AJR* 1984; 143:115–122.

59. Coleman DL, Haltner RS, Luce JM, et al: Correlation between gallium lung scans and fiberoptic bronchoscopy in patients with suspected *Pneumocystis carinii* pneumonia and the acquired immune deficiency syndrome. *Am Rev Respir Dis* 1984; 130:1166–1169.

60. Comstock C, Wolson AH: Roentgenology of sporotrichosis. *AJR* 1975; 125:651–655.

61. Connell JV, Muhm JR: Radiographic manifestations of pulmonary histoplasmosis: A 10 year review. *Radiology* 1976; 121:281–285.

62. Conte P, Heitzman ER, Markarian B: Viral pneumonia: Roentgen pathological correlations. *Radiology* 1970; 95:267–272.

63. Costello P, Rose RM: CT findings in pleural aspergillosis. *J Comput Assist Tomogr* 1985; 9:760–762.

64. Cross AS, Steigbigel RT: *Pneumocystis carinii* pneumonia presenting as localized nodular densities. *N Engl J Med* 1974; 291:831–832.

65. Curry WA: Human nocardiosis: A clinical review with selected case reports. *Arch Intern Med* 1980; 140:818–826.

66. Curtis A McB, Walker Smith GJ, Ravin CE: Air crescent sign of invasive aspergillosis. *Radiology* 1979; 133:17–21.

67. Cuthbert R: Sylvatic pulmonary hydatid disease: A radiological survey. *J Can Assoc Radiol* 1974; 26:132–138.

68. Danner PK, McFarland DR, Felson B: Massive pulmonary gangrene. *AJR* 1968; 103:548–554.

69. Davies SF, McKenna RW, Sarosi GA: Trephine biopsy of the bone marrow in disseminated histoplasmosis. *Am J Med* 1979; 67:617–622.

70. Dee P, Teja K, Korzeniowski O, et al: Miliary tuberculosis resulting in adult respiratory distress syndrome: A surviving case. *AJR* 1980; 134:569–572.

71. Dee P, Winn W, McKee K: *Pneumocystis carinii* infection of the lung: Radiologic and pathologic correlation. *AJR* 1979; 132:741–746.

72. Degregorio MW, Lee WMF, Linker CA, et al: Fungal infections in patients with acute leukemia. *Am J Med* 1982; 73:543–548.

73. de Leon EP, Pardo de Tavero MP: Pulmonary schistosomiasis in the Philippines. *Dis Chest* 1968; 53:154–161.

74. Demos TC, Studlo JD, Puczynski M: *Mycoplasma* pneumonia: Presentation as a mediastinal mass. *AJR* 1984; 143:981–982.

75. Dennis JM, Bondreau RP: Pleuropulmonary tularemia: Its roengten manifestations. *Radiology* 1957; 68:25–30.

76. Dietrich PA, Johnson RD, Fairbank JT, et al: The chest radiograph in Legionnaire's disease. *Radiology* 1978; 127:577–582.

77. di Sant' Agnese PA, Davis PB: Cystic fibrosis in adults: 75 cases and a review of 232 cases in the literature. *Am J Med* 1979; 66:121–132.

78. Donohue JF: Lower respiratory tract involvement in Rocky Mountain spotted fever. *Arch Intern Med* 1980; 140:223–226.

79. Doppman JL, Geelhoed GW, DeVita VT: Atypical radiographic features in *Pneumocystis carinii* pneumonia. *Radiology* 1975; 114:39–44.

80. Drutz DJ, Catanzaro A: Coccidioidomycosis: State of the art. Parts 1 and 2. *Am Rev Respir Dis* 1978; 117:559–585; 727–771.

81. Dubois PJ, Myerowitz RL, Allen CM: Pathoradiologic correlation of pulmonary candidiasis in immunosuppressed patients. *Cancer* 1977; 40:1026–1036.

82. Duperval R, Hermans PE, Brewer NS, et al: Cryptococcosis, with emphasis on the significance of isolation of *Cryptococcus neoformans* from the respiratory tract. *Chest* 1977; 72:13–19.

83. Eastridge CE, Young JM, Cole F, et al: Pulmonary aspergillosis. *Ann Thorac Surg* 1972; 13:397–403.

84. Edelman RR, Hann LE, Simon M: *Chlamydia trachomatosis* pneumonia in adults: Radiographic appearance. *Radiology* 1984; 152:279–282.

85. Edelstein G, Levitt RG: Cavitary coccidioidomycosis

presenting as spontaneous pneumothorax. *AJR* 1983; 141:533–534.

86. Edwards LB, Acquaviva FA, Livesay VT, et al: An atlas of sensitivity to tuberculin, PPD-B and histoplasmin in the United States. *Am Rev Respir Dis* 1969; 99(suppl 4):1–32.

87. Evans AF, Oakley RH, Whitehouse GH: Analysis of the chest radiograph in Legionnaire's disease. *Clin Radiol* 1981; 32:361–365.

88. Everett ED, Nelson RA: Pulmonary meliodosis: Observations in thirty-nine cases. *Am Rev Respir Dis* 1975; 112:331–340.

89. Faulkner SL, Vernon R, Brown PP, et al: Hemoptysis and pulmonary aspergilloma: Operative versus non-operative treatment. *Ann Thorac Surg* 1978; 25:389–392.

90. Fawcitt J, Parry HE: Lung changes in pertussis and measles in childhood: A review of 1894 cases with a follow up study of the pulmonary complications. *Br J Radiol* 1957; 30:76–82.

91. Feigin DS: Pulmonary cryptococcosis: Radiologic-pathologic correlates of its three forms. *AJR* 1983; 141:1263–1272.

92. Feigin DS: Nocardiosis of the lung: Chest radiographic findings in 21 cases. *Radiology* 1986; 159:9–14.

93. Felson B, Rosenberg LS, Hamburger M: Roentgen findings in acute Friedlander's pneumonia. *Radiology* 1949; 53:559–565.

94. Fine NL, Smith LR, Sheedy PF: Frequency of pleural effusions in mycoplasma and viral pneumonias. *N Engl J Med* 1970; 283:790–793.

95. Finegold SM, Will D, Murray JF: Aspergillosis. *Am J Med* 1959; 27:463–482.

96. Finnegan OC, Fowler SJ, White RJ: Radiographic appearances of *Mycoplasma* pneumonia. *Thorax* 1981; 36:469–472.

97. Fisher MS: "Miliary" actinomycosis. *J Can Assoc Radiol* 1980; 31:149–150.

98. Flynn MW, Felson B: The roentgen manifestations of thoracic actinomycosis. *AJR* 1970; 110:707–716.

99. Forrest JV: Common fungal diseases of the lungs: II. Histoplasmosis. *Radiol Clin North Am* 1973; 11:163–168.

100. Forrest JV: Radiographic findings in *Pneumocystis carinii* pneumonia. *Radiology* 1972; 103:539–544.

101. Foy HM, Loop J, Clarke ER, et al: Radiographic study of *Mycoplasma pneumoniae* pneumonia. *Am Rev Respir Dis* 1973; 108:469–474.

102. Frank P, Strickland B: Pulmonary actinomycosis. *Br J Radiol* 1974; 47:373–378.

103. Frazier AR, Rosenow EC, Roberts GD: Nocardiosis: A review of 25 cases occurring during 24 months. *Mayo Clin Proc* 1975; 50:657–663.

104. Freundlich IM, Israel HL: Pulmonary aspergillosis. *Clin Radiol* 1973; 24:248–253.

105. Friedman PJ, Hellekant CAG: Radiologic recognition of bronchopleural fistula. *Radiology* 1977; 124:289–295.

106. Frommhold W, Lagemann K, Wolf KJ: Die akute Klebsiellen—pneumonie (in German—summary in English). *Fortschr Geb Roentgenstr* 1974; 121:25–34.

107. Gale AM, Kleitsch WP: Solitary pulmonary nodule due to phycomycosis (mucormycosis). *Chest* 1972; 62:752–755.

108. Galloway RW, Miller RS: Lung changes in the recent influenza epidemic. *Br J Radiol* 1959; 32:28–31.

109. Gamsu G, Hecht ST, Birnberg FA, et al: *Pneumocystis carinii* pneumonia in homosexual men. *AJR* 1982; 139:647–651.

110. Garcia-Palmieri MR, Marcial-Rojas RA: The protean manifestations of *Schistosomiasis mansoni:* A clinicopathologic correlation. *Ann Intern Med* 1962; 57:763–775.

111. Gedroyc WMW, Reidy JF: The early chest radiographic changes of *Pneumocystis pneumonia. Clin Radiol* 1985; 36:331–334.

112. Gefter WB, Albeda SM, Talbot GH, et al: Invasive pulmonary aspergillosis and acute leukemia. Limitations in the diagnostic utility of the air crescent sign. *Radiology* 1985; 157:605–610.

113. Gefter WB, Weingrad TR, Epstein DM, et al: "Semi-invasive" pulmonary aspergillosis: A new look at the spectrum of *Aspergillus* infections of the lung. *Radiology* 1981; 140:313–321.

114. Gelpi AP, Mustafa A: *Ascaris* pneumonia. *Am J Med* 1968; 44:377–389.

115. George RB, Mogabgab WJ: Atypical pneumonia in young men with rhinovirus infections. *Ann Intern Med* 1969; 71:1073–1078.

116. George RB, Weill H, Rasch JR, et al: Roentgenographic appearances of viral and mycoplasmal pneumonias. *Am Rev Respir Dis* 1967; 96:1144–1150.

117. George RB, Ziskind MM, Rasch JR, et al: Mycoplasma and adenovirus pneumonias: Comparison with other atypical pneumonias in a military population. *Ann Intern Med* 1966; 65:931–942.

118. Geppert EF, Leff A: The pathogenesis of pulmonary and miliary tuberculosis. *Arch Intern Med* 1979; 139:1381–1383.

119. Gold R, Wilt JC, Adhikari PK, et al: Adenoviral pneumonia and its complications in infants and childhood. *J Can Assoc Radiol* 1969; 20:218–224.

120. Gonzalez CL, Calia FM: Bacteriologic flora of aspiration-induced pulmonary infections. *Arch Intern Med* 1975; 135:711–714.

121. Goodman PC, Daley C, Minagi H: Spontaneous pneumothorax in AIDS patients with *Pneumocystis carinii* pneumonia. *AJR* 1986; 147:29–31.

122. Goodwin RA, Des Prez RM: Histoplasmosis: State of the art. *Am Rev Respir Dis* 1977; 117:929–956.

123. Goodwin RA, Loyd JE, Des Prez RM: Histoplasmosis in normal hosts. *Medicine* 1981; 60:231–266.

124. Goodwin RA, Owens FT, Snell JD, et al: Chronic pulmonary histoplasmosis. *Medicine* 1976; 55:413–452.

125. Goodwin RA, Shapiro JL, Thurmann GH, et al: Disseminated histoplasmosis: Clinical and pathological correlations. *Medicine* 1980; 59:1–33.

126. Goodwin RA, Snell JD: The enlarging histoplasmoma. *Am Rev Respir Dis* 1969; 100:1–12.

127. Gordon JD, McKeen AD, Maric TJ, et al: The radiographic features of epidemic and sporadic Q fever pneumonia. *J Can Assoc Radiol* 1984; 35:293–296.

128. Gordonson J, Birnbaum W, Jacobson G, et al: Pulmonary cryptococcosis. *Radiology* 1974; 112:557–561.

129. Grayston JT, Alexander ER, Kenny GE, et al: *Mycoplasma pneumoniae* infections: Clinical and epidemiologic studies. *JAMA* 1965; 191:369–374.

130. Greene R: Pulmonary aspergillosis: Three distinct entities or a spectrum of disease. *Radiology* 1981; 140:527–530.

131. Greendyke WH, Resnick DL, Harvey WC: Roentgen manifestations of coccidioidomycosis. *AJR* 1970; 109:491–499.

132. Gremillion DH, Crawford GE: Measles pneumonia in young adults. *Am J Med* 1981; 71:539–542.

133. Grix A, Giammona ST: Pneumonitis with pleural effusion in children due to *Mycoplasma* pneumonia. *Am Rev Respir Dis* 1974; 109:665–671.

134. Gross BH, Spitz HB, Felson B: The mural nodule in cavitary opportunistic pulmonary aspergillosis. *Radiology* 1982; 143:619–622.

135. Grossman CB, Bragg DG, Armstrong D: Roentgen manifestations of pulmonary nocardiosis. *Radiology* 1970; 96:325–330.

136. Gutman E, Pongdee O, Park YS: Massive pulmonary gangrene. *Radiology* 1973; 107:293–294.

137. Halde C: Basic mycology for the clinician. *Semin Respir Med* 1987; 9:117–122.

138. Halvorsen RA, Duncan JD, Merten DF, et al: Pulmonary blastomycosis: Radiologic manifestations. *Radiology* 1984; 150:1–5.

139. Hammerman KJ, Powell KE, Christianson CS, et al: Pulmonary cryptococcosis: Clinical forms and treatment. *Am Rev Respir Dis* 1973; 108:1116–1123.

140. Harrison BDW: Community-acquired pneumonia in adults in British hospitals in 1982–1983: A survey of aetiology, mortality, prognosis factors and outcome. *Q J Med* 1987; 62(239):195–220.

141. Hawley C, Felson B: Roentgenographic aspects of intrathoracic blastomycosis. *AJR* 1956; 75:751–757.

142. Hebert DH: The roentgen features of Eaton agent pneumonia. *AJR* 1966; 98:300–304.

143. Henkle JQ, Nair SV: Endobronchial pulmonary nocardosis. *JAMA* 1986; 256:1331–1332.

144. Heppleston AG: The fibrogenic action of silica. *Br Med Bull* 1969; 25:282–287.

145. Herbert PA, Bayer AS: Fungal pneumonia (part 4). Invasive pulmonary aspergillosis. *Chest* 1981; 80:220–225.

146. Herlinger H: Pulmonary changes in tropical eosinophilia. *Br J Radiol* 1963; 36:889–901.

147. Heron CW, Hine AL, Pozniak AL, et al: Radiographic features in patients with pulmonary manifestations of the acquired immune deficiency syndrome. *Clin Radiol* 1985; 36:583–588.

148. Holmes RB: Friedlander's pneumonia. *AJR* 1956; 75:728–747.

149. Hulnick DH, Naidich DP, McCauley DI: Pleural tuberculosis evaluated by computed tomography. *Radiology* 1983; 149:759–765.

150. Hyde L: Coccidioidal pulmonary cavitation. *Chest* 1968; 54(suppl 1):273–277.

151. Iannini PB, Claffey T, Quintiliani R: Bacteremic pseudomonas pneumonia. *JAMA* 1974; 230:558–561.

152. Ibarra-Perez C: Thoracic complications of amoebic abscess of the liver: Report of 501 cases. *Chest* 1981; 79:672–677.

153. Irwin A: Radiology of aspergillosis. *Clin Radiol* 1966; 18:432–438.

154. Israel HL, Ostrow A: Sarcoidosis and aspergilloma. *Am J Med* 1960; 47:243–250.

155. Jacobs LG: Pulmonary torulosis. *Radiology* 1958; 71:398–403.

156. James AE, Dixon GD, Johnson HF: Melioidosis: A correlation of the radiologic and pathologic findings. *Radiology* 1967; 89:230–235.

157. Jamison HW: A roentgen study of chronic pulmonary coccidioidomycosis. *AJR* 1946; 55:396–412.

158. Janower ML, Weiss EB: Mycoplasmal, viral, and rickettsial pneumonias. *Semin Roentgenol* 1980; 15:25–34.

159. Jawahiry KI, Karpas L: Pulmonary schistosomiasis: A detailed clinicopathologic study. *Am Rev Respir Dis* 1963; 88:517–527.

160. Jewkes J, Kay PH, Paneth M, et al: Pulmonary aspergilloma: Analysis of prognosis in relation to hemoptysis and survey of treatment. *Thorax* 1983; 38:572–578.

161. Johnson JS: Pulmonary aspergillosis. *Semin Respir Med* 1987; 9:187–199.

162. Johnson PC, Sarosi GA: Histoplasmosis. *Semin Respir Med* 1987; 9:145–151.

163. Johnson RJ, Johnson JR: Paragonimiasis in Indochinese refugees: Roentgenographic findings with clinical correlations. *Am Rev Respir Dis* 1983; 128:534–538.

164. Jones TC: Cestodes (tapeworms), in Mandell GL, Douglas RG, Bennett JE (eds): *Principles and Practice of Infectious Diseases*. New York, John Wiley & Sons, 1985.

165. Kantor HG: Many radiologic facies of pneumococcal pneumonia. *AJR* 1981; 137:1213–1220.

166. Kaplan MH, Armstrong D, Rosen P: Tuberculosis complicating neoplastic diseases: A review of 201 cases. *Cancer* 1974; 33:850–858.

167. Karas A, Hankins JR, Attar S, et al: Pulmonary aspergillosis: An analysis of 41 patients. *Ann Thorac Surg* 1976; 22:1–7.

168. Katzenstein ALA, Askin FB: Interpretation and significance of pathologic findings in transbronchial lung biopsy. *Am J Surg Pathol* 1980; 4:223–234.

169. Kaufman JM, Cuvelier CA, Van der Straeten M: Mycoplasma pneumonia with fulminant evolution into diffuse interstitial fibrosis. *Thorax* 1980; 35:140–144.

170. Kauffman CA, Israel KS, Smith JW, et al: Histoplasmosis in immunosuppressed patients. *Am J Med* 1978; 64:923–932.

171. Kerkering TM, Duma RJ, Shadomy S: The evolution of pulmonary cryptococcosis: Clinical implications from a study of 41 patients with and without compromising host factors. *Ann Intern Med* 1981; 94:611–616.

172. Khan FA, Rehman M, Marcus P, et al: Pulmonary gangrene occurring as a complication of pulmonary tuberculosis. *Chest* 1980; 77:76–80.

173. Khoury MB, Godwin JD, Ravin CE, et al: Thoracic cryptococcosis: Immunologic competence and radiologic appearance. *AJR* 1984; 142:893–896.

174. Klein BS, Kuritsky JN, Chappell WA, et al: Comparison of enzyme immunoassay, immunodiffusion, and complement fixation tests in detecting antibody in human serum to the A antigen of blastomyces dermatitidis. *Am Rev Respir Dis* 1986; 133:144–148.

175. Koletsky RJ, Weinstein AJ: Fulminant *Mycoplasma pneumoniae* infection. *Am Rev Respir Dis* 1980; 122:491–496.

176. Kovacs JA, Kovacs AA, Polis M, et al: Cryptococcosis in acquired immunodeficiency syndrome. *Ann Intern Med* 1985; 103:533–538.

177. Kroboth FJ, Yu VL, Reddy SC, et al: Clinicoradiographic correlation with the extent of Legionnaire's disease. *AJR* 1983; 141:263–268.

178. Krowka MJ, Rosenow EC, Hoagland HC: Pulmonary complications of bone marrow transplantation. *Chest* 1985; 87:237–246.

179. Kuhlman JE, Fishman EK, Siegelman SS: Invasive pulmonary aspergillosis in acute leukemia: Characteristic finding on CT, the CT halo sign and the role of CT in early diagnosis. *Radiology* 1985; 157:611–614.

180. Kulczycki LL, Murphy TM, Bellanti JA: *Pseudomonas* colonization in cystic fibrosis: A study of 160 patients. *J Am Med Assoc* 1978; 240:30–34.

181. Landay MJ, Christensen EE, Bynum LJ, et al: Anaerobic pleural and pulmonary infections. *AJR* 1980; 134:233–240.

182. Landen P, Palayew MJ: Infectious mononucleosis. A review of chest roentgenographic manifestations. *J Can Assoc Radiol* 1974; 25:303–306.

183. Laskey W, Sarosi GA: The radiological appearance of pulmonary blastomycosis. *Radiology* 1978; 126:351–357.

184. Lee REJ, Terry SI, Walker TM, et al: The chest radiograph in leptospirosis in Jamaica. *Br J Radiol* 1981; 54:939–943.

185. Lees RF, Harrison RB, Williamson BRJ, et al: Radiographic findings in Rocky Mountain spotted fever. *Radiology* 1978; 129:17–20.

186. Leff A, Geppert EF: Public health and preventive aspects of pulmonary tuberculosis. Infectiousness, epidemiology, risk factors classification and preventive therapy. *Arch Intern Med* 1979; 139:1405–1410.

187. Leight GS, Michaelis LL: Open lung biopsy for the diagnosis of acute diffuse pulmonary infiltrates in the immunosuppressed patient. *Chest* 1978; 73:477–482.

188. Levine BE: Coccidioidomycosis. *Semin Respir Med* 1987; 9:152–158.

189. Lewis JL, Rabinowich S: The wide spectrum of cryptococcal infections. *Am J Med* 1972; 53:315–322.

190. Libshitz HI, Atkinson EW, Israel HI: Pleural thickening as a manifestation of *Aspergillus* superinfection. *AJR* 1974; 120:883–886.

191. Libshitz HI, Pagani JJ: Aspergillosis and mucormycosis: Two types of opportunistic fungal pneumonia. *Radiology* 1981; 140:301–306.

192. Light RW: *Pleural Disease.* Philadelphia, Lea & Febiger, 1983.

193. Light RW: Parapneumonic effusions and empyema. *Clin Chest Med* 1985; 6:55–62.

194. Light RW: Management of parapneumonic effusions. *Arch Intern Med* 1981; 141:1339–1341.

195. Light RW, Girard WM, Jenkinson SG, et al: Parapneumonic effusions. *Am J Med* 1980; 69:507–511.

196. Lipinski JK, Weisbrod GL, Saunders DE: Unusual manifestations of pulmonary aspergillosis. *J Can Assoc Radiol* 1978; 29:216–220.

197. Littman ML, Zimmerman LE: *Cryptococcosis, Torulosis or European Blastomycosis.* New York, Grune & Stratton, 1956.

198. Loewen DF, Procknow JJ, Loosli CG: Chronic active pulmonary histoplasmosis. *Am J Med* 1960; 28:252–280.

199. Long RF, Berens SV, Shambhag GR: An unusual manifestation of pulmonary cryptococcosis. *Br J Radiol* 1972; 45:757–759.

200. Luce JM, Ostenson RC: Invasive aspergillosis presenting as pericarditis and cardiac tamponade. *Chest* 1979; 76:703–705.

201. MacPherson RI, Cumming GR, Chernick V: Unilateral hyperlucent lung: A complication of viral pneumonia. *J Can Assoc Radiol* 1969; 20:225–231.

202. Maile CW, Moore AV, Ulreich S, et al: Chest radiographic-pathologic correlation in adult leukemia patients. *Invest Radiol* 1983; 18:495–499.

203. Makanjuola D: Fluid levels in pulmonary tuberculosis cavities in a rural population of Nigeria. *AJR* 1983; 141:519–520.

204. Martin W, Choplin R, Shertzer ME: The chest radiograph in Rocky Mountain spotted fever. *AJR* 1982; 139:889–893.

205. Mashburn TD, Dawson DF, Young JM: Pulmonary calcifications and histoplasmosis. *Am Rev Respir Dis* 1961; 84:208–216.

206. Mays BB, Thomas GD, Leonard JS, et al: Gram-negative bacillary necrotizing pneumonia: A bacteriologic and histopathologic correlation. *J Infect Dis* 1969; 120:687–697.

207. McCarthy DS, Pepys J: Pulmonary aspergilloma—clinical immunology. *Clin Allergy* 1973; 3:57–70.

208. McCauley DI, Naidich DP, Leitman BS, et al: Radiographic patterns of opportunistic lung infections and Kaposi sarcoma in homosexual men. *AJR* 1982; 139:653–658.

209. McGahan JP, Graves DS, Palmer PES, et al: Classic and contemporary imaging of coccidioidomycosis. *AJR* 1981; 136:393–404.

210. McPhail JL, Arora TS: Intrathoracic hydatid disease. *Dis Chest* 1967; 52:772–781.

211. Meenhorst PL, Mulder JD: The chest in *Legionella* pneumonia (legionnaires' disease). *Eur J Radiol* 1983; 3:180–186.

212. Meighan JW: Pulmonary cryptococcosis mimicking carcinoma of the lung. *Radiology* 1972; 103:61–62.

213. Meredith HC, Cogan BM, McLaulin B: Pleural aspergillosis. *AJR* 1978; 130:164–166.

214. Meyer RD, Rosen P, Armstrong D: Phycomycosis complicating leukemia and lymphoma. *Ann Intern Med* 1972; 77:871–879.

215. Millar JK: The chest film findings in Q fever—a series of 35 cases. *Clin Radiol* 1978; 29:371–375.

216. Miller RP, Bates JH: Pleuropulmonary tularemia: A review of 29 patients. *Am Rev Respir Dis* 1969; 99:31–34.

217. Mohr JA, Patterson CD, Eaton BG, et al: Primary pulmonary sporotrichosis. *Am Rev Respir Dis* 1972; 106:260–264.

218. Moore WR, Scannell JG: Pulmonary actinomycosis simulating cancer of the lung. *J Thorac Cardiovasc Surg* 1968; 55:193–195.

219. Moskowitz PS, Sae JY, Gooding CA: Tracheal coccidioidomycosis causing upper airway obstruction in children. *AJR* 1982; 139:596–600.

220. Murray HW: Pulmonary mucormycosis: One hundred years later. *Chest* 1977; 72:1–2.

221. Murray HW, Masur H, Senterlit LB, et al: The protean manifestations of *Mycoplasma pneumoniae* infection in adults. *Am J Med* 1975; 58:229–242.

222. Murray JF, Finegold SM, Froman S, et al: The changing spectrum of nocardiosis. *Am Rev Respir Dis* 1961; 83:315–330.

223. Murray JF, Lurie HI, Kaye J, et al: Benign pulmonary histoplasmosis (cave disease) in South Africa. *S Afr Med J* 1957; 31:245–253.

224. Naraqi S, McDonnell G: Hematogenous staphylococcal pneumonia secondary to soft tissue infection. *Chest* 1981; 79:173–175.

225. Neu HC, Silva M, Hazen E, et al: Necrotizing nocardial pneumonitis. *Ann Intern Med* 1967; 66:274–284.

226. Neva FN, Ottesen EA: Current concepts in parasitology: Tropical (filarial) eosinophilia. *New Engl J Med* 1978; 298:1129–1131.

227. Ogakwu M, Nwokolo C: Radiological findings in pulmonary paragonimiasis as seen in Nigeria: A review based on one hundred cases. *Br J Radiol* 1973; 46:669–705.

228. Oldham SAA, Castello M, Jacobson FL, et al: HIV-associated lymphocytic interstitial pneumonia: Radiologic manifestation and pathologic correlation. *Radiology* 1989; 170:83–87.

229. O'Reilly GV, Dee PM, Otteni GV: Gangrene of the lung: Successful medical management of three patients. *Radiology* 1978; 126:575–579.

230. Ort S, Ryan JL, Barden G, et al: Pneumococcal pneumonia in hospitalized patients. *JAMA* 1983; 249:214–218.

231. Osborne D: Radiologic appearance of viral disease of the lower respiratory tract in infants and children. *AJR* 1978; 130:29–33.

232. Osborne D, White P: Radiology of epidemic adenovirus 21 infection of the lower respiratory tract in infants and young children. *AJR* 1979; 133:397–400.

233. Overholt EL, Tiggert WE: Roentgenographic manifestations of pulmonary tularemia. *Radiology* 1960; 74:758–765.

234. Pagani JJ, Kangarloo H, Gyepes MT, et al: Radiographic manifestations of bone marrow transplantation in children. *AJR* 1979; 132:883–890.

235. Pagani JJ, Libshitz HI: Opportunistic fungal pneumonias in cancer patients. *AJR* 1981; 137:1033–1039.

236. Palayew MJ, Frank H: Benign progressive multinodular pulmonary histoplasmosis. *Radiology* 1974; 111:311–314.

237. Palayew MJ, Frank H, Sedlezky I: Our experience with histoplasmosis: An analysis of seventy cases with follow up study. *J Can Assoc Radiol* 1966; 17:142–150.

238. Palmer DL, Harvey RL, Wheeler JK: Diagnostic and therapeutic considerations in *Nocardia asteroides* infections. *Medicine* 1974; 53:391–401.

239. Parker JD, Sarosi GA, Doto IL, et al: Treatment of chronic pulmonary histoplasmosis: A national communicable disease center cooperative mycoses study. *N Engl J Med* 1970; 283:225–229.

240. Paul R: Pulmonary "coin" lesion of unusual pathology. *Radiology* 1960; 75:118–120.

241. Pearlberg J, Haggar AM, Saravolatz L, et al: Hemophilus influenzal pneumonia in the adult. *Radiology* 1984; 151:23–26.

242. Pfister AK, Goodwin AW, Squire EW, et al: Pulmonary blastomycosis: Roentgenographic clues to the diagnosis. *South Med J* 1966; 59:1441–1447.

243. Pierce AK, Sandford JP: Aerobic gram-negative bacillary pneumonias: State of the art. *Am Rev Respir Dis* 1974; 110:647–658.

244. Pitchenik AE, Rubinson HA: The radiographic appearance of tuberculosis in patients with the acquired immune deficiency syndrome (AIDS) and pre-AIDS. *Am Rev Respir Dis* 1985; 131:393–396.

245. Pope TL, Armstrong P, Thomas R, et al: Pittsburgh pneumonia agent: Chest film manifestations. *AJR* 1983; 138:237–241.

246. Pratt PC: Pathology of tuberculosis. *Semin Roentgenol* 1979; 14:196–203.

247. Proto AV, Merhar GL: Central bronchial displacement with large posterior pleural collections. Findings on the lateral chest radiograph and CT scans. *J Can Assoc Radiol* 1984; 35:128–132.

248. Purtilo DT, Meyers WM, Connor DH: Fatal strongyloidiasis in immunosuppressed patients. *Am J Med* 1974; 56:488–493.

249. Putman CE, Curtis A McB, Simeone JF, et al: Mycoplasma pneumonia: Clinical and roentgenographic patterns. *AJR* 1975; 124:417–422.

250. Quinn JL: Measles pneumonia in an adult. *AJR* 1964; 91:560–563.

251. Quinn SF, Erickson S, Oshman D, et al: Lobar collapse with respiratory syncytial virus pneumonitis. *Pediatr Radiol* 1985; 15:229–230.

252. Rabinowitz JG, Busch J, Buttram WR: Pulmonary manifestations of blastomycosis. *Radiology* 1976; 120:25–32.

253. Radkowski MA, Kranzler JK, Beem MO, et al: *Chlamydia* pneumonia in infants: Radiography in 125 cases. *AJR* 1981; 137:703–706.

254. Rafferty P, Biggs BA, Crompton GK, et al: What happens to aspergilloma? Analysis of 23 cases. *Thorax* 1983; 38:579–583.

255. Rakower J, Milwidsky H: Primary mediastinal echinococcus. *Am J Med* 1960; 29:73–83.

256. Randolph KA, Beckman JF: Legionnaire's disease presenting with empyema. *Chest* 1979; 75:404–406.

257. Rasmussen FO: Om haemoptyse, navnlig den lethale, i anatomisk og klinisk henseende. *Hospitalstidende* 1868; 11:49–52.

258. Recht LD, Davies SF, Eckman MR, et al: Blastomycosis in immuno-compromised patients. *Am Rev Respir Dis* 1982; 125:359–362.

259. Record NB, Ginder DR: Pulmonary phycomycosis without obvious predisposing factors. *JAMA* 1976; 235:1256–1257.

260. Reed WP: Indolent pulmonary abscess associated with *Klebsiella* and *Enterobacter*. *Am Rev Respir Dis* 1973; 107:1055–1059.

261. Reed WP, Palmer DL, Williams RC, et al: Bubonic plague in the southwestern United States: A review of recent experience. *Medicine* 1970; 49:465–468.

262. Reich J, Renzetti AD: Pulmonary phycomycosis. Report of a case of bronchocutaneous fistula formation and pulmonary arterial mycothrombosis. *Am Rev Respir Dis* 1970; 102:959–964.

263. Renner RR, Coccaro AP, Heitzman ER, et al: *Pseudomonas* pneumonia: A prototype of hospital-based infection. *Radiology* 1972; 105:555–562.

264. Rice RP, Loda F: A roentgenographic analysis of respiratory syncytial virus pneumonia in infants. *Radiology* 1966; 87:1021–1027.

265. Riggs W, Nelson P: The roentgenographic findings in infantile and childhood histoplasmosis. *AJR* 1966; 97:181–185.

266. Ripstein CB, Spain DM, Bluth I: Scar cancer of the lung. *J Thorac Cardiovasc Surg* 1968; 56:362–370.

267. Rivkin LM, Winn DF, Salyes JM: The surgical treatment of pulmonary coccidioidomycosis. *J Thorac Cardiovasc Surg* 1961; 42:402–412.

268. Roberts CM, Citron KM, Strickland B: Intrathoracic aspergilloma: Role of CT in diagnosis and treatment. *Radiology* 1987; 165:123–128.

269. Rohlfing BM, White EA, Webb WR, et al: Hilar and mediastinal adenopathy caused by bacterial abscess of the lung. *Radiology* 1978; 128:289–293.

270. Rohwedder JJ: Pulmonary sporotrichosis. *Semin Respir Med* 1987; 9:176–179.

271. Rose HD, Sheth NK: Pulmonary candidiasis. A clinical and pathological correlation. *Arch Intern Med* 1978; 138:964–965.

272. Rose RW, Ward BH: Spherical pneumonias in children simulating pulmonary and mediastinal masses. *Radiology* 1973; 106:179–182.

273. Rosenow EC, Wilson WR, Cockerill FR: Pulmonary disease in the immunocompromised host. *Mayo Clin Proc* 1985; 60:473–487.

274. Rossiter SJ, Miller C, Churg AM, et al: Open lung biopsy in the immunosuppressed patient. Is it really beneficial? *J Thorac Cardiovasc Surg* 1979; 77:338–345.

275. Rubin E, Weisbrod GL, Sanders DE: Pulmonary alveolar proteinosis: Relationship to silicosis and pulmonary infection. *Radiology* 1980; 135:35–41.

276. Rubin SA: Radiographic spectrum of pleuropulmonary tularemia. *AJR* 1978; 131:277–281.

277. Sadrieh M, Dutz W, Navabpoor MS: Review of 150 cases of hydatid cyst of the lung. *Dis Chest* 1967; 52:662–666.

278. Sagel SS: Common fungal diseases of the lungs. *Radiol Clin North Am* 1973; 11:153–161.

279. Saksouk FA, Fahl MH, Rizk GK: Computed tomog-

raphy of pulmonary hydatid disease. *J Comput Assist Tomogr* 1986; 10:226–232.

280. Sargent EN, Balchum E, Freed AL, et al: Multiple pulmonary calcifications due to coccidioidomycosis. *AJR* 1970; 109:500–504.

281. Sargent EN, Carson MJ, Reilly ED: Roentgenographic manifestations of varicella pneumonia with postmortem correlation. *AJR* 1966; 98:305–317.

282. Sarosi GA, Davies SF: Blastomycosis: State of the art. *Am Rev Respir Dis* 1979; 120:911–938.

283. Sarosi GA, Parker JD, Doto IL, et al: Chronic pulmonary coccidioidomycosis. *N Engl J Med* 1970; 283:325–329.

284. Scheld WM: North American blastomycosis. *Va Med* 1983; 110:240–248.

285. Schwarz J, Baum GL: Actinomycosis. *Semin Roentgenol* 1970; 5:58–63.

286. Schwarz J, Baum GL: Blastomycosis. *Am J Clin Pathol* 1951; 21:999–1029.

287. Schwarz J, Baum GL: Coccidioidomycosis. *Semin Roentgenol* 1970; 5:29–39.

288. Schwarz J, Baum GL: Nocardiosis. *Semin Roentgenol* 1970; 5:64–68.

289. Schwarz J, Baum GL: North American blastomycosis. *Semin Roentgenol* 1970; 5:40–48.

290. Schwarz J, Baum GL: Pulmonary histoplasmosis. *Semin Roentgenol* 1970; 5:13–28.

291. Schwarz J, Baum GL, Straub M: Cavitary histoplasmosis complicated by fungus ball. *Am J Med* 1961; 31:692–700.

292. Shaffner W, Drutz DJ, Duncan GW, et al: The clinical spectrum of endemic psittacosis. *Arch Intern Med* 1967; 119:433–443.

293. Shin MS, Ho KJ: Broncholithiasis: Its detection by computed tomography in patients with recurrent hemoptysis of unknown etiology. *J Comput Tomogr* 1983; 7:189–193.

294. Shin MS, Ho KJ: Computed tomographic characteristics of pleural empyema. *J Comput Tomogr* 1983; 7:179–182.

295. Sider L, Davis T: Pulmonary aspergillosis: Unusual radiographic appearance. *Radiology* 1987; 162:657–659.

296. Simila S, Ylikorkala O, Wasz-Hockert O: Type 7 adenovirus pneumonia. *J Pediatr* 1971; 79:605–611.

297. Simmons JT, Suffredini AF, Lack EE: Nonspecific interstitial pneumonitis in patients with AIDS: Radiologic features. *AJR* 1987; 149:265–268.

298. Simpson W, Hacking PM, Court SDM, et al: The radiological findings in respiratory syncytial virus infection in children. *Pediatr Radiol* 1974; 2:155–160.

299. Smith CB, Overall JC: Clinical and epidemiologic clues to the diagnosis of respiratory infections. *Radiol Clin North Am* 1973; 11:261–278.

300. Smith LJ, Katzenstein ALA: Pathogenesis of massive pulmonary hemorrhage in acute leukemia. *Arch Intern Med* 1982; 142:2149–2152.

301. Spencer H: *Pathology of the Lung,* ed 4. Oxford, UK, Pergamon Press, 1985.

302. Spiro HM, in *Clinical Gastroenterology,* ed 3. New York, Macmillan Publishing Co, 1983, p 706.

303. Stark DD, Federle MP, Goodman PC, et al: Differentiating lung abscess and empyema: Radiography and computed tomography. *AJR* 1983; 141:163–167.

304. Stead WW: Pathogenesis of the sporadic case of tuberculosis. *N Engl J Med* 1967; 277:1008–1012.

305. Stelling CB, Woodring JH, Rehm SR, et al: Miliary pulmonary blastomycosis. *Radiology* 1984; 150:7–13.

306. Stenstrom R, Jansson E, von Essen R: Mycoplasma pneumonias. *Acta Radiol [Diagn]* (Stockh) 1972; 12:833–841.

307. Stephen SJ, Uragoda CG: Pleuro-pulmonary amebiasis: A review of 40 cases. *Br J Dis Chest* 1970; 64:96–106.

308. Stevens D, Swift PG, Johnston PG, et al: *Mycoplasma pneumoniae* infection in children. *Arch Dis Child* 1978; 53:38–42.

309. Strutman HR, Rettig PJ, Reyes S: *Chlamydia trachomatis* as a cause of pneumonitis and pleural effusion. *J Pediatr* 1984; 104:588–591.

310. Suster B, Akerman M, Orenstein M, et al: Pulmonary manifestations of AIDS: Review of 106 episodes. *Radiology* 1986; 161:87–93.

311. Sweet RS, Wilson ES, Chandler BF: Melioidosis manifested by cavitary lung disease. *AJR* 1968; 103:543–547.

312. Taryle DA, Potts DE, Sahn SA: The incidence and clinical correlates of parapneumonic effusions in pneumococcal pneumonia. *Chest* 1978; 74:170–173.

313. Taylor CR, Swett HA: Pulmonary paragonimiasis in Laotion refugees. *Radiology* 1982; 143:411–412.

314. Tenholder MF, Hooper RG: Pulmonary infiltrates in leukemia. *Chest* 1980; 78:468–473.

315. Tew J, Calenoff L, Berlin BS: Bacterial or nonbacterial pneumonia: Accuracy of radiographic diagnosis. *Radiology* 1977; 124:607–612.

316. Tillotson JR, Lerner AM: Characteristics of pneumonias caused by bacillus proteus. *Ann Intern Med* 1968; 68:287–294.

317. Tillotson JR, Lerner AM: Characteristics of nonbacteremic pseudomonas pneumonia. *Ann Intern Med* 1968; 68:295–307.

318. Tillotson JR, Lerner AM: Characteristics of pneumonias caused by *Escherichia coli. N Engl J Med* 1967; 277:115–122.

319. Triebwasser JH, Harris RE, Bryant RE, et al: *Varicella* pneumonia in adults: Report of seven cases and a review of the literature. *Medicine* 1967; 46:409–423.

320. Turbiner EH, Yeh HD, Rosen PP, et al: Abnormal gallium scintigraphy in *Pneumocystis carinii* pneumo-

nia with a normal chest radiograph. *Radiology* 1978; 127:437–438.

321. Udwadia FE: Tropical eosinophilia. *Prog Respir Res* 1975; 7:35–155.

322. Unger JD, Rose HD, Unger GF: Gram-negative pneumonia. *Radiology* 1973; 107:283–291.

323. Vessal K, Yeganehdoust J, Dutz W, et al: Radiological changes in inhalational anthrax: A report of radiological and pathological correlation in two cases. *Clin Radiol* 1975; 26:471–474.

324. Vianna NJ: Nontuberculous bacterial empyema in patients with and without underlying diseases. *JAMA* 1971; 215:69–75.

325. Vix VA: Radiographic manifestations of broncholithiasis. *Radiology* 1978; 128:295–299.

326. von Lichtenberg F: Infectious diseases, in Robbins SL, Cotran RS, Kumar V (eds): *Pathologic Basis of Disease*, ed 3. Philadelphia, WB Saunders Co, 1984, pp 349–350.

327. Ward JI, Weeks M, Allen D, et al: Acute histoplasmosis: Clinical, epidemiologic and serologic findings of an outbreak associated with exposure to a fallen tree. Am J Med 1979; 66:587–595.

328. Webb WR, Sagel SS: Actinomycosis involving the chest wall: CT findings. *AJR* 1982; 139:1007–1009.

329. Weber AL, Bird KT, Janower ML: Primary tuberculosis in childhood with particular emphasis on changes affecting the tracheobronchial tree. *AJR* 1968; 103:123–132.

330. Webster BH: Pleuropulmonary amebiasis: A review with an analysis of ten cases. *Am Rev Respir Dis* 1960; 81:683–688.

331. Weese WC, Shindler ER, Smith IM, et al: Empyema of the thorax, then and now. *Arch Intern Med* 1973; 131:516–520.

332. Wenzl RP, McCormick DP, Beam WC: Parainfluenza pneumonia in adults. *JAMA* 1972; 221:294–295.

333. Wheat LJ, Kohler RB, Tewari RP: Diagnosis of disseminated histoplasmosis by detection of *Histoplasma capsulatum* antigen in serum and urine specimens. *N Engl J Med* 1986; 314:83–88.

334. Whitehouse WM, Davey WN, Engelke OK, et al: Roentgen findings in histoplasmin-positive school children. *J Mich State Med Soc* 1959; 58: 1266–1269.

335. Wiita RM, Cartwright RR, Davis JG: Staphylococcal pneumonia in adults: A review of 102 cases. *AJR* 1961; 86:1083–1091.

336. Williams DM, Krick JA, Remington JS: Pulmonary infection in the compromised host: State of the art. *Am Rev Respir Dis* 1976; 114:359–394.

337. Williford ME, Godwin JD: Computed tomography of lung abscess and empyema. *Radiol Clin North Am* 1983; 21:575–583.

338. Wilson ES: Pleuropulmonary amebiasis. *AJR* 1971; 111:518–524.

339. Witorsh P, Utz JP: North American blastomycosis: A study of 40 patients. *Medicine* 1968; 47:169–200.

340. Wolfe JN, Jacobson G: Roentgen manifestations of torulosis (cryptococcosis). *AJR* 1958; 79:216–227.

341. Woodring JH, Vandiviere JH, Fried AM, et al: Update: The radiographic features of pulmonary tuberculosis. *AJR* 1986; 146:497–506.

342. Woolfenden JM, Carrasquilo JA, Larson SM, et al: Acquired immunodeficiency syndrome: Ga-67 citrate imaging. *Radiology* 1987; 162:383–387.

343. Young RC, Bennett JE, Vogel CL, et al: Aspergillosis—the spectrum of the disease in 98 patients. *Medicine* 1970; 49:147–173.

344. Young EJ, Hirsch DD, Fainstein V, et al: Pleural effusions due to cryptococcus neoformans: A review of the literature and report of two cases with cryptococcal antigen determinations. *Am Rev Respir Dis* 1980; 121:743–747.

345. Young WB: Actinomycosis with involvement of the vertebral column: Case report and review of the literature. *Clin Radiol* 1960; 11:175–182.

346. Young LW, Smith DI, Glasgow LA: Pneumonia of atypical measles: Residual nodular lesions. *AJR* 1970; 110:439–448.

347. Zagoria RJ, Choplin RH, Karstaedt N, et al: Pulmonary gangrene as a complication of mucormycosis. *AJR* 1985; 144:1195–1196.

348. Zimmerman RA, Miller WT: Pulmonary aspergillosis. *AJR* 1970; 109:505–515.

7

Neoplasms of the Lungs, Airways, and Pleura

BRONCHIAL CARCINOMA

Bronchial carcinoma continues to show a striking increase in incidence. It is by far the most common fatal malignant neoplasm in men and is threatening to overtake carcinoma of the breast as the most common cancer in women.[339]

Primary carcinoma of the lung is classified by its histologic appearances. The most widely used histologic classifications are based on that recommended by the World Health Organization (WHO)[210] and include the following[190]:

1. Epidermoid (squamous cell) carcinoma, which comprises 30% to 50% of cases. Its relative incidence appears, however, to be falling.[367]

2. Small (oat) cell carcinoma, which comprises 20% to 30% of cases.

3. Adenocarcinoma, which in older series comprised 10% to 20% of cases but now appears to be rising, and probably accounts for 30% to 35% of cases.[367] Bronchioloalveolar carcinoma (alveolar cell carcinoma) is sometimes classed separately and at other times included under adenocarcinoma. It comprised 2.8% of all cases of lung cancer in the large series of Vincent et al.[367]

4. Large cell anaplastic carcinoma (including the giant cell variety), which comprises 10% to 15% of cases.

Epidermoid and adenocarcinomas are further subdivided into poorly differentiated and well-differentiated varieties. The mixed tumors with features of both adenocarcinoma and epidermoid carcinomas may be classified separately. (Three rare varieties of growth do not fit neatly into the above classification: clear cell carcinoma, carcinosarcoma, and basal cell carcinoma of the bronchus.) The histologic distinction between these various categories is not always clear-cut, and pathologists may differ in their interpretations. Indeed, different portions of the same tumor may warrant different classifications.

Primary carcinoma of the lung is usually solitary. Multiple primary tumors are surprisingly rare.[62] The precise incidence depends on the rigidity of the criteria used to define whether or not two tumors in the lung can be regarded as both being primary lesions.[43] Synchronous tumors may be of the same histologic type but should be physically quite separate. Metachronous lesions are, in general, accepted as primary lesions only if they show unique histologic features. In one large survey comprising 1,381 patients with bronchial carcinoma, only 10 presented with multiple primaries: 5 with synchronous and 5 with metachronous tumors.[348]

Bronchial carcinoma, particularly adenocarcinoma, may develop in scarred lung or within an area of lipoid pneumonia.[117] Scar carcinomas develop in conditions such as old tuberculosis or old infarcts, as well as in the various forms of interstitial pulmonary fibrosis[15, 128, 235] (see Fig 7–6). It may be that the regenerating epithelium at the edges of a scar predisposes to malignant transformation[262] or, as suggested recently, that the fibrous tissue may be a desmoplastic response to the cancer; in other words the scar may follow, rather than precede, the carcinoma.[18, 243]

Approximately 25% of patients with bronchial carcinoma are asymptomatic at the time of diagnosis.[319] Cough, wheezing, hemoptysis, and paraneoplastic syndromes (Table 7–1) are the cardinal symptoms of the disease at a stage where it may still prove possible to resect the tumor, whereas hoarseness, chest pain, brachial plexus neuropathy, and Horner's syndrome (Pancoast's tumor), superior vena cava obstruction, dysphagia and the problems of pericardial tamponade indicate invasion of the mediastinum or chest wall.[190] Bone and brain metastases are often symptomatic at initial presentation, whereas liver, lymph nodes, and adrenal gland metastases are often asymptomatic.

Symptoms and signs vary with cell type.[86, 120] Epidermoid carcinoma, a relatively slow growing and late metastasizing tumor, often arises centrally and usually presents with obstructive atelectasis and pneumonia, hemoptysis, or the signs and symptoms of invasion of adjacent structures such as the recurrent laryngeal nerve. When epidermoid tumors arise peripherally in the lung, they may grow to substantial size before presentation. In one large review, about two-thirds were greater than 4 cm, and most of the remainder were 8 cm or more in diameter. Also, chest wall invasion and Pancoast's syndrome are seen more frequently with epidermoid carcinomas than with the other cell types. Hypercalcemia resulting from parathormone production by the tumor may be an early manifestation.

Large cell anaplastic carcinoma is similar to epidermoid carcinoma in that the tumor may grow to a large size, but dissimilar in that it metastasizes early, particularly to the mediastinum and brain.[335] Small (oat) cell carcinoma also metastasizes early and widely. The whole course of the disease is compressed, and metastases are usually present at initial diagnosis. Hormone production, notably adrenocorticotropic hormone, antidiuretic hormone, and melanocyte-stimulating hormone production, is a feature of small (oat) cell tumors.[305]

Adenocarcinoma most often arises as a peripheral pulmonary nodule and is frequently first discovered on the chest radiograph in the absence of chest symptoms. Nevertheless, hilar and mediastinal node involvement and distant metastases, particularly in the brain and adrenal glands, are frequently present at or soon after presentation. Pancoast's syndrome and dyspnea resulting from pleural effusion are particular features of adenocarcinoma. Bronchioloalveolar carcinoma, unlike other bronchial adenocarcinomas, is often an indolent tumor that metastasizes late.

TABLE 7–1

Classification of Extrapulmonary Manifestations of Carcinoma of the Lung*

Endocrine and metabolic	Dermatologic
Cushing's syndrome	Acanthosis nigricans
Excessive antidiuretic hormone	Scleroderma
Carcinoid syndrome	Other dermatoses
Hypercalcemia	Vascular
Ectopic gonadotropin	Migratory thrombophlebitis
gynecomastia	Nonbacterial verrucous endocarditis
Insulin-like activity	Arterial thrombosis
Neuromuscular	Hematologic
Carcinomatous myopathy	Anemia
Peripheral neuropathies	Red cell aplasia
Subacute cerebellar degeneration	Fibrinolytic purpura
Encephalomyelopathy	Nonspecific leukocytosis
Skeletal	Polycythemia
Clubbing	Eosinophilia
Pulmonary hypertrophic-	Leukoerythroblastic reaction
osteoarthropathy	
Osteomalacia	

*Filderman AE, Shaw C, Matthay RA: Lung cancer: Part I. Etiology, pathology, natural history, manifestations, and diagnostic techniques. *Invest Radiol* 1986; 21:80-90. Used by permission.

Imaging Features

The imaging appearances are best considered in the following framework:

1. The peripheral tumor (i.e., a tumor arising beyond the hilus).
2. The central tumor (i.e., a tumor arising at or close to the hilus).
3. Intrathoracic spread of tumor.

The Peripheral Tumor

Approximately 40% of bronchial carcinomas arise beyond the larger segmental bronchi, and in 30% a peripheral mass is the sole radiographic finding.[58–61, 218, 362] The fact that peripheral tumors may enlarge most in the direction of the hilus[133, 229, 313] may explain the variable proportions of peripheral versus central tumors reported in large surveys and the unexpectedly high number of "peripheral" masses visible at bronchoscopy. The mass can be virtually any size, but it is rare for a bronchial carcinoma to be seen on plain chest radiographs unless it is more than 1 cm in diameter.[146, 212, 273, 349, 362]

Computed tomography (CT), because of its better contrast resolution, will detect smaller lesions and virtually eliminate the problem of the tumor being hidden by normal overlying structures. The subject of early diagnosis is considered further in the section "Early Diagnosis of Bronchial Carcinoma" later in this chapter.

Shape.— In general, peripheral bronchial carcinomas (except for certain bronchioloalveolar carcinomas) assume an approximately spherical configuration, though an oval shape is not uncommon (Fig 7–1, A), and even a dumbbell shape is sometimes encountered. Bronchogenic carcinoma is, therefore, one of the major diagnostic considerations in adults with a solitary pulmonary nodule—a subject discussed in detail in Chapter 5. Occasionally, two nodules are seen next to one another (Fig 7–1, B). The overall shape and details of the edge of lung carcinomas are usually seen as well with plain film techniques as with conventional CT examinations. High-

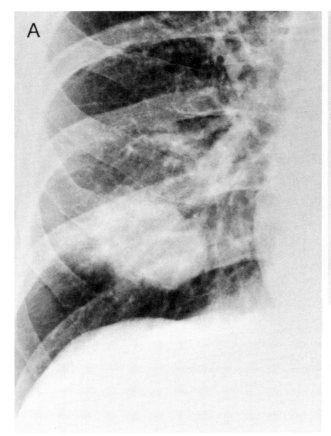

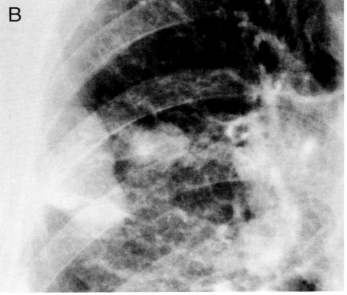

FIG 7–1.
A, squamous cell bronchial carcinoma presenting as a solitary oval lobular peripheral mass. **B,** two adjacent nodules due to a bronchial carcinoma. The more lateral lesion shows distinct notching.

resolution thin-section (1.5 to 3 mm) CT will show the features more clearly,[213] though it is rarely needed in clinical practice.

Lobulation, a sign that indicates uneven growth rates for differing portions of the tumor, is common[362] (see Fig 7–1, A). An equally frequent finding is a notch, or umbilication, a sign that is the counterpart of lobulation because it indicates relatively slow growth of a particular portion of the tumor (see Fig 7–1, B).[314]

Sometimes, the edge of the tumor is irregular, with one or more strands radiating into the surrounding lung (Fig 7–2). The term "corona radiata"[170] indicates the passage of multiple strands extending into the surrounding lung owing to tumor extension or a fibrotic response to the tumor. Such stranding is best seen with tomography, particularly thin-section CT[213] (Fig 7–3). A well-developed corona radiata is a useful sign in the differential diagnosis of a solitary pulmonary nodule because it makes the diagnosis of bronchogenic carcinoma highly likely. It is not, however, entirely specific and has been encountered in a variety of lesions, including benign processes, notably chronic pneumonia and granuloma. A single linear or bandlike shadow may connect the lesion to the pleura (Fig 7–4). This so-called pleural tail sign is seen with both benign and malignant nodules (see Chapter 5).

Careful observation of the pattern of vessels in the neighboring lung parenchyma may show convergence of peripheral blood vessels leading to and entering the cancerous mass (see Fig 7–3), a sign that is best appreciated with thin-section CT.[213]

Regardless of the irregularity of the border, the nodules or masses described thus far can be regarded as having a well-defined edge. Some peripheral cancers, 25% in one series,[362] show a very poorly defined edge similar to that seen in pneumonia (Figs 7–5 and 7–6, A and B). In such cases the spherical shape and relatively slow enlargement seen with carcinomas usually permit their distinction from infectious processes.

Occasionally, bronchial carcinoma arising in segmental or subsegmental bronchi presents radiographically as mucoid impaction (Fig 7–7).[116] The shadow then, to a greater or lesser extent, results from dilated bronchi filled with inspissated secretions, the shape corresponding to branching ectatic bronchi. Another rare pattern is an infarct shadow extending from the primary tumor, giving two contiguous but distinct components to the opacity, the distal one being based on the pleura.[248]

Cavitation.—Approximately 16% of peripheral carcinomas will show cavitation,[76, 362] squamous cell carcinoma being much more likely to cavitate than the other cell types. Adenocarcinoma and large cell carcinoma cavitate infrequently, and small cell carcinoma not at all.[59–61, 76]

Cavitation may be seen in any size of tumor. The cavity is frequently eccentric, the walls are often very irregular, and tumor nodules may be visible (Fig 7–8). The wall is usually 8 mm thick or greater, but on rare occasions it is notably thin, 4 mm or less[381] (Figs 7–9 and 7–10). Cavitary bronchial carcinoma may even have smooth inner and outer margins. It

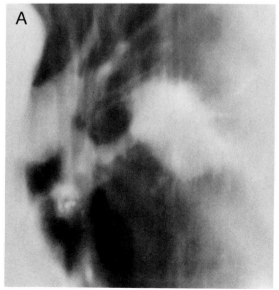

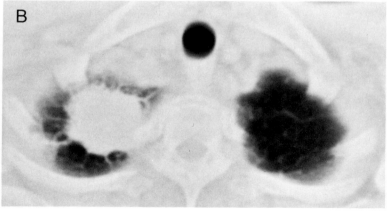

FIG 7–2.
Bronchial carcinoma showing irregular infiltrating edge. **A,** conventional tomogram. **B,** CT scan in a different patient.

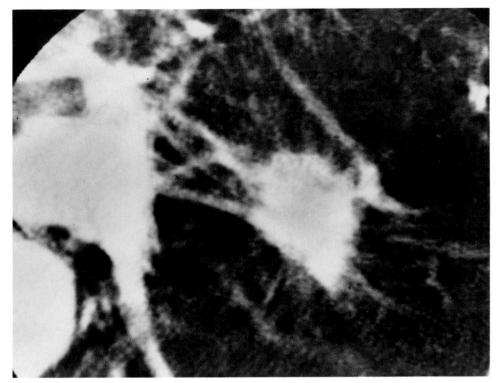

FIG 7–3.
High-resolution thin-section CT scan of bronchial carcinoma showing infiltrating edges and distortion of adjacent vessels.

FIG 7–4.
Bronchial adenocarcinoma showing pleural tail sign *(arrow).*

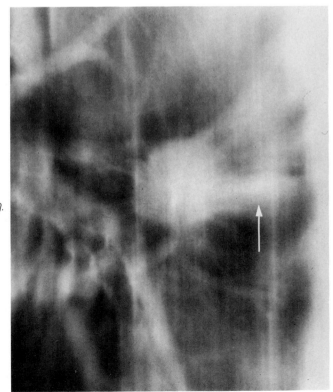

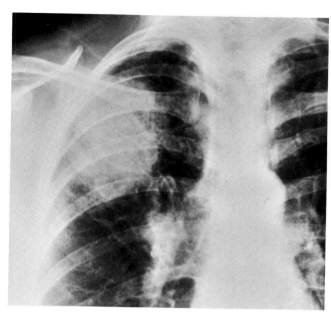

FIG 7–5.
Poorly differentiated squamous cell carcinoma of the lung with ill-defined edge resembling pneumonia.

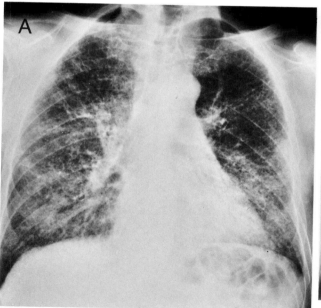
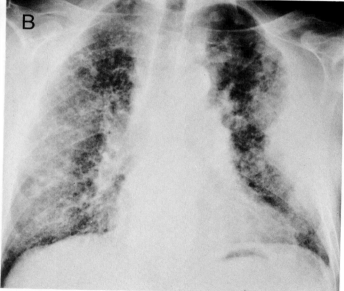

FIG 7–6.
A and **B,** adenocarcinoma of the bronchus developing in a patient with diffuse interstitial pulmonary fibrosis (rheumatoid lung). Note that, in this case, the tumor has a very ill-defined edge re-

sembling pneumonia. The two examinations were acquired 6 months apart.

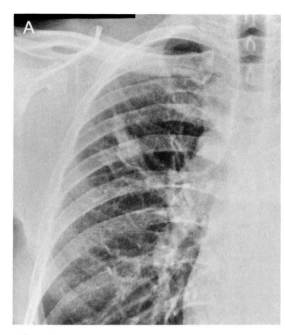

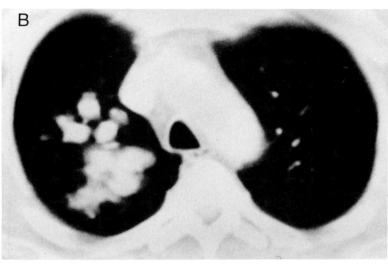

FIG 7—7.

A, dilated, mucus-filled bronchi (mucoid impaction) beyond a small cell bronchial carcinoma. Hilar and paratracheal nodal me- tastases are also present. **B,** CT scan in another patient showing mucoid impaction beyond a bronchial carcinoma.

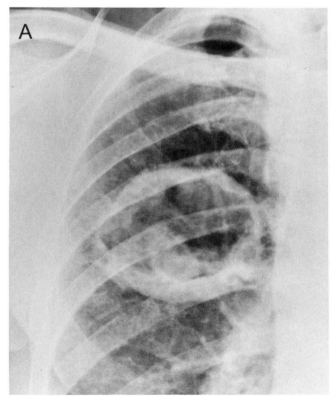

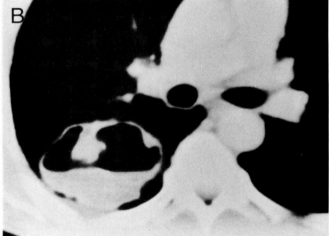

FIG 7—8.

Squamous cell carcinoma of the bronchus showing cavitation. The cavity wall is of variable thickness and shows a mural nodule as well as an air-fluid level. **A,** PA radiograph. **B,** CT scan.

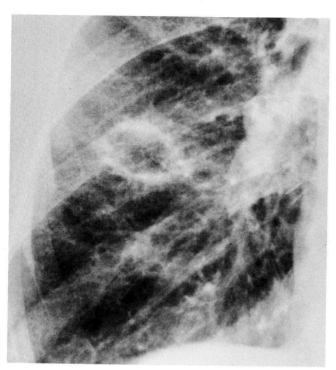

FIG 7–9.
Squamous cell carcinoma of the bronchus showing uniform thinness of the cavity wall, a rare finding.

has been suggested that such very thin walled cavities represent tumor cells lining bullae rather than true cavitation.[76]

Calcification.—Pathologists have long recognized calcification of necrotic tumors in bronchial carcinomas. Such calcification can be demonstrated with specimen radiography[286] and, on rare occasions, with CT (Fig 7–11),[147, 352, 386] but almost never with conventional techniques during the patient's life.[150]

In some cases the tumor may engulf preexisting calcified granulomata. Such granulomatous calcifications are likely to be eccentric in location (Fig 7–12), but focal central calcifications are occasionally seen (Fig 7–13). Concentric laminated calcification centered on the middle of the mass or diffuse calcification throughout the nodule virtually excludes the diagnosis of bronchial carcinoma. The detection of such calcification is the underlying principle behind the use of CT in evaluating solitary pulmonary nodules, which is discussed in detail in Chapter 5.

Rate of Growth.—It is difficult to obtain a large series of cases in which the rate of growth of primary lung carcinoma can be observed, because nod-

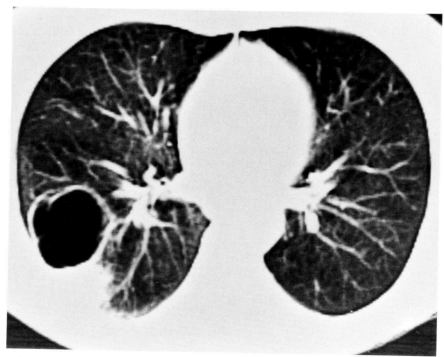

FIG 7–10.
Bronchial adenocarcinoma showing that most of the cavity has a uniform very thin cavity wall. (Courtesy of Dr. John Pitman, Williamsburg, Va.)

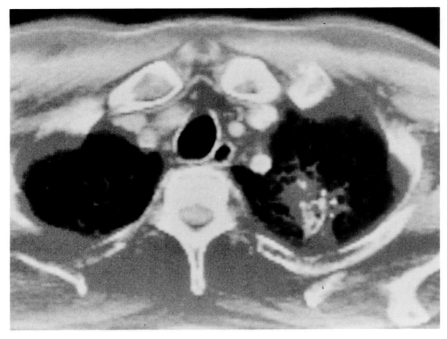

FIG 7–11.
Adenocarcinoma of the bronchus showing widespread calcification, which on histologic study was dystrophic calcification in necrotic areas of the tumor, not preexisting granulomatous calcification. (Courtesy of Dr. John Pitman, Williamsburg, Va.)

FIG 7–12.
Bronchial adenocarcinoma engulfing preexisting calcified granuloma. Note the eccentric location of the calcification in this conventional tomogram and the small size of the calcification in comparison to the shadow of the tumor.

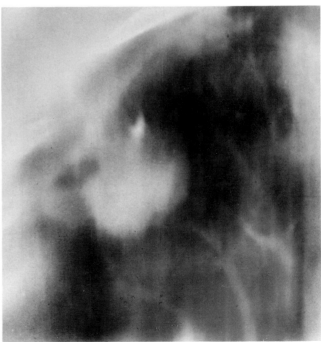

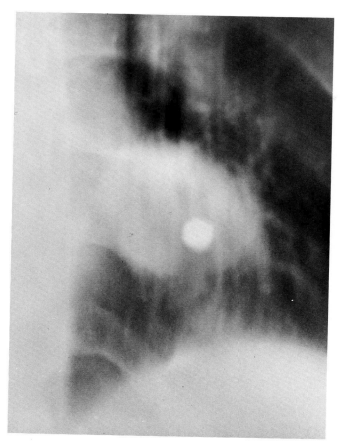

FIG 7–13.
Calcified granuloma engulfed by bronchial carcinoma. This case is unusual in that the granuloma is relatively central.

ules that might be bronchial carcinoma are rarely left untreated. There is, therefore, as Geddes found in his review, surprisingly little information about the growth rate of lung cancer.[135] The volume doubling time for most bronchial carcinomas appears to be between 1 month and 18 months[161, 279, 354]; a 26% increase in diameter is equivalent to a doubling of volume. The primary tumors that grow more slowly are likely to be bronchioloalveolar carcinoma.[177] In one large series, the average doubling time was 4.1 months for undifferentiated carcinomas, 4.2 months for squamous cell carcinoma, and 7.3 months for adenocarcinoma.[132]

One point to bear in mind is that, because tumors close to 1 cm are usually invisible on plain chest radiographs, it is impossible to calculate or infer growth rate if a lesion close to 1 cm in diameter is seen on a film in an area previously shown to be normal in appearance.

Central Tumors

The cardinal imaging signs of a central tumor are collapse/consolidation of the lung beyond the tumor and the presence of a hilar mass, signs which may be seen in isolation or in conjunction with one another.

Collapse/Consolidation.—Obstruction of a major bronchus leads to atelectasis as a result of reduced ventilation of the affected segments or lobes. Collateral air drift may partially or completely prevent this loss of volume. The inability to evacuate secretions leads to consolidation, and pneumonia often supervenes. The pneumonia beyond obstructing tumors often has a high lipid content and is referred to by pathologists as "golden pneumonia" or as endogenous lipoid pneumonia.

As might be expected, the most frequent cell type to present with collapse/consolidation is squamous cell carcinoma, partly because it is a common cell type and partly because a larger proportion of squamous carcinomas originate centrally. In the Mayo Clinic series, over half the patients with squamous cell carcinoma had collapse, consolidation, or obstructive pneumonitis.[59] The incidence of these signs with the other cell types was between 15% and 37%.[60, 61, 218]

Collapse and consolidation, both of which can be patchy (Fig 7–14) or homogeneous, are readily recognizable radiographically. Loss of volume is usual with central tumors, but patchy or homogeneous consolidation without loss of volume is not infrequent. Air bronchograms visible on plain chest radiographs are uncommon, particularly prior to antibiotic therapy. If the tumor regresses with therapy, a previously invisible air bronchogram may become visible. Air bronchograms are seen much more frequently at CT scanning (Fig 7–15), and dilated, fluid-filled bronchi beyond an obstructing tumor may also be visible at CT (Fig 7–16).

The following features suggest that a pneumonia is secondary to an obstructing neoplasm.

1. The shape of the collapsed or consolidated lobe may be altered because of the bulk of the underlying tumor. The fissure in the region of the mass is unable to move in the usual manner, with the result that the fissure appears bulged ("Golden S" sign) (Fig 7–17). The importance of the sign is that it indicates that the collapse is the result of an underlying mass and predicts that the mass will be suffi-

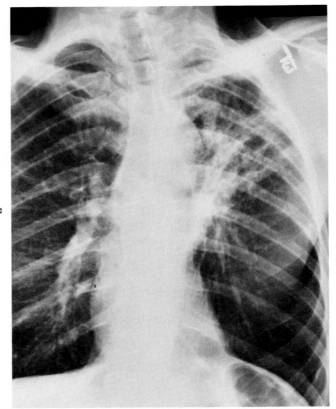

FIG 7−14.
Collapse/consolidation beyond an obstructing bronchial carcinoma in the left upper lobe.

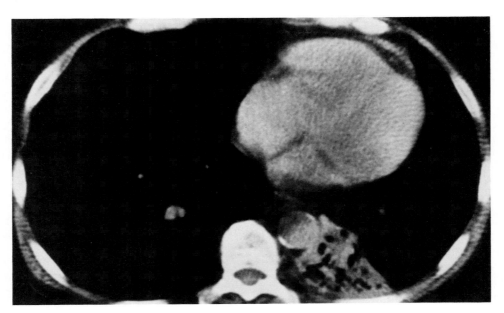

FIG 7−15.
Air bronchogram in the left lower lobe, which had collapsed as a result of a bronchial carcinoma in the left lower lobe bronchus.

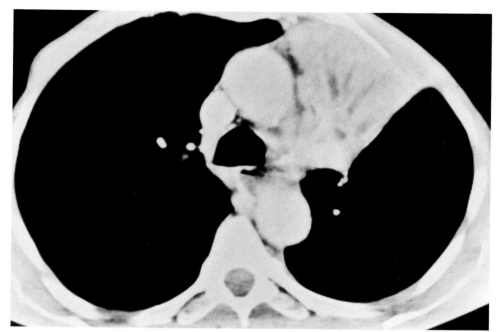

FIG 7–16.
Dilated, fluid-filled bronchi in a collapsed left upper lobe beyond a centrally obstructing bronchial carcinoma. (The plain chest radiograph of this patient is shown in Fig 7–18.)

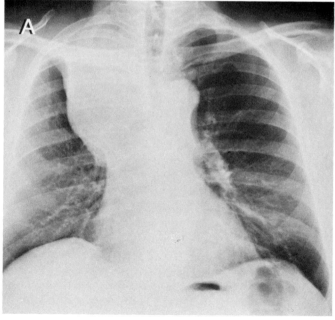
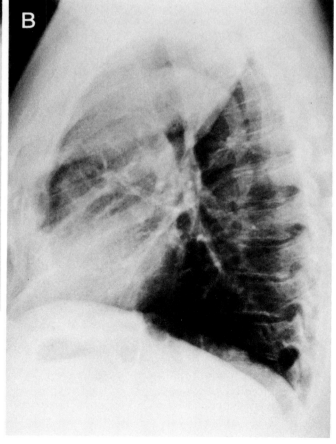

FIG 7–17.
Golden S sign in right upper lobe collapse. The lobe has collapsed around a large, obstructing, centrally positioned bronchial carcinoma in the right upper lobe bronchus. **A,** PA view. **B,** lateral view.

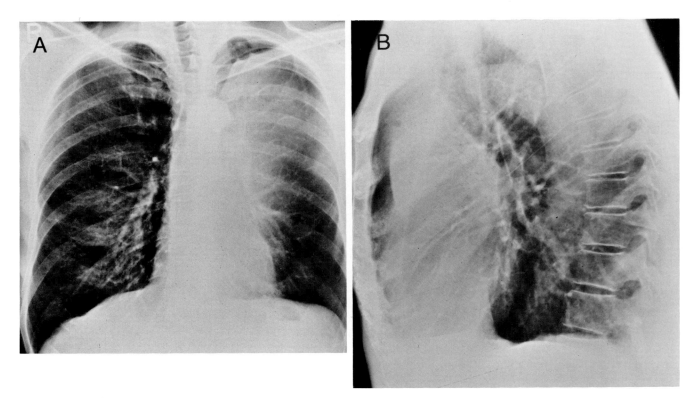

FIG 7–18.
Left upper lobe collapse shown on PA **(A)** and lateral **(B)** chest radiographs beyond a centrally obstructing bronchial carcinoma. (One image from the CT scan of this patient is shown in Fig 7–16.)

ciently central that successful bronchoscopic biopsy should be readily achievable. Thus, the presence of the "S" sign eliminates any doubt as to whether diagnostic bronchoscopy should be undertaken.

2. The presence of pneumonia is confined to one lobe (or more lobes if there is a common bronchus supplying these lobes), with loss of volume, in patients over the age of 35 years, particularly if the lobe shows substantial loss of volume and no air bronchograms (Fig 7–18). Occasionally, the opacified lobe will appear larger than normal because of the buildup of secretions and infection behind the obstructing carcinoma (Fig 7–19). This appearance has been labeled the "drowned lobe." In cases of obstructive pneumonitis or atelectasis, the tumor should be readily visible at bronchoscopy, an investigation that is usually performed without delay in patients with these radiographic findings.

3. The presence of a visible mass or irregular stenosis in a main stem or lobar bronchus.

4. The presence of an associated hilar mass (Fig 7–20). Simple pneumonia rarely causes radiographically visible hilar adenopathy. Bacterial lung abscess can, however, be confused with bronchial carcinoma because it not uncommonly results in hilar or mediastinal adenopathy.[316]

5. A localized pneumonia that persists for more than 2 weeks. Simple pneumonia often clears or spreads to other segments during this time interval. Although consolidation may improve partially on appropriate antibiotic therapy, it virtually never resolves completely if it is secondary to an underlying carcinoma. Complete resolution of pneumonia, in practice, excludes an obstructing neoplasm as the cause of infection.

Overinflation.—Recognizable overinflation by check valve obstruction is very unusual[87]; no such condition was found in the 600 case reports from the Mayo Clinic.[58–61, 218] Expiration films to detect air trapping, though occasionally positive, have not proved useful in the early diagnosis of bronchial carcinoma. Fraser and Pare[127] found only one case of carcinoma in which air trapping was evident in the 6 years that inspiratory-expiratory films were obtained as a routine in their institution.

Hilar Mass.—Hilar enlargement is a common presenting feature in patients with bronchial carcinoma. In the Mayo Clinic series,[58–61, 218] 38% of patients had a hilar or perihilar mass, and in 12%, the central mass was the only radiographic abnormality

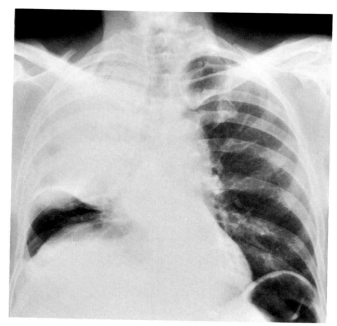

FIG 7–19.
"Drowned lobe" beyond a bronchial carcinoma in the right upper lobe bronchus. The right upper lobe shows extensive consolidation and expansion.

(Fig 7–21). Such enlargement may result from the tumor itself or from enlargement of hilar nodes containing metastatic tumor. It can be very difficult to decide from plain films how much of the mass is tumor and how much is enlarged nodes. The distinction may be easier with CT. In general, the more lobular the shape, the more likely it is that adenopathy is present.

A mass superimposed on the hilus will lead to increased density of the hilus, due to summation, when the opacity of the mass is added to the density of the normal hilar shadows (Fig 7–22). Usually hilar enlargement is recognizable on one or other view, but on rare occasions, the increased density of the hilus is the only sign of the tumor mass.[127]

Spread of Tumor

Bronchial carcinoma invades locally by endobronchial and transbronchial growth,[170] spreads by way of the lymphatics to hilar and mediastinal nodes, and also spreads by means of the bloodstream to remote sites, including other thoracic structures. Only those features visible at chest imaging are discussed here. (Lymphangitis carcinomatosa is discussed on p. 335.)

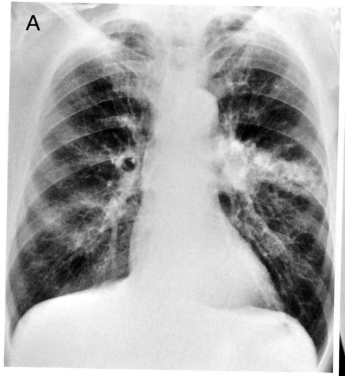

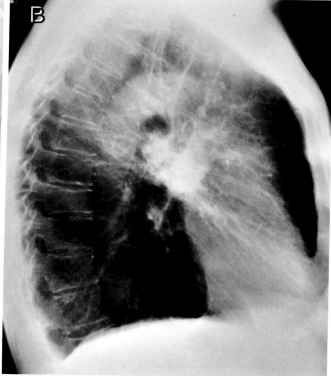

FIG 7–20.
Collapse/consolidation beyond a hilar mass, which resulted from bronchial carcinoma. **A,** PA view. **B,** lateral view.

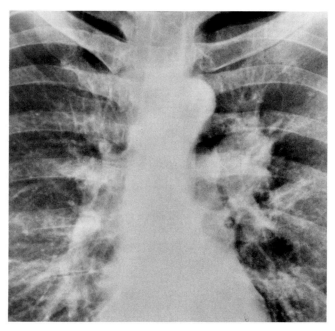

FIG 7–21.
Small cell carcinoma of the bronchus presenting as a hilar mass. As is so often the case, it is not possible to tell whether the mass is all tumor, all enlarged nodes, or a mixture of the two.

Staging

Until 1986 the system of staging developed for the American Joint Committee (AJC) for Cancer Staging and End-Results Reporting was widely used.[347] A new International Staging System for lung cancer has now been introduced, designed to meet more closely the needs of thoracic surgeons considering patients for surgical resection, and radiation therapists and oncologists trying to treat widespread disease.[270] The TNM system is used (Table 7–2) to describe the findings, and the stage (Table 7–3) is then derived from the TNM description (T signifies the primary tumor; N, the regional lymph nodes; and M, distant metastases).

In essence:

- *Stage I* consists of T1 or T2 lesions with no hilar, mediastinal, or distant metastases. These lesions are eminently resectable surgically.
- *Stage II* consists of the same lesions as stage I, but with hilar nodal involvement. These lesions are also resectable for cure, but the prognosis will not be as good.
- *Stage III* has been divided into substages. *Stage IIIA* designates those patients with locally extensive intrathoracic disease which may be surgically resectable. *Stage IIIB* identifies patients

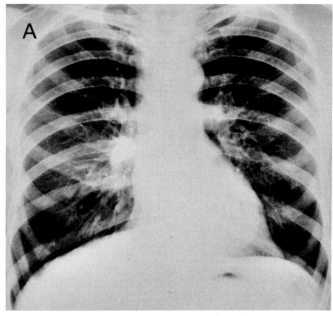

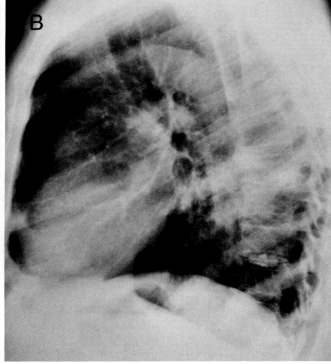

FIG 7–22.
Dense hilus sign. The most obvious sign in the PA view of carcinoma in the superior segment of the right lower lobe is an increase in the density of the right hilus resulting from superimposition of the mass, the distal pneumonia, and the hilar structures. **A,** PA view. **B,** lateral view.

TABLE 7—2

TNM Definitions for Proposed International Staging System for Lung Cancer*

Primary Tumor (T)

TX	Tumor proved by the presence of malignant cells in bronchopulmonary secretions but not visualized roentgenographically or bronchoscopically, or any tumor that cannot be assessed as in a retreatment staging.
T0	No evidence of primary tumor
T1S	Carcinoma in situ
T1†	A tumor that is 3.0 cm or less in greatest dimension, surrounded by lung or visceral pleura, and without evidence of invasion proximal to a lobar bronchus at bronchoscopy
T2	A tumor more than 3.0 cm in greatest dimension, or a tumor of any size that either invades the visceral pleura or has associated atelectasis or obstructive pneumonitis extending to the hilar region. At bronchoscopy the proximal extent of demonstrable tumor must be within a lobar bronchus or at least 2.0 cm distal to the carina. Any associated atelectasis or obstructive pneumonitis must involve less than an entire lung
T3	A tumor of any size with direct extension into the chest wall (including superior sulcus tumors), diaphragm, or the mediastinal pleura or pericardium without involving the heart, great vessels, trachea, esophagus or vertebral body; or a tumor in the main bronchus within 2 cm of the carina without involving the carina
T4‡	A tumor of any size with invasion of the mediastinum or involving the heart, great vessels, trachea, esophagus, vertebral body, or carina; or presence of malignant pleural effusion

Nodal involvement (N)

N0	No demonstrable metastasis to regional lymph nodes
N1	Metastasis to lymph nodes in the peribronchial or the ipsilateral hilar region, or both, including direct extension
N2	Metastasis to ipsilateral mediastinal lymph nodes and subcarinal lymph nodes
N3	Metastasis to contralateral mediastinal lymph nodes, contralateral hilar lymph nodes, ipsilateral or contralateral scalene, or supraclavicular lymph nodes

Distant metastasis (M)

M0	No (known) distant metastasis
M1	Distant metastasis present—specify sites

*From Mountain CF: A new international staging system for lung cancer. *Chest* 1986; 89(suppl):225S-233S. Used by permission.

†T1 The uncommon superficial tumor of any size with the invasive component limited to the bronchial wall which may extend proximal to the main bronchus is classified as T1.

‡T4 Most pleural effusions associated with lung cancer are due to tumor. There are, however, some few patients in whom cytopathologic examination of pleural fluid (on more than one specimen) is negative for tumor, the fluid is nonbloody, and it is not an exudate. In such cases in which these elements and clinical judgment dictate that the effusion is not related to the tumor, the patients should be staged T1, T2, or T3, excluding effusion as a staging element.

with locally extensive intrathoracic invasion beyond the limits of conventional surgical resection. *Stage IIIB* tumors may, however, be considered localized in terms of planning radiation therapy.

- *Stage IV* includes all patients with distant metastatic disease.

Patients who seem to survive better than their stage might suggest[121] include those with (1) intracapsular lymph node metastasis rather than extracapsular matted nodes,[250] (2) localized areas of nodal disease amenable to surgical resection,[250] (3) positive mediastinal nodes discovered only at surgery after a negative mediastinoscopy,[297] and (4) involvement of the mediastinum by squamous cell carcinoma rather than adenocarcinoma or large cell carcinoma.[204, 324]

Currently, the standard imaging tests used to stage the intrathoracic spread of lung cancer are the plain chest radiograph and the CT scan of the chest. The role of magnetic resonance imaging (MRI) remains to be seen. So far, it has not demonstrated enough advantages to replace chest CT as the stan-

TABLE 7-3
Stages for Proposed International Staging System for Lung Cancer*

Stage	Definition†
I	T1, N0, M0
	T2, N0, M0
II	T1, N1, M0
	T2, N1, M0
IIIA	T3, N0, M0
	T3, N1, M0
	T1-3, N2, M0
IIIB	Any T, N3, M0
	T4; any N, M0
IV	Any T; any N, M1

*From Moutain CF: A new international staging system for lung cancer. *Chest* 1986; 89 (suppl):225S-233S. Used by permission.
†See Table 7-1.

dard procedure, though it can, as discussed later, prove useful in selected cases.

A related but distinct issue is the preoperative decision whether a lobectomy or a pneumonectomy will be required for centrally situated tumors. The decision depends on whether or not the tumor has crossed fissures, invaded central vessels, or spread centrally within the bronchial tree. Plain radiography, CT scanning, and bronchoscopy all provide important information with which to make these decisions, but CT scanning has not proved sufficiently accurate in predicting whether or not a pneumonectomy will be required in patients with central tumors; therefore, the surgeon is still often called on to make this decision at the time of thoracotomy.[308]

Even with tumors amenable to surgical resection, a major decision in many patients is whether or not lung function would be adequate if a pneumonectomy proves necessary. Pulmonary perfusion scans have a role to play here. The relative perfusion of each lung is quantitated by the number of radioactive counts in the combined anterior and posterior scans. The percentage contribution of each lung to the total counts is then multiplied by the overall forced expiratory volume in one second (FEV_1) to predict the postoperative FEV_1 of the lung that is to remain.[45]

Intrathoracic Lymph Node Metastases

Hilar and mediastinal nodal metastases are often present at the time of initial diagnosis, particularly with adenocarcinoma and small cell tumors. Primary tumors greater than 3 cm in diameter have a higher incidence of nodal involvement than tumors of smaller diameter. Also, the more central the primary tumor, the more likely it is to be accompanied by nodal metastasis.

Currently, the only useful sign of hilar/mediastinal lymph node metastases is enlargement. Low-density necrotic areas within a node, a sign that has proved so useful in differentiating metastases from head and neck tumors in cervical lymph nodes, has not proved to be common enough to be of value in diagnosing mediastinal nodal involvement by lung cancer. Radionuclide scanning, even with gallium 67, has proved to be both insensitive and nonspecific in diagnosing the spread of bronchial carcinoma[3, 101] and MRI using standard T1- and T2-weighted spin-echo sequences has not yet permitted the recognition of tumor involvement based on signal intensity alone.[131, 139, 275, 321, 373]

Hilar node enlargement is recognizable on plain chest radiography, conventional tomography, CT, and MRI. The advantages of CT over conventional tomography in evaluating the hilar nodes is moderate or slight. In practice, however, CT has replaced conventional tomography even for hilar assessment because it shows the mediastinal nodes in addition to the hilar nodes. The recognition of mediastinal node metastasis has more impact on the decision as to whether or not to operate, because the presence of hilar node enlargement does not preclude surgery, whereas recognizable mediastinal disease usually prevents curative resection.

Hilar nodes are easier to identify at MRI than at CT because, on the MR images, they stand out against the signal void of flowing blood in hilar vessels and air in the bronchi.[371] Thus, it is to be expected that MRI will be a more sensitive technique than either CT or hilar tomography for identifying enlarged hilar nodes, and early reports have confirmed this prediction.[139, 275]

Mediastinal nodal enlargement must be substantial if it is to be recognizable with conventional techniques. Plain chest radiography and conventional tomography have repeatedly been found to be relatively insensitive tests compared with CT scanning in the detection of mediastinal nodal metastases.[84, 112, 223, 288] There are three CT series to date in which normal mediastinal lymph node size has been measured.[136, 140, 328] These show that nodes smaller than 10 mm in transverse diameter fall within the 95th percentile and should, therefore, be considered normal. In 5% to 7% of normal subjects, nodes between 10 and 15 mm in diameter will be found in certain sites, notably the subcarinal and

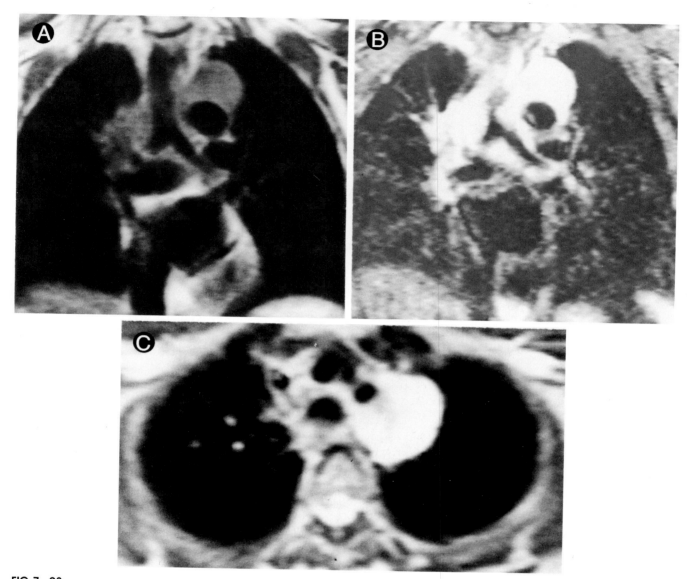

FIG 7–23.
MR images of the mediastinum showing extensive mediastinal adenopathy owing to involvement by small cell carcinoma of the lung. **A,** T1-weighted coronal section. **B,** T2-weighted coronal section at same level. **C,** T2-weighted axial section above the level of the aortic arch. The tumor tissue can be clearly distinguished from the signal void of air in the bronchi and of flowing blood in the major vessels. (Courtesy of Dr. William C. Black, Washington, D.C.)

tracheobronchial regions. MRI (Fig 7–23, A–C) appears to provide information comparable to that of CT regarding the presence and size of mediastinal lymph nodes, provided multiple sequences are performed.* One advantage of MRI over CT is that it may be easier to distinguish lymph nodes from blood vessels, owing to the signal void in areas of fast-flowing blood. This advantage is offset, however, by greater image degradation by motion artifact and the inability of MRI to demonstrate calcification in nodes. Extensive calcification of a large node is an excellent indication that the node is enlarged because of a benign cause, such as granulomatous disease, rather than metastasis.

The problem with using size as the only criterion for malignant involvement is that intrathoracic lymph node enlargement has many nonmalignant causes (Fig 7–24) including reactive inflammation to the tumor or to pneumonia distal to it, previous tuberculosis or histoplasmosis, and coincidental pneu-

*References 167, 220, 251, 275, 303, and 373.

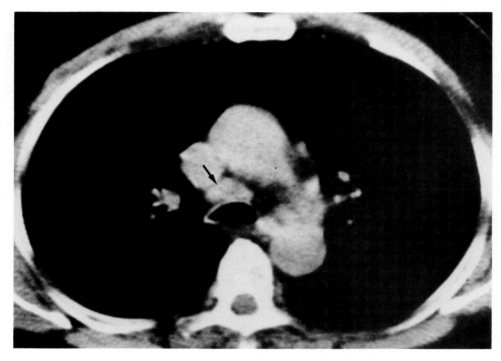

FIG 7–24.
Enlarged mediastinal lymph node in a patient with bronchial carcinoma. This was a false positive CT study for metastasis. The node *(arrow),* which measures 1.7 cm in short axis diameter, showed only reactive hyperplasia on histologic examination.

moconiosis and sarcoidosis. Conversely, microscopic involvement by tumor can be present without causing enlargement of the node. It will therefore be clear that there is no measurement above which all nodes can be assumed to be malignant and below which all can be considered benign. Many centers have provided estimates of the sensitivity and specificity of CT in the staging of bronchial carcinoma. Such figures are difficult to obtain because, ideally, one requires a large series of patients in whom all the mediastinal nodes, whether enlarged or not, are examined histologically and correlated with their size at CT scanning. Such information is rarely available.[227, 228] As can be seen from Table 7–4, the sensitivity and specificity of CT for the diagnosis of metastases in mediastinal lymph nodes has varied greatly, and there is no clear explanation for this variability.

As with all survey techniques where there are no clear-cut criteria for abnormality, sensitivity varies inversely with specificity as the criterion for abnormality is relaxed or tightened. For example, if a short axis diameter of 2 cm is chosen as the cutoff between benign and malignant (Fig 7–25), the specificity will be reasonably high, but many nodes which in fact contain tumor will be diagnosed as tumor

free, because the criterion is so generous. The opposite applies when a small diameter is chosen. If 6 mm is used as the diameter above which nodes are regarded as positive,[288] then virtually all cases of tumor involvement will be diagnosed as positive by CT (high sensitivity); however, many patients whose mediastinal nodes are free of tumor will be falsely diagnosed as having metastatic disease (low specificity). In practice, the CT examination is largely used to decide whether to perform mediastinoscopy or mediastinotomy and to demonstrate which nodes should undergo biopsy.[110] For this purpose, nodes less than 10 mm in short-axis diameter are unlikely to contain tumor and, therefore, do not warrant preoperative biopsy, whereas nodes above this size should probably be subjected to some form of biopsy. Thus, few patients are denied thoracotomy for an otherwise resectable lung cancer solely because of enlarged nodes found at mediastinal CT.

The accuracy of CT in diagnosing nodal involvement varies significantly according to the site of the nodes. Left hilar and aortopulmonary window nodal enlargements are particularly difficult to detect,[119, 307] but nevertheless, in one large survey,[300] cancers of the left lung were staged by CT at least as accurately as cancers of the right lung. This some-

TABLE 7-4

CT in the Evaluation of Mediastinal Node Involvement by Bronchial Carcinoma

Authors (Reference)	No. of Patients	Criterion (mm)	Sensitivity (%)	Specificity (%)	Positive Predictive Value (%)	Negative Predictive Value (%)
Brion et al[52]	153	5	89	46	47	89
Osborne et al.[289]	42	6	94	62	65	94
Backer et al.[13]	87	10	96	92	84	98
Baron et al.[17]	98	10	74	98	84	97
Conte et al.[90]	75	10	85	89	74	94
Eckholm et al.[107]	35	10	29	46	13	72
Glazer et al.[141]	49	100 mm^2	95	64	67	95
Khan et al.[199]	50	10	83	90	83	90
Lewis et al.[222]	75	10	91	94	88	95
Libshitz et al.[227]	86	10	67	66	39	86
Martini et al.[251]	34	10	87	79	76	88
Musset et al.[275]	44	10	91	82	91	82
Osborne et al.[288]	42	10	72	83	76	80
Richey et al.[312]	48	10	95	68	68	95
Baron et al.[17]	98	15	92	80	76	94
Daly et al.[94]	146	15	80	91	77	92
Faling et al.[112]	51	15	88	94	88	88
Goldstraw et al.[148]	41	15	57	85	67	79
Libshitz and McKenna[227]	86	15	38	83	42	81
Libshitz and McKenna[227]	86	20	24	97	71	80

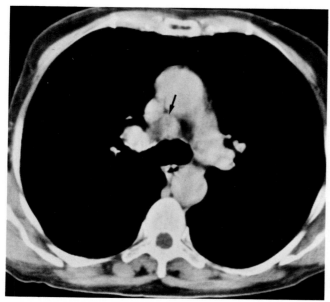

FIG 7-25.
Enlarged mediastinal lymph node in a patient with bronchial carcinoma—a true positive CT scan for lymph node involvement by tumor. The node identified by the *arrow* has a short axis diameter in excess of 2 cm.

what surprising observation was explained by the high incidence of spread to subcarinal and right-sided lymph nodes from left-sided tumors, so that the poor sensitivity of CT in detecting left-sided nodal enlargement was not of great practical significance in the surgical management of the patient.[300]

The utility of chest CT in T1N0M0 cancers by clinical and plain chest radiographic criteria is controversial. The prevalence of mediastinal nodal involvement with such small tumors is less than 20%[165] and may be much less.[296] Therefore, the problem of false positive test results becomes a major factor. A cost-effectiveness analysis showed that with current surgical techniques, chest CT would be both clinically useful and cost-saving, provided the CT examination was readily available and the prevalence of nodal involvement was 12.5% or greater.[35]

Mediastinal Invasion

Direct invasion of the mediastinum can often be detected by CT and MRI, but is only occasionally diagnosable by conventional techniques. Radionuclide perfusion scanning will demonstrate reduced perfusion in cases in which the central pulmonary arteries are invaded by the tumor, but the test is too insensitive and too nonspecific to be of practical value in routine staging.

Plain film evidence relies on demonstrating phrenic nerve paralysis. Caution is needed, however, before deciding that a high hemidiaphragm is caused by phrenic nerve invasion, because lobar collapse can also lead to elevation of a hemidiaphragm, and subpulmonary effusion may mimic it. Fluoroscopy can be helpful in distinguishing between these possibilities. Barium swallow studies may show esophageal invasion; the appearance closely resembles that of esophageal carcinoma, with irregular narrowing of the lumen and a soft tissue mass surrounding both the esophagus and the adjacent tracheobronchial tree. Barium may enter the bronchial tree by way of the fistula through the tumor.

The CT and MRI signs of mediastinal invasion are visible tumor surrounding the mediastinal vessels, esophagus, or proximal main stem bronchi (Figs 7–26 and 7–27). Mere contact with the mediastinum is not enough for the diagnosis of invasion, and apparent interdigitation with mediastinal fat can be a misleading sign on both CT and MRI[251] (Fig 7–28). Baron et al.[17] suggested that if one-third of the circumference of any of these structures was in direct contact with the tumor, then mediastinal invasion could be diagnosed. Tumors that are in contact with the mediastinum but show no firm evidence of invasion have to be regarded as indeterminate. Asso-

ciated pneumonia or atelectasis may make it difficult to determine whether mediastinal contact is present. Currently, MRI does not appear to offer any advantages over CT in the diagnosis of mediastinal invasion. The signs are basically the same, and the axial imaging plane is the standard projection for both tests.[251, 275]

Chest Wall Invasion

A peripheral lung carcinoma may cross the pleura and invade the chest wall. Rib or spinal destruction is sometimes visible on plain films (Fig 7–29), but confirmatory tomography or CT may be necessary (Fig 7–30). Soft tissue invasion is best detected by CT or MRI. The presence of bone destruction in the vicinity of a pulmonary shadow, whatever the shape of the shadow, is virtually diagnostic of primary carcinoma of the lung. With the rare exception of fungal disease, notably actinomycosis, neither pulmonary infection nor any other non-neoplastic pulmonary process invades the adjacent bone.

Diagnosing visceral or parietal pleural involvement adjacent to the tumor is difficult even at CT in cases without bone destruction or a definite chest wall mass.[143, 298] Local chest pain remains the single most specific indicator of whether or not the tumor has spread to the parietal pleura or chest wall. Contact with the pleura on CT examination, even if the pleura is thickened, does not necessarily indicate in-

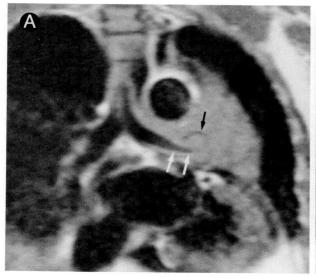
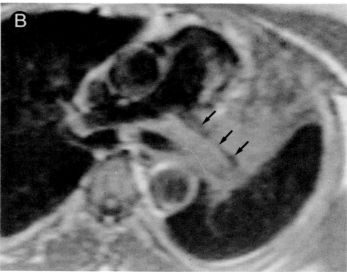

FIG 7–26.

MR image of central squamous cell carcinoma causing left upper lobe collapse. The invasion of tumor into the mediastinum, and the severe narrowing of the left pulmonary artery *(black arrows)* and the left upper lobe bronchus *(white arrows)* are well demon-

strated. **A,** sagittal section TR = 680 ms TE = 26 ms. **B,** axial section TR = 680 ms TE = 26 ms. (Courtesy of Dr. William C. Black, Washington, D.C.)

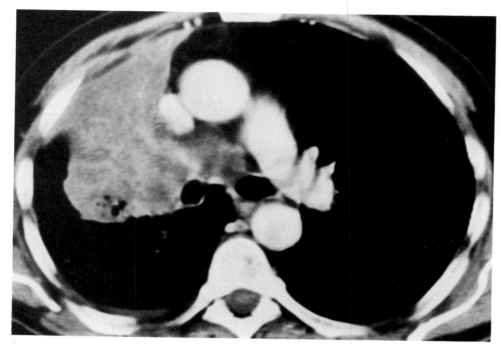

FIG 7–27.
Mediastinal invasion by lung cancer. Note that the tumor crosses the mediastinum to contact the opposite main stem bronchus.

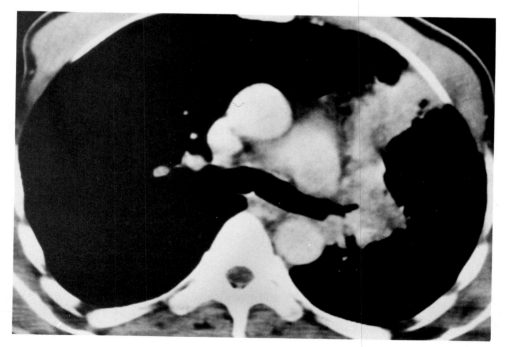

FIG 7–28.
Mediastinal contact by bronchial carcinoma that proved to be surgically resectable and not invading the mediastinum. Preoperatively, it was not possible to say whether the tumor had invaded the mediastinum.

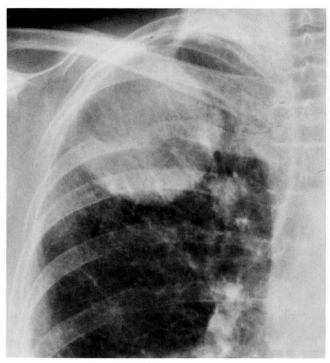

FIG 7–29.
Bronchial carcinoma showing invasion of the right fifth rib. Note the irregular destruction of the rib. In this case, there is widening of the adjacent rib interspace. Such widening is very unusual in bronchial carcinoma.

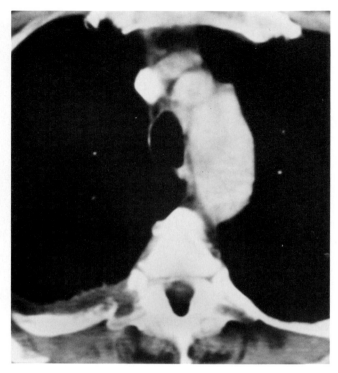

FIG 7–30.
Rib destruction from bronchial carcinoma shown by CT. The destruction, which was questioned on plain film, is shown to be extensive at CT scanning.

vasion. The greater the degree of contact and the greater the pleural thickening, the more likely it is that the parietal pleura has been invaded. A definite chest wall mass that is not explicable by previous chest trauma is highly likely to be the result of invasion by tumor. Conversely, a clear extrapleural fat plane adjacent to the mass may prove to be helpful, though not definitive, in excluding chest wall invasion.

Early reports suggest that MRI is distinctly better than CT in demonstrating chest wall invasion.[275] The advantage stems partly from the ability to image in the sagittal and coronal planes, which are the optimal planes in which to demonstrate invasion of the chest wall or neck by apical tumors or invasion of the diaphragm by basal tumors. The fat and muscle planes of the chest wall are well demonstrated at MRI, and obliteration or distortion of these planes is therefore easy to recognize.

Technetium-99m radionuclide bone scans are a sensitive technique with which to assess bone invasion (see Fig 7–32). They are frequently positive when the plain films still show no bony abnormality.

The Pancoast tumor deserves special mention.

The eponym nowadays refers to the symptom complex of pain in the shoulder and arm that results from apical tumors that invade the lower cords of the brachial plexus and the sympathetic chain. Pancoast's original description included ipsilateral Horner's syndrome, from invasion of the sympathetic chain, and local destruction of bone by the tumor.[291] Because these tumors arise adjacent to the groove for the subclavian artery, they are also called superior sulcus tumors. They may be of any cell type.[12, 293] Radiographically[192] the tumors appear as a mass in approximately one-half to three-quarters of the cases and as an apical cap resembling pleural thickening in the remainder. Bone destruction in the adjacent ribs or spine is seen in approximately one-third of cases (Figs 7–30 and 7–31).[12, 283] These tumors are, however, often difficult to diagnose on standard plain chest radiographs because the lung apex is partly hidden by overlying ribs and clavicle. Even with lordotic apical views the diagnosis can be very difficult because the tumor so often closely resembles benign pleural thickening (see Fig 7–32) and the cardinal plain film sign of the lesion—bone destruction—is either absent or difficult to diagnose with confidence. Asymmetric pleural thickening,

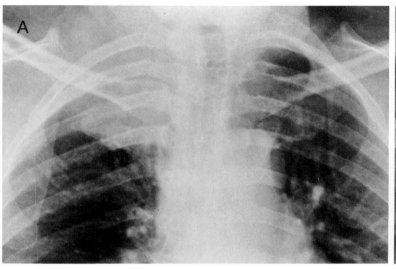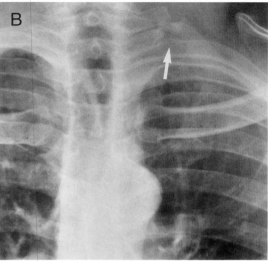

FIG 7–31.
A, superior sulcus carcinoma of the lung destroying the major portion of the right first rib. The patient, a 52-year-old man, complained of chest wall pain and pain in the right arm. **B,** a more subtle example of superior sulcus carcinoma of the lung. The apical cap is slight, and the rib destruction of the neck and head of the first rib *(arrow)* is not easy to see.

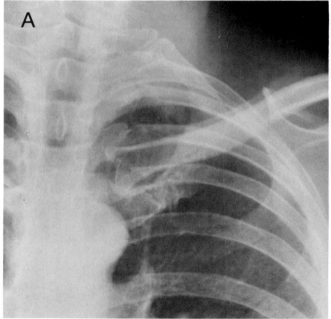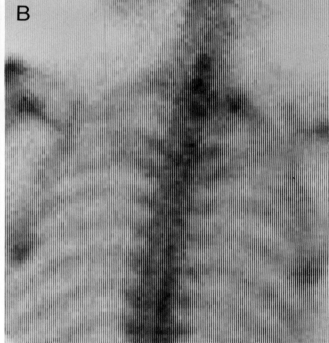

FIG 7–32.
Pancoast's tumor. **A,** on plain film the appearance resembles an apical pleural cap. **B,** ^{99m}Tc bone scan shows increased activity in the invaded left first rib (posterior scan, but aligned to correspond with chest radiograph.)

particularly if associated with appropriate symptoms, should be viewed with suspicion. Clearly, a chronically enlarging unilateral apical cap is highly suspicious for superior sulcus carcinoma; such patients are usually symptomatic.[257]

CT scans can be helpful in diagnosing Pancoast's tumors[159, 283, 372] (Fig 7−33). They may demonstrate an intrapulmonary mass rather than just pleural thickening, thus providing extra confidence that the diagnosis is neoplasm rather than inflammatory pleural thickening. Also, CT scanning is a sensitive technique with which to diagnose the full extent of the tumor, particularly the chest wall invasion. MRI scans may prove to be particularly useful in demonstrating Pancoast's tumors, partly because the coronal plane is the optimal imaging plane for such lesions.

Pleural Involvement

Both peripheral and central bronchial carcinoma may spread to involve the pleura by direct spread, lymphatic permeation, or tumor emboli in the pulmonary arteries.[264, 343] Pleural effusions occur with all cell types of lung carcinoma, but appear to be most frequent with adenocarcinoma.[78] The usual radiographic manifestation of pleural involvement is pleural effusion, which may be free or loculated. Usually there are no radiographic features that allow one to distinguish between pleural fluid resulting from neoplastic invasion of the pleura and fluid from other causes, notably benign diseases such as pneumonia adjacent to the neoplasm. Hemorrhagic effusion on pleural aspiration is a strong indication of direct involvement by tumor.[264]

Occasionally, nodules of tumor are visible as lobular pleural thickening (Fig 7−34). On plain films such nodules are only visible when separate from adjacent fluid. At CT, however, pleural nodules of tumor may be identifiable even when bathed in fluid.

Radiographic Patterns Based on Cell Type

The radiographic pattern of bronchial carcinoma varies with the cell type. The generalizations listed here are based on the series of 600 cases of bronchial carcinoma analyzed at the Mayo Clinic;[58] these observations clearly are no substitute for histologic examination. Bronchioloalveolar carcinoma is considered separately because it shows significant differences from the other major cell types.

Early, and often massive, lymphadenopathy is a well-recognized phenomenon in small cell carcinoma (Figs 7−35 and 7−36) and in giant cell carcinoma. [221, 335] Woodring and Stelling have pointed out that adenocarcinoma appears to be changing its pattern and nowadays it also often shows hilar and

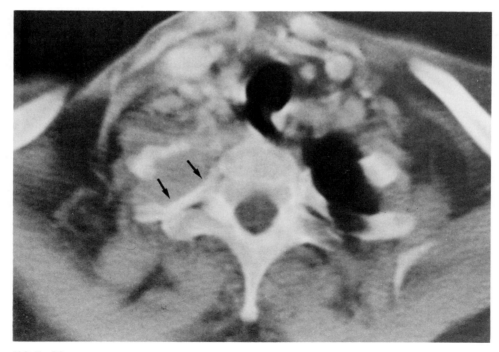

FIG 7−33.
CT scan of Pancoast's tumor showing tumor at the lung apex invading the adjacent rib *(arrows).*

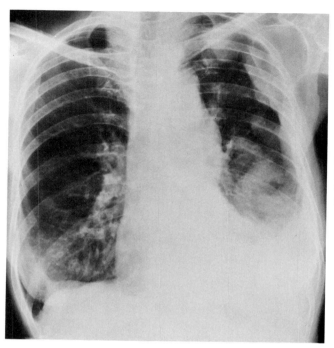

FIG 7–34.
Extensive lobular pleural thickening and pleural effusion as a result of pleural invasion by bronchial adenocarcinoma. Note the resemblance to malignant mesothelioma of the pleura.

mediastinal adenopathy,[382] though the nodal enlargement is not as massive as with the small cell and large cell undifferentiated tumors. A mass in, or adjacent to, the hilus is a particular characteristic of small cell carcinoma, being seen in 78% of cases (see Fig 7–21).

A peripheral nodule (Fig 7–37) is very common in adenocarcinoma (72% of cases) and large cell tumors (63% of cases), with over twice the incidence that is seen with squamous cell or small cell carcinomas. The largest peripheral masses are seen with squamous and large cell tumors, whereas most adenocarcinomas and small cell carcinomas are less than 4 cm in diameter. Squamous cancers may attain great size (Fig 7–38), and they cavitate more frequently than the other cell types; cavitation was seen in 22% of squamous cell carcinomas presenting as a peripheral mass (Fig 7–39), compared with only 6% of peripheral large cell and 2% of peripheral adenocarcinomas.

Collapse-consolidation of the lung beyond the tumor is the most frequent feature seen with squamous cell carcinoma, in keeping with the predominantly central origin of this form of neoplasm.

Bronchioloalveolar Carcinoma

Bronchioloalveolar carcinoma, also known as alveolar cell and bronchiolar carcinoma, is a subtype of adenocarcinoma according to the WHO classification.[210] It accounts for some 2% to 5% of all lung cancers. There are a number of clinical and radiologic features which justify regarding it as a separate clinical entity.[330] The characteristic pathologic feature is a peripheral neoplasm showing lepidic growth with the malignant cells using surrounding alveolar walls as a scaffold. These tumors are believed to arise from type II pneumocytes and probably also from bronchiolar epithelium.[343] The cells produce mucus, sometimes in such large amounts that one of the presenting symptoms may be expectoration of large quantities of mucoid sputum.

The tumors occur equally in both sexes, and the average age at onset is 50 years. Both unifocal and multifocal disease are seen, unifocal being much the more common,[177] and it is a matter of debate whether the multifocal form is merely an extension of the unifocal variety or whether it is a different and more aggressive entity.[265] The prognosis of bronchioloalveolar carcinoma, when resected as a solitary pulmonary nodule, is relatively good.[25, 187] The prognosis of the larger, more ill-defined lesion and of the disseminated form is very bad.[111]

Radiographic Features[32, 177, 237]

Because these tumors arise from the alveoli and the immediately adjacent small airways, they present as peripheral pulmonary opacities rather than with the effects of large airway obstruction. The most common finding is a solitary pulmonary nodule or

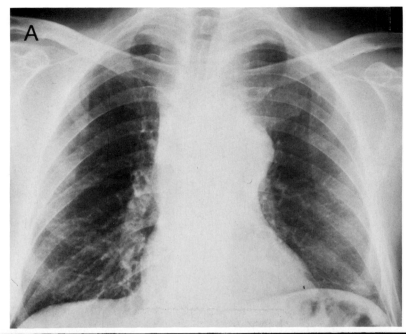

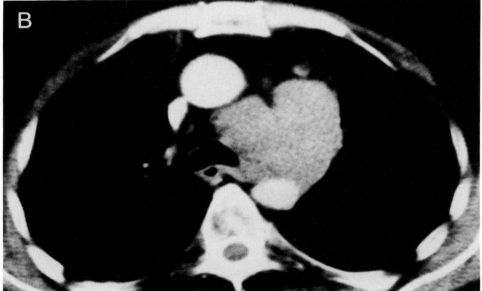

FIG 7–35.
Small (oat) cell carcinoma showing massive mediastinal adenopathy. The primary tumor, which was centrally located in the bronchial tree, is not visible radiographically. **A,** plain film. **B,** CT scan.

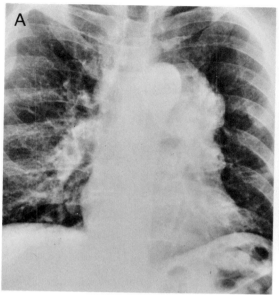
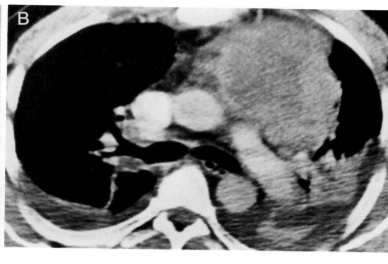

FIG 7–36.

Small (oat) cell carcinoma. **A,** plain film showing lobular widening of the mediastinum due to massive mediastinal adenopathy. **B,** CT scan a few days later showed the partially necrotic lymph node involvement, plus left lower lobe collapse and bilateral pleural effusions.

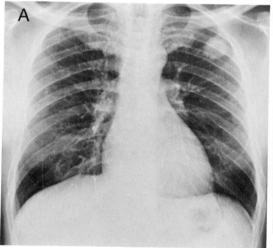
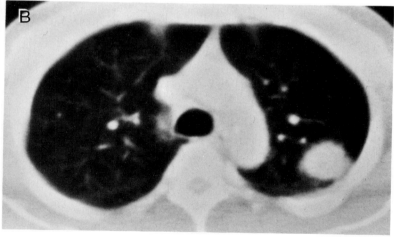

FIG 7–37.

Adenocarcinoma of the bronchus presenting as a peripheral lung nodule. There was no hilar or mediastinal adenopathy in this case. **A,** plain film. **B,** CT scan.

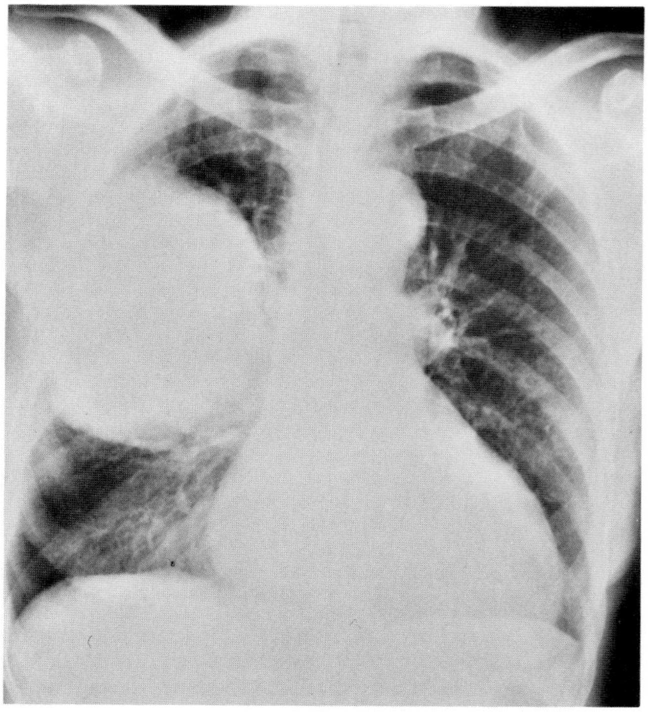

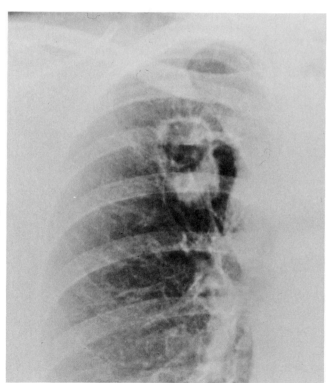

FIG 7–38.
Squamous cell carcinoma of the bronchus, illustrating the huge size that these tumors may attain at initial presentation.

FIG 7–39.
Squamous cell carcinoma of the bronchus presenting as a cavitating nodule. Note that part of the wall is very thin and smooth.

mass that is usually indistinguishable from other types of carcinoma (Fig 7–40). There is, however, a propensity to a subpleural location and the development of a pleuropulmonary tail[177, 211, 334] due to desmoplastic reaction in the peripheral septa of the lung. A few such nodules will have a visible air bronchogram, a phenomenon that is best seen with CT.[211] They may on occasion grow slowly, with doubling times far in excess of the 18 months usually quoted for bronchial carcinoma.[177]

The radiographic presentation that distinguishes bronchioloalveolar carcinoma from the other cell types is when the lesion takes the form of ill-defined opacities or multiple small nodules. Bronchorrhea is a frequent clinical manifestation in this form of the disease. There are a variety of appearances: an ill-defined opacity resembling a patch of pneumonia (Fig 7–41); homogeneous consolidation of one lobe (Fig 7–42);[111]; patchy consolidation; or multiple nodules spread widely through multiple lobes in one or both lungs (Fig 7–43). Both atelectasis and expansile consolidation (Fig 7–44) are reported.[179] Air bronchograms may be an obvious feature (see Fig 7–41). They are particularly well demonstrated by CT, which has been reported to show uniform narrowing of the bronchi within the lung.[184] Thickened septal lines due to lymphatic permeation may also be visible, as may branching tubular densities of mucoid impaction.[179] Pleural effusions are seen in up to a third of patients, and hilar/mediastinal lymphade-

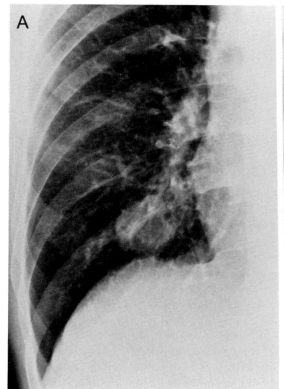

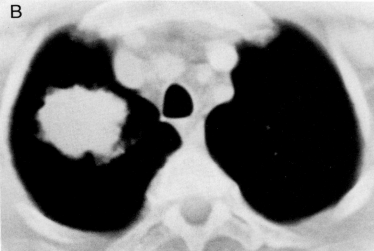

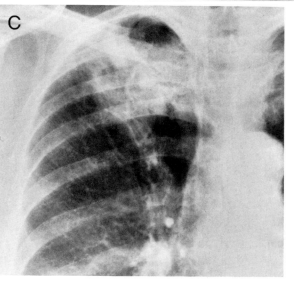

FIG 7–40.
Two examples of bronchioloalveolar cell carcinoma presenting as a solitary pulmonary nodule/mass. **A,** Plain radiograph in a 47-year-old asymptomatic man. **B,** CT scan in a different patient showing a lobular irregular mass. Note that on the plain film **(C),** this tumor was ill-defined in outline and resembled a pneumonia.

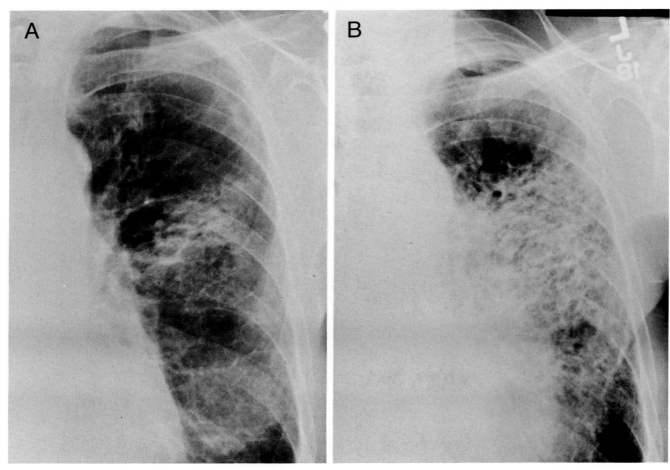

FIG 7–41.
Bronchioloalveolar carcinoma presenting as an ill-defined opacity with air bronchograms. Plain films at presentation **(A)** and 7 months later **(B)**. Note the resemblance of each individual image to pneumonia. The time course is the major clue to the diagnosis of neoplasm.

nopathy is seen in close to a fifth. Cavitation is unusual but has been recorded; one case showed thickening of the wall of a preexisting lung cavity due, presumably, to tumor growing around the wall of a bronchogenic cyst.[179] The differential diagnosis from pneumonia or pulmonary edema depends on knowing the clinical findings and appreciating the more chronic course of the disease. CT scanning has been advocated to make sure that the tumor is confined to one lobe, as CT may show pulmonary foci in areas not appreciated on plain chest radiograph.[261]

Early Diagnosis of Bronchial Carcinoma

The value of any cancer screening program is ultimately assessed by comparing the benefit, namely increased survival and lessened morbidity, to the costs. Costs include both the monetary cost of the screening program and the overall cost of false positive diagnoses, including unnecessary patient morbidity, worry, and expense. At present, only the plain chest radiograph and, to a much lesser extent, sputum cytologic study are of proved value in the detection of asymptomatic lung cancer on a large scale. Comparison with previous normal radiographs allows greater confidence in the diagnosis of small nodules and will, therefore, permit smaller lesions to be reported.[54] Chest radiographs for the detection and evaluation of bronchial carcinoma should be obtained with high-kV techniques, primarily because of the larger volume of lung that can be surveyed (the higher kilovoltage causes less lung to be hidden by ribs, clavicles, heart, or diaphragm).

The basic idea underlying a lung cancer detection program is that more cures will be achieved if small tumors, particularly peripheral ones, are

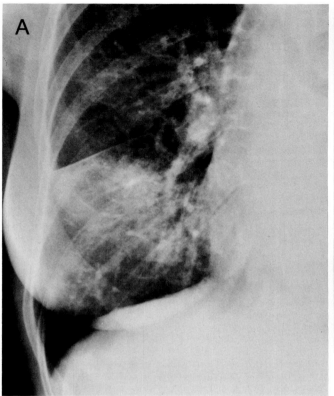

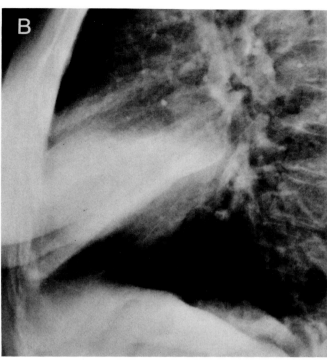

FIG 7−42.
Bronchioloalveolar cell carcinoma presenting as lobar consolidation of the middle lobe. The patient complained of coughing up copious amounts of mucoid suptum. **A,** PA radiograph. **B,** lateral radiograph.

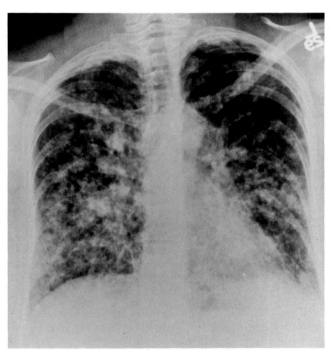

FIG 7−43.
Bronchioloalveolar carcinoma presenting as widespread ill-defined patchy areas of consolidation.

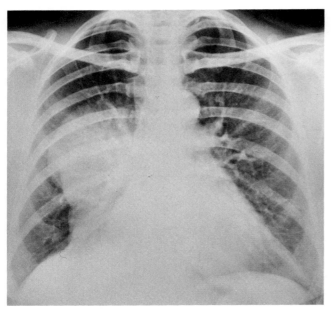

FIG 7–44.
Bronchioloalveolar carcinoma presenting as expansile consolidation of the right lower lobe.

found in asymptomatic individuals, since it is in this category of patients that the best surgical results are obtained.[125, 176, 187, 290] Such presumptions are, however, fraught with difficulties because there are so many variables to consider.[180] The published surgical series refer to selected patients and are not necessarily representative of the population at large. Another problem is "lead time bias"—the extra life expectancy that occurs simply from having a tumor diagnosed earlier, regardless of whether or not treatment is effective. In the series of Huhti et al.,[180] for example, average survival was better in those patients whose tumors were discovered by regular survey; but 5-year survival was not improved. Yet another pitfall is "length bias"—the tendency for tumors with an inherently better prognosis to be found by mass screening, particularly at the first attendance, thereby invalidating comparisons unless the series is carefully controlled. As Garland and co-workers have pointed out,[134] slow-growing tumors, even though large and clinically late-appearing, usually have a better prognosis than rapidly growing tumors, even when the latter are small and ostensibly found early.

Several large screening programs have been undertaken.[33, 44, 51, 162, 180, 278] One that has attracted considerable interest is the multicenter survey conducted by the National Cancer Institute. Hopefully the project, which has a randomized control group,

will in time provide enough data for meaningful statistical analysis to determine the utility of intensive screening programs. Only the briefest outline of the interim results are given here. From a population of approximately 10,000 high-risk patients at each center (men over 45 years of age who were chronic excessive cigarette smokers), 0.5% to 0.8% had lung cancer diagnosed at their initial screening.[124, 126, 129, 166] (By way of comparison, the yield for diagnosing breast carcinoma by large-scale mammography is approximately 0.7% at initial screening.) The rate of cancer diagnosis in the group subsequently assigned to four monthly chest radiographs and sputum cytologic examination was 2% in the ensuing 10 years, approximately half of these tumors being at AJC stage I, and therefore surgically resectable.[259, 273]

There were some disappointments. The initial hope that intensive screening would detect a large proportion of early cases of squamous cell carcinoma, the cell type with the best surgical results, was not fulfilled.[126] Two findings of particular interest to radiologists are that many peripherally located cancers were overlooked initially; 90% of those missed were visible in retrospect for months or even years. Fortunately, peripheral carcinomas may grow slowly, so despite delayed diagnosis, 70% were still within AJC stage I when finally noted.[273] Huhti et al.[180] also noted that wherever the diagnosis was previously missed, the survival rates were better—again a reflection that the rate of tumor growth may be more important than "early" diagnosis. Second, in approximately 20% of the patients in the survey, malignant cells were present in the sputum when the plain chest radiograph was normal. These patients, who all had either centrally situated squamous cell carcinoma or mixed histologic features with squamous carcinoma as one element were, interestingly, more likely to have a favorable prognosis than those who had positive radiographic findings.[125, 273, 383]

Patients with normal chest radiographs but malignant cells in the sputum, or those strongly suspected of having lung carcinoma because of a paraneoplastic syndrome, should have the upper airways examined, and bronchoscopy should be performed. If the tumor is still not found, CT scanning should be undertaken, since it can demonstrate tumors that are too small to be identifiable on plain chest radiographs. CT can regularly demonstrate peripheral tumors less than 0.5 cm in size, whereas it is very unusual to identify bronchial carcinoma on plain chest radiograph until the tumor is 1 cm or more in diameter. Even then, the tumor may be very difficult to see because its edge may be very ill-defined, and more often than not it will be partly obscured by overlying ribs.

In summary, the utility of routine surveys in the detection of lung carcinoma is still unclear. Survival from the time of diagnosis is likely to be prolonged, but whether a true reduction in mortality is achievable has yet to be proved.

BRONCHIAL CARCINOID, ADENOID CYSTIC CARCINOMA, AND MUCOEPIDERMOID CARCINOMA

These neoplasms, which used to be grouped under the name bronchial adenoma, show a spectrum of microscopic appearances and clinical behavior ranging from locally invasive to a malignant metastasizing tumor. Even an individual tumor may show widely different patterns in different portions of the lesion. Local lymph node spread is common, but blood-borne metastasis is rare.

These lesions form 1% to 2% of all pulmonary tumors. The patient age range is wide and includes children, the peak incidence occurring in the patients' 5th or 6th decades.[215] They are divided histologically into bronchial carcinoid (90%), adenoid cystic carcinoma (cylindroma) (8%), and mucoepidermoid adenoma/carcinoma (2%); adenoid cystic carcinoma is the most frequent variety in the trachea.[83] There is an atypical form of bronchial carcinoid with cellular and clinical features intermediate between those of typical carcinoid and small cell carcinoma of the lung.[81] Bronchial carcinoid, atypical bronchial carcinoid, and small cell bronchial carcinoma are believed to be of neuroendocrine origin and are thought to form a spectrum with varying degrees of malignancy. Typical bronchial carcinoids are vascular tumors and frequently present with hemoptysis. Most arise centrally in the main, lobar, or segmental bronchi and therefore cause cough, pneumonia, atelectasis, or occasionally wheezing. Atypical carcinoids of the lung usually arise peripherally in the lung, and both hemoptysis and pneumonitis are rare. Carcinoid syndrome is very rare with bronchial carcinoids.

The central tumor may be predominantly intraluminal, assuming a polypoid configuration, or predominantly extraluminal, in which case it is known as an "iceberg" lesion. The surface is usually smooth; only rarely is it ulcerated to any degree.

Both calcification and ossification within the neoplasm may be seen at pathologic study and identified radiologically (Fig 7–45, A–C).[21, 215]

The chest radiograph appears abnormal in most cases.[215] Tumors in the larger bronchi cause partial or complete obstruction and consequent atelectasis (Figs 7–45 and 7–46). Repetitive bouts of pneumonia are common, and bronchiectasis and lung abscess may occur beyond the obstruction.[301] Collateral air drift may keep segments aerated when the lesion is in a segmental bronchus; even whole lobes can be kept fully aerated despite complete occlusion of a lobar bronchus.[127] The consequent hypoxia of the affected lung leads occasionally to recognizable local vasoconstriction on plain film and perfusion scintigraphy.[255] The tumor itself is visible on plain film as a hilar mass (Fig 7–47) in about 25% of those instances with a central lesion,[6, 138] but it can be demonstrated on conventional (Figs 7–48 and 7–49) or computed tomography (Fig 7–50) in many other instances. The appearance differs from carcinoma in that the adjacent bronchial wall is smooth and there is no narrowing of the bronchus above the lesion; indeed, the bronchus may widen slightly as it approaches the mass (Fig 7–51). Bronchography shows these features very well but is unnecessary as bronchoscopy provides more specific information.[360]

Approximately 20% to 25% of bronchial carcinoids appear roentgenographically as a solitary pulmonary nodule. Multiple lesions are a frequent finding pathologically,[343] but almost invariably they are tiny and too small to be recognized radiologically. The nodules are well-defined and are round, oval, or lobulated, usually with a smooth edge, though spiculation is reported.[81] Two large series have been reported from the Mayo Clinic.[6, 149] In the earlier series of 23 peripheral bronchial adenomas, the average diameter of the nodule was 4 cm; however, the later report on 20 similarly located tumors showed none with a diameter greater than 4 cm.

Small tumors in segmental or subsegmental bronchi may result in mucous distention of the bronchi beyond the obstruction. The resulting bronchocele (mucoid impaction) may then be the dominant radiographic sign (Fig 7–52) on plain chest radiograph or CT, because the surrounding lung remains aerated by collateral air drift.[116, 306]

In approximately 10% of cases, the chest radiograph is normal, and the diagnosis is established only by bronchoscopy.[6, 138]

CT scanning provides superb anatomic localization of both the intraluminal and extraluminal components of the tumors in the major bronchi,[277] but usually does not permit distinction from carcinoma (see Fig 7–50) unless the lesion is demonstrably cal-

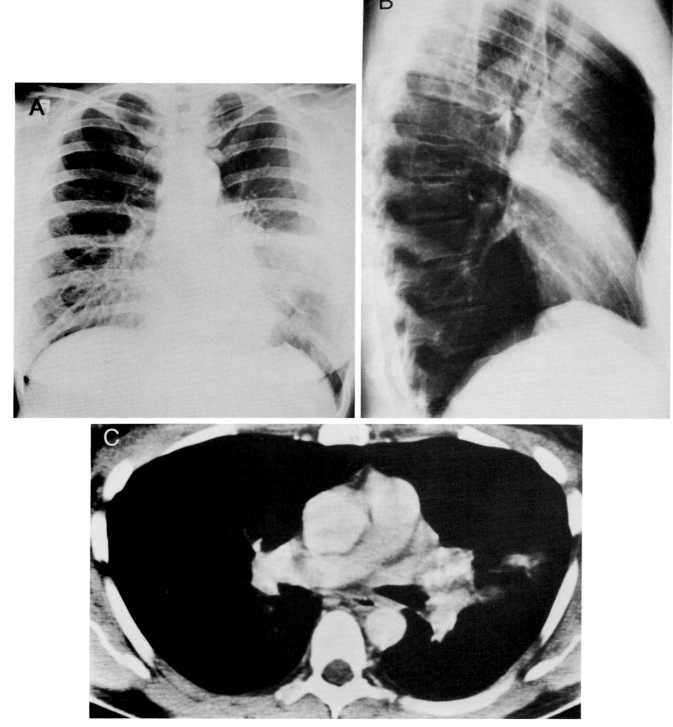

FIG 7–45.
Bronchial carcinoid in the lingular bronchus causing atelectasis of the lingular segments. In this instance, the tumor is partially calci-fied, but the calcification was only visible on the CT examination. **A,** PA radiograph. **B,** lateral radiograph. **C,** CT scan.

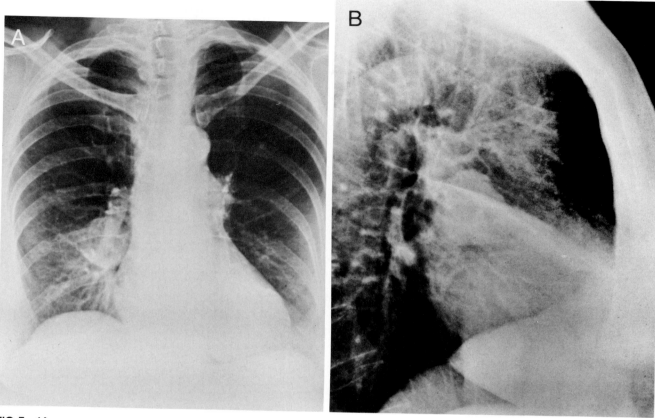

FIG 7—46.
Bronchial carcinoid causing right middle lobe collapse. The tumor itself is visible as a hilar mass. **A,** PA radiograph. **B,** lateral radiograph.

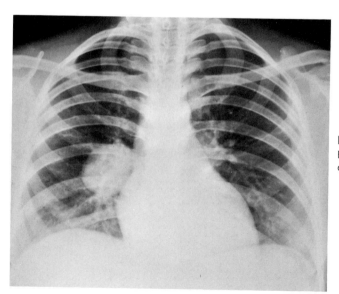

FIG 7—47.
Bronchial carcinoid presenting as a hilar mass without distal atelectasis. (Courtesy of Dr. Peter Hacking, Newcastle, England.)

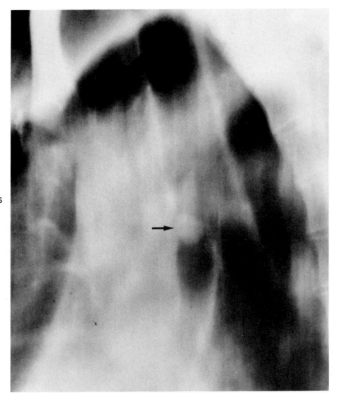

FIG 7–48.
Small endobronchial carcinoid in the right main stem bronchus *(arrow)* shown on tomography.

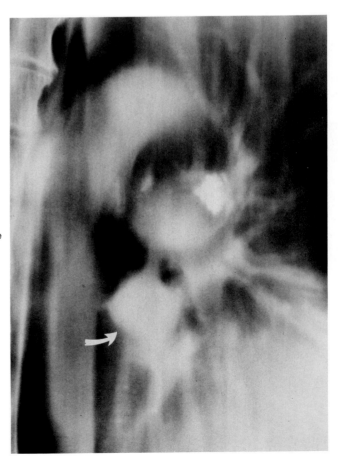

FIG 7–49.
Bronchial carcinoid of the right lower lobe bronchus with a large extrabronchial *(arrow)* and small endobronchial component.

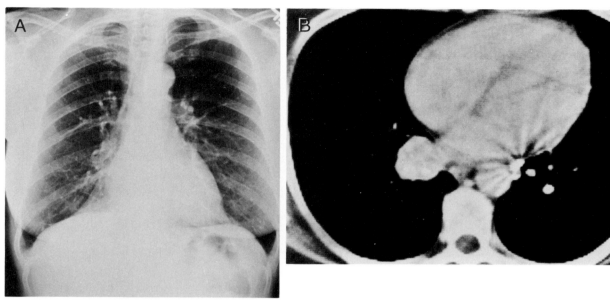

FIG 7–50.
A, bronchial carcinoid causing right lower lobe collapse. **B,** CT scan showing the central mass of tumor.

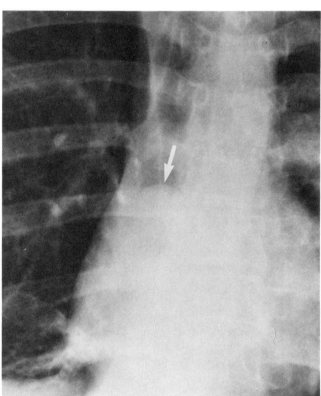

FIG 7–51.
Bronchial carcinoid in intermediate stem bronchus showing widening of the bronchus immediately above the tumor *(arrow).*

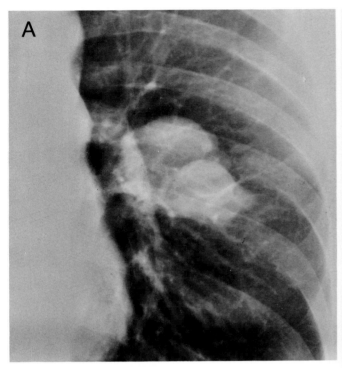

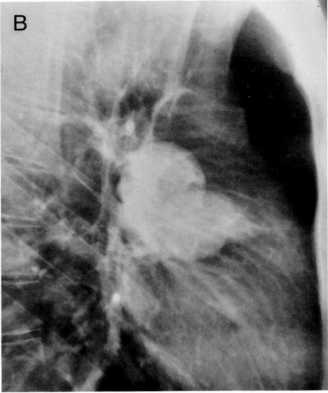

FIG 7-52.
Bronchial carcinoid causing mucoid impaction. The mucus-filled, dilated bronchi (bronchoceles) beyond the obstruction resemble a bilobed mass, but their tubular configuration can be recognized, particularly on the lateral view. **A,** PA view. **B,** lateral view.

cified (see Fig 7–45). In tumors of the trachea, however, although CT shows the extraluminal component of the tumor, it is poor at predicting whether or not mediastinal structures, such as the esophagus and aorta, are invaded. Obliteration of the fat planes between the tumor and these structures is sometimes due to invasion, but at other times, no invasion is found when the patient finally comes to surgery.[345] Marked contrast enhancement is seen in some cases of bronchial carcinoid,[11] a feature that must be very rare with bronchogenic carcinoma.

HAMARTOMAS

Hamartomas are defined pathologically as tumor-like malformations composed of an abnormal mixture of the normal constituents of the organ in which they are found. Most pulmonary hamartomas contain masses of cartilage with clefts lined by bronchial epithelium, and they may also contain fat[19] or cystic collections of fluid within the lesion. Some authors prefer the term hamartochondromas or chondromatous hamartoma to distinguish these lesions from the much rarer vascular hamartomas that do not contain cartilage.[20, 302] Although the precise nature of pulmonary hamartomas is debatable, they are usually classified as benign neoplasms. They grow slowly and are usually solitary, though there are a few case reports of multiple pulmonary hamartomas.[29] Malignant transformation is either nonexistent or extremely rare,[304] but in one series a higher than expected incidence of lung carcinoma was observed in the vicinity of a hamartoma.[195]

The average age of the patient at presentation is 45 to 50 years[302]; hamartomas are rarely seen in children. Over 90% are situated peripherally with 8% or less arising in central bronchi.[302] The peripheral lesions are asymptomatic; the endobronchial hamartomas present because of the consequences of bronchial obstruction or, occasionally, hemoptysis.

On plain chest radiograph and CT scans, the peripheral lesion is seen as a spherical, lobulated, or notched pulmonary nodule with a very well defined edge surrounded by normal lung (Fig 7–53). Pulmonary hamartomas can range in size up to 10 cm

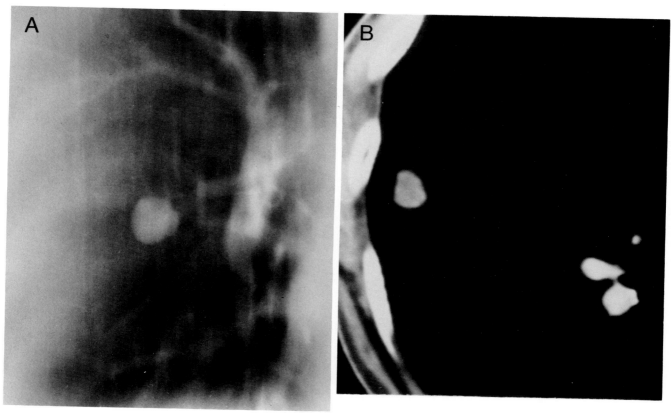

FIG 7–53.
Hamartoma of the lung presenting as a small, noncalcified, very well defined, slightly lobulated solitary pulmonary nodule. **A,** conventional tomogram. **B,** CT scan.

in diameter[95]; large lesions are unusual, however, and most are less than 4 cm.[302] The larger the lesion, the more likely it is to calcify. Most show homogeneous density. Definite calcification is seen on plain film in 10% to 15% of patients in most series.[302] In some series, however, the incidence of calcification is less than 4%.[36] The calcification may show the typical popcorn configuration of cartilage calcification, in which case the diagnosis is virtually certain (Figs 7–54 and 7–55). The presence of fat density within the mass is another important diagnostic feature (see Fig 7–55). Radiologically detectable air within the tumors is exceedingly uncommon,[104] but central lucency due to fat can be confused with cavitation. The signs at CT scanning are similar to those at plain radiography, but, because of the better contrast resolution, calcium and, particularly, fat are more easy to identify.[216, 338] In a series of 47 patients with pulmonary hamartomas it was possible to identify fat, or calcium plus fat, in the nodule in 28 patients using thin-section CT, a combination that appears to be specific for hamartoma,

at least in nodules under 2.5 cm in diameter.[338] In 17 of the cases the hamartomas showed neither calcification nor fat and, in the remaining two, there was diffuse calcification throughout the nodule.

Endobronchial hamartomas lead to airway obstruction, the radiologic features being identical to those seen with bronchial carcinoid.

RARE MALIGNANT PULMONARY NEOPLASMS

Primary pulmonary sarcomas are usually fibrosarcomas or leiomyosarcomas.[26, 65, 310] In a large review from the Armed Forces Institute of Pathology,[156] endobronchial leiomyosarcomas and fibrosarcomas exhibited, for the most part, a relatively benign behavior compared to that of intrapulmonary tumors, which showed great variability in their degree of malignancy, with a significant incidence of highly aggressive tumors. Chondrosarcomas, fibroleiomyosarcomas, rhabdomyosarcomas, myxosarcomas, and neurofibrosarcomas may also arise primarily in the

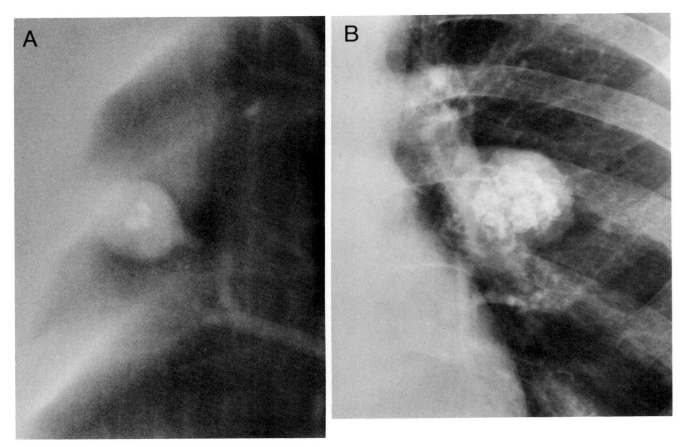

FIG 7–54.
Hamartoma. **A,** a smooth edge and central cartilage calcification are seen on conventional tomography. **B,** plain radiograph in another patient shows extensive popcorn calcification.

lung. Most sarcomas of the lung, however, are metastases from extrathoracic primaries.

Pulmonary blastoma and *carcinosarcoma* are very rare. The carcinosarcoma is composed of mixed malignant epithelial and connective tissue components, whereas the blastoma is a malignant tumor of a multipotential mesodermal cell, which histologically resembles embryonic bronchial structures in a background of abundant immature sarcoma.[343, 346] The peak age at presentation for pulmonary blastoma is in the patients' 3rd and 4th decades; 20% to 25% of reported cases have been in children.[285] Carcinosarcoma is often endobronchial in origin,[346] whereas pulmonary blastoma generally arises peripherally in the lung.[160, 174, 294]

Hemangiopericytoma, which may be benign or malignant, may also very occasionally arise primarily in the lung.[258]

Radiologically, all these lesions present as solitary pulmonary nodules or as an endobronchial mass indistinguishable from bronchial carcinoma (Fig 7–56).

Plasmacytoma of the lungs or major airways is an exceedingly rare tumor, even in patients with multiple myeloma. With solitary lesions, the sheets of plasma cells may be difficult to distinguish histologically from the benign plasma cell granuloma, and some of the cases in the literature may well have been wrongly categorized. The most common form of intrathoracic plasmacytoma is inward extension from a rib. Rarely, plasmacytoma may be seen radiographically as a mass arising within the trachea,[102] the bronchi,[252] or the lung, or as greatly enlarged intrathoracic lymph nodes.[137, 194, 201] A single case with extensive ossification of a solitary pulmonary plasmacytoma has been reported,[203] though this particular case may well have been a plasma cell granuloma, a condition in which calcification is not so rare.[194]

Kaposi sarcoma is a rare tumor of uncertain cell

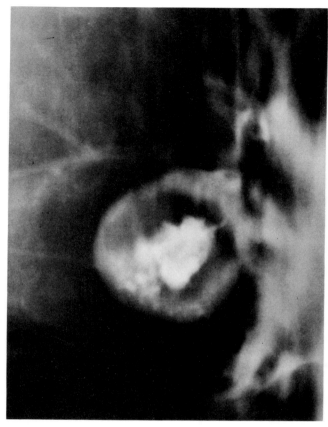

FIG 7—55.
Hamartoma. Conventional tomogram shows central cartilage calcification and surrounding fat density within the lesion.

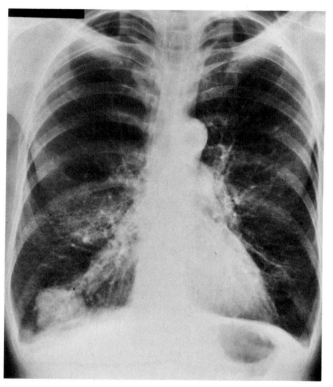

FIG 7—56.
Primary rhabdomyosarcoma of the lung. The right lower lobe mass was surgically resected on the preoperative assumption that it was a bronchial carcinoma.

origin. Until the recent epidemic of acquired immune deficiency syndrome (AIDS), Kaposi sarcoma was regarded primarily as a skin tumor of the lower extremities. The tumor is now being encountered with increased frequency in patients with AIDS. It usually affects multiple organs, and widespread lymph node involvement is particularly common. Involvement of the lung is fairly frequent.[96] Histologically,[342] the pulmonary interstitium shows an expansile invasive angiomatous proliferation of irregular slitlike vessels with atypical endothelial cells, a finding that correlates with linear shadowing on the chest radiographs. There are also nodular lesions composed of prominent fascicles of spindle cells with atypical mitotic figures and pleomorphism corresponding to nodular opacities on chest radiographs.

The radiographic appearance* can be categorized into disease that (1) is localized to one lobe or (2) is widespread (Fig 7—57). Widespread disease is much more common; only three of 22 patients in one review showed localized disease.[342] Two of these showed consolidation of an entire lobe and the other one showed segmental consolidation. When widespread, the shadows may be nodular or linear in configuration. The nodules are ill-defined and increase in size on follow-up. An alternative pattern is areas of ill-defined consolidation resembling pneumonia. Pleural effusion is seen in one-third to one-half the cases, and hilar/mediastinal lymphadenopathy is common and may be substantial.[342] The diagnosis is difficult to make because the amount of tumor in the lungs is often small and the nodular shadows that result are either obscured by adjacent infection or are so nonspecific in appearance that they are confused with one of the many pneumonias that these patients are so likely to suffer from. In one series of 24 patients with AIDS whose pulmonary Kaposi sarcomas were diagnosed at autopsy, only three showed nodular shadows that

*References 55, 96, 206, 253, and 342.

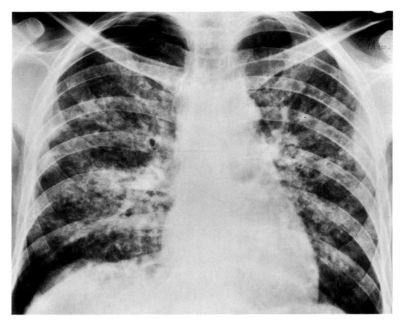

FIG 7–57.
Kaposi sarcoma in a patient with AIDS. There are multiple, small, ill-defined nodular shadows patchily distributed throughout both lungs.

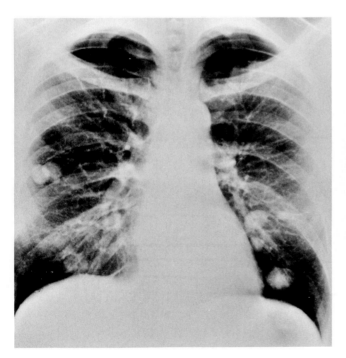

FIG 7–58.
Multiple pulmonary nodules as a result of amyloidosis. Several of the nodules contain a central core of calcification.

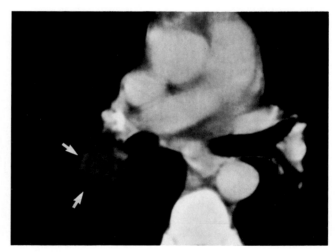

FIG 7–59.
Endobronchial lipoma *(arrows)*. The fat density of the mass is well shown by CT. (Courtesy of Dr. Ted A. Glass, Fredericksburg, Va.)

could have fairly definitively suggested the diagnosis during the patient's life.[96]

RARE BENIGN PULMONARY NEOPLASMS

Amyloidoma is one of the forms of amyloidosis in which one or more nodular masses are seen in the lung parenchyma or tracheobronchial tree (Fig 7–58). The lesions occur in the elderly and are frequently asymptomatic. The nodules are round or slightly lobulated, may contain visible calcification, and may cavitate.[379] (Other manifestations of intrathoracic amyloidosis are discussed in Chapter 12.)

Granular cell myoblastoma is a benign tumor that is most commonly found in subcutaneous tissues but may very rarely occur in the larger bronchi and even more rarely in the lung parenchyma or trachea.[242] Radiologically, it usually presents as postobstructive atelectasis/pneumonia beyond the lesion itself, occasionally as a small solitary pulmonary nodule, or as a polypoid lesion arising in a bronchus.[57, 361]

Fibroma, chondroma, lipoma, hemangioma, neurofibroma, and *neurilemmoma* may arise in the walls of the bronchi or in the lung parenchyma. Those arising in the lung parenchyma present as a nonspecific solitary pulmonary nodule; those that arise in the larger bronchi are indistinguishable from the more common bronchial carcinoid,[329] except that it may be possible to distinguish the fat in a lipoma by CT[260] (Fig 7–59). Hemangiomas frequently present with hemoptysis. A triad of pulmonary chondroma (often multiple), gastric epithelioid leiomyosarcoma, and functioning extra-adrenal paraganglioma has been described.[67] The importance of the condition, which is mostly seen in women under 35 years of age, is that if multiple slow-growing cartilage tumors are found in the lung, the other tumors in the triad should be searched for, since the other neoplasms are potentially lethal.

Leiomyoma of the lung may be a solitary lesion, radiographically indistinguishable from the other benign connective tissue neoplasms. *Multiple leiomyomas* are also encountered. These present as multiple nodular lesions in the lung. They are given a wide variety of names, including *benign metastasizing leiomyoma*.[249] Their behavior varies from that of a benign lesion to that of low-grade sarcoma. In women these tumors may be metastases from the uterus; the lesions are often hormone-sensitive and,

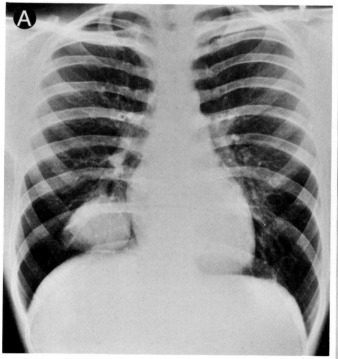 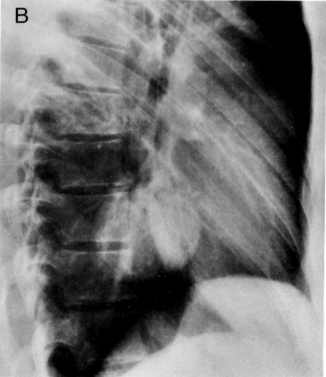

FIG 7–60.
Plasma cell granuloma in the right lower lobe. The mass shows no distinguishing features. **A,** PA view. **B,** lateral view.

if they are treated, the patient's prognosis appears good.[249]

Chemodectomas, benign clear cell tumors, and endometriosis are very occasionally encountered in the lung parenchyma, as are the extremely rare intrapulmonary *teratomas,* either benign or malignant. All these lesions present radiologically as nonspecific pulmonary nodules.

Plasma cell granuloma of the lung is the name given to what is presumed to be reactive granulomatous inflammation. Numerous other terms have been applied, notably inflammatory pseudotumor, sclerosing hemangioma, and histocytoma. Many of the patients are children or young adults. Macroscopically, the lesions are firm, sharply circumscribed, pale-colored masses. Histologically, there is a localized benign proliferation of plasma cells within a background of granulation or fibrocollagenous tissue.[173] The lesion may histologically resemble plasmacytoma. Most patients are asymptomatic, the lesion being discovered incidentally on plain chest radiographs as a solitary pulmonary nodule (Fig 7–60) or as a larger ill-defined area of consolidation. Cavitation and calcification have both been described,* and an air-meniscus sign may be seen (Fig 7–61).[14] The occasional one arises in a central bronchus[10] and is radiologically indistinguishable from bronchial carcinoid. CT scanning shows all these features to advantage but does not allow a specific diagnosis to be made.[333]

Squamous papillomas of the bronchi and lungs are most commonly associated with *laryngeal papillomatosis,* a disease that usually commences in childhood and is believed to be viral in origin.[208] The risk of malignant change is uncertain; clearly it is exceedingly low. Papillomatosis is almost invariably confined to the larynx, but in a small minority of patients, one or more papillomas are found in the trachea and bronchi, where they may cause atelectasis and bronchiectasis. Rarely, they are present in the lung and are seen on plain chest radiographs or CT scans as multiple small, widely scattered, well-defined round pulmonary nodules, frequently with cavitation[142, 208, 317] (Fig 7–62). The cavities, which may become several centimeters in diameter, are often thin-walled. Secondary infection may lead to air-fluid levels. Atelectasis is surprisingly infrequent. Squamous cell papilloma of the trachea without laryngeal papillomatosis has been described in adults.[154]

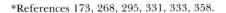

*References 173, 268, 295, 331, 333, 358.

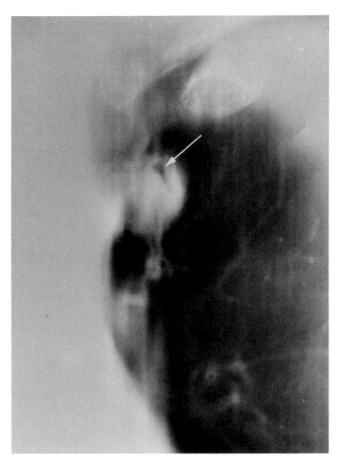

FIG 7–61.
Plasma cell granuloma showing an air-meniscus sign *(arrow).*

INTRATHORACIC MALIGNANT LYMPHOMA

The lymphomas are malignant neoplasms of lymphocytes and histiocytes together with precursors and derivatives of these two cell types, set in a background of non-neoplastic, presumably normal, inflammatory cells.[315] Hodgkin's disease is separated from the more common and more frequently fatal non-Hodgkin's lymphomas by the presence of a distinctive histologic feature, the Sternberg-Reed giant cell, a large reticulum cell with a tendency to form large, densely staining nuclei.

Hodgkin's disease is classified into four subtypes in the Rye classification[239]: nodular sclerosing, which comprises 40% to 75% of cases; and three further categories based on the relative proportion of Sternberg-Reed cells (and their mononuclear counterparts) to reactive elements. These latter are lymphocyte predominant (5% to 15% of cases), mixed cell (20% to 40% of cases), and lymphocyte depleted (5%

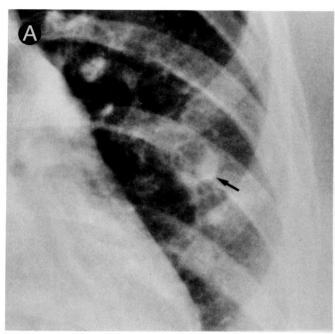

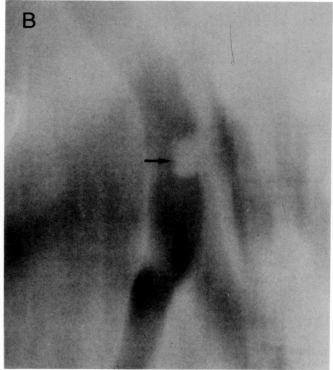

FIG 7–62.
Laryngeal papillomatosis. **A,** in a 7-year-old child who showed multiple small cavitary nodules. The *arrow* points to one of the thin-walled nodules. **B,** in another patient who shows just one polypoid lesion *(arrow)* in the trachea.

to 15% of cases).[47, 315] The disease may progress through the latter three types to become lymphocyte-depleted, the variety with the worst prognosis. The lymphocyte-predominant form tends to be localized and has a less aggressive clinical course.

Most patients present in their 2nd or 3rd decade with a secondary peak in the 5th or 6th decade. At initial presentation there is usually lymph node enlargement on either physical examination or the plain chest radiograph. The enlarged nodes are firm and nontender on palpation, the cervical nodes being the most frequently affected at initial presentation. Systemic symptoms such as fever, night sweats, anorexia, fatigue, weight loss, and pruritus usually appear late. The so called Pel-Ebstein pattern of fever, with recurrent episodes of diurnal waxing and waning of fever, is characteristic of the disease, but is only occasionally encountered. Bone pain following alcohol intake is another well-known pointer to the diagnosis. Anemia may be seen, but is usually absent at initial presentation. The blood may show leukocytosis or leukopenia. Eosinophilia is occasionally seen.

The disease is staged using the Ann Arbor classification (Table 7–5). Staging of intrathoracic disease utilizes the plain chest radiograph and chest CT (or possibly MRI in the future), with biopsy where indicated.

Hodgkin's disease spreads predictably from one lymph node group to the next contiguous group.[318] Knowing the pattern of spread is useful when considering imaging procedures for staging and when designing radiation therapy ports. The ports usually include both the areas of known disease and the adjacent node groups. Direct invasion from affected nodes into the lung or bone is another characteristic form of spread.[68]

The classification of the non-Hodgkin's lymphomas, unlike that of Hodgkin's disease, is in a constant state of flux.[64] The most recent classification, the Working Formulation for Clinical Usage, was devised by the National Cancer Institute[280] as a compromise between histologic classification and the need to classify according to prognosis. It divides the non-Hodgkin's lymphomas on morphologic grounds into three grades that correspond to prognosis: low, intermediate, and high. The dividing lines are not clear-cut, and conversion from one grade to a more malignant grade often occurs. It is still uncertain

TABLE 7—5
Ann Arbor Staging Classification for Hodgkin's Disease*

Stage	Definition†
I	Involvement of a single lymph node region (I) or of a single extralymphatic organ or site (I$_E$)
II	Involvement of two or more lymph node regions on the same side of the diaphragm (II) or localized involvement of an extralymphatic organ or site and of one or more lymph node regions on the same side of the diaphragm (II$_E$)
III	Involvement of lymph node regions of both sides of the diaphragm (III), which may also be accompanied by involvement of the spleen (III$_S$) or by localized involvement of an extralymphatic organ or site (III$_E$) or both (III$_{SE}$)
IV	Diffuse or disseminated involvement of one or more extralymphatic organs or tissues, with or without associated lymph node involvement

*Adapted from Carbone PP, Musshoff HS, Smithers EW, et al: Report of the committee on Hodgkin's disease staging. *Cancer Res* 1971; 31:1860–1861.
†The absence or presence of fever, night sweats, and/or unexplained loss of 10% or more of body weight in the 6 months preceding admission are to be denoted in all cases by the suffix letters A or B, respectively.

how successful the classification will prove to be.[48] Before the introduction of the Working Formulation, the Rappaport classification was the one most widely used. (The interrelationship between the Working Formulation and the Rappaport classification is shown in Table 7–6). The Rappaport classification,[311] which is based purely on histologic appearances at light microscopy, characterizes non-Hodgkin's lymphomas as nodular (follicular) or diffuse, depending on whether or not the lymphomatous tissue clusters into distinct nodules. They are then divided further into well- or poorly differentiated forms, and finally classified according to the dominant cell type: lymphocytic, histiocytic, or undifferentiated. The nodular varieties, which occur in approximately 40% of adults, are seen predominantly in older people and, in general, have a better prognosis. The nodular form may progress to the diffuse form. The prognosis also varies with the cell type and the degree of differentiation. The best outcome is seen with the well-differentiated lymphocytic form; the worst, with the undifferentiated varieties. The prognosis of histiocytic lymphoma lies between these two.

Well-differentiated lymphocytic lymphoma exists only in the diffuse form, giving rise to few symptoms despite being widely distributed in the body. A similar histology and protracted clinical course is seen with chronic lymphocytic leukemia and Waldenstrom's macroglobulinemia.

Immunological classifications based on surface marker immunophenotyping of T-cell, B-cell, or non–T-, non–B-cell origin may provide greater insights into the behavior of the lymphomas and may also provide a guide to which conditions should be included under the term lymphoma.[238] It is believed that true lymphomas arise as a proliferation from a single clone of cells. Polyclonal origins suggest one

TABLE 7—6
Classification of Non-Hodgkin's Lymphomas*

Working Formulation	Incidence† (%)	Rappaport Classification
Low-grade		
Small lymphocytic	3.6	Lymphocytic, well differentiated
Follicular, predominantly small cleaved cell	22.5	Nodular, poorly differentiated lymphocytic
Follicular, mixed small cleaved and large cleaved cells	7.7	Nodular, mixed lymphocytic histiocytic
Intermediate-grade		
Follicular, predominantly large cell	3.8	Nodular, histiocytic
Diffuse, small cleaved cell	6.9	Diffuse, poorly differentiated lymphocytic
Diffuse, mixed large and small cell	6.7	Diffuse, mixed lymphocytic and histiocytic
Diffuse, large cell	19.7	Diffuse histiocytic
High-grade		
Large cell, immunoblastic	7.9	Diffuse histiocytic
Lymphoblastic	4.2	Lymphoblastic lymphoma
Small noncleaved cell	5.0	Undifferentiated, Burkitt's and non-Burkitt's lymphoma

*Modified from Robbins SL, Cotran RS, Kumar V: *Pathologic Basis of Disease*, ed. 3. Philadelphia, WB Saunders, 1984.
†Relative incidences are from National Cancer Institute–sponsored study of classifications of non-Hodgkin lymphomas: Summary and description of a working formulation for clinical usage. *Cancer* 1982; 49:2112-2135. This study reviewed 1,041 patients with non-Hodgkin lymphomas. Used by permission.

of the nonlymphomatous reactive hyperplasias.[27] These conditions have features in common with the non-Hodgkin's lymphomas and may convert to a true lymphoma. Included in the list[144] are plasma cell granuloma, pseudolymphoma, lymphocytic interstitial pneumonia, and lymphomatoid granulomatosis. These entities, though they may involve lymph nodes, are essentially extranodal processes. They are discussed separately in later sections of this chapter.

The non-Hodgkin's lymphomas vary greatly in their initial presentation and aggressiveness. Low-grade non-Hodgkin's lymphomas often produce widespread adenopathy at initial diagnosis, and the patient frequently has no systemic symptoms. Provided their grades do not change, these lymphomas are relatively nonaggressive. Treatment may induce a temporary remission, but these tumors usually recur. The aim of treatment is palliation of symptoms rather than cure. One-fifth to one-half of patients with low-grade non-Hodgkin's lymphoma progress

to a more aggressive form, and one-quarter undergo spontaneous remission.[178]

Intermediate and high-grade non-Hodgkin's lymphomas both present with enlargement of lymph nodes, but frequently show extranodal disease. Most are treated for cure or at least long-term control, but unfortunately many will relapse within 2 years of initial treatment.

Radiologic Features of the Malignant Lymphomas

Lymph Node Enlargement.—The cardinal feature of the malignant lymphomas on chest radiographs and CT is mediastinal and hilar node enlargement, which may be accompanied by pulmonary or pleural involvement. Very rarely, Hodgkin's disease, particularly the nodular sclerosing type, may arise primarily in the thymus.[114] Lymph node calcification prior to therapy is very rare indeed, even at CT,[356, 384] but may be seen occasionally following

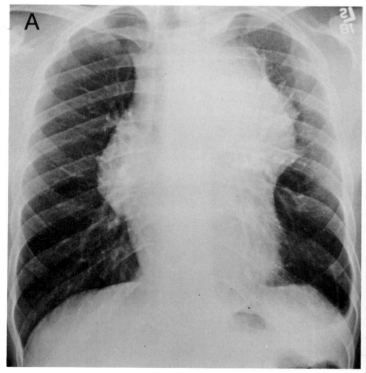

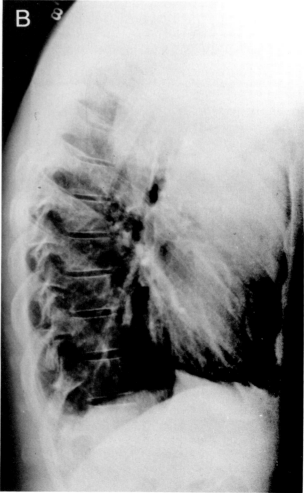

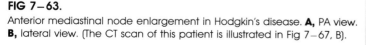

FIG 7–63.
Anterior mediastinal node enlargement in Hodgkin's disease. **A,** PA view. **B,** lateral view. (The CT scan of this patient is illustrated in Fig 7–67, B).

therapy. Irregular, eggshell and diffuse patterns of calcification may be seen.[356, 385] Except for their location and large size, these calcified nodes resemble the more commonly seen granulomatous nodes in the mediastinum. They are larger than granulomatous calcified nodes and are usually limited to the anterior mediastinum.[46]

The appearances on examinations of the chest are similar in both Hodgkin's disease and in the non-Hodgkin's lymphomas, but there are differences in the frequency and distribution of the abnormalities. Filly and co-workers reviewed the plain chest radiographs of patients with untreated malignant lymphomas.[122] Sixty-seven percent of the 164 patients with Hodgkin's disease had visible intrathoracic disease, and all but one of these had mediastinal or hilar adenopathy. The proportions are higher still with CT,[68] and as Bragg has pointed out in his review article, it is important for the radiologist to remember that virtually all patients with nodular sclerosing Hodgkin's disease will have disease in the mediastinum.[46] In the non-Hodgkin's lymphomas, the proportion of patients showing intrathoracic abnormality on plain chest radiograph was somewhat less (43%), as was the incidence of mediastinal/hilar adenopathy (87%).

The incidence of mediastinal adenopathy in younger patients with malignant lymphomas is lower. In patients under 10 years of age, approximately one-third of those with Hodgkin's disease and one-quarter of those with non-Hodgkin lymphoma will show mediastinal hilar node enlargement on plain chest radiographs.[69, 155, 292]

Any intrathoracic nodal group may be enlarged and the possible combinations are legion, but the following generalizations regarding plain film and CT/MRI findings may be useful[71, 122]:

1. The anterior mediastinal and paratracheal nodes are the most frequently involved groups (see Fig 7–63). The tracheobronchial and subcarinal nodes are also enlarged in many cases. In most cases, the lymphadenopathy is bilateral, but asymmetric. Hodgkin's disease has a propensity to involve the anterior mediastinal and paratracheal nodes. The incidence of nodular sclerosing Hodgkin's disease in the anterior mediastinum is particularly striking (Fig 7–63). In fact, evidence of intrathoracic disease without concomitant enlargement of these nodes at CT should prompt the radiologist either to question the diagnosis of Hodgkin's disease or to raise the possibility of a second disease process.[68]

2. The great majority of cases of Hodgkin's disease show enlargement of two or more nodal groups, whereas only one nodal group is involved in about half the cases of non-Hodgkin's lymphoma.

3. Hilar node enlargement is rare without accompanying mediastinal node enlargement, particularly in Hodgkin's disease.

4. The posterior mediastinum is infrequently involved. The enlarged nodes are often low down, and contiguous retroperitoneal disease is likely[155] (Fig 7–64).

5. The paracardiac nodes are rarely involved but become important as sites of recurrence because they may not be included in the radiation field[70, 191] (Fig 7–65, A). They may be visibly enlarged on plain

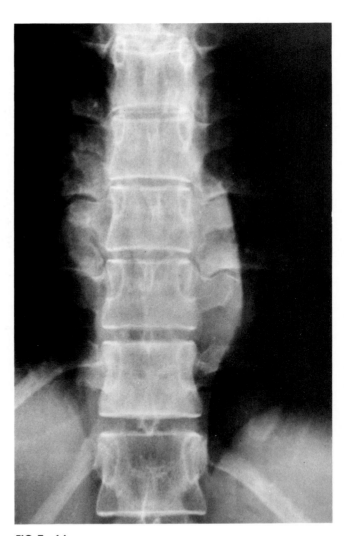

FIG 7–64.
Posterior mediastinal nodal enlargement in Hodgkin's disease. The left paraspinal line is displaced by the enlarged nodes. Note the sclerosis of the body of T-11 resulting from lymphomatous involvement of the bone.

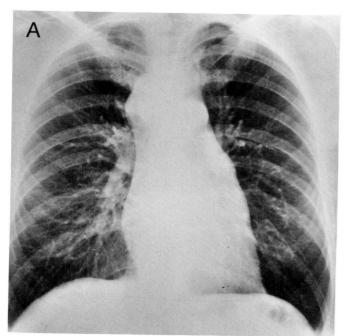

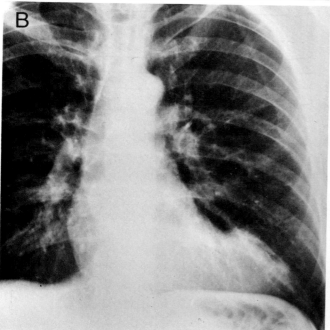

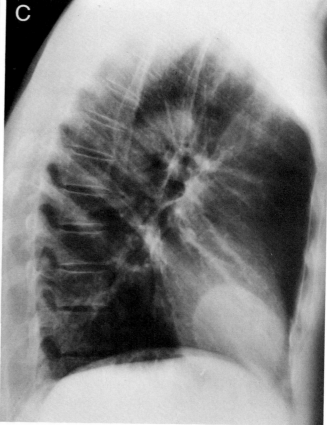

FIG 7–65.
Paracardiac node enlargement in Hodgkin's disease. **A,** plain film prior to radiation therapy. There is enlargement of paratracheal nodes bilaterally and of nodes along the left border of the heart. The nodes in the left cardiophrenic angle are not enlarged. **B** and **C,** four years later at time of recurrence, the PA and lateral films show massive enlargement of the left cardiophrenic angle nodes but no detectable enlargement of the mediastinal nodes in the original radiation field.

chest radiographs, but frequently CT is needed for their demonstration[80] (Fig 7–66, B).

6. Compression of the pulmonary arteries[122] and major bronchi[340] within the mediastinum by enlarged nodes may be seen, particularly with CT.

7. At CT scanning the enlarged nodes in any of the malignant lymphomas may be discrete or matted together, and their edges may be well-defined or ill-defined[37] (Fig 7–67,A). In general, they do not enhance following use of intravenous contrast material. Low-density areas (Fig 7–67,B) resulting from cystic degeneration may be seen in both Hodgkin's and non-Hodgkin's lymphoma. The cystic areas may persist following therapy, when the rest of the nodal masses shrink away.

8. MRI shows much the same features as CT, but does allow vascular compression to be demonstrated without the use of intravascular contrast media (Fig 7–68).

CT is considered useful for demonstrating mediastinal/hilar adenopathy in Hodgkin's disease because radiation therapy to enlarged nodes is either the only treatment or a major component of it.[71, 263, 322] Inadequate radiation therapy portals are believed to be a major cause of treatment failure; accurate demonstration of the extent of disease is, therefore, of great importance. Castellino et al.[71] compared CT scans of the chest with the findings on plain chest radiographs in 203 patients with Hodgkin's disease at initial presentation: 84% had intrathoracic disease, and of this 84%, all had mediastinal/hilar adenopathy. The authors also found that the incremental information obtained from chest CT scans prompted a change in treatment in almost 10% of these patients.[71] As expected, the impact was greatest in the 65 patients being treated with radiation therapy alone. In nine of these, the CT findings of more extensive mediastinal/hilar adenopathy or the presence of pericardial or chest wall involvement resulted in a change in management. Chest CT scanning is most useful in patients in whom the appearance of the mediastinum on plain chest radiograph is normal or equivocal.

In general, CT scanning of the chest is more useful in the initial staging of Hodgkin's disease than it is for non-Hodgkin's lymphoma.[68, 322] With disseminated non-Hodgkin's lymphoma, demonstrating the full extent of intrathoracic sites of disease with CT may not change management because the basic treatment is chemotherapy, not radiation therapy. If there is definite lymphadenopathy on plain chest radiograph but the disease is confined to the thorax, the main use of CT is to demonstrate pericardial disease, which would necessitate chemotherapy, and paracardiac node enlargement, which would alter the radiation portals. In patients with apparently localized extrathoracic disease and a normal plain

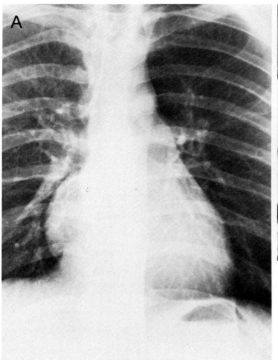

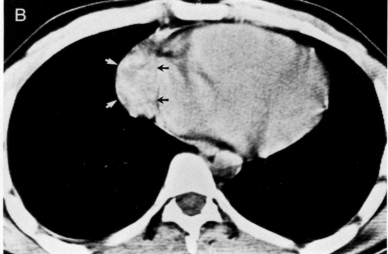

FIG 7–66.
Paracardiac node enlargement in immunoblastic lymphoma. **A,** the distortion of the right mediastinal border is difficult to distinguish from right atrial enlargement on plain film (the lateral projection was unremarkable). **B,** the CT scan demonstrates enlarged lymph nodes (*arrows*) to advantage.

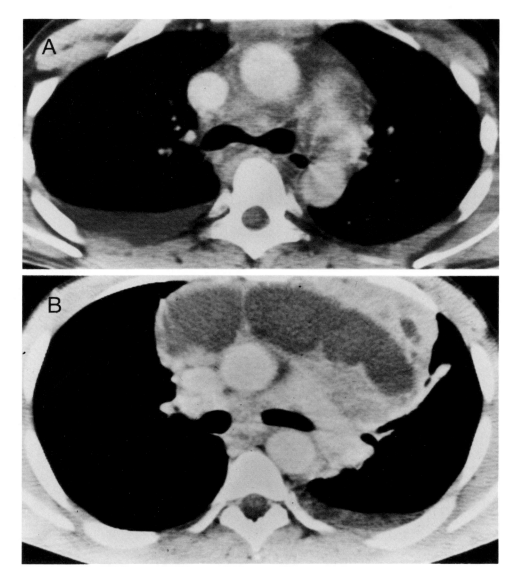

FIG 7–67.
CT scans of enlarged lymph nodes. **A,** in a patient with high-grade large-cell lymphoma. The nodes are matted together and appear as ill-defined conglomerate soft tissue densities. **B,** in a patient with Hodgkin's disease, showing multiple fluid density areas of presumed necrosis.

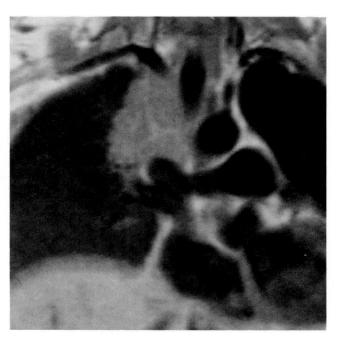

FIG 7–68.
Hodgkin's disease showing large lymph node masses that have compressed the right brachiocephalic vein and superior vena cava. The MRI study (T1-weighted coronal image) shows the venous compression without the need for contrast medium. (Courtesy of Dr. William C. Black, Washington, D.C.)

chest radiograph, CT scanning may reveal enlarged mediastinal/hilar nodes.[200] CT can also be used to exclude adenopathy in patients with a questionably abnormal mediastinal contour on plain chest radiograph.

It is important to realize that although successfully treated nodes may return to normal size, bulky disease, particularly that due to nodular sclerosing or to acellular forms of Hodgkin's disease, is often slow to resolve and may leave residual masses of sterilized fibrous tissue (Fig 7–69). This occurs, presumably, because these particular lymphomas consist chiefly of fibrous tissue to start with.[46]

Another post-treatment non-neoplastic radiographic abnormality that can cause confusion is cystic degeneration of the thymus. It is presumed that the thymus gland undergoes cystic degeneration after radiation therapy for anterior mediastinal Hodgkin's disease, and this condition should not be confused with recurrent Hodgkin's disease. Either CT or MRI can be used to confirm its presence.[46]

Parenchymal involvement of the lung in malignant lymphoma is comparatively rare, occurring in 10% to 15% of cases at initial presentation,[122] though as the disease takes hold it becomes more common.[240] In Filly's series of plain chest radiographs in untreated cases,[122] parenchymal involvement was seen three times more frequently in Hodgkin's disease than in non-Hodgkin's lymphoma. Parenchymal involvement in Hodgkin's disease is almost invariably accompanied by visible intrathoracic adenopathy,

whereas in the non-Hodgkin's lymphoma, isolated pulmonary involvement occurs with some frequency, more than 50% of the time according to Jenkins et al.[189] Well-differentiated lymphocytic lymphoma (low-grade small lymphocytic) is the most frequently encountered primary (i.e., isolated) lymphoma of the lung.[198] If the mediastinal and hilar nodes have been previously irradiated, then recurrence confined to the lungs may be seen in both Hodgkin's and non-Hodgkin's lymphoma (Fig 7–70).

The pulmonary opacities in both Hodgkin's disease* and non-Hodgkin's lymphoma[16, 56, 122, 336] are varied and resist easy classification. One pattern is focal or patchy consolidation (Figs 7–70 and 7–71), which resembles pneumonia and may even show air bronchograms. Another pattern is one or more discrete nodules resembling primary or metastatic carcinoma, but usually rather less well defined (Fig 7–72).[56, 122, 355] Such nodules may, on occasion, cavitate[122, 340] (Fig 7–73). Sometimes, there is focal, streaky shadowing, perhaps reflecting spread by way of the bronchopulmonary lymphatics. Widespread, reticulonodular shadowing (Fig 7–74) resembling diffuse interstitial lung disease is also seen, but is an uncommon pattern.

The pulmonary involvement is frequently perihilar or juxtamediastinal in location,[240] in keeping with the concept that extension into the lungs is by direct invasion from involved hilar/mediastinal

*References 122, 123, 240, 336, 340, 353, and 377.

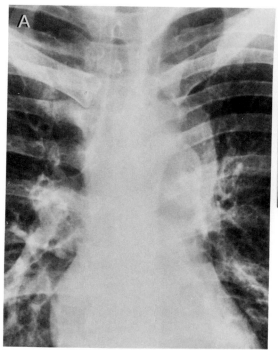

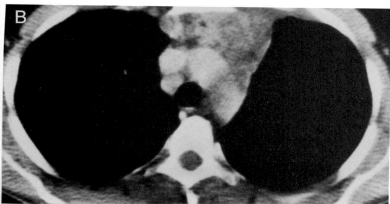

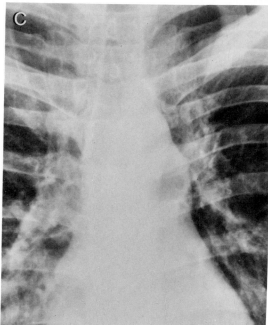

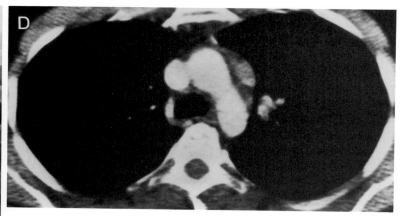

FIG 7–69.
Residual fibrous tissue following successful radiation treatment for Hodgkin's disease. **A** and **B,** enlarged nodes in the aortopulmonary window and left paratracheal area. **C** and **D,** residual mass of fibrous tissue in the aortopulmonary window. This residual mass remained unchanged over 3 years with no further treatment.

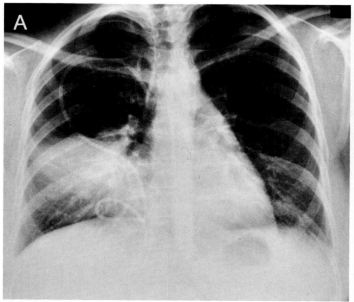

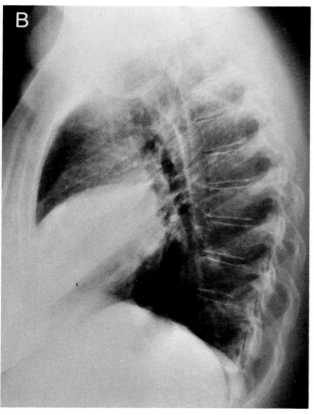

FIG 7–70.
Hodgkin's disease of the lung. The pulmonary involvement has taken the form of lobar consolidation. This young woman had previously had radiation therapy to enlarged mediastinal lymph nodes. **A,** PA radiograph. **B,** lateral radiograph.

FIG 7–71.
Histiocytic lymphoma of the lung in an elderly man. The multifocal ill-defined consolidations in the lung were originally thought to result from pneumonia because of accompanying fever and chills, but at autopsy they were shown to result from lymphoma.

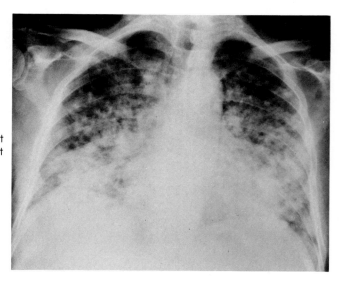

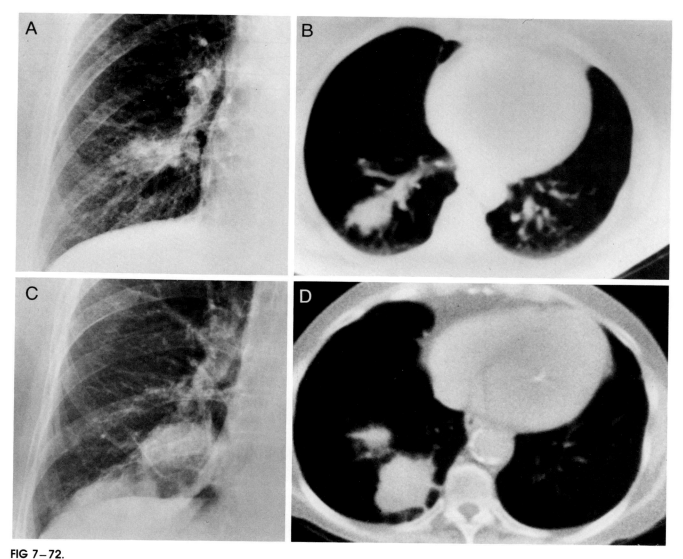

FIG 7–72.

Lymphoma presenting as a solitary pulmonary nodule. **A** and **B,** primary poorly differentiated lymphocytic lymphoma of the lung presenting as a solitary pulmonary nodule in a 53-year-old woman. The diagnosis was only made following surgical resection. There was no evidence of lymphoma elsewhere in the body. **C** and **D,** primary large cell lymphocytic lymphoma of the lung, again showing the nonspecificity of the appearance of the pulmonary mass.

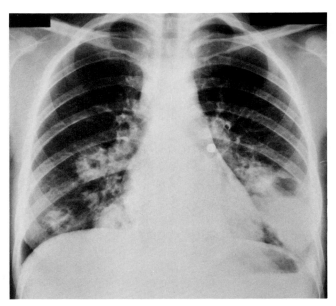

FIG 7-73.
Hodgkin's disease showing multiple cavitating pulmonary nodules (and right paratracheal nodal enlargement).

nodes (Fig 7–75). However, peripheral subpleural masses or consolidations without visible connection to the mediastinum and hilus (Fig 7–76) are not uncommon in both Hodgkin's disease and non-Hodgkin's lymphoma.[123, 336, 353] These lesions are particularly well demonstrated by CT.[336] Chest wall invasion and rib destruction are seen on occasion, suggesting that the lesions must either arise extrapleurally or cross the pleural cavity[336] (Fig 7–77).

Rapid growth of the pulmonary lesions may be seen with histiocytic lymphoma.[16, 72, 105] The development of large opacities or widespread disease in under 4 weeks and even in as little as 7 days may cause great diagnostic confusion with pneumonia.

Because Hodgkin's disease is believed to spread from nodal sites, it has been suggested that if an individual presents with Hodgkin's lymphoma and a lung nodule but no evidence of hilar or mediastinal disease, it can be assumed that the lung nodule represents something other than Hodgkin's lymphoma.[46] A caveat here is that the patient should not previously have received radiation therapy to the mediastinum.

Endobronchial disease is rare, particularly in non-Hodgkin's lymphoma,[202] but so is bronchial occlusion by neighboring lymph node enlargement. Therefore, when atelectasis is encountered, the pos-

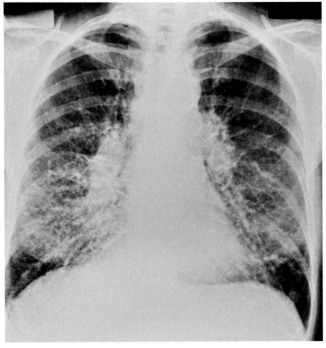

FIG 7-74.
Histiocytic lymphoma showing widespread reticulonodular shadowing in both lungs (and enlargement of hilar and right paratracheal nodes).

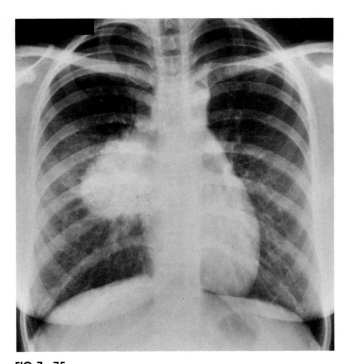

FIG 7-75.
Pulmonary invasion in nodular sclerosing Hodgkin's disease in a 15-year-old girl.

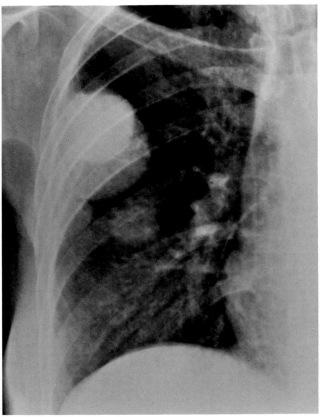

FIG 7—76.
Histiocytic lymphoma of the lung, showing subpleural deposits of
tumor.

sibility of endobronchial lymphoma should be seriously considered.

Pleural effusion is usually, but not quite always,
accompanied by mediastinal adenopathy visible on
plain chest radiographs[122] and sometimes also by
pulmonary involvement. With the more sensitive
technique of CT, mediastinal adenopathy appears to
be an invariable accompaniment of pleural effusion
in patients with Hodgkin's disease.[71] Pleural effusion
was seen in up to a quarter of patients in several
larger series,[71, 122, 189, 240, 377] being uncommon at
presentation. Most pleural effusions are unilateral.
They are usually exudates and may disappear with
irradiation of the mediastinal nodes.[66] Such effusions are presumed to result from venous or lymphatic obstruction by enlarged mediastinal nodes
rather than neoplastic involvement of the pleura.[71]

Pericardial effusions are presumptive evidence of
pericardial involvement. For practical purposes,
pericardial effusion requires ultrasound, CT, or
MRI for its recognition. In Castellino's series of 203
patients with Hodgkin's disease who had CT on ini-

tial presentation,[71] 6% had pericardial effusion, and
in all these patients there was coexistent large mediastinal adenopathy extending over the cardiac margins. A nodular mass within the pericardium was
seen in just one case.

MRI may provide useful information in the staging of the patient with intrathoracic lymphoma. It is
capable of imaging in anatomic planes that may be
more useful to the radiation oncologist than those
available with CT. Whether signal changes in patients undergoing treatment will prove either useful
or specific in monitoring tumor response must await
further trials.[46]

Mycosis Fungoides

Mycosis fungoides is a T-cell lymphoma that
originates in the skin and may disseminate to multiple sites, the lungs being the most frequently involved internal organ.[236, 247] Such dissemination was
previously thought to be a transition to another
form of lymphoma, e.g., histiocytic lymphoma, lym-
phosarcoma, or Hodgkin's disease, but it is now believed that the neoplastic cells in both the cutaneous
and the extracutaneous forms of the disease are distinctive to mycosis fungoides.[247] Abnormal cells
known as Sézary cells are frequently found in the
peripheral blood of patients with disseminated mycosis fungoides.

Radiologically,[247, 323] the lungs may show (1) one
or more pulmonary nodules resembling metastases,
(2) multiple areas of consolidation resembling pneumonia, a resemblance that may be very striking,
since in some cases the consolidations show rapid increase in size,[185, 323] and/or (3) bilateral reticulonodular shadowing, hilar/mediastinal adenopathy, or
pleural effusion.

Pseudolymphoma and Lymphocytic Interstitial Pneumonitis

Pseudolymphoma is a term coined by Saltzstein[326] in 1963 to describe a localized pulmonary lesion which, up until that time, had been classified as
a primary lymphoma, but with a better prognosis.
Lymphocytic interstitial pneumonitis (LIP) has microscopic features similar to those of pseudolymphoma, so much so that Spencer in his textbook of
pathology says, "It appears that pseudolymphoma
and LIP merge and are identical, pseudolymphoma
being the name applied when there is a localized tumor mass and LIP when it affects the lung diffusely."[343] Even though the two conditions are similar histologically, clinically they are different.[193] In

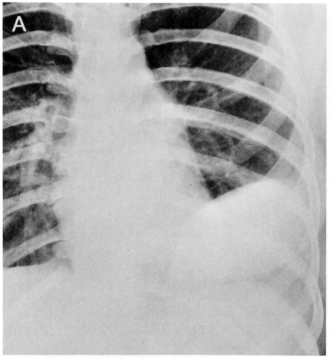

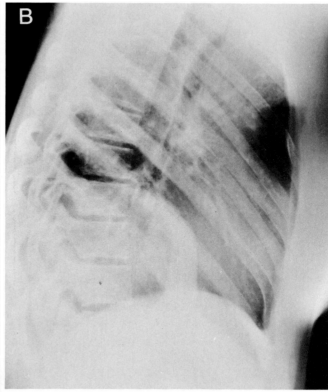

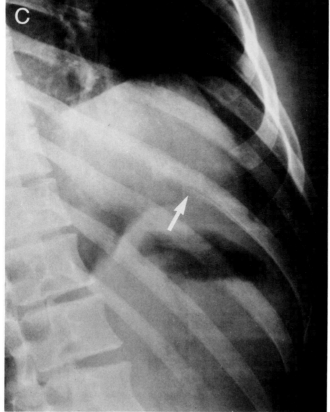

FIG 7–77.
Solitary histiocytic lymphoma. There is a large pleural/extrapleural mass of tumor tissue. The rib view shows bone destruction and periosteal reaction of the adjacent left ninth rib *(arrow* in **C**). **A,** PA view. **B,** lateral view. **C,** oblique view of the rib.

pseudolymphoma, the pulmonary nodule is usually an asymptomatic isolated finding, though it can be seen in patients with collagen vascular diseases and may be associated with dysgammaglobulinemia.[207] Patients with LIP are typically middle aged—though the range extends from childhood to 77 years[357]—and there is about a 2:1 female preponderance. The symptoms are primarily cough, chest pain, and fatigue, sometimes accompanied by low-grade fever and loss of weight. The physical signs are often unimpressive: with bilateral basal crackles in the chest, occasional finger clubbing, and evidence of peripheral lymphadenopathy and salivary gland enlargement in those patients who have associated Sjögren's disease.[357] The onset is often insidious,[35, 231] but the disease is frequently progressive and has a significant mortality. Like pseudolymphoma, LIP may be associated with Sjögren's syndrome.[193] Other associations are much less common and include myasthenia gravis,[267] systemic lupus erythematosis,[28] pernicious anemia,[98] autoerythrocyte sensitization syndrome,[98, 219] chronic active hepatitis,[172] Hashimoto thyroiditis,[193] diphenylhydantoin therapy,[73] and AIDS.[269] Dysproteinemia, usually a diffuse polyclonal gammopathy but sometimes a monoclonal gammopathy or hypogammaglobulinemia, is commonly present in LIP,[207, 219, 365] being found in three-quarters of cases in one series[357].

Histologically, in both conditions, there is an infiltrate consisting mainly of mature small lymphocytes in the interstitium of the lung.[196] This cellular infiltration may so expand the interstitium that the adjacent alveoli are compressed, thus explaining the presence of air bronchograms on radiologic studies. Active germinal centers are frequently, though not invariably, present. The number of plasma cells is variable. They may be the predominant cell, and then confusion with solitary pulmonary plasmacytoma may arise. The number of plasma cells in the infiltrate correlates roughly with the presence and degree of the gammopathy.[207] Some patients also have amyloid deposits.[41, 357] Pseudolymphoma and LIP are morphologically inseparable from small (well-differentiated) lymphocytic lymphoma, though the cells in small lymphocytic lymphoma do show a higher incidence of plasmacytoid features and a greater degree of mast cell infiltration.[198]

Immunologic surface markers may help to separate small lymphocytic lymphoma from pseudolymphoma and LIP. Pseudolymphoma and lymphocytic interstitial pneumonitis are believed to be reactive hyperplasia, showing the polyclonality of surface markers to be expected of reactive hyperplasia,

whereas monoclonality is found in the neoplastic condition of small lymphocytic lymphoma.[198] Indeed, Kradin and Mark[207] have suggested that pseudolymphoma be renamed "nodular lymphoid hyperplasia" and that LIP be renamed "diffuse lymphoid hyperplasia," as they believe that the term pseudolymphoma is vague and confusing.

Pseudolymphoma and LIP have been considered premalignant conditions, because in some reported cases, they have behaved ultimately as malignant lymphomas.[343] According to the extensive review by Kradin and Mark,[207] the reported incidence of conversion to malignant lymphoma ranges from a small percentage to more than 50%. Since the diagnoses in these reported cases did not involve the use of immunocytologic techniques, doubt has been cast on the accuracy of the initial diagnosis. Therefore, the comments of Blank and Castellino[38] remain as valid as ever: "Does pseudolymphoma transform into lymphoma, or is it simply that the pathologist's interpretation transforms after viewing biopsy specimens obtained at different times, or from different areas of the same lesion?"

Radiologically,[115, 183, 193] pseudolymphoma of the lung presents as a round or segmental-shaped opacity, which can be solitary or multifocal (Fig 7-78). There is no lobar predilection, and the lesion may be placed centrally or peripherally in the lung parenchyma. Visible air bronchograms are frequent and may be a striking feature. A few of the lesions show cavitation, but calcification does not occur. Pseudolymphomas are rarely associated with pleural effusions despite contact with the pleura.[198]

The typical radiologic appearance of LIP* is that of bilateral reticulonodular opacities, the linear component of which may be quite coarse; septal lines may also be seen (Fig 7-79, A and B). The nodular component may be fine or may show the features of acinar nodules. This latter pattern shades into multifocal, patchy consolidations that may be flame-shaped and contain air bronchograms. These consolidations may be transient. Mixed alveolar and interstitial patterns are common. The shadowing, while usually predominant in the lower zone, may be more uniform in distribution and may even show upper zone predominance. The disease may progress into an end-stage lung with honeycomb shadowing. As with other predominantly interstitial processes, pathologic changes may be present when the chest radiograph is still normal in appearance.[158] Lymph node

---

*References 73, 115, 144, 153, 158, 169, 193, 231, 241, and 357.

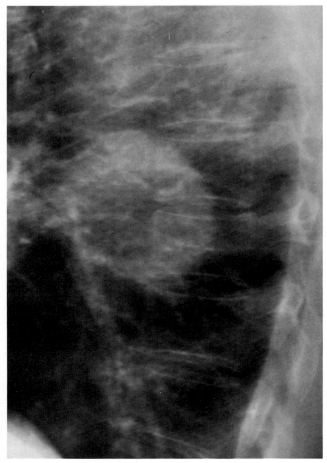

FIG 7–78.
Pseudolymphoma. Lateral close-up view of one of three similar nodules in an asymptomatic 68-year-old man. (The lesion was behind the heart in the frontal view.)

enlargement is not seen[115] and, if present, should suggest the development of lymphoma.[153] Pleural effusions occur in about 15% of patients.[115, 231]

Waldenstrom's Macroglobulinemia

Waldenstrom's macroglobulinemia is a malignant proliferation of cells with lymphoplasmacytic morphology which secrete an atypical IgM immunoglobulin indistinguishable, except by immunoelectrophoresis, from the monoclonal IgM peak found in the serum in multiple myeloma. The reticuloendothelial system is diffusely infiltrated by the atypical lymphoid cells, leading to anemia, hemorrhagic phenomena, hepatosplenomegaly, and palpable lymphadenopathy. The disease, therefore, may resemble multiple myeloma and chronic lymphocytic leukemia clinically. Other features include osteopenia

of the bones as well as thickening of the folds of the small bowel. The patient's symptoms commonly reflect the anemia and the high serum viscosity, which can cause headache, dizziness, drowsiness, and even coma. Bulges and constrictions of the veins of the optic fundus are a characteristic finding on physical examination.

Histologically,[380] the lung, the pleura, and the intrathoracic lymph nodes show a patchy cellular infiltrate consisting of sheets of lymphocytes and plasmacytoid forms. Histologically, the condition may need to be differentiated from LIP. In Waldenstrom's macroglobulinemia the cellular infiltration of the lung is accompanied by destruction of lung architecture, whereas in LIP the lung architecture is preserved.

Lung involvement is unusual; it was seen in 4 of the 20 patients in one series.[380] When seen, it may be accompanied by dyspnea and cough, or it may be asymptomatic. The major chest radiographic finding[130, 380] is diffuse reticulonodular shadowing (Fig 7–80), which may be asymmetric; less commonly, there is focal homogeneous consolidation that can be round in shape[246] and resemble a neoplasm, even to the extent of compressing a major airway and causing atelectasis. The masslike consolidations can be single or multiple. Pleural effusion is seen in about half the cases. The pleural fluid may contain the same monoclonal IgM immunoglobulin peak that is found in the serum.

Lymphomatoid Granulomatosis

Lymphomatoid granulomatosis is a complex entity that has proved difficult to classify. It was defined by Liebow et al. in 1972 as "an angiocentric, angiodestructive, lymphoreticular, proliferative and granulomatous disease involving predominantly the lungs."[232] The infiltrate, which is intensely cellular, is composed of small lymphocytes, plasma cells, histiocytes, and atypical lymphoreticular cells.[197] Necrosis and fibrosis may be present.

In 1973, Liebow grouped five entities including lymphomatoid granulomatosis under the heading "pulmonary angiitis and granulomatosis."[230] These conditions* all showed necrosis of tissue accompanied by a granulomatous reaction and a vasculitis. The grouping was based on morphologic similarities, and it was felt that the five conditions might be

---

*The five conditions were: classic Wegener's granulomatosis, limited angiitis and granulomatosis of the Wegener type, lymphomatoid granulomatosis, necrotizing "sarcoid" angiitis and granulomatosis, and bronchocentric granulomatosis.

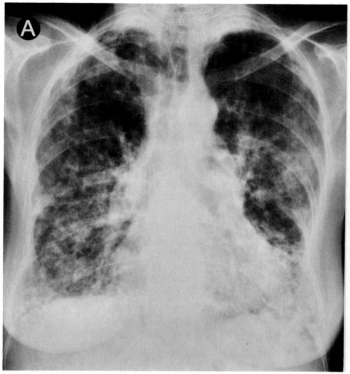

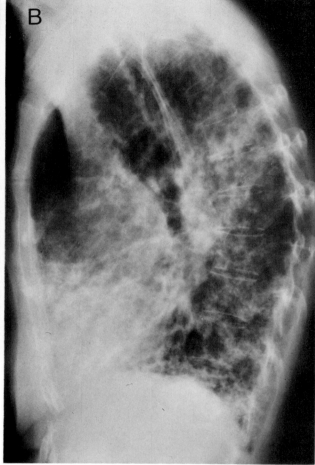

FIG 7–79.
Lymphocytic interstitial pneumonitis showing widespread coarse reticulonodular shadowing in the lungs. **A,** PA view. **B,** lateral view.

variants of one another, although Liebow and co-workers seriously considered that lymphomatoid granulomatosis may be some form of lymphoma.[232] Subsequently, lymphomatoid granulomatosis was usually considered to be a vasculitis with an exuberant lymphoid reaction related to, and treated similarly to, Wegener's granulomatosis. More recent reviews, however, have emphasized that lymphomatoid granulomatosis should be regarded as a heterogeneous group of pulmonary lymphomas.[27, 82, 88, 144, 198, 207] The reasons given are the similarity of the cellular elements to lymphoma, the tendency to follow lymphatic routes (a feature of lymphoma), and a high incidence of progression to true malignant lymphomas.

Vasculitis is now regarded as a feature that may be seen in lymphoma.[89] The high rate of progression to malignant lymphoma has been repeatedly observed, occurring in up to 50% of patients.[113, 144, 197, 232]

Diagnosing lymphomatoid granulomatosis is difficult because of the variability in the histologic findings from area to area and at different times in the patient's course. It is therefore clear that in many series, patients labeled as having lymphomatoid granulomatosis, Wegener's granulomatosis, and lymphoma will have been wrongly assigned.[375]

Men predominate in a ratio of 2 to 1, and most patients are in early middle age (range, 7 to 85 years).[232] Most complain of some combination of cough, often productive; fever; and dyspnea. Massive hemoptysis from cavitating pulmonary lesions was the cause of death in three of Liebow's 40 patients.[232] Cutaneous involvement occurs in nearly half of the subjects. Central nervous system involvement occurs at least 20% of the time, with peripheral neuritis occurring with almost equal frequency.[232] The kidneys show focal nodular collections of lymphomatoid granulomatosis at autopsy, not the generalized glomerulonephritis seen with Wegener's granulomatosis; thus, renal failure is not a feature of the disease. This latter feature, together with the rarity of upper airway involvement and the common

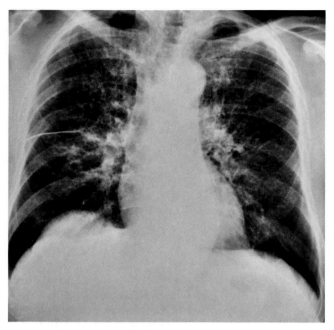

FIG 7–80.
Waldenstrom's macroglobulinemia, showing widespread coarse reticulonodular shadowing in the lung.

presence of skin and nervous system lesions, helps to distinguish lymphomatoid granulomatosis from Wegener's granulomatosis. Surprisingly, the disease usually spares lymph nodes, spleen, and bone marrow.

Radiographically,[100, 144, 175, 232] the most frequent appearance, occurring in some 80% of patients, is multiple pulmonary nodules, which are usually bilateral but may be unilateral; occasionally, only a solitary pulmonary mass is seen (Fig 7–81, A). The nodules, which closely resemble metastases, are usually round in shape and have ill-defined margins, though a small proportion have a well-defined edge. They may be very large, and nodules of up to 10 cm in diameter have been reported. Multiple, ill-defined areas of consolidation resembling pneumonia are a less common radiographic manifestation. Coalescence of the nodules or consolidations is a feature that may help in the radiographic differential diagnosis from pulmonary metastases. The lesions show a predisposition for the mid and lower lung zones, with a tendency to spare the apices. At least some of the nodules seen on plain chest radiograph are a result of infarcts related to the angiodestructive nature of the disease.[100, 186] Dee et al.[100] showed on histologic examination in three cases that the bulk of the lesion was an infarct, the cellular infiltrate of lymphomatoid granulomatosis being confined to the periphery and contributing little to the radiographic shadow. Cavitation was seen in approximately 10% of patients in one review of the literature.[175] In individual series, the rate of cavitation is as high as 25%.[232, 375] The cavities are usually thick-walled, but a thin-walled cystlike cavity was reported by Wechsler et al.[375] Cavitation appears to be associated with a poor prognosis.[232] Air bronchograms are seen in some cases, the highest reported incidence of air bronchograms being 40%.[232] Widely distributed reticulonodular shadowing has been reported in a few cases.[100, 375] When examined at biopsy, these lesions proved to result from cellular infiltration without infarction.[100]

Visible hilar and mediastinal adenopathy are very unusual. Pleural effusion does not appear to be a major feature of the disease, though small pleural effusions are seen on plain chest radiograph in up to one-third of patients. The plain chest radiograph may be normal in patients diagnosed as having lymphomatoid granulomatosis of the sinuses or skin.

LEUKEMIA

Several abnormalities may be seen at chest imaging in leukemic patients. These can be divided into three categories.

1. Leukemic infiltration of the lung, defined as extravascular leukemic cells in regions of the lung parenchyma not involved by infection, infarction or hemorrhage. Leukostasis is a separate category that may or may not be accompanied by leukemic infiltration of the lung parenchyma.

2. Intrathoracic lymph node enlargement due to leukemia.

3. Non-neoplastic complications of leukemia or its treatment, notably pulmonary infection, pulmonary hemorrhage (Fig 7–82), pulmonary edema, and drug reactions. The differential diagnosis of non-neoplastic pulmonary shadowing in leukemic patients is discussed on page 238.

The incidence of leukemic infiltration of the lungs, mediastinal lymph nodes, and pleura varies with the course of the disease. Clearly the highest incidence will be shown in autopsy series. Several large series of autopsies in patients who died from leukemia have been published.[40, 205, 244, 320] In most of these series, regardless of whether the patients were reviewed during or before the era when chemotherapy for leukemia was well-developed, the incidence

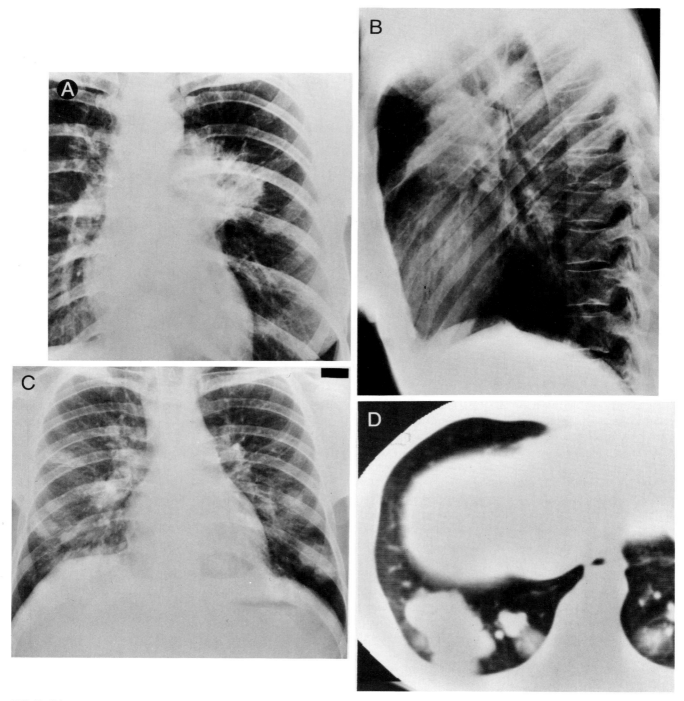

FIG 7–81.

Lymphomatoid granulomatosis. **A,** and **B,** an example showing a large irregular, lobular mass adjacent to the left hilus. **C,** an example showing multiple well-defined pulmonary nodules resembling pulmonary metastases. **D,** CT scan in another patient showing multiple lobular pulmonary masses.

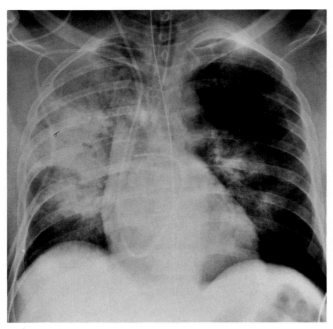

FIG 7–82.
Acute pulmonary hemorrhage in a 39-year-old man with acute myloid leukemia; the bilateral air-space shadowing is from intrapulmonary bleeding.

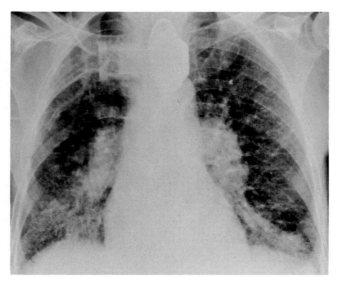

FIG 7–83.
Leukemic infiltrates in the lungs. Note also the bilateral hilar adenopathy resulting from leukemic involvement of the lymph nodes.

of leukemic infiltration of the lungs on microscopic examination was high (31% to 64%), but only rarely was this infiltration radiographically visible. The most recently published series is typical.[244] Forty-one percent of the patients showed leukemic infiltrates of the lung histologically (ranging from 67% of patients with chronic lymphatic leukemia to 35% of patients with acute myloid leukemia); however, the leukemic infiltration was almost never visible radiographically. Ninety percent of the patients in the study had pulmonary shadows on the chest radiographs immediately prior to death. In all except two, the shadowing was the result of a complication of the disease, not the leukemic infiltration per se. One study of chest radiographs in 33 leukemic patients who died showed a higher incidence of radiographically visible leukemic infiltrates; chest radiographs in seven of the patients (21%) showed widespread ill-defined peribronchial shadowing (Fig 7–83) that was demonstrated at autopsy to result from leukemic infiltration of the lungs. Multiple small nodular opacities due to focal collections of leukemic cells have also been occasionally encountered.[244] In summary, provided those patients with leukostasis are considered separately, leukemic infiltration of the lungs, though very common pathologically, does not appear to be a cause of pulmonary symptoms and is

rarely a cause of significant pulmonary opacities on chest radiographs. Indeed, the chest film is frequently normal in appearance. When respiratory impairment is present, the leukemic infiltrates are accompanied by pulmonary infection, edema, or hemorrhage, and these are the likely cause of the patient's symptoms.[320]

Leukostasis is a condition seen in patients with acute myeloid leukemia who have very high white blood cell counts, on the order of 100,000 to 300,000 cells/mm^3, together with accumulations of leukemic cells in small blood vessels, especially of the lungs, heart, brain, and testes. Central nervous system symptoms are frequent, and the patients may be dyspneic because of obliteration of small pulmonary blood vessels by the leukemic cells.[366] The chest radiograph may be normal or may show air-space shadowing (Fig 7–84). In a report on radiographic findings in a series of 10 patients who died with leukostasis, four had a normal appearing chest film, four showed widespread air-space disease attributed to superimposed pulmonary edema, and one showed a small area of pulmonary consolidation.[364] The radiographic shadowing in leukostasis appears to be due to pulmonary edema rather than directly due to the accumulation of leukemic cells in the lungs.[276, 364, 366]

Radiographically visible hilar and/or mediastinal lymph node enlargement is seen in up to 17% of adult patients who come to autopsy.[205, 244] The distribution of nodal enlargement closely resembles the

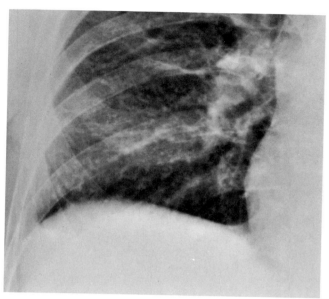

FIG 7–84.
Leukostasis in a 43-year-old man in blast crisis, showing hazy opacity in the lungs. The shadows cleared with leukophoresis therapy.

lymphomas. The incidence of leukemic infiltration of the nodes on pathologic examination is very high, 50% in the large series of Klatte et al.;[205] however, most involved nodes show little or no enlargement and are therefore not diagnosable by radiographic means.

T-cell leukemias may show massive mediastinal adenopathy that responds rapidly to chemotherapy or radiation treatment. Huge mediastinal masses of T-cell leukemia may disappear within a few days with appropriate treatment (Fig 7–85, A and B).

Pleural effusion is common in leukemia. Subpleural deposits of leukemic cells are often found at autopsy, but pulmonary infection, infarction, hemorrhage, and edema so frequently coexist with these leukemic deposits that it is not usually possible to state the cause of the effusion with any confidence.

MESOTHELIOMA

Localized Pleural Mesothelioma

Localized mesothelioma has a variety of synonyms including pleural fibroma and fibrous mesothelioma. Most patients are between 45 and 65 years.[109] In a recent literature review of 360 cases, the mean age at presentation was 51 years (range, 5 to 87 years), with no significant sex difference.[53] Unlike diffuse mesothelioma, the localized tumor is not asbestos-related.[53] Histologically, the lesion consists of spindle-shaped cells separated by collagen.[109] It exists in benign and malignant forms in a ratio of about 7:1.[53] Some workers consider that the distinction between benign and malignant forms can be made on histologic grounds,[287] but others

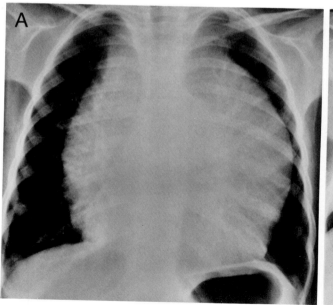

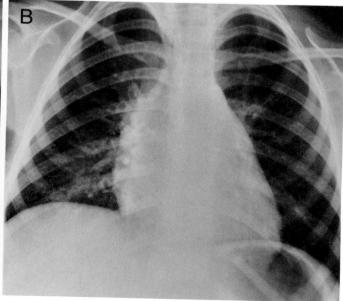

FIG 7–85.
T-cell leukemia/lymphoma, in a 4-year-old girl **A,** massive mediastinal adenopathy. **B,** following a very rapid response to chemotherapy. The films were obtained 9 days apart.

think this distinction is not possible and consider that pedunculation is the best evidence of benignity.[53]

Macroscopically the tumor is seen as a mass in contact with the pleura, but a small number appear to be totally encased within lung.[287] Three-quarters arise from visceral pleura and one-quarter from parietal pleura.[53] An origin from within a fissure is fairly common.[182, 344] Pedunculation is present in about 50%.[34] The stalk can be up to 9 cm in length.[157]

About half the patients with localized mesothelioma are asymptomatic, the tumor being detected incidentally at chest radiography.[53] The commonest symptoms, each present in about 50% of symptomatic patients, are cough, chest pain, and dyspnea. Although hypertrophic osteoarthropathy was common in earlier series, its prevalence in series reported since 1972 has been about 12%[53]; it appears to be more common in tumors over 7.0 cm in diameter. Other reported symptoms include chills and fevers, weight loss and debility, and a sensation of something rolling around in the chest.[343] Symptomatic hypoglycemia is seen in about 4% of patients.[53]

Radiologically, the usual finding is a rounded or oval, often lobulated, homogeneous mass in contact with a pleural surface.[109, 168] The lesions vary in size from less than 1 cm up to 30 cm diameter (Figs 7–86; 7–87). Occurrence is slightly more common in the lower half of the chest.[109] When lesions are very large, their origin from the pleura may not be obvious.[109] The wall usually shows an obtuse angle at the margin, a finding that was present in 94% of 17 cases in one series.[182] Lesions with acute angles are, however, reported.[99, 109] As previously mentioned, some 50% of localized mesotheliomas have pedicles which confer mobility on the tumors, so that they may change in shape and position on images taken on different occasions and with the patient in different postures.* (Similar changes in shape, particularly with different phases of respiration, may also be seen with chest wall lipomas.[151]) If the lesion is not pedunculated, inspiration/expiration imaging will show whether the mass is in the lung or is attached to the chest wall.[109] The malignant forms of localized mesothelioma may spread into soft tissue and destroy bone.[287] On CT, the lesions are usually homogeneous and sharply marginated, though the occasional one is inhomogeneous as a result of necrosis.[99] Calcification is uncommon but recorded.[109, 182] Pleural effusions are occasionally present[99, 109, 157]

*References 34, 109, 163, 222, and 376.

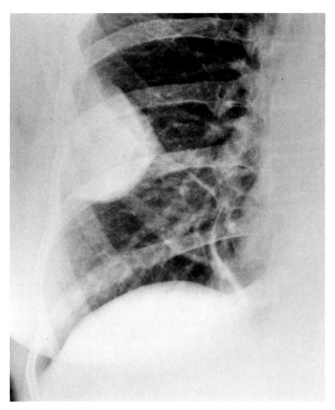

FIG 7–86.
Localized mesothelioma of the pleura in a 61-year-old woman. At surgery, this lesion lay in the minor fissure and was benign.

and are sometimes large enough to obscure the underlying mass.[39, 287]

Benign mesothelial tumors behave in a very indolent fashion, and some have been known to be present for 20 years before removal.[327] The malignant form of localized mesothelioma may recur after removal,[109] and in one series 86% of those with malignant histology were dead within 2 years of surgery.

Diffuse Mesothelioma

Diffuse (malignant) mesothelioma is a rare tumor. However, the incidence, approximately one to two cases per million population per year,[50, 254] is expected to increase because of the increasing exposure of the population to asbestos. The etiologic role of asbestos was first suggested by Wagner et al. in a group of 33 patients with malignant mesothelioma, 32 of whom had had possible contact with asbestos.[369] Some patients were asbestos miners, but most just lived and worked in the mining community without entering the mines themselves. Asbestos

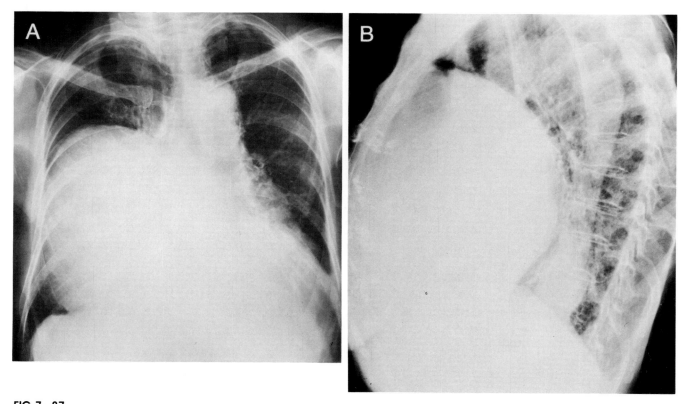

FIG 7–87.

A and **B,** huge localized mesothelioma of the pleura in an elderly woman. Despite the size of the tumor, the patient had no chest symptoms. The tumor was benign on histologic examination.

contact is now documented in about half of all patients,[8] but the incidence of exposure ranges in various series from under 25%[50, 284] to almost 90%.[9] The contribution of asbestos in the usual urban environment is unknown. Of the various forms of asbestos (chrysotile, crocidolite, amosite, and anthophyllite), crocidolite appears to be the most carcinogenic form, followed by chrysotile and then by amosite, but because chrysotile is the most widely used form of asbestos, it is believed to account for most of the cases of diffuse mesothelioma.[217] The interval between first exposure to asbestos and presentation with the tumor is in the order of 20 to 40 years.[2] Prior thoracic irradiation has occasionally been noted[50] and is thought to play an etiologic role.

Pathologically, diffuse malignant mesothelioma appears as plaques and nodules on the visceral or parietal pleura that eventually form a lobular sheet of tumor up to several centimeters thick, encasing the lungs, extending through the pleural cavity and growing into the interlobar fissures. Invasion into the adjacent chest wall, diaphragm, and mediastinal structures usually occurs relatively late[233] but may be seen early.[9] Lymphatic and hematogeneous me-

tastases are usually late manifestations which, though present in 50% of patients at autopsy, are generally clinically silent.[8] Occasionally, a malignant mesothelioma will form a localized mass and macroscopically resemble the benign (fibrous) mesothelioma. Histologically, malignant mesotheliomas are divided into epithelial, mesenchymal (fibrous or sarcomatous), or mixed tumors. The relative prevalence of the mesothelioma cell types varies considerably from series to series and also varies according to the diligence with which the entire tumor is examined for mixed cell-types. In Legha and Muggia's compilation of 382 cases from the literature,[217] 54% were epithelial, 21% were fibrosarcomatous, and 25% were mixed, and in the recently reported Mayo Clinic series, the proportions were very similar.[1] The epithelial type consists of cuboidal cells in various arrangements, whereas the mesenchymal type shows sheets of parallel spindle-shaped cells similar to many soft tissue sarcomas. The epithelial type can be very difficult to differentiate from bronchial adenocarcinoma that has spread to the pleura. Because bronchial carcinoma also shows a higher than expected incidence in patients exposed to asbestos, the

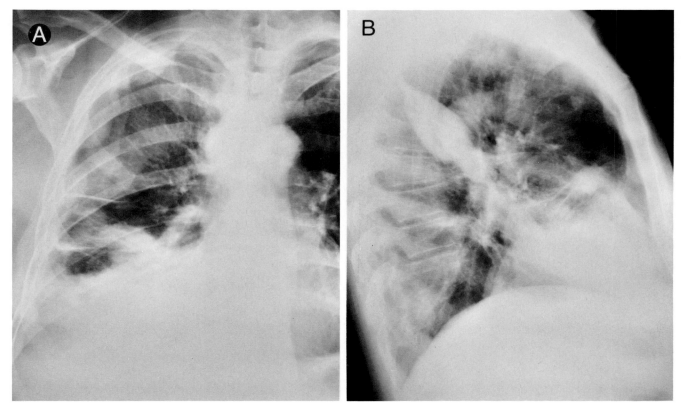

FIG 7–88.
Malignant mesothelioma of the pleura, showing lobular pleural masses. Note the lobular thickening of the major fissures. **A,** PA view. **B,** lateral view.

confusion between these tumors can be very real. The complex subject of the histologic differential diagnosis of malignant mesothelioma has recently been reviewed by Antman.[9]

The pleural fluid associated with malignant mesothelioma is an exudate that is serosanguinous in half the cases.[42] With large tumors, the glucose and pH levels are low. On cytologic examination, the fluid may contain malignant mesothelial cells together with varying numbers of lymphocytes and polymorphonuclear leukocytes,[217] but the cytologic distinction between benign and malignant mesothelial cells is difficult,[1] and pleural biopsy is usually needed to establish the diagnosis. Open rather than percutaneous needle biopsy is strongly recommended[233] because needle biopsy is often falsely negative or equivocal.[1]

The peak age at presentation is between 40 and 70 years; the male-to-female ratio is 2-4:1.[1, 50, 217, 254] The usual symptoms are chest pain, shortness of breath, and cough, followed by dyspnea and weight loss.[1, 9, 50, 217] There may be intermittent low-grade fever. Clubbing of the fingers and hypertrophic pul-

monary osteoarthropathy are seen, but are much less common than with benign mesothelioma.[8]

The radiologic features of diffuse malignant mesothelioma* are essentially similar on plain chest radiographs and CT scans (Figs 7–88 through 7–90). CT shows the extent of the tumor with greater accuracy and the accompanying pleural fluid with greater sensitivity,[214] but because the tumor is usually so extensive at initial presentation, CT provides little advantage over conventional radiology in the management of most patients.[214] The findings consist of nodular thickening of the pleura, which may conglomerate to form a lobular sheet of soft tissue density encasing the lung, accompanied by varying amounts of pleural fluid. Calcification of the tumor is extremely rare, though reported.[282] The nodularity of the pleural thickening is an important diagnostic feature and is frequently easiest to identify on the lateral projection (see Fig 7–88). The tumor is usually more prominent posteriorly, and the adja-

*References 1, 5, 109, 152, 171, 209, 214, 224, 266, and 374.

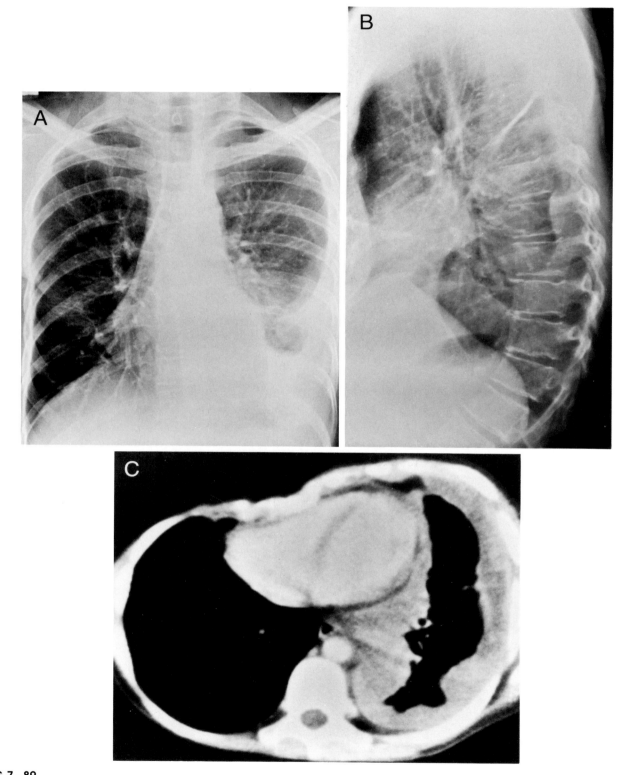

FIG 7–89.
Malignant mesothelioma of the pleura. There is lobular pleural thickening encasing the left lung and thickening of the major fissure. The patient, a 28-year-old woman, had received radiation therapy to the opposite thorax for a Wilm's tumor in childhood, hence the contracted right thorax. The etiologic role of radiation therapy in this case of mesothelioma is conjectural. **A,** PA radiograph. **B,** lateral radiograph. **C,** CT scan.

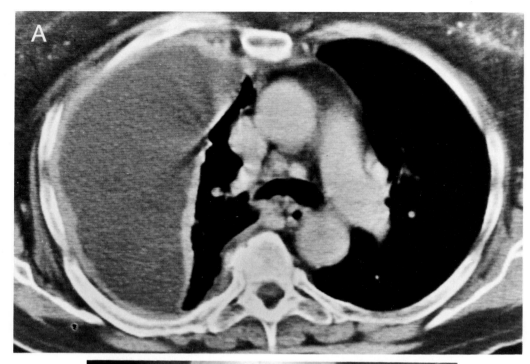

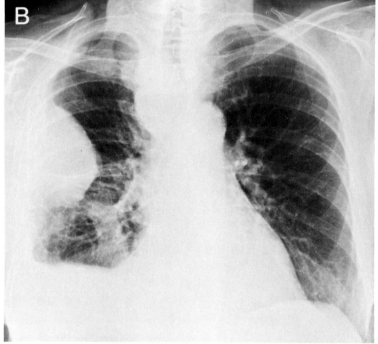

FIG 7–90.
A, CT appearance of malignant mesothelioma. In this 72-year-old woman, there is a relatively thin rind of nodular pleural thickening and a large loculus of pleural fluid. **B,** plain film study of same patient for comparison.

cent lung often shows evidence of invasion.[209] Sometimes the accompanying pleural effusion is very large (Fig 7–91), and it may be so predominant that it obscures the pleural masses on plain chest radiograph. In such cases, the chest radiographic appearances may be indistinguishable from other causes of pleural effusion. One point of distinction from other large pleural effusions is that this neoplastic encasement of the lung may fix the position of the mediastinum, so that shift away from the side of the effusion is not seen as often in patients with malignant mesothelioma as it is with other causes of large pleural effusion.[182] The tumor nodules may become evident only on plain chest radiographs following thoracentesis, particularly if air enters the pleural space through the needle. At CT scanning, the soft tissue density of the tumor tissue can be readily distinguished from the adjacent pleural effusion. Turning the patient into a prone or decubitus position can help decide between fluid and tumor when doubt exists.[209] The hemithorax is frequently contracted owing to encasement of the lung by the pleural tumor.

Chest wall invasion, bone destruction and direct extension to the pericardium and other mediastinal structures, and invasion through the diaphragm into the upper abdomen are seen in approximately 11% of patients at initial presentation, increasing to 30% or more during the course of the disease.[50, 152, 214, 224, 266] Extension to the contralateral thoracic cavity is common in advanced cases.[5, 152, 224]

Asbestos-related pleural plaques may be seen in either pleural cavity, and calcified plaques may be engulfed by the tumor.[209, 224]

The differential diagnosis includes pleural involvement by other malignant tumors, notably bronchial adenocarcinoma, breast carcinoma, malignant thymoma and subpleural lymphoma, as well as benign conditions such as tuberculous pleural thickening, and asbestos-related pleural plaques together with round atelectasis. Unless there are other features to indicate the primary tumor, the distinction between adenocarcinoma of the lung and malignant mesothelioma cannot be made radiographically from the appearance of the pleural involvement alone. This is hardly surprising in view of the difficulty that pathologists experience when trying to distinguish between these two tumors. Although pleural involvement by breast carcinoma can also appear identical, there is usually no diagnostic difficulty because the primary tumor will have been diagnosed previously or be clinically obvious. Pleural deposits of lymphoma and thymoma usually appear as more discrete localized masses than malignant mesothelioma. The distinction from benign pleural thickening due to conditions such as previous tuberculosis or old hemothorax is usually readily made by noting the smoothness of the pleural shadowing in these disorders.[1]

The differential diagnosis of early malignant pleural mesothelioma from noncalcified or partially calcified asbestos-related plaques can be difficult. Rabinowitz et al.[309] found that pleural plaques associated with advanced asbestosis were large and irregular and resembled mesothelioma. However, nodular involvement of the pleural fissures and ipsilateral volume loss with a fixed mediastinum suggested mesothelioma, as did pleural effusion. Pleural effusion can, however, be seen in asbestos-related pleural disease without malignant change. These authors cautioned that determining the growth of the pleural plaque may be of little value because benign plaques may also enlarge on serial examinations.

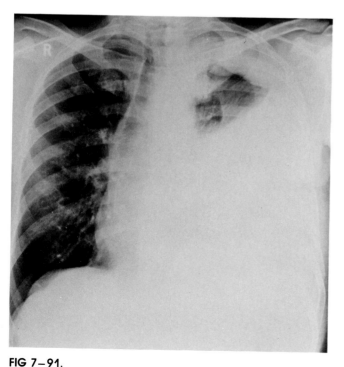

FIG 7–91.
Malignant mesothelioma. A very large pleural effusion partially hides the lobular neoplastic thickening of the pleura.

METASTASES

Pulmonary Metastases

The lungs are more often affected by metastatic tumors than they are by primary neoplasms. Any carcinoma or sarcoma may spread to the lungs, usually by way of the bloodstream, but sometimes through the lymphatics or by direct extension.

The incidence of pulmonary metastases varies with the primary tumor and the stage of the disease. In autopsy series, the most common sources of metastases to the lungs include tumors of the breast, colon, kidney, uterus, prostate, head, and neck.[91] Tumors such as choriocarcinoma, osteosarcoma, Ewing's sarcoma, testicular tumors, melanoma, and thyroid carcinoma have a high incidence of pulmonary metastases, but because they are not as prevalent in the population, lung deposits from these tumors are encountered less frequently.[91]

The hallmark of blood-borne metastases to the lungs is one or more discrete pulmonary nodules, maximal in the outer portions of the lungs (Figs 7–92 and 7–93).[92] They vary in size from microscopic to many centimeters in diameter, are usually multiple, and have well or moderately well defined outlines. On occasion, they show very irregular edges; this is particularly true of metastatic adenocarcinoma (Fig 7–94). Cavitation is seen from time to time. It occurred in some 4% to 6% of Dodd and Boyle's large series,[103] squamous cell carcinoma showing cavitation twice as often as adenocarcinoma, though other similar sized series have shown a more even distribution between the two cell types (Fig

7–95).[75] The most common sites of origin of cavitary neoplasms appear to be the uterine cervix, colon, and head and neck.[75, 103] The presence of cavitation is unrelated to the size of the metastasis,[75, 103] thus making it unlikely that cavitation is caused by the neoplasm outstripping its blood supply. The process seems more related to cell type, dependent perhaps on processes such as liquefaction of keratin in squamous cell carcinomas, or mucin/mucoid degeneration in adenocarcinomas.[103] The thickness of the wall is variable. In general, metastases originating in the head and neck undergo cavitation when quite small and may have strikingly thin walls,[103] though many other cell types also show thin walls.[145] When multiple, it is usual for cavitary lesions to coexist with solid nodules.[97]

In general, pulmonary metastases that respond to treatment with chemotherapy disappear and are no longer visible radiographically as nodules. Rarely, however, a residual nodule of sterilized fibrous tissue may remain, and in this case there can be a major dilemma in deciding whether treatment should be continued.[226] This phenomenon has been observed particularly with choriocarcinoma[225, 359] and with testicular cancer.[368]

Detectable calcification in metastases is very unusual indeed, except in metastases from sarcomas, notably osteosarcoma and chondrosarcoma, in which

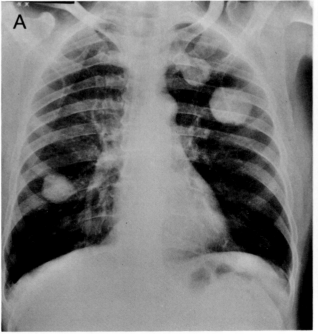
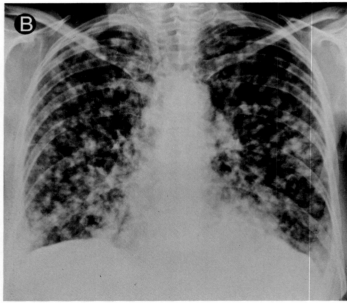

FIG 7–92.
Typical hematogenous metastases. **A,** from colon carcinoma. **B,** from rhabdomyosarcoma of the anterior abdominal wall.

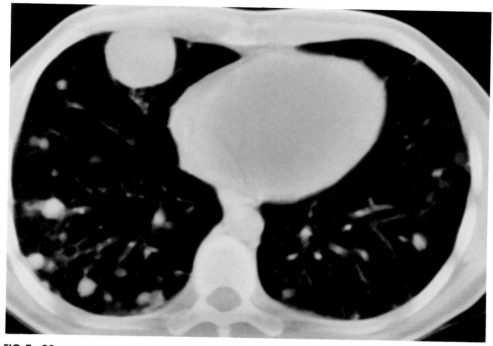

FIG 7–93.
CT scan showing the peripheral distribution of hematogenous metastases—in this case from a germ cell tumor of the testis.

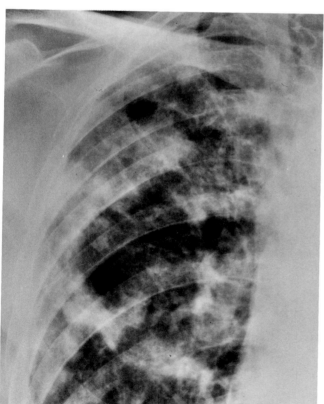

FIG 7–94.
Metastases from adenocarcinoma of the colon showing irregular outline of the pulmonary nodules.

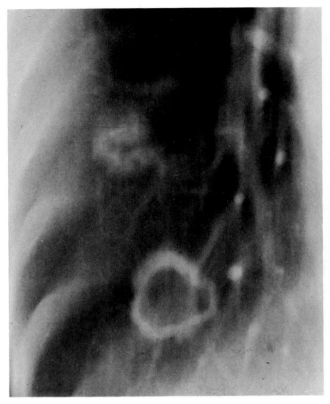

FIG 7−95.
Cavitating metastatic carcinoma, in this case from squamous cell carcinoma of the tonsil.

it is relatively common (Figs 7−96; 7−97,A and B).[245, 388] The calcification is then part of the tumor matrix just as it is in the primary tumor. Even in those tumors such as breast, ovarian, colon, and thyroid carcinomas where calcification can be seen in the primary tumor, calcification in pulmonary metastases has only been recognized in a few isolated cases.[245] Calcification may, however, be seen in successfully treated metastases.[85, 245]

Miliary nodulation, a pattern of innumerable tiny nodules resembling miliary tuberculosis, is occasionally encountered but is decidedly rare (Fig 7−98). Miliary metastases are most likely to be due to thyroid or renal carcinoma, bone sarcoma, trophoblastic disease,[127] or melanoma.[370]

Very occasionally, metastases present radiographically as myriads of tiny shadows which summate to resemble pulmonary consolidation and may then be confused with infection, edema, or drug reaction. This pattern has been seen particularly with melanoma.[77, 106, 370]

Parenchymal metastases occur at least ten times as often as intrathoracic nodal metastases, and nodal

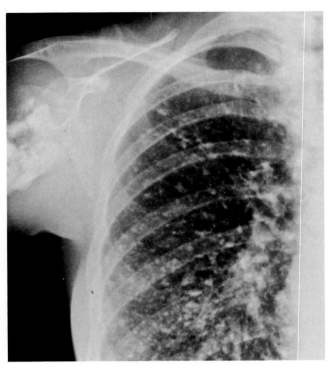

FIG 7−96.
Calcified metastases in a case of osteosarcoma (the primary tumor is visible in the upper right humerus).

disease alone is quite unusual, except in seminoma of the testis.[378] McLeod et al. reviewed 1,071 cases of extrathoracic malignant neoplasms.[256] Only 2% to 3% had evidence of hilar or mediastinal lymph node metastases, and concomitant pulmonary metastases were present in almost half these cases (Fig 7−99). They found that the primary neoplasms consisted chiefly of tumors of the head and neck, tumors of the genitourinary system, breast cancer, and malignant melanoma.

The Role of Tomography in Metastasis Detection

The standard initial test for the detection of pulmonary metastases is the plain chest radiograph. High-kV technique (kilovoltages of over 125) will show more lesions than low-kV films, and whole lung tomography will enable detection of more lesions than plain films, particularly if the tomograms are taken at 1-cm intervals.[24, 281, 341] Nodules in the posterior costophrenic sulci are often obscured by the upper abdominal structures and, therefore, a plain film "diaphragm view" exposed with the same factors as an abdominal film has been recommended when whole lung tomography is undertaken.[23] In Bein's large series,[23] additional metastases were

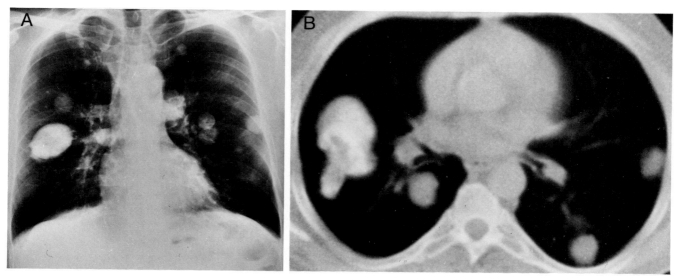

FIG 7–97.
Calcification/ossification in metastases from osteosarcoma of the leg. **A,** PA radiograph. **B,** CT scan.

found in 8% of patients when this film was added to the tomographic series. CT is currently the most sensitive technique available for the detection of pulmonary metastases. There are two principal reasons: better contrast resolution and fewer blind spots. The better contrast resolution of CT allows smaller nodules to be demonstrated. Individual nodules as small as 3 mm in diameter may be visible on CT, whereas

the lower limit for uncalcified nodules on plain film is somewhere between 7 mm and 9 mm. The increased sensitivity in detecting metastases carries with it a decrease in specificity, since some of the smaller nodules discovered by CT are benign granulomas, particularly in those parts of the world where fungal granulomas such as histoplasmomas are common. An early series[74, 332] suggested that a large proportion of the nodules shown only by CT would prove to be benign; however, other surveys[272, 299]

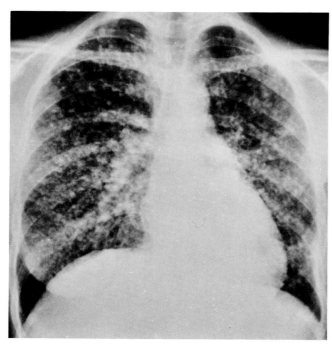

FIG 7–98.
Miliary metastases from breast carcinoma.

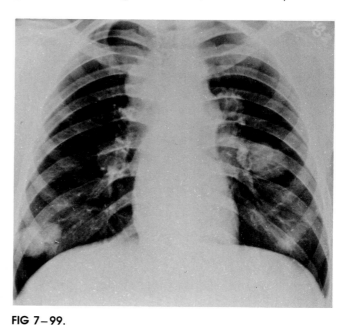

FIG 7–99.
Concomitant pulmonary and mediastinal metastases in a 17-year-old boy with seminoma of the testis.

indicate that over 80% of nodules seen with CT which are not visible on plain chest radiographs or conventional whole lung tomograms will turn out to be metastases. In countries such as the United Kingdom, where fungal granulomas are virtually nonexistent, the specificity of CT rises. In a study of 100 adult patients without known malignant disease, only two nonmetastatic nodules were encountered, both of which were calcified,[108] but even in the United Kingdom caution is needed because in a series of 200 patients with seminoma of the testis 6% of the noncalcified nodules revealed by CT were nonmetastatic in nature;[378] presumably they were tuberculous granulomas. Another advantage of CT is that blind areas are to a large extent eliminated, owing to the cross-sectional technique and the lack of artifact from adjacent levels, an advantage that is particularly important because hematogenous metastases tend to occur in the outer one-third of the lung and are often subpleural in location (see Fig 7–93).[92] These areas, particularly the subpleural regions against the chest wall, mediastinum, and posterior costophrenic recesses, are the most difficult to assess with whole lung tomography or plain chest radiography. An additional advantage of CT is that it can demonstrate disease in the mediastinum, an anatomic region for which whole lung tomography is relatively insensitive. CT will also show the axillae, the root of the neck, and the upper abdomen on routine chest images. CT does, however, have one disadvantage: so-called contiguous sections are often not truly contiguous because, if the patient breathes during the examination, small nodules may be out of section every time and therefore are not imaged at all.

CT is used only in selected cases because it is rarely necessary to demonstrate further metastases once the presence of definite pulmonary metastatic disease has been established. General indications for CT include:

1. *Patients with a normal chest radiograph in whom the presence of pulmonary metastases would significantly alter patient management.* With tumors such as osteosarcoma, choriocarcinoma, and testicular germ cell tumors,[181] all of which have a significant incidence of pulmonary metastases at presentation but which may have no detectable metastatic spread to other sites, it seems reasonable to obtain CT scans of the chest to find neoplastic deposits not visible on plain chest radiograph. The incidence of pulmonary metastases from seminoma is low, but since the incidence of mediastinal nodal disease can be as high as

12.5%, chest CT is still recommended for initial staging as well as follow-up for potential relapse.[92]

Locally advanced melanoma is cited as an example of a tumor that metastasizes early to the lungs, but whether routine chest CT is justified in cases with a normal chest radiograph is far from clear. In one series of 42 patients with locally advanced melanoma and either a solitary pulmonary nodule or no abnormality on chest radiographs, CT scanning showed further nodules believed to be metastases in approximately one-third of patients.[164] The authors did, however, point out that in only one of the 42 patients did the discovery of an additional nodule by CT alter the management of the patient.

The incidence of pulmonary metastases in patients with head and neck carcinoma, superficial melanoma, and with carcinomas of the kidney, bladder, and female genital tract is relatively low. Chiles and Ravin[79] recommended that in patients with these tumors CT should be reserved for those with advanced local disease and thoracic symptoms.

Similarly, patients with carcinomas of the gastrointestinal tract, breast, or prostate are unlikely to have pulmonary metastases in the absence of metastases to such organs as the liver and bones, and CT should, therefore, be reserved for those patients in whom thoracic involvement is uncertain on plain chest radiograph or is suspected clinically.[79, 93]

2. *Patients who are being considered for surgical resection of known pulmonary metastasis to look for further occult lesions.* CT is clearly indicated to demonstrate all pulmonary metastases in those patients for whom surgical resection of the pulmonary lesions is being considered. Currently, such surgery is recommended when the primary tumor has (or can be) definitively treated and all known metastatic disease can be encompassed by the projected pulmonary resection.[271] Resection of pulmonary metastases appears most beneficial for tumors of the urinary tract, testicular and uterine neoplasms, colon and rectal carcinoma, tumors of the head and neck, and various sarcomas, notably osteogenic sarcoma.[271] How many other tumors should be added to this list is debatable.

3. *Distinguishing solitary from multiple pulmonary nodules where the diagnostic dilemma is metastasis versus new primary bronchial carcinoma.* A truly solitary pulmonary nodule may represent a primary bronchogenic carcinoma rather than a metastasis, even in patients with a known extrathoracic primary tumor. Clearly, the relative probabilities depend on the likelihood of the specific tumor metastasizing to the lungs and such factors as the smoking habits of the

patient and the interval between the original diagnosis and the appearance of the nodule. A rule of thumb suggested by Cahan and co-workers[63] states that:

> . . .for patients over 35, if a patient has a squamous cancer elsewhere in the body, the solitary lung lesion is usually a separate primary (and most likely squamous cancer as well). If the patient has an adenocarcinoma elsewhere, there is an equal chance that the solitary shadow is a primary lung cancer as it is a metastasis. If there is a soft tissue or skeletal sarcoma or a melanoma elsewhere, the solitary lung lesion is most often a metastasis.

Endobronchial Metastases

Metastases to the walls of a large bronchus are unusual. Bramman and Whitcomb found the incidence to be only 2% in a very large series of patients who had died from solid neoplasms.[49] The most common primary sites appear to be kidney, breast, colon, and rectum.[22] The clinical and radiologic features are indistinguishable from those produced by other central tumors, namely cough, wheezing, hemoptysis, atelectasis, and obstructive pneumonitis[4, 22] (Fig 7–100).

Lymphangitis Carcinomatosa

Lymphangitis carcinomatosa is the name given to permeation of pulmonary lymphatics by neoplastic cells. The most common tumors that spread in this manner are carcinomas of the bronchus, breast, pancreas, stomach, colon, and prostate. The route by which tumor cells reach the intrapulmonary lymphatics is debated. Spencer,[343] when reviewing the subject, concluded that some cases are caused by blood-borne emboli that lodge in smaller pulmonary arteries and subsequently spread through the vessel walls into the lymphatic vessels. Other tumors, notably upper abdominal cancers, spread by way of lymph vessels to hilar nodes and thence in retrograde fashion into the pulmonary lymphatics. Primary carcinoma of the lung can invade the pulmonary lymphatics directly and may give rise to segmental or lobar lymphangitis carcinomatosa as well as involving one or both lungs diffusely.

Histologically, there is interstitial thickening of the interlobular septa due to a combination of tumor cells, desmoplastic response, and dilated lymphatics. The lymphatic obstruction can lead to interstitial edema. The hilar lymph nodes may, or may not, show histologic evidence of tumor involvement.

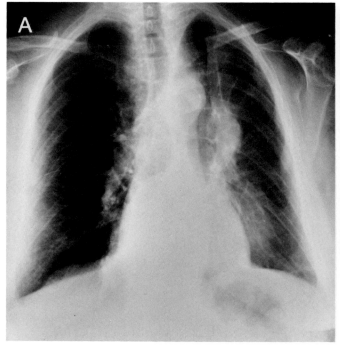

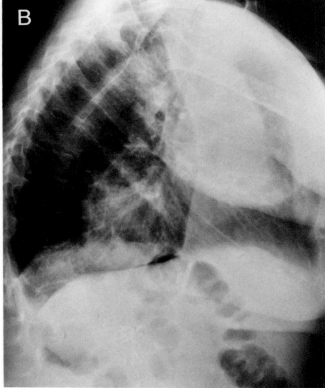

FIG 7–100.
Endobronchial metastasis from carcinoma of the kidney causing left upper lobe collapse. **A,** PA view. **B,** lateral view.

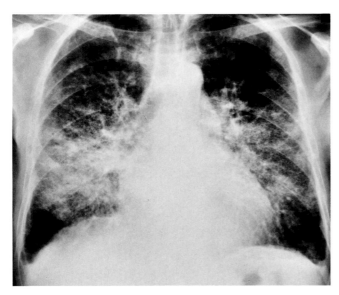

FIG 7 – 101.
Lymphangitis carcinomatosa from carcinoma of the prostate showing bilateral centrally predominant reticulonodular shadows.

The radiologic findings are fine reticulonodular shadowing and/or thickened septal lines (Figs 7 – 101 and 7 – 102). These signs occur because of a combination of dilated lymphatics and interstitial edema, together with shadows due to the tumor cells themselves and any desmoplastic response which may have been induced by the tumor.[168, 188, 363] Another

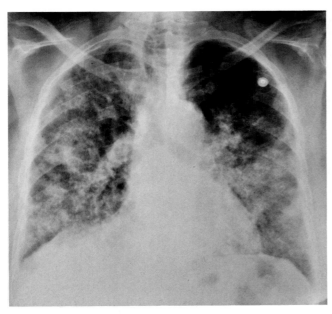

FIG 7 – 102.
Lymphangitis carcinomatosa from carcinoma of the breast showing randomly distributed reticulonodular shadowing with areas of confluence.

useful sign of lymphangitis carcinomatosa is subpleural edema resulting from lymphatic obstruction by tumor cells, a feature that is most readily visible as thickening of the fissures.[168] These changes can be unilateral (Fig 7 – 103), particularly in cases resulting from bronchial carcinoma. More often the pulmonary shadowing is bilateral, and symmetrical. Pleural effusion is common.

As would be expected, CT scanning is more sensitive than plain radiography in the detection of lymphangitic spread and may show of changes in patients whose chest film is normal. CT scans, particularly thin-section (2 mm or less) scans reconstructed with high-resolution algorithms, show numerous linear shadows 1 to 2 cm in length (Fig 7 – 104).[31, 274, 350, 387] The lines, which are seen throughout the parenchyma, are arranged in Y, U, or polygonal configurations, or may be seen simply as lines that contact the pleural surface. They almost certainly represent thickened interlobular septa. Small, peripherally located, wedge-shaped densities were also seen in some of the patients, which may represent volume averaging of the thickened septa. Nodular densities are present in addition to the linear shadows,[31, 274, 387] and it may be possible to ap-

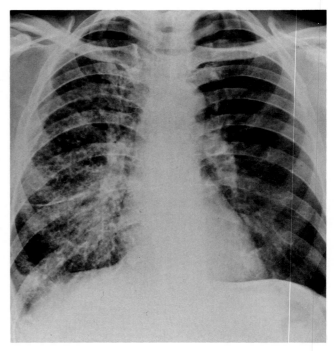

FIG 7 – 103.
Unilateral lymphangitis carcinomatosa from bronchial carcinoma. Note the reticulonodular shadows and the subpleural thickening of the minor fissure and of the lung in the right cardiophrenic angle. Septal lines are also present.

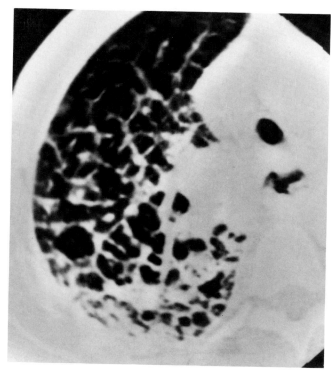

FIG 7–104.
Lymphangitis carcinomatosa. Thin-section, high-resolution CT scan reveals 1- to 2-cm linear shadows which are believed to correspond to thickening of the interlobular septa. Note also the nodular thickening, particularly at points of intersection. (Courtesy of Dr. Elias A. Zerhouni, Baltimore, Md.)

preciate thickening of the bronchovascular bundles in the central portions of the lungs.[31, 274]

Hilar lymph node enlargement is seen in only some of the patients, five of the 12 cases in one series, supporting the supposition that lymphangitis carcinomatosa is sometimes the result of hematogeneous spread of tumor to the interstitium.[188]

The major differential diagnosis of lymphangitis carcinomatosa is pulmonary edema. The nodularity of the septal thickening at thin-section CT is very helpful but on plain chest radiographs, at least in those cases without visible lung cancer or adenopathy, the findings may be similar to pulmonary edema, and distinguishing between the two conditions can be impossible. Clearly, knowledge of the clinical or radiographic progression of disease is very helpful and is frequently decisive.

Malignant Pleural Effusion and Pleural Metastases

Carcinomatous metastases to the pleura can originate from almost any organ, but the lung appears to be the most frequent primary site, followed by breast, pancreas, stomach, and ovary.[7, 78, 264] Carcinoma of the lung and breast, together with lymphoma, accounts for approximately 75% of malignant pleural effusions.[7] Leukemia and sarcoma are rare causes of pleural effusion,[325] as is malignant

mesothelioma. The responsible neoplasm usually involves both the visceral and parietal pleura; isolated involvement of the parietal pleura was not seen in any case in the series reported by Meyer.[264]

A malignant tumor can lead to a pleural effusion in several different ways.[233] Decreased lymphatic drainage due to blockage of the small lymphatic stomas that drain the pleura is the probable mechanism in many cases, and obstruction to lymphatic drainage through mediastinal nodes which have been infiltrated by tumor is also believed to play a significant role. Another, probably less common, mechanism is increased permeability of the pleural surfaces because of the presence of metastases so that more protein enters the pleural cavity than can be removed. Malignant tumors can also produce pleural effusions by obstructing the thoracic duct, in which case the resulting pleural effusion will be chylous.

Not all patients with pleural metastases have pleural effusions. Meyer found that only 60% of autopsy patients with pleural metastases had pleural effusions and that the presence of a pleural effusion was more closely related to neoplastic invasion of the mediastinal lymph nodes than to the extent of pleural involvement by nodal metastases.[264]

Clinically, the most frequent symptom of pleural effusion resulting from metastases is dyspnea on ex-

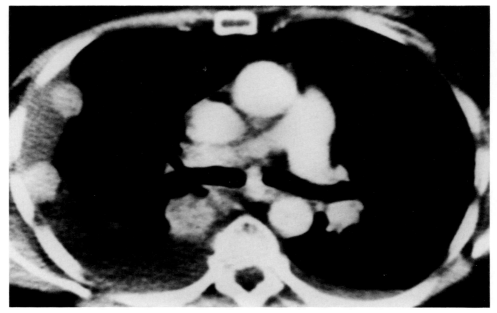

FIG 7–105.
Pleural metastases shown as tumor nodules by CT in a case of metastatic melanoma. The tumor was widely metastatic, involving not only the pleura bilaterally but also mediastinal lymph nodes.

FIG 7–106.
Pleural metastases from carcinoma of the uterus. This case is unusual in that the lesion was solitary and there is no pleural effusion.

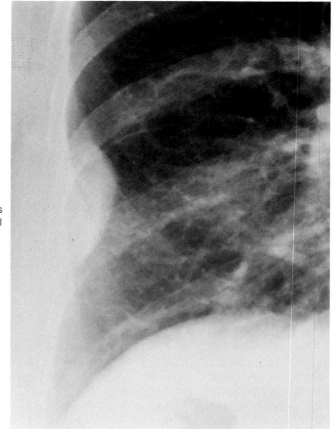

ertion. Chest pain is relatively uncommon, being seen in less than a quarter of patients.[78]

Pleural effusions resulting from malignant tumor[30, 78] contain high levels of protein and may show a low pH, a low glucose level, and a high lactic acid dehydrogenase level. Approximately 10% of patients with malignant pleural effusion have an elevated level of amylase in the pleural fluid, even though the primary tumor is usually not in the pancreas.[234] Bleeding may occur into the effusion, and typically the fluid contains a large number of lymphocytes. The reason for the high lymphocyte count is not entirely clear, but it is known that any chronic pleural effusion in the absence of active inflammation will generally be lymphocyte predominant. Unlike tuberculous effusions, which are also lymphocyte predominant, malignant effusions often contain mesothelial cells. The presence of definite malignant cells on cytologic examination or pleural biopsy removes all doubt about the diagnosis. The percentage of cases in which cytologic study of the pleural fluid establishes the diagnosis ranges from 40% to 80%. The rate varies with the cell type, the yield being low with squamous tumors.[233] In general, cytologic study of the pleural fluid establishes the diagnosis more frequently than pleural biopsy, presumably because pleural biopsy samples are from the parietal pleura and parietal pleural involvement is often spotty.[233]

Usually the findings on plain chest radiography, CT, and ultrasound are those of free or loculated pleural effusion without any specific features to the effusion itself. There may be recognizable tumor nodules in the pleura on CT (Fig 7–105), ultrasound,[351] or even, occasionally, on chest radiographs (Fig 7–106). Other features of bronchogenic carcinoma or lymphoma are often present in patients whose effusion results from one of these diseases. For example, enlarged intrathoracic lymph nodes are seen in about 10% of patients with pleural effusion due to breast cancer.[118]

REFERENCES

1. Adams VI, Unni KK, Muhm JR, et al: Diffuse malignant mesothelioma of pleura: Diagnosis and survival in 92 cases. *Cancer* 1986; 58:1540–1551.
2. Aisner J, Wiernik PH: Malignant mesothelioma: Current status and future prospects. *Chest* 1978; 74:438–444.
3. Alazraki NP, Ramsdell JW, Taylor A: Reliability of gallium scan chest radiography compared to mediastinoscopy for evaluating mediastinal spread in lung cancer. *Am Rev Respir Dis* 1978; 117:415–420.
4. Albertini RE, Ekberg NL: Endobronchial metastasis in breast cancer. *Thorax* 1980; 35:435–440.
5. Alexander E, Clark RA, Colley DP, et al: CT of malignant mesothelioma. *AJR* 1981; 137:287–291.
6. Altman RL, Miller WE, Carr DT, et al: Radiographic appearance of bronchial carcinoid. *Thorax* 1973; 28:433–434.
7. Anderson CB, Philpott GW, Ferguson TB: The treatment of malignant pleural effusions. *Cancer* 1974; 33:916–922.
8. Antman KH: Clinical presentation and natural history of benign and malignant mesothelioma. *Semin Oncol* 1981; 8:313–320.
9. Antman KH, Corson JM: Benign and malignant pleural mesothelioma. *Clin Chest Med* 1985; 6:127–140.
10. Armstrong P, Elston C, Sanderson M: Endobronchial histiocytoma. *Br J Radiol* 1975; 48:221–222.
11. Aronchick JM, Wexler JA, Christen B, et al: Computed tomography of bronchial carcinoid. *J Comput Assist Tomogr* 1986; 10:71–74.
12. Attar S, Miller SE, Satterfield J, et al: Pancoast's tumor: Irradiation or surgery? *Ann Thorac Surg* 1979; 28:578–586.
13. Backer CL, Shields TW, Lockhart CG, et al: Selective preoperative evaluation for possible N2 disease in carcinoma of the lung. *J Thorac Cardiovasc Surg* 1987; 93:337–343.
14. Bahk YW, Shinn KS, Choi BS: The air meniscus sign in sclerosing hemangioma of the lung. *Radiology* 1978; 128:27–29.
15. Bakris, Mulopulos GP, Korchik, et al: Pulmonary scar carcinoma: A clinicopathologic analysis. *Cancer* 1983; 52:493–497.
16. Balikian JP, Herman PG: Non-Hodgkin's lymphoma of the lungs. *Radiology* 1979; 132:569–576.
17. Baron RL, Levitt RG, Sagel SS, et al: Computed tomography in the preoperative evaluation of bronchogenic carcinoma. *Radiology* 1982; 145:727–732.
18. Barsky SH, Huang SJ, Bhuta S: The extracellular matrix of pulmonary scar carcinoma is suggestive of a desmoplastic origin. *Am J Pathol* 1986; 124:412–419.
19. Bateson EM: Relationship between intrapulmonary and endobronchial cartilage containing tumours, so called hamartomata. *Thorax* 1965; 20:447–461.
20. Bateson EM, Abbot EK: Mixed tumours of the lung, or hamartochondromas. *Clin Radiol* 1960; 11:232–247.
21. Bateson EM, Whimster WF, Woo-Ming M: Ossified bronchial adenoma. *Br J Radiol* 1970; 43:570–573.
22. Baumgartner WA, Mark JBD: Metastatic malignancies from distant sites to the tracheobronchial tree. *J Thorac Cardiovasc Surg* 1980; 79:499–503.
23. Bein ME: Plain film diaphragm view as adjunct to full lung tomography. *AJR* 1979; 133:217–220.
24. Bein ME, Greenberg M, Liu PY, et al: Pulmonary nodules: Detection in 1 and 2 cm full lung linear tomography. *AJR* 1980; 135:513–520.

25. Belgrad R, Good CA, Woolner LB: Alveolar cell carcinoma (terminal bronchiolar carcinoma): A study of surgically excised tumors with special emphasis on localized lesions. *Radiology* 1962; 79:789–798.

26. Beluffi G, Bertolotti P, Mietta A, et al: Primary leiomyosarcoma of the lung in a girl. *Pediatr Radiol* 1986; 16:240–244.

27. Bender BL, Jaffe R: Immunoglobulin production in lymphomatoid granulomatosis and relation to other "benign" lymphoproliferative disorders. *Am J Clin Pathol* 1980; 73:41–47.

28. Benisch B, Peison B: The association of lymphocytic interstitial pneumonia and systemic lupus erythematosus. *Mt Sinai J Med* 1979; 46:398–401.

29. Bennett LL, Lesar MSL, Tellis CJ: Multiple calcified chondrohamartomas of the lung: CT appearance. *J Comput Assist Tomogr* 1985; 9:180–182.

30. Berger HW, Maher G: Decreased glucose concentration in malignant pleural effusions. *Am Rev Respir Dis* 1971; 103:427–429.

31. Bergin CJ, Muller NL: CT of interstitial lung disease: A diagnostic approach. *AJR* 1987; 148:8–15.

32. Berkmen YM: The many faces of alveolar cell carcinoma of the lung. *Semin Roentgenol* 1977; 12:207–214.

33. Berlin NI, Buncher CR, Fontana RS, et al: The National Cancer Institute Cooperative early lung cancer detection program. Results of initial screen (prevalence). Early lung cancer detection: Introduction. *Am Rev Respir Dis* 1984; 130:545–549.

34. Berne AS, Heitzman ER: The roentgenologic signs of pedunculated pleural tumors. *AJR* 1962; 87:892–895.

35. Black WC, Armstrong P, Daniel TM: Cost-effectiveness of chest CT in T1N0M0 lung cancer. *Radiology* 1988; 167:373–378.

36. Blair TC, McElvein: Hamartoma of the lung: A clinical study of 25 cases. *Dis Chest* 1963; 44:296–302.

37. Blank N, Castellino RA: The mediastinum in Hodgkin's and non-Hodgkin's lymphomas. *J Thorac Imag* 1987; 2(1):66–71.

38. Blank N, Castellino RA: The intrathoracic manifestations of malignant lymphomas and the leukemias. *Sem Roentgenol* 1980; 15:227–245.

39. Blount HC: Localized mesothelioma of the pleura. *Radiology* 1956; 67:822–834.

40. Bodey GP, Powell RD, Hersh EM, et al: Pulmonary complications of acute leukemia. *Cancer* 1966; 19:781–793.

41. Bonner H, Ennis RS, Geelhoed GW, et al: Lymphoid infiltration and amyloidosis of the lung in Sjögren's syndrome. *Arch Pathol* 1973; 95:42–44.

42. Borrow M, Couston A, Livornese L, et al: Mesothelioma following exposure to asbestos: A review of 72 cases. *Chest* 1973; 64:641–646.

43. Bower SL, Choplin RH, Muss HB: Multiple primary carcinomas of the lung. *AJR* 1983; 140:253–258.

44. Boucot KR, Weiss W: Is curable lung cancer detected by semiannual screening? *JAMA* 1973; 224:1361–1365.

45. Boysen PG, Harris JO, Block AJ, et al: Prospective evaluation for pneumonectomy using perfusion scanning: Follow up beyond one year. *Chest* 1981; 80:163–166.

46. Bragg DG: Radiology of the lymphomas. *Curr Probl Diagn Radiol* 1987; 16:183–206.

47. Bragg DG: The clinical, pathologic and radiographic spectrum of the intrathoracic lymphomas. *Invest Radiol* 1978; 13:2–11.

48. Bragg DG, Colby TV, Ward JH: New concepts in the non-Hodgkin lymphomas: Radiologic implications. *Radiology* 1986; 159:289–304.

49. Bramman SS, Whitcomb ME: Endobronchial metastasis. *Arch Intern Med* 1975; 135:543–547.

50. Brenner J, Sordillo PP, Magill GB, et al: Malignant mesothelioma of the pleura: Review of 123 patients. *Cancer* 1982; 49:2431–2439.

51. Brett GZ: Earlier diagnosis and survival in lung cancer. *Br Med J* 1968; 2:260–262.

52. Brion JP, Depauw L, Francquen PDe, et al: Role of computed tomography and mediastinoscopy in preoperative staging of lung carcinoma. *J Comput Assist Tomogr* 1985; 9:480–484.

53. Briselli M, Mark EJ, Dickersin GR: Solitary fibrous tumors of the pleura: Eight new cases and review of 360 cases in the literature. *Cancer* 1981; 47:2678–2689.

54. Brogdon BG, Kelsey CA, Moseley RD: Factors affecting perception of pulmonary lesions. *Radiol Clin North Am* 1983; 21:633–654.

55. Brown RJK, Huberman RP, Vanley G: Pulmonary features of Kaposi sarcoma. *AJR* 1982; 139:659–660.

56. Burgener FA, Hamlin DJ: Intrathoracic histiocytic lymphoma. *AJR* 1981; 136:499–504.

57. Butchart EG, Urquhart W, Porteous IB, et al: Granular cell myoblastoma of the bronchus. *Br J Radiol* 1976; 49:87–90.

58. Byrd RB, Carr DT, Miller WE, et al: Radiographic abnormalities in carcinoma of the lung as related to histological cell type. *Thorax* 1969; 24:573–575.

59. Byrd RB, Miller WE, Carr DT, et al: The roentgenographic appearance of squamous cell carcinoma of the bronchus. *Mayo Clin Proc* 1968; 43:327–332.

60. Byrd RB, Miller WE, Carr DT, et al: The roentgenographic appearance of large cell carcinoma of the bronchus. *Mayo Clin Proc* 1968; 43:333–336.

61. Byrd RB, Miller WE, Carr DT, et al: The roentgenographic appearance of small cell carcinoma of the bronchus. *Mayo Clin Proc* 1968; 43:337–341.

62. Caceres J, Felson B: Double primary carcinomas of the lung. *Radiology* 1972; 102:45–50.

63. Cahan WG, Castro EB, Hajdu SI: The significance of a solitary lung shadow in patients with colon carcinoma. *Cancer* 1974; 33:414–421.

64. Callihan TR, Beard CW: The classification and pathology of the lymphomas and the leukemias. *Semin Roentgenol* 1980; 15:203–218.

65. Cameron EWJ: Primary sarcoma of the lung. *Thorax* 1975; 30:516–520.

66. Carmel RJ, Kaplan HS: Mantle radiation and Hodgkin's disease. *Cancer* 1976; 37:2813–2825.

67. Carney JA: The triad of gastric epithelioid leiomyosarcoma, pulmonary chondroma and functioning extra-adrenal paraganglioma: A five year review. *Medicine* 1983; 62:159–169.

68. Castellino RA: Hodgkin disease: Practical concepts for the diagnostic radiologist. *Radiology* 1986; 159:305–310.

69. Castellino RA, Bellani F, Gasparini M, et al: Radiographic findings in previously untreated children with non-Hodgkin's lymphoma. *Radiology* 1975; 117:657–663.

70. Castellino RA, Blank N: Adenopathy of the cardiophrenic angle (diaphragmatic) lymph nodes. *AJR* 1972; 114:509–515.

71. Castellino RA, Blank N, Hoppe RT, et al: Hodgkin disease: Contributions of chest CT in the initial staging evaluation. *Radiology* 1986; 160:603–605.

72. Cathcart-Rake W, Bone RC, Sobonya RE, et al: Rapid development of diffuse pulmonary infiltrates in histiocytic lymphoma. *Am Rev Respir Dis* 1978; 117:587–593.

73. Chamberlain DW, Hyland RH, Ross DJ: Diphenylhydantoin-induced lymphocytic interstitial pneumonia. *Chest* 1986; 90:458–460.

74. Chang AE, Shaner EG, Conkle DM, et al: Evaluation of computed tomography in the detection of pulmonary metastasis: A prospective study. *Cancer* 1979; 43:913–916.

75. Chaudhuri MR: Cavitary pulmonary metastases. *Thorax* 1970; 25:375–381.

76. Chaudhuri MR: Primary pulmonary cavitating carcinomas. *Thorax* 1973; 28:354–366.

77. Chen JTT, Dahmash NS, Ravin CE, et al: Metastatic melanoma to the thorax: Report of 130 patients. *AJR* 1981; 137:293–298.

78. Chernow B, Sahn SA: Carcinomatous involvement of the pleura. *Am J Med* 1977; 63:695–702.

79. Chiles C, Ravin CE: Intrathoracic metastases from an extrathoracic malignancy; radiographic approach to patient evaluation. *Radiol Clin North Am* 1985; 23:427–438.

80. Cho CS, Blank N, Castellino RA: CT evaluation of cardiophrenic angle lymph nodes in patients with malignant lymphoma. *AJR* 1984; 143:719–721.

81. Choplin RH, Rawamoto EH, Dyer RB, et al: Atypical carcinoid of the lung: Radiographic features. *AJR* 1986; 146:665–668.

82. Churg A: Pulmonary angiitis and granulomatosis revisited. *Hum Pathol* 1983; 14:868–883.

83. Cleveland RH, Nice CM, Ziskind J: Primary adenoid cystic carcinoma (cylindroma) of the trachea. *Radiology* 1977; 122:597–600.

84. Clinical staging of primary lung cancer. Official statement of the American Thoracic Society. *Am Rev Respir Dis* 1983; 127:659–664.

85. Cockshott WP, Hendrickse JP: Pulmonary calcification at the site of trophoblastic metastases. *Br J Radiol* 1969; 42:17–20.

86. Cohen MH: Signs and symptoms of bronchogenic carcinoma. *Semin Oncol* 1974; 3:183–189.

87. Cohen S, Hossain S: Primary carcinoma of the lung: A review of 417 histologically proved cases. *Dis Chest* 1966; 49:67–74.

88. Colby TV, Carrington CB: Pulmonary lymphomas: Current concepts. *Hum Pathol* 1983; 14:884–887.

89. Colby TV, Carrington CB: Pulmonary lymphomas simulating lymphomatoid granulomatosis. *Am J Surg Pathol* 1982; 6:19–32.

90. Conte CC, Bucknam JCA: Role of computerized tomography in assessment of the mediastinum in patients with lung carcinoma. *Am J Surg* 1985; 149:449–452.

91. Coppage L, Shaw C, Curtis AM: Metastatic disease to the chest in patients with extrathoracic malignancy. *J Thorac Imag* 1987; 2(4):24–37.

92. Crow J, Slavin G, Kreel L: Pulmonary metastasis: A pathologic and radiologic study. *Cancer* 1981; 47:2595–2602.

93. Curtis AM, Ravin CE, Collier PE, et al: Detection of metastatic disease from carcinoma of the breast: Limited value of full lung tomography. *AJR* 1980; 134:253–255.

94. Daly BDT, Faling LJ, Pugatch RD, et al: Computed tomography: An effective technique for mediastinal staging in lung cancer. *J Thorac Cardiovasc Surg* 1984; 88:486–494.

95. Darke CS, Day P, Grainger RG, et al: The bronchial circulation in a case of giant hamartoma of the lung. *Br J Radiol* 1972; 45:147–150.

96. Davis SD, Henschke CI, Chamides BK, et al: Intrathoracic Kaposi sarcoma in AIDS patients: Radiographic-pathologic correlation. *Radiology* 1987; 163:495–500.

97. Deck FW, Sherman RS: Excavation of metastatic nodules in the lungs. *Radiology* 1959; 72:30–34.

98. De Coteau WE, Tourville D, Ambrus JL, et al: Lymphoid interstitial pneumonia and autoerythrocyte sensitization syndrome: A case with deposition of immunoglobulins on the alveolar basement membrane. *Arch Intern Med* 1974; 134:519–522.

99. Dedrick CG, McLoud TC, Shepard JP, et al: Computed tomography of localized pleural mesothelioma. *AJR* 1985; 144:275–280.

100. Dee PM, Arora NS, Innes DI: The pulmonary man-

ifestations of lymphomatoid granulomatosis. *Radiology* 1982; 143:613–618.

101. DeMeester TR, Golomb HM, Kirchner P: The role of gallium-67 scanning in the clinical staging and pre-operative evaluation of patients with carcinoma of the lung. *Ann Thorac Surg* 1979; 28:451–464.

102. Dines DE, Lillie JC, Henderson LL, et al: Solitary plasmacytoma of the trachea. *Am Rev Respir Dis* 1965; 92:949–951.

103. Dodd GD, Boyle JS: Excavating pulmonary metastases. *AJR* 1961; 85:277–293.

104. Doppman J, Wilson G: Cystic pulmonary hamartoma. *Br J Radiol* 1965; 38:629–631.

105. Dunnick NR, Parker BR, Castellino RA: Rapid onset of pulmonary infiltration due to histiocytic lymphoma. *Radiology* 1976; 118:281–285.

106. Dwyer AJ, Reichart CM, Woltering EA, et al: Diffuse pulmonary metastasis in melanoma: Radiographic pathologic correlation. *AJR* 1984; 143:983–984.

107. Eckholm S, Albrechtsson U, Krugelberg J, et al: Computed tomography in preoperative staging of bronchogenic carcinoma. *J Comput Assist Tomogr* 1980; 4:763–765.

108. Edwards SE, Kelsey-Fry I: Prevalence of nodules on computed tomography of patients without known malignant disease. *Br J Radiol* 1982; 55:715–716.

109. Ellis K, Wolff M: Mesotheliomas and secondary tumors of the pleura. *Semin Roentgenol* 1977; 12:303–311.

110. Epstein DM, Stephenson LW, Gefter WB, et al: Value of CT in the preoperative assessment of lung cancer: A survey of thoracic surgeons. *Radiology* 1986; 161:423–427.

111. Epstein DM, Gefter WB, Miller WT: Lobar bronchioloalveolar cell carcinoma. *AJR* 1982; 139:463–468.

112. Faling LJ, Pugatch RD, Jung Legg Y, et al: Computed tomographic scanning of the mediastinum in the staging of bronchogenic carcinoma. *Am Rev Respir Dis* 1981; 124:690–695.

113. Fauci AS, Haynes BF, Costa J, et al: Lymphomatoid granulomatosis, prospective clinical and therapeutic experience over ten years. *N Engl J Med* 1982; 306:68–74.

114. Federle MP, Callen PW: Cystic Hodgkin's lymphoma of the thymus: Computed tomography appearance. *J Comput Assist Tomogr* 1979; 3:542–544.

115. Feigin DS, Siegelman SS, Theros EG, et al: Nonmalignant lymphoid disorders of the chest. *AJR* 1977; 129:221–228.

116. Felson B: Mucoid impaction (inspissated secretions) in segmental bronchial obstruction. *Radiology* 1976; 133:9–16.

117. Felson B, Ralaisomay G: Carcinoma of the lung complicating lipoid pneumonia. *AJR* 1983; 141:901–907.

118. Fentiman IS, Millis R, Sexton S, et al: Pleural effusion in breast cancer: A review of 105 cases. *Cancer* 1981; 47:2087–2092.

119. Ferguson MK, MacMahon H, Little AG, et al: Regional accuracy of computed tomography of the mediastinum in staging of lung cancer. *J Thorac Cardiovasc Surg* 1986; 91:498–504.

120. Filderman AE, Shaw C, Matthay RA: Lung cancer: Part I. Etiology, pathology, natural history, manifestations, and diagnostic techniques. *Invest Radiol* 1986; 21:80–90.

121. Filderman AE, Shaw C, Matthay RA: Lung cancer: Part II. Staging and therapy. *Invest Radiol* 1986; 21:173–185.

122. Filly R, Blank N, Castellino RA: Radiographic distribution of intrathoracic disease in previously untreated patients with Hodgkin's disease and non Hodgkin's lymphoma. *Radiology* 1976; 120:277–281.

123. Fisher AMH, Kendal B, Van Leuven BD: Hodgkin's disease: A radiological survey. *Clin Radiol* 1962; 13:115–127.

124. Flehinger BJ, Melamed MR, Zaman MB, et al: Early lung cancer detection: Results of the initial (prevalence) radiologic and cytologic screening in the Memorial Sloan-Kettering study. *Am Rev Resp Dis* 1984; 130:555–560.

125. Fontana RS: Early diagnosis of lung cancer, editorial. *Am Rev Respir Dis* 1977; 116:399–402.

126. Fontana RS, Sanderson DR, Taylor WF, et al: Early lung cancer detection: Results of the initial (prevalence) radiologic cytologic screening in the Mayo Clinic study. *Am Rev Respir Dis* 1984; 130:561–565.

127. Fraser RG, Pare JAP: *Diagnosis of Diseases of the Chest*, ed 2. Philadelphia, WB Saunders Co, 1979.

128. Freant LJ, Joseph WL, Adkins PC: Scar carcinoma of the lung: Fact or fantasy? *Ann Thorac Surg* 1974; 17:531–537.

129. Frost JK, Ball WC, Levin ML, et al: Early lung cancer detection: Results of initial (prevalence) radiologic and cytologic screening in the Johns Hopkins study. *Am Rev Respir Dis* 1984; 130:549–554.

130. Furgerson WB, Bachman LB, O'Toole WF: Waldenstrom's macroglobulinemia with diffuse pulmonary infiltration: Lung biopsy and response to chlorambucil therapy. *Am Rev Respir Dis* 1963; 88:689–697.

131. Gamsu G, Webb WR, Sheldon P, et al: Nuclear magnetic resonance imaging of the thorax. *Radiology* 1983; 147:473–480.

132. Garland LH: The rate of growth and natural duration of primary bronchial cancer. *AJR* 1966; 96:604–611.

133. Garland LH, Beier RL, Coulson RL, et al: The apparent sites of origin of carcinoma of the lung. *Radiology* 1962; 78:1–11.

134. Garland LH, Coulson W, Wollin E: The rate of growth and apparent duration of untreated primary bronchial carcinoma. *Cancer* 1963; 16:694–707.

135. Geddes DM: The natural history of lung cancer: A review based on rates of tumor growth. *Br J Dis Chest* 1979; 73:1–17.

136. Genereux GP, Howie JL: Normal mediastinal lymph node size and number: CT and anatomic study. *AJR* 1984; 142:1095–1100.

137. Gilroy JA, Adams AB: Extraosseus infiltration in multiple myeloma. *Radiology* 1959; 78:406–409.

138. Giustra PE, Stassa G: The multiple presentations of bronchial adenoma. *Radiology* 1969; 93:1013–1019.

139. Glazer GM, Gross BH, Aisen AM, et al: Imaging of the pulmonary hilum: A prospective comparative study in patients with lung cancer. *AJR* 1985; 145:245–248.

140. Glazer GM, Gross BH, Quint LE, et al: Normal mediastinal lymph nodes: Number and size according to American Thoracic Society mapping. *AJR* 1985; 144:261–265.

141. Glazer GM, Orringer MB, Gross BH, et al: The mediastinum in non-small cell lung cancer: CT-surgical correlation. *AJR* 1984; 142:1101–1105.

142. Glazer G, Webb WR: Laryngeal papillomatosis with pulmonary spread in a 69-year-old man. *AJR* 1979; 132:820–822.

143. Glazer HS, Duncan-Meyer J, Aronberg DJ, et al: Pleural and chest wall invasion in bronchogenic carcinoma: CT evaluation. *Radiology* 1985; 157:191–194.

144. Glickstein M, Kornstein MJ, Pietra GG, et al: Non-lymphomatous lymphoid disorders of the lung. *AJR* 1986; 147:227–237.

145. Godwin JD, Webb WR, Savoca CJ, et al: Multiple, thin walled cystic lesions of the lung. *AJR* 1980; 135:593–604.

146. Goldmeier E: Limits of visibility of bronchogenic carcinoma. *Am Rev Respir Dis* 1965; 91:232–239.

147. Goldstein MS, Rush M, Johnson P, et al: A calcified adenocarcinoma of the lung with very high CT numbers. *Radiology* 1984; 150:285–286.

148. Goldstraw P, Kurzer M, Edwards D: Preoperative staging of lung cancer: Accuracy of computed tomography versus mediastinoscopy. *Thorax* 1983; 38:10–15.

149. Good CA: Asymptomatic bronchial adenoma. *Mayo Clin Proc* 1953; 28:577–586.

150. Good CA: The solitary pulmonary nodule: A problem of management. *Radiol Clin North Am* 1963; 1:429–438.

151. Gramiak R, Koerner HJ: A roentgen diagnostic observation in subpleural lipoma. *AJR* 1966; 98:465–467.

152. Grant DC, Seltzer SE, Antman KH, et al: Computed tomography of malignant pleural mesothelioma. *J Comput Assist Tomogr* 1983; 7:626–632.

153. Greenberg SD, Haley MD, Kenkins DE, et al: Lymphoplasmacytic pneumonia with accompanying dysproteinemia. *Arch Pathol* 1973; 96:73–80.

154. Greenfield H, Herman PC: Papillomatosis of the trachea and bronchi. *AJR* 1963; 89:45–50.

155. Grossman H, Winchester PH, Bragg DG, et al: Roentgenographic changes in childhood Hodgkin's disease. *AJR* 1970; 108:354–364.

156. Guccion JG, Rosen SH: Bronchopulmonary leiomyosarcoma and fibrosarcoma. A study of 32 cases and review of the literature. *Cancer* 1972; 30:836–847.

157. Hahn PF, Novelline RA, Mark EJ: Arteriography in the localization of massive pleural tumors. *AJR* 1982; 139:814–817.

158. Halprin GM, Ramirez RJ, Pratt PC: Lymphoid interstitial pneumonia. *Chest* 1972; 62:418–423.

159. Hamlin DJ, Burgener FA: CT including sagittal and coronal reconstruction in the evaluation of Pancoast tumors. *J Comput Tomogr* 1982; 6:35–40.

160. Han S, Wills JS, Allen O: Pulmonary blastoma: Case report and literature review. *AJR* 1976; 127:1048–1049.

161. Hayabuchi N, Russell WJ, Murakami J: Slow-growing lung cancer in a fixed population sample: Radiologic assessments. *Cancer* 1983; 52:1098–1104.

162. Hayabuchi N, Russell WJ, Murakami J, et al: Screening for lung cancer in a fixed population by biennial chest radiography. *Radiology* 1983; 148:369–373.

163. Hayward RH: Roentgenogram of the month. Migrating lung tumor. *Chest* 1974; 66:77–78.

164. Heaston DK, Putman CE, Rodan BA, et al: Solitary pulmonary metastases in high risk melanoma patients: A prospective comparison of conventional and computed tomography. *AJR* 1983; 141:169–174.

165. Heavey LR, Glazer GM, Gross BH, et al: The role of CT in staging radiographic T1N0M0 lung cancer. *AJR* 1986; 146:285–290.

166. Heelan RT, Flehinger BJ, Melamed MR, et al: Non-small-cell lung cancer: Results of New York screening program. *Radiology* 1984; 151:289–293.

167. Heelan RT, Martini N, Westcott JW, et al: Carcinomatous involvement of the hilum and mediastinum: Computed tomographic and magnetic resonance evaluation. *Radiology* 1985; 156:111–115.

168. Heitzman ER: *The lung: Radiologic-Pathologic Correlations,* ed 2. St Louis, CV Mosby Co, 1984.

169. Heitzman ER, Markarian B, DeLise CT: Lymphoproliferative disorders of the thorax. *Semin Roentgenol* 1975; 10:73–81.

170. Heitzman ER, Markarian B, Raasch BN, et al: Pathways of tumor spread through the lung: Radiologic correlations with anatomy and pathology. *Radiology* 1982; 144:3–14.

171. Heller RM, Janower ML, Weber AL: The radiological manifestations of malignant pleural mesothelioma. *AJR* 1970; 108:53–59.

172. Helman CA, Kieton GR, Benatar SR: Lymphoid interstitial pneumonia with associated chronic active

hepatitis and renal tubular acidosis. *Am Rev Respir Dis* 1977; 115:161–164.

173. Herman PG, Hillman B, Pinkus G, et al: Unusual noninfectious granulomas of the lung. *Radiology* 1976; 121:287–292.

174. Herzog KA, Putman CE: Pulmonary blastoma. *Br J Radiol* 1974; 47:286–288.

175. Hicken P, Dobie JC, Frew E: The radiology of lymphomatoid granulomatosis in the lung. *Clin Radiol* 1979; 30:661–664.

176. Higgins GA, Shields TW, Keehn RJ: The solitary pulmonary nodule: Ten-year follow up of Veterans Administration–Armed Forces cooperative study. *Arch Surg* 1975; 110:570–575.

177. Hill CA: Bronchioloalveolar carcinoma: A review. *Radiology* 1984; 150:15–20.

178. Horning SJ, Rosenberg SA: The natural history of initially untreated low-grade non-Hodgkin's lymphoma. *N Engl J Med* 1984; 311:1471–1475.

179. Huang D, Weisbrod GL, Chamberlain DW: Unusual radiologic presentations of bronchioloalveolar cell carcinoma. *J Can Assoc Radiol* 1986; 37:94–99.

180. Huhti E, Saloheimo M, Sutinen S: The value of roentgenologic screening in lung cancer. *Am Rev Respir Dis* 1983; 128:395–398.

181. Husband JE, Barrett A, Peckham MJ: Evaluation of computed tomography in the management of testicular teratoma. *Br J Urol* 1981; 53:179–183.

182. Hutchinson WB, Friedenberg MJ: Intrathoracic mesothelioma. *Radiology* 1963; 80:937–945.

183. Hutchinson WB, Friedenberg MJ, Saltzstein SL: Primary pulmonary pseudolymphoma. *Radiology* 1964; 82:48–56.

184. Im JG, Choi BI, Park JH, et al: CT findings of lobar bronchioloalveolar carcinoma—a case report. *J Comput Assist Tomogr* 1986; 10:320–322.

185. Israel RH: Mycosis fungoides with rapidly progressive pulmonary infiltration. *Radiology* 1977; 125:10.

186. Israel HL, Patchefsky AS, Saldana MJ: Wegener's granulomatosis, lymphomatoid granulomatosis, and benign lymphocytic angiitis and granulomatosis: Recognition and treatment. *Ann Intern Med* 1977; 87:691–699.

187. Jackman RJ, Good CA, Clagett OT, et al: Survival rates in peripheral bronchogenic carcinoma up to four centimeters in diameter presenting as solitary pulmonary nodules. *J Thorac Cardiovasc Surg* 1969; 57:1–8.

188. Janower ML, Blennerhassett JB: Lymphangitic spread of metastatic cancer to the lung: A radiologic-pathologic classification. *Radiology* 1971; 101:267–273.

189. Jenkins PF, Ward MJ, Davies P, et al: Non-Hodgkin's lymphoma, chronic lymphocytic leukaemia and the lung. *Br J Dis Chest* 1981; 75:22–30.

190. Jett JR, Cortese DA, Fontana RS: Lung cancer: Current concepts and prospects. *CA* 1983; 33:74–86.

191. Jochelson MS, Balikian JP, Mauch P, et al: Peri- and paracardial involvement in lymphoma in a radiographic study of 11 cases. *AJR* 1983; 140:483–488.

192. Johnson DH, Hainsworth JD, Greco FA: Pancoast's syndrome and small cell lung cancer. *Chest* 1982; 82:602–606.

193. Julsrud PR, Brown LR, Li CY, et al: Pulmonary processes of mature-appearing lymphocytes: Pseudolymphoma, well differentiated lymphocytic lymphoma, and lymphocytic interstitial pneumonitis. *Radiology* 1978; 127:289–296.

194. Kaplan JO, Morillo G, Weinfeld A, et al: Mediastinal adenopathy in myeloma. *J Can Assoc Radiol* 1980; 31:48–49.

195. Karasik A, Modam M, Jacob CO, et al: Increased risk of lung cancer in patients with chondromatous hamartoma. *J Thorac Cardiovasc Surg* 1980; 80:217–220.

196. Katzenstein AL, Askin FB: *Surgical Pathology of Nonneoplastic Lung Disease.* Philadelphia, WB Saunders Co, 1982.

197. Katzenstein AA, Carrington CB, Liebow AA: Lymphomatoid granulomatosis. A clinicopathologic study of 152 cases. *Cancer* 1979; 43:360–373.

198. Kennedy JL, Nathwani BN, Burke JS, et al: Pulmonary lymphomas and other pulmonary lymphoid lesions: A clinicopathologic and immunologic study of 64 patients. *Cancer* 1985; 56:539–552.

199. Khan A, Gersten KC, Garvey J, et al: Oblique hilar tomography, computed tomography, and mediastinoscopy for prethoracotomy staging of bronchogenic carcinoma. *Radiology* 1985; 156:295–298.

200. Khoury MB, Godwin JD, Halvorsen R, et al: Role of chest CT in non-Hodgkin's lymphoma. *Radiology* 1986; 158:659–662.

201. Kilburn KH, Schmidt AM: Intrathoracic plasmacytoma: Report of a case and review of the literature. *Arch Intern Med* 1960; 106:862–869.

202. Kilgore TL, Chasen MH: Endobronchial non-Hodgkin's lymphoma. *Chest* 1983; 84:58–61.

203. Kinare SG, Parulkar GB, Panday SR, et al: Extensive ossification in a pulmonary plasmacytoma. *Thorax* 1965; 20:206–210.

204. Kirsch MM, Kahn DR, Gago O, et al: Treatment of bronchogenic carcinoma with mediastinal metastases. *Ann Thorac Surg* 1971; 12:11–21.

205. Klatte EC, Yardley J, Smith EB, et al: The pulmonary manifestations and complications of leukemia. *AJR* 1963; 89:598–609.

206. Kornfeld H, Axelrod JL: Pulmonary presentation of Kaposi's sarcoma in a homosexual patient. *Am Rev Respir Dis* 1983; 127:248–249.

207. Kradin RL, Mark EJ: Benign lymphoid disorders of the lung with a theory regarding their development. *Hum Pathol* 1983; 14:857–867.

208. Kramer SS, Wehunt WD, Stocker JT, et al: Pulmo-

nary manifestations of juvenile laryngotracheal papillomatosis. *AJR* 1985; 144:687–694.

209. Kreel L: Computed tomography in mesothelioma. *Semin Oncol* 1981; 8:302–312.

210. Kreyberg L: *Histological Typing of Lung Tumors.* Vol 1. *International Histological Classification of Tumors.* Geneva, World Health Organization, 1967.

211. Kuhlman JE, Fishman EK, Kuhajda FP, et al: Solitary bronchioloalveolar carcinoma: CT criteria. *Radiology* 1988; 167:379–382.

212. Kundel HL: Predictive value and threshold detectability of lung tumors. *Radiology* 1981; 139:25–29.

213. Kuriyama K, Tateishi R, Doi O, et al: CT-pathologic correlation in small peripheral lung cancers. *AJR* 1987; 149:1139–1143.

214. Law MR, Gregor A, Husband JE, et al: Computed tomography in the assessment of malignant mesothelioma of the pleura. *Clin Radiol* 1982; 33:67–70.

215. Lawson RM, Ramanathan L, Hurley G, et al: Bronchial adenoma: Review of an 18 year experience at the Brompton Hospital. *Thorax* 1976; 31:245–252.

216. Ledor K, Fish B, Chaise L, et al: CT of pulmonary hamartomas. *J Comput Tomogr* 1981; 5:343–344.

217. Legha SS, Muggia FM: Pleural mesothelioma: Clinical features and therapeutic implications. *Ann Intern Med* 1977; 87:612–613.

218. Lehar TJ, Carr DT, Miller WE, et al: Roentgenographic appearance of bronchogenic adenocarcinoma. *Am Rev Respir Dis* 1967; 96:245–248.

219. Levinson AI, Hopewell PC, Stites DP, et al: Coexistent lymphoid interstitial pneumonia, pernicious anemia and agammaglobulinemia. *Arch Intern Med* 1976; 136:213–216.

220. Levitt RG, Glazer HS, Roper CL, et al: Magnetic resonance imaging of mediastinal and hilar masses: Comparison with CT. *AJR* 1985; 145:9–14.

221. Lewis E, Bernadino ME, Farha P, et al: Computed tomography and routine chest radiography: oat cell carcinoma of the lung. *J Comput Assist Tomogr* 1982; 6:739–745.

222. Lewis MI, Horak DA, Yellin A, et al: Roentgenogram of the month. The case of the moving intrathoracic mass. *Chest* 1985; 88:897–898.

223. Lewis JW, Madrazo BL, Gross SC: The value of radiographic and computed tomography in the staging of lung carcinoma. *Ann Thorac Surg* 1982; 34:553–558.

224. Libshitz HI: Malignant pleural mesothelioma: The role of computed tomography. *J Comput Tomogr* 1984; 8:15–20.

225. Libshitz HI, Baber CE, Hammond CB: The pulmonary metastases of choriocarcinoma. *Obstet Gynecol* 1977; 49:412–416.

226. Libshitz HI, Jing BS, Wallace S, et al: Sterilized metastases: A diagnostic and therapeutic dilemma. *AJR* 1983; 140:15–19.

227. Libshitz HI, McKenna RJ: Mediastinal lymph node size in lung cancer. *AJR* 1984; 143:715–718.

228. Libshitz HI, McKenna RJ, Haynie TP, et al: Mediastinal evaluation in lung cancer. *Radiology* 1984; 151:295–299.

229. Liebow AA: Pathology of carcinoma of the lung as related to the roentgen shadow. *AJR* 1955; 74:383–401.

230. Liebow AA: The J. Burns Amberson lecture—pulmonary angiitis and granulomatosis. *Am Rev Respir Dis* 1973; 108:1–18.

231. Liebow AA, Carrington CB: Diffuse pulmonary lymphoreticular infiltrations associated with dysproteinemia. *Med Clin North Am* 1973; 57:809–843.

232. Liebow AA, Carrington CB, Friedman PJ: Lymphomatoid granulomatosis. *Hum Pathol* 1972; 3:457–558.

233. Light RW: *Pleural Disease.* Philadelphia, Lea & Febiger, 1983.

234. Light RW, Ball WB: Glucose and amylase in pleural effusions. *JAMA* 1973; 225:257–260.

235. Limas C, Japaze H, Garcia-Bunuel R: "Scar" carcinoma of the lung. *Chest* 1971; 59:219–222.

236. Long JC, Mihm MC: Mycosis fungoides with extracutaneous dissemination: A distinct clinicopathologic entity. *Cancer* 1974; 34:1745–1755.

237. Luddington LG, Verska JJ, Howard T, et al: Bronchiolar carcinoma (alveolar cell), another great imitator: A review of 41 cases. *Chest* 1972; 61:622–628.

238. Lukes RJ, Collins RD: Immunological characterization of human malignant lymphomas. *Cancer* 1974; 34:1488–1503.

239. Lukes RJ, Craver LF, Hall TC, et al: Report of the nomenclature committee. *Cancer Res* 1966; 26:1311.

240. MacDonald JB: Lung involvement in Hodgkin's disease. *Thorax* 1977; 32:664–667.

241. MacFarlane A, Davies D: Diffuse lymphoid interstitial pneumonia. *Thorax* 1973; 28:768–776.

242. Madewell JE, Feigin DS: Benign tumors of the lung. *Semin Roentgenol* 1977; 12:175–186.

243. Madri JA, Carter D: Scar cancers of the lung: Origin and significance. *Hum Pathol* 1984; 15:625–631.

244. Maile CW, Moore AV, Ulreich S, et al: Chest radiographic-pathologic correlation in adult leukemia patients. *Invest Radiol* 1983; 18:495–499.

245. Maile CW, Rodan BA, Godwin JD, et al: Calcification in pulmonary metastases. *Br J Radiol* 1982; 55:108–113.

246. Major D, Meltzer MH, Nedwich A, et al: Waldenstrom's macroglobulinemia presenting as a pulmonary mass. *Chest* 1973; 64:760–762.

247. Marglin SI, Soulen RL, Blank N, et al: Mycosis fungoides: Radiographic manifestations of extracutaneous intrathoracic involvement. *Radiology* 1979; 130:35–37.

248. Marriott AE, Weisbrod G: Bronchogenic carcinoma associated with pulmonary infarction. *Radiology* 1982; 145:593–597.

249. Martin E: Leiomyomatous lung lesions: A proposed classification. *AJR* 1983; 141:269–272.

250. Martini N, Beattie EJ, Flehinger BJ, et al: Prospective study of 455 lung carcinomas with mediastinal lymph node metastasis. *J Thorac Cardiovasc Surg* 1980; 80:390–397.

251. Martini N, Heelan R, Westcott J, et al: Comparative merits of conventional computed tomographic and magnetic resonance imaging in assessing mediastinal involvement in surgically confirmed lung carcinoma. *J Thorac Cardiovasc Surg* 1985; 90:639–648.

252. Mazumdar P, Abraham S, Damodaran VN, et al: Pulmonary plasmacytoma: A case report. *Am Rev Respir Dis* 1969; 100:866–869.

253. McCauley DI, Naidich DP, Leitman BS, et al: Radiographic patterns of opportunistic lung infections and Kaposi's sarcoma in homosexual men. *AJR* 1982; 139:653–658.

254. McDonald AD, Harper A, EL Attar OA, et al: Epidemiology of primary malignant mesothelial tumors in Canada. *Cancer* 1970; 26:914–919.

255. McGuinnis EJ, Lull RJ: Bronchial adenoma causing unilateral absence of pulmonary perfusion. *Radiology* 1976; 120:367–368.

256. McLeod TC, Kalisher L, Stark P, et al: Intrathoracic lymph node metastases from extrathoracic neoplasm. *AJR* 1978; 131:403–407.

257. McLoud TC, Isler RJ, Novelline RA, et al: The apical cap. *AJR* 1981; 137:299–306.

258. Meade JB, Whitwell F, Bickford BJ, et al: Primary haemangiopericytoma of lung. *Thorax* 1974; 29:1–15.

259. Melamed MR, Flehinger BJ, Zaman MB, et al: Screening for early lung cancer: Results of the Memorial Sloan-Kettering study in New York. *Chest* 1984; 86:44–53.

260. Mendelsohn SL, Fagelman D, Zwanger-Mendelsohn S: Endobronchial lipoma demonstrated by CT. *Radiology* 1983; 148:790–792.

261. Metzger RA, Mulhern CB, Arger PH, et al: CT differentiation of solitary from diffuse bronchioloalveolar carcinoma. *J Comput Assist Tomogr* 1981; 5:830–833.

262. Meyer EC, Liebow AA: Relationship of interstitial pneumonia, honeycombing and atypical epithelial proliferation to cancer of the lung. *Cancer* 1965; 18:322–351.

263. Meyer JA, Linggood RM, Lindfors KK, et al: Impact of thoracic computed tomography on radiation planning in Hodgkin's disease. *J Comput Assist Tomogr* 1984; 8:892–894.

264. Meyer PC: Metastatic carcinoma of the pleura. *Thorax* 1966; 21:437–443.

265. Miller WT, Husted J, Freiman D, et al: Bronchioloalveolar carcinoma: Two clinical entities with one pathological diagnosis. *AJR* 1978; 130:905–912.

266. Mirvis S, Dutcher JP, Haney PJ, et al: CT of malignant pleural mesothelioma. *AJR* 1983; 140:665–670.

267. Montes M, Tomasi TB, Noehren TH, et al: Lymphoid interstitial pneumonia with monoclonal gammopathy. *Am Rev Respir Dis* 1968; 98:272–280.

268. Monzon CM, Gilchrist GS, Burgert EO, et al: Plasma cell granuloma of the lung in children. *Pediatrics* 1982; 70:268–274.

269. Morris JC, Rosen MJ, Marchevsky A, et al: Lymphocytic interstitial pneumonia in patients at risk for the acquired immune deficiency syndrome. *Chest* 1987; 91:63–67.

270. Mountain CF: A new international staging system for lung cancer. *Chest* 1986; 89(suppl):225S–233S.

271. Mountain CF, McMurtrey MJ, Hermes KE: Surgery for pulmonary metastasis: A 20 year experience. *Ann Thorac Surg* 1984; 38:323–330.

272. Muhm JR, Brown LR, Crowe JK, et al: Comparison of whole lung tomography and computed tomography for detecting pulmonary nodules. *AJR* 1978; 131:981–984.

273. Muhm JR, Miller EW, Fontana RS, et al: Lung cancer detected during a screening program using four month chest radiographs. *Radiology* 1983; 148:609–615.

274. Munk PL, Muller NL, Miller RR, et al: Pulmonary lymphangitic carcinomatosis: CT and pathologic findings. *Radiology* 1988; 166:705–709.

275. Musset D, Grenier P, Carette MF, et al: Primary lung cancer staging: Prospective comparative study of MR imaging with CT. *Radiology* 1986; 160:607–611.

276. Myers TJ, Cole SR, Klatsky AU, et al: Respiratory failure due to pulmonary leukostasis following chemotherapy of acute nonlymphocytic leukemia. *Cancer* 1983; 51:1808–1813.

277. Naidich DP, McCauley DI, Siegelman SS: Computed tomography of bronchial adenomas. *J Comput Assist Tomogr* 1982; 6:725–732.

278. Nash FA, Morgan JM, Tomkins JC: South London lung cancer study. *Br Med J* 1968; 2:715–721.

279. Nathan MH, Collins VP, Adams RA: Differentiation of benign and malignant pulmonary nodules by growth rate. *Radiology* 1962; 79:221–232.

280. National Cancer Institute–sponsored study of classifications of non-Hodgkin's lymphomas: Summary and description of a working formulation for clinical usage. *Cancer* 1982; 49:2112–2135.

281. Neifeld JP, Michaelis LL, Doppman JL: Suspected pulmonary metastases. *Cancer* 1977; 39:383–387.

282. Nichols DM, Johnson MA: Calcification in a pleural mesothelioma. *J Can Assoc Radiol* 1983; 34:311–313.

283. O'Connell RS, McLoud TC, Wilkins EW: Superior sulcus tumor: Radiographic diagnosis and workup. *AJR* 1983; 140:25–30.

284. Oels HC, Harrison EG, Carr DT, et al: Diffuse ma-

lignant mesothelioma of the pleura: A review of 37 cases. *Chest* 1971; 60:664–670.

285. Ohtomo K, Araki T, Yashiro N, et al: Pulmonary blastoma in children. *Radiology* 1983; 147:101–104.

286. O'Keefe ME, Good CA, McDonald JR: Calcification in solitary nodule of the lung. *AJR* 1957; 77:1023–1033.

287. Okike N, Bernatz PE, Woolner LB: Localized mesothelioma of the pleura: Benign and malignant variants. *J Thorac Cardiovasc Surg* 1978; 75:363–372.

288. Osborne DR, Korobkin M: Detection of intrathoracic lymph node metastases from lung carcinoma, letter. *Radiology* 1982; 144:187–188.

289. Osborne DR, Korobkin M, Ravin CE, et al: Comparison of plain radiography, conventional tomography and computed tomography in detecting intrathoracic metastases from lung carcinoma. *Radiology* 1982; 142:157–161.

290. Overholt RH, Neptune WB, Ashraf MM: Primary cancer of the lung. A 42 year experience. *Ann Thorac Surg* 1975; 20:511–519.

291. Pancoast HK: Superior sulcus tumor: Tumor characterized by pain, Horner's syndrome, destruction of bone and atrophy of hand muscles. *JAMA* 1932; 99:1391–1396.

292. Parker BR, Castellino RA, Kaplan HS: Pediatric Hodgkin's disease: I. Radiographic evaluation. *Cancer* 1976; 37:2430–2435.

293. Paulson DL: Carcinomas in the superior pulmonary sulcus. *J Thorac Cardiovasc Surg* 1975; 70:1095–1104.

294. Peacock MJ, Whitwell F: Pulmonary blastoma. *Thorax* 1976; 31:197–204.

295. Pearl M: Post inflammatory pseudotumor of the lung in children. *Radiology* 1972; 105:391–395.

296. Pearlberg JH, Sandler MA, Beute GH, et al: T1N0M0 bronchogenic carcinoma: Assessment by CT. *Radiology* 1985; 157:187–190.

297. Pearson FG, DeLarue NC, Ilves R, et al: Significance of positive superior mediastinal nodes identified at mediastinoscopy in patients with resectable cancer of the lung. *J Thorac Cardiovasc Surg* 1982; 83:1–11.

298. Pennes DR, Glazer GM, Wimbish KH, et al: Chest wall invasion by lung cancer: Limitations of CT evaluation. *AJR* 1985; 144:507–511.

299. Peuchot M, Libshitz HI: Pulmonary metastatic disease: Radiologic-surgical correlation. *Radiology* 1987; 164:719–722.

300. Platt JF, Glazer GM, Gross BH, et al: CT evaluation of mediastinal lymph nodes in lung cancer: Influence of the lobar site of the primary neoplasm. *AJR* 1987; 149:683–686.

301. Pock Steen OC: Bronchial adenoma. *Acta Radiol* 1959; 51:266–272.

302. Poirier TJ, Van Ordstrand HS: Pulmonary chondromatous hamartoma: Report of seventeen cases and review of the literature. *Chest* 1971; 59:50–55.

303. Poon PY, Bronskill MJ, Henkelman RM, et al: Mediastinal lymph node metastases from bronchogenic carcinoma: Detection with MR imaging and CT. *Radiology* 1987; 162:651–656.

304. Poulsen JT, Jacobsen M, Francis D: Probable malignant transformation of a pulmonary hamartoma. *Thorax* 1979; 34:557–558.

305. Primack A: The production of markers by bronchogenic carcinoma: A review. *Semin Oncol* 1974; 1:235–244.

306. Pugatch RD, Gale ME: Obscure pulmonary masses: Bronchial impaction revealed by CT. *AJR* 1983; 141:909–914.

307. Quint LE, Glazer GM, Orringer MB, et al: Mediastinal lymph node detection and sizing at CT and autopsy. *AJR* 1986; 147:469–472.

308. Quint LE, Glazer GM, Orringer MB: Central lung masses: Prediction with CT of need for pneumonectomy versus lobectomy. *Radiology* 1987; 165:735–738.

309. Rabinowitz JG, Efremidis SC, Cohen B, et al: A comparative study of mesothelioma and asbestosis using computed tomography and conventional chest radiography. *Radiology* 1982; 144:453–460.

310. Ramanathan T: Primary leiomyosarcoma of the lung. *Thorax* 1974; 29:482–489.

311. Rappaport H: Tumors of the hematopoietic system, in Rappaport H (ed): *Atlas of Tumor Pathology*, section 2, fascicle 8. Washington, DC, Armed Forces Institute of Pathology, 1966.

312. Richey HM, Matthews JI, Helsei RA, et al: Thoracic CT scanning in the staging of bronchogenic carcinoma. *Chest* 1984; 85:218–221.

313. Rigler LG: A roentgen study of the evolution of carcinoma of the lung. *J Thorac Surg* 1957; 34:283–297.

314. Rigler LG: The roentgen signs of carcinoma of the lung. *AJR* 1955; 74:415–428.

315. Robbins SL, Cotran RS, Kumar V: *Pathologic Basis of Disease*, ed 3. Philadelphia, WB Saunders Co, 1984.

316. Rohlfing BM, White EA, Webb WR, et al: Hilar and mediastinal adenopathy caused by bacterial abscess of the lung. *Radiology* 1978; 128:289–293.

317. Rosenbaum HD, Alavi SM, Bryant LR: Pulmonary parenchymal spread of juvenile laryngeal papillomatosis. *AJR* 1968; 90:654–660.

318. Rosenberg SA, Kaplan HS: Evidence for an orderly progression in the spread of Hodgkin's disease. *Cancer Res* 1966; 26:1225–1231.

319. Rosenow EC, Carr DT: Bronchogenic carcinoma. *CA* 1979; 29:233–245.

320. Ross JS, Ellman L: Leukemic infiltration of the lungs in the chemotherapeutic era. *Am J Clin Pathol* 1974; 61:235–241.

321. Ross JS, O'Donovan PB, Noroa R, et al: Magnetic resonance of the chest: Initial experience with imag-

ing and in vivo T1 and T2 calculations. *Radiology* 1984; 152:95–101.

322. Rostock RA, Giangreco A, Wharam MD, et al: CT scan modification in the treatment of mediastinal Hodgkin's disease. *Cancer* 1982; 49:2267–2275.

323. Rubin DL, Blank N: Rapid pulmonary dissemination in mycosis fungoides simulating pneumonia: A case report and review of the literature. *Cancer* 1985; 56:649–651.

324. Rubinstein I, Baum GL, Kalter Y, et al: The influence of cell type and lymph node metastases on survival of patients with carcinoma of the lung undergoing thoracotomy. *Am Rev Respir Dis* 1979; 119:253–262.

325. Sahn SA: Malignant pleural effusions. *Clin Chest Med* 1983; 6:113–125.

326. Saltzstein SL: Pulmonary malignant lymphomas and pseudolymphomas: Classification, therapy and prognosis. *Cancer* 1963; 16:928–955.

327. Scharifker D, Kaneko M: Localized fibrous "mesothelioma" of pleura (submesothelial fibroma). *Cancer* 1979; 43:627–635.

328. Schnyder PA, Gamsu G: CT of the pretracheal retrocaval space. *AJR* 1981; 136:303–308.

329. Schraufnagel D, Morin JE, Wang NS: Endobronchial lipoma. *Chest* 1979; 75:97–99.

330. Schraufnagel D, Peloquin A, Pare JAP, et al: Differentiating bronchioloalveolar carcinoma from adenocarcinoma. *Am Rev Respir Dis* 1982; 125:74–79.

331. Schwartz EE, Katz SM, Mandell GA: Postinflammatory pseudotumors of the lung: Fibrous histiocytoma and related lesions. *Radiology* 1980; 136:609–613.

332. Shaner EG, Chang AE, Doppman JL, et al: Comparison of computed and conventional whole lung tomography in detecting pulmonary nodules: A prospective radiology-pathology study. *AJR* 1978; 131:51–54.

333. Shapiro MP, Gale ME, Carter BL: Variable CT appearance of plasma cell granuloma of the lung. *J Comput Assist Tomogr* 1987; 11:49–51.

334. Shapiro R, Wilson GL, Yasner R, et al: A useful roentgen sign in the diagnosis of localized bronchioloalveolar carcinoma. *AJR* 1972; 114:516–524.

335. Shin MS, Jackson LK, Shelton RW, et al: Giant cell carcinoma of the lung: Clinical and roentgenographic manifestations. *Chest* 1986; 89:366–369.

336. Shuman LS, Libshitz HI: Solid pleural manifestations of lymphoma. *AJR* 1984; 142:269–273.

337. Siegelman SS, Khouri NF, Scott WW, et al: Computed tomography of the solitary pulmonary nodule. *Sem Roentgenol* 1984; 19:165–172.

338. Siegelman SS, Khouri NF, Scott WW, et al: Pulmonary hamartoma: CT findings. *Radiology* 1986; 160:313–317.

339. Silverberg E: Cancer statistics 1986. *CA* 1986; 36:9–25.

340. Simon G: Intrathoracic Hodgkin's disease: I. Less common intrathoracic manifestations of Hodgkin's disease. *Br J Radiol* 1967; 40:926–929.

341. Sindelar WF, Bagley DH, Felix EL, et al: Lung tomography in cancer patients. *JAMA* 1978; 240:2060–2063.

342. Sivit CJ, Schwartz AM, Rockoff SD: Kaposi's sarcoma of the lung in AIDS: Radiologic-pathologic analysis. *AJR* 1987; 148:25–28.

343. Spencer H: *Pathology of the Lung*, ed 4. Philadelphia, WB Saunders Co, 1985.

344. Spizarny DL, Gross BH, Shephard JO: CT findings in localized fibrous mesothelioma of the pleural fissure. *J Comput Assist Tomogr* 1986; 10:942–944.

345. Spizarny DL, Shepard JAO, McLoud TC, et al: CT of adenoid cystic carcinoma of the trachea. *AJR* 1986; 146:1129–1132.

346. Stackhouse EM, Harrison EG, Ellis FH: Primary mixed malignancies of the lung: Carcinosarcoma and blastoma. *J Thorac Cardiovasc Surg* 1969; 57:385–399.

347. *Staging of Lung Cancer 1979*. Chicago, American Joint Committee for Cancer Staging and End-Results Reporting: Task Force on Lung Cancer, 1979.

348. Stark P: Multiple independent bronchogenic carcinomas. *Radiology* 1982; 145:599–601.

349. Steele SD: The solitary pulmonary nodule: Report of a cooperative study of resected asymptomatic solitary pulmonary nodules in males. *J Thorac Cardiovasc Surg* 1963; 46:21–39.

350. Stein MG, Mayo J, Muller N, et al: Pulmonary lymphangitic spread of carcinoma: Appearance on CT scans. *Radiology* 1987; 162:371–375.

351. Steinberg HV, Erwin BC: Metastases to the pleura: Sonographic detection. *J Clin Ultrasound* 1987; 15:276–279.

352. Stewart JG, MacMahon H, Viborny CJ, et al: Dystrophic calcification in carcinoma of the lung: Demonstration by CT. *AJR* 1987; 149:29–30.

353. Stollberg HO, Patt NL, MacEwen KF, et al: Hodgkin's disease of the lung. *AJR* 1964; 92:96–115.

354. Strauss MJ: The growth characteristic of lung cancer and its application to treatment design. *Semin Oncol* 1974; 1:167–174.

355. Strickland B: Intrathoracic Hodgkin's disease: II. Peripheral manifestations of Hodgkin's disease in the chest. *Br J Radiol* 1967; 40:930–938.

356. Strijk SP: Lymph node calcification in malignant lymphoma: Presentation of nine cases and a review of the literature. *Acta Radiol [Diagn]* (Stockh) 1985; 26:427–431.

357. Strimlan CV, Rosenow EC, Weiland LH, et al: Lymphocytic interstitial pneumonitis. Review of 13 cases. *Ann Intern Med* 1978; 88:616–621.

358. Strutynsky N, Balthazer EJ, Klein RM: Inflamma-

tory pseudotumours of the lung. *Br J Radiol* 1974; 47:94–96.

359. Swett HA, Wescott JL: Residual nonmalignant pulmonary nodules in choriocarcinoma. *Chest* 1974; 65:560–562.

360. Templeton AW, Moffat R, Nelson D: Bronchography and bronchial adenoma. *Chest* 1971; 59:59–61.

361. Teplick JG, Teplick SK, Haskin ME: Granular cell myoblastoma of the lung. *AJR* 1975; 125:890–894.

362. Theros EG: Varying manifestations of peripheral pulmonary neoplasms: A radiologic-pathologic correlative study. *AJR* 1977; 128:893–914.

363. Trapnell DH: The radiological appearances of lymphangitis carcinomatosa of the lung. *Thorax* 1964; 19:251–260.

364. van Buchem MA, Wondergem JH, Kool LJS, et al: Pulmonary leukostasis: Radiologic-pathologic study. *Radiology* 1987; 165:739–741.

365. Vath RR, Alexander CB, Fulmer JD: The lymphocytic infiltrative lung disease. *Clin Chest Med* 1982; 3:619–634.

366. Vernant JP, Brun B, Mannoni P, et al: Respiratory distress of hyperleukocytic granulocytic leukemias. *Cancer* 1979; 44:264–268.

367. Vincent RG, Pickien JW, Lane WW, et al: The changing histopathology of lung cancer: A review of 1682 cases. *Cancer* 1977; 39:1647–1653.

368. Vogelzang NJ, Stenlund R: Residual pulmonary nodules after combination chemotherapy of testicular cancer. *Radiology* 1983; 146:195–197.

369. Wagner JC, Sleggs CA, Marhand P: Diffuse pleural mesothelioma and absestos exposure in North Western Cape Province. *Br J Industr Med* 1960; 17:260–271.

370. Webb WR, Gamsu G: Thoracic metastasis in malignant melanoma: A radiographic survey of 65 patients. *Chest* 1977; 71:176–181.

371. Webb WR, Gamsu G, Stark DD, et al: Magnetic resonance imaging of the normal and abnormal pulmonary hila. *Radiology* 1984; 152:89–94.

372. Webb WR, Jeffrey RB, Godwin JD: Thoracic computed tomography in superior sulcus tumors. *J Comput Assist Tomogr* 1981; 5:361–365.

373. Webb WR, Jensen BG, Sollitto R, et al: Bronchogenic carcinoma: Staging with MR compared with staging with CT and surgery. *Radiology* 1985; 156:117–124.

374. Wechsler RJ, Rao VM, Steiner RM: The radiology of malignant mesothelioma. *CRC Crit Rev Diagn Imaging* 1984; 20:283–310.

375. Wechsler RJ, Steiner RM, Israel HL, et al: Chest radiograph in lymphomatoid granulomatosis: Comparison with Wegener granulomatosis. *AJR* 1984; 142:79–83.

376. Weisbrod GL, Yee AC: Computed tomographic diagnosis of pedunculated fibrous mesothelioma. *J Can Assoc Radiol* 1983; 34:147–148.

377. Whitcomb ME, Schwartz MJ, Keller AR, et al: Hodgkin's disease of the lung. *Am Rev Respir Dis* 1972; 106:79–85.

378. Williams MP, Husband JE, Heron CW: Intrathoracic manifestations of metastatic testicular seminoma: A comparison of chest radiographic and CT findings. *AJR* 1987; 149:473–475.

379. Wilson SR, Sanders DE, Delarie NC: Intrathoracic manifestations of amyloid disease. *Radiology* 1976; 102:283–289.

380. Winterbauer RH, Riggins RCK, Griesman FA, et al: Pleuropulmonary manifestations of Waldenstrom's macroglobulinemia. *Chest* 1974; 66:368–375.

381. Woodring JH, Fried AW, Chuang VP: Solitary cavities of the lung: Diagnostic implications of cavity wall thickness. *AJR* 1980; 135:1269–1271.

382. Woodring JH, Stelling CB: Adenocarcinoma of the lung: A tumor with a changing pleomorphic character. *AJR* 1983; 140:657–664.

383. Woolner LB, Fontana RS, Cortese DA, et al: Roentgenographically occult cancer: Pathologic findings and frequency of multicentricity during a 10 year period. *Mayo Clin Proc* 1984; 59:453–466.

384. Wycoco D, Raval B: An unusual presentation of mediastinal Hodgkin's lymphoma on computed tomography. *J Comput Tomogr* 1983; 7:187–188.

385. Wyman S, Weber AL: Calcification in intrathoracic nodes in Hodgkin's disease. *Radiology* 1969; 93:1021–1024.

386. Zerhouni EA, Stitik FP: Controversies in computed tomography of the thorax: The pulmonary nodule—lung cancer staging. *Radiol Clin North Am* 1985; 23:407–426.

387. Zerhouni EA, Naidich DP, Stitik FP, et al: Computed tomography of the pulmonary parenchyma: Part 2. Interstitial disease. *J Thorac Imaging* 1985; 1:54–64.

388. Zollikofer C, Casteñeda-Zuñiga W, Stenlund R, et al: Lung metastases from synovial sarcoma simulating granulomas. *AJR* 1980; 135:161–163.

Pulmonary Vascular Diseases and Pulmonary Edema

PULMONARY THROMBOEMBOLISM

Pulmonary thromboembolism is generally considered to be the third most common cause of death in hospitalized patients in the United States; only myocardial infarction and strokes result in a higher mortality rate.[58] Accurate incidence figures are difficult to obtain because they depend on how carefully embolism is searched for,[88] but pulmonary thromboembolism appears to be the sole or major cause of death in 10% to 15% of adults dying in the acute-care wards of general hospitals. It is particularly common in patients who die after severe burns or trauma.

Almost all emboli lodge within the branches of the pulmonary arteries, a few straddle the bifurcation of the main pulmonary artery (saddle emboli), and the occasional one lodges in the right side of the heart. Their effects[168, 272] are due primarily to mechanical obstruction. Reflex responses by the vessels and bronchi are transient and are believed to be clinically unimportant.[203] Virchow demonstrated, and it has since been repeatedly confirmed, that the bronchial circulation alone can sustain the lung parenchyma without infarction occurring.[60] Exactly why some pulmonary emboli cause infarction whereas others do not is uncertain, but it would appear that infarction occurs only when the combined bronchial and pulmonary arterial circulation is inadequate, a situation that applies particularly when emboli lodge peripherally in the pulmonary arterial tree and also when emboli occur in patients with heart failure or circulatory shock.[60, 251] It has been estimated that fewer than 15% of thromboemboli cause true infarction.[168]

Pathologically, pulmonary infarction is characterized by ischemic necrosis of alveolar walls, bronchioles, and blood vessels within an area of hemorrhage. Most infarcts occur in the lower lobes, and the majority are multiple. Usually they are cone-shaped areas of hemorrhage and edema that point toward the hilus and are based on the pleura, the pleura often being covered by a fibrinous exudate. Following infarction, fibrous replacement converts the infarct into a contracted scar with in-drawing of the pleura. In some cases hemorrhage is the dominant finding and there is no evidence of tissue necrosis. These lesions resolve without residual scar formation.

Pulmonary edema is a rare consequence of pulmonary embolism. Such patients usually have heart disease as well, and it seems probable that, in these patients, the pulmonary emboli precipitate left ventricular failure.[276] In massive pulmonary embolism, the edema may be due to over-perfusion of non-occluded portions of the pulmonary circulation.[121]

Emboli usually resolve, and the vessel lumen is restored.[58, 85, 152, 168] The main mechanism is presumed to be intravascular lysis and fragmentation.[208] In a few patients, the emboli do not lyse,[43, 247] and the presence of repeated, unresolved emboli may lead to chronic pulmonary hypertension.[58, 82, 204]

Clinically, the manifestations of pulmonary embolism are protean and often nonspecific. They range from no symptoms to sudden death. The symptoms and signs include dyspnea, chest pain that is often pleuritic but is sometimes anginal, cough, hemoptysis, tachypnea, hypotension, tachycardia, fever, and a pleural friction rub.[22, 272] Most patients have an underlying disorder, such as congestive heart failure, recent surgery, or carcinomatosis, or are immobilized.[22, 272] Because so many of the symptoms and signs of pulmonary embolism are nonspecific, the diagnosis is frequently overlooked.[200]

The standard laboratory tests are nonspecific. Arterial pO_2 values are usually, but not always, low. Serum lactic dehydrogenase values tend to be high, and although the electrocardiogram may show right axis shift, $S_1Q_3T_3$ pattern, or a new incomplete right bundle branch block, the test is often within normal limits or shows only preexisting or nonspecific changes.[93]

Accurate diagnosis is important because anticoagulant therapy, which is highly beneficial in patients with pulmonary emboli, carries significant risks[149, 187] that would not be justified in the absence of pulmonary embolism.

Imaging of Pulmonary Emboli

Plain chest radiography, radionuclide lung scanning, and pulmonary angiography are the major methods of establishing the diagnosis of pulmonary embolism. In most instances, plain chest films and radionuclide lung scans are obtained first, pulmonary angiography being reserved for those cases in which the risks of misdiagnosis outweigh the risks of the procedure.

Plain Chest Radiography

Many plain film signs of pulmonary embolism and infarction have been described.* Before discussing these signs, it is important to state clearly that none is specific and that the sensitivity of the signs is poor.[98, 241, 242] Even in patients with life-threatening pulmonary embolism, the plain chest radiograph can appear normal.[262] In one large series of 152 patients suspected to have pulmonary emboli, the overall sensitivity of the plain chest radiograph was 0.33 and the overall specificity was 0.59.[98] Therefore, the major role of the chest film is to exclude other diagnoses that might mimic pulmonary embolism, such

*References 47, 80, 133, 138, 158, 170, 180, 213, 218, 242, 243, 248, 265, 267.

as pneumothorax, pneumonia, or rib fractures, and to provide information that helps in interpreting the radionuclide scans. There will, however, be some cases in which the chest radiograph will suggest the diagnosis, and it is therefore important to appreciate the plain film signs, despite their low sensitivity and specificity. A useful framework for discussing the radiographic abnormalities in acute pulmonary emboli is to divide them into (1) pulmonary embolism without infarction, and (2) pulmonary embolism with infarction.[47]

Acute Pulmonary Embolism Without Infarction.—As discussed earlier, most emboli do not cause infarction. The few plain film signs of acute pulmonary embolism without infarction or hemorrhage are: oligemia of the lung beyond the occluded vessel (Westermark's sign) (Fig 8–1), increase in the size of the main pulmonary artery or of one of the descending pulmonary trunks, and elevation of a hemidiaphragm.* The nonspecificity of these signs is self-evident; emphysema and previous inflammatory disease may cause similar pulmonary vascular changes, and the position of the diaphragm is influenced by numerous factors, pulmonary embolism being just one.

Linear or disk-shaped densities[83] may be seen in patients with pulmonary emboli (Fig 8–2). These shadows represent discoid atelectases, not pulmonary infarcts,[252, 264] and are secondary to elevation of the diaphragm and inhibition of ventilation, features that are frequently encountered in patients with pulmonary emboli.[17]

Repetitive emboli may cause pulmonary arterial hypertension, a phenomenon which can be recognized radiologically (see the section "Pulmonary Arterial Hypertension" later in this chapter).

Acute Pulmonary Embolism With Infarction.—Pulmonary infarction gives rise to radiographically detectable consolidation, which is usually multifocal in distribution and predominant in the lower lung fields.[60] Such shadows usually occur 12 to 24 hours after the embolic episode, although their appearance may be delayed for several days.[256] The resulting opacity (Fig 8–3) may assume a variety of shapes depending on the location and underlying lobular architecture of the lung.[103, 112] Lobar consolidation is, however, unusual,[125] and a pattern resembling pulmonary edema is only occasionally encountered.

Hampton and Castleman described their famous

*References 48, 80, 133, 138, 180, 213, 243, and 265.

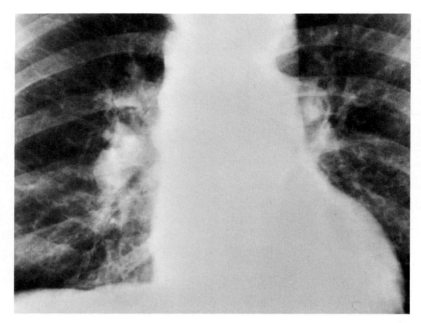

FIG 8–1.
Westermark's sign of pulmonary embolism. The right hilus is large, and the vessels beyond the hilus in the right lower lobe are small.

"hump" in an early paper which correlated the pathologic findings with the postmortem chest radiograph.[103] They emphasized that "infarcts are always in contact with pleural surfaces and that the shadows are rarely, if ever, triangular in shape." They noticed that the central margin of the infarct shadow may be rounded, hence the term "hump" (see Fig 8–3). In fact, a Hampton's hump is unusual[111] and is, in any event, a nonspecific finding. Air bronchograms are rarely seen on plain films,[13] an observation that could help in the differential diagnosis from pneumonia and other causes of consolidation.

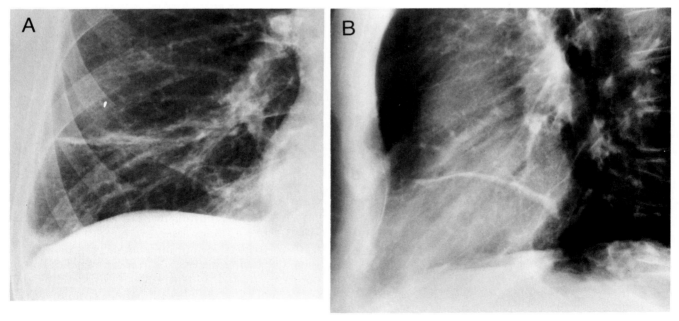

FIG 8–2.
A and **B,** PA and lateral radiographs showing discoid atelectasis in a patient with pulmonary embolism.

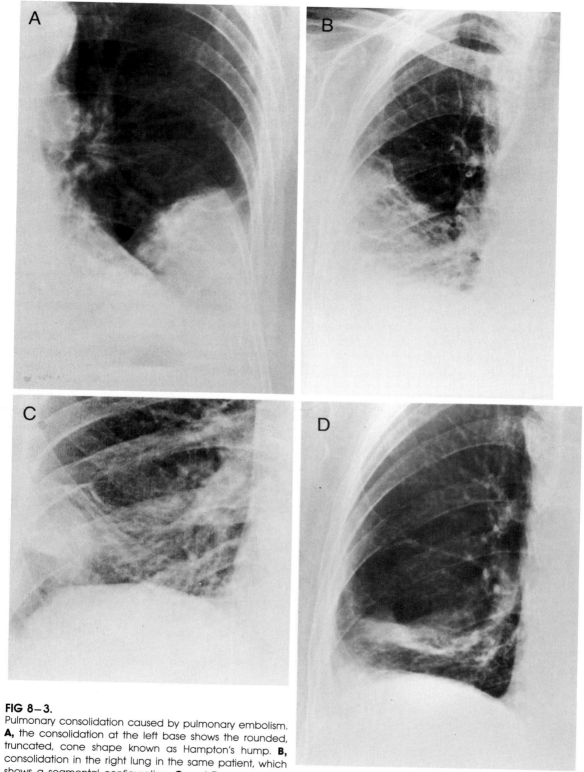

FIG 8–3.
Pulmonary consolidation caused by pulmonary embolism.
A, the consolidation at the left base shows the rounded, truncated, cone shape known as Hampton's hump. **B,** consolidation in the right lung in the same patient, which shows a segmental configuration. **C** and **D,** appearance of the right-sided consolidation **(C)** 2½ weeks later and **(D)** 5½ weeks later showing the gradual resolution "from the periphery."

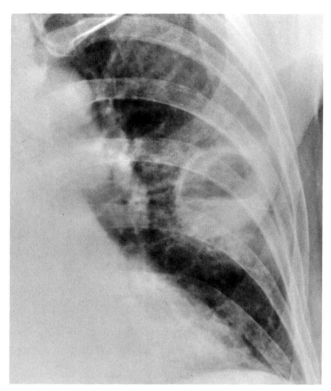

FIG 8–4.
Cavitating pulmonary infarct.

Frequently, the clinical features point to one or other diagnosis; if they do not, the radiographic appearance of the opacity cannot be relied upon to offer a distinction between the various causes of consolidation.

Where the consolidation is the result of pulmonary hemorrhage without true infarction, radiographic clearing will occur quickly, often within a week, whereas infarction takes several months to resolve[76] and frequently leads to the development of permanent linear scars.[219] By 3 months, infarct shadows are either totally resolved or show no more than linear scarring or pleural thickening.[156] As infarcts resolve they may "melt away like an ice-cube" (see Fig 8–3), whereas acute pneumonia disappears in a patchy fashion.[270] It may, therefore, be possible to suggest the diagnosis retrospectively, but this sign is, of course, of no value at the time when it is most needed.

Cavitation within the infarct is rare (Figs 8–4 and 8–5). It may be seen in the absence of infection, particularly in larger lesions,[99, 214] but usually cavitary infarcts are either secondarily infected or result from septic emboli.

Pleural effusions commonly accompany pulmonary embolism.[35, 76, 170, 241] In a carefully conducted prospective study, Bynum and Wilson showed that approximately 50% of patients with pulmonary embolism also had pleural effusion, often bloody.[40] In one-third of their cases, the effusion was an isolated finding, and, in the remaining two-thirds, it was ac-

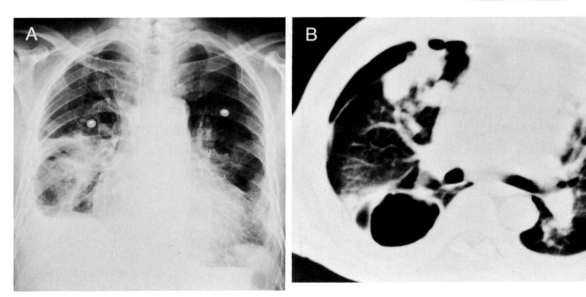

FIG 8–5.
Cavitating pulmonary infarcts. **A,** plain film. **B,** CT scan showing a mixture of cavitating and noncavitating infarcts, which on autopsy were not infected.

companied by radiographic evidence of pulmonary infarction or hemorrhage. Typically, the effusions are small and unilateral and appear soon after the onset of symptoms, but occasionally the effusions are bilateral and large.[242] It is interesting to note that almost all patients who had pleural effusion had chest pain on the same side as the effusion.[40] It appears probable that pleural effusions following pulmonary embolism are caused by infarction of the lung and that, in those cases in which no infarct shadow is visible on plain chest radiograph, the infarct is there but is either hidden from view or is not identifiable on the plain radiograph.[40]

Radionuclide Imaging

Perfusion Lung Scanning.—The most widely practiced methods of performing perfusion lung scanning involve injecting particles of approximately 10 to 60 μm in diameter into a peripheral vein. Most centers use either human albumin microspheres or macroaggregated albumin (MAA) labeled with technetium-99m (^{99m}Tc). These particles are similar in density to red blood cells, and they travel in the bloodstream to lodge in the pulmonary arterioles or capillaries. Imaging their distribution reflects regional blood flow provided there is uniform mixing of the particles in the right side of the heart (Fig 8–6). Some 200,000 to 500,000 particles are injected, but since there are approximately 300 million pulmonary arterioles with a diameter small enough to trap the particles, there is a large safety factor. The particles are biodegradable and leave the lung, with a biological half time of 6 to 8 hours.

It is the practice in some laboratories to reduce the number of particles in patients with severe pulmonary hypertension or known severe embolic disease. However, at least 50,000 particles are required to produce an image unblemished by visualization of the individual particles.[109] If there is right-to-left cardiac shunting, the particles will appear in the systemic arterial circulation. In the past, quantitation of the activity in the kidneys has been used as a crude index of the amount of shunting. There have been no apparent functional deficits resulting from the deposition of particles in areas such as the brain, but it would seem that caution should be exercised in cases of known right-to-left shunting.

The distribution of pulmonary blood flow is highly dependent on gravitational forces. In the supine patient blood flow is reasonably uniform from lung apex to lung base. Thus, if the injection of the radionuclide particles is done with the patient supine, the images will show a reasonably uniform distribution of activity. The gradient of activity from ventral to dorsal is of minor importance. To avoid clumping of the particles and possible nonuniform distribution of activity within the lungs, it is also recommended that the radionuclide should not be drawn back into the syringe. High-resolution gamma camera images are obtained with the patient upright, if possible, because the examination is usually easier to perform with the patient erect. Six views are generally recommended[173, 228, 229]: anterior, posterior, both laterals, and both posterior obliques (see Fig 8–5). Some centers add anterior oblique views to this routine. The role of single-photon emission computed tomography (SPECT) scanning in the diagnosis of pulmonary emboli[144] has yet to be evaluated. SPECT holds out the promise of quantitative images.[177]

The injected dose of ^{99m}Tc particles ranges from 1 to 4 mCi and over 90% of the activity is trapped in the lung capillaries. Aggregated albumin particles disappear from the lungs with a half-life of about 5.6 hours, while 20% of the injected activity is excreted in 24 hours. The particles break up into even smaller particles which are phagocytized by the liver and spleen. The aggregated albumin gives a radiation dose to the lung in the order of 0.250 rads/mCi and less than 30 mrads to any other major organ. The dose from microspheres is greater because the spheres are less easily eliminated from the lung capillaries. The need for radionuclide imaging in pregnant women should always be considered carefully. When indicated, an adequate examination can be performed with as little activity as 0.5 mCi to reduce the radiation dose. The ^{99m}Tc is also excreted in human milk, so nursing mothers should express their milk and save it for 3 or 4 days until the radionuclide has decayed to a safe level.

Ventilation Scanning.—The images obtained with ventilation scanning reflect the regional distribution of an inhaled radioactive tracer. Radioactive xenon gas, either ^{133}Xe or ^{127}Xe, is by far the most widely used agent. Krypton-81m gas is an alternative to xenon, and aerosol ventilation agents are also being developed.[2]

Xenon 133 is cheap and widely available. It is a reactor-produced beta-minus emitter with a half-life of 5.3 days and a low photon energy of 81 keV. Ventilation studies with ^{133}Xe usually consist of an image taken after inhalation of a single breath, which can be followed by serial images. Intervals will vary but a typical routine would be to take images at 15-second

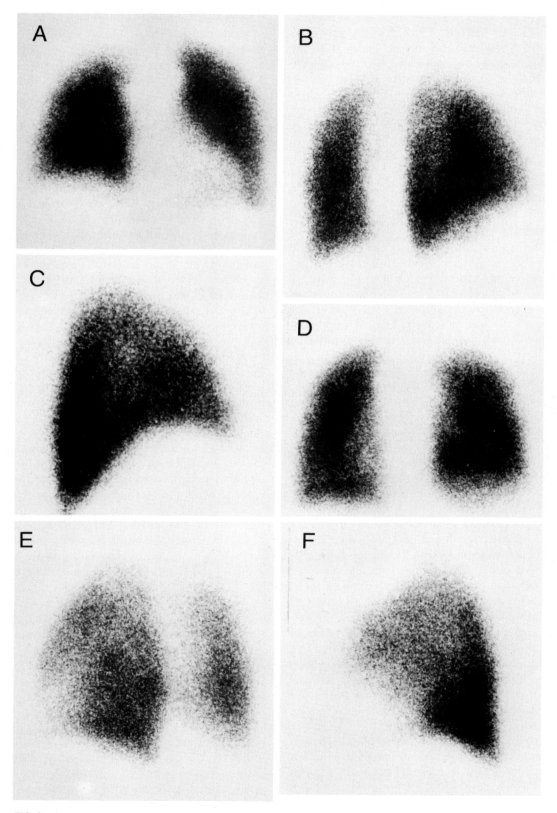

FIG 8–6.
Normal ⁹⁹ᵐTc perfusion scans of lungs. **A,** anterior. **B,** right posterior oblique. **C,** right lateral. **D,** posterior. **E,** left posterior oblique. **F,** left lateral view.

intervals during a rebreathing period of 3 to 5 minutes, which allows the gas to enter abnormally ventilated lung by way of collateral air drift. The images, therefore, represent both the normally and abnormally ventilated lung.[68] Further 15-second images can be obtained during yet another period of breathing room air or oxygen, during which time the tracer washes out of the lungs, enabling areas of retention caused by partial airway obstruction to be identified. The standard projection is the posterior view (Fig 8–7), but if a perfusion scan has already been obtained, the projection is the one that shows the perfusion defects to advantage. Because ^{99m}Tc emits photons with a peak energy of 140 keV, well above that of ^{133}Xe, the Compton scatter of the

^{99m}Tc emissions produces photons at various energies below 140 keV. These photons degrade the image of a ^{133}Xe scan. Thus, from the technical point of view, the best ^{133}Xe examinations are obtained either before the perfusion scan or after a delay of several hours to allow the ^{99m}Tc radioactivity to decay. But there are disadvantages to routinely performing ^{133}Xe ventilation scans before the perfusion scan: (1) in patients who subsequently prove to have normal perfusion scans or whose perfusion defects correspond to a radiographic abnormality, the ventilation scan is unnecessary and could therefore have been omitted altogether; and (2) a standard projection, not necessarily one that corresponds to any perfusion defect, has to be used, since the position

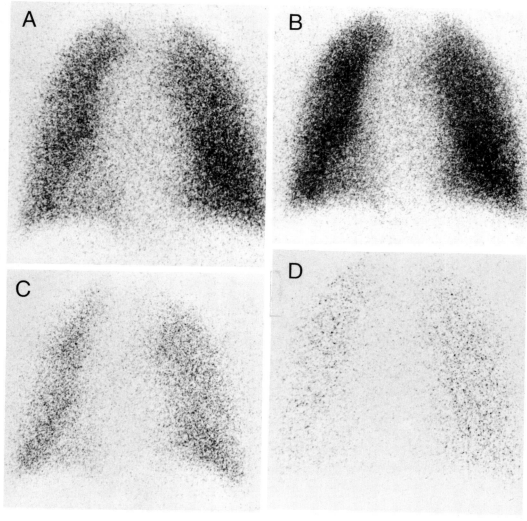

FIG 8–7.

Normal ^{133}Xe ventilation scan. Posterior scans: 0.5 to 1 minute after beginning of wash-in **(A)**; 2 to 2.5 minutes after beginning of wash-in (equilibrium) **(B)**; 1 to 1.5 minutes after beginning of wash-out **(C)**; and 2 to 2.5 minutes after beginning of wash-out **(D)**.

of the perfusion defects cannot be known beforehand. If it is decided to obtain the ^{99m}Tc perfusion scan first and follow it with a ^{133}Xe ventilation scan, the inevitable degradation of the resulting images due to the overlap in energies from ^{133}Xe and ^{99m}Tc can be minimized by computer processing. The image degradation is greatest during the wash-in phase and moderate during the wash-out phase.[134]

Between 2 and 30 mCi of ^{133}Xe is administered in a ventilation study; the absorbed dose is 0.011 rads/mCi for a dose administered in 5 L of air.[9]

Because it is produced in a cyclotron, Xenon 127 is less readily available and considerably more expensive than ^{133}Xe; it decays by electron capture without beta-minus decay and gives a lower radiation dose to the respiratory mucosa than ^{133}Xe: 0.0047 rads/mCi for a dose administered in 5 L of air. Xenon 127 emits a 203-keV photon and has a half life of 36.4 days; consequently, it has a very long shelf life. The technique for ^{127}Xe ventilation images is basically the same as that described for ^{133}Xe except that the images can be made immediately after the perfusion scans. This procedure has the major advantage of allowing a projection corresponding to the most readily visualized perfusion defects. The gamma camera is adjusted to disregard all counts below 150 keV in order to avoid significant counts due to the ^{99m}Tc.

Krypton 81m has a very short physical half-life of 13 seconds. It is produced by a rubidium-81 generator with a half-life of only 4.7 hours. A cyclotron is required for its manufacture, thus limiting the use of ^{81m}Kr to those centers close to a cyclotron unit. Its photon energy of 190 keV allows ^{81m}Kr to be used after the perfusion scan. The patient breathes the agent through a face mask. No radiation precautions are required for the exhaled gas, because the radioactivity decays within seconds. Because little patient cooperation is required, it is a suitable technique in patients who cannot follow instructions, including young children. Ventilation scans can be performed immediately after each of the perfusion projections (see Fig 8–11). Thus, paired ventilation/perfusion (V/Q) scans can be obtained in all desired projections. It is, however, not possible to diagnose retention of tracer in areas of airway obstruction using ^{81m}Kr.

Radioactive aerosol ventilation is an alternative to gaseous ventilation (see Fig 8–12). The most commonly used radiopharmaceutical is ^{99m}Tc-DTPA (diethylenetriaminepentaacetic acid), and a nebulizer is prepared with about 60 mCi of ^{99m}Tc. The esti-

mated radiation dose for 0.500 mCi of ^{99m}Tc-DTPA aerosol is 0.025 rads. The patient rebreathes from the apparatus until a specified count rate is achieved. Because clearance causes changes in the distribution of the tracer, imaging should take place immediately if it is to reflect ventilation. The aerosol distribution is stable for the time required for imaging and clears by diffusion of the label through the epithelial membrane into the plasma. A normal value for clearance is about 2%/minute, with increased values in various chronic lung diseases. Because the amount of activity from the aerosol is usually much less than that from the ^{99m}Tc perfusion study, some laboratories routinely begin with the aerosol study and then proceed to the perfusion study. Others begin with the perfusion study, using perhaps 1 mCi of ^{99m}Tc MAA, then proceed to the aerosol and observe whether areas of perfusion deficit fill in following the administration of aerosol. The computer can be used to great advantage to match and compare similar views, but accurate repositioning can be difficult. The use of another radionuclide, such as indium 111, to label the aerosols eliminates the difficulties of using ^{99m}Tc for both ventilation and perfusion. Aerosols can only be administered to compliant patients, so gases may have to be kept on hand for the more difficult patients.

Positron-emitting radionuclides, such as ^{15}O, ^{13}N and ^{11}C, have been used in various compounds for pulmonary examinations. The imaging of distributions of positron-emitting nuclides must be carried out with special equipment. If dynamic examinations are desired, then the instrument must have a large active surface, as a camera does. For static imaging, it is possible to use an instrument that collects data from a few slices at a time. Ventilation with a number of insoluble positron-emitting gases, such as ^{13}N with a 10-minute half-life, produces results similar to those of ^{133}Xe, and leaves the patient without radioactivity. Perfusion can be studied by having the patient breathe a single breath of a soluble gas, followed by breathholding. The disappearance of the gas from the lungs indicates perfusion. Such examinations can be performed with oxygen labeled with ^{15}O, or carbon monoxide/dioxide labeled with ^{11}C or ^{15}O. Multiple views can be performed with these short-lived materials.

Interpretation of Radionuclide Lung Scanning in Suspected Pulmonary Embolism.— For practical management purposes, a normal perfusion scan excludes the diagnosis of pulmonary embolism.[135] The cardinal sign of pulmonary embolism on radionuclide lung scanning is a perfusion defect. But the presence of a perfusion defect does not necessarily mean that pulmonary embolism has taken place, because reduction in blood flow can be the result of reflex vasoconstriction in response to such processes as pneumonia, atelectasis, pulmonary edema, and asthma. Reduction in blood flow can also be caused by diseases that destroy or obstruct the pulmonary vasculature such as emphysema, tuberculosis, and vasculitis. All these phenomena can cause perfusion defects indistinguishable from those of pulmonary emboli. In other words, though the perfusion scan is 100% sensitive for clinically significant pulmonary embolism, its specificity is significantly lower.[231] The specificity can be increased when the appearances on plain chest radiography and the findings of radionuclide ventilation studies are taken into account.[3, 52] Perfusion defects that correspond to a ventilation defect or to an opacity on a chest radiograph, though they may be due to areas of infarction or hemorrhage beyond emboli, are less likely to be the result of embolism than perfusion defects in areas that are normally ventilated and show no visible abnormality on chest radiography.

Perfusion defects due to pulmonary emboli are usually segmental in shape and extend to the pleural surface (Fig 8–8). There are two signs which significantly reduce the probability that a perfusion defect is the result of a pulmonary embolus. If a stripe of activity is seen forming the peripheral boundary between a perfusion defect and the pleura, then the probability of that defect being due to pulmonary embolism is very low. This finding has been termed the "stripe sign."[227] The second sign is the so-called fissure sign, which may represent multiple microemboli but is more usually due to pleural fluid in a fissure (Fig 8–9).

Abnormal V/Q scan results should be expressed in terms which indicate the probability that the diagnosis of pulmonary embolism is correct or, put in statistical terminology, some estimate of positive predictive value should be given. As discussed in Chapter 3, positive and negative predictive values are highly dependent on the prevalence (or likelihood) of disease. From the imager's point of view the probability of a particular patient's actually having pulmonary embolism is related to two factors: the clinical likelihood of disease, and the diagnostic test result. As McNeil so rightly says, "on the one hand, are patients whose clinical histories are so suggestive of pulmonary embolism that no diagnostic test result can, or perhaps should, alter significantly this clinical diagnosis. At the other extreme are patients whose

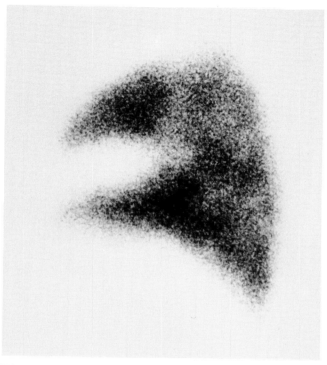

FIG 8–8.
Perfusion defect. ^{99m}Tc scan; right lateral view. Typical segmental-shaped perfusion defect is pointing to the hilus and based on the pleura. The defect in this case corresponds to the whole of the middle lobe and is due to a pulmonary embolus. The ventilation scan was normal.

likelihood of disease is so low that even the most abnormal of diagnostic test results should be viewed with some caution."[160]

The standard methods of expressing the probability of pulmonary embolism are "low probability" (corresponding in most series to less than 10% likelihood in the general hospital population) and "high probability" (corresponding to more than 85% likelihood in the general hospital population), together with the categories "normal" and "intermediate." The term "indeterminate" has been used, but has created considerable confusion. It was used to describe patients with perfusion defects and radiographic abnormalities in the same areas[28] because, when a matched perfusion defect corresponds to consolidation on the chest radiograph, the cause could be any one of the many reasons for segmental consolidation, including of course infarction. Because the more recent classifications do not use the term, we will dispense with it. Although the terms low, intermediate, and high probability imply the post-test probability, they are in fact used to describe the scan findings and applied to an assumed pretest

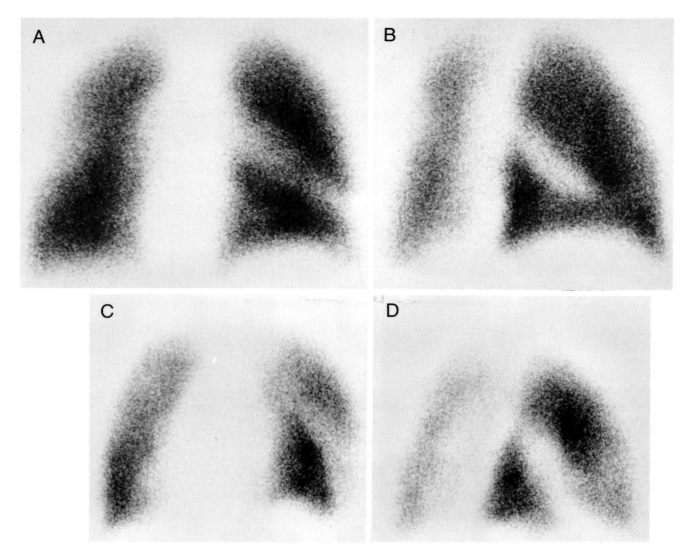

FIG 8–9.
Two examples of the fissure sign on ^{99m}Tc perfusion scans. **A** and **B,** the only perfusion defect in this 43-year-old man, for whom there was a strong clinical suspicion of pulmonary emboli, was a linear band of low activity corresponding to the position of the right major fissure. A right pleural effusion was present on the chest radiograph. The pulmonary angiogram was normal. **A,** posterior. **B,** right posterior oblique. **C** and **D,** similar findings in a 78-year-old woman with congestive cardiac failure. In this example, the pleural effusion produces a strikingly large perfusion defect. **C,** posterior. **D,** right posterior oblique.

TABLE 8– 1.

Criteria for Diagnosing Pulmonary Embolism at Radionuclide V/Q Scanning

Probability of Pulmonary Embolism	Biello et al.[79,87]	PIOPED[229]
Normal	No perfusion defects	No perfusion defects
Low probability	Small V/Q mismatches Focal V/Q matches with no corresponding radiographic abnormalities Perfusion defects substantially smaller than radiographic abnormalities	Small perfusion defects regardless of number and regardless of ventilation or CXR abnormalities Perfusion defect substantially smaller than CXR abnormality (V scan findings irrelevant) V/Q match in ≤50% of one lung or ≤75% of one lung zone. CXR normal or nearly normal* Single moderate perfusion defect with normal CXR* (V scan findings irrelevant) Nonsegmental perfusion defects
Intermediate probability	Diffuse severe airway obstruction Matched perfusion defects and radiographic abnormalities (i.e., of same size) Single medium or large V/Q mismatch	Abnormality that is not defined by either "high" or "low" probability
High probability	Two or more medium or large V/Q mismatches with no corresponding radiographic abnormalities Perfusion defect(s) substantially larger than radiographic abnormality(s)	Two or more large perfusion defects with ventilation scan and CXR normal* Two or more large perfusion defects in which the perfusion defects are substantially larger than either the matching ventilation defects or the CXR abnormality Two or more moderate perfusion defects and one large perfusion defect when the ventilation scan and the CXR are normal* Four or more moderate perfusion defects when the ventilation scan and the CXR are normal*
Definitions	Small defect = <25% of a segment Medium defect = 25% to 90% of a segment Large defect = >90% of a segment	Small defect = <25% of area of segment Moderate defect =25% to 75% of area of segment Large defect = >75% of area of segment

*CXR normal means chest x-ray normal in the area of the ventilation or perfusion defect and need not necessarily mean that the entire radiograph is normal in appearance.

probability. This assumed pretest probability is based on the prevalence of pulmonary emboli in the published series of patients who had undergone both radionuclide scanning and pulmonary angiography. In clinical practice, however, the pretest probability of embolism in a particular patient may be significantly higher or lower than these selected cases. This important concept is often overlooked. A review of 566 consecutive patients with suspected pulmonary embolism showed physicians placed a very strong reliance on the lung scan results when deciding patient management.[84] Patients with high-probability scans invariably received anticoagulant therapy without further study, whereas most pa-

tients with low- or intermediate-probability scans were not treated and did not undergo pulmonary angiography. Thus, it would appear that the limitations of test interpretation are in practice being ignored and that the clinician's estimate of the probability of disease is not being taken into account.

High, low, and intermediate probabilities of pulmonary embolus (Table 8–1) are based on several large series of patients in whom the results of V/Q scanning were correlated with the findings at pulmonary angiography.* Unfortunately, differing criteria have been used, and these criteria are in a state of

*References 29, 32, 36, 52, 118, 159, 231.

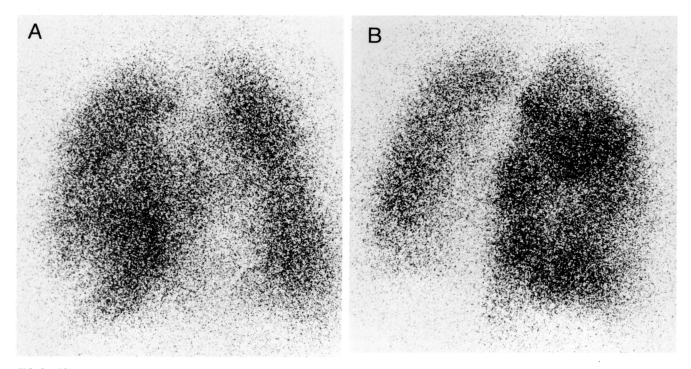

FIG 8–10.
Low-probability scan. The scattered perfusion defects are all smaller than 25% of a segment. The images are ^{99m}Tc perfusion scans. **A,** left posterior oblique. **B,** right posterior oblique.

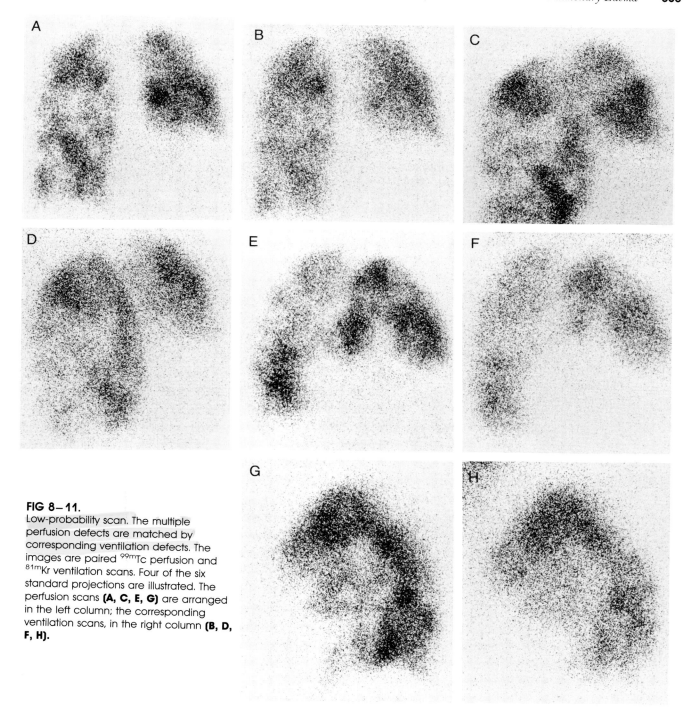

FIG 8–11.
Low-probability scan. The multiple perfusion defects are matched by corresponding ventilation defects. The images are paired ⁹⁹ᵐTc perfusion and ⁸¹ᵐKr ventilation scans. Four of the six standard projections are illustrated. The perfusion scans **(A, C, E, G)** are arranged in the left column; the corresponding ventilation scans, in the right column **(B, D, F, H).**

flux.[238] Even with agreed-upon criteria, there is the very real problem of how one decides what proportion of the segment has reduced perfusion. Because our aim is to clarify, we will emphasize the basic principles of test interpretation and the points of agreement.

A *low probability* scan refers to:

1. Perfusion defects that are small, regardless of whether or not there is a matched ventilation defect and regardless of the findings on the chest x-ray. (Biello et al.[26, 29] defined small as less than 25% of a segment, and the National Heart, Lung, and Blood Institute prospective study of pulmonary embolism diagnosis (PIOPED) groups[229] are using the same definition.) (Fig 8–10).

2. Perfusion defects that are equivalent in size (Fig 8–11) to the corresponding ventilation defect with no corresponding radiographic abnormalities.

3. Perfusion defects that are substantially smaller than the matching ventilation defects or the radiographically demonstrated abnormalities (Fig 8–12).

4. Perfusion defects that are readily accountable for by, for example, a large hilus, a large aorta, or previous surgery.

5. Smith et al. added to the above items the criterion that the matched defects should occupy less than 50% of the visible lung.[225]

A *high probability* scan refers to:

1. Two or more moderate or large defects which are not matched by either a corresponding ventilation defect or an abnormality on the plain chest radiograph (Fig 8–13). It is worth noting that when the diagnosis is clinically likely and when there are multiple segmental or larger than segmental defects, with a normal ventilation scan, the probability of pulmonary embolism exceeds 90%.[52, 160, 231] The presence of a stripe sign or a fissure sign can be used to remove perfusion defects from the high-probability category, as can the existence of a comparable defect on a scan taken prior to the clinical episode.

2. Perfusion defects that are substantially larger than the matching radiographic abnormalities or the matching ventilation defects.

An *intermediate* probability scan refers to all the patients who do not fit into either high- or low-probability categories. In essence, the probability of thromboembolism in patients placed in this category is likely to be similar to what it was prior to the test. In other words a change in management would probably be unwarranted. In general terms, intermediate probability refers to:

1. Perfusion defects, even though matched, which correspond in size and shape to an area of consolidation on the chest radiograph.

2. Perfusion defects in areas of severe obstructive lung disease, pulmonary edema, or pleural effusion.

Solitary perfusion defects, even if not matched, must be viewed with great caution. Such a defect indicates vascular obstruction, but not necessarily one that is embolic in nature. When the perfusion defect corresponds reasonably closely to the size of a radiographic abnormality, the probability of embolism drops well into the intermediate range.[29] For example, pneumonia and infarction may both give the same pattern. Similarly, when a perfusion defect is associated with a pleural effusion one cannot tell if an embolus caused the effusion or whether the effusion, regardless of cause, is compressing the lung and, therefore, reducing perfusion.

Symmetric perfusion defects, even if not matched, should also be viewed with caution. Biello and Kumar reported two such patients who, on angiography, did not have pulmonary emboli. The rea-

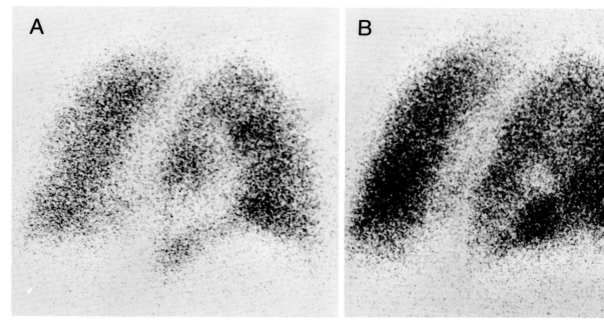

FIG 8–12.
Low-probability scan. The perfusion defect in the posterior segment of the right lower lobe is smaller than the ventilation defect.

A, ^{99m}Tc perfusion scan; right posterior oblique. **B,** ^{99m}Tc aerosol ventilation scan; right posterior oblique.

son for the findings on the radionuclide studies was unclear.[27]

Differential Diagnosis of Pulmonary Thromboembolism.—Phenomena other than recent pulmonary thromboemboli can produce perfusion defects without disturbing ventilation or producing local abnormalities in the radiograph.[139, 173] These include:

1. Previous pulmonary emboli.
2. Nonthrombotic embolism.
3. Pulmonary vasculitis/radiation therapy/sickle cell disease.
4. Neoplastic (Fig 8–14), inflammatory, or mechanical occlusion of blood vessels (e.g., Swan-Ganz catheter, *Dirofilaria immitis*).

5. Benign or malignant mediastinal tumors/adenopathy.
6. Fibrosing mediastinitis.
7. Primary pulmonary arterial hypertension.
8. Pulmonary veno-occlusive disease.
9. Systemic arterial blood flow to a portion of the lung, (e.g., surgical shunt, pulmonary sequestration, hypogenetic lung [scimitar] syndrome, agenesis of pulmonary artery).
10. Pulmonary-systemic shunt such as pulmonary arteriovenous malformation.
11. Shifting pleural effusions when comparisons are made between images taken with the patient in different positions.
12. Emphysema and pneumonia. Though they usually give matched defects, these conditions can, on occasion, cause mismatched defects.

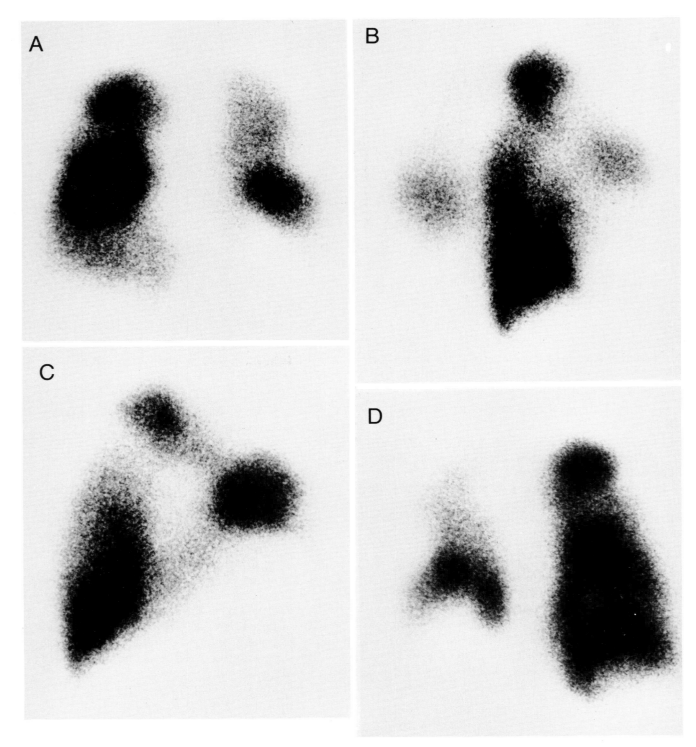

FIG 8–13.
High-probability scan. Six views of a ^{99m}Tc perfusion scan. **A,** anterior. **B,** right posterior oblique. **C,** right lateral. **D,** posterior.

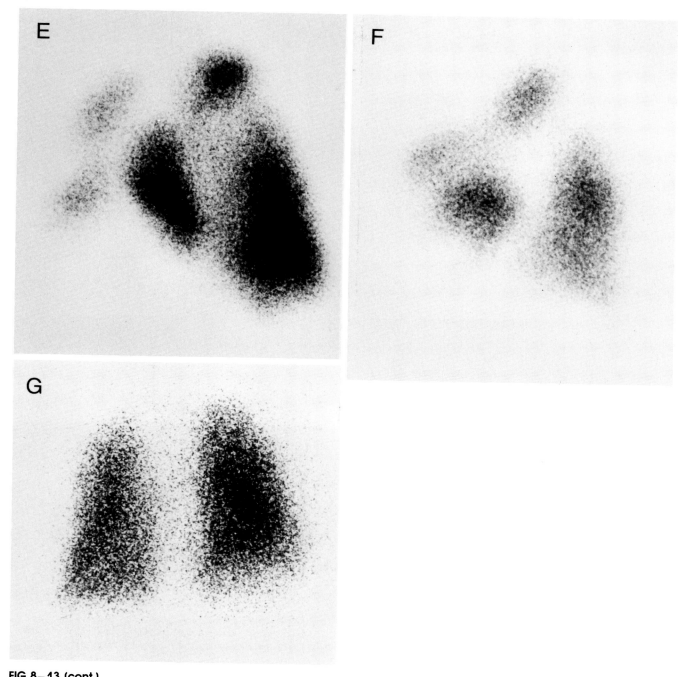

FIG 8–13 (cont.).
E, left posterior oblique. **F,** left lateral. The ventilation scan was a normal study. A selected image of the posterior ¹³³Xe scan at 1 minute after the beginning of wash-in is illustrated in **G.**

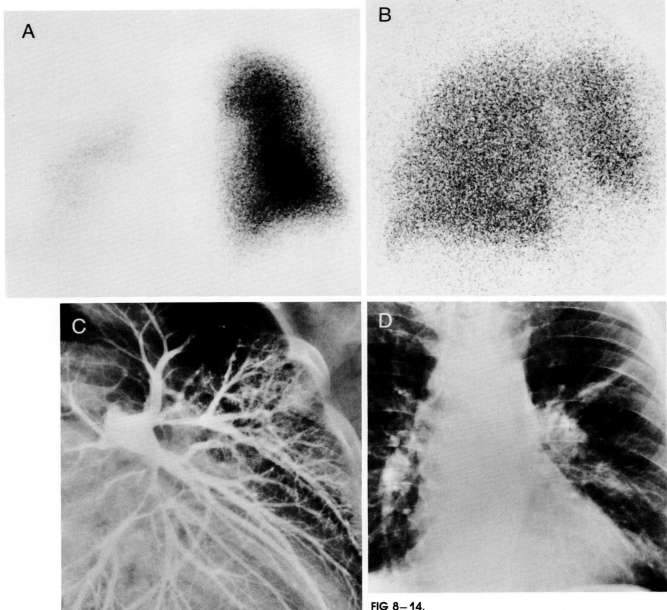

FIG 8–14.
Mismatched perfusion defect resulting from carcinoma of the bronchus involving the major divisions of the left pulmonary artery. **A,** ^{99m}Tc scan, posterior view. **B,** ^{133}Xe ventilation scan, left posterior oblique. **C,** pulmonary arteriogram illustrates the involvement of the central pulmonary arteries by the tumor. **D,** posteroanterior radiograph.

Pulmonary Angiography

Accurate morbidity and mortality statistics for pulmonary angiography are difficult to obtain. In many large series, there are no deaths,[52, 174, 191, 254] and in others the rate is less than 1%, usually under 0.5%.[21, 59, 86, 150, 163, 170] When all these series were combined, ten deaths, in a total of 4,209 patients, were attributed to pulmonary angiography.[94] Pulmonary hypertension was a major predisposing factor; of the ten patients, nine had proved or presumed pulmonary hypertension. Of the nonfatal complications, arrhythmias are the most common, followed by cardiac perforation. Cardiac perforation, though it may lead to pericardial tamponade, frequently resolves without incident, particularly if there is no associated myocardial intravasation. Such nonfatal complications can be expected in 1% to 2% of patients.[94] It should be borne in mind that patients subjected to angiography tend to be more acutely ill and are therefore less likely to recover from physical insults. When a perfusion lung scan has been performed, the angiographic examination can be tailored to search for emboli in the areas of perfusion defect. Thus, the perfusion scan helps in performing the study and may also reduce complications by justifying a more limited examination than would otherwise be necessary.[68]

Interpretation.—The two major angiographic signs of acute pulmonary embolism are[59, 75, 236, 267] (Figs 8–15 and 8–16):

1. Intraluminal filling defects within the opacified arterial tree seen on two or more films during the angiographic study. Filling defects are caused by opacified blood flowing around the thrombus. Sometimes, the contrast medium flows past the thrombus to opacify the distal vessels. At other times, only the trailing edge of a thrombus impacted in a downstream arterial branch is seen.
2. Occlusion of a pulmonary artery branch. Occlusion is a nonspecific sign and may be seen in a variety of conditions including congenital malformations, organized thrombus from previous embolus, in situ thrombosis, mediastinal fibrosis, occlusion from direct involvement by neoplasm, inflammatory disease (e.g., lung abscess or granulomatous infection), progressive massive fibrosis, or pneumoconiosis.

The other arteriographic sign of pulmonary embolism is focal reduction or delay in the opacification of the pulmonary arterial branches,[59] equivalent to the perfusion defect seen at radionuclide imaging. Clearly, reduced perfusion, regardless of how it is demonstrated, is a less specific sign than an intraluminal filling defect or an abrupt occlusion of a vessel.[33, 205] It will be seen in any condition which destroys lung parenchyma, notably emphysema, bronchiectasis, or pulmonary scarring, and in any condition which leads to focal hypoxia with secondary reduction of blood flow, for example, fibrothorax and pneumonia.

Pulmonary thromboemboli usually lyse following the embolic episode. In dogs, experimentally produced emboli can disappear within days,[61, 169] and rapid resolution has also been recorded in humans.[209] But, in general, it would appear that thromboemboli are detectable angiographically for weeks or months following the acute event. Goodman recently reviewed the literature on the subject and warned that pulmonary angiography should not be withheld simply because of a few days' delay in the onset of symptoms.[94]

Some emboli do not lyse completely. They may leave residual webs, which can be seen angiographically,[137, 182] or they may form permanent occlusions. When multiple vessels are occluded, pulmonary arterial hypertension results.[273] In chronic pulmonary embolism, the occlusion of vessels dominates the picture; the filling defects of recent emboli are then often more difficult to find and may not be detectable.

Indications for Pulmonary Angiography.—Which patients should have angiography? Practice varies,[52, 197, 200, 230] but, in general, pulmonary angiography is recommended for patients suspected of having pulmonary embolism:

1. When the V/Q scan is abnormal but cannot be placed into either high- or low-probability categories. This is a particularly common dilemma in patients with underlying chronic obstructive lung disease.[141]
2. When the V/Q scan result is significantly at variance with the clinical probability of pulmonary embolism.

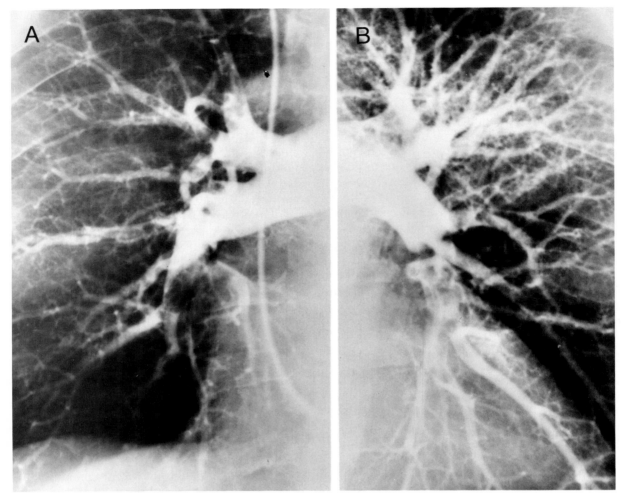

FIG 8–15.
Pulmonary emboli. There are multiple filling defects and occlusions of the branches of the pulmonary arteries at pulmonary angiography. Right **(A)** and left **(B)** pulmonary arteriograms.

3. When long-term anticoagulation is contemplated, or when drug therapy would carry a high risk.

4. Prior to embolectomy, vena caval interruption, or filter insertion.

In practice these criteria are not strictly adhered to. It has been argued that physicians should realize that the risks of pulmonary angiography performed by experienced operators, though not negligible, are often less than those of anticoagulant therapy, particularly in patients whose V/Q scan findings are nonspecific,[52] and that pulmonary angiography should, therefore, be performed more readily, not just as a last resort.[197] The fact that practice varies so much reflects the inherent difficulties of assigning

risks and benefits in the common, but nevertheless poorly documented, entity of pulmonary embolism.

Pulmonary angiography is the currently accepted "gold standard" for the diagnosis of pulmonary embolism during life.[21, 59, 197] It is self-evident, however, that there must be both false positive and false negative interpretations. It would appear, however, that life-threatening emboli are not missed. Novelline et al.[174] and Cheely et al.[52] each followed a large group of patients clinically suspected of having pulmonary embolism who had normal pulmonary angiograms. Had significant pulmonary emboli been overlooked, it seems likely that some of these patients would have had further embolic episodes in the ensuing years. In fact, none of Novelline's 167 patients did, even though they were not receiving

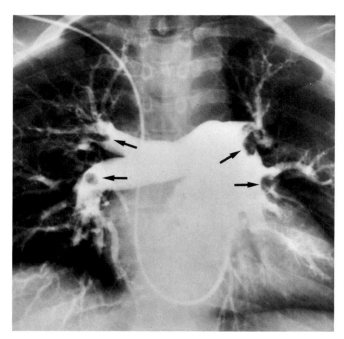

FIG 8–16.
Pulmonary emboli. Pulmonary angiogram shows multiple filling defects. The trailing ends of the occluding thromboemboli are particularly well shown *(arrows)*.

anticoagulant therapy; in three cases, small incidental emboli were found in patients dying for other reasons.[174] In Cheely's series, four of 144 patients with angiograms negative for disease subsequently developed emboli, but in none were they the cause of death.[52] The problem of false positive diagnoses is more difficult to evaluate.[236] In those patients who die, presumably the most severe cases, there appears to be a good correlation between the angiographic diagnosis of pulmonary embolism and the findings at autopsy.[4]

Digital Subtraction Angiography

Digital subtraction angiography may eventually prove to be a less invasive alternative to conventional pulmonary angiography for detecting pulmonary emboli. The advantages are increased contrast resolution and greater safety, but these advantages are currently offset by the poor spatial resolution of the imaging system and, particularly, motion artifact from misregistration of mask frames.[31, 74, 116] The technique is not widely used in clinical practice, though it has its advocates.[136, 186] It appears to be significantly more accurate in the diagnosis of emboli in the proximal two thirds of the pulmonary arterial tree than for emboli lodged distally, and

may be a good alternative to radionuclide imaging, particularly in patients with chronic obstructive lung disease.[145]

Computed Tomography and Magnetic Resonance Imaging

Large thrombi in the main pulmonary arteries and their major branches may be visible at both contrast-enhanced computed tomography (CT) (Figs 8–17 and 8–18)[132] and at electrocardiographically gated magnetic resonance imaging (MRI).[89, 167, 235, 246] Most reports have concentrated on the detection of central emboli in patients with pulmonary arterial hypertension. Neither technique is currently used on a routine basis, and there are no data on sensitivity and specificity. MRI would appear to be the more promising of the two techniques, because no contrast agents are needed and because blood clots in the pulmonary arteries generate signal, whereas fast-flowing blood creates a signal void. Care must be taken not to misinterpret the signal generated from slow-flowing blood on MR images, a phenomenon that is particularly prevalent in patients with pulmonary arterial hypertension. The distinction between slow-flowing blood and thrombus is best made by comparing the change in signal intensity during the cardiac cycle.[77, 266] Intraluminal clot produces focal moderate to moderately high signal intensity that remains fixed in distribution during the cardiac cycle and demonstrates little or no increase in relative intensity from first to second echo,[266] whereas the signal from slow-flowing blood varies with the cardiac cycle and increases in relative intensity from first to second echo. At its current stage of development MRI does not appear to be clinically useful in the diagnosis of peripheral pulmonary emboli.[266]

Infarct shadows in the lung may show a pleural-based truncated cone or triangular configuration on CT scans—a shape that corresponds to the Hampton's hump described earlier in this chapter (Fig 8–19).

Tumor Emboli

Tumor emboli sufficiently large to be hemodynamically significant are also sometimes seen[45, 102, 269] and can, on occasion, be the presenting feature of the neoplastic disease.[38, 63] They occlude small pulmonary vessels and can give rise to severe dyspnea, which usually develops over a matter of days, but sometimes builds up over several

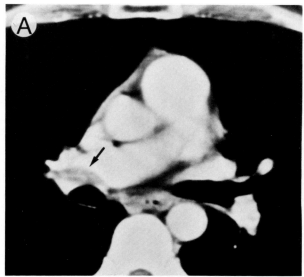

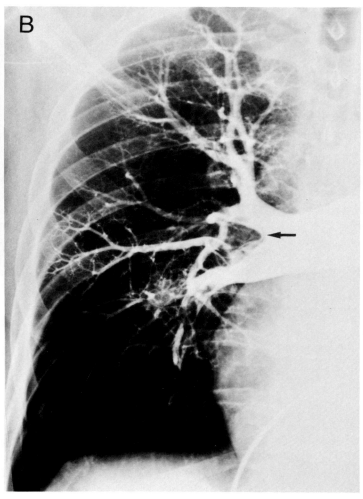

FIG 8–17.
Pulmonary emboli. **A,** arrow points to intraluminal defect in the right pulmonary artery on the contrast enhanced CT scan. **B,** corresponding pulmonary angiogram shows a large embolus straddling the bifurcation of the right pulmonary artery *(arrow)* and multiple emboli occluding the right lower lobe artery and its branches.

weeks. Pleuritic chest pain is relatively common, and fatigue, weight loss, cough, hemoptysis, and syncope are seen in a few patients.

On physical examination, most patients show signs of right ventricular overload but, just as with pulmonary thromboembolism, there may be relatively few respiratory findings. The condition differs from widespread, blood-borne metastases in that a metastasis represents tumor that has invaded the vessel wall and acquired its own blood supply, whereas tumor emboli are clumps of cells lodged within the lumen of the pulmonary vessels, which have not yet invaded the vessel wall but are acting as obstructing emboli similar to thromboemboli. The patients are hypoxemic, have increased alveolar-arterial oxygen gradients, and have pulmonary arterial hypertension, sometimes severe.[44] Tumor emboli are a fairly frequent finding at autopsy, but the condition is rarely diagnosed antemortem. Chan et al.,[45] in their extensive review of the literature on the subject, found a wide distribution of responsible malignancies. The primary tumor frequently associated with tumor embolism are hepatoma, breast and renal carcinoma,[63] gastric and prostatic cancers, and choriocarcinoma.[72, 95]

The plain chest radiographs are usually normal. Pulmonary arterial hypertension is rarely recognizable. A few patients show nonspecific pulmonary shadows. Radionuclide lung scans show multiple, small, peripheral, subsegmental perfusion defects with a normal ventilation scan, corresponding to a low-probability or intermediate probability scan for pulmonary embolism. Pulmonary angiography shows delayed filling of segmental arteries, reduction in number of branch vessels, and occasionally 1- to 2-mm filling defects.

The mortality of the condition is very high, and the role of intervention is not clear. Surgical resection of the primary tumor without specific treatment of the emboli has been attempted, and good results

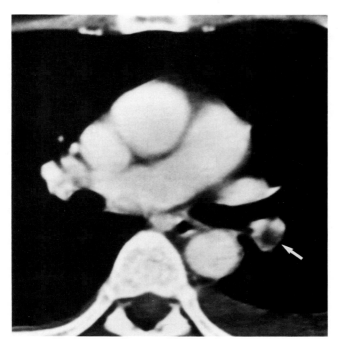

FIG 8–18.
CT scan (contrast enhanced) showing filling defect as a result of an embolus lodged in the left lower lobe artery *(arrow)*.

have been claimed.[63] Whether these emboli will respond to chemotherapy has not yet been investigated; the number of patients diagnosed antemortem is too low.

PULMONARY ARTERIAL HYPERTENSION

Pulmonary artery pressure is a function of blood flow and the resistance across the pulmonary vascular system, the resistance to flow depending predominantly on the cross-sectional area of the perfused vascular bed. The pulmonary vascular bed has a much lower resistance than the systemic circuit and can respond to increasing flow by opening up additional vascular channels. Pulmonary arterial hypertension occurs when the flow increases to such an extent that the available extra channels are saturated, or because of vasoconstriction or structural change in the small pulmonary vessels. It is defined as pulmonary artery pressures above the normal systolic value of 30 mm Hg or above the mean value of 18 mm Hg.

The basic radiographic features of pulmonary arterial hypertension will be discussed before the

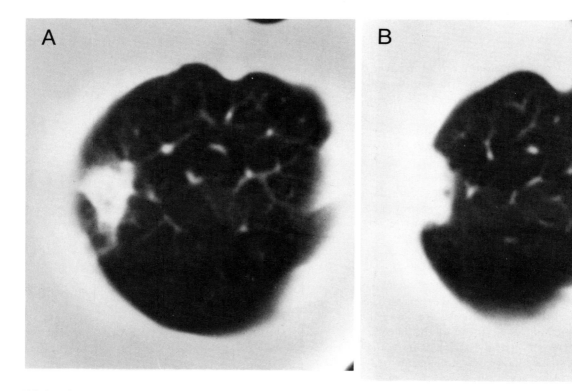

FIG 8–19.
CT scans of pulmonary infarct in the left upper lobe. **A** and **B,** adjacent sections illustrating the truncated cone shape based on the pleura (same patient as Fig 8–17).

various causes are described (Table 8–2), because the same signs are seen regardless of the cause of the hypertension. The basic signs are cardiac enlargement, right ventricular enlargement, and enlargement of the central pulmonary arteries with rapid tapering of the vessels as they proceed distally (Fig 8–20). The distal vessels may be large, normal, or reduced in caliber. The important point is the disparity in the relative size of the central and distal vessels. The terms "central" and "distal" are inevitably vague, as there is no precise anatomic definition of central and distal (peripheral) vessels, but the term "central arteries" refers to the main pulmonary artery and its branches approximately down to segmental level. The term "distal vessels" refers to vessels beyond the segmental level. The criteria of central vessel dilation on plain chest radiographs are, with one exception, also poorly defined. On plain film, the main pulmonary artery is border-forming for less than half of its circumference, and this border represents a portion of the vessel that is traveling obliquely upward and backward. Thus, diagnosing dilation based on increased prominence or convexity of the main pulmonary artery segment of the cardiac contour is at best a crude measurement. CT scanning provides a more accurate indication of size. One well-documented measurement of the size of the pulmonary arterial tree on plain films is that of the right descending pulmonary artery.[46] The upper limit of normal for transverse diameter at the midpoint of this vessel is 16 to 17 mm. Thus, measurements of 17 mm or greater indicate dilation (Fig 8–21).

The degree of dilation of the central pulmonary arteries varies considerably, not only among the various entities that cause pulmonary arterial hypertension, but also from patient to patient with the same condition. Therefore, although the radiographic changes are reasonably specific, they are neither sensitive nor well correlated with the severity of the hypertension. Indeed, severe pulmonary arterial hypertension can be present in patients with a normal appearing chest radiograph.

Prolonged severe pulmonary arterial hypertension may lead to atheroma formation in the central pulmonary arteries or their branches (Fig 8–22). (Atheroma is not seen in the pulmonary circuit with normal pulmonary artery pressures.) The atheroma reveals itself radiographically by curvilinear calcification identical to that seen with atheromatous change in the aorta and its branches. In practice, atheromatous calcification of the pulmonary artery is very rare and is seen only in Eisenmenger's syndrome

TABLE 8–2.
Classification of Pulmonary Hypertension

Increased resistance to pulmonary venous drainage:
Congenital narrowing of pulmonary veins
Mediastinal fibrosis
Pulmonary veno-occlusive disease
Left atrial obstruction – mitral valve disease, cor triatriatum, left atrial myxoma
Left ventricular dysfunction
Constrictive pericarditis

Increased resistance due to disease in the arterial/arteriolar wall or lumen:
Emboli: thrombotic and other
Primary pulmonary hypertension
Eisenmenger's syndrome
Persistence of fetal circulation
Arteriopathy in hepatic cirrhosis
Drug or chemically induced
Pulmonary vasculitis
Schistosomiasis
Congenital stenosis
Hypogenesis or aplasia
Surgical resection of lung

Increased pulmonary vascular resistance secondary to pleuropulmonary disease:
Chronic obstructive pulmonary disease
Interstitial fibrosis of the lungs
Sarcoidosis
Pneumoconioses
Granulomatous infections
Pleural fibrothorax

Increased pulmonary blood flow:
Left-to-right shunts (atrial septal defect, ventricular septal defect, patent ductus arteriosus)

Hypoventilation:
Obesity hypoventilation syndrome
Pharyngeal/tracheal obstructions
High altitude
Neuromuscular disorders of breathing
Chest wall deformity/kyphoscoliosis

and in a few patients with very prolonged pulmonary hypertension.

Pulmonary Hypertension Secondary to Increased Resistance to Pulmonary Venous Drainage

Restriction of flow through the pulmonary venous system or through the left atrium and mitral valve raises pulmonary venous pressure, which in turn leads to elevation of pulmonary arterial pressure. With a healthy right ventricle, increases in mean left atrial pressure up to 25 mm Hg are accompanied by a proportional increase in pulmonary

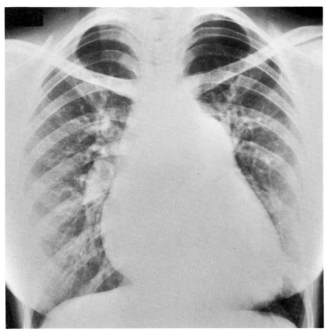

FIG 8–20.
Pulmonary arterial hypertension illustrating cardiomegaly and enlargement of the main pulmonary artery and hilar arteries. The vessels beyond the hilus are normal or small, notably in the lower zones. The patient, a 19-year-old woman, had severe primary pulmonary hypertension.

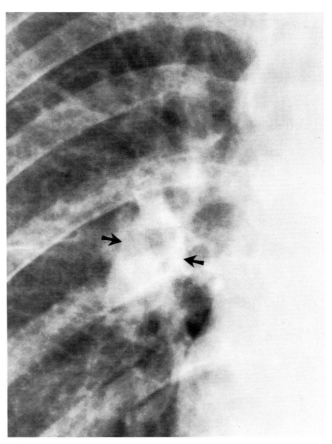

FIG 8–21.
Pulmonary arterial hypertension due to chronic pulmonary thromboembolism showing method of measuring the size of the lower lobe arteries. The transverse diameter of the right lower artery in this patient *(arrows)* measures 19 mm.

artery pressure to maintain a constant mean gradient of approximately 10 mm Hg. When the mean venous pressure is chronically above 25 mm Hg, a disproportionate elevation of pulmonary arterial pressure is observed, indicating an increase in pulmonary arteriolar resistance. (Mitral stenosis is a good example; just under one-third of patients with stenosis sufficiently severe to chronically elevate pulmonary venous pressure above 25 mm Hg will develop systolic pressures of 80 mm Hg or greater.) The mechanism for the elevation of pulmonary arterial pressure is unclear. Both vasoconstriction and structural changes play a part. Microscopic examination shows distention of the pulmonary capillaries, thickening and rupture of the basement membranes of the endothelial cells, and minor degrees of hemorrhage into the alveoli. The appearance of the arteries depends on whether the venous obstruction has been present since birth or was acquired later in life. In adult-onset pulmonary arterial hypertension, there is medial hypertrophy and intimal fibrosis of the smaller pulmonary arteries and arterioles. Necrotizing arteritis may occasionally be seen.

The changes of pulmonary arterial hypertension secondary to chronic impedance of pulmonary venous drainage are only visible radiologically when the pulmonary arterial pressures are very high. Such high pressures are almost never encountered in left ventricular failure, reduced left ventricular compliance, or constrictive pericarditis. Thus, when pulmonary arterial hypertension is diagnosable radiologically in an adult, the conditions to be considered in the category of increased impedance to pulmonary venous drainage are mitral valve disease, left atrial myxoma, cor triatriatum (which may present first in adult life) and pulmonary veno-occlusive disease. (Pulmonary veno-occlusive disease has been grouped by the World Health Organization [WHO] with primary pulmonary hypertension and is therefore discussed in the section "Pulmonary Veno-occlusive Disease" later in this chapter).

The radiographic changes reflect a combination of pulmonary arterial and pulmonary venous hypertension together with the features of the primary

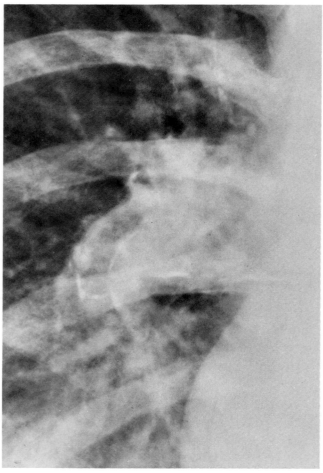

FIG 8–22.
Atheromatous calcification in the pulmonary arteries in a case of prolonged severe pulmonary hypertension due to patent ductus arteriosus with Eisenmenger's syndrome.

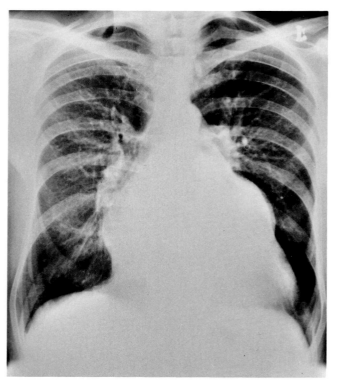

FIG 8–23.
Pulmonary arterial hypertension secondary to mitral stenosis. Note the large hilar arteries and the small arteries beyond the hili. The upper zone vessels are large due to elevation of the pulmonary venous pressure, and the left atrium is massively dilated.

condition (Figs 8–23 and 8–24). The central pulmonary arteries are dilated, tapering to normal caliber at or beyond segmental level. The peripheral lower zone arteries may even be reduced in caliber. The upper zone vessels are enlarged due to upper zone blood diversion. In mitral stenosis, the left atrium will be enlarged and may show calcification either in its wall or in left atrial thrombus. Although the left atrium is almost invariably enlarged in cases of mitral valve disease with pulmonary arterial hypertension, it may not be strikingly big, and enlargement should, therefore, be looked for carefully on the plain chest radiograph. The chest radiograph in left atrial myxoma is identical to that of mitral stenosis except that, on occasion, it may be possible to recognize focal calcifications within the tumor mass.

Pulmonary Hypertension Secondary to Thromboembolism

Pulmonary hypertension follows acute pulmonary embolism when the emboli occlude enough of the pulmonary arterial bed. The mechanisms are complex, consisting of a mixture of mechanical obstruction and vasoconstriction. These acute changes in pulmonary artery pressure do not produce radiographically visible pulmonary arterial hypertension, in part because a previously normal right ventricle can only produce right ventricular systolic pressures up to 45 to 55 mm Hg. Higher pressures require preexisting right ventricular hypertrophy.

Repetitive thromboemboli without intervening lysis of thrombi may lead to chronic elevation of pulmonary artery pressure. The condition is rare, being seen in less than 1% of patients following acute emboli. Infarction is not usually a feature, and the patients frequently do not present clinically until the progressive occlusion of the pulmonary vascular bed has led to symptomatic pulmonary arterial hyperten-

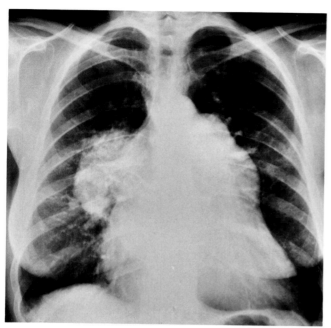

FIG 8–24.
Pulmonary arterial hypertension due to mitral stenosis. The dilation of the central pulmonary arteries is particularly striking in this 59-year-old woman with systemic pressures in her pulmonary circuit. Note the enlarged left atrium.

sion.[105] It is these patients who may show the radiographic changes of pulmonary arterial hypertension. Surgical thromboendarterectomy has been undertaken in a few patients with substantial success.[204]

At pathologic study, organized thrombi are seen in both elastic and muscular arteries. The thrombi in the smaller vessels show recanalization, forming a lattice of fibrous trabeculae lined by endothelium. New blood vessels may form within the thrombi, and medial hypertrophy occurs secondarily. Plexiform lesions (see the description in the following section) are absent, though organizing thrombi may, on occasion, be difficult to distinguish from plexiform lesions.[70]

The plain chest radiograph shows cardiomegaly and central vessel dilation, with patchy peripheral oligemia in the majority of patients[6, 273] (Fig 8–25). Oligemic areas correspond well with the distribution of emboli, though normal vascularity may be seen in areas perfused by vessels that contain sizable emboli.[273] A few patients have normal or near-normal studies; others show only changes such as atelectasis, pleural thickening, or pleural effusion, the radiographic signs of pulmonary hypertension being absent.

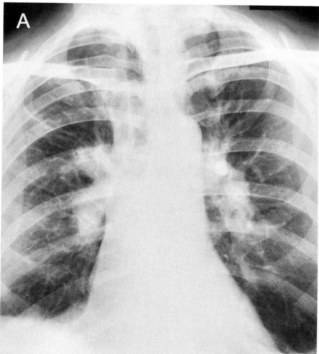

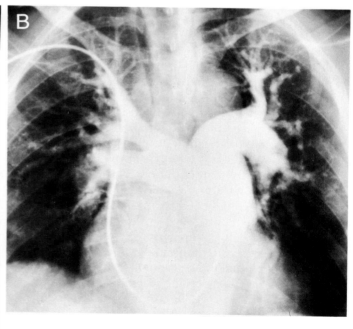

FIG 8–25.
Pulmonary arterial hypertension due to chronic thromboemboli. **A,** plain film showing enlargement of the hilar arteries with patchy peripheral oligemia. **B,** pulmonary angiogram showing the central vessel dilation with occlusion of multiple branch vessels and increase in size of the unobstructed pulmonary arterial branches.

Radionuclide perfusion scans show a pattern consistent with high probability of pulmonary embolism in all cases.[62, 78, 142, 273]

Pulmonary angiography[6, 273] reveals filling defects due to thrombi in the lobar or segmental arteries, with occlusions of large and medium-size vessels. The central vessels are frequently dilated, with rapid distal tapering. Web-shaped filling defects are occasionally seen.

Primary Pulmonary Hypertension

The term "unexplained" or "primary pulmonary hypertension" refers to a group of patients who have pulmonary arterial hypertension with no clinically discernible cause, a normal pulmonary arterial wedge pressure, and no evidence of left-to-right shunt on cardiac catheterization. Patients with major emboli are excluded from the designation primary pulmonary hypertension.[70, 105, 258] Primary pulmonary hypertension was classified by the WHO[107] into three subtypes based on the histologic appearances of the vascular bed: (1) plexogenic arteriopathy, (2) recurrent pulmonary thromboembolism, and (3) pulmonary veno-occlusive disease. In this chapter we have treated recurrent pulmonary thromboembolism and pulmonary veno-occlusive disease separately because they often, though by no means always, have distinguishing features on imaging tests.

Prolonged vasoconstriction is believed to be the first stage of plexogenic pulmonary arteriopathy (classic primary pulmonary hypertension); the next stage is structural change in the arterial wall. Pathologically,[30, 70, 258] the initial structural manifestations are medial hypertrophy of the muscular pulmonary arteries and muscularization of the arterioles. This is followed by concentric laminar fibrosis in the so-called "onion skin" configuration. The walls of the muscular pulmonary arteries may show necrotizing arteritis with fibrinoid necrosis. Plexiform lesions are a striking and diagnostically important finding, consisting of a network of capillary-like channels within a dilated segment of a muscular pulmonary artery. The lesions are seen only in patients with severe pulmonary arterial hypertension. Plexiform lesions are not specific to primary pulmonary hypertension, being seen also in patients with pulmonary hypertension secondary to left-to-right shunts, both natural and postsurgical, as well as in those with pulmonary hypertension secondary to liver disease; but they are not seen in pulmonary veno-occlusive disease or in recurrent pulmonary thromboemboli.

A number of theories have been proposed to explain the etiology of classic primary pulmonary hypertension.[258] These include recurrent venous thromboembolism, in situ thrombosis secondary to a coagulation defect, effect of drugs, a congenital defect of the arterial walls, and an arteritis or some form of collagen vascular disease. Venous thromboemboli are considered an unlikely cause of the plexogenic form,[105, 258] partly because of the absence of plexiform lesions in cases which show definite histologic features of large thromboemboli, and also because of the predominance of children and young adults, an unlikely age group to predominate if venous thromboembolism were the cause. *Aminorex fumarate*, an appetite suppressant, produced an identical picture to primary pulmonary hypertension in those few subjects who used the drug, as does the "bush tea" of native West Indians in which *Crotolaria fulva* is believed to be responsible. The striking female-to-male ratio and the fact that the disease is often encountered shortly after puberty suggest that female sex hormones may be important in the etiology of the condition. Familial cases of primary pulmonary hypertension have also been reported, and it has been postulated that the disease may be related to an inherited tendency to increased pulmonary vascular reactivity.

The age range is wide; most patients are adults or older children, but cases have been described in young children and infants. In a large series of 156 patients, the average age was 33 (range, 16 to 69) and the female-to-male ratio was 4:1.[258] The patients complain of weakness, dyspnea, and chest pain. Hemoptysis may occur. Arrhythmias are common in the later stages. Physical examination reveals all the expected signs of right ventricular pressure overload and elevated systemic venous pressure. Pulmonary regurgitation may be heard on auscultation. Cyanosis is a late finding.

The radiographic features of primary pulmonary hypertension (Figs 8–20 and 8–26)[6, 101, 129] (excluding pulmonary veno-occlusive disease) are dilation of the main pulmonary artery and the other central arteries with rapid tapering to oligemic peripheral lung, the peripheral lung vessels being narrow and inconspicuous. The average width of the right descending pulmonary artery was twice the diameter of normal controls in one review of 54 patients with primary pulmonary hypertension,[129] but as with all types of pulmonary hypertension, the plain film studies may show relatively little dilation of central vessels (Fig 8–27).

The radionuclide perfusion patterns in primary pulmonary hypertension have been extensively

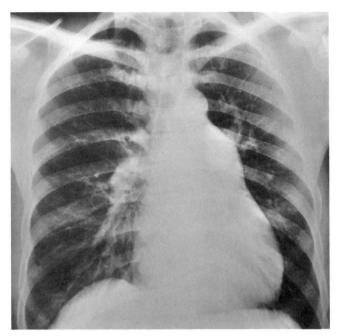

FIG 8–26.
Primary pulmonary hypertension in a 37-year-old man. There is cardiomegaly, an enlarged main pulmonary artery, and enlarged hilar arteries. In this instance, the arteries beyond the hili are normal in size.

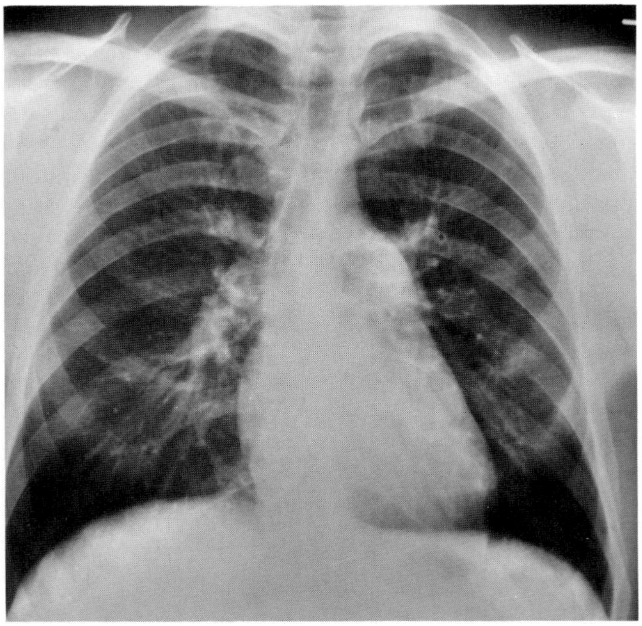

FIG 8–27.
Primary pulmonary hypertension in a 25-year-old man. The chest is almost normal despite a pulmonary artery pressure of 93 mm Hg systolic and a mean pressure of 62 mm Hg. The heart is normal in size and shape. The only abnormal finding is enlargement of the main pulmonary artery.

studied.* The usual pattern is either normal perfusion or patchy, peripheral, nonsegmental, perfusion defects. A few patients with primary pulmonary hypertension, three out of 13 in one series, showed segmental defects consistent with high probability for pulmonary embolism.[188]

In one recent study of primary pulmonary hypertension, the patients were divided into plexogenic and microthromboembolic on histologic criteria. In the plexogenic group, the lung scans showed a normal distribution of tracer, whereas in the microthromboembolic group there was patchy distribution of the radionuclide in the lung periphery in all but one patient.[194] The patchy distribution of tracer in the thromboembolic group was thought to result probably from occlusion of some of the larger pulmonary arterioles. This separation between the histologic subtypes of primary pulmonary hypertension by radionuclide perfusion scanning was not confirmed in another large study.[188]

Cardiac catheterization is required for the diagnosis. The pulmonary vascular resistance is extremely high. The pulmonary capillary wedge pressure, if it can be measured, is normal and the left-

*References 62, 78, 142, 188, 194, and 268.

sided pressures are also normal. Right-to-left shunting through a patent foramen ovale may be present. Pulmonary arteriography is mainly used to exclude intraluminal filling defects due to thromboemboli. The pulmonary arterial tree shows dilatation of the central vessels. The peripheral vessels taper to an abnormal degree[34] and are reduced in number. Delayed clearance of contrast material from the arterial tree was seen in 22 of 25 patients in one series.[101]

Pulmonary Veno-occlusive Disease

Pulmonary veno-occlusive disease is a very rare disorder, and its cause is unknown. The entity was included by the WHO as one of the subtypes of primary pulmonary hypertension along with plexogenic pulmonary arteriopathy (classic primary pulmonary hypertension) and recurrent pulmonary thromboembolism.[107] The pulmonary veins thrombose and develop intimal fibrosis. It is often suggested that the initial pulmonary venous thromboses follow infection, presumably by a yet unidentified virus.[244, 257, 259] Occlusion of the pulmonary veins leads to pulmonary venous and capillary congestion, pulmonary edema, alveolar hemosiderin deposits, and pulmonary arterial hypertension which may be very severe.[259] The muscular pulmonary arteries develop medial hypertrophy, and there is muscularization of the small pulmonary veins and arterioles.[105] Thrombi, either recent, organized, or recanalized, may be seen in these vessels, but plexiform lesions are absent. Patchy interstitial fibrosis and interstitial pneumonia are often present, though honeycomb lung is not a feature.[70, 105] The pulmonary arteriolar wedge pressure is usually normal—and if abnormal, is only mildly elevated.[41, 51, 190, 201, 212] It is primarily for this reason that pulmonary veno-occlusive disease is included in the category of primary pulmonary hypertension.

The chest radiographic appearances[190, 212] are those of pulmonary arterial hypertension together with, in some cases, signs of pulmonary edema. Both alveolar edema and interstitial edema are commonly seen in this condition (Fig 8–28). In one review of the radiographic features of 26 cases, 20 patients showed pulmonary edema.[190] The left atrium is not enlarged, an important point of difference with mitral valve disease, left atrial myxoma and cor triatriatum. Surprisingly, there is usually no evidence of upper zone blood diversion.

Radionuclide lung scans are either normal or show small bilateral wedge-shaped perfusion defects.[244] Pulmonary angiography shows dilatation of the proximal pulmonary arteries and slow circulation through the pulmonary vascular bed.[244] The venous phase does not help in making the diagnosis, but does help exclude other causes of pulmonary arterial hypertension, such as congenital stenosis of the pulmonary veins, left atrial myxoma, and cor triatriatum.[212]

Pulmonary Hypertension Secondary to Pulmonary Vasculitis

Pulmonary arterial hypertension may be caused by a large variety of pulmonary vasculitides. Mostly these conditions affect the small vessels and these are discussed in Chapter 11. Large vessel vasculitis is much less common. Takayasu's disease is the best known example of a large vessel vasculitis causing pulmonary hypertension.

Takayasu's arteritis (Takayasu's disease, pulseless disease) is an arteritis of medium/large arteries that most commonly affects segments of the aorta and its main branches. The vessel wall becomes fibrosed and thickened, usually causing luminal stenosis rather than aneurysm. Takayasu's arteritis occurs chiefly in women, with 75% of patients presenting between 10 and 20 years of age.[147] The presenting features are constitutional symptoms, fever, arthralgia, and symptoms of local ischemia with absent pulses or bruits. Moderate systemic hypertension is common, usually due to renal ischemia.[147] The

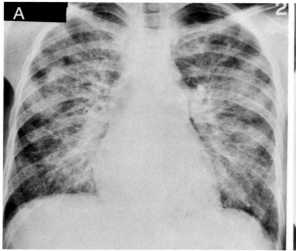
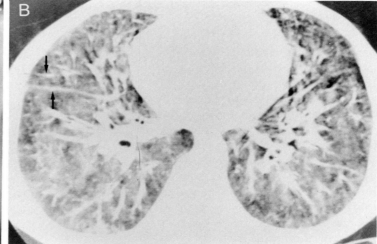

FIG 8–28.
Pulmonary veno-occlusive disease in a 16-year-old boy with a 4-month history of increasing dyspnea. The patient died 3 days later. Note the alveolar and interstitial edema and the signs of pulmonary arterial hypertension. The CT scan shows the septal lines *(downward pointing arrow)* and subpleural pulmonary edema *(upward pointing arrow)* to advantage. **A,** PA radiograph. **B,** CT scan. (Courtesy of Dr. Ian Kerr, London.)

course is variable, with episodic remissions, or progression; death occurs in about 25% of cases.

Involvement of pulmonary arteries occurs in approximately half the patients.[131, 146] The pulmonary hypertension is usually mild, and pulmonary symptoms are unusual.[146] The plain chest radiograph, in addition to showing the features of pulmonary arterial hypertension, may reveal oligemic areas beyond the obstructed arteries.[274] The plain chest radiograph may also show the features of aortic arteritis, namely irregular outline to the aorta, aortic ectasia, calcification of the aortic wall, or even rib notching.[24, 274] Abnormal perfusion scans, resembling the pattern in pulmonary embolism, are seen in up to 80% of patients.[131] Angiography reveals obstructions or stenoses of the lobar and segmental branches of the pulmonary arteries, and there may also be focal areas of dilatation.[146, 274]

Pulmonary Hypertension Secondary to Pleuropulmonary Disease

Pulmonary hypertension is a common phenomenon in chronic pulmonary diseases, notably in chronic bronchitis, emphysema, and interstitial fibrotic lung disease (Figs 8–29 and 8–30). Fibrothorax and lung destruction resulting from infection are less frequent causes of pulmonary hypertension.

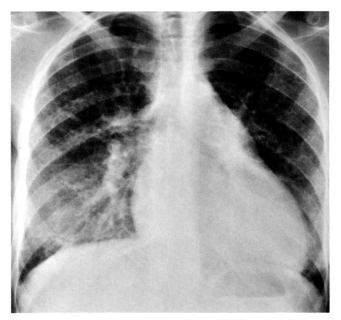

FIG 8–29.
Pulmonary arterial hypertension secondary to interstitial fibrosis, in this instance due to polymyositis/dermatomyositis.

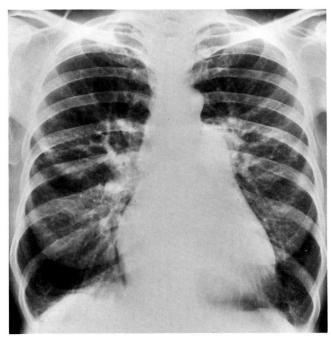

FIG 8–30.
Pulmonary arterial hypertension secondary to chronic bronchitis and emphysema showing the signs of pulmonary hypertension, namely, cardiomegaly, central arterial dilatation, and upper zone vessel enlargement, and the signs of emphysema, namely, overly inflated lungs and patchy vessel deficiency.

The common factor responsible for the elevated pulmonary vascular resistance in all these conditions is probably hypoxia, the most efficient known vasoconstrictor. Hypercapnea, acidemia, erythrocytemia, and increased blood volume may all contribute to the pulmonary hypertension. In disorders such as emphysema and interstitial fibrosis, there is the added possibility that destruction of the lung vasculature may play a role.[154] The relationship between lung destruction and raised pulmonary vascular resistance is not simple. No direct correlation between the severity of the emphysema and the degree of right ventricular hypertrophy at autopsy has been shown.[57, 115] (Right ventricular hypertrophy is the pathologist's criterion of long-standing pulmonary arterial hypertension.) Also, more lung can be destroyed by pan-acinar emphysema than by centrilobular emphysema without raising pulmonary arterial pressure. Yet, centrilobular emphysema is associated with particularly severe forms of cor pulmonale (the blue bloater).

The radiologic features consist of a combination of the signs of the responsible pleuropulmonary disease and the signs of pulmonary arterial hypertension, often with evidence of associated biventricular cardiac failure.

Pulmonary Hypertension Secondary to Increased Pulmonary Blood Flow

Pulmonary artery pressure can be elevated even without a rise in pulmonary vascular resistance if the pulmonary arterial blood flow is large enough. Sustained very high flows of this order are seen only with left-to-right shunts. The increased vessel size due to the massive blood flow dominates the radiographic picture. The elevations of pulmonary artery pressure are mild and do not contribute in a recognizable fashion to the radiographic appearances.

The term "Eisenmenger reaction" refers to raised pulmonary vascular resistance secondary to left-to-right shunting of blood, the usual causes of which are atrial septal defect (ASD), ventricular septal defect (VSD), and patent ductus arteriosus (PDA). The appearances on histologic examination are identical to those seen in primary pulmonary hypertension. The arterial changes consist of varying degrees of hypertrophy of the media of the small muscular arteries and arterioles, together with intimal cellular proliferation in the more severe cases. Plexiform lesions and necrotizing arteritis may also be seen in the advanced cases. The medial hypertrophy and any vasoconstrictive element that may be present are potentially reversible, whereas necrotizing arteritis and the plexiform lesions are regarded as irreversible.

The radiographic features of left-to-right shunt are cardiac enlargement and enlargement of all the pulmonary vessels, both central and peripheral, in all lung zones. With normal pulmonary vascular resistance, the distention of the pulmonary vascular tree is approximately proportional to the increased flow. With a fully established Eisenmenger's syndrome (reversal of shunt owing to elevation of pulmonary vascular resistance) the central vessels show disproportionate enlargement with rapid tapering at segmental level and beyond. It can be difficult to recognize mild or moderate elevation of pulmonary vascular resistance, because the diagnosis depends on evaluating the relative size of the vessels, and there are no acceptable measurements or ratios on which to base this decision. The pattern varies according to the defect. Rees and Jefferson[192] showed that in Eisenmenger ASD the chest radiograph shows massive enlargement of the central vessels

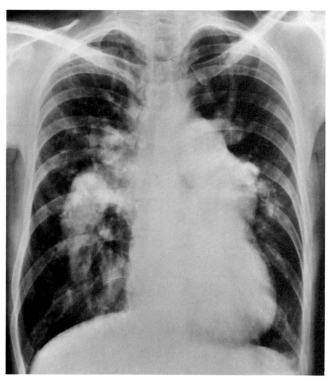

FIG 8–31.
Pulmonary arterial hypertension in a middle-aged man due to atrial septal defect with Eisenmenger's syndrome, showing the truly massive enlargement of the central pulmonary arteries in this condition.

with rapid tapering beyond hilar level (Fig 8–31), whereas with Eisenmenger VSD the degree of dilatation of the central vessels is usually mild and sometimes even unrecognizable (Fig 8–32). Thus, with ventricular septal defect, even in cases with systemic pressures in the pulmonary circuit, the rapid tapering of vessel size is often not present. In fact, the appearances are often similar to a mild or moderate left-to-right shunt with no recognizable evidence of pulmonary arterial hypertension. It is even possible to see a normal or near normal radiograph in Eisenmenger VSD. Eisenmenger PDA shows moderate dilatation of the aortic arch and the main pulmonary artery, and mild dilatation of the right and left hilar arteries. (The ductus itself may calcify.) The explanation for the different appearances of Eisenmenger ASD, VSD, and PDA is conjectural. In the fetus the arterioles have a relatively thick muscular wall and a small lumen. In the normal individual, the thickness of the muscle layer decreases and the relative size of the lumen increases after birth. In a patient with an ASD, even a sizable one, the pulmonary vascular resistance drops to normal and only rises again much

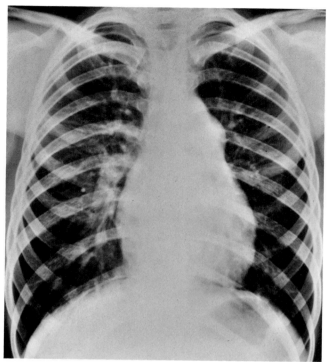

FIG 8–32.
Pulmonary arterial hypertension in a 14-year-old boy due to ventricular septal defect with Eisenmenger's syndrome, illustrating the relatively mild dilatation of the main pulmonary artery and hilar arteries seen with this condition even when, as in this case, the pulmonary arterial pressure is at systemic levels.

later in life, whereas in a patient with a large VSD, the pulmonary vascular resistance remains high from early infancy on. It seems likely that, in such patients, the constant pulmonary hypertension during early life prevents the involution of elastic tissue in the main pulmonary artery and its proximal branches. These arteries are, therefore, less distensible than in patients with ASD.[105]

Pulmonary Hypertension Due to Alveolar Hypoventilation Without Underlying Lung Disease

Alveolar hypoventilation can lead to hypoxia, and hypoxia is the most potent known stimulus for pulmonary vasoconstriction.[79] Hypoxic pulmonary vasoconstriction normally helps match blood flow and ventilation, diverting blood flow away from poorly ventilated areas.[161] When only a small portion of the lung is hypoxic, this response improves arterial oxygen saturation by reducing blood flow to the poorly ventilated segments without increasing pulmonary artery pressure. However, with wide-spread alveolar hypoxia, this normally protective response causes a large fraction of the pulmonary vasculature to constrict, thereby increasing pulmonary artery pressure.[161]

Alveolar hypoventilation without underlying disease is seen in morbid obesity—an entity that used to be called "the Pickwickian syndrome," but is now more frequently labeled the alveolar hypoventilation syndrome. (The term "Pickwickian syndrome" was coined in 1956 by Burwell et al.[39] when describing an obese middle-aged executive with fatigue and somnolence; they likened the syndrome to the fat boy in Charles Dickens' novel *The Pickwick Papers*.) The effects of morbid obesity on lung ventilation are complex, consisting of (1) obstructive sleep apnea, and (2) hypoventilation (hypoxemia and hypercarbia) even while awake and breathing room air. The mechanisms of hypoventilation include a marked increase in abdominal contents which push the diaphragm up, increased chest wall compliance, weakness of inspiratory muscles, and altered hypoxic and hypercapnic responsiveness.[199, 237, 279] Most patients with the sleep apnea and alveolar hyperventilation syndromes are markedly obese, but there are exceptions. Conversely, many very obese patients do not suffer from either syndrome.

Radiographically, the appearances are those of pulmonary arterial hypertension with cardiomegaly and dilatation of the central pulmonary arteries in an obese subject.

PULMONARY ARTERY ANEURYSM

Pulmonary artery aneurysms are rare. They may be congenital in origin or acquired. Mycotic aneurysms are the most frequently encountered.[193] Those that develop in the walls of tuberculous cavities are known as Rasmussen's aneurysms.[10] Mycotic aneurysms may also occur in association with lung abscess or septicemia, particularly in drug addicts. Post-traumatic false aneurysm,[65, 240] dissecting aneurysm of a pulmonary artery,[217] and myxomatous emboli from a right atrial myxoma[91] are all very rare causes of pulmonary artery aneurysm.

Hemoptysis is the principal complication and is frequently fatal. The largest series were reported before the advent of antituberculous therapy. In one autopsy series,[10] rupture of the aneurysm was the immediate cause of death in 38 of the 45 tuberculosis patients examined. In only two cases were the aneurysms believed to be incidental. Even today, fatalities occur.[193]

It is rare to see the aneurysm as a discrete mass in an otherwise normal lung. Usually, the aneurysm is adjacent to, or surrounded by, the infection that caused it and it may, therefore, be very difficult to appreciate. On plain radiographs and conventional tomograms, Rasmussen's aneurysms may closely resemble mycetomas growing in cavities. Because both cause hemoptysis, the true diagnosis is easily overlooked. The clue may be the rapid change in size of a mass due to an aneurysm. CT scanning clearly showed the vascular nature of the mass in one of the cases reported by Remy et al.[193]

ANGIODYSPLASIA IN HEPATIC CIRRHOSIS

Patients with severe, long-standing hepatic cirrhosis of any cause may develop an angiodysplasia of the lungs. These lesions, which have been likened to spider nevi, are spidery vessels randomly distributed through the lungs with a predilection for the subpleural regions.[25, 175, 198] They are believed to be responsible for right-to-left shunting of blood with consequent hypoxia. The mechanism of hypoxia in patients with hepatic cirrhosis is not always certain. Shunting of blood from the portal system to the pulmonary veins has been suggested as one possibility,[105, 206] but this would not explain all the cases.[175] Most of the reports in the literature consist of small groups of patients,* but one prospective study of 170 patients with various types of liver disease showed gas transfer defects in 20%. The patients may develop severe enough hypoxemia to be cyanosed, and clubbing of the fingers and toes may be evident. Most of the patients, but not all, have spider nevi of the skin.[16]

The chest radiograph may be normal or may show increased vascular markings and/or small nodular shadows (Fig 8–33).[25, 198] In the 170 patients reported by Stanley and Woodgate, mottled shadowing was found on the chest radiograph in 6%.[233] Radionuclide perfusion lung scanning shows extensive extrapulmonary uptake due to the bypassing of the pulmonary arteriolar bed.[5, 16] The percentage shunt can be calculated from the radionuclide counts. Shunt calculations may reveal large shunts, with more than 50% of the pulmonary blood flow bypassing the alveoli.[271] In one reported case, substantial fluctuation in the degree of right-to-left shunting was observed which corresponded to changes in arterial oxygen tension.[53] Pulmonary angiography

*References 16, 25, 71, 104, 130, 175, and 202.

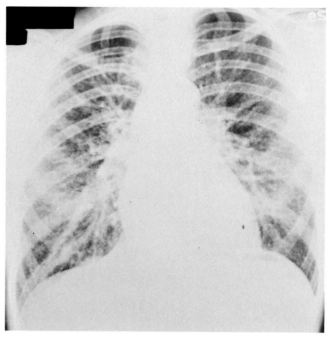

FIG 8–33.
Angiodysplasia of the lungs in a 20-year-old man with juvenile cirrhosis who was very hypoxic. The lungs show widespread increase in vessel size.

shows dilatation of the large and medium-sized arteries, with a myriad of abnormal spidery branches in the lung periphery and rapid filling of enlarged pulmonary veins. It is noteworthy that lung biopsy may be negative for disease, even in patients with very abnormal radiographic findings.[71] The lungs do not show interstitial fibrosis, nor is there any thickening of the alveolar walls.[25] The best way to demonstrate the angiodysplasia at pathologic study is with latex or gelatin casts of the vascular tree.[25, 175]

THE CHEST RADIOGRAPH IN SICKLE CELL DISEASE

Patients with sickle cell anemia are at increased risk for pneumonia and pulmonary infarction. Distinguishing between these two entities both clinically and radiologically can be very difficult.[19] Because of this difficulty, the more general term "acute chest syndrome" is now applied to describe fever, clinical findings of a pulmonary process, and radiologic evidence of new pulmonary consolidation in a patient with sickle cell hemoglobinopathy.[185] The acute chest syndrome is one of the most common reasons for hospitalization and is a significant cause of mortality in these patients.[18, 185]

A large survey of children who required hospital admission during the period 1958 to 1968[18] showed that bacterial pneumonia, particularly pneumococcal pneumonia, was responsible for the acute event in some 40% of patients, and the authors speculated that the true incidence of bacterial pneumonia was much higher. A recent survey revealed a similar incidence of pulmonary infections but a much lower proportion of bacterial pneumonia and relatively few cases of pneumococcal pneumonia.[185] Viral pneumonia and mycoplasmal pneumonia were about as frequent as bacterial pneumonia. The lower incidence of bacterial pneumonia in the more recent study may have reflected the use of penicillin prophylaxis and pneumococcal immunization.[185] In both of these series, the precise cause of more than half the episodes could not be determined, and they were presumed to result from pulmonary infarction, atelectasis, or missed infection.

Pulmonary infarction, which is much more frequent in adults than in children,[49, 64] is often associated with other evidence of sickle cell crisis such as abdominal or musculoskeletal pain.[18] Pulmonary infarction is rare in children under 12 years of age. Autopsy series, which clearly represent the severe end of the spectrum of pulmonary disease, show a high prevalence of pulmonary infarcts, even in infants and young children.[176] The autopsy findings consist of (1) pneumonia, (2) pulmonary infarction with necrosis of alveolar walls, (3) pulmonary vascular thrombosis with pulmonary hypertension, and (4) bone marrow embolization from areas of ischemic bone necrosis.[108]

Radiographically,[224] there are confluent lobar or segmental consolidations that may be accompanied by pleural effusion (Fig 8–34). The consolidations resolve more slowly than in the general population, and recurrence is common. Distinguishing consolidation resulting from infection from that due to infarction is often impossible. Pulmonary angiography is not recommended, and radionuclide lung scanning is of limited diagnostic value because so many of the scans will fall into the intermediate probability category. One clue to the diagnosis of infarction may be the late development of a pulmonary shadow; consolidation resulting from pneumonia is likely to be present on the initial film. If the shadowing is clearly interstitial in character and the patient has fever, then viral or mycoplasmal pneumonia are the likely diagnoses. Pulmonary edema, either interstitial or alveolar, may be present and can be confused with pneumonia/infarction. The edema may be the result of treatment with analge-

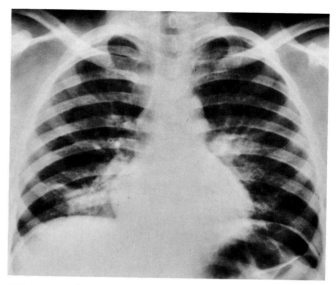

FIG 8–34.
Sickle cell disease, with probable pulmonary infarcts, in a 17-year-old boy with left-sided chest pain. Radionuclide scan showed mismatched ventilation/perfusion defects in lung regions that were clear on this chest radiograph.

sics such as morphine or may be the consequence of heart failure.

In addition to the pulmonary features of the acute chest syndrome, the heart may show nonspecific enlargement and the pulmonary blood vessels are frequently enlarged. Several hemodynamic factors are at work, and the relative role of each may be difficult to unravel in an individual case. Chronic anemia of any cause gives rise to a sustained increase in cardiac output even when the patient is at rest.[255] Chronic high cardiac output can be recognized on plain chest radiographs as nonspecific cardiomegaly and increase in the size of the pulmonary blood vessels. Increased left ventricular mass has been well documented by echocardiography.[14] Myocardial damage or ischemia from sickle cell disease may also contribute to the cardiac enlargement and to cardiac dysfunction, though the evidence for this is tenuous.[140] Finally, and very rarely, pulmonary hypertension similar to that seen in primary pulmonary hypertension may develop secondary to obstruction of the pulmonary vascular bed.[56]

PULMONARY EDEMA

Pulmonary edema is usually due to one of two mechanisms[11, 123, 153, 232]: elevated pulmonary venous pressure or increased permeability of the alveolar-capillary membrane. Occasionally, the edema is related to decreased plasma oncotic pressure or lymphatic insufficiency. Finally there are those disorders in which the mechanism is unknown or incompletely understood; even here, increased vascular permeability is often a major factor.

This division of pulmonary edema into "cardiogenic" and "noncardiogenic," though convenient, is not always clear-cut,[232] nor is there general agreement about all the conditions to be included in these catch-all terms. Despite the imprecision, the concept of dividing pulmonary edema into those conditions in which the cause is primarily hydrostatic and those in which the cause is primarily capillary damage (e.g., adult respiratory distress syndrome; see discussion in a later section) has considerable merit for the clinician, since the treatment is fundamentally different.

Raised Pulmonary Venous Pressure

Because the signs of raised pulmonary venous pressure frequently precede or accompany cardiogenic pulmonary edema, they will be described first.

Normally, in the upright subject, particularly on a film taken with deep inspiration, the vessels in the lower zones are larger than the equivalent vessels in the upper zones. With elevation of the pulmonary venous pressure, the upper zone vessels enlarge.[221] If, when the patient is erect, the upper zone vessels have a diameter equal to or larger than the equivalent lower zone vessels, then elevation of the pulmonary venous pressure should be strongly considered (Fig 8–35).[253]

It would be ideal to have well documented criteria for vessel size in various parts of the lungs, but so far none are available. The following may, however, be helpful. (1) Jefferson and Rees suggest that vessels in the first intercostal space on standard upright films should not exceed 3 mm in diameter.[126] (2) In some patients one can measure the diameter of the vessels that accompany a bronchus. For example, the anterior segmental bronchus of one or other upper lobe can often be identified end-on as a ring shadow. The accompanying artery is normally much the same diameter as the bronchus. A marked disparity, say greater than 1½ times the diameter of the bronchus, is taken to represent vessel enlargement.

The sign of upper zone vessel dilatation is believed to reflect increased blood flow to the upper zones.[87, 196, 263] The most widely accepted explanation for redistribution of pulmonary blood flow in subjects with elevated pulmonary venous pressure is that of West et al.,[263] who suggested that in the up-

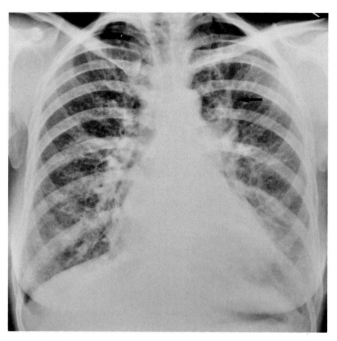

FIG 8–35.
Raised pulmonary venous pressure in a patient with mitral stenosis. Note that the vessels in the first and second rib interspace *(arrow)* are large compared with equivalent vessels in the lower zones.

right subject, there is preferential development of pulmonary edema in the lower lobes. This basal interstitial edema, though not visible radiographically, is believed to form a perivascular cuff, which acts as a buffer between the vessels and the distending forces being transmitted through the lungs, with resultant redistribution of blood flow to the upper zones.[263] This explanation has, however, been disputed.[100, 196, 239]

The assessment of the signs of redistribution of blood flow requires technically good radiographs and is therefore easier when one uses films obtained with fixed equipment, though acceptable interpretations can often be made from images taken with portable equipment. Two essentials are that the patient be upright and that the film be exposed on inspiration. In normal supine subjects, blood flow is fairly equal in the upper and lower zones, and redistribution of blood flow is, therefore, much more difficult to recognize on examinations with the patient supine. Also, it should be realized that a similar pattern of redistribution occurs in several other conditions, notably raised pulmonary arteriolar resistance;[100] basal lung disease, particularly emphysema;[164, 165] and basal pulmonary emboli.

The radiographic sign of upper zone redistribution of blood flow has proved very accurate in predicting the pulmonary venous pressure in chronic valvular heart disease[20, 220] and reasonably accurate in acute and chronic ischemic heart disease.[20, 23, 110, 157] The sign is, however, of limited value in the differential diagnosis of pulmonary shadows, when pulmonary edema is just one of several diagnoses being considered. In one large series, only 50% of the patients with pulmonary edema resulting from heart disease showed redistribution of flow.[166] We too have seen many examples of cardiogenic pulmonary edema in which the vascular redistribution could not be recognized. Sometimes the vessels cannot be adequately seen because of surrounding edema; sometimes they can be readily identified, but no redistribution is present.

Cardiogenic Pulmonary Edema

Under normal circumstances, the pulmonary interstitium and alveoli are kept relatively dry. Increased quantities of tissue fluid resulting from elevated pulmonary venous pressure lead at first to increased lymphatic drainage. Once the capacity of the pulmonary lymphatics is exceeded, pulmonary edema results. Fluid collects first in the interstitium and then spills into the air spaces.

The major causes of cardiogenic (hydrostatic) pulmonary edema are cardiac disease, overhydration, and fluid retention as a result of renal failure. Clinically, the major effect is dyspnea and tachypnea. With the development of alveolar flooding, severe hypoxemia and hypocapnea or hypercapnea occur. In extreme cases, blood-tinged foam is expectorated. Wheezing, the demand for an upright posture, and sweating are all prominent symptoms.

The radiologic signs of cardiogenic pulmonary edema are usually divided into interstitial and alveolar patterns, even though these phenomena are in reality a continuum. Interstitial edema may be seen without alveolar fluid, but if alveolar edema is present, the interstitium must also be edematous, whether or not one can see it on the radiograph.

Plain chest films are highly sensitive for the diagnosis of pulmonary edema, and can even demonstrate edema in patients who have not yet developed symptoms.[42, 106] Conversely, it should be realized that pulmonary edema may be visible radiographically long after the hemodynamic factors have returned to normal.[184]

Cardiogenic Interstitial Pulmonary Edema

Interstitial pulmonary edema causes a variety of radiographic signs,[96, 113, 183] the most readily recognized of which are septal lines, bronchial wall thickening, and subpleural pulmonary edema (see Fig 8–36).

Septal Lines.— The appearance of septal lines is discussed in detail in Chapter 5. Because thickened septal lines occur in few conditions (see Table 5–9, Chapter 5), their identification is an extremely useful indicator of pulmonary edema. If transient or rapid in development, they are virtually diagnostic of interstitial pulmonary edema. Septal lines are not, however, a particularly frequent finding even in florid pulmonary edema.[42, 106] On occasion they may persist after pulmonary edema has resolved.

Bronchial Wall Thickening.— In normal chest radiographs the walls of the bronchi within the lung substance are invisible unless end-on to the x-ray beam, when they are seen to have a very thin and well-defined ringlike wall. If edema collects in the peribronchial interstitial space, the combined shadow of the edematous bronchial wall and the thickened interstitium results in visible bronchial wall thickening.[67] Not only do the end-on bronchial walls become much thicker, those that are not end-on may now have visible walls. The posterior wall of the bronchus intermedius, as seen in the lateral chest radiograph, is another useful site at which to assess thickening due to edema; it should normally measure less than 3 mm.[210]

Subpleural Pulmonary Edema.— Fluid can accumulate in the loose connective tissue beneath the visceral pleura. The pulmonary septa communicate freely with this space, and edema can therefore flow peripherally to dissect beneath the pleura. Subpleural edema is seen radiographically as a sharply defined band of increased density which, when adjacent to a fissure, makes the fissure appear thick[111] (Fig 8–36), and when in the costophrenic angles, produces a lamellar-shaped fluid collection resembling pleural effusion. It is the lamellar shape with the shadow conforming to the pleural boundary that suggests pulmonary rather than pleural fluid (Fig 8–37).

Lack of Clarity of the Intrapulmonary and Hilar Vessels (Hilar Haze).— The hilar and pulmonary blood vessels may appear indistinct because of surrounding edema. This sign, which is one of the most consistent findings with interstitial pulmonary edema,[106, 183] may be very difficult to evaluate. Comparison with previous radiographs in order to establish the normal appearance for a particular patient is

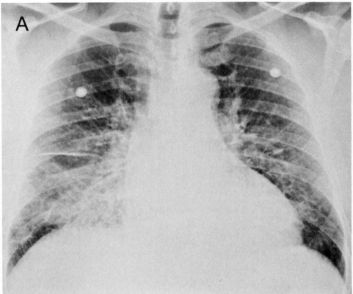

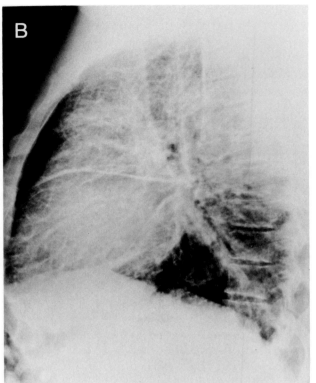

FIG 8–36.
Cardiogenic pulmonary edema following myocardial infarction in a 52-year-old man, illustrating widespread fissural thickening, and lack of clarity of intrapulmonary vessels and septal lines. There is frank alveolar edema in the right lower zone. The fissural thickening due to subpleural edema is particularly striking. **A,** frontal view. **B,** lateral view.

frequently needed. Often the sign can only be appreciated retrospectively on follow-up films once the edema has resolved.

Generalized Increase in Density of the Lung Parenchyma.—This is another subtle feature of pulmonary edema. The density of the lung on a plain chest radiograph is dependent on so many anatomic and technical factors that the sign is of little use in clinical management, though it has been used in experimental animals.[226] Density measurement by CT and signal characteristics at MRI both promise to be very useful in quantitating the amount of fluid present in the lungs.[222, 223]

Cardiogenic Alveolar Edema

Alveolar edema represents spill of fluid from the interstitium into the alveolar air spaces. The cardinal radiographic sign is, therefore, shadowing with the characteristics of air-space filling (Fig 8–38). The margins are poorly defined, though larger collections may show a well-defined boundary. The distribution is patchy and widespread, and the shadows tend to coalesce. Usually the shadowing is bilateral, occasionally unilateral, and rarely lobar. When unilateral, there is a striking and unexplained predispo-

sition for the right lung[172, 275] (Fig 8–39). Air bronchograms or air alveolograms may be evident, particularly when the edema is confluent. The acinar shadow of pulmonary edema has been emphasized. The appearance is due to the contrast between fluid-filled acini surrounded by aerated acini. The resulting shadow is a 5- to 10-mm moderately ill-defined nodule. Sometimes the nodules are smaller and resemble the miliary pattern seen in miliary tuberculosis.

The terms "bat's wing"[117] and "butterfly" shadowing were coined to describe the appearance of perihilar shadowing that is predominantly in the central portions of the lobes and fades out peripherally, leaving an aerated outer "cortex" (see Fig 8–38). This pattern is best seen on frontal views, the distribution being less easy to define on the lateral views.[92] The mechanism responsible for this characteristic distribution is uncertain. One suggestion is that lymphatic drainage is better in the outer portions of the lungs. Another is that the greater change in volume of the outer lung during each respiratory cycle in some way helps prevent edema.[81] Despite the emphasis given to the bat's wing pattern, it should be realized that most patients show a more diffuse and random distribution, with some lobes more severely affected than others. True, the shad-

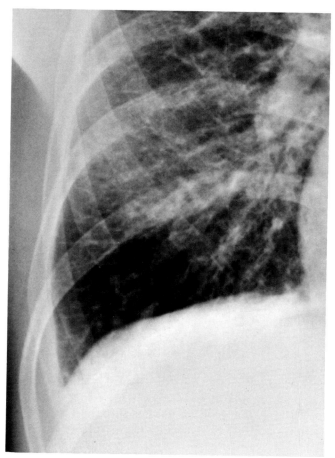

FIG 8–37.
Subpleural pulmonary edema producing a lamellar-shaped homogeneous density parallel to the chest wall in the costophrenic angle.

owing often spares the extreme upper and lower zones, but the classic bat's wing pattern is seen in the minority of patients.

Whatever the pattern, a striking feature of cardiogenic pulmonary edema is rapid change on films taken over short intervals; rapid clearing is particularly suggestive of the diagnosis. An extension of this phenomenon is the change in distribution of pulmonary edema when patients alter their position for a few hours, for example, by lying on one side.[277]

Adult Respiratory Distress Syndrome

Adult respiratory distress syndrome (ARDS), often referred to as noncardiogenic pulmonary edema, is a common disorder with a very high mortality.[66] It is due to increased pulmonary vascular permeability, and develops in response to lung injury. A large variety of insults may precipitate the

disorder, particularly bacterial sepsis, pneumonia, aspiration of gastric contents, circulatory shock, trauma, burns, and drug overdose. A full list of causes is given in Table 8–3.

The clinical syndrome[15, 66, 97] is characterized by acute, severe, progressive respiratory distress, widespread pulmonary opacity on chest radiographs, significant hypoxemia despite high inspired oxygen concentration, and decreased compliance of the lungs. In most cases, these features are present within 12 to 24 hours of the inciting events, and in 90% of patients the syndrome is evident within 72 hours.

The mechanism of damage to the pulmonary vascular endothelium is under intensive investigation, but the factors mediating ARDS have proved frustratingly difficult to unravel.[195] It appears clear that the inciting condition activates an injurious cascade.[97] The neutrophil appears to be an important agent in producing increased capillary permeability, but the inciting and inhibiting forces are unclear. Complement byproducts, alveolar macrophages, platelets, arachidonic acid metabolites, free radicals of oxygen, proteolytic enzymes, and inflammatory mediators such as prostaglandins, may all play a part,[7, 97] but no known pathogenetic sequence completely accounts for the acute alveolar damage that characterizes ARDS.[97]

Whatever the mechanism, the end result is damage to the alveolar capillary membrane leading to increased permeability to protein and interstitial edema. As the process continues, proteinaceous fluid spills into the alveoli. Eventually alveolar disruption and hemorrhage occur; surfactant is reduced and the alveoli tend to collapse. Unlike cardiogenic pulmonary edema, the edema is prolonged because the oncotic forces for reabsorption of fluid are not present.

Pathologically,[12] the alveoli and the perivascular and peribronchial spaces are congested and edematous. The alveoli are inhomogeneously filled with proteinaceous fluid, white cells, debris, and often hemorrhage. Greene, in his review article, divided the morphologic features into the following three stages[97]:

1. In stage 1 (first 12 to 24 hours), there is capillary congestion, endothelial cell swelling, and extensive microatelectasis. During this stage fluid leakage is minimal and limited to the interstitium, the respiratory distress being largely due to decreased pulmonary compliance.

2. In stage 2 (1 to 5 days), there is fluid leakage

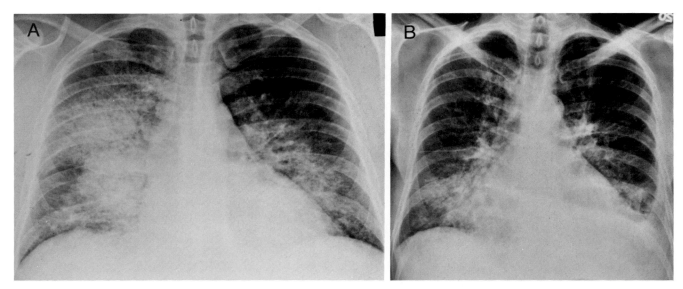

FIG 8–38.
Cardiogenic alveolar edema. **A,** butterfly pattern. **B,** bibasilar edema in a different patient showing septal lines and left pleural effusion. Note also the bronchial wall thickening and the thickening of the minor fissure.

and fibrin deposition and hyaline membranes develop. Alveolar consolidation by hemorrhagic fluid becomes extensive, and severe hypoxemia develops.

3. In stage 3 (after 5 days), there is alveolar cell proliferation, collagen deposition and microvascular destruction. The type II pneumonocytes become hyperplastic in an attempt to cover the denuded alveolar surfaces.

The roentgenographic changes may be delayed by 12 hours or more following the onset of clinical symptoms,[122, 128, 178] an important difference from

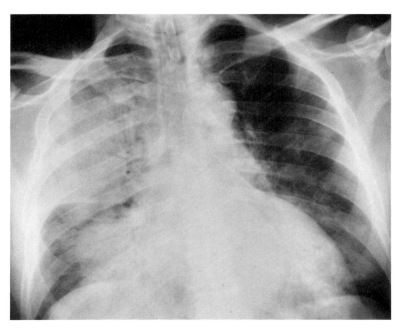

FIG 8–39.
Unilateral pulmonary edema following overtransfusion with intravenous fluids, showing an alveolar filling process almost entirely confined to the right lung. Note the air bronchograms.

TABLE 8–3.

Clinical Disorders Associated With the Adult Respiratory Distress Syndrome*

Septicemia—notably bacterial and viral pneumonia, gram-negative septicemia
Hemodynamic shock of any cause
Circulating toxins or vasoactive substances—notably bacterial endotoxins
Trauma, including radiation damage
Major surgery, notably following cardiopulmonary bypass
Burns
Bowel infarction
Fat embolism
Amniotic fluid embolism
Aspiration of liquids:
   Gastric contents
   Near drowning
   Hydrocarbon fluids
Inhaled toxins, notably:
   Smoke
   Oxygen
   Chemicals (NO_2, NH_3, war gases)
   Metal fumes (cadmium, mercury)
Metabolic disorders:
   Acute pancreatitis
   Diabetic ketoacidosis
   Uremia
Hematologic disorders, notably:
   Disseminated intravascular coagulation
   Leukoagglutinin reactions of drugs
Drug related, notably:
   Heroin
   Salicylates
   Methadone
   Ethchlorvynol

*Modified from Balk R, Bone RC: The adult respiratory distress syndrome. *Med Clin North Am* 1983; 67:685–700, and Matthay MA: Pathophysiology of pulmonary edema. *Clin Chest Med* 1985; 6:301–314.

cardiogenic pulmonary edema, where the chest radiograph is frequently abnormal before or coincident with the onset of symptoms. Some patients never develop significant pulmonary shadowing even though they become profoundly hypoxemic.[261]

The major features on plain chest radiograph (Figs 8–40 and 8–41)[69, 122, 128, 184, 189] are bilateral widespread patchy ill-defined densities resembling cardiogenic pulmonary edema, usually without cardiomegaly, upper zone blood diversion, or pleural effusion. The densities progress in severity to produce confluent opacification, the distribution of which is variable, but usually all lung zones are involved both centrally and peripherally, and air bronchograms may be a prominent feature. CT scans, however, show that the distribution of the pulmonary shadowing is patchy with preservation of normal lung regions,[155] the density being mostly in the posterior, or dependent, portions of the lungs.[90]

Signs of interstitial edema, namely hilar haze and lack of clarity of lung vessels, may also be present. Occasionally, the shadowing appears exclusively interstitial,[69] but septal lines are very rare.[184] Pistolesi et al.[184] have pointed out that the main pulmonary artery may appear bulged and that enlargement of the right side of the heart is frequently seen.

Patients with abnormal radiographs are all severely hypoxic and require assisted ventilation. There is usually a good correlation between the radiographic severity of the pulmonary edema and the arterial PO_2, except during the early phase of the disorder, when the chest radiograph may show only mild abnormality, or may even be normal.

Distinguishing Cardiogenic and Noncardiogenic Pulmonary Edema

The distinction between cardiogenic and noncardiogenic pulmonary edema on radiographic grounds alone can be difficult, but certain features may point in one direction or another.[184] In cardiogenic edema, the shadows due to pulmonary edema are present coincident with the onset of symptoms, show a central predominance, and may be associated with peribronchial cuffing and septal lines. Air bronchograms are relatively rare, occurring one-third as frequently as in ARDS. The severity of the shadows changes rapidly on serial films. The pulmonary vascular pedicle is often enlarged, and upper zone diversion of blood flow may be visible. Pleural effusions are common.

In noncardiogenic pulmonary edema, the shadows may be delayed compared with the onset of symptoms, and show relatively uniform zonal distribution. ARDS is rarely associated with septal lines, and peribronchial cuffing is less common than with the cardiogenic pulmonary edema. Air bronchograms are common in ARDS. The central and peripheral pulmonary vascular pattern is normal, though the main pulmonary artery may appear large. Pleural effusions are small and are only occasionally seen.

Complications of Adult Respiratory Distress Syndrome

ARDS results in high mortality and, as might be expected, many complications are seen. Septicemia is common and, in many instances, results from a pneumonia which complicates the ARDS. Multiple organ failure is a major cause of death. It is not clear whether organs such as the kidney, liver, and central nervous system are damaged by the same process that initiates the ARDS or whether multiple organ

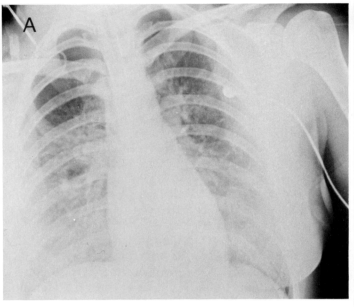

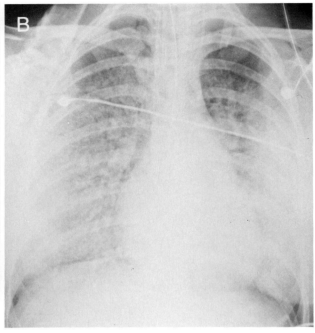

FIG 8–40.
Adult respiratory distress syndrome in a 19-year-old woman. **A,** early phase showing perihilar air space shadowing. **B,** 24 hours later there is widespread, fairly uniformly distributed air-space shadowing.

failure results from complications that follow the pulmonary injury, but it would appear that with modern critical care facilities, death from respiratory failure is less common than death from multiple organ failure.

Diagnosing pneumonia[8] from the chest radiograph in the presence of extensive pulmonary edema is clearly very difficult (see Fig 8–41). Increasing consolidation in one area of the lung in a patient with clinical features to indicate pneumonia is the important radiographic finding. The distinction from edema and atelectasis is often impossible. Cavitation is fairly specific to pneumonia, but even here there is still the difficulty of distinguishing abscess formation from pneumatocele formation. CT scanning may be very helpful in this regard (see Fig 8–41). Pulmonary hemorrhage resulting from trauma, for example, the balloon of a Swan-Ganz catheter, has to be included in the differential diagnosis.

During the acute phase, many patients will suffer barotrauma due to positive pressure ventilation with relatively noncompliant lungs. Pneumothorax and pneumomediastinum are very common, and in severe cases air will dissect from the mediastinum into the neck and chest wall and even into the retroperitoneum or peritoneal cavity (Fig 8–42). Interstitial emphysema is common, and pneumatoceles may develop within the lungs (Fig 8–43).

The long-term outlook for survivors of ARDS is poorly documented. Alberts et al.[1] in their review of the literature could find descriptions of follow-up chest radiographs in only 81 patients. In the great majority, the chest radiograph returned to normal, a few showed some degree of hyperinflation, and 11% showed residual interstitial shadowing. The true rate of conversion of ARDS to interstitial fibrosis is unknown, since follow-up lung biopsy is so rarely performed. It would appear to be very low.

Pulmonary Edema From Neurogenic Causes, High Altitude, and Acute Airway Obstruction

These three forms of pulmonary edema are considered separately because the edema in these conditions shows certain differences from the other varieties of noncardiogenic pulmonary edema.

Neurogenic Pulmonary Edema

A number of intracranial conditions including head trauma, seizures, intracranial hemorrhage, and tumors can be associated with acute pulmonary

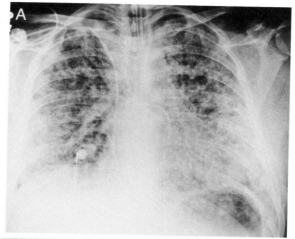

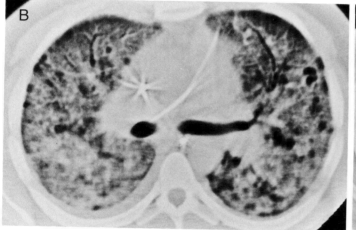

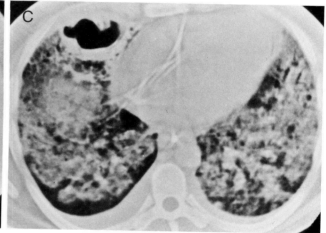

FIG 8–41.

Lung abscess complicating ARDS. **A,** plain chest radiograph shows the features of ARDS, but the complicating pneumonia with abscess formation is difficult to recognize. **B,** CT scan shows widespread but patchy distribution of air-space shadows. **C,** CT section at a lower level reveals a large abscess in the middle lobe. Sputum cultures revealed mixed gram-positive and gram-negative bacteria.

edema, even in patients who have no detectable heart or lung disease. The mechanism of the edema is debated.[55, 245] Because the edema can occur within a minute, it has been suggested that a sudden burst of neural activity stimulates the sympathetic nervous system, increasing the pulmonary blood volume and raising the pulmonary venous pressure.[245] The edema becomes proteinaceous, suggesting that endothelial damage also plays a part, but the cause of this damage is obscure.

The radiographic picture[73] is indistinguishable from that of cardiogenic pulmonary edema except that the heart is not enlarged (Fig 8–44). Although the edema may appear quickly, it may take up to 24 hours to be radiologically apparent. Unlike the usual forms of noncardiogenic pulmonary edema, the lungs usually clear within 24 to 48 hours.[55]

High Altitude Pulmonary Edema

High altitude pulmonary edema (mountain sickness) is seen predominantly in children or young adults who rapidly ascend to heights of 2,700 to 3,500 meters or greater. The entity is seen more frequently in individuals who undertake heavy physical exercise shortly after arrival at altitude, and there seems to be an individual susceptibility.[143] Symptoms of pulmonary edema develop 3 to 48 hours after achieving high altitude, the majority of patients experiencing the symptoms within 24 hours.[151] The most frequent early symptoms are dyspnea, short-

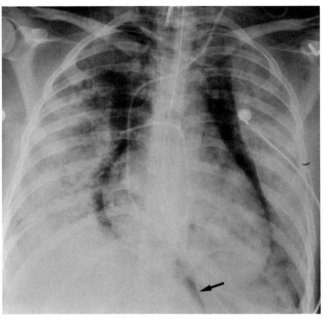

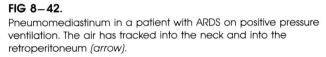

FIG 8–42.
Pneumomediastinum in a patient with ARDS on positive pressure ventilation. The air has tracked into the neck and into the retroperitoneum *(arrow).*

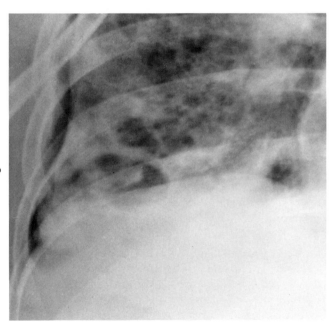

FIG 8–43.
Pneumatoceles that developed in a patient with ARDS. (There is also a right pneumothorax and chest drainage tube.)

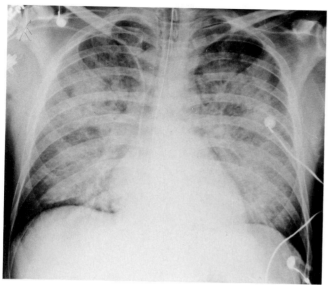

FIG 8–44.
Pulmonary edema due to raised intracranial pressure following subarachnoid hemorrhage caused by a ruptured aneurysm.

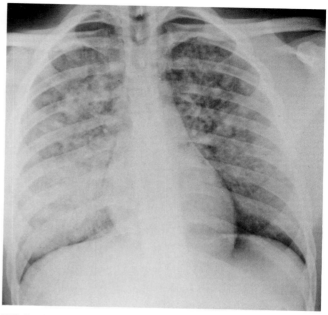

FIG 8–45.
Pulmonary edema due to acute severe laryngospasm following general anesthesia for a meniscectomy.

ness of breath, dry cough, and restlessness. The edema is extremely responsive to treatment with oxygen and return to lower altitudes.[151]

The mechanism is debated. Lockhart and Saiag, in their review, while acknowledging that the pathogenesis was elusive, divided the potential causes into the consequences of high pulmonary arterial pressure secondary to hypoxia, and the effect of increased capillary permeability.[143] Pulmonary capillary wedge pressures are near normal,[119] though transient elevations at the time of edema cannot be excluded. The protein content of the edema which, if high, would indicate increased vascular permeability, is not known, but the presence of hyaline membranes and fibrin-like material in the alveoli at autopsy suggests a protein-rich edema fluid.[151, 171]

The chest radiographic appearances are those of acute alveolar edema.[148] The heart remains normal in size, but the main pulmonary artery becomes prominent, decreasing in size with recovery.[151]

Pulmonary Edema Associated With Upper Airway Obstruction

Pulmonary edema can, on rare occasions, be associated with acute upper airway obstruction due to conditions such as laryngospasm[124] (Fig 8–45), croup,[250] epiglottitis,[250] sleep apnea,[50] or strangulation.[179] The mechanism is not clear. The possibilities include hypoxia, sympathomimetic overactivity, and negative intrapleural pressure. Clearly these processes may act in concert with one another.[250] The

extremely negative intrathoracic pressures in a patient struggling to overcome upper airway obstruction may lead to transudation of fluid on a mechanical basis, whereas severe hypoxemia may damage the small intrapulmonary vessels directly or may act by means of extreme vasoconstriction, elevation of pulmonary pressure, and excess sympathomimetic activity.

Reexpansion Pulmonary Edema

Following drainage of a pneumothorax the reexpanded lung may become acutely edematous. A similar sequence of events can follow drainage of a pleural effusion. The mechanism is obscure, some authors suggesting it is related to surfactant depletion[162, 181, 211, 249] and others that it results from anoxic capillary damage, leading to increased capillary permeability.[211] The edema usually develops within 2 hours of reexpansion and can progress for 1 or 2 days, resolving within 5 to 7 days. Reexpansion edema generally causes little morbidity, but patients can become hypotensive and hypoxic,[114, 127] and at least one death has been recorded.[207] It is generally held that complete pneumothoraces with gross lung collapse, chronicity of the pneumothorax, and high negative aspiration pressures are predisposing factors. Most pneumothoraces have been complete and present for at least 3 days,[162, 249] but exceptions of

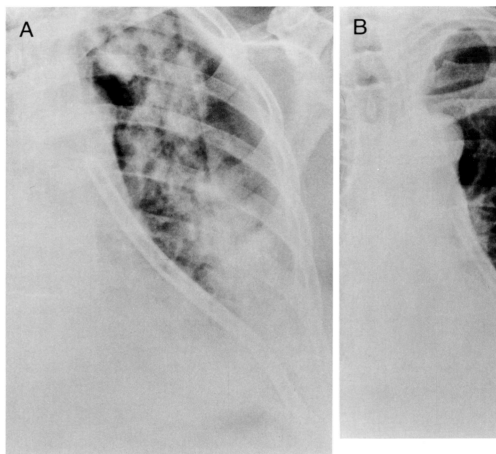

FIG 8–46.
Reexpansion pulmonary edema. **A,** plain chest radiograph showing acute pulmonary edema that developed after a large left pleural effusion was drained. **B,** 25 hours later, the pulmonary edema has cleared.

shorter duration have been reported.[216] In many patients expansion has been rapid because negative aspiration pressure was used,[54, 207, 278] but this has by no means been universal.[37, 120, 249, 260] The chest radiograph shows ipsilateral air space shadowing (Fig 8–46). Exceptional cases are reported with contralateral edema[114, 234] and recurrent edema with recurrent pneumothorax.[215]

Amniotic Fluid Embolism

Under normal circumstances no amniotic fluid enters the maternal circulation during pregnancy or during labor. Amniotic fluid contains fetal cellular debris and mucin and it is the squames from the fetal skin, and the mucin from fetal meconium, that appear to be responsible for the syndrome of amniotic fluid embolism.[181] On reaching the lungs, these materials incite hemodynamic shock with dyspnea, frothy blood-tinged sputum, cyanosis, and central nervous system irritability. Right heart catheterization characteristically shows elevated central venous pressure, elevated pulmonary arterial pressure, and elevated capillary wedge pressure, and it may be possible to identify amniotic fluid debris in blood samples taken through the right heart catheter.[171]

The condition is rare but frequently fatal (in a recent review of the literature the fatality rate was found to be 86%[171]) and is responsible for approximately 10% of maternal deaths.[171] Peterson and Taylor[181] suggested that in the majority of patients the amniotic fluid gains access through the site of placental attachment, the placenta having prematurely separated. In some cases uterine laceration is present. There is a high correlation with intrauterine death and fetal distress, suggesting that it is the amniotic fluid contents—particularly mucin—that do the harm. In patients who die from amniotic fluid embolism, labor is usually rapid with evidence of strong uterine contractions, implicating uterine hypertonicity as an important etiologic factor.[171, 181] The condition is most often seen late in the course of pregnancy, the babies rarely being premature, though the syndrome has recently been found to be an important cause of illegal abortion−related deaths.[171] At autopsy, the lungs are edematous with widespread atelectasis. It is not possible on gross examination to recognize that amniotic fluid embolism has occurred, but histologic examination with special stains will reveal fetal squames and/or mucin in all cases.[181]

Radiologically, the appearances are those of pulmonary edema, indistinguishable from the two other conditions that need to be considered in women during labor, namely acute cardiogenic edema and massive gastric aspiration.

REFERENCES

1. Alberts WM, Priest GR, Moser KM: The outlook for survivors of ARDS. *Chest* 1983; 84:272−274.
2. Alderson PO, Biello DR, Gottshalk A, et al: Tc^{99m}-DTPA aerosol and radioactive gases compared as adjuncts to perfusion scintigraphy in patients with suspected pulmonary embolism. *Radiology* 1984; 153:515−521.
3. Alderson PO, Rujanavech N, Secker-Walker RH, et al: The role of ^{133}Xe ventilation studies in the scintigraphic detection of pulmonary embolism. *Radiology* 1976; 120:633−640.
4. Alexander JK, Gonzalez DA, Fred HL: Angiographic studies in cardiorespiratory diseases: Special reference to thromboembolism. *JAMA* 1966; 198:575−578.
5. Andersen BL, Gordon L, Buse MG: Intrapulmonary shunting associated with cirrhosis: Incidental diagnosis by perfusion lung scan. *Clin Nucl Med* 1982; 7:108−110.
6. Anderson G, Reid L, Simon G: The radiographic appearances in primary and in thromboembolic pulmonary hypertension. *Clin Radiol* 1973; 24:113−120.
7. Andreadis NA, Petty TL: New basic and clinical science in adult respiratory distress syndrome. *Semin Respir Med* 1986; 8(Suppl):1−74.
8. Andrews CP, Coalson JJ, Smith JD, et al: Diagnosis of nosocomial bacterial pneumonia in acute diffuse lung injury. *Chest* 1981; 80:254−258.
9. Atkins HL, Robertson JS, Croft BY, et al: Estimates of radiation absorbed doses from radioxenons in lung imaging. *J Nucl Med* 1980; 21:459−465.
10. Auerbach O: Pathology and pathogenesis of pulmonary arterial aneurysm in tuberculous cavities. *Am Rev Tuberc* 1939; 39:99−115.
11. Ayres SM: Mechanisms and consequences of pulmonary edema: Cardiac lung, shock lung, and principles of ventilatory therapy in adult respiratory distress syndrome. *Am Heart J* 1982; 103:97−112.
12. Bachofen M, Wiebel ER: Structural alterations of lung parenchyma in the adult respiratory distress syndrome. *Clin Chest Med* 1982; 3:35−56.
13. Bachynski JE: Absence of air bronchogram sign. A reliable finding in pulmonary embolism with infarction or hemorrhage. *Radiology* 1971; 100:547−552.
14. Balfour IC, Covitz W, Davis H, et al: Cardiac size and function in children with sickle cell anemia. *Am Heart J* 1984; 108:345−350.
15. Balk R, Bone RC: The adult respiratory distress syndrome. *Med Clin North Am* 1983; 67:685−700.
16. Bank ER, Thrall JH, Dantzker DR: Radionuclide demonstration of intrapulmonary shunting in cirrhosis. *AJR* 1983; 140:967−969.
17. Baron MG: Fleischner lines and pulmonary emboli. *Circulation* 1972; 45:171−178.
18. Barrett-Connor E: Acute pulmonary disease and sickle cell anemia. *Am Rev Respir Dis* 1971; 104:159−165.
19. Barrett-Connor E: Pneumonia and pulmonary infarction in sickle cell anemia. *JAMA* 1973; 224:997−1000.
20. Baumstark A, Swensson RG, Hessel SJ, et al: Evaluating the radiographic assessment of pulmonary venous hypertension in chronic heart disease. *AJR* 1984; 141:877−884.
21. Bell WR, Simon TL: Current status of pulmonary thromboembolic disease: Pathophysiology, diagnosis, prevention and treatment. *Am Heart J* 1982; 103:239−262.
22. Bell WR, Simon TL, deMetz DL: The clinical features of submassive and massive pulmonary emboli. *Am J Med* 1977; 62:355−360.
23. Bennett ED, Rees S: The significance of radiological changes in the lungs in acute myocardial infarction. *Br J Radiol* 1974; 47:879−881.
24. Berkmen YM, Lande A: Chest roentgenography as a window to the diagnosis of Takayasu's arteritis. *AJR* 1975; 125:842−846.
25. Berthelot P, Walker JG, Sherlock S, et al: Arterial changes in the lungs in cirrhosis of the liver—lung spider nevi. *N Engl J Med* 1966; 274:291−298.
26. Biello DR: Radiological (scintigraphic) evaluation of patients with suspected pulmonary thromboembolism. *JAMA* 1987; 257:3257−3259.
27. Biello DR, Kumar B: Symmetrical perfusion defects without pulmonary embolism. *Eur J Nucl Med* 1982; 7:197−199.
28. Biello DR, Mattar AG, Achaw OW, et al: Interpretation of indeterminate lung scintigrams. *Radiology* 1979; 133:189−194.
29. Biello DR, Mattar AG, McKnight RC, et al: Ventilation-perfusion studies in suspected pulmonary embolism. *AJR* 1979; 133:1033−1037.
30. Bjornsson J, Edwards WD: Primary pulmonary hypertension: A histopathologic study of 80 cases. *Mayo Clin Proc* 1985; 60:16−25.

31. Blinder RA, Coleman RE: Evaluation of pulmonary embolism. *Radiol Clin North Am* 1985; 23:391–405.

32. Bogren HG, Berman DS, Vismara LA, et al: Lung ventilation-perfusion scintigraphy in pulmonary embolism: Diagnostic specificity compared to pulmonary angiography. *Acta Radiol* [Diagn] (Stockh) 1978; 19:933–944.

33. Bookstein JJ, Silver TM: The angiographic differential diagnosis of acute pulmonary embolism. *Radiology* 1974; 110:25–33.

34. Boxt LM, Rich S, Fried R, et al: Automated morphologic evaluation of pulmonary arteries in primary pulmonary hypertension. *Invest Radiol* 1986; 21:906–909.

35. Branch WT, McNeil BJ: Analysis of the differential diagnosis and assessment of pleuritic chest pain in young adults. *Am J Med* 1983; 75:671–679.

36. Braun SD, Newman GE, Ford K, et al: Ventilation-perfusion scanning and pulmonary angiography: Correlation in clinical high-probability pulmonary embolism. *AJR* 1984; 143:977–980.

37. Brennan NJ, FitzGerald MX: Anatomically localised re-expansion pulmonary oedema following pneumothorax drainage. *Respiration* 1979; 38:233–237.

38. Burchard KW, Carney WI: Tumor embolism as the first manifestation of cancer. *J Surg Oncol* 1984; 27:26–30.

39. Burwell CS, Robin ED, Whaley RD: Extreme obesity associated with alveolar hypoventilation—a Pickwickian syndrome. *Am J Med* 1956; 21:811–818.

40. Bynum LJ, Wilson JE: Radiographic features of pleural effusions in pulmonary embolism. *Am Rev Respir Dis* 1978; 117:829–834.

41. Carrington CB, Liebow AA: Pulmonary veno-occlusive disease. *Human Pathol* 1970; 1:322–324.

42. Chait A, Cohen HE, Meltzer LE, et al: The bedside chest radiograph in the evaluation of incipient heart failure. *Radiology* 1972; 105:563–566.

43. Chait A, Summers D, Krasnow N, et al: Observation on the fate of large pulmonary emboli. *AJR* 1967; 100:364–373.

44. Chakeres DW, Spiegel PK: Fatal pulmonary hypertension secondary to intravascular metastatic tumor emboli. *AJR* 1982; 139:997–1000.

45. Chan CK, Hutcheon MA, Hyland RH, et al: Pulmonary tumor embolism: A critical review of clinical, imaging and hemodynamic features. *J Thorac Imag* 1987; 2:4–14.

46. Chang CH: The normal roentgenographic measurement of the right descending pulmonary artery in 1,085 cases. *AJR* 1962; 87:929–935.

47. Chang CH: Radiological considerations in pulmonary embolism. *Clin Radiol* 1967; 18:301–309.

48. Chang CH, Davis WC: A roentgen sign of pulmonary infarction. *Clin Radiol* 1965; 16:141–147.

49. Charache S, Scott JC, Charache P: "Acute chest syndrome" in adults with sickle cell anemia: Microbiology, treatment, and prevention. *Arch Intern Med* 1979; 139:67–69.

50. Chaudhary BA, Ferguson DS, Speir WA: Pulmonary edema as a presenting feature of sleep apnea syndrome. *Chest* 1982; 82:122–124.

51. Chawla SK, Kittle CF, Faber LP, et al: Pulmonary veno-occlusive diseases. *Ann Thorac Surg* 1976; 22:249–253.

52. Cheely R, McCartney WH, Perry JR, et al: The role of noninvasive tests versus pulmonary angiography in the diagnosis of pulmonary embolism. *Am J Med* 1981; 70:17–22.

53. Chen NS, Barnett CA, Farrer PA: Reversibility of intrapulmonary arteriovenous shunts in liver cirrhosis documented by serial radionuclide perfusion lung scans. *Clin Nucl Med* 1984; 9:279–282.

54. Childress ME, Moy G, Mottram M: Unilateral pulmonary edema resulting from treatment of spontaneous pneumothorax. *Am Rev Respir Dis* 1971; 104:119–121.

55. Colice GL, Matthay MA, Bass E, et al: Neurogenic pulmonary edema: Clinical commentary. *Am Rev Respir Dis* 1984; 130:941–948.

56. Collins FS, Orringer EP: Pulmonary hypertension and cor pulmonale in the sickle hemoglobinopathies. *Am J Med* 1982; 73:814–821.

57. Cromie JB: Correlation of anatomic pulmonary emphysema and right ventricular hypertrophy. *Am Rev Respir Dis* 1961; 84:657–662.

58. Dalen JE, Alpert JS: Natural history of pulmonary embolism. *Prog Cardiovasc Dis* 1975; 17:259–270.

59. Dalen JE, Brooks HL, Johnson LW, et al: Pulmonary angiography in acute pulmonary embolism: Indications, techniques, and results in 367 patients. *Am Heart J* 1971; 81:175–185.

60. Dalen JE, Haffajee CI, Alpert JS, et al: Pulmonary embolism, pulmonary hemorrhage and pulmonary infarction. *N Engl J Med* 1977; 296:1431–1435.

61. Dalen JE, Mathur VS, Evans H, et al: Pulmonary angiography in experimental pulmonary embolism. *Am Heart J* 1966; 72:509–520.

62. D'Alonzo GE, Bower JS, Dantzkes DR: Differentiation of patients with primary and thromboembolic hypertension. *Chest* 1984; 85:457–461.

63. Daughtry JD, Stewart BH, Golding LAR, et al: Pulmonary embolus presenting as the initial manifestation of renal cell carcinoma. *Ann Thorac Surg* 1977; 24:178–181.

64. Davies SC, Luce PJ, Win AA, et al: Acute chest syndrome in sickle-cell disease. *Lancet* 1984; 1:36–38.

65. Dillon WP, Taylor AT, Mineau DE, et al: Traumatic pulmonary artery pseudoaneurysm simulating pulmonary embolism. *AJR* 1982; 139:818–819.

66. Divertie MB: The adult respiratory distress syndrome: Subject review. *Mayo Clin Proc* 1982; 57:371–378.

67. Don C, Johnson R: The nature and significance of peribronchial cuffing in pulmonary edema. *Radiology* 1977; 125:577–582.

68. Dunnick NR, Newman GE, Perlmutt LM, et al: Pul-

monary embolism. *Curr Prob Diagn Radiol* 1988; 6:197–229.

69. Dyck DR, Zylak CJ: Acute respiratory distress in adults. *Radiology* 1973; 106:407–501.
70. Edwards WD, Edwards JE: Clinical primary pulmonary hypertension: Three pathologic types. *Circulation* 1977; 56:884–888.
71. El Gamal M, Stoker JB, Spiers EM, et al: Cyanosis complicating hepatic cirrhosis. *Am J Cardiol* 1970; 25:490–494.
72. Evans KT, Cockshott WP, Hendrickse P de V, et al: Pulmonary changes in malignant trophoblastic disease. *Br J Radiol* 1965; 38:161–171.
73. Felman AH: Neurogenic pulmonary edema: Observations in 6 patients. *AJR* 1971; 112:393–396.
74. Ferris EJ, Holder JC, Lim WN, et al: Angiography of pulmonary emboli: Digital studies and balloon-occlusion cineangiography. *AJR* 1984; 142:369–373.
75. Ferris EJ, Steinzler RM, Rowke JA, et al: Pulmonary angiography in pulmonary embolic disease. *AJR* 1967; 100:355–363.
76. Figley MM, Gerdes AJ, Ricketts HJ: Radiographic aspects of pulmonary embolism. *Semin Roentgenol* 1967; 2:389–405.
77. Fisher MR, Higgins CB: Central thrombi in pulmonary arterial hypertension detected by MR imaging. *Radiology* 1986; 158:223–226.
78. Fishman AJ, Moser KM, Fedullo PF: Perfusion lung scans vs. pulmonary angiography in evaluation of suspected primary pulmonary hypertension. *Chest* 1983; 84:679–683.
79. Fishman AP: Chronic cor pulmonale: State of the art. *Am Rev Respir Dis* 1976; 114:775–794.
80. Fleischner FG: Pulmonary embolism. *Clin Radiol* 1962; 13:169–182.
81. Fleischner FG: The butterfly pattern of acute pulmonary edema. *Am J Cardiol* 1967; 20:39–46.
82. Fleischner FG: Recurrent pulmonary embolism and cor pulmonale. *N Engl J Med* 1967; 176:1213–1220.
83. Fleischner FG, Hampton AO, Castleman B: Linear shadows in the lung. *AJR* 1941; 46:610–618.
84. Frankel N, Coleman RE, Pryor DB, et al: Utilization of lung scans by clinicians. *J Nucl Med* 1986; 27:366–369.
85. Fred HL, Axelrad MA, Lewis JM, et al: Rapid resolution of pulmonary thromboemboli in man. *JAMA* 1966; 196:1137–1140.
86. Fred HL, Burdine JA, Gonzales DA, et al: Arteriographic assessment of lung scanning in the diagnosis of pulmonary embolism. *N Engl J Med* 1966; 275:1025–1032.
87. Friedman WF, Braunwald E: Alterations in regional blood flow in mitral valve disease studied by radioisotopic scanning. *Circulation* 1966; 34:363–376.
88. Freiman DG, Suyemoto J, Wessler S: Frequency of pulmonary thromboembolism in man. *N Engl J Med* 1965; 272:1278–1280.
89. Gamsu G, Hirji M, Moore EH, et al: Experimental pulmonary emboli detected using magnetic resonance. *Radiology* 1984; 153:467–470.
90. Gattinoni L, Presenti A, Thorresin A, et al: Adult respiratory distress syndrome profiles by computed tomography. *J Thorac Imag* 1986; 1(3):25–30.
91. Geddes DM, Kerr IH: Pulmonary arterial aneurysms in association with a right ventricular myxoma. *Br J Radiol* 1976; 49:374–376.
92. Gleason DC, Steiner RE: The lateral roentgenogram in pulmonary edema. *AJR* 1966; 98:279–290.
93. Goldhaber SZ, Braunwald E: Pulmonary embolism, in Braunwald E (ed): *Heart Disease: A Textbook of Cardiovascular Medicine*, ed 3. Philadelphia, WB Saunders, 1988.
94. Goodman PC: Pulmonary angiography. *Clin Chest Med* 1984; 5:465–477.
95. Graham JP, Rotman HH, Weg JG: Tumor emboli presenting as pulmonary hypertension. *Chest* 1976; 69:229–230.
96. Grainger RG: Interstitial pulmonary oedema and its radiological diagnosis. A sign of pulmonary venous and capillary hypertension. *Br J Radiol* 1958; 31:201–217.
97. Greene R: Adult respiratory distress syndrome: Acute alveolar damage. *Radiology* 1987; 163:57–66.
98. Greenspan RH, Ravin CE, Polansky SM, et al: Accuracy of the chest radiograph in diagnosis of pulmonary embolism. *Invest Radiol* 1982; 17:539–543.
99. Grieco MH, Ryan SF: Aseptic cavitary pulmonary infarction. *Am J Med* 1968; 45:811–816.
100. Guintini C, Mariani M, Barsotti A, et al: Factors affecting regional pulmonary blood flow in left heart valvular disease. *Am J Med* 1974; 57:421–436.
101. Gupta BD, Moodie DS, Hodgman JR: Primary pulmonary hypertension in adults: Clinical features, catheterization findings and long-term follow-up. *Cleve Clin Q* 1980; 47:275–284.
102. Hadfield JW, Sterling JC, Wraight EP: Multiple tumour emboli simulating a massive pulmonary embolus. *Postgrad Med J* 1982; 58:792–793.
103. Hampton AO, Castleman B: Correlations of post mortem chest teleroentgenograms with autopsy findings with special reference to pulmonary embolism and infarction. *AJR* 1940; 43:305–326.
104. Hansoti RC, Shah NJ: Cirrhosis of liver simulating congenital cyanotic heart disease. *Circulation* 1966; 32:71–77.
105. Harris P, Heath D: *The Human Pulmonary Circulation*, ed 3. Edinburgh, Churchill Livingston, 1986.
106. Harrison MO, Conte PJ, Heitzman ER: Radiological detection of clinically occult cardiac failure following myocardial infarction. *Br J Radiol* 1971; 44:265–272.
107. Hatano S, Strasser T (eds): *Primary Pulmonary Hypertension: WHO Committee Report*. Geneva, World Health Organization, 1975.
108. Haupt HM, Moore W, Bauer TW, et al: The lung in sickle cell disease. *Chest* 1982; 81:332–337.

109. Heck LL, Duley JW: Statistical considerations in lung imaging with Tc-99m albumin particles. *Radiology* 1974; 113:675–679.

110. Heikkila J, Hugenholtz PG, Tabakin BS: Prediction of left heart filling pressure and its sequential change in acute myocardial infarction from the terminal force of the P wave. *Br Heart J* 1973; 35:142–151.

111. Heitzman ER: *The Lung: Radiologic-Pathologic Correlations*, ed 2. St Louis, CV Mosby Co, 1984.

112. Heitzman ER, Markarian B, Dailey ET: Pulmonary thromboembolic disease: A lobular concept. *Radiology* 1972; 103:529–537.

113. Heitzman ER, Ziter FM: Acute interstitial pulmonary edema. *Radiology* 1966; 98:291–299.

114. Henderson AF, Banham SW, Moran F: Re-expansion pulmonary oedema: A potentially serious complication of delayed diagnosis of pneumothorax. *Br Med J* 1985; 291:593–594.

115. Hicken P, Heath D, Brewer D: The relation between the weight of the right ventricle and the percentage of abnormal air space in the lung in emphysema. *J Pathol Bacteriol* 1966; 92:519–528.

116. Hirji M, Gamsu G, Webb WR, et al: EKG-gated digital subtraction angiography in the detection of pulmonary emboli. *Radiology* 1984; 152:19–22.

117. Hodson CJ: Pulmonary oedema and bats-wing shadows. *J Fac Radiol* 1950; 1:176–186.

118. Hull RD, Hirsh J, Carter CJ, et al: Pulmonary angiography, ventilation lung scanning, and venography for clinically suspected pulmonary embolism with abnormal perfusion lung scan. *Ann Intern Med* 1983; 98:891–899.

119. Hultgren HN, Lopez CE, Lundberg E, et al: Physiologic studies of pulmonary edema at high altitude. *Circulation* 1985; 29:393–408.

120. Humphreys RL, Berne AS: Rapid re-expansion of pneumothorax. A cause of unilateral pulmonary edema. *Radiology* 1970; 96:509–512.

121. Hyers TM, Fowler AA, Wicks AB: Focal pulmonary edema after massive pulmonary embolism. *Am Rev Respir Dis* 1981; 123:232–233.

122. Iannuzzi M, Petty TL: The diagnosis, pathogenesis, and treatment of adult respiratory distress syndrome. *J Thorac Imag* 1986; 1(3):1–10.

123. Ingram RH, Braunwald E: Pulmonary edema: Cardiogenic and noncardiogenic, in Braunwald E (ed): *Heart Disease: A Textbook of Cardiovascular Medicine*, ed 3. Philadelphia, WB Saunders, 1988.

124. Jackson FN, Rowland V, Corssen G: Laryngospasm-induced pulmonary edema. *Chest* 1980; 78:819–821.

125. Jacoby CG, Mindell HJ: Lobar consolidation in pulmonary embolism. *Radiology* 1976; 118:287–290.

126. Jefferson K, Rees S: *Clinical Cardiac Radiology*. London, Butterworths, 1973.

127. Jenkinson SG: Pneumothorax. *Clin Chest Med* 1985; 6:153–161.

128. Joffe N: The adult respiratory distress syndrome. *AJR* 1974; 122:719–732.

129. Kanemoto N, Furuya H, Etoh T, et al: Chest roentgenograms in primary pulmonary hypertension. *Chest* 1979; 76:45–49.

130. Karlish AJ, Marshall R, Reid L, et al: Cyanosis with hepatic cirrhosis: A case with pulmonary arteriovenous shunting. *Thorax* 1967; 22:555–561.

131. Kawai C, Ishikawa K, Kato M, et al: "Pulmonary pulseless disease": Pulmonary involvement in so-called Takayasu's disease. *Chest* 1978; 73:651–657.

132. Kereiakes DJ, Herfkens RJ, Brundage BH, et al: Computerized tomography in chronic thromboembolic pulmonary hypertension. *Am Heart J* 1983; 106:1432–1436.

133. Kerr IH, Simon G, Sutton GC: The value of the plain radiograph in acute massive pulmonary embolism. *Br J Radiol* 1971; 44:751–757.

134. Kipper MS, Alazraki N: The feasibility of pulmonary ^{133}Xe ventilation imaging following the perfusion study. *Radiology* 1982; 144:581–586.

135. Kipper MS, Moser KM, Kortman KE, et al: Long term follow-up of patients with suspected pulmonary embolism and a normal lung scan. *Chest* 1982; 82:411–415.

136. Kollath J, Riemann H: Pulmonary digital subtraction angiography. *Cardiovasc Intervent Radiol* 1983; 6:233–238.

137. Korn D, Gore I, Blenke A, et al: Pulmonary arterial bands and webs; an unrecognised manifestation of organised pulmonary emboli. *Am J Pathol* 1962; 40:129–151.

138. Laur A: Roentgen diagnosis of pulmonary embolism and its differentiation from myocardial infarction. *AJR* 1963; 90:632–637.

139. Li DK, Seltzer SE, McNeil BJ: V/Q mismatches unassociated with pulmonary embolism: Case report and review of the literature. *J Nucl Med* 1978; 19:1331–1333.

140. Lindsay J, Meshel JC, Patterson RH: The cardiovascular manifestations of sickle cell disease. *Arch Intern Med* 1974; 133:643–651.

141. Lippmann M, Fein A: Pulmonary embolism in the patient with chronic obstructive pulmonary disease: A diagnostic dilemma. *Chest* 1981; 79:39–42.

142. Lisbona R, Kreisman H, Novales-Diaz J, et al: Perfusion lung scanning: Differentiation of primary from thromboembolic pulmonary hypertension. *AJR* 1985; 144:27–30.

143. Lockhart A, Saiag B: Altitude and the human pulmonary circulation. *Clin Sci* 1981; 60:599–605.

144. Loken MK: *Pulmonary Nuclear Medicine*. Norwalk, Conn, Appleton & Lange, 1987.

145. Ludwig JW, Verhoeven LAJ, Kersbergen JJ, et al: Digital subtraction angiography of the pulmonary arteries for the diagnosis of pulmonary embolism. *Radiology* 1983; 147:639–645.

146. Lupi EH, Sanchez GT, Horwitz S, et al: Pulmonary artery involvement in Takayasu's arteritis. *Chest* 1975; 67:69–74.

147. Lupi-Herrera E, Sanchez-Torres G, Marcushamer J,

et al: Takayasu's arteritis: Clinical study of 107 cases. *Am Heart J* 1977; 93:94–103.

148. Maldonado D: High altitude pulmonary edema. *Radiol Clin North Am* 1978; 16:537–549.

149. Mant MJ, O'Brien BD, Thony KL, et al: Haemorrhagic complications of heparin therapy. *Lancet* 1977; 1:1133–1135.

150. Marsh JD, Glynn M, Torman HA: Pulmonary angiography: Application in a new spectrum of patients. *Am J Med* 1983; 75:763–770.

151. Marticorena E, Tapia FA, Dyer J, et al: Pulmonary edema by ascending to high altitudes. *Dis Chest* 1964; 45:273–283.

152. Mathur VS, Dalen JE, Evans H, et al: Pulmonary angiography one to seven days after experimental pulmonary embolism. *Invest Radiol* 1967; 2:304–312.

153. Matthay MA: Pathophysiology of pulmonary edema. *Clin Chest Med* 1985; 6:301–314.

154. Matthay RA, Berger HJ: Cardiovascular function in cor pulmonale. *Clin Chest Med* 1983; 4:269–295.

155. Maunder RJ, Shuman WP, McHugh JW, et al: Preservation of normal lung regions in the adult respiratory distress syndrome: Analysis by computed tomography. *JAMA* 1986; 255:2463–2465.

156. McGoldrick PJ, Rudd TG, Figley MM, et al: What becomes of pulmonary infarcts? *AJR* 1979; 133:1039–1045.

157. McHugh TJ, Forrester JS, Adler L, et al: Pulmonary vascular congestion in acute myocardial infarction: Hemodynamic and radiologic correlations. *Ann Intern Med* 1972; 76:29–33.

158. McLeod JG, Grant IWB: A clinical, radiographic, and pathological study of pulmonary embolism. *Thorax* 1954; 9:71–83.

159. McNeil BJ: A diagnostic strategy using ventilation-perfusion studies in patients suspect for pulmonary embolism. *J Nucl Med* 1976; 17:613–616.

160. McNeil BJ: Ventilation perfusion studies and the diagnosis of pulmonary embolism: Concise communication. *J Nucl Med* 1980; 21:319–323.

161. Michael JR, Summer WR: Pulmonary hypertension. *Lung* 1985; 163:65–82.

162. Miller WC, Toon R, Palat H, et al: Experimental pulmonary edema following re-expansion of pneumothorax. *Am Rev Respir Dis* 1973; 108:664–666.

163. Mills SR, Jackson DC, Older RA, et al: Incidence, etiologies and avoidance of complications of pulmonary angiography in a large series. *Radiology* 1980; 136:295–299.

164. Milne ENC: Some new concepts of pulmonary blood flow and volume. *Radiol Clin North Am* 1978; 16:515–536.

165. Milne ENC, Bass H: Roentgenologic and functional analysis of combined chronic obstructive pulmonary disease and congestive cardiac failure. *Invest Radiol* 1969; 4:129–147.

166. Milne ENC, Pistolesi M, Miniati M, et al: The radio-logic distinction of cardiogenic and noncardiogenic edema. *AJR* 1985; 144:879–894.

167. Moore EH, Gamsu G, Webb WR, et al: Pulmonary embolus: detection and follow-up using magnetic resonance. *Radiology* 1984; 153:471–472.

168. Moser KM: Pulmonary embolism: State of the art. *Am Rev Respir Dis* 1977; 115:829–852.

169. Moser KM, Guisan M, Bartimmo EE: In vivo and post mortem dissolution rates of pulmonary emboli and venous thrombi in the dog. *Circulation* 1973; 48:170–178.

170. Moses DC, Silver TM, Bookstein JJ: The complementary roles of chest radiography, lung scanning, and selective pulmonary angiography in the diagnosis of pulmonary embolism. *Circulation* 1974; 49:179–188.

171. Mulder JI: Amniotic fluid embolism: An over view and case report. *Am J Obstet Gynecol* 1985; 152:430–435.

172. Nessa CB, Rigler LG: The roentgenological manifestations of pulmonary edema. *Radiology* 1941; 37:35–46.

173. Neumann RD, Sostman HD, Gottschalk A: Current status of ventilation-perfusion imaging. *Semin Nucl Med* 1980; 10:198–217.

174. Novelline RA, Baltarowich OH, Athanasoulis CE, et al: The clinical course of patients with suspected pulmonary embolism and a negative pulmonary arteriogram. *Radiology* 1978; 126:561–567.

175. Oh KS, Bender TM, Bowen A, et al: Plain radiographic, nuclear medicine and angiographic observations of hepatogenic pulmonary angiodysplasia. *Pediatr Radiol* 1983; 13:111–115.

176. Oppenheimer EH, Esterly JR: Pulmonary changes in sickle cell disease. *Am Rev Respir Dis* 1971; 103:858–859.

177. Osborne D, Jaszczak RJ, Greer K, et al: SPECT quantification of technetium-99m microspheres within the canine lung. *J Comput Assist Tomogr* 1985; 9:73–77.

178. Ostendorf P, Brizle H, Vogel W, et al: Pulmonary radiographic abnormalities in shock. *Radiology* 1975; 115:257–263.

179. Oswalt CE, Gates GA, Holmstrom FMG: Pulmonary edema as a complication of acute airway obstruction. *JAMA* 1977; 238:1833–1835.

180. Palla A, Donnamaria V, Petruzzelli S, et al: Enlargement of the right descending pulmonary artery in pulmonary embolism. *AJR* 1983; 141:513–517.

181. Peterson EP, Taylor HB: Amniotic fluid embolism. *Obstet Gynecol* 1970; 35:787–793.

182. Peterson KL, Fred HL, Alexander JK: Pulmonary arterial webs: A new angiographic sign of previous thromboembolism. *N Engl J Med* 1967; 277:33–35.

183. Pistolesi M, Giuntini C: Assessment of extravascular lung water. *Radiol Clin North Am* 1978; 16:551–574.

184. Pistolesi M, Miniati M, Milne ENC, et al: The chest

roentgenogram in pulmonary edema. *Clin Chest Med* 1985; 6:315–344.

185. Poncz M, Kane E, Gill FM: Acute chest syndrome in sickle cell disease: Etiology and clinical correlations. *J Pediatr* 1985; 107:861–866.

186. Pond GD: Pulmonary digital subtraction angiography. *Radiol Clin North Am* 1985; 23:243–260.

187. Porter J, Jick H: Drug-related deaths among medical in-patients. *JAMA* 1977; 237:879–881.

188. Powe JE, Palevsky HI, McCarthy KE, et al: Pulmonary arterial hypertension: Value of perfusion scintigraphy. *Radiology* 1987; 164:727–730.

189. Putman CE, Minagi H, Blaisdell FW: Roentgen appearance of disseminated intravascular coagulation (DIC). *Radiology* 1972; 109:13–18.

190. Rambihar VS, Fallen EL, Cairns JA: Pulmonary veno-occlusive disease: Antemortem diagnosis from roentgenographic and hemodynamic findings. *Can Med Assoc J* 1979; 120:1519–1522.

191. Ranniger K: Pulmonary arteriography: A simple method for demonstration of clinically significant pulmonary emboli. *AJR* 1962; 106:588–592.

192. Rees RSO, Jefferson KE: The Eisenmenger syndrome. *Clin Radiol* 1967; 18:366–371.

193. Remy J, Lemaitre L, Lafitte JJ, et al: Massive hemoptysis of pulmonary artery origin: Diagnosis and treatment. *AJR* 1984; 143:963–969.

194. Rich S, Pietra GG, Kieras K, et al: Primary pulmonary hypertension: Radiographic and scintigraphic patterns of histologic subtypes. *Ann Intern Med* 1986; 105:499–502.

195. Rinaldo JE, Rogers RM: Adult respiratory distress syndrome. *N Engl J Med* 1986; 315:578–580.

196. Ritchie BC, Schauberger G, Staub NC: Inadequacy of perivascular edema hypothesis to account for distribution of pulmonary blood flow in lung edema. *Circ Res* 1969; 24:801–814.

197. Robin ED: Overdiagnosis and overtreatment of pulmonary embolism: The emperor may have no clothes. *Ann Intern Med* 1977; 87:775–781.

198. Robin ED, Horn B, Goris ML, et al: Detection, quantitation and physiology of lung spiders. *Trans Assoc Am Physicians* 1975; 88:202–216.

199. Rochester DF, Enson Y: Current concepts in the pathogenesis of the obesity hypoventilation syndrome. *Am J Med* 1974; 57:402–420.

200. Rosenow EC III, Osmundson PJ, Brown ML: Pulmonary embolism: Subject review. *Mayo Clin Proc* 1981; 56:161–178.

201. Rosenthal A, Vawter G, Wagenvoort CA: Intrapulmonary veno-occlusive disease. *Am J Cardiol* 1973; 31:78–83.

202. Rydell R, Hoffbauer FW: Multiple arteriovenous fistulas in juvenile cirrhosis. *Am J Med* 1956; 21:450–460.

203. Sabiston DC: Pathophysiology, diagnosis, and management of pulmonary embolism. *Am J Surg* 1979; 138:384–391.

204. Sabiston DC, Wolfe WG, Oldham HN, et al: Surgical management of chronic pulmonary embolism. *Ann Surg* 1977; 185:699–712.

205. Sagel SS, Greenspan RH: Nonuniform pulmonary arterial perfusion: Pulmonary embolism? *Radiology* 1970; 99:541–548.

206. Sano A, Kuroda Y, Moriyasu F, et al: Porto-pulmonary venous anastomosis in portal hypertension demonstrated by percutaneous transhepatic cine-portography. *Radiology* 1982; 144:479–484.

207. Sautter RD, Dreher WH, MacIndoe JH, et al: Fatal pulmonary edema and pneumonitis after reexpansion of chronic pneumothorax. *Chest* 1971; 60:399–401.

208. Sautter RD, Fletcher FW, Emanuel DA, et al: Complete resolution of massive pulmonary thromboembolism. *JAMA* 1964; 189:948–949.

209. Sautter RD, Fletcher FW, Ousley JL, et al: Extremely rapid resolution of a pulmonary embolus: Report of a case. *Dis Chest* 1967; 52:825–827.

210. Schnur MJ, Winkler B, Austin JHM: Thickening of the posterior wall of the bronchus intermedius. *Radiology* 1981; 139:551–559.

211. Sewell RW, Fewel JG, Grover FL, et al: Experimental evaluation of reexpansion pulmonary edema. *Ann Thorac Surg* 1978; 26:126–132.

212. Shackleford GD, Sacks EJ, Mullins JD, et al: Pulmonary veno-occlusive disease: Case report and review of the literature. *AJR* 1977; 128:643–648.

213. Shapiro R, Rigler LE: Pulmonary embolism without infarction. *AJR* 1948; 60:460–465.

214. Scharf J, Nahir AM, Munk J, et al: Aseptic cavitation in pulmonary infarction. *Chest* 1971; 59:456–458.

215. Shaw TJ, Caterine JM: Recurrent re-expansion pulmonary edema. *Chest* 1984; 86:784–786.

216. Sherman S, Ravikrishnan KP: Unilateral pulmonary edema following reexpansion of pneumothorax of brief duration. *Chest* 1980; 77:714.

217. Shilkin KB, Low LP, Chen BTM: Dissecting aneurysm of the pulmonary artery. *J Pathol* 1969; 98:25–29.

218. Short DS: A radiological study of pulmonary infarction. *Q J Med* 1951; 79:233–245.

219. Simon G: Further observations on the long line shadow across a lower zone of the lung. *Br J Rad* 1970; 43:327–332.

220. Simon G: The value of radiology in critical mitral stenosis—an amendment. *Clin Radiol* 1972; 23:145–146.

221. Simon M: The pulmonary vessels: Their hemodynamic evaluation using routine radiographs. *Radiol Clin North Am* 1963; 1:363–376.

222. Skalina S, Kundel HL, Wolf G, et al: The effect of pulmonary edema on proton nuclear magnetic resonance relaxation times. *Invest Radiol* 1984; 19:7–9.

223. Slutsky RA, Long S, Peck WW, et al: Pulmonary density distribution in experimental noncardiac ca-

nine pulmonary edema evaluated by computed transmission tomography. *Invest Radiol* 1984; 19:168–173.

224. Smith JA: Cardiopulmonary manifestations of sickle cell disease in childhood. *Sem Roentgenol* 1987; 22:160–167.

225. Smith R, Maher JM, Miller RI, et al: Clinical outcomes of patients with suspected pulmonary embolisms and low-probability aerosol-perfusion scintigrams. *Radiology* 1987; 164:731–733.

226. Snashall PD, Keyes SJ, Morgan BM, et al: The radiographic detection of acute pulmonary oedema. A comparison of radiographic appearances, densitometry and lung water in dogs. *Br J Radiol* 1981; 54:277–288.

227. Sostman HD, Gottschalk A: The stripe sign: A new sign for diagnosis of nonembolic defects in pulmonary perfusion scintigraphy. *Radiology* 1982; 142:731–741.

228. Sostman HD, Rapoport S, Glickman MG, et al: Problems in noninvasive imaging of pulmonary embolism. *Radiol Clin North Am* 1983; 21:759–774.

229. Sostman HD, Rapoport S, Gottschalk A, et al: Imaging of pulmonary embolism. *Invest Radiol* 1986; 21:443–454.

230. Sostman HD, Ravin CE, Sullivan DC, et al: Use of pulmonary angiography for suspected pulmonary embolism: Influence of scintigraphic diagnosis. *AJR* 1982; 139:673–677.

231. Spies WG, Burstein SP, Dillchan GL, et al: Ventilation-perfusion scintigraphy in suspected pulmonary embolism: Correlation with pulmonary angiography and refinement of criteria for interpretation. *Radiology* 1986; 159:383–390.

232. Sprung CL, Rackow EC, Fein IA, et al: The spectrum of pulmonary edema: Differentiation of cardiogenic, intermediate and non-cardiogenic forms of pulmonary edema. *Am Rev Respir Dis* 1981; 124:718–722.

233. Stanley NN, Woodgate DJ: Mottled chest radiograph and gas transfer defect in chronic liver disease. *Thorax* 1972; 27:315–323.

234. Steckel RJ: Unilateral pulmonary edema after pneumothorax. *N Engl J Med* 1973; 289:621–622.

235. Stein MG, Crues JV, Bradley WG, et al: MR imaging of pulmonary emboli: An experimental study in dogs. *AJR* 1986; 147:1133–1137.

236. Stein PD, O'Connor JF, Dalen JE, et al: The angiographic diagnosis of acute pulmonary embolism: Evaluation of criteria. *Am Heart J* 1967; 73:730–741.

237. Sugerman JH: Pulmonary function in morbid obesity. *Gastroenterol Clin North Am* 1987; 16:225–237.

238. Sullivan DC, Coleman RE, Mills SR, et al: Lung scan interpretation: Effect of different observers and different criteria. *Radiology* 1983; 149:803–807.

239. Surrette GD, Muir AL, Hogg JC, et al: Roentgeno-

graphic study of blood flow redistribution in dogs. *Invest Radiol* 1975; 10:109–114.

240. Symbas P, Scott HW: Traumatic aneurysm of the pulmonary artery. *J Thorac Cardiovasc Surg* 1963; 45:645–649.

241. Szucs MM, Brooks HL, Grossman W, et al: Diagnostic sensitivity of laboratory findings in acute pulmonary embolism. *Ann Intern Med* 1971; 74:161–166.

242. Talbot S, Worthington BS, Roebuck EJ: Radiographic signs of pulmonary embolism and infarction. *Thorax* 1973; 28:198–203.

243. Teplick JG, Haskin ME, Steinberg SB: Changes in the main pulmonary artery segment following pulmonary embolism. *AJR* 1964; 92:557–560.

244. Thadani V, Burrow C, Whitaker W, et al: Pulmonary veno-occlusive disease. *Q J Med* 1975; 173:133–159.

245. Theodore J, Robin ED: Editorial: Speculations on neurogenic pulmonary edema (NPE). *Am Rev Respir Dis* 1976; 113:405–411.

246. Thickman D, Kressel HY, Axel L: Demonstration of pulmonary embolism by magnetic resonance imaging. *AJR* 1984; 142:921–922.

247. Tilkian AG, Schroeder JS, Robin ED: Chronic thromboembolic occlusion of main pulmonary artery or primary branches: Case report and review of the literature. *Am J Med* 1976; 60:563–570.

248. Torrance DJ: Roentgenographic signs of pulmonary artery occlusion. *Am J Med Sci* 1959; 237:651–662.

249. Trapnell DH, Thurston JGB: Unilateral pulmonary oedema after pleural aspiration. *Lancet* 1970; 1:1367–1369.

250. Travis KW, Tordres ID, Shannon DC: Pulmonary edema associated with croup and epiglottitis. *Pediatrics* 1977; 59:695–698.

251. Tsao MS, Schraufnagel D, Wang NS: Pathogenesis of pulmonary infarction. *Am J Med* 1982; 72:599–606.

252. Tudor J, Maurer BJ, Wray R, et al: Lung shadows after acute myocardial infarction. *Clin Radiol* 1973; 24:365–369.

253. Turner AF, Lau FYK, Jacobson G: A method for the estimation of pulmonary venous and arterial pressures from the routine chest roentgenograms. *AJR* 1972; 116:97–106.

254. Urokinases Pulmonary Embolism Trial: A national cooperative study. *Circulation* 1973; 47(suppl II):38–45.

255. Varat MA, Adolph RJ, Fowler NO: Cardiovascular effects of anemia. *Am Heart J* 1972; 83:415–426.

256. Vix VA: The usefulness of chest radiographs obtained after a demonstrated perfusion scan defect in the diagnosis of pulmonary emboli. *Clin Nucl Med* 1983; 8:497–500.

257. Wagenvoort CA: Pulmonary veno-occlusive disease: Entity or syndrome? *Chest* 1976; 69:82–86.

258. Wagenvoort CA, Wagenvoort N: Primary pulmo-

nary hypertension: A pathologic study of the lung vessels in 156 clinically diagnosed cases. *Circulation* 1970; 42:1163–1184.

259. Wagenvoort CA, Wagenvoort N: The pathology of pulmonary veno-occlusive disease. *Virchows Arch [Pathol Anat]* 1974; 364:69–79.

260. Waqaruddin M, Bernstein A: Re-expansion pulmonary oedema. *Thorax* 1975; 30:54–60.

261. Wegenius G, Erikson U, Borg T, et al: Value of chest radiography in adult respiratory distress syndrome. *Acta Radiol* 1984; 25:177–184.

262. Wenger NK, Stein PD, Willis PW: Massive acute pulmonary embolism: The deceivingly nonspecific manifestations. *JAMA* 1972; 220:843–844.

263. West JB, Dollery CT, Heard BE: Increased pulmonary vascular resistance in the dependent zone of isolated dog lung caused by perivascular edema. *Circ Res* 1965; 17:191–206.

264. Westcott JL, Cole S: Plate atelectasis. *Radiology* 1985; 155:1–9.

265. Westermark N: On the roentgen diagnosis of lung embolism. *Acta Radiol* 1938; 19:357–372.

266. White RD, Winkles ML, Higgins CB: MR imaging of pulmonary arterial hypertension and pulmonary emboli. *AJR* 1987; 149:15–21.

267. Wiener SN, Edelstein J, Charms B: Observations on pulmonary embolism and the pulmonary angiogram. *AJR* 1966; 98:859–873.

268. Wilson AG, Harris CN, Lavender JP, et al: Perfusion lung scanning in obliterative pulmonary hypertension. *Br Heart J* 1973; 35:917–930.

269. Winterbauer RH, Elfenbein IB, Ball WC: Incidence and clinical significance of tumor embolisation to the lungs. *Am J Med* 1968; 45:271–290.

270. Woesner ME, Sanders I, White GW: The melting sign in resolving transient pulmonary infarction. *AJR* 1971; 111:782–790.

271. Wolfe JD, Taskkin DP, Holly FE, et al: Hypoxemia of cirrhosis: Detection of abnormal pulmonary vascular channels by a quantitative radionuclide method. *Am J Med* 1977; 63:746–754.

272. Wolfe WG, Sabiston DC: *Pulmonary Embolism.* Philadelphia, WB Saunders Co, 1980.

273. Woodruff WW, Hoeck BE, Chitwood WR, et al: Radiographic findings in pulmonary hypertension from unresolved embolism. *AJR* 1985; 144:681–686.

274. Yamato M, Lecky JW, Hiramatsu K, et al: Takayasu arteritis: Radiographic and angiographic findings in 59 patients. *Radiology* 1986; 161:329–334.

275. Youngberg AS: Unilateral diffuse lung opacity. *Radiology* 1977; 123:277–281.

276. Yuceoglu YZ, Rubler S, Eshwar K, et al: Pulmonary edema associated with pulmonary embolism: A clinicopathological study. *Angiology* 1971; 22:501–510.

277. Zimmerman JE, Goodman LR, St. Andre AC, et al: Radiographic detection of mobilizable lung water: The gravitational shift test. *AJR* 1982; 138:59–64.

278. Ziskind MM, Weill H, George RA: Acute pulmonary edema following the treatment of spontaneous pneumothorax with excess negative intrapleural pressure. *Am Rev Respir Dis* 1965; 92:632–636.

279. Zwillich CW, Sutton FO, Pierson DJ, et al: Decreased hypoxic ventilatory drive in the obesity-ventilation syndrome. *Am J Med* 1975; 59:343–348.

Inhalational Diseases of the Lungs

PNEUMOCONIOSIS

The term "pneumoconiosis" means "dusty lungs." Nowadays, it is used to describe the non-neoplastic reactions of the lungs to inhaled dust particles. By definition, the term "pneumoconiosis" excludes asthma, bronchitis, and emphysema,[94] all of which may, in some instances, be due to dust inhalation. Although some authors include organic as well as mineral dust,[94] many limit the term to inorganic dust—notably coal, silica, and asbestos.

The character and severity of the reaction of lung tissue are determined by three basic factors[94]:

1. The nature and properties of the inhaled dust, particularly the size of the particles and the degree to which the dust is fibrogenic.

2. The amount of dust retained in the lungs and the duration of exposure to it.

3. Individual idiosyncrasy and immunological reactivity of the subject.[14, 86] Individuals with positive circulating rheumatoid factor show a response different from that normally encountered.

The pneumoconioses are best classified according to the mineral dust responsible. This classification is not always easy because the industrial exposure may involve more than one dust known to be fibrogenic. Silica is so plentiful in the rocks of the earth's crust that some exposure to silica is inevitable in many forms of mining. The pneumoconioses are therefore classified according to the predominant dust responsible.

Roentgenographic Classification of the Pneumoconioses

The need for standard interpretations of plain chest radiographs of subjects with pneumoconiosis led to the development of the International Labour Office/University of Cincinnati (ILO/UIC) international classification. The ILO/UIC classification, which is now the standard internationally recognized descriptive system, is modified periodically, the latest revision having been made in 1980.[20, 65] It is accompanied by a set of standard radiographs because the primary aim is to encourage reproducible radiographic interpretation. The system does not take clinical features into account.

The ILO/UIC classification is complex. Put simply, opacities resulting from dust inhalation are divided into two major groups: multiple small opacities up to 1 cm in diameter, and opacities larger than 1 cm in diameter. The multiple small opacities are subdivided into categories 1, 2, and 3 according to the profusion of small opacities in the lungs. Those radiographs in which the number of opacities is too small to justify inclusion in category 1 are relegated to category 0.

- Category 1—small opacities definitely seen but few in number.
- Category 2—numerous small opacities with normal lung vasculature still visible.
- Category 3—very numerous opacities where the lung vasculature is partly or totally obscured.

A system with 12 categories has been introduced in order to help overcome the difficulty of deciding between categories 1, 2, and 3. It uses two numbers. The first number is the category finally chosen, the second is the alternate category considered (e.g., 1/2 would indicate that category 2 was considered but that the final choice was category 1).

The opacities in categories 1, 2, and 3 are further subdivided according to whether they are round or irregular in shape. Those that are round are classified according to size as p, q, or r (p = up to about 1.5 mm in diameter, q = about 1.5 to 3 mm in diameter, and r = about 3 to 10 mm in diameter). Those that are classified as irregular cannot be meaningfully measured, so they are designated as fine, medium, or coarse using the letters s, t, and u, respectively. As might be expected, the interobserver variability in categorizing small opacities is great.[4]

Opacities larger than 1 cm in diameter are categorized as A, B, and C according to the size of the opacity.

- Category A—one or more opacities whose combined diameter(s) is 1 to 5 cm.
- Category B—one or more opacities whose combined diameters are greater than 5 cm but whose combined area does not exceed the equivalent of the right upper zone.
- Category C—one or more opacities whose combined area is larger than the equivalent of the right upper zone (i.e., greater than category B).

Where opacities of different categories are present on a single radiograph, one category is usually predominant, and this is the one quoted.

Additional descriptors are given for pleural thickening and calcification as well as for lack of definition of the diaphragm and cardiac outline.

It is important to realize that the ILO/UIC classification is a method of describing chest radiographs. Small opacities, particularly those in category 1, will be seen in diseases other than the pneumoconioses and even on a proportion of routine radiographs in patients with no exposure to dust.

Silicosis

Free silica (silicon dioxide) is present in many rocks in the earth's crust. It occurs in amorphous and crystalline forms, quartz being the most important crystal. The entity "silicosis" refers to lung disease due primarily to free silica; it should not be used to describe coal pneumoconiosis, or other pneumoconioses, even if free silica plays some part in the pathogenesis.[94]

The incidence of silicosis has fallen since its peak during the Second World War. Exposed individuals usually work in quarries, drill or tunnel quartz-containing rocks, cut or polish masonry, clean boilers or castings in iron and steel foundries (Fettlers), or are exposed to sandblasting. The usual chronic form of the disease requires 20 years' or more exposure to high dust concentrations before radiographic abnormalities are visible.[142] With very high concentrations of dust, radiographic changes may be visible in 4 to 8 years.[142] Acute silicosis is a somewhat different entity which occurs with very severe exposure, particularly in enclosed spaces (see below).

Dust particles of appropriately small size are deposited on the alveolar walls and ingested by macrophages. They may enter the pulmonary lymphatics, or may be transported to bronchioles by the mucociliary escalator. The macrophages die and produce fibrosis by releasing their contents, including the particulate silica. The precise mechanism of fibrogenesis is debatable, as is the role of autoimmunity.[94, 142]

The basic lesion of silicosis is the hyalinized nodule.[75] The silica particles, nearly all of which are 1 to 2 μm in diameter, are found fixed within the silicotic nodules. These nodules are usually more prominent in the upper zones and lie close to the bronchioles, small vessels, and lymphatics. They consist of concentric layers of collagen, containing silica particles surrounded by a fibrous capsule. The outer zone is made up of irregularly dispersed connective tissue which also contains crystalline silica. Silica in this peripheral zone sets up further reaction resulting in enlargement of nodules and the creation of new nodules. The fibrosis seen with silicosis is both more abundant and more collagenous than that seen with other mineral dusts, such as coal. The airways are not usually involved, provided that most of the nodules are smaller than 5 mm.[142] Silica-laden macrophages that reach the hilar and mediastinal nodes form granuloma-like lesion in the nodes.

Silicosis is often complicated by the massive fibrotic lesions which are the result of the conglomeration of nodules matted together by fibrosis. These masses, which contain obliterated blood vessels and bronchi, may cavitate. Tuberculous infection coexists in some cases.

Radiographic Appearance[8, 98]

An exposure of 10 to 20 years is usually necessary before the subject's chest radiograph becomes

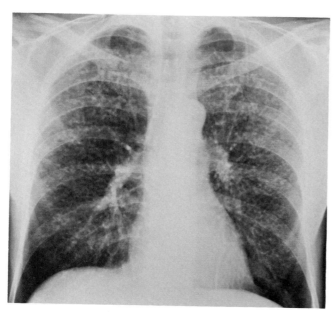

FIG 9—1.
Silicosis. There is widespread 2- to 3-mm nodulation in the lungs, with mid-zone and upper zone predominance.

abnormal.[142] Early in the course of the disease 1- to 3-mm nodules are seen, maximal in the posterior portions of the upper two-thirds of the lungs (Fig 9–1). A reticular pattern may also be seen, either alone or in combination with the nodules. As the process advances, the nodules increase in size and number and become more widespread, involving all zones. Usually the nodulation is symmetrical. Sometimes the nodules are calcified.[38]

Progressive massive fibrosis is defined as nodules greater than 1 cm in diameter. These masses, which are identical to those seen with coal worker's pneumoconiosis (see Fig 9–4), develop when the silicotic nodules coalesce. As the nodules coalesce, contraction of the upper lobes is observed and bullae are seen in the vicinity of the conglomerate masses. Emphysematous changes are also seen in the lower lobes.[142]

The conglomerate nodules may have sharp margins, but more often are irregular in shape, with strands of density extending into the surrounding lung. They usually appear in the periphery of the lungs and either remain there or slowly migrate towards the hili[48] leaving emphysematous lung between the fibrotic mass and the chest wall.[98] Cavitation may be visible, and the cavities may empty and fill over a period of time.[48] Pleural thickening is frequently seen in association with progressive massive fibrosis.

Hilar and mediastinal lymph node enlargement are not uncommon. Calcification, sometimes of the eggshell type, may be seen in the nodes (Fig 9–2).[68]

Computed tomography (CT)[8] shows all these features more definitively than does the plain chest radiograph and shows coalescence of nodules earlier than the plain film. CT also shows the accompanying emphysema to advantage. Bergin et al. suggested that the deterioration of pulmonary function in patients with silicosis correlated with the extent of associated emphysema and not with the profusion of silicotic nodules.[8] CT scanning does not appear to identify more patients with minimal parenchymal disease.[8]

Acute Silicoproteinosis

Extremely intense exposure to silica dust may result in lung damage after a period of only weeks or months: so-called acute silicosis. In these cases, there is a marked cellular and exudative alveolar reaction,[127] and death may ensue within 2 to 3 years of exposure. Usually, such a patient has worked as a sandblaster. The dominant feature is the presence of an alveolar proteinaceous exudate, hence the term "acute silicoproteinosis."[13]

Radiographically, there is widespread alveolar shadowing which progresses rapidly over a period of months.[28] There is reasonable side-to-side symmetry, but a tendency to central and upper zone predominance is frequent (Fig 9–3). Air bronchograms may be noted, and contraction of the lungs may be minimal at first, suggesting consolidation of the lungs. Hilar and mediastinal adenopathy may be seen, but the hili are often obscured by the parenchymal shadows. Peripheral air trapping, bulla formation, lung volume loss, and distortion of mediastinal structures all indicate increasing fibrosis. Pneumothorax may occur.

Coal Worker's Pneumoconiosis

The factors that govern the degree of lung damage caused by inhalation of coal dust are not fully understood. An important factor, probably the most important, is the amount of dust of suitable particle size that is inhaled.[63, 94] What is less certain is the importance of the silica content of the dust. That coal dust alone could cause classic progressive massive fibrosis (PMF) was shown many years ago in coal trimmers who, because they worked in the hulls of ships, were exposed only to coal dust containing virtually no free silica. At postmortem investigation, their disease was attributable to coal dust alone.[44] Later epidemiologic studies have shown that the radiographic changes in miners are closely related to coal dust ex-

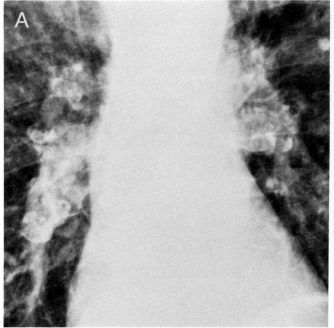

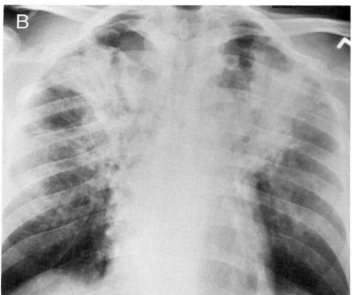

FIG 9–2.
Eggshell calcification in silicosis. **A,** AP view. **B,** lateral view.

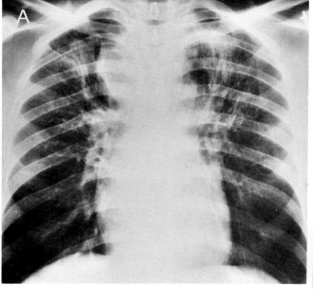

FIG 9–3.
Acute silicoproteinosis in a young man employed for 2 years as a sandblaster. **A,** note the mediastinal adenopathy and upper zone shadowing after 2 years of exposure. **B,** 1 year later there is dense consolidation of the upper zones with air bronchograms. Death ensued shortly thereafter.

posure,[102] but poorly related to the silica content of the coal. It is generally agreed that silica plays little part in simple pneumoconiosis,[63, 86] although some dispute this.[67, 117] The role of silica in the production of PMF remains uncertain.[86, 94] Suffice it to say that there is reasonable evidence that silica plays a part in the development of PMF in some cases[88, 89, 97] and that PMF can develop in miners exposed to coal dust with negligible quantities of silica.[90]

Pathology[27, 86]

With excessive dust load of appropriate size, clearance by the mucociliary escalator is overwhelmed, and dust-laden macrophages aggregate in the respiratory bronchioles and alveoli. After a time, fibroblasts lay down reticulin. The aggregation of dust and fibroblasts leads to the basic lesion of simple pneumoconiosis: the coal macule. If silica is released, collagenous fibrosis is stimulated. The coal macule develops around bronchioles, weakening the bronchiolar wall and leading to a form of centrilobular emphysema known as proximal acinar or focal emphysema,[54, 111] a form of emphysema believed to be clinically unimportant.[86] The extent to which clinically important panacinar emphysema is caused by coal dust is debated.[18, 79, 81, 94, 111]

Despite the similarity of their radiographic appearances, coal worker's pneumoconiosis and silicosis are different pathologically. The coal macule does not have a hyaline center, nor does it show the laminated collagen typical of the silicotic nodule.

The massive nodules (defined as those with a diameter greater than 1 cm) in coal worker's pneumoconioses are ill-defined, amorphous, inhomogeneous collections of proteinaceous material, mineral dust, and calcium phosphates. The mass lesions may cavitate with or without infection.

The pathogenesis of PMF in coal workers is poorly understood. PMF is related to the severity of dust exposure, and it has recently been postulated that the fibrosis occurs in response to dust-laden macrophages that have ruptured from the mediastinal lymph nodes into the bronchi or pulmonary vessels.[116]

Coal worker's pneumoconiosis in patients with rheumatoid arthritis (Caplan's syndrome) is considered separately in Chapter 11.

Clinical Features

It has been stated that simple coal worker's pneumoconiosis is symptom-free.[86, 94] It should be remembered, however, that bronchitis and emphy-sema, features that are so frequently encountered in miners, are excluded from the definition of pneumoconiosis. The extent to which these two processes are due to coal dust exposure or to other factors such as smoking is a highly contentious issue. The interested reader is referred to the reviews by Parkes[94] and Morgan and Lapp.[86]

PMF category A appears not to cause symptoms or signs. PMF categories B and C may be associated with respiratory disability and deterioration in ventilatory function tests.[86] Cough and sputum are sometimes seen. Hemoptysis is rare. Jet-black sputum following ischemic rupture of PMF into a bronchus may occasionally be reported.

Radiographic Appearance

The chest radiograph reflects fairly well the extent and severity of the macules and masses found pathologically and is thus a good tool for diagnosing and following the progression of coal worker's pneumoconiosis.* The radiographic findings correlate well with the amount of dust to which the worker was exposed,[67] and the quantity of dust found in the lungs at postmortem examination.[105] Except in the grossest cases—namely those in categories B and C—the correlation between the chest radiograph and lung function is, however, poor,[92] probably because the radiograph substantially underdiagnoses the associated emphysema.[89, 111] This latter point is of great importance, because the degree of functional disability appears to correlate far better with the severity of emphysema than it does with the presence of macules or PMF.[53, 81, 111]

The radiographic signs of coal worker's pneumoconiosis are similar to, and often indistinguishable from, those described for silicosis. Like silicosis, coal worker's pneumoconiosis is divided into simple and complicated forms based on the chest radiograph. Nodules, at first barely visible, appear in the upper two-thirds of the lungs. A reticular pattern may also be seen, either in combination with the nodules or in isolation, and septal (Kerley) lines may be seen.[132] The significance of the reticular or linear shadows has been debated over the years.[3] Recent work has suggested that the irregular opacities (s, t, u) may be a better guide to disablement in simple coal worker's pneumoconioses than the purely rounded opacities, because they correlate better with the extent of emphysema.[80]

PMF is uncommon in coal workers with less than 20 years' experience in and around the mines.[139]

*References 17, 41, 45, 52, 53, 102, 109.

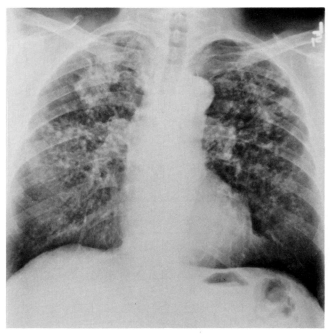

FIG 9—4.
Coal worker's pneumoconiosis. Typical example shows widespread mid-zone and upper zone small nodules with category A PMF. The PMF shadows are larger on the right than on the left.

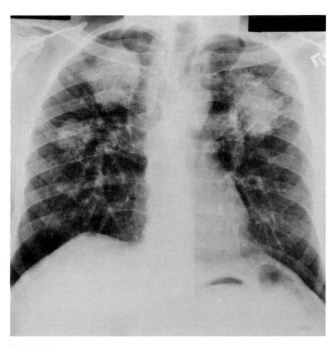

FIG 9—5.
Category B PMF in a coal miner in whom the background lung nodulation is minimal.

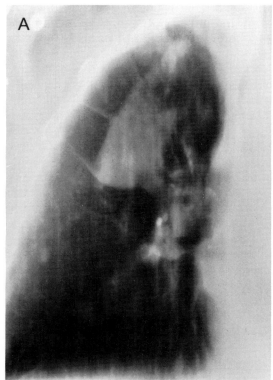

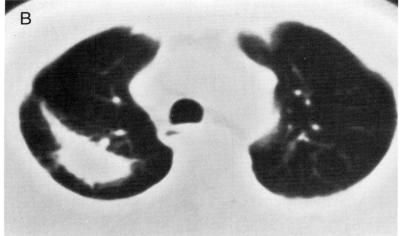

FIG 9—6.
A case of PMF. **A,** tomogram shows the well-defined outer margin paralleling the chest wall. **B,** CT scan in a different patient shows the characteristic shape, with the outer margin parallel to the chest wall and the axis of the density parallel to the major fissure.

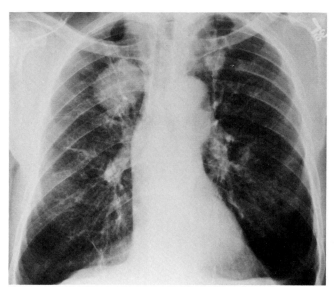

FIG 9—7.
PMF in a coal miner, showing predominantly unilateral opacity in the right upper lobe. There is a small area of PMF in the left upper lobe. Note the accompanying emphysema and relative lack of background nodulation in the lungs.

Typically, (Fig 9—4) PMF starts as a mass near the periphery of the lung. The shape varies. It may be round or oval with lobular or irregular edges (Fig 9—5). There is often a well-defined lateral border that parallels the lateral chest wall (Fig 9—6). In contrast the medial border is frequently ill-defined. The depth of the mass may be significantly less than the side-to-side diameter; in other words, it may show a lens-shaped opacity, a feature that is best appreciated in a lateral or oblique view or at CT scanning (Fig 9—6). Because PMF is frequently bilateral and accompanied by widespread nodulation in the remainder of the lungs (see Fig 9—4), the diagnosis is rarely in doubt. There are cases, however, in which the mass is completely or predominantly unilateral (Fig 9—7), and background nodulation may or may not exist or may be difficult to appreciate. In such cases, the differential diagnosis from lung carcinoma becomes particularly important. In a patient with a long history of exposure to coal dust, a lens-shaped density is virtually diagnostic of PMF if it is peripherally situated in an upper lobe close to and parallel to the major fissure, and has a well-defined outer margin paralleling the chest wall.[139] Another important feature that distinguishes PMF from bronchial carcinoma is that small, irregular calcifications may be seen in PMF and sometimes the mass has a calcified rim. PMF masses may cavitate (Fig 9—8).

PMF masses, as the name implies, enlarge over time. The rate of growth is, however, very slow—an observable increase in diameter taking years, not months, as is the case with carcinoma. In some cases, PMF lesions migrate medially toward the hilus (Fig 9—9). The migration is slow, taking 10 or more years to reach the hilus. Severe emphysema accompanies such migration (Fig 9—10).

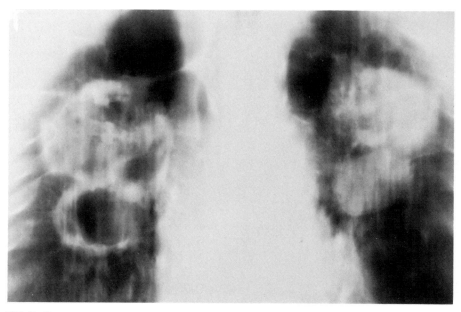

FIG 9—8.
Cavitation in PMF. Tomogram shows the bilateral masses with thick-walled irregular cavitation, worse on the right than the left.

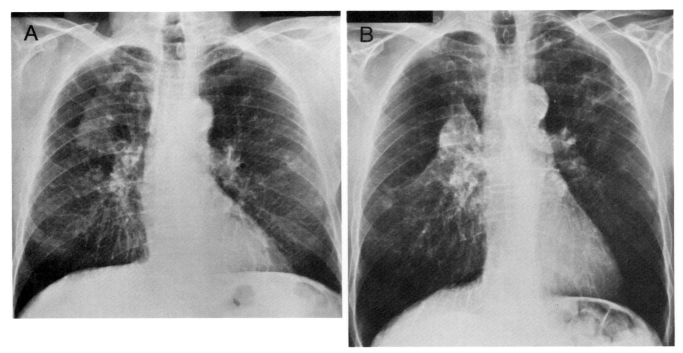

FIG 9–9.
Coal worker's pneumoconiosis showing medial migration of PMF (same patient as Fig 9–6, A). **A** was obtained 7 years before **B.**

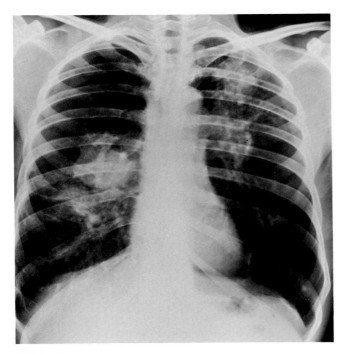

FIG 9–10.
Coal worker's pneumoconiosis with PMF. There has been substantial medial migration of the right PMF shadow. Note the punctate calcification in the left-sided masses and the accompanying severe emphysema.

Asbestos-Related Diseases

Asbestos is composed of a group of fibrous silicates with differing chemical and physical properties but with the notable common property of heat resistance. Chemical differences such as solubility and acid resistance, and physical differences such as fiber length, brittleness, and texture, are probably important determinants of the distribution and severity of the deleterious effects on the lungs and pleura. Asbestos is divided into two principal subgroups based on the physical properties of the fibers: the serpentines and the amphiboles. Serpentine asbestos has long, curly, flexible, smooth fibers composed of fibrillary subunits. The only serpentine asbestos used commercially is chrysotile. This form of asbestos accounts for over 90% of the asbestos used in the United States today, having made considerable inroads on the amphibole asbestos forms since World War II.[26] The amphiboles have straight, needle-like fibers of varying length, diameter, brittleness and texture. The main types in use are crocidolite (blue asbestos), amosite (brown asbestos), and anthophyllite. A major reason for the decline in the use of the amphiboles was the recognition of the fact that the amphiboles, particularly crocidolite, have a much greater fibrogenic and carcinogenic potential than the serpentine form chrysotile.[136]

World production and use of asbestos has expanded to an extraordinary degree over the past century. Production expanded from 50 tons/yr in the 1860s to a peak of over 5 million tons/yr in the early 1970s.[7] Asbestos production has now declined somewhat as alternative materials have become available. At the same time, there has been a distinct switch to the white asbestos chrysotile as more information about the different health hazards of the various forms of asbestos has become available. Nevertheless, with the long time lags known to exist before the adverse effects of asbestos exposure become manifest and with the vast tonnages of the material now in place or in use, asbestos is likely to remain one of the major environmental hazards well into the 21st century.

Benign Asbestos Pleural Effusion

The association of asbestos exposure with benign, possibly recurrent, pleural effusions was firmly established only in the last 25 years.[34, 35, 42] The transient, often asymptomatic, nature of these effusions and the lack of specific markers to indicate their cause undoubtedly accounted for the delayed recognition of this condition. Indeed, the diagnosis is one of exclusion and should conform to the following criteria: (1) a history of occupational or environmental asbestos exposure; (2) no other cause for the effusion; (3) no evidence of malignancy within 3 years of the detection of the effusion.

In the noteworthy epidemiologic study of Epler et al.,[35] the overall incidence of benign pleural effusion was 3.1%, with a 7% incidence among individuals with a heavy occupational exposure and a 0.2% incidence in environmentally exposed individuals. Effusions may be unilateral or bilateral and tend to recur. The amount of fluid is usually small; effusions greater than 500 cc are uncommon. The fluid has the characteristics of an exudate and may be blood-tinged. Clinically, there may be pleuritic pain, fever, and an elevated white blood cell count, but many patients have only mild symptoms or no symptoms at all.

Benign pleural effusion is the most common abnormality seen within 10 years of the onset of asbestos exposure. No direct causal relationship between benign effusions and the subsequent development of malignant pleural effusion has been postulated, but in one study of 70 cases of malignant mesothelioma,[29] five cases were preceded by what were regarded as successive benign pleural effusions for up to 7 years. A long latent period taken together with a history of heavy exposure should, in general, make

one less ready to accept a diagnosis of a benign effusion without thorough investigation and extended follow-up. In the series of Cookson et al.,[24] 12 years was the shortest latent period for the development of an effusion related to a malignant pleural mesothelioma. On the other hand, these authors do record a latent period of 22 years in one patient with a benign, asbestos-related effusion.

Benign pleural effusions are associated with the subsequent development of diffuse pleural thickening (Fig 9–11). McLoud et al.[82] found that just over 50% of their cases with benign pleural effusions subsequently developed diffuse basal pleural thickening, an association also emphasized by Cookson et al.[24] As will be discussed later, there is possibly an association between benign pleural effusions and the subsequent development of rounded atelectasis.[84] On rare occasions, the degree and extent of the subsequent pleural thickening may be such that the resultant impairment of lung function necessitates a decortication procedure.[41]

Pleural Thickening and Calcification Related to Asbestos Exposure

Irregular pleural thickening and calcification was first positively related to exposure to asbestos in 1955[66] and the occurrence of noncalcified asbestos-induced plaques was first reported in 1967.[5] Considerable attention has since been paid to these changes which, in fact, represent the most frequent radiographic manifestation of exposure to asbestos. Pleural plaques are usually first identified more than 20 or 30 years after the initial asbestos exposure. Asbestos-induced pleural plaques occur on the parietal pleura, especially over the diaphragm and along the posterolateral chest wall. The apices and the costophrenic sulci tend to be spared. The plaques are composed of hyalinized fibrous tissue and frequently underlie ribs. Although often isolated pleural elevations, they may enlarge, spread, and coalesce. Dystrophic calcification within plaques is common and is more frequent as the plaques age and enlarge. Electron microscopy studies have allowed identification of asbestos fibers in the plaques on the parietal pleura, indicating that transpleural migration and assimilation of inhaled asbestos fibers must occur.[70] There is evidence that the widely used, more benign form of asbestos, chrysotile, is particularly associated with this transpleural migration, while the more fibrogenic and carcinogenic amphiboles, crocidolite and amosite, tend to get held up in the lung parenchyma.[118] This may account for the widespread finding of asbestos-related pleural disease unassoci-

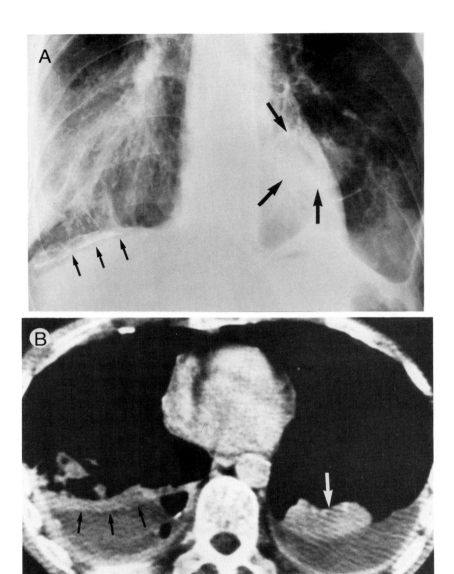

FIG 9–11.
A, diffuse basal pleural thickening in an asbestos exposed individual. Note also the pleural calcification *(small arrows)* and the left basal rounded atelectasis *(large arrows).* **B,** CT scan shows bilateral pleural effusions with a rind of pleural thickening on the right *(black arrows).* There is also an area of rounded atelectasis on the left *(white arrow).*

ated with parenchymal fibrosis or intrathoracic malignancy. Population surveys in industrial regions and in asbestos-mining areas have revealed a surprisingly high incidence of pleural plaques even in individuals with only a remote connection with asbestos.[2, 60, 121] The use of asbestos is so widespread that many individuals are exposed unwittingly and unknowingly and, therefore, accurate data are difficult to obtain. In some 20% of cases with autopsy-proved plaque formation, Hillerdal[55] was not able to find any association with asbestos. One should not discount the possibility of other, as yet unidentified,

environmental agents as a cause of pleural plaque formation. In an exhaustive study of pleural plaque formation in a rural region of Czechoslovakia, Rous and Studeny[107] were adamant that asbestos could not be implicated in their cases.

Radiographically, pleural plaques are irregular, smooth elevations of the pleura most easily identified in profile along the margins of the lungs or over the diaphragm (Fig 9–12). Plaques are less easily seen *en face* unless they are larger. Plaques seen *en face* are relatively flat in relation to their width and the density of the shadow projected over the lungs

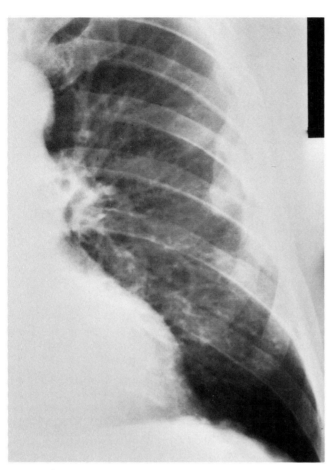

FIG 9–12.
Typical noncalcified pleural plaques in an asbestos-exposed individual. Note the sparing of the costophrenic sulcus.

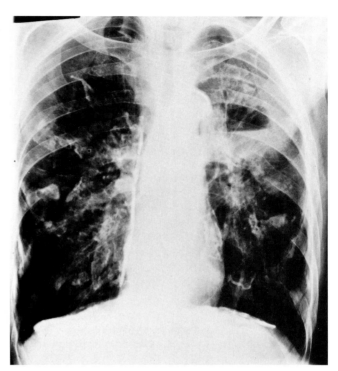

FIG 9–13.
Linear calcification in pleural plaques over the diaphragm and in the right paravertebral region. There is also calcified plaque formation seen *en face* as well as a left upper lobe bronchial carcinoma.

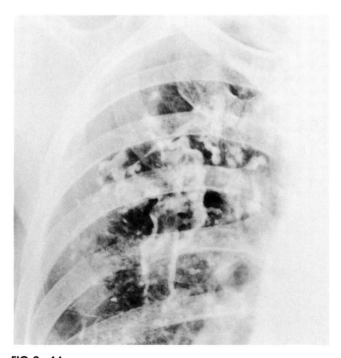

FIG 9–14.
"Holly leaf" calcification in asbestos-related plaques seen *en face*.

is, therefore, less than would be expected for a parenchymal lesion of equivalent size. Furthermore, one margin of the lesion is likely to be indistinct as it smooths off into normal pleura. Plaques are multiple, and there is reasonable side-to-side symmetry. Sparing of the costophrenic sulci and the mediastinal contours is characteristic. Calcification is linear when the plaques are seen in profile (Fig 9–13) but, when seen *en face,* the appearance is variable, the most common type being so-called holly leaf calcification (Fig 9–14). Extensive pleural calcification in association with parenchymal fibrosis may be lacelike (Fig 9–15). Enlargement and spreading of plaques will result in thick, irregular sheets of pleural thickening, which are often calcified (Fig 9–16). Pleural plaques do occur on the visceral pleura, especially in association with parenchymal fibrosis,[104, 135] a position that can be inferred by identifying pleural thickening or calcification in an interlobar fissure (Fig 9–17).

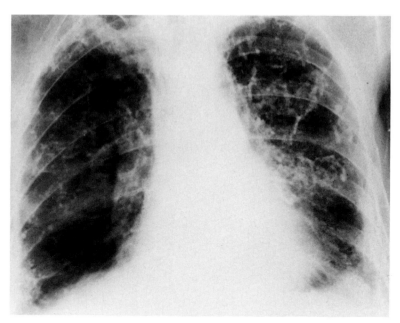

FIG 9–15.
Lacelike asbestos-related pleural plaque formation seen *en face*.

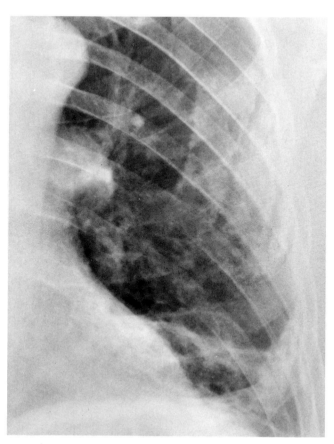

FIG 9–16.
Extensive calcifications in sheetlike pleural plaque formation.

Visualization of pleural plaques is improved by optimal radiographic technique. Oblique views can substantially increase the rate of plaque detection by throwing posterolateral plaques into profile.[6] CT scanning further increases plaque detection rates, both by virtue of the axial nature of the images and greater sensitivity in the detection of calcification (Fig 9–18).[76] The differential diagnosis of pleural plaques includes extrapleural fat deposition in obesity,[112] extrapleural thickening in relation to multiple rib fractures, postinflammatory pleural thickening (especially when calcified), pleural metastases, and overprojected densities representing unusually prominent costal insertions of the serratus anterior muscle.[22, 43]

It is important to differentiate pleural plaque from diffuse pleural thickening related to previous benign asbestos-induced pleural effusions, because diffuse posteffusion thickening is more likely to be associated with parenchymal fibrosis and intrathoracic malignancy. Diffuse pleural thickening involves and obliterates the costophrenic sulci, whereas pleural plaques tend to spare these regions. Extensive sheetlike plaque formation may, however, simulate diffuse posteffusion thickening. McLoud et al.[82] found evidence to suggest that diffuse pleural thickening could be attributed to extensive sheetlike plaque formation in approximately half the cases in which it was found.

The pleural changes associated with exposure to

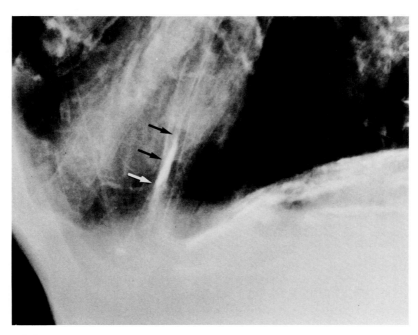

FIG 9–17.
Calcified plaque formation in a major fissure *(arrows).* The calcification must be in the visceral pleura.

asbestos have attracted inordinate interest, possibly because of their epidemiologic implications, but from a purely practical clinical standpoint, isolated asbestos-related pleural changes have only minor significance.[115] The changes are rarely confused with more significant disease processes, and indeed in many cases, the changes are either overlooked or are below the limits of radiographic visibility. Studies have shown that only 12.5% of asbestos-related pleural changes found at autopsy are identified on plain

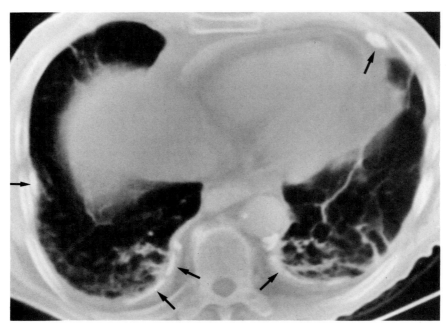

FIG 9–18.
CT scan showing calcified pleural plaques *(arrows).* Note the parenchymal fibrosis in the underlying lung.

chest films even by trained observers using the strictest criteria.[59]

There are three fundamental questions related to pleural plaques and associated disease.

1. Does pleural plaque formation in environmentally exposed individuals still raise the possibility of potentially significant fibrosis even in the absence of radiographic evidence of parenchymal disease? Studies of such individuals identified through health surveys indicate that minor lung function abnormalities suggestive of inhomogeneously distributed fibrosis may occur.[19] However, it has not been suggested that these changes progress to become clinically significant. It should be mentioned in passing that although patients with asbestos-induced fibrosis frequently have pleural plaques and calcifications, these changes are not invariable. Indeed, in 20% to 25% of such cases, pleural changes are conspicuously absent.[40] Two parallel processes, both related to asbestos exposure but of differing clinical and pathologic significance may, therefore, be operating.

2. Do pleural plaques ever degenerate into malignant mesotheliomas or, alternatively, are pleural plaques an indicator of an increased risk of mesothelioma? There is no evidence of the former, although there is certainly evidence to support a small, but statistically significant, incidence of mesothelioma in individuals with occupational exposure and radiographically detectable pleural plaques.[32, 39] On the other hand, pleural plaques are not invariably found in patients with mesotheliomas. An autopsy study by Scully et al.[114] found pleural plaques in 27 of 47 (58%) mesothelioma cases. On balance it would appear that the environmentally exposed individual with pleural plaques and calcification is not at significant risk for the development of mesothelioma.

3. Is there increased incidence of bronchogenic carcinoma in patients with asbestos-related pleural plaque formation? Again analysis is distorted because two parallel processes may be under comparison. In occupationally exposed individuals, Fletcher[39] found a mortality from bronchogenic carcinoma 2.4 times greater than expected in individuals with plaques as opposed to a 1.2 times incidence in individuals without plaques. However, in environmentally exposed individuals, Kiviluoto et al.[74] could find no such association. Data from autopsy studies relating the incidence of bronchial carcinoma to coincident pleural plaques are conflicting.[56, 115, 131] A prospective study with controls matched for age, occupational exposure, and smoking habits is lacking.

Again, it appears that the environmentally exposed individual with pleural plaques and calcification is not at significant risk for the development of bronchogenic carcinoma.

Benign Asbestos-Related Parenchymal Masses

Rounded atelectasis is an unusual form of a juxtapleural lung collapse that may simulate a pulmonary neoplasm. There is a definite association between this condition and asbestos exposure, and it has been widely accepted that benign, asbestos-induced effusions are an essential precursor in such cases.[84] However, Hillerdal and Hemmingsson[58] have challenged this concept; hence, the mechanism of origin of rounded atelectasis must remain conjectural. The condition was first described in patients who had undergone therapeutic pneumothorax for tuberculosis.[103] Other conditions such as pulmonary infarction, Dressler's syndrome, congestive cardiac failure, and nonspecific pleurisy can precede the formation of rounded atelectasis.[126] Alternative designations for rounded atelectasis include folded lung,[10] atelectatic pseudotumor,[77] and pleuroma.[122]

Hanke and Kretzschmar[51] have proposed a sequence of events to account for the development and the appearance of rounded atelectasis. First, a pleural effusion causes atelectasis in the underlying lung. An infolding of the visceral pleura isolates an area of atelectasis, which floats in the effusion and is, thereby, elevated and tilted. The development of fibrous adhesions suspends the rounded atelectatic area in the elevated and tilted position. The pleural effusion resorbs and the lung reexpands except for the now sequestered, rounded area of atelectasis. Kretzschmar[77] added that organization and contraction of the fibrinous pleural exudate together with fibrous contraction in the surrounding lung parenchyma produced additional distortion. Hillerdal and Hemmingsson[58] suggest that, at least in asbestos-related cases, the condition may result from contraction of diffuse visceral pleural thickening, plus retraction caused by parenchymal fibrosis. These authors point out that rounded atelectasis may arise long after the normal time during which benign asbestos-related pleural effusions occur.

The radiographic findings are characteristic (Figs 9–11 and 9–19). Rounded atelectasis is usually a single, masslike lesion although more than one lesion is occasionally seen in a lung.[119] The mass lesion is juxtapleural in position and is most commonly found in one of the lower lobes posteriorly or posteromedially. The upper lobes, particularly the lin-

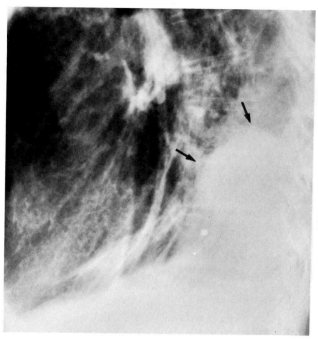

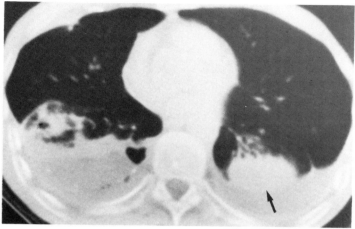

FIG 9–19.
Rounded atelectasis. **A,** lateral chest radiograph shows pleural thickening at the lung bases plus a rounded juxtapleural mass *(arrows).* **B,** CT scan shows the juxtapleural mass *(arrow)* with underlying pleural thickening and fluid. Note the characteristic "parachute cord" divergence of the pulmonary vessels as they merge into the rounded atelectasis.

gula, may be involved.[58] Rounded atelectasis forms a rounded or oval mass 2.5 to 5.0 cm in diameter in contact with the pleural surface. Acute angles are usually visible at the pleural margins and indicate an intraparenchymal location. The mass is usually separated from the diaphragm by interposed lung. Thickening of the pleura will be present, particularly in the vicinity of the lesion, and the costophrenic sulci are usually blunted or obliterated. The pathognomonic feature, however, is the characteristic pattern of distortion of the vessels in the vicinity of the lesion (and the bronchi too if these are demonstrated by bronchography). The vessels leading towards the mass are crowded but, as they reach the mass, they tend to diverge and arc round the under surface of the mass before merging with it. This appearance has been variously described as the "vacuum cleaner effect,"[122] the "comet tail,"[119] and the helical effect. Conventional tomography is an excellent method of demonstrating this vital sign (Fig 9–20), although it can be appreciated on CT scans (see Fig 9–19). On CT the juxtapleural mass is readily identified and there is a characteristic pattern of divergence of vessels as they approach and merge with the atelectatic mass. The appearance simulates the cords of a parachute. It is essential to clearly demonstrate this finding before excluding a peripheral bronchogenic carcinoma on the basis of appearances alone (Fig 9–21). Rounded atelectasis is ordinarily a static process, as can be readily determined by serial radiographs.

Asbestosis

Asbestosis was identified with some certainty as a disease at the turn of the century.[23] By the mid 1980s, an estimated 65,000 persons in the United States had clinically diagnosable asbestosis.[134] The

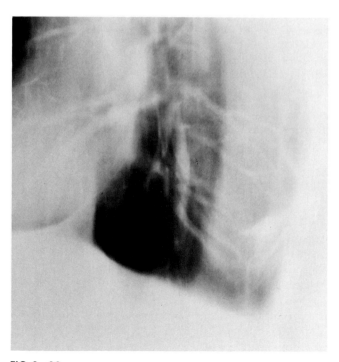

FIG 9–20.
Tomogram demonstrates rounded atelectasis at the lung base posteriorly, showing the characteristic arching of the vessels as they merge into the density.

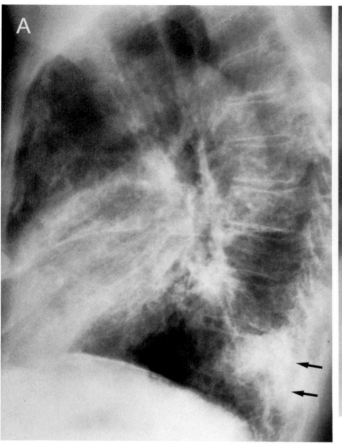

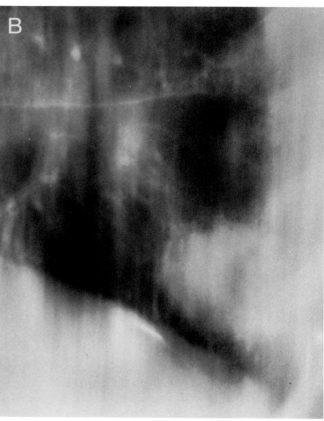

FIG 9–21.
A, radiograph of shipyard worker with asbestosis and a postero-basal mass *(arrows).* Note also pleural calcification and plaque formation. **B,** conventional tomogram showing a juxtapleural mass *without* distortion of the lung vessels. Biopsy proved bronchogenic carcinoma.

term "asbestosis" is generally reserved for asbestos-induced pulmonary fibrosis and associated visceral pleural fibrosis. Thus, the commonly found parietal pleural changes associated with asbestos exposure are excluded, being regarded more as an indication of such exposure than a significant disease entity. Asbestosis is related to cumulative dust exposure, whereas the parietal pleural changes are more related to the length of time elapsed from the initial exposure.[19] The time interval between the initial exposure and the development of evidence of asbestosis is extremely variable, but 20 to 30 years is usual. Intense exposures can cause asbestosis in as short a period as 3 years, but this is exceptional. The most fibrogenic form of asbestos is crocidolite and, in descending order of fibrogenicity, are amosite, anthophyllite, and chrysotile.

Pathologically, asbestos causes interstitial pulmonary fibrosis that spreads centrifugally from the region of the terminal bronchioles and the alveolar ducts,[26] with histologic features that are indistinguishable from those of idiopathic pulmonary fibrosis. The changes predominate in the subpleural portions of the lungs and at the lung bases. Visceral pleural thickening does occur, particularly over the regions of maximum fibrosis. Mild to moderate fibrosis correlates broadly with increasing cumulative exposure. Established asbestos-induced pulmonary fibrosis tends to progress with time even after cessation of exposure.[49, 108]

Radiographically, asbestosis presents the following features on plain chest radiographs.

1. A ground-glass haze over the lower portions of the lungs may be appreciated.[123] The early changes at the level of the terminal bronchioles are far below the resolving power of the x-ray beam, but the resulting diffuse thickening can summate, attenuating the x-ray beam in much the same way as a layer of pleural fluid along the posterior chest wall

with the patient supine affects the chest radiograph. This radiographic feature is nonspecific and its interpretation is highly subjective.

2. Interstitial shadowing develops, particularly at the lung bases and in a subpleural location (Figs 9–22 and 9–23). The shadows, a mixture of opacities, pinpoint to 4 mm in diameter. These are interspersed with linear opacities, some of which represent septal lines. The subpleural location of the fibrosis over the diaphragm and the mediastinum tends to obscure these soft tissue contours. Laterally, the fibrotic changes may be seen to extend up the chest wall toward the axillae. The fibrotic changes may become severe, with upper lobe involvement, progressive lung volume loss, and even "honeycombing," which is indicative of severe end-stage fibrosis. The fibrotic changes are in no way specific for asbestosis, and comparable changes may be seen, for example, in idiopathic pulmonary fibrosis. However, pleural changes suggestive of asbestos exposure are present in all but some 20% of cases of asbestosis, providing an important clue to the underlying cause (see Fig 9–21).

3. Pleural plaques, diffuse pleural thickening, and pleural calcification are to be found in 80% of patients with asbestosis. The radiographic features of these pleural changes have been dealt with earlier

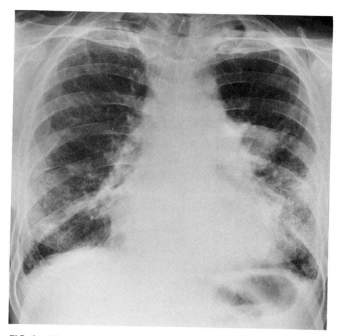

FIG 9–23.
Asbestosis with a bronchogenic carcinoma in the left lung. Note the basally predominant pulmonary fibrosis. There is slight blunting of the costophrenic sulci; otherwise, pleural changes are lacking in this case.

in this chapter. Plain radiographs cannot allow one to distinguish visceral from parietal pleural thickening and calcification except when these occur in the interlobar fissures. At CT, parenchymal fibrosis may be patchy, and pleural thickening is often seen in relation to regions of increased fibrosis. Conceivably, at least part of this thickening involves the visceral pleura.

4. Conglomerate shadowing akin to progressive massive fibrosis in silicosis has been reported.[47, 57] However, such changes may, in fact, relate to concomitant exposure to silica or talc.[37] Caplan's syndrome (multiple rheumatoid necrobiotic nodules associated with occupational exposure to dust) has also been reported.[46, 130] These two causes of benign pulmonary masses must be exceedingly uncommon in asbestosis, even if a true association could be proved.

CT scanning offers an alternative method of evaluating patients with asbestosis (Figs 9–18 and 9–24). CT has been shown to be extremely sensitive in the detection of both asbestos-induced pleural changes and parenchymal fibrosis.[71, 76, 133] Tylen and Nilsson,[133] for example, detected pulmonary fibrosis on the CT scans of 9 of 12 individuals with a

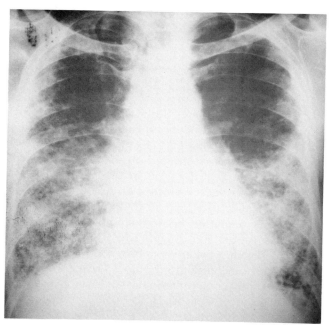

FIG 9–22.
Radiograph of shipyard worker with asbestosis showing the basal predominance of the fibrosis. The subpleural fibrosis is obscuring the contours of the heart and the diaphragm and extending up along the lateral margins of the lungs towards the apices.

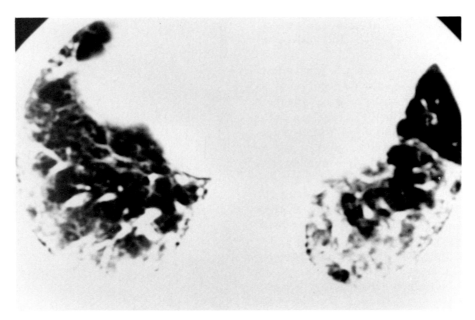

FIG 9–24.
CT scan of patient with asbestosis. Note the predominantly subpleural location of the pulmonary fibrosis.

history of asbestos exposure, whereas the plain radiographs enabled detection of fibrosis in only 2 of these 9 patients. Katz and Kreel[71] compared CT scans and plain chest films in 36 individuals exposed to asbestos. Pleural changes were detected in 27 cases (75%) and parenchymal changes in 12 cases (33%) by CT, whereas the corresponding figures for plain chest films were 24 cases (66%) and 6 cases (16%). The value of CT in the investigation of possible pulmonary pseudotumors has been emphasized.[58, 133]

Plaques are advantageously demonstrated by CT, particularly in areas difficult to examine by plain radiography such as the paravertebral regions and the posterior aspects of the diaphragm. CT is more sensitive in the detection of calcification in plaques than are plain radiographs.[124] The plaques may be focal or diffuse with diffuse plaques being much more likely to be associated with asbestos-related pleural fibrosis.[1] High-resolution CT is superior to both chest radiography and conventional CT in the detection of asbestos-related disease.[1] High-resolution CT is capable of resolution to submillimeter levels and volume-averaging artifacts are less of a problem than with conventional CT. The CT changes are predominantly seen in the subpleural portions of the lungs, particularly at the lung bases posteriorly. These changes consist of thickened short interstitial lines, often with a perivascular ori-

entation, interspersed with longer, thicker parenchymal bands 2-5 cm in length extending to the pleural surface.[1] Associated pleural thickening, either focal or diffuse, is common but not invariable. In more advanced cases the changes may progress to honeycombing in which air spaces some 1 cm in diameter with thickened walls develop in the involved areas.

The diagnosis of asbestoses requires consideration of the patient's occupational history or possible environmental exposure, the clinical features (breathlessness, clubbing, lung crackles), the results of pulmonary function tests, and the chest radiographs. CT is undoubtedly an excellent method of investigation for asbestosis, but—for practical reasons and because of the costs involved—CT should be reserved for special studies or for those cases in which particular problems in diagnosis arise. There is a better correlation between pulmonary function and radiographic abnormalities in asbestosis than in silicosis or coal worker's pneumoconiosis.[42] Nevertheless, the chest radiograph may appear normal despite CT, clinical, or pulmonary function indications of the presence of asbestosis. Pulmonary function tests are more sensitive than chest radiography in the detection of early or subclinical asbestosis,[42, 96] but they lack specificity. Chest radiography remains an essential tool in grading the severity of asbestosis and is clearly of vital importance in the diagnosis of the benign and malignant complications of this condition.

Talcosis

Talc is a hydrated magnesium silicate that has widespread uses as a cosmetic, an industrial lubricant, and as a filling agent, for example, in the tire and pharmaceutical industries. Geologically, talc is often associated with asbestos and silica, and this has resulted in problems in determining the extent to which radiographic and pathologic changes can be attributed to an exposure to talc. Feigin[37] correlated the radiographic and pathologic findings in a series of individuals exposed to talc of varying degrees of purity. Mineralogic analysis of the talc gave an estimate of the extent of contamination by asbestos and silica. Feigin described four categories of disease, namely, talcoasbestosis, talcosilicosis, pure talcosis, and intravenous talcosis.[37] Intravenous talcosis is considered separately on p. 455. Talcoasbestosis and talcosilicosis show the classic features discussed earlier in this chapter that result from exposure to asbestos and silica, the changes attributable to talc being completely overshadowed. Pure talcosis presents radiographically as a reticulonodular infiltration of the lungs, either diffuse or predominant in the lower zone. Hilar adenopathy may occur. Pleural thickening and calcification are not features of pure talcosis, contrary to previous description.

Kaolinosis

Kaolin, a hydrated aluminum silicate, causes a pneumoconiosis with features similar to those of coal worker's pneumoconiosis, including the tendency for progressive massive fibrosis and even Caplan's syndrome.[137] The radiographic changes of kaolinosis occur in a minority of exposed workers, and progression of the lesions is slow.[72, 93] The most frequent abnormality is a fine nodulation of the lungs with some basal predominance (Fig 9–25). The nodules become larger and more numerous with prolonged exposure, and a reticular element may become apparent. Enlargement and condensation of the nodules into progressive massive fibrosis occurs in only a very small minority of cases, some 1% in Oldham's estimate (Fig 9–26).[93]

The Inert Dust Pneumoconioses

A number of inorganic dusts are inert and fail to excite any fibrous response when taken up into the

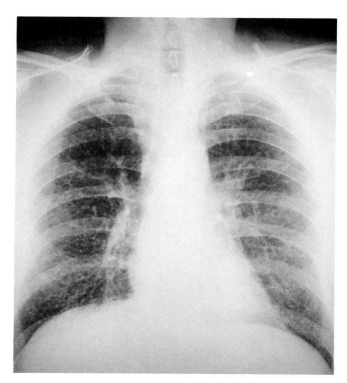

FIG 9–25.
Uncomplicated kaolinosis in a Cornish china clay worker. (Courtesy of Dr. Irving Wells, Plymouth, England.)

lung parenchyma. The dust accumulations in the lung parenchyma may become radiographically visible, often dramatically so. The most frequently encountered inert dusts are:

1. *Iron* (siderosis). This is classically found in electric arc welders, oxyacetylene cutters, and silver polishers (Fig 9–27).
2. *Tin* (stannosis). The main occupational exposure occurs during the smelting of tin ores (Fig 9–28).
3. *Barium* (baritosis). This condition is encountered in miners and handlers of the ore baryta.
4. *Antimony.* Antimony pneumoconiosis is encountered as a result of the mining, milling, and refining of antimony ores (Fig 9–29).

Pathologically some dust is seen at alveolar level, but the major accumulations are seen in aggregations of dust-laden macrophages in the interstitium of the lung and along the lymphatic pathways. Radiographic visibility is dependent on the atomic number of the dust and the severity of dust accumulation. Relatively small dust accumulations may be visible as a very fine low-density stippling of the lung

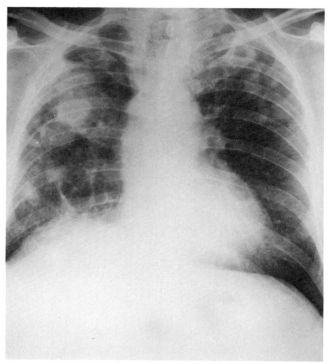

FIG 9–26.
Kaolinosis with progressive massive fibrosis in a patient from the same region as the patient in Fig 9–25. (Courtesy of Dr. Irving Wells, Plymouth, England.)

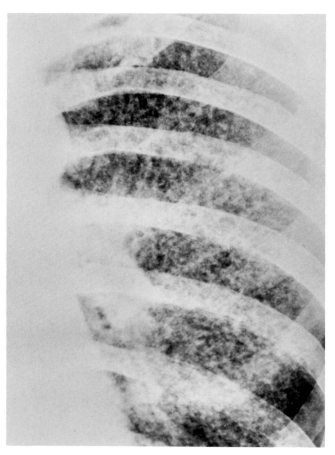

FIG 9–27.
Siderosis in a hematite miner from Cumberland, England. (Courtesy of Dr. Peter Hacking, Newcastle upon Tyne, England.)

parenchyma, which may be vaguely referred to as "dirty looking lungs." Dusts of high atomic number, such as iron, may result in much more remarkable radiographic changes if the dust accumulation is considerable. The pattern tends to be reticulonodular, with the nodular element predominating. The changes are most pronounced in the central portion of the lungs reflecting, perhaps, the greater amount of interstitial tissue in the perihilar regions. The unusually high radiographic density of the nodules may be more evident if comparison is made with the density of the ribs.

In many industrial circumstances the workers receive a concomitant exposure to silica dust, and changes of silicosis may also be present. An example of this is the siderosilicosis of hematite miners illustrated in Figure 9–30.

Aluminosis

The inhalation of aluminum and its oxides has been associated with the development of pulmonary fibrosis in workers in the aluminum industry. Only a few workers are affected, and these are usually involved with particular processes. For example,

Shaver and Riddel described a form of pulmonary fibrosis in workers who were involved in the smelting of aluminum ore (bauxite) to produce corundum.[120] The pneumoconiosis resulting from the smelting of bauxite, frequently known as Shaver's disease, is basically the prototype of the condition termed aluminosis.

The role of aluminum and aluminum oxides in causing pulmonary disease is difficult to assess because workers are also exposed to silica and mineral oils in dusts and fumes. This complex subject is well reviewed by Brooks.[11] Exposure to the fumes may be acute and intense, the result being acute tracheobronchitis and possibly even pulmonary edema. The pulmonary edema pattern in such individuals usually evolves over subsequent weeks or months into a diffuse reticulonodular pattern indicative of diffuse lung damage with fibrosis. Shaver's cases were subjected to chronic exposure to fumes over periods ranging from 3 to 15 years, and the result was a

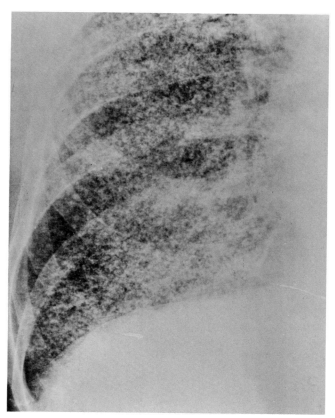

FIG 9–28.
Stannosis in an apparently healthy middle-aged man.

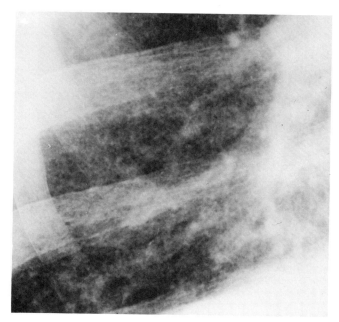

FIG 9–29.
Detailed view of the right lung base in a antimony refiner. Note the fine diffuse increase in the lung markings, representing antimony dust deposition.

coarse interstitial pulmonary fibrosis with reduced lung volumes. The upper zones were more severely involved, and honeycombing and bleb formation were frequent findings (Fig 9–31). Pneumothorax was strikingly common. Widening of the mediastinum with distortion of the tracheobronchial structures was common and was presumably related to the fibrosis (Fig 9–32). Less intense exposures may cause an asthma-like syndrome after single or repeated exposures.

Berylliosis

Awareness of the serious toxic effects of beryllium has restricted its use and brought about improved industrial hygiene. The condition of berylliosis is, therefore, much less common today, although sporadic cases continue to be reported.[25, 61]

The lesions of berylliosis are characterized by the presence of noncaseating granulomata indistinguishable from those of sarcoidosis. Indeed, there are many striking clinical and radiographic similarities between these two conditions.[125] Thus, one finds

granulomatous skin lesions, lymphadenopathy, nephrocalcinosis and hypercalcemia, granulomatous involvement of the liver and spleen, and diffuse lung disease in both diseases. However, involvement of the salivary glands, eyes, bones, and the central

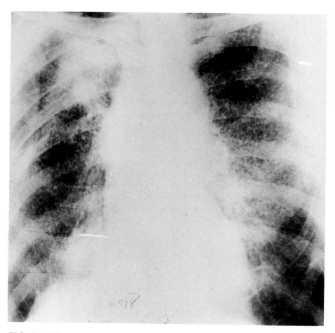

FIG 9–30.
Siderosilicosis in a hematite miner from Cumberland, England.

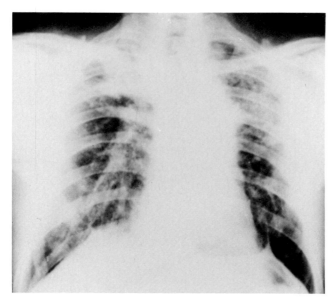

FIG 9–31.
Aluminosis in a bauxite smelter showing dense upper zone pulmonary fibrosis.

as miliary nodulation of the lungs rather than the patchy alveolar filling pattern of pulmonary edema. In the majority of cases the radiographic findings resolve over a period of 2 to 4 weeks, and only in some 10% of cases is there a transition to chronic berylliosis.

In chronic pulmonary berylliosis, hilar and mediastinal adenopathy is a very frequent finding. The parenchymal lesions may be miliary in type in the early stages, although this stage may go unobserved (Fig 9–33). Symmetrical reticulonodular parenchymal infiltration without zonal predominance is characteristic. With progression of disease the lungs lose volume, and the fibrosis becomes coarser and more honeycombed. Bleb formation occurs, and pneumothorax is a potential complication (Figs 9–34 and 9–35). With further progression of the disease, the hilar shadows become increasingly prominent, reflecting a combination of central pulmonary artery dilatation and adenopathy. The patient eventually succumbs from respiratory failure or cor pulmonale.

nervous system is not found in berylliosis. Berylliosis is encountered in two forms: acute and chronic.

Acute berylliosis results from a single intense exposure and manifests as an acute tracheobronchitis and pulmonary edema. In some cases the pulmonary parenchymal changes are seen radiographically

INHALATION OF NOXIOUS GASES, VAPORS, AND FUMES

The deleterious effects of noxious gases and fumes are mediated by several different physiologic

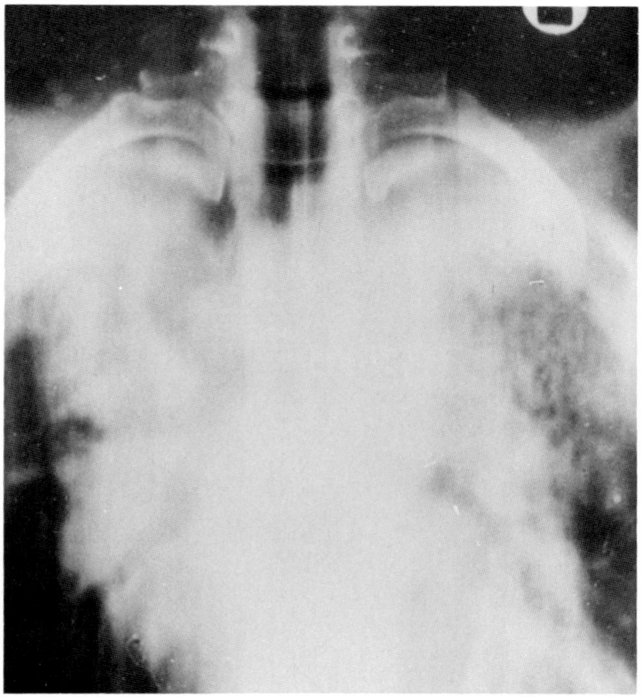

FIG 9–32.
Chest tomogram in patient with aluminosis showing dense apical fibrosis, mediastinal widening, and marked distortion of the trachea.

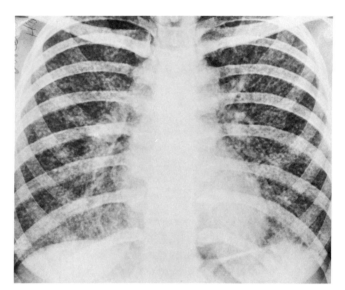

FIG 9–33.
Chronic berylliosis. There is diffuse, finely nodular, interstitial infiltration of the lungs with hilar and mediastinal adenopathy.

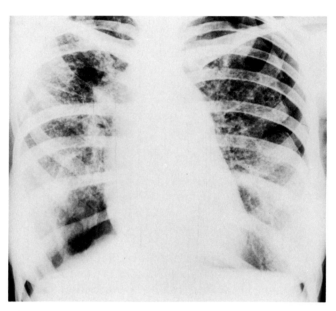

FIG 9–35.
Same patient as in Figure 9–34. The bulla at the right base has been excised. Note the left pneumothorax and the increase in heart size from the previous radiograph.

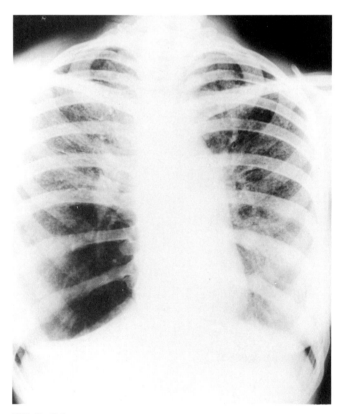

FIG 9–34.
Radiograph of a young female metallurgist with chronic berylliosis. Note the large bulla at the right base, the enlarged main pulmonary artery and hili, and the diffuse interstitial infiltration of the lungs.

mechanisms. These mechanisms include asphyxiation, absorption of toxins, allergic reaction, and surface irritation.

1. *Asphyxiation.* When the oxygen in the ambient air is displaced by gas or vapor, the subject suffers from acute lack of oxygen. Examples include asphyxiation by carbon dioxide, nitrogen, methane, and freon. Alternatively the transport of oxygen may be interfered with as, for example, in carbon monoxide or cyanide poisoning. There are no radiographic features.

2. *Toxic absorption.* Absorption of toxic materials may affect the lung directly or affect more distant body systems. Aluminum and beryllium are examples of substances that may damage the lungs acutely.

3. *Allergy.* Certain (inorganic) substances, notably compounds of platinum, may excite an allergic response, resulting in an occupational asthma without specific radiographic features. Many inhaled organic substances are responsible for allergic manifestations, a subject discussed in Chapter 11.

4. *Surface irritants.* Many substances, when inhaled, have a direct irritating or damaging effect on the airways and lungs. The resulting inflammatory and edematous changes can be life-threatening. Notable examples were seen following the use of chlorine and other gases during World War I. In indus-

trial accidents a single identifiable agent is usually involved. The list of potentially hazardous substances is long and includes sulphur dioxide, zinc chloride, hydrogen fluoride, ammonia, osmium tetroxide, vanadium pentoxide, chromates, nitrogen dioxide, phosgene, and many others. The principal cause of nonindustrial inhalational injury is fire.

Acute Inhalational Injury

Injury to the airways and the lung parenchyma may result from the inhalation of a variety of noxious substances. The result may be chemical pulmonary edema and pneumonia severe enough in some cases to cause death. Fire accidents are the most frequent cause of severe acute inhalational injury. The injury results from a combination of physical (heat) and chemical damage. The composition of the smoke may be complex and may include volatilized plastics and their breakdown products as well as simpler noxious agents such as oxides of nitrogen, carbon monoxide, cyanides, and aldehydes.[30] In other cases the changes may be attributed to a single noxious agent such as beryllium (acute berylliosis, discussed earlier) or nitrogen dioxide (as in silo-filler's disease, discussed in the following section). One

should not overlook the possibility that patients who are perhaps suffering from other external trauma might have aspirated gastric contents during the course of rescue and resuscitation (see the section "Aspiration of Gastric Contents" later in this chapter).

The patient will have an acute tracheobronchitis, which may be membranous and ulcerative. Damage to the pulmonary parenchyma tends to be central—with edema and later, in many instances, pneumonitis. However, the patient may recover from the toxic tracheobronchitis and pulmonary edema without ever developing secondary pneumonitis (Fig 9–36). However, in spite of this rapid clearing, there may be delayed sequelae in silo-filler's disease and other inhalational injuries. After an interval of 10 to 14 days, a bronchiolitis obliterans may become manifest with recrudescence of symptoms (Fig 9–37). The degree of residual disability will depend on the nature of the exposure, its severity, and the degree of residual fibrosis and scarring.

The radiographic features reflect the severity of the insult and the extent of the response to this insult. Patients with airway damage only may never develop radiographic changes—or, if changes do occur, the radiographs may simply show nondescript

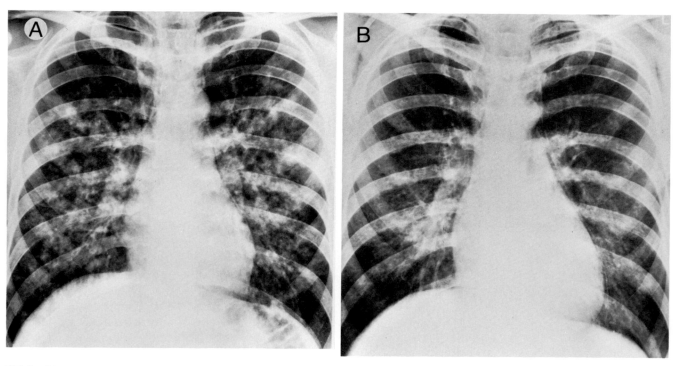

FIG 9–36.
A, radiograph of a young man admitted after accidentally setting his kitchen on fire while intoxicated. **B,** prompt recovery after 72 hours. (Courtesy of Dr. K. Simpkins, Leeds, England.)

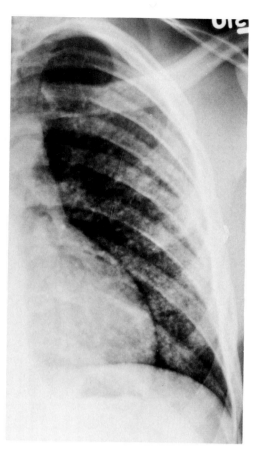

FIG 9–37.
Bronchiolitis obliterans (biopsy proven) in a young man who had made a heroic attempt to rescue a person from a burning car 3 weeks previously.

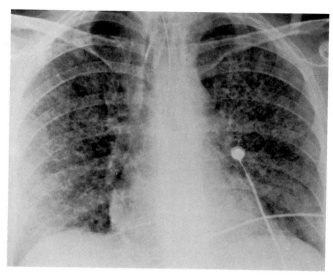

FIG 9–38.
Radiograph of a patient who had sustained severe thermal burns to the lungs 36 hours previously.

areas of atelectasis or consolidation, reflecting the results of airway obstruction and pneumonitis. Severe inhalational injury involving the pulmonary parenchyma produces more diffuse change. These radiographic changes may be present on the patient's admission, or may develop during the first 12 to 24 hours.[129] The basic pattern in severe inhalational injury is that of perihilar infiltration, which may be indistinguishable from cardiogenic edema (Fig 9–38). Inhalation of vapors and gases will generally result in fairly symmetric changes, whereas inhalation of fluids may predominantly affect one lung, depending on the position of the patient at the time of inhalation. However, cardiogenic edema may also be remarkably asymmetric on occasion. The problems may only compound if the patient goes on to develop renal failure or the shock lung syndrome. Heart size is not a reliable guide; patients with acute heart failure following a myocardial infarction may initially have a normal heart size. Serial radiographs

after inhalational injury with pulmonary edema should not, however, reveal any tendency of the heart to dilate. Equally, there should not be any tendency for pleural effusions to be a prominent feature in the radiographic picture. It is particularly in the more severe and more critical cases being followed in intensive care units that one has difficulty "fractionating" the various components of the radiographic picture. Even with the aid of various clinical data (such as pulmonary artery wedge pressures, the nature of the tracheal aspirates, ventilatory pressures, blood gas data, and so on), it may not be possible for one to make more than an educated guess. The various processes and factors that can contribute to the final radiographic picture include[69, 128]:

1. Reaction to the initial insult;
2. The severity and extent of secondary pneumonitis;
3. The development of noncardiogenic edema (adult respiratory disease syndrome);
4. Fluid imbalances in severe burn patients or patients with secondary renal failure;
5. Patchy atelectasis resulting from bronchial mucosal damage and mucous plugging;
6. The patient's preexisting medical status (e.g., preexisting chronic obstructive pulmonary disease).

In general, the more rapid the radiographic improvement, the more favorable the prognosis. As previously indicated this does not rule out the later development of a bronchiolitis obliterans. Such cases may manifest a fine patchy pulmonary interstitial process—mainly peripheral in location and fairly symmetric in distribution. These changes will gradually wane over a period of days or weeks leaving no visible sequelae, although the patient may continue to have respiratory deficits.

Silo-filler's Disease

Silo-filler's disease has been given its own particular designation in part because of the circumstances of exposure and in part because it tends to have a characteristic two-phase pattern of disease.[87, 101, 113] The patients are exposed to oxides of nitrogen produced from silage in the closed environment of a silo. The initial phase occurs immediately following exposure. The patient develops cough and dyspnea, and the radiographic features vary from normal to those of classic pulmonary edema (Fig 9–39). The patient recovers steadily, only to develop a recrudescence of symptoms some 2 to 3 weeks later, at which time a diffuse miliary or fine nodular pattern develops in the lungs. This appearance corresponds to diffuse bronchiolitis obliterans. In certain instances death may ensue during this secondary phase; in these individuals the pulmonary infiltrates may become coarser and confluent. In the majority of cases

there is a gradual clearing of the infiltrates, leaving no visible sequelae.

Drowning or Submersion Injury

It is estimated that some 150,000 persons lose their lives annually worldwide as a result of drowning.[140] The number of episodes of near drowning cannot be estimated. Unless prevented by laryngeal spasm, the fluid penetrates into the lungs of the drowning victim, where it may be radiographically demonstrable as pulmonary edema (Fig 9–40). Laryngeal spasm, which is particularly frequent in children, may prevent ingress of fluid, but this may be fatal because of cerebral hypoxia from inadequate ventilation. In one series of 12 children requiring mechanical ventilation, 4 did not have radiographic evidence of pulmonary edema on admission;[36] nevertheless, 2 of these 4 children subsequently died.

The initial radiographic appearances, therefore, may vary from complete normality through varying degrees of pulmonary edema (see Fig 9–40).[62] It should be emphasized, however, that an initially normal chest radiograph may be associated with significant hypoxia and, furthermore, that radiographic deterioration may occur in any case in the first 48 to 72 hours.[99] Mechanical ventilation, aspiration of gastric contents during resuscitation, neurologic damage, prolonged hypoxia, and similar factors may modify the radiographic picture during subsequent

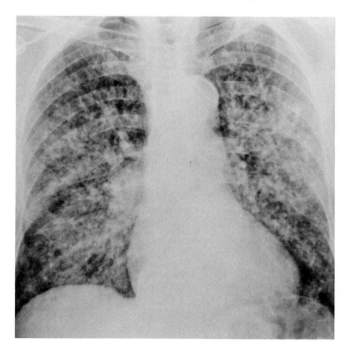

FIG 9–39.
Radiograph of a patient overcome by fumes in a silo several hours previously.

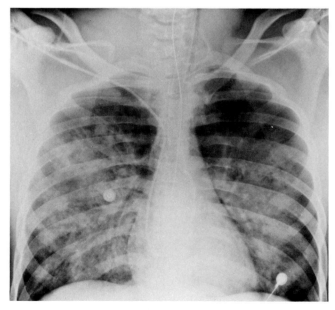

FIG 9–40.
Radiograph of a young man just after an episode of near drowning shows a pulmonary edema pattern.

examinations. The aspiration of gastric contents could, for example, lead to a secondary aspiration pneumonia. Pneumothorax and pneumomediastinum are frequent in victims of near drowning who are on ventilator support. Neurogenic pulmonary edema, or even a frank adult respiratory distress syndrome, may supervene.[33] Although the common drowning fluids (fresh water or saltwater) are capable of damaging the pneumocytes and dispersing or inactivating lung surfactant, there may be no demonstrable effect in very many cases of near drowning, and the aspirated fluid may be promptly absorbed or otherwise dispersed.[95] Nevertheless, in more severe cases, there may be a significant decrease in lung compliance and alterations in ventilation/perfusion matching, necessitating mechanical ventilation. It is in just this type of case that the secondary pulmonary problems and more severe neurologic defects are most likely to be encountered.

Aspiration of Gastric Contents

Massive aspiration of gastric contents is sometimes known as Mendelson's syndrome. Mendelson,[83] in fact, described massive aspiration of gastric contents in a particular patient group, namely women during parturition. A number of factors make pregnant patients more liable to aspiration. During pregnancy, the volume and acidity of gastric secretions increases, and there is relative atony of the stomach with delayed emptying. The gastroesophageal sphincter is relatively lax, and the administration of some form of anesthesia, often with the patient in an "unprepared" state, is common. However, massive aspiration of gastric contents may occur in other patients, almost invariably during periods of altered consciousness. The clinical features are abrupt in onset—consisting of cough, wheezing, cyanosis, dyspnea, and tachypnea. Initially, the pathologic changes consist of a chemical tracheobronchitis and pneumonia. Secondary bacterial infection, however, is common, and the clinical course may be further complicated by pulmonary embolism and the adult respiratory distress syndrome.

The classic radiographic findings are those of diffuse perihilar alveolar consolidation very similar to that of cardiogenic pulmonary edema (Fig 9–41). Landay et al. reviewed the records of 60 patients who had suffered acute aspiration of gastric contents and found a remarkable variability in the radiographic findings.[78] It was apparent from this study that the severity of the pulmonary changes depended on the volume of fluid aspirated, and there is experimental evidence to indicate that the severity of the process is also related to the pH of the aspirate.[15] Almost all patients have abnormalities of the chest radiograph following an episode of massive aspiration, and some worsening is usual in the first 24 to 36 hours following such an episode. Uncomplicated cases will subsequently clear over the next 4 to 5 days. Secondary bacterial pneumonia with severe underlying pulmonary disease and the development of the adult respiratory distress syndrome are adverse features which may lead to a fatal outcome even after an initial period of improvement. The parenchymal densities are often ill-defined acinar airspace shadows, which are frequently confluent. Small irregular shadows are, however, common. The distribution of the densities is generally perihilar or bibasilar, although there is considerable variation, possibly dependent on the position of the patient during the episode of aspiration. The pulmonary shadows may even be entirely unilateral[141] (Fig 9–42). Pleural effusions are uncommon, presumably a reflection of the more central location of the inflammatory process. The more severe and extensive the shadowing on the initial examination, the worse the prognosis. However, relatively minor initial changes may progress to a fatal outcome. In cases with minor changes or rather nondescript patchily distributed densities, consideration of the clinical circumstances is particularly important in determining the cause of radiographic changes.

Hydrocarbon Pneumonia

Volatile hydrocarbons, when aspirated, may result in a widespread chemical pneumonia. There has, in the past, been debate as to whether ingested hydrocarbons cause pneumonia in the absence of aspiration. Volatile hydrocarbons, when absorbed from the gut, are excreted by way of the lungs, and it has been suggested that this excretion may result in toxic damage to the lungs. However, the present consensus of opinion is that ingested hydrocarbons have minimal or no effect on the lungs, the pulmonary toxic effects being overwhelmingly caused by aspirated hydrocarbons.[31] The low pulmonary toxicity of ingested hydrocarbons may result because these products are poorly absorbed from the gut and may also undergo some detoxification during their transit through the liver. Toxic lung damage caused by intravenously administered hydrocarbons has, however, been observed both experimentally[64] and in clinical practice.[91]

Radiographic abnormalities are commonly

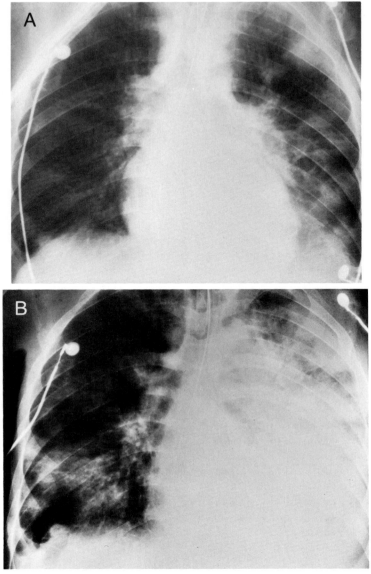

FIG 9–41.
A, radiograph taken shortly after an episode of massive aspiration that occurred during cardiac resuscitation. **B,** radiograph 10 hours later shows marked deterioration, especially in the left lung.

present on admission or develop within the first 12 hours. There is a poor correlation of these radiographic abnormalities with clinical symptoms and signs. Many patients with radiographic abnormalities have no symptoms, or symptoms resolve before the radiographic changes clear. Chest radiographs show scattered pulmonary densities which are almost invariably bilateral, with mid and lower zone predominance (Fig 9–43). Initially, the densities are often mottled but, with time, they may become confluent. The pulmonary shadowing commonly worsens somewhat over the first 48 to 72 hours following aspiration. The pulmonary densities, in the average case, then clear over the next few days. On occasion, however, radiographic changes may take weeks or months to clear, particularly in adults. Obstructive emphysema with air trapping peripherally may be seen, and pneumatoceles are also occasionally observed. Segmental or subsegmental atelectasis is frequent.

The majority of cases of hydrocarbon pneumonia occur in children, particularly young children.

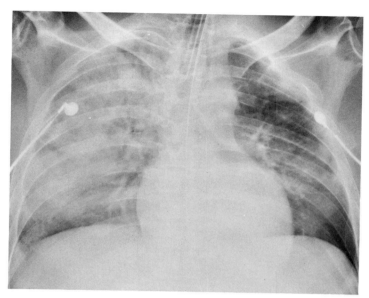

FIG 9–42.
Predominantly unilateral shadowing following an episode of massive gastric aspiration in a 43-year-old man.

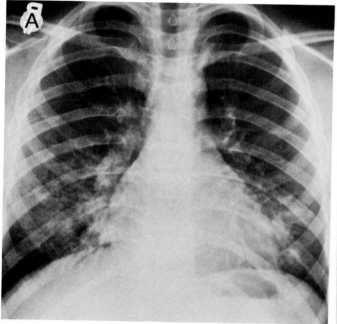

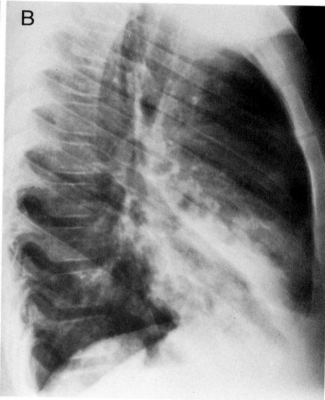

FIG 9–43.
Kerosene pneumonia in a 12-year-old boy shows extensive patchy bibasilar infiltration. **A,** PA view. **B,** lateral view.

The prognosis, both immediate and in the long term, is good. Few of these children have any damage to the lungs although there may be minor residual pulmonary function abnormalities.[50] Some adults may suffer permanent damage, such as chronic organizing pneumonia, fibrosis, and bronchiectasis.

INHALATION OF FOREIGN BODIES

The usual foreign materials inhaled into the airways are food and broken fragments of teeth; a nut represents the single most common object. Inhalation of foreign bodies occurs most frequently during the first 3 years of life, with a peak incidence between 1 and 2 years. It is a rare occurrence before 6 months of age. The usual site of lodgment of the foreign body is the left or right main bronchus; neither side is involved significantly more often than the other. The next most common site is the trachea, followed by a lobar bronchus.[9, 21, 73]

Although most individuals who aspirate foreign bodies are diagnosed within 2 to 3 days of the event, the diagnosis may not be made for weeks or sometimes even months after the initial aspiration, as was the case in approximately one-third of children in two large series.[9, 21] In over 80% of cases[9, 12, 73, 106] a definite event of aspiration or choking is followed by

cough and/or wheezing. After these initial symptoms, the cough and wheezing may persist, usually without respiratory distress. In time, the cough may disappear. It is important to note, however, that an interval of hours, months, or years may occur during which the child is asymptomatic following the initial event.[100]

The most common complication of foreign body aspiration is pneumonia or atelectasis, which occurs in approximately one-fourth of the cases when the foreign body lodges in a bronchus, but is rare when the object lodges in the trachea. Bronchiectasis may follow prolonged retention of a bronchial foreign body.

Bronchoscopy is the usual method of final diagnosis and also permits removal of the foreign body in almost all cases. Thoracotomy or other surgical intervention is rarely required. Blazer et al.[9] emphasized that 15% of their patients who had inhaled foreign bodies required a second or third bronchoscopy, demonstrating that foreign bodies may be missed at bronchoscopy and that the finding of one foreign body does not exclude the presence of another.

The plain chest film will show a radiopaque foreign body in 5% to 15% of cases. Occasionally, the foreign body is seen as a shadow of soft tissue density in one of the larger airways.

The cardinal sign of inhalation soon after aspira-

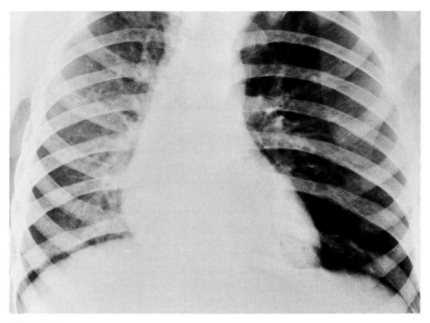

FIG 9–44.
Inhaled foreign body lodged in the left main bronchus in a young child is causing obstructive air-trapping in the left lung.

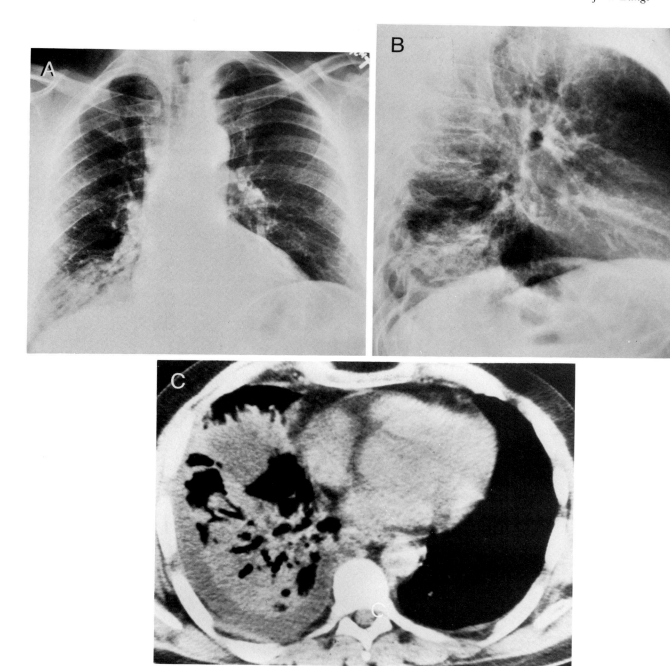

FIG 9–45.
An inhaled peanut lodged in the bronchus intermedius in an adult causing postobstructive collapse and consolidation of the right middle and lower lobes, which had been present for 2 months.

The prebronchoscopic diagnosis was carcinoma of the lung. **A,** PA radiograph. **B,** lateral radiograph. **C,** CT scan.

tion is obstructive overinflation or air trapping of the affected lobe or lobes[9, 12, 106] (Fig 9–44). Air trapping, with or without contralateral shift of the mediastinum, is best demonstrated on radiographs taken during expiration. Such studies can be difficult to obtain in young children, and it is often easier to

demonstrate both air trapping and mediastinal shift with fluoroscopy.

Alternative techniques that do not require fluoroscopy include assisted expiratory films and lateral decubitus examinations.[16] An assisted expiratory film consists of a chest radiograph exposed while gentle pressure is being applied to the epigastrium with a lead-gloved hand;[138] air trapping is demonstrated by the contrast between the relatively lucent affected lobe and the more opaque normal lobes. The idea behind lateral decubitus studies to detect inhaled foreign bodies is that the dependent lung is normally less inflated than the uppermost lung regardless of the degree of inspiration, whereas air trapping renders the dependent lung hyperlucent. Radionuclide perfusion scanning of the lungs has been used to demonstrate reduced blood flow to areas of the lung whose airway has been partially occluded by a foreign body.[85, 110]

The other major feature of foreign body aspiration into the airway is atelectasis or pneumonia distal to the obstructing foreign body (Fig 9–45). These signs were seen in 20% to 45% of patients in the larger series.[9, 73, 12, 106] A pneumothorax or a pneumomediastinum may be present, but both are surprisingly uncommon following aspiration of a foreign body, being seen in less than 2% of patients.[9, 106]

Normal inspiratory and expiratory chest radiographs can be expected in about one-fourth of cases. In the 200 patients described by Blazer and coworkers, 15.6% of those with bronchial foreign bodies and 60.6% of those with tracheal foreign bodies, showed no abnormalities on inspiratory and expiratory films; and even with fluoroscopy, almost half the patients with tracheal foreign bodies showed no abnormality.[9]

REFERENCES

1. Aberle DR, Gamsu G, Ray CS: High-resolution CT of benign asbestos-related diseases: clinical and radiographic correlation. *AJR* 1988; 151:883–891.
2. Albeda SM, Epstein DM, Gefter WB, et al: Pleural thickening: Its significance and relationship to asbestos dust exposure. *Am Rev Respir Dis* 1982; 126:621–624.
3. Amandus HE, Lapp NL, Jacobson G, et al: Significance of irregular small opacities of coal miners in the USA. *Br J Ind Med* 1976; 33:13–17.
4. Amandus HE, Prendergrass EP, Dennis JM, et al: Pneumoconiosis: Interreader variability in the classification of the type of small opacities in the chest roentgenogram. *AJR* 1974; 122:740–743.
5. Anton HC: Multiple pleural plaques. *Br J Radiol* 1967; 40:685–690.
6. Baker EL, Greene R: Incremental value of oblique chest radiographs in the diagnosis of asbestos-induced lung disease. *Am J Ind Med* 1982; 3:17–22.
7. Becklake MR: Asbestos-related diseases of the lung and other organs: Their epidemiology and implications for clinical practice. *Am Rev Respir Dis* 1976; 114:187–227.
8. Bergin CJ, Muller NL, Vedal S, et al: CT in silicosis: Correlation with plain films and pulmonary function tests. *AJR* 1986; 146:477–483.
9. Blazer S, Naveh Y, Friedman A: Foreign body in the airway. *Am J Dis Child* 1980; 134:68.
10. Blesovsky A: The folded lung. *Br J Dis Chest* 1966; 60:19–22.
11. Brooks SM: Lung disorders resulting from the inhalation of metals. *Clin Chest Med* 1981; 2:235–254.
12. Brown BSTJ, Ma H, Dunbar JS, et al: Foreign bodies in the tracheobronchial tree in childhood. *J Can Assoc Radiol* 1963; 14:158–171.
13. Buechner HA, Ansari A: Acute silico proteinosis. A new pathologic variant of acute silicosis in sandblasters, characterized by histologic features resembling alveolar proteinosis. *Dis Chest* 1969; 55:274–278.
14. Burrell R: Immunological aspects of coal worker's pneumoconiosis. *Ann NY Acad Sci* 1972; 200:94–105.
15. Bynum LJ, Pierce AK: Pulmonary aspiration of gastric contents. *Am Rev Respir Dis* 1976; 114:1129–1136.
16. Capitanio MA, Kirkpatrick JA: The lateral decubitus film, an aid in determining air trapping in children. *Radiology* 1972; 103:460–462.
17. Caplan A: Correlation of radiological category with lung pathology in coal worker's pneumoconiosis. *Br J Ind Med* 1962; 19:171–179.
18. Caplan A, Simon G, Reid L: The radiological diagnosis of widespread emphysema and categories of simple pneumoconiosis. *Clin Radiol* 1966; 17:68–70.
19. Casey KR, Rom WN, Moatamed F: Asbestos-related diseases. *Clin Chest Med* 1981; 2:179–202.
20. Classification of radiographs of the pneumoconioses. *Med Radiogr Photogr* 1981; 57:2–17.
21. Cohen SR, Herbert WI, Lewis GB, et al: Foreign bodies in the airway: Five-year retrospective study with special reference to management. *Ann Otol Rhinol Laryngol* 1980; 89:437–442.
22. Collins JD, Brown RKT, Batra P: Asbestosis and the serratus anterior muscle. *J Natl Med Assoc* 1983; 75:296–300.
23. Cooke WE: Pulmonary asbestosis. *Br Med J* 1927; 2:1024–1025.
24. Cookson WO, Deklerk NH, Musk AW, et al: Benign and malignant pleural effusions in former Wittenoom crocidolite millers and miners. *Aust NZ J Med* 1985; 15:731–737.
25. Cotes E, Gibson JC, McKerrow CB, et al: A long term follow-up of workers exposed to beryllium. *Br J Ind Med* 1983; 40:13–21.
26. Craighead JE, Mossman BT: The pathogenesis of asbestos-associated diseases. *N Engl J Med* 1982; 306:1446–1455.
27. Davis JMG, Chapman J, Collings P, et al: *Autopsy*

Study of Coal Miner's Lungs, Report No. TM/79/9 (Eur. P27). Edinburgh, Institute of Occupational Medicine, 1979.

28. Dee PM, Suratt P, Winn W: The radiographic findings in acute silicosis. *Radiology* 1978; 126:359–363.

29. DeLajartre M, DeLajartre AY: Mesothelioma on the coast of Brittany, France. *Ann NY Acad Sci* 1979; 330:323–332.

30. Demling RH: Smoke inhalation injury. *Postgrad Med* 1987; 82:63–68.

31. Eade NR, Taussig LM, Marks MI: Hydrocarbon pneumonitis. *Pediatrics* 1974; 54:351–357.

32. Edge JR: Incidence of bronchial carcinoma in shipyard workers with pleural plaques. *Ann NY Acad Sci* 1979; 330:289–294.

33. Effmann EL, Merten DF, Kirks DR, et al: Adult respiratory distress syndrome in children. *Radiology* 1985; 157:69–74.

34. Eisenstadt HB: Asbestos pleurisy. *Dis Chest* 1964; 46:78–81.

35. Epler GR, McCloud TC, Gaensler EA: Prevalence and incidence of benign asbestos pleural effusion in a working population. *JAMA* 1982; 247:617–622.

36. Fandel I, Bancalari E: Near drowning in children: Clinical aspects. *Pediatrics* 1976; 58:573–579.

37. Feigin DS: Talc: Understanding its manifestations in the chest. *AJR* 1986; 146:295–301.

38. Felson B: *Chest Roentgenology.* Philadelphia, WB Saunders Co, 1973.

39. Fletcher DE: A mortality study of shipyard workers with pleural plaques. *Br J Ind Med* 1972; 29:142–145.

40. Freundlich IM, Greening R: Asbestosis and associated medical problems. *Radiology* 1967; 89:224–229.

41. Gaensler EA, Carrington CB, Coutre RE, et al: Pathological, physiological and radiological correlations in the pneumoconioses. *Ann NY Acad Sci* 1972; 200:574–607.

42. Gaensler EA, Kaplan AI: Asbestos pleural effusion. *Ann Intern Med* 1971; 74:178–191.

43. Gilmartin D: The serratus anterior muscle on chest radiographs. *Radiology* 1979; 131:629–635.

44. Gough J: Pneumoconiosis of coal trimmers. *J Pathol Bacteriol* 1940; 51:277–285.

45. Gough J, James WRL, Wentworth JE: A comparison of the radiological and pathological changes in coal worker's pneumoconiosis. *J Fac Radiol* 1949; 1:28–60.

46. Greaves IA: Rheumatoid "pneumoconiosis" (Caplan's syndrome) in an asbestos worker: A 17 years' follow-up. *Thorax* 1979; 34:404–405.

47. Green RA, Dimcheff DG: Massive bilateral upper lobe fibrosis secondary to asbestos exposure. *Chest* 1974; 65:52–55.

48. Greening RR, Heslep JH: The roentgenology of silicosis. *Semin Roentgenol* 1967; 2:265–275.

49. Gregor A, Parkes RW, duBois R, et al: Radiographic progression of asbestosis: Preliminary report. *Ann NY Acad Sci* 1979; 330:147–156.

50. Gurwitz D, Kaltan M, Levison H, et al: Pulmonary function abnormalities in asymptomatic children after hydrocarbon pneumonitis. *Pediatrics* 1978; 62:789–794.

51. Hanke R, Kretzschmar R: Round atelectasis. *Semin Roentgenol* 1980; 15:174–182.

52. Heitzman ER: in, *The Lung: Radiologic and Pathologic Correlations.* St Louis, CV Mosby Co, 1984.

53. Heitzman ER, Naeye RL, Markarian B: Roentgen pathological correlations in coal worker's pneumoconiosis. *Ann NY Acad Sci* 1972; 200:510–526.

54. Heppleston AG: The pathological recognition and pathogenesis of emphysema and fibrocystic disease of the lung with special reference to coal workers. *Ann NY Acad Sci* 1972; 200:347–369.

55. Hillerdal G: Pleural plaques in a health survey material. Frequency, development and exposure to asbestos. *Scand J Respir Dis* 1978; 59:257–263.

56. Hillerdal G: Pleural plaques and risk for cancer in the county of Uppsala. *Eur J Respir Dis* 1980; 61(suppl 107):111–118.

57. Hillerdal G: Asbestos exposure and upper lobe involvement. *AJR* 1982; 139:1163–1166.

58. Hillerdal G, Hemmingsson A: Pulmonary pseudutumors and asbestos. *Acta Radiol [Diagn] (Stockh)* 1980; 21:615–620.

59. Hillerdal G, Liadgren A: Pleural plaques: Correlation of autopsy findings to radiographic findings and occupational history. *Eur J Respir Dis* 1980; 61:315–319.

60. Hilt B, Lien JT, Lund-Larsen PG, et al: Asbestos-related findings in chest radiographs of the male population of the county of Telemark, Norway—a cross-sectional study. *Scand J Work Environ Health* 1986; 12:567–573.

61. Hooper WF: Acute beryllium lung disease. *NC Med J* 1981; 42:551–553.

62. Hunter TB, Whitehouse WH: Fresh water drowning: Radiological aspects. *Radiology* 1974; 112:51–56.

63. Hurley JF, Burns J, Copland L, et al: Coal worker's simple pneumoconiosis and exposure to dust at 10 British coalmines. *Br J Ind Med* 1982; 39:120–127.

64. Huxtable KA, Bolande RP, Klaus M: Experimental furniture polish pneumonia in rats. *Pediatrics* 1964; 34:228–235.

65. International Labour Office: *Guidelines for the Use of the ILO International Classification of Radiographs of Pneumoconiosis,* International Labor Office Occupational Safety and Health series no. 22 (rev 80). Geneva, Switzerland, International Labour Office, 1980.

66. Jacob B, Bohlig H: Die rontgenologische komplikationen der lungen asbestose. *Fortschr Geb Roentgenstr* 1955; 83:515–525.

67. Jacobsen M: New data on the relationship between simple pneumoconiosis and exposure to coal mine dust. *Chest* 1980; 78:408–410.

68. Jacobson GJ, Felson B, Pendergrass EP, et al: Eggshell calcifications in coal and metal miners. *Semin Roentgenol* 1967; 2:276–282.

69. Kangarloo H, Beachley MC, Ghahremani GG: The radiographic spectrum of pulmonary complications in burn victims. *AJR* 1977; 128:441–445.

70. Kannerstein M: Recent advances and perspectives relevant to the pathology of asbestos-related diseases in man, in Wagner JC (ed): *Biological Effects of Mineral Fibers.* Lyon, France, International Agency for Research on Cancer 1980, vol 1, pp 149–162.

71. Katz D, Kreel L: Computed tomography in pulmonary asbestosis. *Clin Radiol* 1979; 30:207–213.

72. Kennedy T, Rawlings W, Baser M, et al: Pneumoconiosis in Georgia kaolin workers. *Am Rev Respir Dis* 1983; 127:215–220.

73. Kim IG, Brummitt WM, Humphry A, et al: Foreign body in the airway: A review of 202 cases. *Laryngoscope* 1973; 83:347.

74. Kiviluoto R, Meurman LO, Hakama M: Pleural plaques and neoplasia in Finland. *Ann NY Acad Sci* 1979; 330:31–33.

75. Kleinerman J: The pathology of some familiar pneumoconioses. *Semin Roentgenol* 1967; 2:244–264.

76. Kreel L: Computer tomography in the evaluation of pulmonary asbestosis. *Acta Radiol* [Diagn] (Stockh) 1976; 17:405–412.

77. Kretzschmar R: Über atelektatische pseudotumoren der lunge. *Fortschr Geb Roentgenstr* 1975; 122:19–29.

78. Landay MJ, Christensen EE, Bynum LJ: Pulmonary manifestations of acute aspiration of gastric contents. *AJR* 1978; 131:587–592.

79. Leigh J, Outhred KG, McKenzie HI, et al: Quantified pathology of emphysema, pneumoconiosis, and chronic bronchitis in coal workers. *Br J Ind Med* 1983; 40:258–263.

80. Lyons JP, Ryder RC, Campbell H, et al: Significance of irregular opacities in the radiology of coal worker's pneumoconiosis. *Br J Ind Med* 1974; 31:36–44.

81. Lyons JP, Ryder R, Campbell H, et al: Pulmonary disability: Coal worker's pneumoconiosis. *Br Med J* 1972; 1:713–716.

82. McLoud TC, Woods BO, Carrington CB, et al: Diffuse pleural thickening in an asbestos-exposed population: Prevalence and causes. *AJR* 1985; 144:9–18.

83. Mendelson CL: The aspiration of stomach contents into the lungs during obstetric anesthesia. *Am J Obstet Gynecol* 1946; 52:191–205.

84. Mintzer RA, Cugell DW: The association of asbestos-induced pleural disease and rounded atelectasis. *Chest* 1982; 81:457–460.

85. Moncada R, Baker D, Kenny J, et al: Reversible unilateral pulmonary hypoperfusion secondary to acute check-valve obstruction to a main bronchus. *Radiology* 1973; 106:361–362.

86. Morgan WKC, Lapp NC: Respiratory disease in coal miners: State of the art. *Am Rev Respir Dis* 1976; 113:531–559.

87. Morrissey WL, Gould IA, Carrington CB, et al: Silo-filler's disease. *Respiration* 1975; 32:81–92.

88. Naeye RL: Rank of coal and coal worker's pneumoconiosis. *Am Rev Respir Dis* 1971; 103:350–355.

89. Naeye RL, Dellinger WS: Coal worker's pneumoconiosis: Correlation of roentgenographic and post mortem findings. *JAMA* 1972; 220:223–227.

90. Nagelschmidt G, Rivers D, King EJ, et al: Dust and collagen content of lungs of coal workers with progressive massive fibrosis. *Br J Ind Med* 1963; 20:181–191.

91. Neeld EM, Limacher MC: Chemical pneumonitis after the intravenous injection of hydrocarbon. *Radiology* 1978; 126:36.

92. Newell DJ, Browne RC: Symptomatology and radiology in pneumoconiosis: A survey in the Durham Coalfield. *J Fac Radiol* 1955; 7:20–28.

93. Oldham PD: Pneumoconiosis in Cornish china clay workers. *Br J Ind Med* 1983; 40:131–137.

94. Parkes WR: *Occupational Lung Disorders,* ed 2. London, Butterworths, 1982.

95. Pearn J: Pathophysiology of drowning. *Med J Aust* 1985; 142:586–588.

96. Picado C, Roisin RR, Sala H, et al: Diagnosis of asbestosis: Clinical, radiological and lung function data in 42 patients. *Lung* 1984; 162:325–335.

97. Pratt PC: Role of silica in progressive massive fibrosis in coal worker's pneumoconiosis. *Arch Environ Health* 1968; 16:734–737.

98. Prendergrass EP: Silicosis and a few of the other pneumoconioses: Observations on certain aspects of the problem with emphasis in the role of the radiologist. *AJR* 1958; 80:1–41.

99. Putman CE, Tummillo AM, Myerson DA, et al: Drowning: Another plunge. *AJR* 1975; 125:543–548.

100. Pyman C: Inhaled foreign bodies in childhood: A review of 230 cases. *Med J Aust* 1971; 1:62–68.

101. Ramirez J, Dowell AR: Silo-filler's disease: Nitrogen dioxide–induced lung injury. Long-term follow-up and review of the literature. *Ann Intern Med* 1971; 74:569–576.

102. Rivers D, Wise ME, King ES, et al: Dust content, radiology, and pathology in simple pneumoconiosis of coal workers. *Br J Ind Med* 1960; 17:87–108.

103. Roche G, Parent J, Daumet P: Atelectasis parcellaires du lobe inferieur et du lobe moyen au cours

du pneumothorax thérapeutique. *Rev Tuberc (Paris)* 1956; 20:87–93.

104. Rockoff SD, Kagan E, Schwartz A, et al: Visceral pleural thickening in asbestos exposure: The occurrence and implications of thickened interlobar fissures. *J Thorac Imag* 1987; 2:58–66.

105. Rossiter CE: Relation of lung dust content to radiological changes in coal workers. *Ann NY Acad Sci* 1972; 200:465–477.

106. Rothmann BG, Boeckman CR: Foreign bodies in the larynx and tracheobronchial tree in children. *Ann Otol Rhinol Laryngol* 1980; 89:434–442.

107. Rous V, Studeny J: Aetiology of pleural plaques. *Thorax* 1970; 25:270–284.

108. Rubino GF, Newhouse M, Murray R, et al: Radiologic changes after cessation of exposure among chrysotile asbestos miners in Italy. *Ann NY Acad Sci* 1979; 330:157–161.

109. Ruckley VA, Fernie JM, Chapman JS, et al: Comparison of radiographic appearances with associated pathology and lung dust content in a group of coal workers. *Br J Ind Med* 1984; 41:459–467.

110. Rudavsky AZ, Leonidas JC, Abramson AL: Lung scanning for the detection of endobronchial foreign bodies in infants and children. *Radiology* 1973; 108:629–633.

111. Ryder R, Lyons JP, Campbell H, et al: Emphysema in coal worker's pneumoconiosis. *Br Med J* 1970; 3:481–487.

112. Sargent EN, Boswell WD, Ralls PW, et al: Subpleural fat pads in patients exposed to asbestos: Distinction from noncalcified pleural plaques. *Radiology* 1984; 152:273–277.

113. Scott EG, Hunt WB: Silo-filler's disease. *Chest* 1973; 63:701–706.

114. Scully RE, Mark EJ, McNeely BV: Case records of the Massachusetts General Hospital, Case 27—1982. *N Engl J Med* 1982; 307:104–112.

115. Seal RME: Current views on pathological aspects of asbestos (the unresolved questions and problems), in Wagner JC (ed): *Biological Effects of Mineral Fibers.* Lyon, France, International Agency for Research on Cancer, 1980, vol 1, pp 217–235.

116. Seal RME, Cockcroft A, Kung I, et al: Central lymph node changes and progressive massive fibrosis in coal workers. *Thorax* 1986; 41:531–537.

117. Seaton A, Dick JA, Dodgson J, et al: Quartz and pneumoconiosis in coalminers. *Lancet* 1981; 2:1272–1275.

118. Sebastien P, Parson X, Gaudichet A, et al: Asbestos retention in human respiratory tissues: Comparative measurements in lung parenchyma and in parietal pleura, in Wagner JC (ed): *Biological Effects of Mineral Fibers.* Lyon, France, International Agency for Research on Cancer, 1980, vol 1, pp 237–246.

119. Schneider HJ, Felson B, Gonzalez LL: Rounded atelectasis. *AJR* 1980; 134:225–232.

120. Shaver CG, Riddell AR: Lung changes associated with the manufacture of alumina abrasive. *J Ind Hyg* 1947; 29:145–157.

121. Sider L, Holland EA, Davis TM, et al: Changes on radiographs of wives of workers exposed to asbestos. *Radiology* 1987; 164:723–726.

122. Sinner WN: Pleuroma—a cancer-mimicking atelectatic pseudotumor of the lung. *Fortschr Geb Roentgenstr* 1980; 133:578–585.

123. Solomon A: The radiology of asbestos-related diseases with special reference to diffuse mesothelioma. *Semin Oncol* 1981; 8:290–301.

124. Sperber M, Mohan KK: Computer tomography—a reliable diagnostic modality in pulmonary asbestosis. *Comput Radiol* 1984; 8:125–132.

125. Sprince NL, Kazemi H, Hardy HL: Current (1975) problems of differentiating between beryllium disease and sarcoidosis. *Ann NY Acad Sci* 1976; 278:654–664.

126. Stark P: Round atelectasis: Another pulmonary pseudotumor. *Am Rev Respir Dis* 1982; 125:248–250.

127. Suratt PM, Winn WC Jr, Brody AR, et al: Acute silicosis in tombstone sandblasters. *Am Rev Respir Dis* 1977; 115:521–529.

128. Teixidor HS, Novick GS, Rubin E: Pulmonary complications in burn patients. *J Can Assoc Radiol* 1983; 34:264–270.

129. Teixidor HS, Rubin E, Novick GS, et al: Smoke inhalation. Radiologic manifestations. *Radiology* 1983; 149:383–387.

130. Tellesson WG: Rheumatoid pneumoconiosis (Caplan's syndrome) in an asbestos worker. *Thorax* 1961; 16:372–377.

131. Thiringer G, Blomqvist N, Brolin I: Pleural plaques in chest x-rays of lung cancer patients and matched controls (preliminary results). *Eur J Respir Dis* 1980; 61(suppl 107):119–122.

132. Trapnell DH: Septal lines in pneumoconiosis. *Br J Radiol* 1964; 37:805–810.

133. Tylen U, Nilsson U: Computed tomography in pulmonary pseudotumors and their relation to asbestos exposure. *J Comput Assist Tomogr* 1982; 6:229–237.

134. Walker AM, Loughlin JE, Friedlander ER, et al: Projections of asbestos-related disease, 1980–2009. *J Occup Med* 1983; 25:409–425.

135. Webb RW, Cooper C, Gamsu G: Interlobar pleural plaque mimicking a lung nodule in a patient with asbestos exposure. *J Comput Assist Tomogr* 1983; 7:135–136.

136. Weill H, Hughes JM: Asbestos as a public health risk: Disease and policy. *Annu Rev Public Health* 1986; 7:171–192.

137. Wells IP, Bhatt RCV, Flanagan M: Kaolinosis: A radiological review. *Clin Radiol* 1985; 36:579–582.

138. Wesenberg RL, Blumhagen JD: Assisted expiratory

chest radiography: Effective technique for the diagnosis of foreign body aspiration. *Radiology* 1979; 130:538–539.

139. Williams JL, Moller GA: Solitary mass in the lungs of coal miners. *AJR* 1973; 117:765–770.

140. Wunderlich P, Rupprecht E, Trefftz R, et al: Chest radiographs of near-drowned children. *Pediatr Radiol* 1985; 15:297–299.

141. Youngberg AS: Unilateral diffuse lung opacity. *Radiology* 1977; 123:277–281.

142. Ziskind M, Jones RN, Weill H: Silicosis: State of the art. *Am Rev Respir Dis* 1976; 113:647–665.

Drug- and Radiation-Induced Diseases of the Lungs

At the present time some 40 commonly used drugs have been shown to affect the lungs adversely. Prominent among these are the cytotoxic drugs used in the treatment of cancer and hematologic malignancies. Since the toxic effects of busulfan were first described over 30 years ago,[13] approximately 20 cytotoxic agents have been found to cause lung damage. This finding is perhaps not surprising when one realizes that cancer chemotherapy is essentially a form of controlled cellular poisoning. Pulmonary toxicity caused by noncytotoxic drugs occurs less frequently and less predictably.

The mechanisms by which drugs produce their deleterious effects are complex and are far from understood. A number of clinicopathologic syndromes have been identified and linked to various drugs (Table 10–1). A grasp of these syndromes and their possible underlying mechanisms helps in understanding the various radiographic manifestations of toxic lung disease.

There is a great deal of overlap both clinically and radiographically in the toxic effects of different drugs. One must realize, however, that the radiographic manifestations of drug-induced disease are entirely nonspecific. There are, basically, only a limited number of radiographic patterns to reflect the changes in drug-induced disease and other diseases. Hence any particular basic pattern can result from numerous different disease processes. The chest radiograph is simply one factor in a diagnostic equation that will include the clinical features, the nature of the drug therapy, the responses to alterations in

therapy, hematologic and biochemical data, microbiological testing, biopsy results, and so on.

PRINCIPAL MECHANISMS IN DRUG EFFECTS

Direct Toxic Action on Lung Tissue

The mechanisms of direct toxic action of drugs on the lung are numerous and poorly understood.[7] The production of excessive reactive oxygen metabolites and a disturbance of the complex oxidant/antioxidant system may result in damage to cells and cell membranes. Alveolar macrophages, polymorphonuclear leucocytes, and lymphocytes may be damaged, resulting in the release of leukokines, lymphokines, and other humoral factors with chemotactic, cytotoxic, or immune system–modulating effects. The balance between collagenosis and collagenolysis may be altered, causing excess collagen deposition that leads to pulmonary fibrosis. The collagen itself may be disordered either by damage to the fibroblasts or by action of anticollagen antibodies. Inflammatory cells release proteolytic enzymes, and a complex antiprotease system exists to combat the effects of these enzymes. Any inhibition of the antiprotease systems could lead to damage.

Histologically there is swelling of the endothelial cells, fibrinous exudation in the interstitium and the alveoli, inflammatory cell infiltration and necrosis of type I alveolar epithelial cells.[49] Hyaline membranes may form. Later, dysplastic type II alveolar epithelial cells proliferate and, depending on the extent of

TABLE 10–1.

Clinicopathologic Syndromes Associated With Adverse Drug Reactions

Direct toxic action on lung tissue with pulmonary infiltration and fibrosis
Hypersensitivity reactions
Systemic lupus erythematosus
Drug-induced phospholipidoses
Pulmonary edema
Pulmonary vasculitis
Pulmonary hemorrhage
Pulmonary thromboembolism
Pulmonary calcification
Pleural effusions/fibrosis
Mediastinal and hilar lymphadenopathy
Pulmonary granulomas
Mediastinal lipomatosis

damage, fibroblast proliferation and collagen deposition also occur. It is apparent that pathologically the toxic effects cause both interstitial lung disease and, to a variable extent, an acinar filling process. These processes will be variably reflected on the chest radiographs depending on the extent of the reaction and the degree of permanent damage and fibrosis.

Direct toxic action on lung tissue usually takes some time to reach a clinically appreciable threshold, and the effects may not be manifest for weeks or months after treatment has begun. In many cases the effect is dose-related, a relationship that is most apparent with the cytotoxic agents bleomycin, busulfan, and carmustine. The toxic effects may be enhanced by other factors such as increasing patient age, decreased renal function, radiation therapy, oxygen therapy, and other cytotoxic drug therapy.[7]

Hypersensitivity Reactions

Because the molecular size of drugs is too small to provoke an immune response, it is therefore likely that the drug molecules act as haptenes in combination with endogenous protein. The immune responses provoked are most commonly type I (immediate hypersensitivity) or type III (immune complex) reactions. The airways show bronchial constriction, mucous hypersecretion and inspissation, and mucosal edema with eosinophilic infiltration. The lung parenchyma may show patchy areas of edema and inflammatory reaction with a preponderance of eosinophils in the cellular infiltrate.

Hypersensitivity reactions are usually immediate and may become clinically apparent within hours or days of beginning therapy with the offending drug. Predominant airway involvement causes an asthma-like syndrome, whereas pulmonary parenchymal in-

volvement results in patchy eosinophilic infiltrates. These infiltrates are often fleeting, and eosinophilia may be present in the peripheral blood. Withdrawal of the offending drug and administration of corticosteroids usually result in prompt and complete clearing.

Neural or Humoral Mechanisms

Neurogenic noncardiac pulmonary edema is the most common response in this category and is encountered particularly with certain central nervous system depressants. The pulmonary capillary permeability for proteins is altered either by a direct toxic action on the lung or by impulses emanating from the brain stem and hypothalamus.[12, 44] Fluid exudes into the pulmonary interstitium and alveoli, and the result may be completely analogous to cardiogenic edema in the rapidity of onset and the radiographic features. However, not all cases of drug-induced pulmonary edema operate through this central neurogenic mechanism. A number of drugs cause water and salt retention, leading to fluid imbalances. A direct toxic action on the pulmonary capillary bed is also possible.[32]

Asthma may result from other less conspicuous neurohumoral mechanisms. Certain drugs may cause asthma by directly effecting bronchial innervation, for example beta-adrenergic antagonists such as propranolol and parasympathetico-mimetics such as neostigmine. Aspirin may cause asthma by inhibiting prostaglandin synthesis.[20]

Autoimmune Mechanisms

An extensive series of drugs cause a systemic lupus erythematosus syndrome, presumably by triggering an autoimmune response. The pleural and pulmonary manifestations of the drug-induced syndrome are indistinguishable from those of the spontaneous form of the disease. Antinuclear factors are biochemically detectable in the serum and may be present in many patients taking these drugs, even in the absence of clinical or radiographic evidence of systemic lupus erythematosus.

Vasculitis, Thromboembolism, Pulmonary Vasospasm, and Pulmonary Hemorrhage

The association between pulmonary vasculitis and drugs is perhaps strongest with the sulfonamides, although the list of potential causative drugs is extensive. Pulmonary involvement is usually associated with and often overshadowed by systemic vasculitis, particularly involving the skin, kidneys, and liver. The result of the pulmonary vasculitis is patchy pulmonary infarction and hemorrhage that may cause acute interstitial infiltration or patchy airspace consolidation. The vasculitis may be an expression of a type III (immune complex) or a type IV (cell mediated) hypersensitivity response.

Intravenous administration of illicit drugs may cause a granulomatous vasculitis with resultant pulmonary hypertension. The vasculitis in these cases is caused by contaminants or suspending agents such as talc, starch, or cellulose and is more like a foreign body reaction.[39] On occasion the granulomatous response may be so extensive and severe as to resemble that of the progressive massive fibrosis seen in silicosis.[9]

Thromboembolism is particularly associated with the use of oral contraceptives and estrogens.[36] It is important to identify this group of patients because the individuals are young and otherwise healthy. They are at risk for developing secondary pulmonary arterial hypertension.

Oil embolism occurs to a greater or lesser extent in all properly conducted lymphangiogram examinations. Only when patients have poor pulmonary reserve or when one inadvertently administers excessive amounts of the contrast medium is there any potential for harm. A transient miliary infiltration accompanied, on occasion, by slight fever and slight dyspnea on exertion is the most that should be expected under normal circumstances.[31]

Pulmonary vasospasm appears to be rare. The best documented instance of this complication was noted in the 1960s with aminorex, an over-the-counter appetite supressant marketed in Europe. The pulmonary arteriolar vasospasm caused pulmonary arterial hypertension and enlargement of the right side of the heart, leading to cor pulmonale.[11]

Pulmonary hemorrhage is usually secondary to a disorder of the clotting mechanisms. In some cases the coagulopathy is unexpected and idiosyncratic as in oxyphenbutazone- or quinidine-induced thrombocytopenia. Most commonly, however, the hemorrhage is the result of anticoagulant therapy and is, therefore, not entirely unexpected. In rare instances penicillamine may cause a syndrome of pulmonary hemorrhage with or without renal failure similar to Goodpasture's syndrome and idiopathic pulmonary hemosiderosis, respectively.[30] Penicillamine-induced pulmonary hemorrhage is presumed to be an immune complex disorder. The predominant effect of pulmonary hemorrhage is patchy air space consolidation of variable severity that is generally rapid in onset and clears fairly quickly. Hemoptysis and a falling hematocrit may be the only clinical clues to the nature of the process.

Drug-Induced Phospholipidoses

The lungs have a number of metabolic functions other than respiration and acid-base balance. These include the inactivation of various endogenous amines such as norepinephrine, 5-hydroxytryptamine, serotonin, and certain prostaglandins. Certain drugs are capable of entering and saturating these carrier mechanisms. These drugs form complexes with phospholipids that are resistant to breakdown by phospholipases. This process results in an abnormal accumulation of phospholipids within the cells. A notable example of a drug-induced phospholipidosis is that caused by the antiarrhythmic drug amiodarone.[19, 25]

THE RADIOGRAPHIC FEATURES OF ADVERSE DRUG REACTIONS IN THE LUNG

Diffuse Alveolar Damage

In the early stages of toxicity the chest radiograph may be normal in appearance even when gallium scans, computed tomographic (CT) scans, pulmonary function testing, or lung biopsies give direct or indirect evidence of diffuse alveolar damage. The radiographic shadows of diffuse alveolar damage are variably interstitial, alveolar, or mixed in type, and it is usually clear that one is dealing with a generalized pulmonary process (Figs 10–1; 10–2). Segmental or lobar consolidations are not a feature of diffuse toxic lung damage. The shadowing tends to be more apparent in the lung bases. Pleural effusions are rarely found, except in some cases of procarbazine or methotrexate toxicity. However, such effusions could well be part of a hypersensitivity response. On rare occasions diffuse alveolar damage caused, for example, by cytoxan, bleomycin, and methotrexate may present as single or multiple pulmonary masses or nodules, a potent source of diagnostic confusion with neoplasm in a patient being treated for a malignant process.[16]

Most cases of diffuse alveolar damage secondary to drugs develop in patients undergoing chemotherapy for various malignant processes, a group in whom diffuse pulmonary shadowing could develop from causes other than drug toxicity (Table 10–2). These include lymphangitis carcinomatosa, leukemic

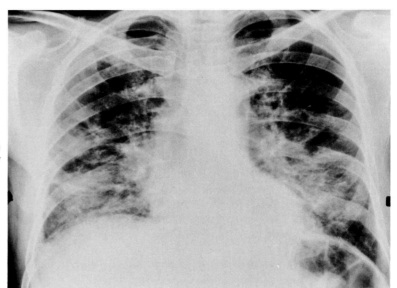

FIG 10—1.
Diffuse alveolar damage resulting from bleomycin treatment showing basally predominant pulmonary infiltration.

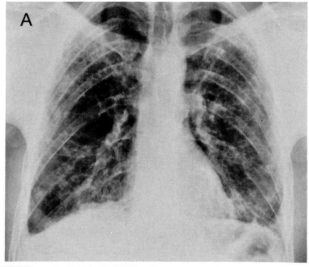

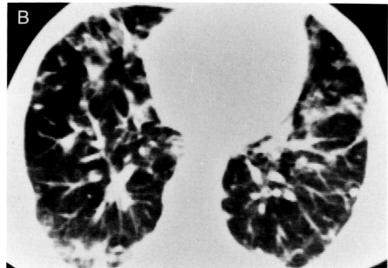

FIG 10—2.
Diffuse alveolar damage from bleomycin. **A,** diffuse coarse pulmonary infiltration. **B,** CT scan of the same patient showing scattered irregular parenchymal densities. (Courtesy of Dr. Elizabeth Bellamy, London.)

TABLE 10—2.
Drugs Causing Diffuse Alveolar Damage

Cytotoxic Agents	Noncytotoxic Agents
Azathioprine	Antibacterial
Bleomycin	Nitrofurantoin
Busulfan	Sulfasalazine
Carmustine (BCNU)	Antiarrhythmics
Chlorambucil	Amiodarone
Chlorozotocin	Tocainide
Cyclophosphamide	Antimigraine
Cytosine arabinoside	Methysergide
Lomustine (CCNU)	Antidepressant
Melphalan	Amitriptyline
6-Mercaptopurine	Gold salts
Methotrexate	Hexamethonium
Methyl CCNU	Mecamylamine
Mitomycin	Oxygen
Neocarzinostatin	Penicillamine
Teniposide (VM 26)	Pentolinium
Vinblastine	
Vindesine	

TABLE 10—3.
Drugs Causing Hypersensitivity Lung Disease

Antiarthritic	Antihypertensives
Aurothioglucose	Mecamylamine
Antiasthmatic	Hydrolazine
Cromolyn sodium	Central nervous system stimulant
Antibacterials	Methylphenidate
Erythromycin	Cytotoxic agents
Nitrofurantoin	Bleomycin
Paraaminosalicylic	Methotrexate
acid	Procarbazine
Isoniazid	Hypoglycemic agent
Penicillin	Chloropropamide
Sulfonamides	Muscle relaxant
Antidepressant	Dantrolene
Imipramine	

or lymphomatous infiltration of the lung, and opportunistic infections, such as *Pneumocystis carinii* pneumonia and pulmonary hemorrhage. The clinical circumstances, the sequence of events, and the radiographic appearances may provide circumstantial evidence that one is dealing with diffuse toxic alveolar damage. Recourse to lung biopsy may, however, be necessary on occasion. The radiographic appearances alone do not permit a firm diagnosis of diffuse alveolar damage.

Hypersensitivity Reactions

Hypersensitivity reactions are often apparent within hours or days of beginning treatment (Table 10—3). Fever and peripheral eosinophilia are features of these reactions and provide useful diagnostic clues. Predominant involvement of the airways produces an asthma-like syndrome which lacks specific radiographic features. Parenchymal involvement may result in a condition similar to idiopathic acute or chronic pulmonary eosinophilia (see Chapter 11). Focal patchy consolidations develop, often in the periphery of the lung (Fig 10—3). The extent of consolidation varies, and the distribution is random. The shadows themselves represent an acinar filling

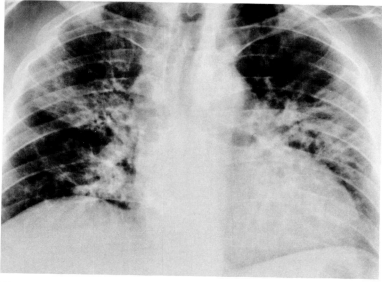

FIG 10—3.
Hypersensitivity pneumonia (biopsy proved) secondary to the administration of desipramine. The shadowing in this case is more central than is usual.

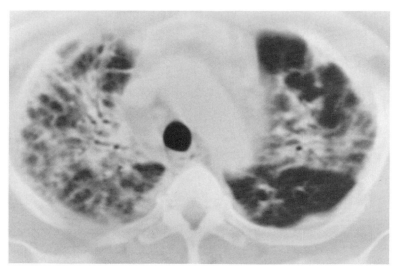

FIG 10−4.
CT scan of the patient in Figure 10−3. Peripheral infiltrates are seen in the right lung, whereas these are less pronounced in the left lung.

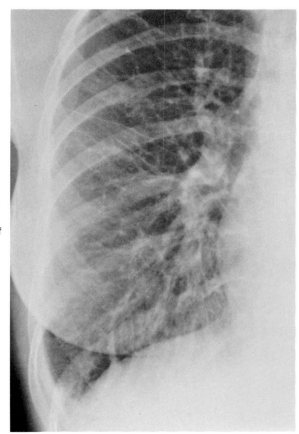

FIG 10−5.
Hyperacute hypersensitivity reaction to nitrofurantoin showing interstitial edema and a small pleural effusion. The patient, a young woman, developed dyspnea and tachypnea a few hours after a single dose of nitrofurantoin.

process and are usually subsegmental in size (Fig 10–4). They tend to be fleeting—in other words, they may resolve in one area of the lung only to appear in another. Particularly following previous exposure, the hypersensitivity reaction is hyperacute and presents as pulmonary edema with interstitial or even alveolar densities (Fig 10–5). On other occasions a diffuse reticulonodular pattern may be encountered, a reaction exemplified by the hypersensitivity response to methotrexate. The response to discontinuation of the offending drug is usually prompt. If rechallenge with the drug is attempted, the same hypersensitivity reaction may be expected. It should be noted that only three cytotoxic agents—bleomycin, methotrexate, and procarbazine—are associated with the hypersensitivity reaction and, with bleomycin, this form of toxicity occurs far less frequently than diffuse alveolar damage.

Pulmonary Edema

The edema resulting from the toxic effect of drugs (Table 10–4) is indistinguishable from cardiogenic edema both in radiographic appearance and in rapidity of onset and clearing (Figs 10–6; 10–7).

Systemic Lupus Erythematosus

The systemic lupus erythematosus (SLE) syndrome that results from the toxic effects of drugs

TABLE 10–4.
Drugs Causing Pulmonary Edema

Analgesics	Diuretics
Acetylsalicylic acid	Hydrochlorothiazide
Codeine	Sedatives
Pentazocine	Chlordiazepoxide
Antibacterials	Ethchlorvynol
Nitrofurantoin	Opiates
Antidepressants	Heroin
Amitriptyline	Propoxyphene
Anti-inflammatories	Methadone
Phenylbutazone	Miscellaneous
Oxyphenbutazone	Iodinated ionic
Beta-adrenergic antagonists	radiographic contrast
Ritodrine	media
Terbutaline	Dextran
Cytoxic agents	Colchicine
Cyclophosphamide	Epinephrine
Methotrexate	
Cytosine arabinoside	

(Table 10–5) does not differ in its pleural or pulmonary manifestations from the idiopathic form of the disease. Pleural effusions are by far the most common manifestation of this condition, and there may be a concomitant pericardial effusion (Fig 10–8). The fact that some of the most common drugs causing this condition are used in the treatment of cardiac disease may delay the realization that pleuropericardial effusions and interstitial lung disease are a complication of therapy rather than a manifesta-

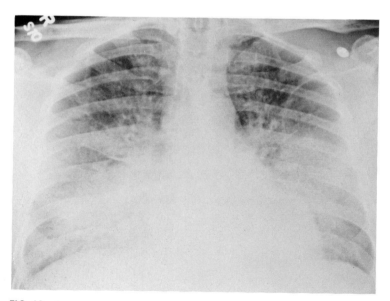

FIG 10–6.
Pulmonary edema secondary to the intravenous administration of "crack" (cocaine). The patient, a young man, recovered promptly with only supportive therapy.

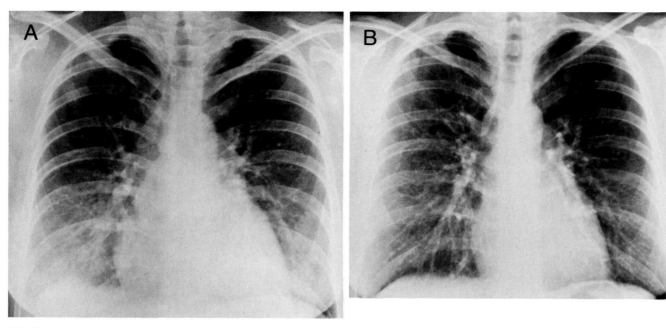

FIG 10—7.
Fluid overload **(A)** following the induction of labor using pitocin. Prompt recovery **(B)** occurred within 24 hours. Note the change in the size of the azygous vein.

tion of primary disease. At least 90% of all cases of drug-induced SLE are associated with procainamide, hydralazine, isoniazid, or phenytoin. When parenchymal shadowing occurs, it is predominantly basal and interstitial. Actual parenchymal involvement is, however, a comparatively unusual manifestation of the SLE syndrome.

TABLE 10—5.
Drug-Induced Systemic Lupus Erythematosus

Antibacterials	Cardiovascular preparations
Griseofulvin	Clofibrate
Isoniazid	Digitalis
Nitrofurantoin	Hydralazine
Paraaminosalicylic	Methyldopa
acid	Procaineamide
Penicillin	Propanolol
Streptomycin	Reserpine
Sulfonamides	Quinidine
Anticonvulsants	Diuretics
Carbamazepine	Chlorthalidone
Diphenyl hydantoin	Thiazides
Ethosuximide	Thyroid blockers
Methsuximide	Thiouracil
Primidone	Propylthiouracil
Trimethadone	Miscellaneous
Anti-inflammatories	Phenothiazines
Phenylbutazone	Penicillamine
Oxyphenbutazone	Methysergide
	Gold salts
	Levodopa

Pulmonary Vasculitis

The radiographic findings in pulmonary vasculitis are variable and nonspecific. Patchy subsegmental infiltrates with a random peripheral distribution may occur, a pattern similar to the hypersensitivity pattern except that fluctuations are not so marked. In other patients, diffuse, coarse, streaky shadows may be seen—which may appear interstitial in some patients and alveolar in others. Pleural effusions are not a feature. Cavitation may occur in areas of infarction caused by the vasculitis. The radiographic findings in this complication are probably the least specific of all adverse reactions to drugs (Table 10—6). A diagnosis of pulmonary vasculitis is unlikely to be made without biopsy evidence of vasculitis in the lungs or other organ systems.

Pulmonary Thromboembolism; Oil Embolism

The radiographic findings in pulmonary thromboembolism are dealt with in Chapter 8.

As previously indicated, some degree of oil embolism is to be expected during lymphangiography. For this reason patients with poor respiratory function should not undergo this form of examination. A very fine miliary pattern may be detected on good quality radiographs taken 24 to 48 hours following

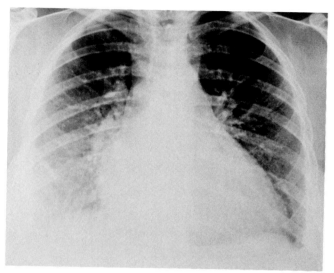

FIG 10—8.
Procainamide-induced SLE showing pleuropericardial effusions.

the administration of contrast material (Fig 10–9). At the same time the patient may experience mild fever and slight shortness of breath on exertion. These clinical and radiographic findings are transient.

Pulmonary Hemorrhage

Pulmonary hemorrhage rarely occurs as a toxic reaction to drug therapy (Table 10–7). It causes diffuse patchy alveolar shadowing, which may be extensive and severe. Depending on the rapidity and severity of the hemorrhage there may be a fall in the hematocrit, and hemoptysis is common. The radiographic findings are confined to the pulmonary parenchyma, and there are no associated pleural, hilar, or mediastinal abnormalities. Drug-induced pulmonary hemorrhage is likely to be an isolated event,

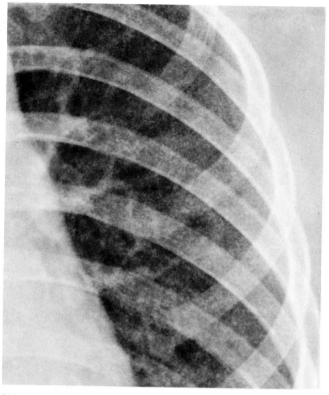

FIG 10—9.
Oil embolization. A radiograph obtained 24 hours following ethiodol lymphography demonstrates a fine diffuse granular infiltration of the lung.

and chronic lung sequelae, such as those found in patients with idiopathic pulmonary hemosiderosis or Goodpasture's syndrome, are not to be expected. Radionuclide studies using red blood cells tagged with technetium-99m offer a method of diagnosing this condition.[50]

Pulmonary Calcification

The most frequent cause of pulmonary parenchymal calcification is hyperparathyroidism, but pulmonary calcification has also been found after prolonged vitamin D and calcium therapy and in the milk-alkali syndrome. The calcification is extremely

TABLE 10—6.
Drugs Associated With Pulmonary Vasculitis

Antiasthmatics	Cardiovascular preparations
Cromolyn sodium	Quinidine
Antibacterials	Hydralazine
Sulfonamides	Cytotoxic agent
Penicillin	Busulphan
Anticonvulsants	Thyroid blockers
Diphenylhydantoin	Thiouracil
Anti-inflammatory	Propylthiouracil
Phenylbutazone	Tranquilizers
	Phenothiazines
	Illicit intravenous drug use
	Talc, starches, and so forth

TABLE 10—7.
Drugs Causing Pulmonary Hemorrhage

Anticoagulants
Estrogens
Penicillamine
Quinidine
Oxyphenbutazone

fine and cannot usually be resolved into distinct microcalculi like those seen in pulmonary microlithiasis. The calcifications are usually patchy and produce cloudlike infiltrates of unusually high radiographic density.

Pleural Effusions and Fibrosis

Pleural effusions most commonly occur in association with the SLE syndrome. Over 50% of patients with drug-induced SLE will develop pleural effusions at some stage of the illness. Effusions may be noted in hypersensitivity reactions to drugs, for example nitrofurantoin, methotrexate, and procarbazine. The effusions associated with SLE and hypersensitivity reactions can be expected to resolve without trace. Administration of methysergide, on the other hand, is associated with the development of pleural fibrosis as well as pleural fluid.[14] Irregular masses of pleural fibrosis may be interspersed with loculated pleural fluid, and there may be associated mediastinal fibrosis. Ergotamine and ergonovine maleate may produce similar effects.

Hilar and Mediastinal Adenopathy

The principal drugs causing hilar and mediastinal adenopathy are phenytoin and methotrexate. The adenopathy caused by methotrexate is part of the hypersensitivity reaction to this drug. Because methotrexate is used in the treatment of malignant processes, the possibility of mistaking the hypersensitivity reaction for tumoral adenopathy is real. Phenytoin-induced adenopathy is usually based on a hypersensitivity reaction. Phenytoin may, however, cause a pseudolymphoma syndrome with generalized adenopathy, fever, skin rashes, eosinophilia, and hepatosplenomegaly. Moreover, there is a slightly increased risk of the development of lymphoma in patients on this drug. Angio-immunoblastic lymphadenopathy is another manifestation of the adverse effects of phenytoin on the hematologic system.

Pulmonary Granulomas

Pulmonary granulomas are aggregations of pulmonary macrophages reacting to certain microorganisms, foreign particles, various drugs such as methotrexate and nitrofurantoin, or other stimuli not as yet defined. A fairly common form of granulomatous reaction is seen following chronic aspiration of mineral oils. These "paraffinomas" are usually seen as chronic bibasilar, often conglomerate, masses (Figs. 10–10 and 10–11). Pulmonary granulomas may develop as a reaction to particulate suspending agents in intravenously administered oral drugs. Talc is the most commonly used filler for many drugs and, because it is a silicate, it produces a granulomatous reaction.[40] A granulomatous angiitis may result in pulmonary hypertension.[39] Alternatively a disseminated granulomatosis may be produced which may become radiographically visible as a diffuse interstitial pulmonary infiltration. More unusually, large conglomerate masses similar to the progressive massive fibrosis of classic silicosis may develop in the upper lung zones.[9]

Mediastinal Lipomatosis

Corticosteroids may cause excessive fat deposition in the mediastinum, a finding rather grandiosely termed mediastinal lipomatosis. Widening of the mediastinum may be noted radiographically and may cause concern, particularly in patients being

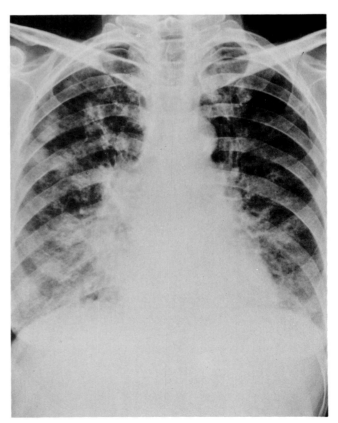

FIG 10–10.
Chronic lipoid pneumonia in an elderly woman with a hiatal hernia and chronic constipation. The patient had used mineral oils for many years and also had esophageal reflux.

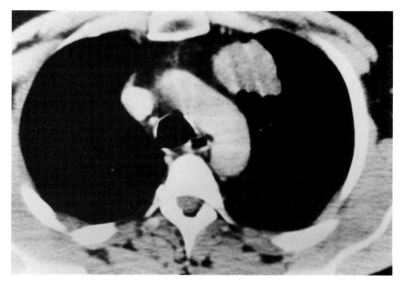

FIG 10–11.
CT scan of a patient with focal lipoid pneumonia. The mass so closely resembled a pulmonary neoplasm that it was resected.

treated for malignant processes. Additional evidence of fat deposition may be seen as extrapleural fat thickening along the lateral chest walls or as increasingly prominent cardiac fat pads (Fig 10–12). CT scanning will readily determine the nature of the process but should scarcely be necessary in practice.

SPECIFIC DRUGS AND THEIR ADVERSE EFFECTS

Certain drugs will be discussed in greater detail here either because their adverse effects are relatively common or serious or because the adverse effects have noteworthy features.

Bleomycin

The cytotoxic antibiotic bleomycin is used in the treatment of squamous cell carcinoma, lymphoma, and testicular neoplasms. This drug is concentrated in the lung which is, therefore, a primary target for adverse effects. Toxicity is related to the cumulative dose and significantly increases when doses exceed a total of 400 mg. The frequency and severity of pulmonary toxicity increases with patient age, prior or concomitant radiation therapy, oxygen therapy, decreased renal function, or other chemotherapy.

An acute hypersensitivity reaction to low doses of bleomycin occurs. However, diffuse alveolar damage is the most common and most significant toxic pulmonary reaction. Bleomycin toxicity ordinarily

becomes manifest within 1 to 3 months after therapy is begun. The chest radiograph is not a sensitive indicator of the toxicity and may be normal in appearance in spite of decreased diffusing capacity, abnormal lung accumulation of gallium 67, increased CT attenuation by the lung, and abnormal pulmonary lavage or biopsy findings.[3, 38] The initial radiographic changes are predominantly basal and reticulonodular in character (see Figs 10–1 and 10–2). Progression may result in conglomerate acinar shadowing. On occasion discrete pulmonary nodules simulating metastases may be seen.[16] The acute hypersensitivity reaction causes a relatively rapid appearance of patchy acinar shadowing with a random distribution, changes which resolve rapidly when therapy is discontinued. Diffuse alveolar damage may, on the other hand, be progressive and lead to irreversible pulmonary fibrosis. The earlier that toxic effects can be detected the greater the likelihood of a favorable response to discontinuation of the drug. Hence strict surveillance of patients under treatment with bleomycin is imperative. This warning, however, applies to all patients undergoing chemotherapy, the incidence of adverse reactions being relatively high with these potent drugs.

Busulfan

Busulfan is used in the treatment of chronic myelogenous leukemia and was one of the earliest chemotherapeutic agents to be used.[13] The reported in-

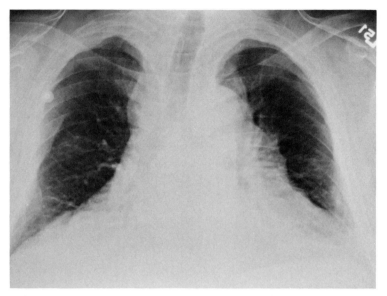

FIG 10–12.
Mediastinal lipomatosis in a patient on long-term steroid therapy. Note the extrapleural fat deposits along the lateral chest wall.

cidence of toxic pulmonary changes with this drug ranges from 2% to 10%. Evidence of pulmonary toxicity may be detected within months of starting treatment, but in some patients several years may elapse before toxic changes become manifest. This variability makes it uncertain as to whether there is a true dose relationship. The pulmonary changes are those of interstitial and intra-alveolar fibrosis, with predominantly a reticular pattern seen on the chest radiograph.

Methotrexate

Methotrexate is used extensively in the treatment of hematologic and other malignancies and is also used to treat a number of benign conditions such as psoriasis. Pulmonary toxicity occurs in some 7% of cases according to the most reliable estimate available.[43]

Methotrexate toxicity differs in certain respects from the toxicity induced by other cytotoxic drugs. The condition under treatment with methotrexate appears to play a role in determining whether toxic reactions occur. For example, patients with acute lymphocytic leukemia have a relatively high incidence of toxic reactions compared with patients with trophoblastic tumors or osteogenic sarcomas.[18] Methotrexate is also unusual in that a hypersensitivity response accompanied by pulmonary infiltrates and peripheral eosinophilia is fairly frequent. Hilar

and mediastinal adenopathy may also occur as part of the hypersensitivity reaction, a unique feature among the cytotoxic drugs. Pleural effusions may occur and may be associated with the development of acute pleuritis.[46] Intrathecal administration of methotrexate has been associated with the development of pulmonary edema.[4]

Despite these atypical effects, diffuse alveolar damage leading to restrictive lung disease remains the significant complication. It has been estimated that fibrosis occurs in approximately 10% of cases of methotrexate-induced pulmonary toxicity.

The prognosis in these patients is generally favorable, with an overall mortality of approximately 1%. Corticosteroids may help in cases of hypersensitivity lung disease. In some cases pulmonary complications may resolve in spite of continued use of the drug, and in other cases rechallenge may not cause a recurrence of toxic manifestations.

Nitrofurantoin

Nitrofurantoin is an antiseptic agent that has been widely used in the treatment of urinary tract infections. Over 80% of cases of nitrofurantoin-induced pulmonary toxicity have been reported in women, probably in large part because of their higher incidence of urinary tract infection.[22] The incidence of adverse reactions is probably not high; the large number of reported cases is more a reflection of the extensive use of the drug in the past.

The pulmonary reaction to nitrofurantoin may be divided into two distinct patterns: an acute form and a chronic form. The acute form is by far the most common reaction, constituting some 90% of all reactions.[22] This is an acute hypersensitivity reaction (a lupus reaction occurs, but is rare). These patients present within 1 month of beginning nitrofurantoin therapy and, if previously sensitized, may present within 24 hours. Symptoms include fever, chest pain, dyspnea, nonproductive cough, arthralgias, and rashes. Peripheral eosinophilia is frequent. The chest radiographs show basally predominant diffuse infiltrates which are interstitial or mixed interstitial/alveolar in character. Pleural effusions are fairly frequent and are usually small. Particularly in hyperacute presentations the pattern resembles cardiogenic edema, especially in the rapidity of its appearance (see Fig 10–5). Response to withdrawal of the drug is prompt and almost invariably complete.

The chronic form of reaction only develops after some 6 months of nitrofurantoin therapy (Fig 10–13). In many instances the patient has had several years of therapy before manifesting pulmonary toxicity. The pulmonary reaction, a fibrosing alveolitis, is reflected on the chest radiograph as a chronic basally predominant interstitial pattern accompanied over time by reduction in lung volume. Improvement usually follows discontinuation of nitrofurantoin therapy, an important diagnostic feature. Depending on the duration and severity of the changes resolution may not be complete, and approximately 10% of cases may have a fatal outcome.[22]

Salicylates

Salicylates probably exert their adverse effects by inhibiting prostaglandin synthesis. In certain patients this leads to bronchospasm. The other principal effect is an alteration in capillary permeability of the lungs, a process leading to noncardiogenic pulmonary edema (Fig 10–14). Salicylate-induced pulmonary edema generally occurs only with blood levels greater than 30 mg/dl and may be related to acute or chronic intoxication.[20] Increasing age and smoking are risk factors. Neurologic disturbances and proteinuria are frequent associated features and possibly indicate alterations in capillary permeability elsewhere. The radiographic features of salicylate-induced pulmonary edema are indistinguishable from those of cardiogenic edema.

Mineral Oil Aspiration

Mineral oils or vegetable oils used as laxatives or lubricants may be chronically aspirated, particularly by elderly patients with swallowing disorders or hiatal hernias. The result is a granulomatous infiltra-

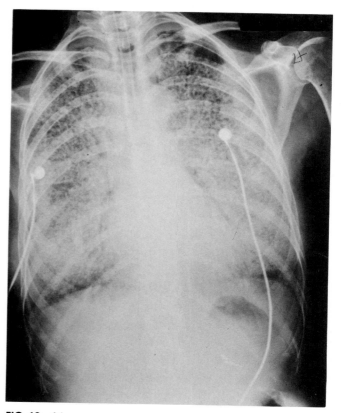

FIG 10–14.
Pulmonary edema in a chronic aspirin abuser. The blood salicylate level exceeded 40 mg/dl.

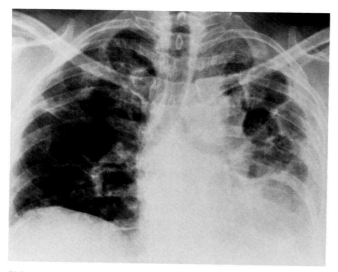

FIG 10–13.
Chronic nitrofurantoin toxicity. There are very coarse linear infiltrates with some reduction in lung volume.

tion of the lung associated with fibrosis. These infiltrates tend to be basal and may be localized or more generalized (see Figs 10–11 and 10–12). In the early stages the infiltrates have the character of alveolar consolidation and may become much more confluent and masslike with the ensuing fibrosis. The changes may be extensive, and the resultant contraction of the lungs severe. An isolated area of chronic lipoid pneumonia is easily mistaken for a primary pulmonary neoplasm (see Fig 10–12). The diagnosis can be difficult because many patients fail to volunteer information about their use of these substances. Too often they regard long-term use of mineral oils as something normal and inconsequential. The diagnosis has been established both by CT examination and percutaneous needle aspiration.[48] With CT the areas of lipoid pneumonia may have a low attenuation, comparable with fat.

Gold Salts

Gold salts used in the treatment of rheumatoid arthritis probably cause pulmonary toxicity in fewer than 1% of patients,[8] although much higher incidences have been quoted. Pulmonary toxicity is overshadowed by the far more frequent complications of stomatitis and dermatitis. Pulmonary toxicity occurs within 3 months of beginning of therapy and is usually gradual in its onset. The most common reaction is a hypersensitivity reaction with a variable combination of diffuse reticulonodular and patchy alveolar densities.[47] Patients may well have evidence of a hypersensitivity response in other systems, for example, fever, proteinuria, or a skin rash. Such manifestations of hypersensitivity may precede the pulmonary abnormalities and be associated with peripheral eosinophilia. Diffuse alveolar damage with fibrosis is also noted on occasion. A lupus reaction is exceptionally uncommon. The major diagnostic problem is that the disease under treatment, rheumatoid arthritis, can itself be associated with diffuse interstitial disease. The shadowing associated with gold-induced toxic reactions can, however, be expected to resolve in most instances on cessation of therapy.

Methysergide

Methysergide is interesting because it may be associated with a syndrome consisting of chronic pleural effusions accompanied by irregular pleural thickening.[14] Rounded atelectasis may also be associated. The syndrome becomes manifest 6 months to several years after therapy begins. Depending on the extent of the fibrosis, a variable degree of regression occurs after cessation of therapy.

Oxygen

Oxygen has significant toxic effects on the lungs, particularly when administered in very high concentrations.[24] It is estimated that 100% inspired oxygen will cause damage within 24 to 48 hours; lesser concentrations, a proportionally longer time. Patients receiving high levels of oxygen for extended periods will almost invariably have significant pulmonary abnormalities from other causes, and it may be difficult or indeed impossible to determine how much additional change one can reasonably attribute to the oxygen therapy.

Oxygen toxicity differs somewhat in the mature and the immature lung. In the mature lung the most significant damage occurs at the alveolar level—with endothelial cell and type I pneumocyte damage, fibrinous exudates with hyaline membranes, and proliferation of type II pneumocytes. This is the classic picture of diffuse alveolar damage, and its onset is rapid. As with diffuse alveolar damage from any cause, pulmonary fibrosis may ensue. Other effects of oxygen include damage to the terminal airways and inhibition of phagocytosis, the result being a predisposition to infection.

The immature lung—in practice, the infant lung—may show a more defined response clinically and radiographically. This is the condition of bronchopulmonary dysplasia (BPD), a fairly common sequel to the treatment of hyaline membrane disease (respiratory distress syndrome). Oxygen therapy plays, of course, a major role in the treatment of these infants. The damage is more apparent in the terminal airways, with epithelial cell necrosis and squamous metaplasia. Damage to the alveoli is less obvious but may in the long run prove more significant because further lung growth and pulmonary vascular development may be seriously affected.

Premature infants with birth weights under 2,000 gm have a high risk of developing hyaline membrane disease and also have a high risk of subsequent BPD. The evolution of BPD may not be fully appreciated in the early stages because of the preexisting pulmonary disease. Many of the features of BPD such as hyperexpansion of the lungs, pulmonary interstitial emphysema, atelectasis, and pneumonias also occur in other diffuse pulmonary diseases involving these infants. The development of progressively coarse reticular infiltration of the lung, irregular cystlike spaces, coarse stranding, and pulmonary hyperexpansion points to BPD (Fig 10–15, A–C). The changes become increasingly "fixed": in other words, the basic radiographic pattern does not show any significant day-to-day variation other than changes related to varying radiographic technique or incidental complications such as atelectasis or barotrauma. The long-term prognosis for survivors is uncertain. Severe cases of BPD are usually fatal but, at the other end of the spectrum, it is possible that mild cases may be clinically and radiographically undetectable.

Talc

The illicit intravenous injection of crushed tablets carries the risk of talc granulomatosis in the lungs. Granulomatous vasculitis may be associated with the development of pulmonary hypertension. The radiographic features vary from a normal lung, through diffuse interstitial shadowing, to the occasional development of conglomerate upper zone mass densities.[9, 39, 41] Signs of coexistent pulmonary hypertension may be present. Biopsy will show giant cell granulomas containing birefringent talc crystals together with a granulomatous arteritis.[40]

Nitrosoureas

Nitrosourea compounds (such as carmustine and lomustine) are used in the treatment of gliomas, lymphomas, and multiple myeloma. There is a significant incidence of diffuse alveolar damage with

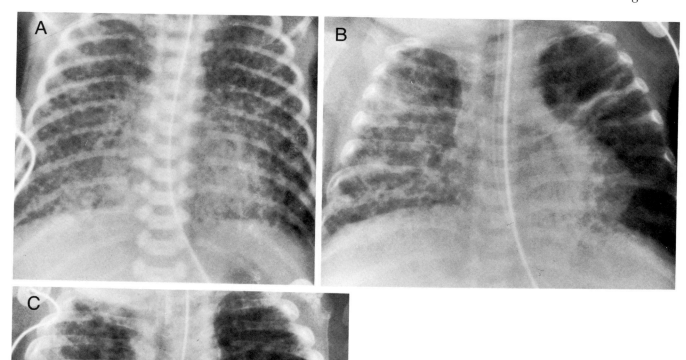

FIG 10–15.
Bronchopulmonary dysplasia in an infant treated for hyaline membrane disease: at 10 days **(A);** at 3 months **(B);** at 7 months **(C).**

nitrosourea therapy, particularly when large doses are administered. The incidence may be as high as 20% to 30% with prolonged aggressive treatment.[1] The pulmonary changes are comparable to those found in cases of diffuse alveolar damage caused by other cytotoxic drugs. The only differences are that the chest radiograph is more likely to remain normal in appearance despite other evidence of pulmonary toxic effects, and that there is an unexplained high incidence of pneumothorax in these patients.

Opiates

Overdoses of heroin, methadone, and propoxyphene are notoriously associated with pulmonary edema. As many as one-third of individuals exhibiting signs of opiate overdose develop pulmonary edema.[42] The mechanism of pulmonary injury has not been elucidated; possible mechanisms include direct effects on the central nervous system—leading to neurogenic edema, hypoxemic or direct drug toxic effects on the alveolar-capillary membrane, allergic responses, and immunologic activation. The radiographic findings are the same as those seen with interstitial or alveolar edema from any other cause (see Fig 10–6).

Penicillamine

Penicillamine is used to treat lead poisoning, Wilson's disease, cystinuria, and, on occasion, connective tissue disorders such as rheumatoid arthritis. Penicillamine is not, however, a commonly used drug, and pulmonary toxic effects are rare. This drug is a recognized cause of diffuse alveolar damage. The primary reason for singling this drug out for special mention is that it may cause a hemorrhagic pneumonitis with acute glomerulonephritis that is clinically and radiographically indistinguishable from Goodpasture's syndrome.[45] In these cases the onset is acute, with the development of widespread patchy alveolar densities in the lungs. Renal dysfunction develops synchronously. Penicillamine may, in rare cases, also cause an obliterative bronchiolitis.[35] The chest radiograph is usually normal in these cases of bronchiolitis.

Amiodarone

The antidysrhythmic drug amiodarone is invaluable in the treatment of refractory cardiac rhythm disturbances. However, amiodarone therapy has a relatively high incidence of pulmonary toxicity—es-

timated to be in the order of 5%.[51] Amiodarone is concentrated in the lung and has a relatively long tissue half-life. This fact accounts for the slow appearance of pulmonary toxic effects (median interval, 6 months) and the slow clearing following cessation of therapy (median interval, 3 months).[15] The mechanisms by which amiodarone exerts its toxic effects have already been discussed (see p 443).

The most common presenting symptom is dyspnea, and patients occasionally have pleuritic chest pain. The most common radiographic appearance is multiple peripheral areas of consolidation resembling those seen in patients with the hypersensitivity reaction (Figs 10–16 and 10–17). There is, however, no evidence of eosinophilia in either the blood or the tissues. The other notable radiographic manifestation is the development of diffuse interstitial shadowing leading to evidence of pulmonary fibrosis (Fig 10–18). Patchy alveolar consolidation frequently coexists with these interstitial changes. The signs resemble those seen in drug-induced diffuse lung damage, for example, with bleomycin or nitrofurantoin. Amiodarone may also, on occasion, cause pleural effusions. Patients being treated with amiodarone have significant cardiac disease, and it may be difficult to distinguish the changes of amiodarone toxicity from changes secondary to congestive cardiac failure. Lack of response to treatment of heart failure and the lack of short-term fluctuations of the pulmonary abnormalities point toward amio-

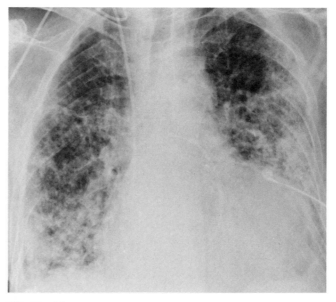

FIG 10–16.
Amiodarone toxicity. There are patchy alveolar infiltrates with a peripheral and basal distribution.

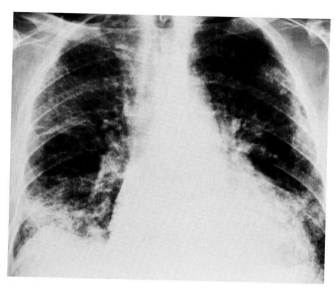

FIG 10–17.
Amiodarone toxicity showing widespread peripheral and basal organized pulmonary infiltrates.

darone toxicity. Stringent control of patients on amiodarone therapy is essential and should include routine follow-up chest radiographs. Any pulmonary toxicity should thereby be detected and reversed by cessation of the drug before fibrosis develops. There are indications that gallium scintigraphy is more sensitive than plain radiography in the diagnosis of amiodarone pulmonary toxicity[33] (Fig 10–19). Amiodarone contains 37% iodine by weight, and there is a

single case report of a patient showing high CT density in the amiodarone-induced infiltrates.[26] Amiodarone pulmonary toxicity is unusual in that it has a specific histologic feature—namely, the accumulation of macrophages with a characteristic foamy cytoplasm in the alveolar spaces.

THE EFFECTS OF RADIATION ON THE LUNG

Radiation therapy is widely used in the treatment of thoracic malignancies and lymphoma of the mediastinum. Normal tissues are inevitably included in the radiation field and subjected to damage to a greater or lesser extent. Radiation effects on the lung are commonly seen on chest radiographs, and abnormalities may also be noted in other structures such as the thoracic skeleton, the pleura, or the heart.

The severity and extent of damage to normal lung tissue depend on a number of factors.[28]

1. The volume of normal lung irradiated is related to field size. Lung damage does not occur outside the field of irradiation, which is purposely kept as small as adequate therapy permits. On average, only one-quarter to one-third of a lung is included in the field; on occasion, however, very large tumors may necessitate irradiation of much larger lung volumes. One should realize that administration of

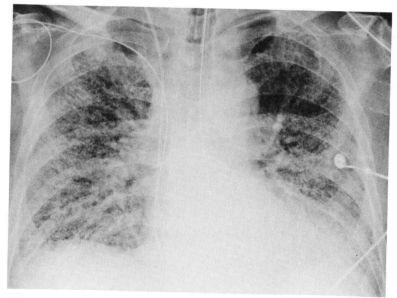

FIG 10–18.
Amiodarone toxicity (biopsy proved). Diffuse mixed interstitial-alveolar infiltrates are in the lungs. The pulmonary wedge pressure was within normal limits.

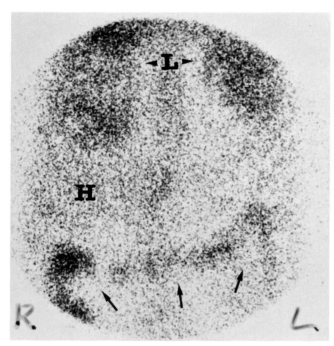

FIG 10–19.
Gallium scan in the patient in Figure 10–18 shows markedly increased uptake in the lungs *(L)* relative to the liver *(H)*. *Arrows* point to colon. *R* = patient's right; *L* = left.

3,000 rads to all of both lungs will kill most individuals, whereas the same or even higher doses administered to a portion of one lung may not even produce symptoms in many cases.

2. The total dose and the fractionation of that dose are of critical importance. The effect of a single large dose is more severe than the effect of the same dose divided into a series of fractions given over 2 to 3 weeks. There is, of course, no threshold at which deleterious effects become manifest; they do, however, become more apparent and inevitable with increasing total doses. With modern radiation therapy, there are no significant differences in the effects of radiation from different sources: for example, from cobalt sources as opposed to linear accelerators.

3. Individual susceptibility to radiation is variable and, at the same time, inexplicable and unpredictable. One patient may develop clinical or radiographic evidence of radiation pneumonitis, whereas another patient receiving comparable treatment may not. The preexisting state of the lungs may also play a role in determining the full clinical effects of radiation. For example, a patient with severe chronic obstructive pulmonary disease and very poor respiratory reserve may be severely affected by even a localized radiation pneumonitis resulting from this supposedly tolerable form of treatment.

4. Previous or concomitant therapy may influence the timing and the severity of the radiation changes. A second course of radiation therapy will produce more severe and earlier changes than the first. Certain cytotoxic agents such as bleomycin heighten the effects of radiation.[27] Other agents, such as actinomycin D and adriamycin that do not in themselves cause pulmonary toxicity accentuate the effects of radiation by a form of synergism.[6] Steroids dampen the effects of irradiation as they do in other inflammatory processes.[37]

Pathology

A knowledge of the underlying pathologic changes is useful in understanding the radiographic manifestations. A series of phases are recognized pathologically, and these have clinical and radiographic counterparts.[34] In the initial 24 to 48 hours there is degeneration of the lymph follicles, the bronchial mucosa becomes hyperemic and edematous, and there is some leukocyte infiltration in the bronchial wall. Ordinarily, these changes are undetectable clinically or radiographically. In rare cases a central tumor may have narrowed the bronchial lumen so critically that the mucosal swelling and reaction may produce clinically and radiographically detectable effects. This reaction subsides, and a latent phase ensues. The phase of acute radiation pneumonitis develops some 1 to 6 months after the therapy. Histologically there is thickening of the alveolar septa by edema and round cell infiltration, hyperplasia and desquamation of the alveolar lining cells, fibrinous alveolar exudation leading to hyaline membrane formation, endothelial cell damage with engorgement and thrombus formation, and evidence of arteritis. Depending on the severity of reaction there is a variable degree of interstitial and alveolar fibrosis. There is a simultaneous reaction in the bronchial mucosa with hyperemia and edema and cessation of mucus gland and ciliary function. These changes peak and merge into a regenerative phase in which the exudates and edema disperse, the alveolar lining cells regenerate, and the capillary endothelial cells become normal. The fibrous changes, however, progress, consolidate, and contract over the following weeks and months. In addition there may be progressive sclerosis of the pulmonary vascular bed and bronchial structural damage. The latter changes may lead to bronchiectasis and altered perfusion of the affected portions of the lung.

Clinical Features

If the patient has any symptoms at all related to pulmonary irradiation these occur during the phase of acute radiation pneumonitis or develop much later as a consequence of fibrosis and lung contraction. The severity of symptoms depends on the extent and severity of the postirradiation changes and also, to a certain extent, on the presence of underlying lung disease. The usual symptoms in the acute phase are dyspnea, cough, production of tenacious sputum and, possibly, some fever and night sweats. These symptoms may persist for several weeks.

In the fibrotic phase the patient is usually asymptomatic. However, if the fibrosis is severe and extensive the patient may be completely disabled. Cough, hemoptysis, dyspnea, orthopnea, clubbing of the fingers, and recurrent infections are all features of such cases.

Radiographic Findings

The single most important observation is that the changes of radiation damage to the lung are con-fined to the field of irradiation. This means that the margins of the abnormal areas in the lung are geometric and correspond to the radiation ports (Fig 10–20). Normal anatomic boundaries such as fissures are crossed with seeming impunity. On frontal radiographs of the chest the involved areas may be clearly delineated, leading one to expect similarly well defined changes on the lateral radiograph. Often the most one can appreciate is that the changes extend fairly uniformly across the chest in the sagittal plane. To observers accustomed to using the lateral radiograph for segmental or lobar localization, this seeming disregard for anatomic boundaries can be quite striking.

The first changes are a diffuse haze in the irradiated region with obscuring of the vascular outlines. Patchy consolidations appear and these areas may coalesce into a nonanatomic, but geometric, area of pulmonary density (Fig 10–21).

The regenerative, fibrotic phase develops almost imperceptibly from the phase of acute pneumonitis. With the passage of time, one may observe that the infiltrates become more linear or reticular or, in other words, "more structured." Fibrous contraction will condense the infiltrates and also distort adjacent structures such as the hilar vessels (Fig 10–22). The fibrosis is often not severe, and the changes can easily be overlooked or attributed to granulomatous scarring. The experienced eye can,

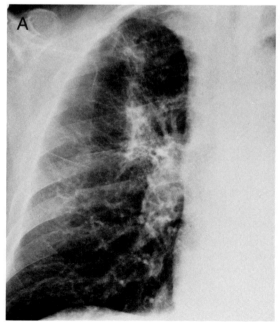
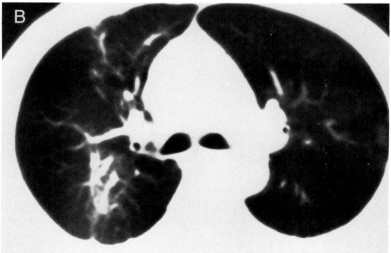

FIG 10–20.
Radiation changes resulting from irradiation of a bronchogenic carcinoma. **A,** note the straight lateral margin to the infiltration in the right upper lobe. **B,** the corresponding CT scan shows that the infiltration extends sagittally across the chest with the same straight lateral margin.

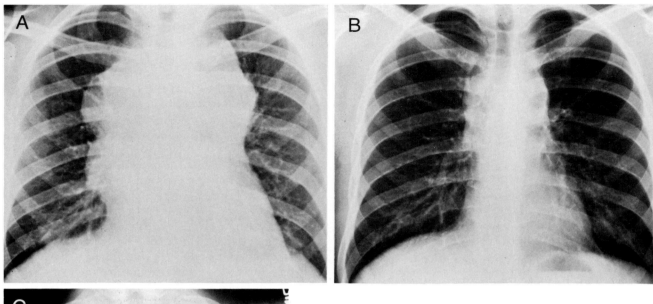

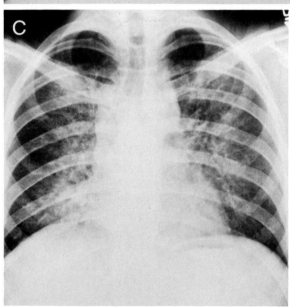

FIG 10–21.
A, radiograph of lymphoma causing massive mediastinal adenopathy. **B,** at 2 weeks there is considerable resolution of the adenopathy following irradiation. **C,** at 10 weeks there is radiation pneumonitis in the necessarily wide field of irradiation.

however, for example, almost instinctively pick up the slight paramediastinal change that may be seen after mediastinal irradiation of patients with lymphoma.

The earliest radiographic changes appear some 6 to 8 weeks after the beginning of therapy, and the peak reaction occurs usually at 3 to 4 months. The ensuing fibrosis and contraction continue over a 12- to 18-month period and then become quiescent. Bronchiectasis may be present within the regions of fibrosis, but this change is usually undetectable on plain films. However, radiation damage to the lung may on occasion be severe, and it is particularly in this type of case that bronchiectasis may be apparent

(Fig 10–23). Fortunately such damage is now rare with modern radiation therapy.

The CT findings following radiation therapy clearly reflect the described pathologic changes.[29] In the phase of acute radiation pneumonitis, patchy and increasingly confluent areas of increased attenuation appear in the irradiated field. The geographic distribution of the changes may be quite striking. Transition to the phase of regeneration and fibrosis is gradual.

Fibrous stranding that merges smoothly with the pleura becomes apparent, and contraction can be appreciated by the distortion of adjacent structures. Bronchiectasis within the contracted portion of lung may be readily apparent on CT scans. CT is more sensitive than plain radiography in the detection of postirradiation changes in the lungs, particularly in peripheral tangential radiation fields.[2] CT scanning may also indicate shrinkage of vessels in lung peripheral to a central field of irradiation. This presumably is a reflection of diminished perfusion resulting from radiation-induced vascular sclerosis. Bell et al.,[2] using scintigraphy, were able to demonstrate significant perfusion abnormalities in lung beyond the field of irradiation. In general, these changes outside the radiation field could not be detected on plain chest radiographs.

Less common manifestations of radiation damage are hyperlucency of a lung,[10] pleural effusions, and spontaneous pneumothorax.[5] Pulmonary hyperlucency presumably results from diminished pulmonary perfusion. Pleural effusions secondary to irradiation are usually coincident with the phase of acute radiation pneumonitis. Calcification in lymphomatous masses or lymph nodes may develop in the years following radiation therapy.[52] In the hilar regions the calcified nodes tend to have an "eggshell" pattern, for which the differential diagnosis includes sarcoidosis, silicosis, amyloidosis, and fungal diseases. In rare cases a second primary tumor such as an osteogenic sarcoma or a bronchial carcinoma

may arise in the field of irradiation and may well be induced by radiation.[21, 23]

The Differential Diagnosis of Radiation Pneumonitis

The two major differential diagnoses to be considered in patients with radiation pneumonitis are infections and tumor recurrence. An infective pneumonitis is not usually confined by the radiation therapy ports and normally runs a less indolent course than radiation pneumonitis. Nevertheless, an area of radiation damage may become secondarily infected and, if it does, the diagnosis cannot be established by radiographic means. Tumor recurrence may be difficult to discern at the height of the postirradiation change, but as these changes stabilize and contraction develops, a focal enlargement should become increasingly apparent. A primary bronchial carcinoma may develop a lymphangitic pattern of spread initially confined to one lung or even one lobe. Lymphangitis carcinomatosa may initially cause diagnostic problems, but the inexorable worsening with the development of septal lines, effusions, and spread to the opposite lung will soon make the situation clear.

CT scanning and magnetic resonance imaging (MRI) have been investigated as means of detecting tumor recurrence. CT, by enabling the detection of

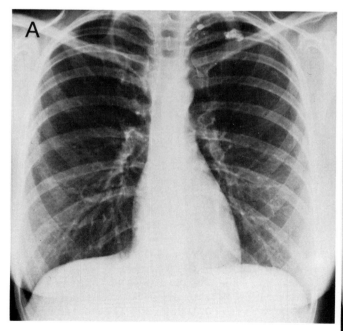

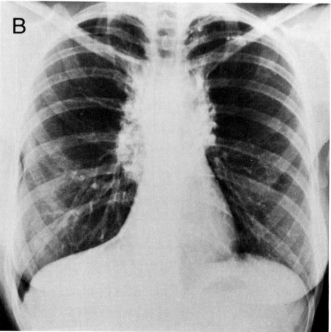

FIG 10–22.
Radiographs taken before **(A)** and approximately 4 months after **(B)** mantle radiation therapy for Hodgkin's disease. Dense geo- metric infiltrates with evidence of fibrous contraction have developed in the radiation portals.

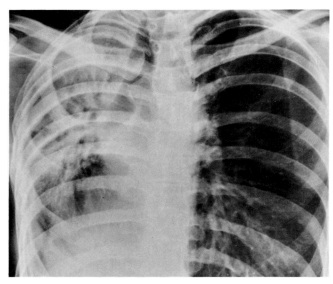

FIG 10–23.
Severe radiation damage to the lungs in a 32-year-old woman who had undergone radiation therapy several years previously for lymphoma.

focal masses or cavitation, may provide some evidence of recurrence. MRI is theoretically capable of tissue differentiation but, at present, the practical results of MRI in postirradiation cases are inconclusive. Radiation fibrosis has low signal intensity on both T1- and T2-weighted sequences.[17] Tumors, on the other hand, have high signal intensity on T2-weighted sequences and can, therefore, be distinguished from pure fibrosis. However, acute radiation pneumonitis, secondary infective pneumonitis, or hemorrhage may have signal intensities similar to tumor and therefore may be confused with recurrent disease.

Radiation Effects on Other Thoracic Structures

One should be aware of the fact that radiation may damage other thoracic structures producing either radiographically visible manifestations or indirect effects on the lungs. Radiation-induced abnormalities in the bony thorax are most commonly seen after therapy for carcinoma of the breast. The bones appear atrophic and osteoporotic, fractures are frequent and may fail to unite, and dystrophic calcifications may be seen in the adjacent soft tissues. Radiation damage to the heart and the pericardium may cause enlargement of the cardiac silhouette and signs of pulmonary vascular congestion and edema. Pericardial effusion is the most common manifestation of radiation damage, but myocardial fibrosis

and coronary artery damage may occur. Radiation damage to the esophagus may cause dysmotility, stricture formation, or fistula development. Any related pulmonary changes are, therefore, likely to be related to chronic aspiration.

REFERENCES

1. Aronin PA, Mahaley MS, Rudnick SA: Prediction of BCNU pulmonary toxicity in patients with malignant gliomas. *N Engl J Med* 1980; 303:183–188.
2. Bell J, McGivern D, Bullimore J, et al: Diagnostic imaging of the post-irradiation changes in the chest. *Clin Radiol* 1988; 39:109–119.
3. Bellamy EA, Husband JE, Blaquiere RM, et al: Bleomycin related lung damage: CT evidence. *Radiology* 1985; 157:155–158.
4. Bernstein ML, Sobel DB, Wimmer RS: Non-cardiogenic pulmonary edema following injection of methotrexate into the cerebro-spinal fluid. *Cancer* 1982; 50:866–868.
5. Blane CE, Silberstein RJ, Sue JY: Radiation therapy and spontaneous pneumothorax. *J Can Assoc Radiol* 1981; 32:153–154.
6. Cassaday JR, Richter MP, Piro AJ, et al: Radiation-adriamycin interactions: Preliminary clinical observations. *Cancer* 1974; 36:946–949.
7. Cooper JAD, White DA, Matthay RA: Drug induced pulmonary diseases: Part 1. Cytotoxic drugs. *Am Rev Respir Dis* 1986; 133:321–340.
8. Cooper JAD, White DA, Matthay RA: Drug-induced pulmonary disease: Part 2: Non-cytotoxic drugs. *Am Rev Respir Dis* 1986; 133:488–505.
9. Crouch E, Chart A: Progressive massive fibrosis of the lung secondary to intravenous injection of talc. A pathologic and mineralogic analysis. *Am J Clin Pathol* 1983; 80:520–526.
10. Farmer W, Ravin C, Schachter EN: Hyperlucent lung after radiation therapy. *Am Rev Respir Dis* 1975; 112:255–258.
11. Follath F, Burkart F, Schweizer W: Drug induced pulmonary hypertension? *Br Med J* 1971; 1:265–266.
12. Frand UI, Shim CS, Williams MK: Methadone induced pulmonary edema. *Intern Med* 1972; 76:975–979.
13. Galton DAG: Myleran in chronic myeloid leukemia. *Lancet* 1953; 1:208–213.
14. Gefter WB, Epstein DM, Bonavita JA, et al: Pleural thickening caused by Sansert and Ergotrate in the treatment of migraine. *AJR* 1980; 135:375–377.
15. Gefter WB, Epstein DM, Pietra GG, et al: Lung disease caused by amiodarone, a new antiarrhythmic agent. *Radiology* 1983; 147:339–344.
16. Glasier CM, Siegel MJ: Multiple pulmonary nodules: Unusual manifestation of Bleomycin toxicity. *AJR* 1981; 137:155–156.

17. Glazer HS, Lee JKT, Levitt RG, et al: Radiation fibrosis: Differentiation from recurrent tumor by MR imaging: Work in progress. *Radiology* 1985; 156:721–726.

18. Gockerman JP: Drug-induced interstitial lung diseases. *Clin Chest Med* 1982; 3:521–536.

19. Heath MF, Costa-Jussa FR, Jacobs JM, et al: The induction of pulmonary phospholipidosis and the inhibition of lysosomal phospholipases by amiodarone. *Br J Exp Pathol* 1985; 66:391–397.

20. Heffner JE, Sahn SA: Salicylate induced pulmonary edema: Clinical features and prognosis. *Ann Intern Med* 1981; 95:405–409.

21. Hill CA, North LB, Osborne BM: Bronchogenic carcinoma in breast carcinoma patients. *AJR* 1983; 140:259–264.

22. Holmberg L, Boman G: Pulmonary reactions to nitrofurantoin: 447 cases reported to the Swedish Adverse Drug Reaction Committee 1966–1976. *Eur J Respir Dis* 1981; 62:180–189.

23. Huvos AG, Woodward HQ, Cahan WB, et al: Post irradiation osteogenic sarcoma of bone and soft tissue. A clinico-pathologic study in 66 patients. *Cancer* 1985; 55:1244–1255.

24. Jackson RM: Pulmonary oxygen toxicity, review. *Chest* 1985; 86:900–905.

25. Kennedy JI, Myers JL, Plumb VJ, et al: Amiodarone pulmonary toxicity. Clinical radiologic and pathologic correlations. *Arch Intern Med* 1987; 147:50–55.

26. Kuhlman JE, Scatarige JC, Fishman EK, et al: CT demonstration of high attenuation pleural-parenchymal lesions due to amiodarone therapy. *J Comput Assist Tomogr* 1987; 11:160–162.

27. Lamoureux K: Increased clinically symptomatic pulmonary radiation reactions with adjuvant chemotherapy: Part 1. *Cancer Chemother Res* 1975; 35:1322–1324.

28. Libshitz HI: Thoracic radiotherapy changes, in Herman PG (ed): *Iatrogenic Thoracic Complications.* New York, Springer-Verlag, 1983; pp 141–160.

29. Libshitz HI, Shuman LS: Radiation-induced pulmonary change: CT findings. *J Comput Assist Tomogr* 1984; 8:15–19.

30. Louie S, Gamble CN, Cross CE: Penicillamine associated pulmonary hemorrhage. *J Rheumatol* 1986; 135:963–966.

31. MacDonald JS: Lymphography, in Ansell G (ed): *Complications in Diagnostic Radiology.* Oxford, Blackwell, 1976, pp 301–316.

32. MacLennan FM, Thomson MAR, Rankin R, et al: Fatal pulmonary oedema associated with the use of Ritodrine in pregnancy. Case report. *Br J Obstet Gynecol* 1985; 92:703–705.

33. Moinuddin M, Rockett J: Gallium scintigraphy in the detection of amiodarone lung toxicity. *AJR* 1986; 147:607–609.

34. Moss WT, Brand WN, Battifora H: *Radiation Oncology: Rationale, Technique, Results,* ed 5. St Louis, CV Mosby Co, 1979, pp 253–288.

35. Murphy KC, Atkins CJ, Offer RC, et al: Obliterative bronchiolitis in two rheumatoid arthritis patients treated with penicillamine. *Arthritis Rheum* 1981; 24:557–560.

36. Oakley C, Somerville J: Oral contraceptives and progressive pulmonary vascular disease. *Lancet* 1968; 1:890–893.

37. Parris TM, Knight JG, Hess CE, et al: Severe radiation pneumonitis precipitated by withdrawal of steroids: A diagnostic and therapeutic dilemma. *AJR* 1970; 132:284–286.

38. Richman SD, Levenson SM, Bunn PA, et al: 67 Ga accumulation in pulmonary lesions associated with Bleomycin toxicity. *Cancer* 1975; 36:1966–1972.

39. Robertson CH, Reynolds RC, Wilson JE: Pulmonary hypertension and foreign body granulomatosis in intravenous drug abusers. *Am J Med* 1976; 61:657–664.

40. Schwartz IS, Basken C: Pulmonary vascular talc granulomatosis. *JAMA* 1986; 256:2584.

41. Sieniewicz DJ, Nidecker AC: Conglomerate pulmonary disease: A form of talcosis in intravenous methadone abusers. *AJR* 1980; 135:697–702.

42. Smith WR, Wells ID, Glauser FL, et al: Immunologic abnormalities in heroin lung. *Chest* 1975; 68:651–653.

43. Sostman HD, Matthay RA, Putman CE, et al: Methotrexate-induced pneumonitis. *Medicine* 1976; 55:371–388.

44. Steinberg AD, Karliner JS: The clinical spectrum of heroin pulmonary edema. *Arch Intern Med* 1968; 122:122–127.

45. Sternbieb I, Bennett B, Scheinberg IH: D-penicillamine induced Goodpasture's syndrome in Wilson's disease. *Ann Intern Med* 1975; 82:673–676.

46. Urban C, Nisenberz A, Caparros B, et al: Chemical pleuritis as a cause of acute chest pain following high-dose methotrexate treatment. *Cancer* 1983; 51:34–37.

47. Weaver LT, Law JS: Lung changes after gold salts. *Br J Dis Chest* 1978; 72:247–250.

48. Wheeler S, Stitik FP, Hutchins GM, et al: Diagnosis of lipoid pneumonia by computed tomography. *JAMA* 1981; 245:65–66.

49. Whimster WF, de Poitiers W: The lung, in Riddell RH (ed): *Pathology of Drug Induced and Toxic Diseases.* New York, Churchill Livingstone, 1982, pp 167–200.

50. Winzelberg GG, Wholey MH, Jarmolowski CA, et al: Patients with hemoptysis examined by Tc-99m sulfur colloid and Tc-99m-labelled red blood cells: A preliminary appraisal. *Radiology* 1984; 153:523–526.

51. Wood DL, Osborn MJ, Rooke J, et al: Amiodarone pulmonary toxicity: Report of two cases associated with rapidly progressive fatal adult respiratory distress syndrome after pulmonary angiography. *Mayo Clin Proc* 1985; 60:601–603.

52. Wyman SM, Weber AL: Calcifications in intrathoracic nodes in Hodgkin's disease in the chest. *Radiology* 1969; 93:1021–1024.

Immunologic Diseases of the Lungs

DIFFUSE INTERSTITIAL PULMONARY FIBROSIS

Diffuse interstitial pulmonary fibrosis may follow acute or chronic insults to the lung. This discussion concerns the chronic interstitial pneumonias (CIP) and, in particular, the idiopathic form.

Chronic interstitial pneumonias are diffuse inflammatory processes that mainly affect the lung interstitium: namely, the alveolar septa and the peribronchial and perivascular sheaths. A large variety of chronic interstitial pneumonias are recognized,[131, 215, 223, 351, 381] and the most important are:

1. Cryptogenic fibrosing alveolitis/idiopathic pulmonary fibrosis
2. CIP associated with collagen vascular disorder, especially rheumatoid disease and progressive systemic sclerosis[177]
3. Drug-related CIP, especially following use of cytotoxic agents and nitrofurantoin[250]
4. Postinfective CIP, particularly following viral,[431, 494] mycoplasmal,[353, 604] and chlamydial infections
5. Pneumoconioses, particularly from inhalation of asbestos, talc, beryllium, tungsten carbide, and the organic dusts that cause extrinsic allergic alveolitis, and also CIP from inhalation of noxious gases[483]
6. Radiation pneumonitis
7. Chronic pulmonary edema
8. Miscellaneous conditions including genetic, metabolic, reactive and inflammatory disorders.[138, 582, 660]

Some authors extend this list to include granulomatous processes such as eosinophilic granuloma and sarcoidosis.[297]

Regardless of the context the pathology and pathogenesis are basically similar,[129, 226] beginning with an injury. This injury may be attributed directly or indirectly to a toxic agent or may be mediated by immune complex deposition or recruitment of inflammatory cells. The result is an acute alveolitis that may arrest at any stage or may go on to fibrosis with restructuring/destruction of air-exchange units, airway distortion, and eventual development of an end-stage lung.[241, 306] Therapy is directed at removal of the inciting agents, suppression of the alveolitis, and palliation of complications. Every effort is made to suppress the alveolitis before it leads to irreversible fibrosis, and steroids are the therapeutic sheet anchor. Because it is important to identify the reversible active alveolitis at a stage when only minor fibrosis is present, much effort has been spent in disease "staging." This is achieved by evaluating lung dysfunction and by assessing the activity of the alveolitis—as indicated by the number, type, and activation of inflammatory cells.[130, 131] In making these assessments, use is made of the patient history; clinical signs; chest radiograph; respiratory function tests; and, most reliably, lung biopsy—which should ideally be an open biopsy. In addition, two other tests have been used to assess activity: gallium-67 scintiscanning[130, 131, 386] and bronchoalveolar lavage.[130, 226, 292]

Most of the chronic interstitial pneumonitides are considered as specific entities elsewhere; the discussion here is limited to the idiopathic variety and to end-stage lung.

Cryptogenic Fibrosing Alveolitis/Idiopathic Pulmonary Fibrosis

This condition is a specific disorder characterized by a combination of clinical, physiologic, morphologic, lavage, and scintigraphic features.[130] Its terminology has been the cause of much confusion, and about 20 synonyms now exist.[226] In much of the literature the terms usual interstitial pneumonia and desquamative interstitial pneumonia have been used, though strictly speaking, these are not specific to the idiopathic form. The term Hamman-Rich syndrome has been used to describe the acute, aggressive form of the disease.[282] In the following discussion, the term introduced by Scadding—cryptogenic fibrosing alveolitis—is used.[384, 546]

Cryptogenic fibrosing alveolitis (CFA) is a disorder of unknown cause. A familial factor has been identified in a few patients,[39, 340, 582] and in one study, the occurrence of eight cases in three generations was consistent with an autosomal dominant inheritance.[47] No definite human lymphocyte antigen (HLA) association has been shown.[228, 636] There is, however, a well-established relationship with autoimmune conditions, particularly rheumatoid arthritis and other connective tissue disorders.[177] It might seem a contradiction in terms to classify such cases as cryptogenic, but several major studies of CFA include such patients. The problem centers on deciding which patients to exclude, because some will have an associated, full-blown collagen vascular disorder, whereas many others will manifest only certain features, such as isolated arthropathy or Raynaud's syndrome. Such difficulties have led to terms like "lone CFA." In the Brompton Hospital series of 220 patients, 70% had lone CFA and 30% had an additional polyarthritis or immunologic disorder. Of the latter group, about a third had rheumatoid arthritis and a third some other collagen vascular disease.[632] Recognized associations of CFA, other than collagen vascular disease, include chronic active hepatitis, primary biliary cirrhosis, ulcerative colitis, adult celiac disease, Sjögren's syndrome, Raynaud's phenomenon, thyroid disorders including Hashimoto's thyroiditis, renal tubular acidosis, pernicious anemia and autoimmune hemolytic anemia.[405, 551, 579, 630, 632] An arthropathy that is not part of a recognized connective tissue disorder is fairly common.

Several large series of CFA have been described in detail.[88, 130, 389, 587, 632] The prevalence rate is about three to five patients per hundred thousand population.[129] The patients are typically adults presenting in their 5th or 6th decades, but the disorder has a wide age range and is even described in infants and children.[311] Most series have shown a slight male preponderance.[632] The most common presenting symptoms are progressive exertional dyspnea and cough, which is usually nonproductive but in one series was productive in just over half of the patients.[632] Less common symptoms include nonspecific chest pain[389]; constitutional symptoms such as fever, weight loss, and fatigue[336]; and joint pains. Some patients date the onset to an influenza-like illness.[336] A small proportion of patients present by way of an abnormal "routine radiograph." In one series, 47% of patients presented in this manner, an exceptionally high frequency for this form of presentation.[676] Late, fine inspiratory crackles at the lung bases are an almost universal finding,[632] and two-thirds to three-fourths of the patients show clubbing of the fingers.[389, 550, 632, 676] Occasionally, there is full-blown hypertrophic osteoarthropathy.[389] In advanced disease cor pulmonale and cyanosis may develop.[336]

On pathologic examination of the lungs the distribution of the alveolitic process is characteristically patchy[88, 130]; therefore, histologic assessment requires open lung biopsy.[231] A definite diagnosis cannot be made from a transbronchial lung biopsy.[649] There is evidence that the histologic changes evolve from an inflammatory alveolitis to an interstitial fibrosis,[156] and it is possible to find the whole range of pathologic changes in the same specimen within a small compass.[351] Early changes consist of infiltration of the alveolar septa by inflammatory cells, made up mainly of lymphocytes and plasma cells with occasional polymorphonuclear leukocytes, eosinophils, and mast cells. Type II pneumocytes proliferate, and there is a loss of type I cells. Intra-alveolar cells, predominantly macrophages, also increase in number. Hyaline membranes are notable by their absence, which helps in differentiating these changes from those of diffuse alveolar damage. Later, interstitial inflammatory cells are replaced by fibrous tissue, with setting down of collagen in the septa and subsequent obliteration of capillaries. Alveoli coalesce and become restructured with the formation of cystlike air spaces, some of which are lined by bronchiolar epithelium that grows into alveoli. There is also focal lymphoid follicle hyperplasia and hyperplasia of smooth muscle, particularly in relation to terminal bronchioles, accounting for the term "muscular cirrhosis" in the older literature.[351] The final appearance is that of an end-stage lung.

A variant on this pattern was described in 1965[383] and called desquamative interstitial pneumonia (DIP). It was distinguished from CFA (usual interstitial pneumonitis) by (1) extensive filling of alveoli with desquamated cells, later shown to be largely macrophages[225]; (2) striking uniformity of the histologic appearance; (3) less interstitial component and fibrosis; (4) the young age of the patients; (5) a characteristic chest radiograph; and (6) a better prognosis, being more responsive to steroids. A number of authors support the contention that DIP is a specific clinicopathologic entity,[88, 232, 351] but others regard it as merely representing an early phase of CFA.[122, 552, 623] On balance, this latter view seems reasonable, especially as some of the original features of DIP such as specific radiologic signs and better prognosis have been shown to be inconstant.[201, 483] In ad-

dition, pathologic changes of DIP can coexist with those of typical CFA.[552]

Changes in respiratory function tests[130, 336, 632] are those that might be expected from a diffuse interstitial process: reduced compliance and lung volumes, particularly vital capacity and total lung capacity with relative sparing of residual volume; altered small airway function; and hyperventilation and arterial desaturation, particularly on exercise. Reduction in diffusing capacity is a particularly early and characteristic change. Laboratory blood tests show raised erythrocyte sedimentation rate (ESR) and immunoglobulin levels in about a third of patients.[632] Overall more than half the patients will have autoantibodies. Antinuclear antibody is positive in 15% to 45% of patients, and rheumatoid factor is found in up to a third.[260, 586, 632, 670]

As in other diffuse interstitial disease,[186, 231] the lungs can be histologically affected despite a normal appearance on the chest radiograph.[231, 383, 389] Such patients with a normal chest radiograph may be both symptomatic and have an abnormal dif-

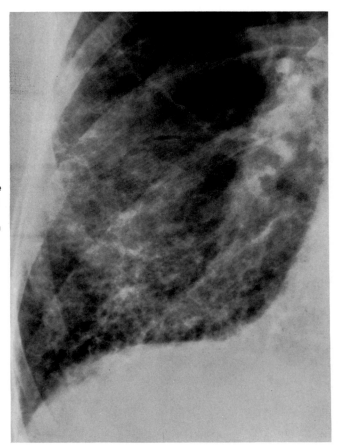

FIG 11–1.
Cryptogenic fibrosing alveolitis. Localized view of the right lung base shows widespread interstitial shadowing. The predominant opacities are small rounded, linear, and irregular shadows. Other less profuse elements include small rounded transradiancies about 1 to 2 mm in diameter and a variety of thin line opacities, some resembling septal lines. In parts, the shadowing has become confluent taking on a ground-glass appearance. Characteristically the shadowing overall is rather fine and uniform.

fusion capacity.[552] In other patients, the radiographic appearance is abnormal before symptoms develop.[586]

A variety of radiographic changes have been described,* the most common being small irregular opacities (Fig 11–1), seen in some three-quarters of the cases, and, less commonly, small rounded opacities, seen in about one-fifth of patients. This reticulonodular shadowing may be basal (Fig 11–2,A) or it may be more generally distributed, with a lower zone accentuation (Fig 11–3).[130] A peripheral accentuation is also a common feature that is much more easily appreciated on computed tomography (Fig 11–4)[35, 454] than on plain radiographs.[389] The shadowing is usually symmetric from side to side, but atypical distributions, such as limitation to a lobe (see Fig 11–4)[130] or apex,[130, 389] may be seen. Another common pattern is hazy, ground-glass opacification, which may be diffuse or patchy and may contain an air bronchogram (Fig 11–5).[130] This pattern is seen

*References 88, 95, 130, 201, 389, 448, 590, and 632.

in up to one-third of patients.[88] At one time this pattern, particularly when confined to the lower zones, was thought to be characteristic of the desquamative interstitial pneumonia variant of CFA,[232, 383] but this is no longer held to be true.[483] Septal lines are occasionally recorded.[130] Volume loss characterized by diaphragmatic elevation[130, 550] is seen in some 25% to 60% of cases,[88, 95, 448] and basal discoid atelectasis may occasionally be seen secondary to elevation of the diaphragm.[201] The loss of volume may be basally predominant or generalized.[355] Although pleural shadowing has been recorded in some series,[95, 156, 632] it is generally not a feature of CFA and should raise the question of other conditions such as asbestosis,[355] rheumatoid disease, or systemic lupus erythematosus. Pneumothorax occurs occasionally and in one series was recorded in four of 45 patients.[389] Pneumomediastinum is also a recognized complication that is probably more common than pneumothorax (Fig 11–6).[355] Ossific nodules recognized pathologically may in rare cases be seen radiologically.[421]

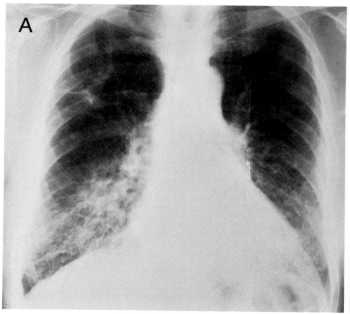

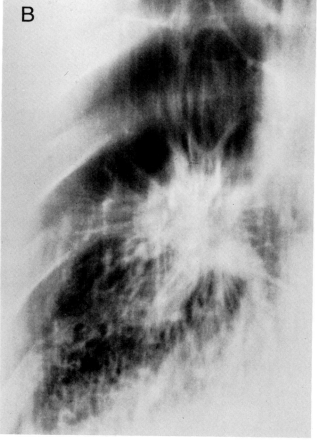

FIG 11–2.
Cryptogenic fibrosing alveolitis. **A,** PA chest radiograph. There is symmetric, basally predominant, shadowing made up of small irregular and rounded opacities. The distribution is characteristic of fibrosing alveolitis. Just below the right hilus there is an area of confluent shadowing 5 cm in diameter. **B,** conventional tomogram of the right lower zone shows a 5-cm, star-shaped, spiculated opacity typical of a bronchial carcinoma. Histologically the lesion was a squamous cell carcinoma.

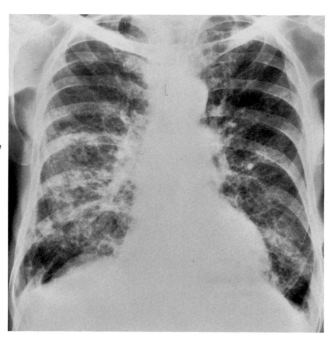

FIG 11—3.
Cryptogenic fibrosing alveolitis. Bilateral changes are more severe on the right than the left. The shadowing is a mixture of small rounded and irregular nodules that are generalized on the right but basally predominant on the left. Lung volume is slightly increased, a recognized but not common finding in fibrosing alveolitis.

With progression of the alveolitis to fibrosis, the initial fine shadowing becomes coarser,[389] and small, cystlike transradiances appear. Initially these are just 2 mm or so in diameter (see Fig 11—4), but later they increase in size until they correspond to the 5- to 7-mm ring opacities of honeycomb lung (Figs 11—6 and 11—7). In several series honeycomb opacities have been present in one-third to one-half of patients.[88, 590] With gross fibrosis, bullae appear (Figs 11—7 and 11—8),[389] and there may be radiographic evidence of pulmonary arterial hypertension (see Fig 11—8).

Attempts have been made to correlate chest radiographic findings with histology, respiratory function tests, symptoms, prognosis, and response to treatment. The literature on the subject is very con-

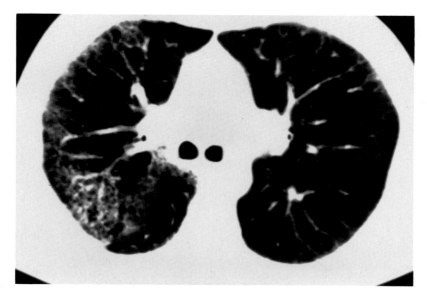

FIG 11—4.
Cryptogenic fibrosing alveolitis. CT scan of chest is at the level of the carina. The chief findings on CT are small (1.5- to 3-mm) reticular opacities. In this patient the opacities are largely confined to the right lung; this degree of asymmetry is unusual. Changes in fibrosing alveolitis are often predominantly subpleural, and the peripheral nature of the opacities is well demonstrated on this CT scan.

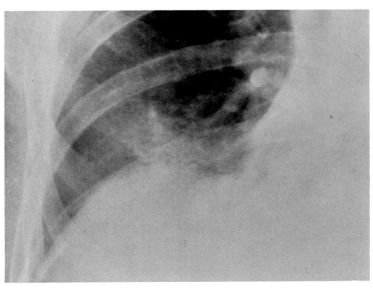

FIG 11—5.
Cryptogenic fibrosing alveolitis. Localized view of the right lung base shows ground-glass opacification. This tends to be an early radiologic change in the natural history of fibrosing alveolitis.

fusing, largely negative, and often inconsistent. Thus, for example, profusion of opacities has been shown both to correlate[632] and not to correlate[590] with dyspnea. The only correlation that appears with any consistency is that coarse reticulation/honey-

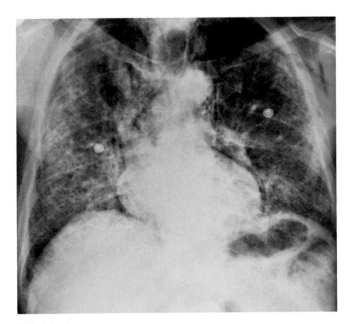

FIG 11—6.
Pneumomediastinum and cryptogenic fibrosing alveolitis. There is long-standing fibrosing alveolitis with changes on the right of aggregated, small, thick-walled ring opacities (honeycomb shadowing). There is also a pneumomediastinum.

comb opacities indicate severe fibrosis.[130, 389, 675] There is weak evidence that alveolar/ground-glass shadowing may correlate with mild fibrosis and/or marked cellularity.[130, 383, 550, 552, 670] However, this is not a universal finding, and other workers find no correlation at all between histologic features and the chest radiograph.[156, 632] In an attempt to overcome the unreliability of the chest radiograph taken on its own, scoring systems that include other variables have been assessed.[655]

A handful of studies have examined the appearance of CFA at CT scanning.[34, 447, 590, 675] CT is a more sensitive examination for CFA and sometimes demonstrates abnormalities when there is a normal appearance on the chest radiograph[355] or shows more abnormalities than does the chest radiograph.[590] To avoid misinterpretation of gravity-induced blood diversion, which can mimic early changes of CFA, scans with the patient prone in addition to supine are recommended.[596] The predominant finding on CT scans are small reticular opacities (1.5 to 3 mm) (see Fig 11—4) with less than 10% small rounded opacities.[590] Others have found no rounded opacities at all[34] and consider the almost universal reticular nature of the shadowing to have diagnostic value in differentiating CFA from other interstitial disorders. Honeycomb shadowing and bullae are particularly well shown on CT (see Fig 11—7).[590] One finding that has emerged from all CT studies is the peripheral nature of the opacities (see

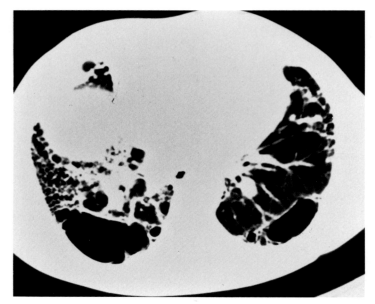

FIG 11–7.
High-resolution thin-section CT scan of long-standing cryptogenic fibrosing alveolitis. On the right there is a mixture of honeycomb reticulation and larger ring opacities, probably bullae. The 6-cm- diameter round opacity anteriorly in the right lung is a complicating adenocarcinoma.

Fig 11–4), which occur particularly posteriorly and basally.[675] This finding contrasts with those of some other interstitial processes, such as extrinsic allergic alveolitis, in which the distribution is predominantly central.[34] CT has shown some promise as a predictor of disease activity.[448]

Gallium-67 is taken up in "active" CFA, and in most series about 70% of patients have had posi- tive scintiscans. In one study, the gallium index (a derivative of the area, intensity, and texture of uptake) correlated with the severity of the alveolitis as assessed by cellularity.[386] The gallium scintiscan is one of the investigations used to stage CFA, but its place in management has yet to be clearly de- fined.

The prognosis in CFA is poor, with mean sur-

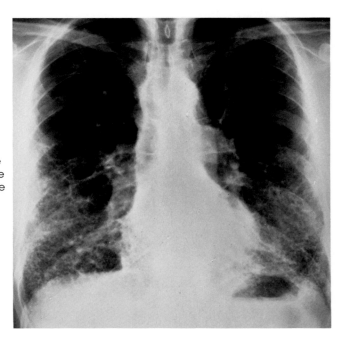

FIG 11–8.
Radiograph of patient with CFA shows typical changes in the middle and lower zones with extensive bullous changes in the middle and upper zones. The proximal pulmonary arteries are large, indicating pulmonary arterial hypertension.

vival after presentation ranging from about 3 years to 6 years.[88, 586, 632] Hidden within these figures, however, is a great variation—ranging, in one series, from 4 months to 20 years.[586] It is well recognized that progression of CFA can be very slow or even come to a halt.[552] The possibility that some cases in which there is rapid progression to death represent diffuse alveolar damage (acute interstitial pneumonitis) rather than CFA should be considered.[351] Features that carry a good prognosis are an age of less than 40 years, short symptomatic history at presentation, a good response to steroids, and a cellular biopsy showing little in the way of fibrosis. The prognosis is the same in fibrosing alveolitis, whether it is cryptogenic or associated with a connective tissue disorder.[626, 632]

The chief treatment for CFA is steroids; occasionally other drugs, such as penicillamine and cytotoxic agents, are tried. Steroids are of some help, with 40% to 60% of patients experiencing subjective improvement and 20% showing objective improvement.[336, 632]

About 50% of patients die of a cause directly related to the CFA, such as respiratory failure. The second most common cause of death is cardiovascular disease,[626] which is four times more common than expected.[586, 632] The third most common cause of death is carcinoma of the lung, which develops 14 times more frequently in these patients than in the general population (see Figs 11–2 and 11–7).[635] Its development is related to the CFA itself, and apart from smoking, no predicting factors for its development, in the presence of CFA, have been identified.[635] An analogous increase in the incidence of bronchial carcinoma in lung fibrosis associated with progressive systemic sclerosis is well recognized.[517] The prevalence of carcinoma in various series of CFA has ranged between 5% and 13%.[586, 626, 635] A review of 62 cases found squamous cell carcinomas in 35%, alveolar cell carcinomas in 27%, adenocarcinomas in 21%, and 11% undifferentiated.[217] This preponderance of adenocarcinoma and alveolar cell carcinoma is not a universal finding, and in some series the pattern of cell types is no different from the usual experience.[635]

End-Stage Lung

Many diffuse diseases such as fibrosing alveolitis that predominantly affect the interstitium of the lung progress to a final nonspecific pattern both pathologically and radiologically termed end-stage lung.[241] The term describes the morphologic change

only and does not imply functional respiratory insufficiency, though this may well be present. A large number of conditions can evolve to produce this pattern. These include fibrosing alveolitis, both cryptogenic and that secondary to collagen vascular disorders; eosinophilic granuloma; drug-induced interstitial pneumonitis; interstitial lymphocytic pneumonitis; extrinsic allergic alveolitis; inorganic dust inhalation (e.g., asbestosis, berylliosis); chronic granulomatous infections (e.g., fungal); sarcoidosis; and lymphangiomyomatosis.[218] End-stage lung is also recognized with chronic venous hypertension, chronic gastric aspiration, and following various forms of diffuse alveolar damage (e.g., toxic inhalations, oxygen, infections, radiation).[351] It is even rarely described with processes considered largely if not entirely alveolar, such as pulmonary alveolar proteinosis.[323]

Pathologically, there is gross distortion and obliteration of lung parenchyma involving both the interstitium and air-spaces.[218] The chief pathologic findings[241, 306, 351] consist of: (1) septal thickening resulting from cellular infiltration and fibrosis; (2) septal dissolution leading to restructuring and coalescence of alveoli; (3) bronchiolectasis and small airway obliteration; (4) obstructive vascular changes and capillary obliteration; (5) smooth muscle proliferation; (6) proliferation of bronchiolar epithelium, which grows along alveolar ducts and alveoli; (7) metaplastic and neoplastic change of bronchiolar epithelium; (8) mesenchymal osseous metaplasia; and (9) endogenous lipid pneumonitis. Grossly, the most characteristic features of end stage lung are small cystic spaces, which give the surface of the lung a bosselated appearance.[241] These cysts vary in size from 1 mm to 2 cm, but are typically in the order of 5 to 10 mm. Three mechanisms account for the formation of cysts: (1) alveolar simplification secondary to septal dissolution; (2) bronchiolectasis; and (3) obstructive emphysema.

Just as the cysts are the most characteristic gross morphologic finding in pathologic specimens, so too are they the most characteristic radiologic feature (Fig 11–9). They appear as aggregated, small, ring opacities that are termed honeycomb shadows when they have diameters of 5 to 10 mm with walls 1- to 2-mm thick (Fig 11–10).[218] There may be additional small rounded and irregular opacities, but these lack the specificity of honeycomb opacities in the diagnosis of end-stage lung. The radiologic changes are usually diffuse, bilateral, and asymmetric. Lung volume may be normal, increased, or decreased—depending on the mix of pathologic processes. There will be fea-

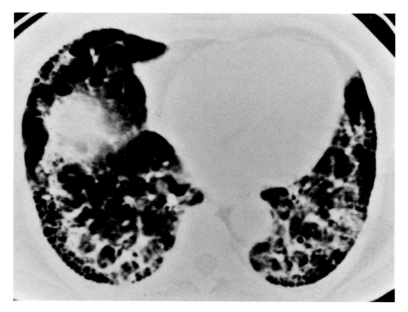

FIG 11—9.
High-resolution thin-section CT study of end-stage lung. The primary process in this patient was fibrosing alveolitis associated with rheumatoid disease. The dominant element is 2- to 10-mm ring opacities separated by band densities of varying thickness produced by fibrosis.

tures of cor pulmonale in advanced cases, and in long-standing cases there may be small calcified nodules[421] as a result of metaplastic ossification.[513] Scar carcinoma is a recognized complication[427] and may appear radiologically as a mass or as consolidation. Multifocal carcinomas are recognized.[351]

Although end-stage lung denotes a nonspecific appearance with a wide variety of causes, it is often possible to limit the differential possibilities on radiologic grounds (see Chapter 5). Radiologic features that help in this way include the zonal distribution of changes, lung volume, pleural changes, and the presence or absence of adenopathy. Zonal distribution is particularly helpful in this regard.[218]

LUNG VASCULITIDES

The vasculitides are a large and varied group of disorders characterized by inflammation and necrosis of blood vessels.[198] They may be localized to one organ or may be disseminated (systemic). Much evidence now indicates that immune complex deposition is of prime pathogenic importance in these disorders, with other mechanisms such as cell-mediated immunity making a contribution.[198, 375]

Several schemes have been used to classify the systemic vasculitides, reflecting the fact that no

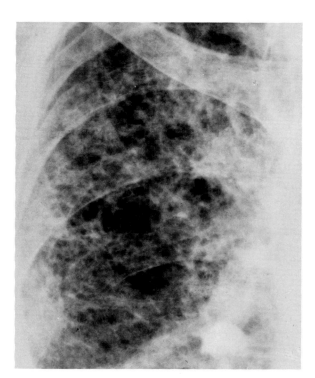

FIG 11—10.
End-stage lung. Localized view, right mid/upper zone. The underlying process in this patient was CFA. Much of the shadowing consists of 2- to 6-mm ring opacities, which in part have the characteristics of honeycomb shadowing. Ring opacities like these are the hallmark of end-stage lung.

one classification is entirely satisfactory. The classification used here is based on several recent reviews[165, 198, 295, 375, 413] (Table 11–1). It is of note that the table does not include polyarteritis nodosa, as this vasculitis characteristically spares the lungs.[198] Several authors discuss the contentious relationship of polyarteritis nodosa, Churg-Strauss syndrome, and the polyangiitis overlap syndrome.[165, 198]

Granulomatous Vasculitis

The pathologic characteristic of granulomatous vasculitis is that the cellular infiltrate consists predominantly of histiocytes (tissue macrophages).

Three vasculitic processes affecting the lungs can be considered granulomatous: (1) Wegener's granulomatosis; (2) allergic granulomatosis and angiitis (Churg-Strauss syndrome); and (3) necrotizing sarcoidal angiitis and granulomatosis.

Wegener's Granulomatosis

Wegener's granulomatosis was first described in the 1930s.[174] It has distinctive clinicopathologic features and can, therefore, be more easily recognized as a distinct entity than most of the other vasculitides.[198] The cause is obscure, but there is accumulating evidence to suggest that the entity is probably an immunologic reaction to a specific antigen and that immune complex formation plays an important role.[375]

Wegener's granulomatosis is characterized pathologically by three features: (1) a necrotizing granulomatous vasculitis of the upper and lower respiratory tracts; (2) a disseminated small vessel vasculitis involving both arteries and veins; and (3) a focal glomerulonephritis.[375] A limited form of the disease has been described as affecting the lung with or without upper respiratory disease but without renal or other systemic involvement.[89, 321] In making the diagnosis of Wegener's granulomatosis, it is important that there be biopsy evidence of a mixed vasculitic and granulomatous process, affecting both arteries and veins.[103]

In most series there has been a slight preponderance of male patients.[199] The mean age at presentation is in the 5th decade,[199] but there is a wide range, 8 to 75 years in one series.[149] Upper airway involvement with sinusitis, rhinitis, and otitis is the most common clinical features at presentation, encountered twice as often as lung and systemic symptoms. Functional renal impairment is unusual at presentation, being seen in only about 10% of patients.[199] Laboratory examination often shows a normochromic, normocytic anemia; absence of leucopenia (which helps distinguish the entity from lymphomatoid granulomatosis); raised ESR; and a positive rheumatoid factor.[199]

Fauci et al.[199] suggest that for a definite diagnosis of Wegener's granulomatosis (1) there should be clinical evidence of disease in at least two of three sites—the so called Wegener's triad: upper airways; lung; and kidney—and (2) biopsy should show disease in at least one and preferably two of these organ systems. In practice, the lung biopsy provides the most useful information. The renal changes are usually nonspecific, rarely showing either vasculitic or granulomatous lesions, and the specific lesions in the upper airways are often masked by the secondary infective changes.

During the course of the illness all patients have lung and/or upper respiratory tract involvement, and the majority (85%) develop renal disease.[199] In about 50% of patients, joint, ear, and eye disorders become manifest, and occasionally the heart and nervous system are affected.[199] Pulmonary or nonpulmonary infection may precipitate clinical relapse, and in some series, such infections have accounted for about 50% of relapses.[492] Untreated Wegener's granulomatosis carries a poor prognosis, with death in about 5 months from renal failure.[174] The outlook has, however, been transformed by treatment with cyclophosphamide and steroids, which can induce and maintain remission in a high percentage of patients.[199] The localized form of the disease has an indolent course.[89]

Pulmonary radiographic changes are found in

TABLE 11–1.
Classification of Pulmonary Vasculitides

Granulomatous vasculitis
  Wegener's granulomatosis
  Allergic granulomatosis and angiitis (Churg-Strauss syndrome)
  Necrotizing sarcoidal angiitis and granulomatosis

Hypersensitivity vasculitis
  Anaphylactoid purpura (Henoch-Schönlein)
  Essential mixed cryoglobulinemia
  Vasculitis associated with connective tissue disease
  Vasculitis associated with malignancy
  Nonspecific hypersensitivity vasculitis

Giant cell vasculitis
  Systemic temporal arteritis
  Other giant cell arteritides

Behçet's disease and Hughes-Stovin syndrome

Polyangiitis overlap syndrome

nearly three-quarters of patients with Wegener's granulomatosis at presentation. These changes may be accompanied by cough, hemoptysis, pain, or dyspnea, but these symptoms are often not a dominant finding. Not infrequently, the patient has no symptoms at all.

Radiologically the most characteristic pulmonary manifestations are discrete focal opacities that vary in character from nodular masses to ill-defined areas of consolidation either of which may cavitate. Nodular shadows are visible at presentation in the majority of patients (62% in one series).[196] In one-third of patients, the nodules are single; in the remaining two-thirds, they are multiple (Fig 11–11). Commonly 2 to 4 cm in diameter,[370] the nodules may range in size from 3 mm to 10 cm.[333, 415] They are round or oval in shape and may be well or poorly defined, sometimes becoming confluent.[415] The nodules are usually few in number but may occasionally be innumerable.[333] There appears to be no strong affinity for any one zone; some series have a preponderance of nodules in the mid/lower zones,[255] while others do not.[251] Nodules commonly resolve with or without treatment over a period ranging from several weeks to 2 months. They may heal without residual abnormality, or they may leave a visible scar.[255]

Focal opacities with the features of pulmonary consolidation occur in some 30% of patients[196] (Fig 11–12). They may be single or multiple and vary from small inhomogeneous patches[415] to homoge-

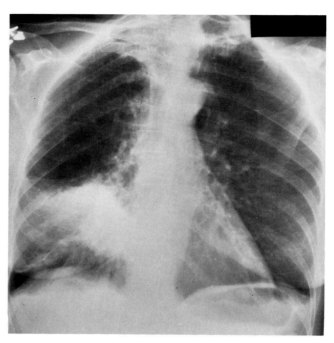

FIG 11–12.
Wegener's granulomatosis. The main finding in this patient is a 10 × 6-cm triangular opacity in the right lower zone. It has the features of consolidation.

neous segmental or lobar consolidations.[196, 251] Sometimes there is a mixed pattern of nodules and consolidation, and the radiographic distinction between the two is not always clear-cut (Fig 11–13).[255] New lung lesions during relapses are often in areas affected in previous episodes even though the radiographic appearance of the lesions may be different from that seen originally.[196]

Cavitation of the nodules and the consolidations is common (Fig 11–14), being seen in approximately 40% of cases at presentation.[196] Cavities may be unilocular or multilocular,[415] and the outer margins of their walls are more commonly irregular than smooth.[370] Wall width varies greatly. Typically, it is thick, with an irregular or smooth inner margin, but when the cavities have been present for some time, there is a tendency for the walls to become thinner.[196] Cavities may have air-fluid levels,[415] and it has been suggested that this is an indication of secondary infection, particularly when accompanied by fever and increasing cavity size.[375] Typical infecting organisms are *Staphylococcus aureus* and anaerobic bacteria.

Ten cases of diffuse pulmonary hemorrhage have been reported in Wegener's granulomatosis,[373] occurring both in patients with established disease[595] and as a presenting feature.[305] The radiologic

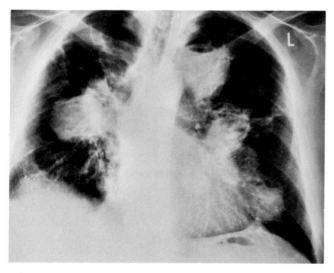

FIG 11–11.
Wegener's granulomatosis. There are multiple well-defined nodules ranging in size from 1 to 7 cm. The lesion in the left upper zone has cavitated and contains a small air-fluid level. *L* = left. (Courtesy of Dr. G.J. Hunter, London.)

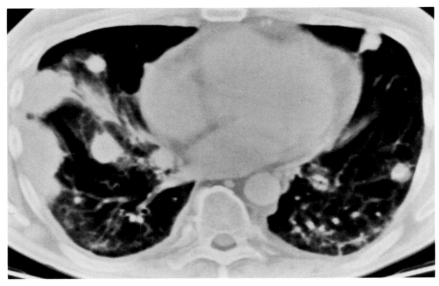

FIG 11–13.
Wegener's granulomatosis. CT scan shows mixed radiologic lesions. There are several nodules, a flame-shaped consolidation anteriorly on the right, and confluent subpleural opacities, also on the right.

changes are similar to those seen in the diffuse pulmonary hemorrhage of Goodpasture's syndrome.

Tracheal narrowing is an infrequent, but important, phenomenon in Wegener's granulomatosis. It was present in 17 of 108 patients with Wegener's granulomatosis in the Mayo Clinic series.[414] It is notable that all but one of these patients were women.

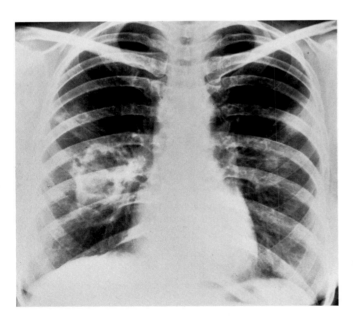

FIG 11–14.
Wegener's granulomatosis. Multiple nodules with a large (6-cm) cavitary lesion adjacent to the right hilus. Its walls are thick and irregular on both aspects. (Courtesy of Dr. G.J. Hunter, London.)

Every patient had nasal involvement, but only four (24%) had pulmonary disease. Hoarseness and stridor usually occurred with, or just after, the onset of nasal symptoms, though in a few patients they were delayed by several years. Half the patients needed tracheostomy.[414]

Stenoses are subglottic and can be well demonstrated by conventional tomography, which shows smooth or irregular circumferential stenoses about 3 to 4 cm long.[113, 414] CT scanning shows abnormal soft tissue within the tracheal rings (Fig 11–15), which themselves may be abnormally thickened and calcified.[592] Stenotic lesions of the more distal airways, usually main stem or lobar, have occasionally been reported. In one series, bronchial stenoses had a frequency of about 7%.[199] They usually become manifest by causing distal collapse/consolidation of a lobe or lung.[195, 397]

Pleural effusions in Wegener's granulomatosis, some of which are quite large, have been reported with a prevalence ranging from 5 to 55%.[251, 255, 397] It seems likely that some of these effusions were only indirectly related to the presence of Wegener's granulomatosis and that, in general, pleural effusions are unusual. Pneumothorax[339] and hydropneumothorax are occasionally seen. In one case they were associated with cavitary lung disease and in another with a bronchopleural fistula, the track of which was lined by Wegener's granulomatosis tissue.[188, 397] Pleural thickening and subpleural masses (see Fig 11–13), have also been reported.[185, 397]

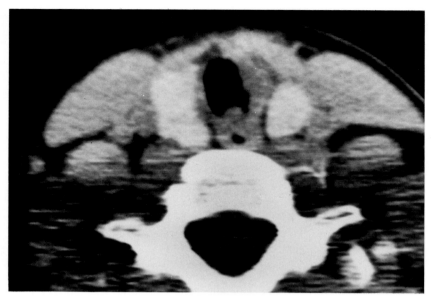

FIG 11–15.
Wegener's granulomatosis. CT scan at the level of the thyroid shows irregular soft tissue thickening of the tracheal wall, posteri- orly and on the left, which compromises the lumen. (Courtesy of Dr. S.C. Rankin, London.)

Churg-Strauss Syndrome

The Churg-Strauss syndrome is a systemic necrotizing vasculitis that occurs in patients with asthma and is characterized by a marked peripheral eosinophilia. It has a variety of synonyms including "allergic granulomatosis and angiitis" and "allergic granulomatosis." It was first described in 1951[105]; since then, three major series have reported the clinical and postmortem features.[102, 371, 529] The criteria for diagnosing the syndrome are: (1) asthma; (2) blood eosinophilia of greater than $1.5 \times 10^9/L$; (3) clinical features of a systemic vasculitis involving two or more extrapulmonary organs; and (4) histologic evidence of necrotizing vasculitis associated with a prominent eosinophilic infiltrate together with vascular and extravascular granulomas. These histologic features may be patchily distributed and therefore may not all be present in the same biopsy specimen.

Patients with the syndrome are commonly middle-aged, the mean age at onset being 38 years,[371] with a range of 15 to 69 years.[102] The sexes are equally affected, and a significant number of patients are atopic.[371]

In many patients, the disease evolves in three stages: (1) asthmatic, (2) eosinophilic, and (3) vasculitic.

Asthma is the first manifestation in all patients and is accompanied in 70% of cases by allergic rhinitis.[102] There is on average a 3-year gap between the onset of asthma and the development of vasculitis,[371] but this interval has ranged from a few months to as long as 30 years. Occasionally, the illness is so telescoped that asthma and vasculitis are simultaneous in onset.[102] A short interval is associated with a poor prognosis.[102] With the onset of the vasculitic phase, the asthma may increase in severity,[371] or it may remit.[105]

An eosinophilic phase commonly follows the asthmatic prodrome. It is characterized by blood eosinophilia and eosinophilic infiltration of tissues, particularly the lungs and gastrointestinal tract. At this stage the disease may relapse and remit for years before ultimately transforming into the final vasculitic phase.[371]

Many different tissues and organs may be involved by the vasculitis, including the myocardium, pericardium, joints, and muscles. The skin may show palpable purpura, erythema, urticaria, or subcutaneous nodules. Vasculitic involvement of the nerves may result in a mononeuritis multiplex and, in the gut, may cause abdominal pain, diarrhea, or intestinal bleeding. The kidneys may show segmental glomerulonephritis similar to that in Wegener's granulomatosis; however, such renal involvement rarely causes significant clinical disease.[102] The vasculitic phase is accompanied by systemic symptoms such as weight loss and fever. The ESR is raised, and there is usually a marked leukocytosis with a striking eosinophilia, which may be as high as $30 \times 10^9/L$. It is possible, however, to have active vasculitis and no blood eosinophilia.[371] The serum IgE value is commonly raised.[371]

Although the diagnosis can readily be made on clinical grounds, histologic confirmation should be obtained by biopsy of involved skin, kidney, or prostate.[371]

The changes on the chest radiograph in the Churg-Strauss syndrome can occur in the eosinophilic or vasculitic phases. The reported frequency of chest radiographic abnormalities varies between 27%[102] and 72%.[371] This variation appears to be related to the frequency of obtaining chest radiographs, the higher figure probably being a better reflection of the true frequency of radiographic abnormalities during the course of the disease. The most common findings are transient, multifocal, nonsegmental consolidations which show no zonal predilection,[105, 119, 371] an appearance which, when combined with blood eosinophilia, sometimes fulfills the criteria for Löffler's syndrome (see p. 506) (Fig 11–16). Multifocal consolidation may take on the appearance of multiple fluffy nodules.[361] The pulmonary consolidation can, however, be unifocal[361] or symmetric or may even show the pattern of chronic eosinophilic pneumonia[110, 365] (see "Eosinophilic Lung Disease" later in this chapter). Widespread symmetric consolidation is seen with diffuse pulmonary hemorrhage.[371] Cavitation is unusual,[144] and it is noteworthy that both large nodule formation and cavitation are much less common than in Wegener's granulomatosis. Less common findings include a diffuse interstitial pattern,[102] diffuse miliary nodulation,[102, 377] and hilar and mediastinal adenopathy, either unilateral or bilateral.[361, 377] Pleural effusions (Fig 11–16) occurred in 29% of patients in one large review of 154 cases,[371] and in many the effusions were eosinophilic. Pleuritic pain may occur without accompanying pleural effusion.[371]

Cardiac involvement causes cardiomegaly resulting from pericarditis or myocarditis as well as signs of raised pulmonary venous pressure, and these signs may complicate the primary pleuropulmonary changes on the radiograph (Fig 11–16).[143, 531]

The radiographic changes may or may not clear with treatment.[102] Churg-Strauss syndrome responds well to steroids, but a small proportion of patients require adjunctive immunosuppressive agents. The vasculitic phase in most treated patients lasts less than a year, and late relapses are uncommon.[371]

Necrotizing Sarcoidal Angiitis

Necrotizing sarcoidal angiitis was first described in 1973 by Liebow,[380] and the problem posed then—as to whether the entity was sarcoidosis with necrosis of the granulomas and vessels, or a necrotizing vasculitis with a sarcoid reaction—still remains unsettled. Some workers, however, consider that the case for its being a form of sarcoidosis is overwhelming.[103] The pathologic findings include (1) many sarcoid-like granulomas with necrosis or hyalinization sometimes associated with an intervening chronic inflammatory infiltrate, (2) a vasculitis of arteries and veins that is often granulomatous, and (3) small-airway obstruction by granulomas, which may cause an endogenous lipid pneumonia.[103, 380]

Much of the information available on this condition comes from four series totaling about 80 cases.[103, 362, 538] The mean age at presentation is about 45 years (range, 12 to 75 years) with a 2.5:1 predominance of female patients.[103, 362, 538] At the time of presentation, between one-quarter and two-thirds of the patients are asymptomatic,[103, 538] and the disease is first discovered because of an abnormal chest radiograph. The remainder of the patients have either systemic symptoms (fever, malaise, weight loss) or respiratory symptoms (cough, chest pain, shortness of breath). Only a few patients have had extrapulmonary lesions that are consistent with sarcoidosis, the chief one being uveitis (9%).[103, 362]

In general, necrotizing sarcoidal angiitis is a benign condition[227] that does not require treatment.[165] When treatment is indicated, steroids are used, and there is little role, at least initially, for cytotoxic agents.[375]

Radiologically, the most common pattern is that of bilateral nodules, occurring in about 75% of patients[103, 380] and ranging up to about 4 cm in diameter. Sometimes the nodules are small enough to be considered miliary.[104, 380] The nodules tend to show a predilection for the lower zones and occasionally cavitate.[210] When followed over years with repeat chest radiographs, the nodules may show a slow increase in size and number[104] and may become confluent.[165] Spontaneous disappearance of nodules has been recorded.[103] When the nodules are unilateral, they are often solitary[104, 210] and resemble a bronchial neoplasm.[594] Less common patterns include bilateral consolidations,[104, 380] basal interstitial shadowing,[362] and pleural effusions, the latter being absent from most series but present in 54% in one study.[362] As with pleural effusions, the prevalence of

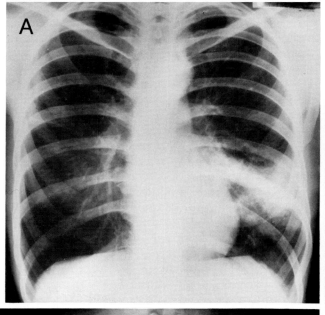

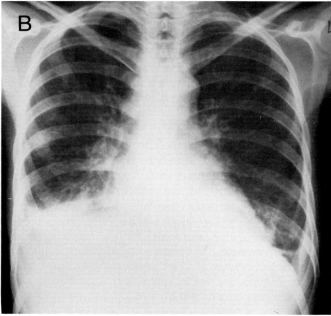

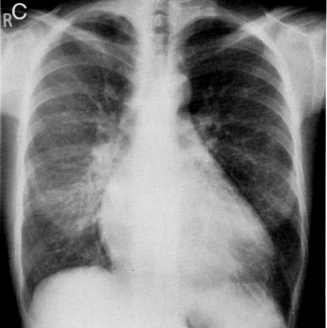

FIG 11–16.

Churg-Strauss syndrome. The patient, a 28-year-old asthmatic woman, presented with colitis which was followed by a Löffler type of syndrome and a blood eosinophilia (10.3 × 10⁹/L). At this stage a few microaneurysms were demonstrated on hepatic and renal arteries. Within a year a cardiomyopathy had developed. **A,** chest radiograph during the Löffler syndrome phase shows consolidation in the left lower zone. This followed right upper zone consolidation. **B,** 6 months later bilateral pleural effusions developed. **C,** 1 year later cardiomegaly has developed on the basis of a cardiomyopathy.

hilar adenopathy has varied considerably from series to series, ranging from 65%[103] to 8%.[362]

Hypersensitivity Vasculitis

The term hypersensitivity vasculitis refers to a heterogeneous group of clinical disorders in which there is a vasculitis of arterioles, capillaries, and venules. There is often a recognized precipitating agent[198, 245, 375] including infectious organisms, par-

ticularly *Streptococcus, Mycobacteria,* viruses, or parasites; foreign proteins; chemicals; drugs; and endogenous antigens, such as those associated with malignant neoplasms.[295] Immune complex formation plays an important role in the pathogenesis of hypersensitivity vasculitis.[198] Skin lesions—classically palpable purpura—tend to be a major finding in these disorders. Systemic involvement also occurs, notably of the kidneys, joints, gastrointestinal tract, lungs, and nervous system,[543] but this is rarely life threatening,[295] usually being self-limiting and responding to conservative treatment.[165]

Hypersensitivity vasculitis embraces a number of well-recognized syndromes, in particular anaphylactoid purpura and essential mixed cryoglobulinemia. Hypersensitivity vasculitis also occurs in collagen vascular diseases and may be cryptogenic.

Anaphylactoid Purpura (Henoch-Schönlein Purpura)

Though found primarily in children, anaphylactoid purpura may occur at any age and frequently follows an upper respiratory tract infection. The virus or bacterium responsible for this infection is the most common source of the inciting antigen. Other antigenic sources include varicella, *Yersinia,* food, drugs, and neoplasms.[304]

Immune complexes containing IgA are found in the walls of blood vessels and distinguish anaphylactoid purpura from other cutaneous vasculitides. The entity is characterized by palpable purpura over the legs and buttocks, abdominal pain, gastrointestinal bleeding, arthralgia and, in 10% to 25% of cases, renal involvement with glomerulonephritis. The prognosis is generally good, although renal disease can progress to chronic renal failure and death. Pulmonary involvement is uncommon; it probably occurs more often in adults than in children.[165] In one series of 64 adults, pulmonary involvement was seen in 6.25%,[125] but in several other large series, lung involvement was absent altogether.[375] The most common abnormalities on plain chest radiographs are pleural effusions and pulmonary consolidations.[125] Patchy, multifocal consolidation[350] and transient consolidation[337] are both reported. When pathologic examination has been available, leukocytoclastic vasculitis and intra-alveolar and septal hemorrhages have been found. It seems likely that the majority of chest radiologic findings are related to alveolar hemorrhage.

Essential Mixed Cryoglobulinemia

In essential mixed cryoglobulinemia (EMC) the vasculitis is usually of the leukocytoclastic type affecting small vessels, but it may also affect medium-sized arteries.[375] The cryoglobulinemia may be primary, or it may be secondary to a variety of disorders such as lymphoma, myeloma, collagen vascular disease, or infectious diseases. In the essential (primary) mixed form, the cryoglobulin is an immune complex commonly made up of IgM rheumatoid factor directed against IgG—hence the term "mixed." EMC is associated with vasculitis, palpable purpura, nephritis, arthralgia, hepatosplenomegaly, and lymphadenopathy.[227] In a series of 23 patients with EMC, there was a high prevalence of small airway disease and impaired gas exchange on respiratory function testing. Nearly 80% of patients had an abnormality in the chest radiograph, with a diffuse, finely nodular interstitial pattern.[45] The pathologic basis for this change is a matter of speculation.[227]

Connective Tissue Disease and Malignancy

Hypersensitivity vasculitis is a recognized finding in some connective tissue diseases and is discussed under the specific disorders. There is also an established association with various malignancies, particularly lymphoid and reticuloendothelial neoplasms.[198]

Nonspecific Hypersensitivity Vasculitis and Disseminated Leukocytoclastic Vasculitis

These conditions are diagnosed by exclusion of those hypersensitivity vasculitides like Henoch-Schönlein purpura that have distinctive clinicopathologic features.[245] Presentation is usually with cutaneous lesions that are polymorphic, but which, early on, are often typical palpable purpura. Systemic involvement may occur, with renal involvement being the most frequent and serious. Other organ/systems that may be affected include the joints, gastrointestinal, respiratory, and the central and peripheral nervous systems. Though death may occur from renal involvement,[543] in general, hypersensitivity vasculitis has a favorable outcome. Up to 25% of patients have pulmonary involvement,[375] but unfortunately descriptions of the radiologic changes have generally lacked detail and histologic material from the lungs has only rarely been available. The radiologic patterns described include air-space shadowing, which is often diffuse or perihilar[399, 543] and probably represents diffuse pulmonary hemorrhage[667]; bilateral basal consolidations on the basis of a hemorrhagic alveolitis[227]; fleeting consolidations[165]; unspecified nodular shadows[543, 667]; and linear interstitial opacities.[134]

Giant Cell Vasculitis

Giant cells are a recognized component of the cellular infiltrate of vasculitic processes and represent a nonspecific response to elastic tissue destruction. In two conditions, Takayasu arteritis (see Chapter 8) and temporal arteritis, the presence of giant cells is a prominent histologic feature.

Systemic Temporal Arteritis

Although this arteritis primarily affects branches of the carotid artery, it may also affect other arteries[359, 379, 467] including the pulmonary. There are few descriptions of radiologic changes in the chest, and their rarity raises the question that such findings may be purely incidental. Described findings include a diffuse interstitial pattern affecting the lower and upper zones, with bullae[227] and multiple nodules up to 3 cm in diameter, together with thick-walled cavities containing air-fluid levels.[54]

Other Giant Cell Arteritides

Patients are described with giant cell arteritis that do not fall into the classic clinicopathologic subgroups of Takayasu or temporal arteritis. Some have had pulmonary involvement including infarctive middle lobe consolidation with segmental pulmonary artery stenosis[645] and main pulmonary artery aneurysm.[147]

Behçet's Disease and Hughes-Stovin Syndrome

Behçet's disease is a rare, multisystem, chronic relapsing vasculitis considered to be secondary to immune complex deposition.[375] It is characterized by recurrent aphthous ulcerations of the mouth or genitalia together with erythema nodosum, various skin infections, and ocular lesions, notably uveitis, choroiditis, retinal vasculitis, and conjunctivitis. Almost one-half of the patients have arthropathy, and one-fifth show thrombophlebitis and neurologic manifestations, particularly meningoencephalitis.[93] Lesser degrees of involvement are described in other organs, including the cardiac, renal, and gastrointestinal systems. Behçet's disease occurs about twice as frequently in men as in women and presents most commonly in the 3rd decade of life.[94] Although worldwide in distribution, it occurs particularly in the Mediterranean, the Middle East, and Japan.

Histologically, the affected vessels show a leukocytoclastic vasculitis. Vasculitis leads to thrombosis, obstruction, aneurysm formation, and rupture of vessels. Arteries, capillaries, and veins of various sizes are affected. Pleuropulmonary involvement, which occurs in about 5% of patients,[141, 572] is usually heralded by hemoptysis, fever, pleuritic pain, or dyspnea. Hemoptysis is frequently a dominant and serious feature; in 40% of cases in one series it led to death.[175]

A variety of radiologic changes in the chest have been described.[75, 93, 141, 175, 269] These are best understood when correlated with the pathologic findings, which consist of (1) pulmonary hemorrhage from vessel rupture or vasculitis; (2) vessel occlusion, nearly always as a result of in situ thrombosis rather than embolism[93]; and (3) proximal pulmonary artery aneurysm.

Pulmonary hemorrhage probably accounts for the radiographically visible consolidations. Areas of consolidation may be focal (Fig 11–17), multifocal (unilateral or bilateral), or diffuse.[75, 269] Sometimes they are fleeting.[93] Some of the consolidations may represent pulmonary infarcts, since some have cavitated,[269] and in one patient at least, the recurrent consolidations were shown to result from pneumonia.[488] Nodular shadows, usually several centimeters in diameter, have also been a common finding. Some have had the appearance of a focal consolidation rather than a mass, some cavitate, and a number have been subpleural in location.[269] The cavitary nodules are almost certainly pulmonary infarcts.[141] They usually resolve in 3 to 9 months.[269] Basal band shadows, possibly also due to infarcts, have also been recorded.[175]

Vascular occlusions may result in hypovascular areas on the plain chest radiograph[269] and cause perfusion defects on radionuclide lung scanning. Just as in pulmonary embolism, these defects will show ventilation/perfusion mismatch.[244] The occlu-

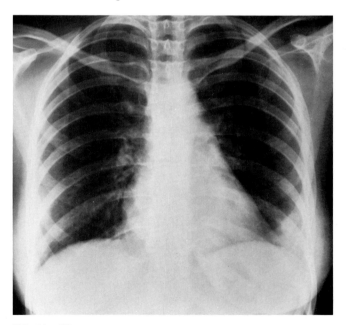

FIG 11–17.
Chest radiograph in a 27-year-old woman with known Behçet's syndrome and hemoptysis. There is an area of consolidation in the left costophrenic angle. It was probably due to pulmonary hemorrhage or infarction and cleared in 2 months without leaving a residuum.

sions have been demonstrated angiographically and are predominantly of lobar or segmental arteries.[269] When widespread, the occlusions can cause pulmonary arterial hypertension, which may be recognizable on the plain chest radiograph or at angiography.[244] Pulmonary artery aneurysms may be visible on plain chest radiographs. They occur in lobar or segmental arteries and are almost invariably proximal to an occlusion.[244] The aneurysms are demonstrable at angiography though, on occasion, thrombus within the aneurysm itself may make it difficult to detect; CT scanning may have an advantage in this situation.[244] Resolution of occlusions and aneurysms has been demonstrated after therapy with steroids and heparin.[269]

Pleural effusions are sometimes present, and these may be serous or bloody. Most are probably secondary to pulmonary infarcts,[269] but some are hemothoraces resulting from rupture of blood vessels.[141] A cavitated infarct in Behçet's disease is a reported cause of a hydropneumothorax.[269]

The Hughes-Stovin syndrome[324] manifests some, but not all, the features of Behçet's disease, and some consider it is a variant.[375] It is even more rare than Behçet's disease, most patients being young adult males in their 2nd to 4th decades (youngest, aged 12 years),[522] with at least one reported description of a female patient.[612] The major features are (1) one or more segmental pulmonary artery aneurysms, (2) pulmonary artery occlusions due to emboli or thrombi, and (3) systemic venous thrombi (limb veins, vena cava, cerebral sinuses). Common presentations are with venous thromboses, fever, or hemoptysis; the latter is caused by erosion of an aneurysm into an airway,[672] and is the major cause of death. Radiologic features are similar to those of Behçet's disease.

Polyangiitis Overlap Syndrome

Polyangiitis overlap syndrome is characterized by a systemic vasculitis with features that overlap the well-defined vasculitic syndromes.[375] In one series of 11 patients there was a pulmonary vasculitis in 54%.[375] Pleuropulmonary radiologic findings are those to be expected from the component conditions. Several overlaps have been reported of the Churg-Strauss syndrome and polyarteritis nodosa, the evidence for the latter being the presence of aneurysms of visceral vasculature. It is felt by some that splitting off such patients from the category of Churg-Strauss syndrome does not serve any useful purpose.[165]

COLLAGEN VASCULAR DISEASE
Rheumatoid Arthritis

Rheumatoid arthritis is a subacute or chronic inflammatory polyarthropathy of unknown cause that particularly affects peripheral joints. It is about three times more common in women than in men and usually has an insidious onset, pursuing a variable course that is typically one of relapses and remissions. The diagnosis of rheumatoid arthritis is based on the presence of certain clinical and laboratory features.[528]

In addition to an arthropathy, many patients have one or more extra-articular manifestations.[326] These tend to be seen in subjects who are seropositive, particularly with high rheumatoid factor titers,[326] and in patients with rheumatoid nodules. Eosinophilia is sometimes seen in rheumatoid arthritis and tends to be associated with vasculitis, pleuropericarditis, pulmonary fibrosis, and subcutaneous nodules.[665]

The association of pulmonary disease and rheumatoid disease was suggested as early as 1948,[180] and although some large early surveys failed to confirm a positive relationship,[634] it is now generally accepted that there are a number of positive associations.* Definite and probable associations are listed (Table 11-2).

Pleural Disease

Pleural involvement is probably the most common thoracic manifestation of rheumatoid disease.[536] At postmortem examination, there are pleural changes in some 50% of cases.[536] However, clinical pleural effusion is much less common, with a 3.3% prevalence in one large series[647] and an annual incidence of effusion of about 1% in patients with rheumatoid disease.[346] Unlike rheumatoid disease in general, but in common with other pulmonary manifestations of the disease, pleural effusion shows a striking preponderance of male patients,[648] and some quite sizable series have recorded virtually no women.[86] Patients are usually middle-aged, with a mean age of about 50 years.[648] The effusions in rheumatoid disease, unlike those seen in systemic lupus erythematosus, are commonly asymptomatic[325]; half the patients in the Mayo Clinic series had no symptoms.[86] When symptoms do occur, the more common are pleuritic pain, dyspnea, cough, and fever.[648]

Pleural effusions most commonly occur in the

*References 325, 326, 345, 571, 634, and 678.

TABLE 11—2.

Pleuropulmonary Lesions in Rheumatoid Disease

Pleural
    Pleuritis
    Effusion
    Empyema
    Bronchopleural fistula/pneumothorax
Fibrosing alveolitis
Parenchymal (necrobiotic) nodules
Caplan's syndrome
Pulmonary arteritis/hypertension
Other associations
    Bronchiolitis obliterans
    Bronchiectasis
    Upper zone fibrosis
    Bronchocentric granulomatosis
    Amyloidosis

setting of established disease and may develop more than 20 years after its onset. They may, however, develop simultaneously with the onset of arthritis or antedate the arthritis by several months.[86, 648, 653] In one series, 4% of effusions developed several months before the arthritis and 20% developed simultaneously with the onset of joint disease.[647] The arthritis in established disease sometimes undergoes an exacerbation as the pleural effusion develops.[78, 86, 346] Effusions are positively associated with the presence of cutaneous nodules in some 50% of patients[86, 648] and with pericarditis,[647] but not with the clinical or radiographic severity of the arthritis.[647] In about one-third of patients there will be other rheumatoid-related abnormalities on the chest radiograph such as fibrosing alveolitis or parenchymal nodules.[648]

Effusions are most commonly small to moderate in size (Fig 11—18),[648] though they can be large.[59] About one-fifth occur bilaterally.[648] Once formed, the effusions behave in a variable fashion, and although some resolve within weeks, more characteristicly they persist for months and indeed sometimes for several years.[648] Effusions may recur on the same or opposite sides of the chest.[400] Once the effusion has cleared, it commonly leaves residual pleural thickening.[86, 346] Fibrothorax and folded lung are recognized complications of rheumatoid pleural thickening[536] that may, on occasion, be severe enough to warrant decortication.[65, 647]

The diagnosis may be strongly suspected or established by the findings in the pleural fluid[536, 634] and sometimes by pleural biopsy which, although frequently nonspecific, may show rheumatoid nodules.[634] The pleural fluid is usually rich in protein and lymphocytes, pale yellow to yellow-green, and occasionally milky. Sometimes in the acute stage it is polymorph predominant and, occasionally, eosinophilic.[498] Its most characteristic features are its low sugar, low pH, and raised lactic dehydrogenase level. Rheumatoid factor is often present with immune complexes and decreased complement levels.

Rheumatoid patients are generally at risk from infection and may develop an empyema either de novo or on top of an established effusion.[155, 342] There are isolated reports of pneumothorax and pyopneumothorax in rheumatoid disease,[400] some associated with diffuse pulmonary fibrosis and others with cavitary nodules and bronchopleural fistula.[126, 139, 155, 567]

Fibrosing Alveolitis

Diffuse interstitial pulmonary fibrosis (IPF) (fibrosing alveolitis, interstitial pneumonitis) was first associated with rheumatoid arthritis by Ellman and Ball in 1948.[180] After the initial case reports, however, there were several large series which failed to show an increased prevalence of IPF in rheumatoid disease.[10, 587, 605] Because it is possible to overlook uncommon associations unless very large numbers are used,[634] it is useful to look at the frequency of the common condition (rheumatoid arthritis) in se-

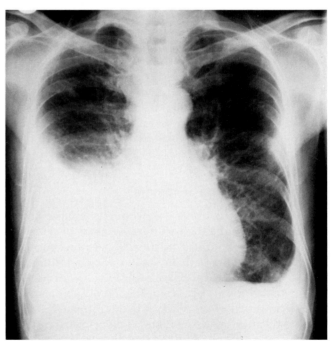

FIG 11—18.
Pleural effusion in rheumatoid disease. Bilateral pleural effusions are present with mild changes of fibrosing alveolitis. The effusions were painless, and that on the right had been present, more or less unchanged, for 5 months.

ries of the more uncommon disorder (IPF/fibrosing alveolitis). When looked at in this way, the prevalence is in the order of 10% to 20%.[159, 632, 634] In a large series of patients with rheumatoid arthritis, eight of the 516 patients (1.6%) had radiologic pulmonary fibrosis.[648]

Histologically, in the early stages, there is interstitial thickening with a lymphocyte and plasma cell rich infiltrate that is replaced by fibrosis and may go on to an end-stage lung pattern.[351] Lymphoid aggregates with germinal centers are commonly seen, and although nonspecific, they are very suggestive of rheumatoid lung. Sometimes the histologic appearance is that of desquamative interstitial pneumonitis.[634]

Rheumatoid IPF is twice as common in men as in women[634]; the mean age of onset is about 50 years.[648] Most cases of alveolitis occurred after the onset of the arthritis, though some 15% to 30% occur before or coincident with the initial joint manifestations.[634, 648] In general, whichever develops first, the gap between the onset of the two conditions is not more than 5 years.[55, 634] Respiratory symptoms can be absent despite radiologic changes[484, 648] but, if present, consist chiefly of exertional dyspnea and cough. The severity and pattern of joint involvement does not differ from that seen generally in rheumatoid arthritis,[634, 648] but an exacerbation of joint symptoms may occur with the onset of alveolitis.[55] The principal physical signs are basal crackles and finger clubbing. It is generally stated that there is a high prevalence of associated subcutaneous nodules,[325] but figures from various series vary considerably, from 75%[621, 648] to 15%,[634] and some consider that the prevalence of subcutaneous nodules is no different from that seen in the general rheumatoid population.[497] Respiratory function tests usually show restriction with impaired carbon monoxide transfer and evidence of hypoxemia at rest or on exercise.[325] Serum rheumatoid factor is elevated in more than two-thirds of patients with alveolitis.[621, 634, 648]

The chest radiograph shows changes that are indistinguishable from cryptogenic fibrosing alveolitis (Fig 11–19) (see p. 467) namely, interstitial shadows. These are largely symmetric and basally predominant,[390] though they can involve all zones[634] and are occasionally midzone predominant.[648] There is a fine nodular pattern, either rounded (q) or irregular (t).[634] When the nodulation is very fine, there is diffuse loss of transradiency giving a "ground-glass" appearance.[390] These small opacities, at least initially, make the vascular shadows appear more prominent, although eventually the vessels become

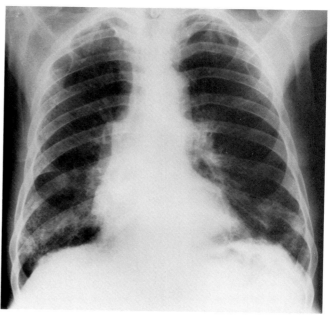

FIG 11–19.
Fibrosing alveolitis in rheumatoid disease. Bilateral basal shadowing consists mainly of small irregular and rounded nodules. The appearances are indistinguishable from other varieties of fibrosing alveolitis.

obscured. Sometimes in the early stage of the alveolitis, there is also evidence of air-space shadowing (soft fluffy opacities).[55] Later on, the reticulonodular pattern becomes coarser and more widespread (Fig 11–20), and honeycomb shadows may appear.[390] Septal lines (Kerley A and B lines) are not features of rheumatoid alveolitis, though the occasional B line will be seen.[390] As fibrosis advances, there is a tendency for lung volume to be lost, a situation reflected in elevation of the diaphragm.[220] Pleural effusion or thickening may coexist with interstitial changes in about 5% to 15% of cases (see Fig 11–18).[634, 648] Cases have been described with interstitial shadowing accompanied by both pleural effusion and intrapulmonary nodules.[613]

Alveolitis in rheumatoid disease probably carries as poor a prognosis as it does in the cryptogenic form,[634] although some authors think it is less severe.[325] In one series, the mean duration of lung disease to death was 5 years, with a range of 1 to 17 years.[634] Treatment with steroids or immunosuppressants helps a proportion of the patients, at least in the short term.[634]

Intrapulmonary Nodules

The third well-recognized pleuropulmonary abnormality associated with rheumatoid disease is the

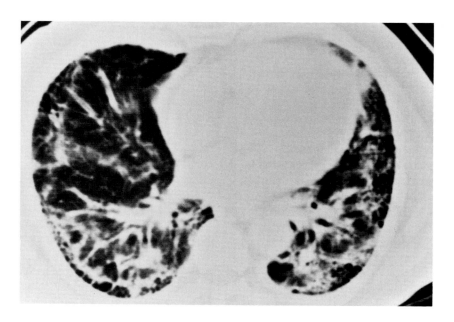

FIG 11–20.
Rheumatoid disease with fibrosing alveolitis. A CT scan through the lower zones in this patient shows multiple bandlike and conglomerate opacities, presumably representing fibrosis, together with a variety of air spaces. Some of these probably represent parasep-tal emphysema and others bullae. There is a tendency for the maximum changes to be peripheral, as with other forms of fibrosing alveolitis.

intrapulmonary (necrobiotic) nodule. These nodules are pathologically identical to subcutaneous nodules[634] and consist of a necrotic center bounded by palisading histiocytes (epithelioid cells) and surrounded by plasma cells and lymphocytes. Peripherally there may be a moderate, nonnecrotizing vasculitis. These lesions need to be distinguished from infectious and noninfectious angiitides and granulomatoses, including Wegener's granulomatosis.[351]

Intrapulmonary nodules are rare; two large series of 955 patients contained no examples[10, 484]; another contained only two cases in 516 patients.[648] Nodules, like pleural effusions and IPF, are more common in men than in women, with about a twofold excess. Mean patient age at presentation is 51 years (range, 24 to 64 years).[476] Nodules usually occur in patients with established disease but may occur with or before the onset of arthritis,[634] as did some 27% of nodules reported by Eraut and coworkers.[190] Should nodules antedate arthritis, the gap is often less than a year,[190, 498, 548] but intervals of up to 11 years are also described.[190] In addition, there are patients with histologically proved necrobiotic nodules followed for 26 years who have failed to develop arthritis. Such nodules are a diagnostic dilemma, since circulating rheumatoid factor is usually absent.[190]

Nodules are usually asymptomatic, but there may be cough or hemoptysis, particularly if a lesion should cavitate.[476] Occasionally, symptoms result from infection,[70] bronchopleural fistula formation, or pneumothorax.[498] Discounting cases in which nodules antedate arthritis, pulmonary necrobiotic nodules usually occur in the context of established and advanced disease,[220] and there are subcutaneous nodules in 80%.[400, 476, 648] Serum rheumatoid factor is found in nearly 90% of patients with nodules,[400, 476] though early on it may be absent or present in low titer.[476] Blood eosinophilia is reported in some cases.[498, 574]

The nodules are usually radiologically discrete, rounded, or occasionally slightly lobulated and subpleural (Fig 11–21).[593] They may be single or, in about three-quarters of patients, they are multiple[648] and show some mid/upper zone predilection (see Fig 11–21).[190] They range in size from a few millimeters[648] to 7 cm. Occasionally when the nodules are small and widely disseminated, a miliary pattern is produced.[400] In about 50% of cases, the nodules cavitate,[400, 648] producing ring opacities with relatively smooth thick walls (Fig 11–22).[220, 390, 400] Occasionally, nodules calcify.[390, 395] Subpleural nodules may erode through the pleura and cause a bronchopleural fistula and hydropneumothorax.[139, 313, 400] Rib erosion by a nodule is rare, but has been described as giving an appearance that resembles an invasive carcinoma.[290] Pleural thickening or effusion is present in 40% to 50% of cases with intrapulmonary

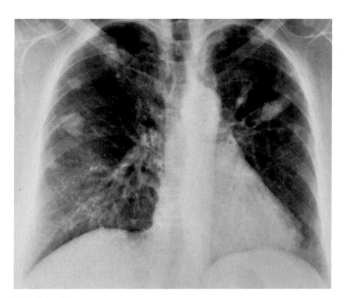

FIG 11–21.
Parenchymal nodules in rheumatoid disease. The patient is a 57-year-old woman with long-standing rheumatoid disease and subcutaneous nodules. The chest radiograph shows multiple 4- to 25-mm nodules distributed bilaterally in the mid and upper zones. The nodules are relatively well demarcated round, oval, or lobulated and had remained essentially unchanged for 6 months. Their distribution and indolent behavior are typical.

nodules.[400, 648] Likewise, alveolitis and pulmonary nodules can coexist.[400] Nodular lesions may increase in size and number, resolve completely, or remain stable for many years[648]; at other times, they wax and wane with the activity of subcutaneous nodules and arthritis.[444, 498]

Caplan's Syndrome

The original description of Caplan's syndrome was of multiple, large (0.5 to 5.0 cm in diameter), rounded nodules seen on the chest radiographs of coal miners with rheumatoid arthritis.[81] Radiographic evidence of simple coal worker's pneumoconiosis was often absent. Since this time the features of the syndrome have been extended to include: (1) individuals exposed to inorganic agents other than silica or coal; (2) those with serologic but not clinical rheumatoid disease; and (3) patients with radiologic patterns other than large nodules.[83] In affected patients, clinical rheumatoid disease may occur before, with, or after the pulmonary changes.[81, 428] Caplan's syndrome—based on broad criteria—has been described with exposure to asbestos,[443, 518, 611] aluminum,[344] dolomite,[7] silica,* and carbon.[654]

Caplan nodules are pathologically similar to

*References 79, 82, 98, 133, 294, and 506.

necrobiotic rheumatoid nodules: a necrotic center surrounded by a cuff of cellular infiltrate consisting of macrophages and polymorphonuclear leucocytes, fibroblasts, and giant cells.[262] Some of the macrophages contain dust, and on macroscopic section these give the characteristic annular ring pattern that distinguishes the Caplan nodules from ordinary rheumatoid nodules. Fibroblasts adjacent to the necrotic area show palisading, which is also a striking feature of subcutaneous rheumatoid nodules. Although the pathogenesis of Caplan's syndrome is incompletely understood, it is apparent that the development of rheumatoid factor seems to be associated with a modified tissue response in coal dust–induced lung disease.[634]

The prevalence rate of Caplan's syndrome in a population of more than 21,000 miners in the United Kingdom, according to the broad criteria,[385] was about 2.5 cases per 1,000 subjects without pneumoco-

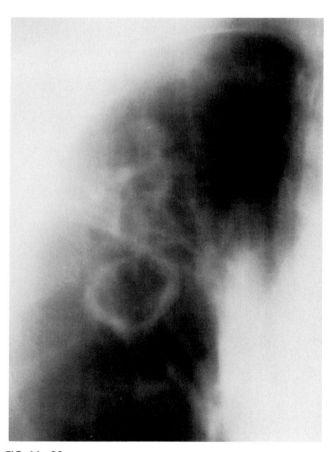

FIG 11–22.
Parenchymal nodules in a patient with rheumatoid disease. Linear tomogram of the right upper zone shows a cluster of nodules that have cavitated. The lowest nodule is 3 cm in diameter with a wall that varies from 1 to 6 mm in thickness.

niosis and between 22 and 62 cases per 1,000 subjects with pneumoconiosis. For an unexplained reason, the prevalence in the United States appears to be low,[479] and no cases were found in a series of 100 Pennsylvania miners with rheumatoid arthritis.[30]

The classic radiologic finding in Caplan's syndrome is bilateral pulmonary nodules, usually 1 to 2 cm in diameter, but ranging from 0.5 to 5 cm (Fig 11–23).[81] Nodules are typically situated at the junction of the outer and middle thirds of the lung and tend to appear in crops of lesions having a similar size and rate of growth.[428] Nodules are not necessarily bilateral, and in one series one-fifth were unilateral.[385] Nodules tend to develop rapidly and grow over a period of months. They then often remain stable or grow slowly for several years. Established nodules occasionally heal by fibrosis and give a stellate scarlike shadow. In East Midlands, United Kingdom coal miners, about 10% of subjects with Caplan's syndrome developed calcification (7/55) or cavitation (4/55) of the nodules.[385] Radiologic changes of coal worker's pneumoconiosis may or may not be present and are not a striking feature. In the original series, in 45% of patients, the radiographic

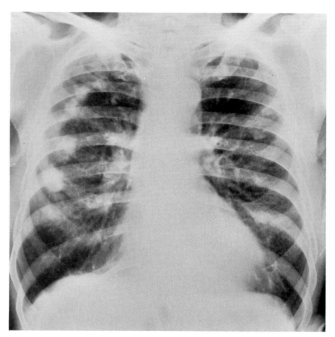

FIG 11–23.
Rheumatoid disease with Caplan's syndrome. This 61-year-old coal miner has multiple peripheral nodules, the majority being on the right. They range between 1 and 2 cm in diameter. Changes of coal worker's pneumoconiosis are characteristically mild. (Courtesy of Dr. P.M. Hacking, Newcastle upon Tyne.)

changes of coal worker's pneumoconiosis were category I or less.[81]

Other radiographic findings are now included in the wider concept of Caplan's syndrome. The most common are (1) 0.3- to 1.0-cm rounded opacities ranging from just a few confined to one lung zone to a "snowstorm" appearance,[83] and (2) mixed nodular and irregular opacities with no background of simple pneumoconiosis.[83]

Pulmonary Arteritis/Hypertension

Systemic vasculitis in rheumatoid disease is usually of the hypersensitivity type and affects chiefly the skin. The lung is rarely involved in a rheumatoid systemic vasculitis,[562] and there are only a few reported cases.* In most of these cases the only radiographic finding has been enlargement of the heart and proximal pulmonary arteries. Although pulmonary arterial hypertension may be due to a vasculitis, it is much more likely to be due to rheumatoid-associated fibrosing alveolitis.[634]

There are also a few case reports of pulmonary consolidations either proved[9] or assumed to be the result of a vasculitis.[26, 395]

Other Associations

There is a recognized association between rheumatoid disease and bronchiolitis obliterans (see Fig 11–24).[238, 310, 395, 409] About half the patients have been on penicillamine therapy, and a cause-and-effect relationship has been proposed.[187, 451]

About ten patients with rheumatoid disease are reported with apical fibrosis and cavitation giving rise to a radiologic appearance that resembles tuberculosis.[395, 396, 487, 598, 679] In some of these patients the pathologic finding reported has been that of confluent necrobiotic nodules.[679]

There is postmortem and clinical evidence that bronchitis and bronchiectasis are more frequent in patients with rheumatoid disease than in matched controls.[10, 646] Thus, in a controlled study, bronchiectasis was ten times more common in patients with rheumatoid disease than in controls with degenerative joint disease.[646] In another review of 13 patients with clinical bronchiectasis and rheumatoid disease, it was noted that bronchiectasis developed after the onset of arthritis in more than half the patients and that hypogammaglobulinemia was present in a number of cases.[118]

A handful of patients with rheumatoid disease have had biopsy proved bronchocentric granuloma-

*References 236, 343, 354, 390, 464, and 644.

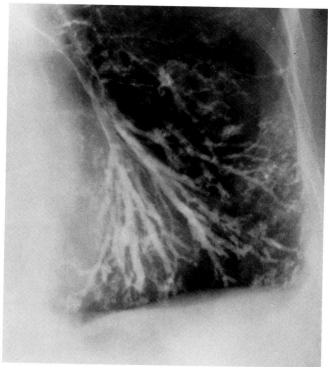

FIG 11–24.
Rheumatoid disease with bronchiolitis obliterans. The patient was a 56-year-old woman whose main complaint was progressive exertional dyspnea. This bronchogram of the left lower lobe shows mild failure of airway tapering and a striking lack of filling of small airways. The patient had not received penicillamine. Pleural thickening is also present.

tosis (see p. 518).[33, 46, 299] Radiologically there were bilateral nodules and focal consolidations ranging in size from 2 to 15 cm, some of which were cavitated.

Systemic Lupus Erythematosus

Systemic lupus erythematosus (SLE) is a multisystem collagen vascular disease characterized by widespread inflammatory changes, particularly in the vessels, serosa, and skin. A characteristic feature is autoantibody production against a wide variety of cellular constituents including nuclear material, particularly deoxyribonucleic acid (DNA). Because the manifestations of the disease are so variable, diagnostic criteria have been drawn up (Table 11–3). Should any four of the criteria be present simultaneously or serially during a period of observation, then SLE can be diagnosed.

The prevalence of the various clinical manifestations in four series[100] was arthropathy, 85%; skin lesions, 80%; nephritis, 53%; pleurisy, 52%; neuropsychiatric disorders, 44%; lymphadenopathy, 43%;

pericarditis, 39%; and mucosal ulceration, 15%. The illness characteristically shows relapses and remissions, with a tendency to progression and eventual multiorgan dysfunction.[100] It is ten times as common in women as in men,[403] and there is an increased prevalence among relatives and blacks. It presents typically during the childbearing period with a wide variety of manifestations, particularly those of joint, skin, and systemic disorders.[168] The reported prognosis has greatly improved over the years, in part due to better therapy but also because subclinical cases have been included in the various studies. In a recent series, the 5-year survival was 98%, and 10-year survival was 89%.[270]

Thoracic involvement is common in SLE, and the lungs, pleura, heart, diaphragm, and intercostal muscles may be affected.[629] The thoracic manifestations (Table 11–4) can be divided into primary changes or secondary complications, but this distinction is by no means always clear-cut. Cardiac and pericardial disease have been recently reviewed[96] and will only be briefly considered here. The lungs and pleura are involved more frequently in SLE than in any other collagen vascular disease,[325] with 50% to 70% of patients developing pleuropulmonary manifestations in the course of the disease.[270, 291, 316, 325, 536] Only 5%, however, will have such changes at presentation.[191, 291, 495]

Primary manifestations

Pleuritis/Pleural Effusion.—Pleuritis is found in 40% to 60% of patients with SLE.[168, 191, 291] It

TABLE 11–3.

Criteria for Diagnosis of Systemic Lupus Erythematosus*

Malar rash
Discoid lupus erythematosus
Photosensitivity
Ulceration of mouth/oropharynx
Arthropathy (nonerosive, nondeforming)
Serositis
Renal disorder (proteinuria or cellular casts)
Neurologic disorder (epilepsy or psychosis)
Hematologic disorder (hemolytic anemia
  or leukopenia or lymphopenia or
  thrombocytopenia)
Immunologic disorder (positive LE cell
  preparation, or antibody to native DNA
  or S$_m$ nuclear antigen, or false positive
  test for syphilis)
Antinuclear antibody

*Modified from Tan EM, Cohen AS, Fries JF, et al: The 1982 revised criteria for the classification of systemic lupus erythematosus. *Arthritis Rheum* 1982; 25:1271–1277.

TABLE 11–4.

Thoracic Manifestations of Systemic Lupus Erythematosus

Primary
 Pleuritis/pleural effusion
 (Acute) lupus pneumonitis
 Fibrosing alveolitis
 Pulmonary hemorrhage
 Diaphragm dysfunction
 Pulmonary arterial hypertension/vasculitis
 Rarities
  Lupus anticoagulant pulmonary embolism
  Lymphocytic pneumonitis/pseudolymphoma
  Bronchiolitis obliterans

Secondary
 Atelectasis
 Pneumonia (simple, opportunistic)
 Cardiac failure/pericarditis
 Renal failure/nephrotic syndrome
 Drug-induced changes

may be a presenting feature[668] but occurs more commonly during an exacerbation of established disease.[325]

The pleuritis is dry 50% of the time,[378] but in the other 50% it is accompanied by a pleural effusion and sometimes also by pericardial effusion (Fig 11–25).[629] Aspirated pleural fluid is usually a clear exudate with white blood cells (granulocytes early on and lymphocytes later) and normal levels of sugar; it often contains antinuclear antibodies. The pleural effusions are usually small or moderate in size[256] but are, on rare occasions, large.[264] Unilateral and bilateral effusions are found with equal frequency.[68, 256, 608, 668] Pleural adhesions are common[608]; therefore, the border of the pleural fluid on chest radiographs may be irregularly angulated. Sometimes the pleural effusions resolve spontaneously, but many require treatment with steroids or immunosuppressive drugs. Clearing may be complete or incomplete, leaving minor pleural thickening.[68, 668] It must be remembered that there are many other causes of pleural effusion in SLE—including the nephrotic syndrome, cardiac and renal failure, pulmonary embolism, and pneumonia.[293, 536] The fact that pleural effusions in SLE are almost always painful[256, 378] is a helpful differentiating feature.

Significant pleural thickening[28] is a nonspecific and common finding at autopsy, being present in 40% to 60% of cases.[274, 432] It is not often recorded as a radiologic finding, probably because of underreporting. It was, however, seen in 12% of patients in one series.[270] Pneumothorax is not a feature of pleuropulmonary SLE.

(Acute) Lupus Pneumonitis.—Pulmonary consolidations in patients with SLE can result from a va-

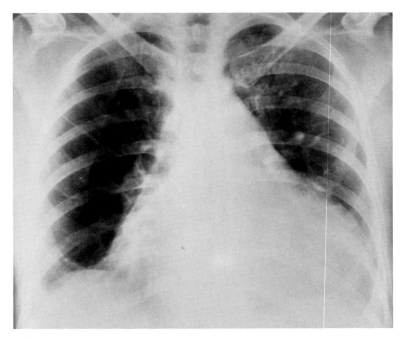

FIG 11–25.
SLE. Chest radiograph shows characteristic appearance, namely a grossly enlarged heart due to a pericardial effusion and small bilateral pleural effusions.

riety of causes including pneumonia, pulmonary edema, pulmonary hemorrhage, and pulmonary infarction. In a small proportion of cases, the consolidation is due to acute lupus pneumonitis. The diagnosis of acute lupus pneumonitis is made in patients with fever, tachypnea, and radiographic consolidation if there is no evidence for one of the other causes of consolidation and if the consolidation responds to steroid therapy. With such poorly defined clinical criteria, it is not surprising that the true incidence of lupus pneumonitis is uncertain. Reports vary from 1% to 12%, with an average of about 4%.[168, 191, 270, 378, 406] In a selected group of 30 patients with *pleuropulmonary* SLE, about one-fifth had probable acute lupus pneumonitis.[318] Histologically, there is diffuse alveolar damage with interstitial edema and inflammation together with intra-alveolar exudation and hyaline membrane formation.[351]

The chest radiograph most commonly shows one or more areas of consolidation, usually bilateral and basal, but sometimes unilateral.[270, 378, 406] A mixed alveolar and interstitial pattern with nodules has also been described.[378] The consolidations are often accompanied by pleural effusions[406] and are sometimes migratory.[332] Cavitation is rare and suggests pneumonia or infarction. Most, but not all patients, respond dramatically to steroids,[325] with complete or partial clearance. In the latter instance, persisting radiographic shadowing often has an interstitial pattern[406] and may be accompanied by a diffusion defect and restrictive abnormality on lung function testing.

Fibrosing Alveolitis.—Fibrosing alveolitis (Fig 11–26) is generally regarded as an unusual manifestation of SLE.[325] However, chronic interstitial infiltrates were present on histologic examination in just over one-third of cases in four autopsy series.[432] In clinical series, diffuse interstitial fibrosis has been notable by its absence.[220] Nevertheless, four patients with pleuropulmonary SLE in a selected group of 30 had radiographic evidence of fibrosing alveolitis (confirmed by biopsy in two)[318]; and in an unselected series of out-patients with SLE, there was a 3% prevalence of pulmonary fibrosis as judged radiologically.[178]

Pulmonary Hemorrhage.—Pulmonary hemorrhage is common in the lungs at postmortem examination in patients with SLE[432] but is not often recognized clinically, only 23 cases having been reported

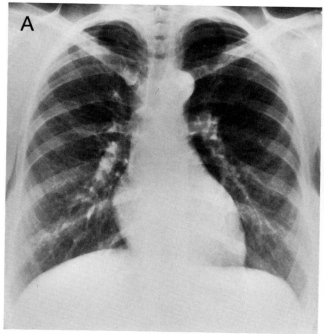

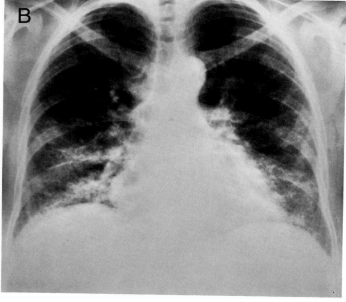

FIG 11–26.
SLE in a 35-year-old woman. **A,** normal PA chest radiograph antedating symptoms. **B,** 4 years later the patient had developed SLE and progressive exertional dyspnea. The chest radiograph now shows bilateral basal reticulonodular and ground-glass opacities consistent with fibrosing alveolitis. In the interval the diaphragm has become elevated. This could be related to decreased lung compliance subsequent to the alveolitis or to diaphragmatic myopathy.

up to 1984.[373] In a large series of more than 400 patients with SLE at the National Institutes of Health, the prevalence of pulmonary hemorrhage was only about 1.5%.[84] On very rare occasions, it may be the mode of presentation of SLE.[73] Pulmonary hemorrhage carries a 70% mortality[373] and is an important diagnosis to make since urgent treatment is needed.[628] The pathogenesis is complex. All of the following factors have been implicated: pulmonary infection; cardiac and renal failure; thrombocytopenia; and, in particular, immune complex deposition in capillaries.[84, 293, 629] Clinically, most patients have rapid onset of severe dyspnea, fever, and hemoptysis, with crepitations on auscultation. Hemorrhage is typically accompanied by signs of active disease elsewhere: fever; arthropathy; and nephritis.[172] Although some patients are in renal failure, this need not be the case.[84, 172] Helpful clinical pointers include hemoptysis and a drop in blood hemoglobin level. Confirmation can be obtained by finding hemosiderin-laden macrophages in the sputum[234] or a rise in carbon monoxide uptake in the lung.[193]

The radiographic appearances are nonspecific. They resemble those of Goodpasture's syndrome (see p. 502) and consist of air-space shadowing that is usually bilateral and diffuse. This results in a variety of patterns: multiple acinar nodules; homogeneous, ill-defined, coalescent patchy shadows; and lobar or segmental consolidations with air bronchograms.[172] The shadowing usually clears within days.[493]

Diaphragm Dysfunction.—Diaphragm dysfunction in SLE may be manifest as elevation of one or both hemidiaphragms and is a cause of dyspnea. Bilateral elevation is a common finding and, in some series, has been the most common radiologic pleuropulmonary abnormality, being seen in as many as 18% of patients (see Fig 11–26).[270] As the diaphragm rises, the lungs lose volume, hence the term "shrinking lungs,"[316] a finding first noted in 1954.[181, 291, 628] The loss of lung volume was initially ascribed to reduction in lung compliance, but it has recently been shown to be due to diaphragmatic weakness presumed to be caused by a myopathy.[243, 401] Pleuritic pain with splinting is an uncommon contributory factor.[243] Treatment with steroids can reverse the process.[493]

Pulmonary Arterial Hypertension/Vasculitis.—A variety of changes are described pathologically in the pulmonary arteries.[200, 351] Chronic lesions consist of intimal thickening, medial hypertrophy, and peri-advential fibrosis. Acute lesions of vasculitis and fibrinoid necrosis are generally regarded as unusual,[293] but a frequency of up to 20% in SLE[200, 274] has been recorded in some autopsy series. Pulmonary arterial hypertension is very uncommon,[629] many reports consisting of small numbers of cases.[13, 364, 493] Some cases of pulmonary arterial hypertension have been associated with the presence of lupus anticoagulant, which predisposes to thrombosis and may be pathogenetically important.[13] Other cases have had features that suggest they would be better classified as an overlap syndrome such as mixed connective tissue disease.[629]

Rarities.—A number of case reports have recorded rare associations with SLE:

1. Pulmonary embolism[42] has been recognized in patients with SLE who have circulating lupus anticoagulant. This antibody is also associated with livedo reticularis, recurrent abortion, and labile hypertension.
2. Lymphocytic interstitial pneumonitis and pseudolymphoma.[493, 680]
3. Obliterative bronchiolitis. This is described pathologically in a few cases[358] without clearly related radiologic changes.

Secondary Manifestations

Atelectasis.—Elevation of the diaphragm may be associated with basal line or band shadows that are usually horizontal, several millimeters wide, and up to 5 or so centimeters long. These shadows are often transient, and it seems most likely that they represent discoid or plate atelectasis,* though some could be due to pulmonary infarcts.[629] There is, in fact, postmortem evidence that pulmonary infarcts are very uncommon and, in two large autopsy series of 138 patients with SLE,[293, 432] they are not recorded. Discoid or plate atelectasis is common following upper abdominal surgery when the diaphragm is elevated and moves poorly, and it seems likely that a similar mechanism is operating in SLE.[325]

Pneumonia.—This is probably the single most common pleuropulmonary abnormality in SLE,[325] occurring in about 50% of patients.[274, 293, 432] Most cases are simple bacterial pneumonias, including tuberculosis, but a few are opportunistic infections.[293] The responsible organisms that have been recorded

---

*References 220, 263, 270, 318, 378, and 608.

include *Cytomegalovirus, Legionella, Pneumocystis, Cryptococcus, Aspergillus,* and *Nocardia.*[84, 293, 378, 432, 629] Cavitary lesions, which are uncommon in SLE, are most often the result of infections.[259, 503, 659]

Pericarditis, Myocarditis, and Renal Disease.— Twenty to thirty percent of all SLE patients develop pericarditis at some time (see Fig 11–25).[96] A reliable figure for myocarditis is not available but is probably in the order of 8%.[168, 191] Myocarditis, however, rarely gives rise to cardiac failure. Renal failure and the nephrotic syndrome may cause pulmonary edema (Fig 11–27) and pleural effusion. The pleural effusions, unlike those due to lupus pleuritis, are pain-free.

Drug-Induced Systemic Lupus Erythematosus

At least 30 drugs can cause an SLE syndrome that differs from the idiopathic variety in that patients are older and without sex or racial predilection. Also renal and central nervous system involvement are rare, and there is restricted antibody specificity.[289] The drugs most frequently implicated are hydralazine and procainamide and, less commonly, isoniazid, chlorpromazine, phenytoin, and *d*-penicillamine.[376] Prolonged and usually high dose drug therapy is associated with a lupus-like syndrome in some 10% of patients taking hydralazine and in 20%

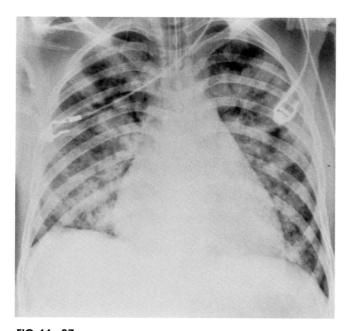

FIG 11–27.
SLE. Chest radiograph shows diffuse patchy air-space shadowing consistent with edema in a patient with an acute nephritic syndrome secondary to SLE.

taking procainamide.[289] Evidence of toxicity usually appears within a couple of years of beginning therapy, but it may be seen within a month or as late as 5 years. Pleuropulmonary involvement occurs in 25% to 30% of those with hydralazine-induced SLE; the percentage is slightly higher in those taking procainamide.[289] Radiologic changes are similar to those in idiopathic SLE.[14]

Polymyositis and Dermatomyositis

Polymyositis (PM) and dermatomyositis (DM) are diffuse inflammatory myopathies of striated muscle. Additionally, in DM there are characteristic skin changes. Several subgroups are identified and these may be classified as in Table 11–5.[43]

Female patients outnumber male about 2:1,[325] and most present at between 40 and 60 years of age, with a second smaller peak in the 5- to 15-year-old age group.[43] Clinical presentation may be with an acute, subacute, or chronic illness[322] characterized by a progressive, symmetric weakness of the girdle and neck muscles. In the acute disease, muscle pain and tenderness are common, and there may also be pharyngeal and respiratory symptoms.[322] In dermatomyositis, additional and characteristic skin changes are present: heliotrope periorbital rash, and violaceous/red papular rash over bony prominences. Associated findings, particularly in the subacute form, include arthropathy, dysphagia, pulmonary disease, and cardiac disease.[77] Five major diagnostic criteria have been suggested, and all should be present to make a definite diagnosis of DM or, if the skin changes are not present, of PM.[43] These criteria are listed in Table 11–6.

Pulmonary involvement is quite common in PM/DM and may occur in up to 50% of patients.[153] It is an important determinant of the clinical course and contributes directly to death in some 10% of patients.[153]

The chest manifestations of PM and DM take on

TABLE 11–5.
Classification of Polymyositis and Dermatomyositis*

Primary, idiopathic polymyositis
Primary, idiopathic dermatomyositis
Polymyositis/dermatomyositis in association with:
    Neoplasia
    Other collagen vascular disorders (overlap
    syndrome)
Polymyositis/dermatomyositis of childhood

*Data from Bohan A, Peter JB: Polymyositis and dermatomyositis. *N Engl J Med* 1975; 292:344–347; 403–407.

TABLE 11–6.
Criteria for Diagnosis of Polymyositis and Dermatomyositis*

Proximal muscle weakness (symmetric, present weeks/months)
Muscle biopsy (necrobiotic and inflammatory change)
Raised serum creatine phosphokinase
Characteristic electromyograph
Characteristic skin rash

*Data from Bohan A, Peter JB: Polymyositis and dermatomyositis. *N Engl J Med* 1975; 292:344–347; 403–407.

a variety of forms: (1) features that are primary to the disease, namely fibrosing alveolitis and, rarely, isolated pulmonary arterial hypertension or diaphragmatic elevation; (2) features that are secondary to muscular dysfunction, namely aspiration pneumonia, simple pneumonia, underinflation, and atelectasis; and (3) predisposing conditions, namely lung carcinoma.

Primary Manifestations

Fibrosing Alveolitis (Interstitial Pneumonitis).—This was first described in DM in 1956 by Mills and Mathews.[434] It is now a well-recognized association[619] that occurs in 5% to 10% of patients.[153, 222, 541] It has been reported slightly more commonly with PM than with DM.[77] Fibrosing alveolitis tends to be associated with joint involvement[560] and, as with alveolitis in other collagen vascular disease, pulmonary change on the chest radiograph can be the first clinical manifestation, even preceding the myositis,[169, 466, 560] although the usual pattern is for the fibrosis to follow soon after the onset of muscle weakness. Biopsy and respiratory function tests are more sensitive than the chest radiograph in the detection of interstitial pneumonitis, and it is possible to have histologic involvement when the plain radiograph shows a normal appearing lung.[153] The clinical manifestations vary greatly. At one extreme is an acute, rapidly fatal illness resistant to therapy[204] in which the muscle disease can be masked by respiratory involvement. At the other is a benign, indolent, and asymptomatic form.[583] It is generally considered that the pneumonitis of PM/DM is more steroid-responsive than that of progressive systemic sclerosis.[325] About half the patients respond with lessening of dyspnea, clearing of the chest radiograph, and improvement in lung function tests.[153, 561]

The radiology is the same as that of cryptogenic fibrosing alveolitis, with symmetric, basally predominant reticulonodular shadowing (Fig 11–28).[222, 561] The more acute cases may show areas of air-space opacities[222] or even widespread ground-glass shadowing superimposed on a reticulonodular background.[153] There is some evidence that the alveolar pattern is due to an organizing pneumonia with bronchiolitis obliterans and alveolar desquamation in addition to the interstitial pneumonitis.[561] Alveolar opacities tend to occur early in the course of lung disease and are more likely to be steroid-responsive. In time, pulmonary shadowing can progress to involve the whole lung, and small circular transradiancies may form (honeycombing),[327, 541, 561] giving the appearance of an end-stage lung. Although pleural inflammatory changes and fibrosis together with small effusions are common pathologically,[561] they have not been described radiologically. The same applies to multifocal dystrophic ossification, which has been demonstrated pathologically[561] but not radiographically. Adenocarcinoma secondary to scarring has not been recorded in PM/DM alveolitis.[153]

Pulmonary arterial hypertension produces large main proximal pulmonary arteries on a chest radiograph. Such hypertension may be seen as a complication of alveolitis[169] or hypoventilation,[212] but it is virtually unrecorded as an isolated thoracic manifestation.[69]

Diaphragmatic Myositis.—When the diaphragm becomes involved in the myositis, functional and radiographic changes are produced similar to those seen with the diaphragmatic myopathy of SLE.

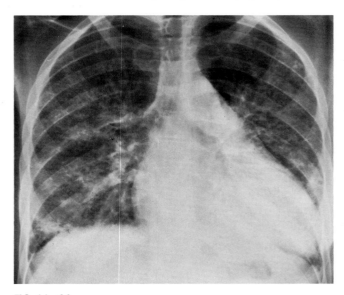

FIG 11–28.
Dermatomyositis. The radiograph of a 21-year-old woman with dermatomyositis shows a large heart secondary to a myocarditis and diffuse reticulonodular shadowing with apical sparing due to fibrosing alveolitis.

Characteristically the myopathy produces bilateral hemidiaphragm elevation, reduced lung volume, and discoid basal atelectasis.[153, 556]

Secondary Manifestations

Aspiration pneumonia is probably the most common finding on chest radiographs in PM/DM. In one series, nearly one-third of patients had radiographic evidence of pneumonia at some stage, and half of these cases were thought to be due to aspiration.[153] Aspiration is caused by cough impairment, pharyngeal dysfunction, and general weakness of body movements. Pharyngeal dysfunction is probably the most important factor, and most patients who aspirate are dysphagic.[153] Since PM/DM affects striated muscle, the upper esophagus and pharynx are selectively involved. These structures are normally closed at rest, but in PM/DM they are hypotonic and often contain air on plain radiographs. A barium swallow will demonstrate vallecular and pyriform pooling, defective bolus propulsion, defective pharyngeal emptying, nasopharyngeal reflux, and tracheal aspiration.[276, 425, 465]

Other pneumonias may be due to compromised defences secondary to muscle weakness and impaired cough.[57, 153] Opportunistic infections have been described in PM/DM, but they are not a common feature.[153]

Underinflation and atelectasis may result from respiratory muscle weakness coupled with stiff lungs and increased chest wall compliance. These factors produce small-volume lungs with diaphragmatic elevation and atelectasis, which is often basal and discoid.[57, 153, 220]

Carcinoma Lung and Polymyositis/Dermatomyositis

There is a five-fold to seven-fold increase in the frequency of malignant disease in PM/DM,[20] especially in older patients. The average prevalence in various series is about 16%,[77] with evidence that the association is almost twice as strong with DM as it is with PM.[76] The carcinomas recorded most commonly in one review were breast, 17%; lung, 15%; ovary, 10%; uterus, 8%; colon, 8%; and stomach, 7%.[77] These figures showed proportionately more carcinoma of the ovary and stomach than expected, but less colonic carcinoma. PM/DM may precede, accompany, or follow the carcinoma. One series found equal numbers in each group,[77] although others have found only 10% of cases to be synchronous.[20] Using Callen's data,[76] one can estimate there is about a 1% to 2% chance that the chest radiograph will show a previously unrecognized lung carcinoma at the time of diagnosis of DM, and the chance of a preceding or subsequent lung carcinoma is similar.

Overlap Syndrome

Overlap of PM/DM with other collagen vascular disorders occurs. It is most common with progressive systemic sclerosis, but is also seen with SLE, rheumatoid arthritis, and Sjögren's syndrome.[44] The chest radiograph will reflect this admixture.

Juvenile Dermato/Polymyositis

Juvenile dermato/polymyositis differs from the adult form in a number of ways.[474, 666] In children, DM occurs much more frequently (10 to 20 times) than PM, calcinosis is common, and widespread vasculitis is a feature, although it does not appear to cause pulmonary complications. A diffuse interstitial pulmonary fibrosis similar to that seen in adults is described.[478] A third of patients have soft tissue calcification, particularly over pressure points.[474] When calcinosis affects the chest wall, it is detectable on the chest radiograph and may occasionally be a striking finding.

Progressive Systemic Sclerosis

Progressive systemic sclerosis (PSS) is a generalized connective tissue disorder characterized by (1) tightening, induration, and thickening of the skin (scleroderma); (2) Raynaud's phenomenon and other vascular abnormalities; (3) musculoskeletal manifestations; and (4) visceral involvement, especially of the gastrointestinal tract, lungs, heart and kidneys.[525] The diagnosis can be made with a high degree of certainty if the single major criterion of proximal scleroderma is present (i.e., proximal to metacarpophalangeal joints) or if there are two or more minor criteria (sclerodactyly, pitting scars or loss of substance of the finger tips, or bilateral basal pulmonary fibrosis).[404]

The pathogenesis is obscure, with lines of evidence pointing to several possibilities that could co-exist: a primary vascular abnormality; an immunologic disorder (both serologic and lymphocyte abnormalities are present); or an inflammatory process.[471] Pathologically there are vascular changes in small vessels (intimal proliferation, medial hypertrophy, myxomatous change, and perivascular fibrosis), inflammatory changes and collagen deposition with atrophy in the skin and a variety of internal organs. At postmortem the lungs are abnormal in more than 80% cases.[137] It is of note that the vascular and fibrotic changes in the lungs do not correlate in degree.[677] Interstitial fibrosis affects all lobes, but is particularly marked peripherally and in lower zones.[657] Pleural fibrosis and adhesions are common, and there are subpleural cysts.[177] Severe cases show extensive parenchymal destruction with the development of honeycomb lung[351] and bronchiolectasis.[657]

PSS has a 3:1 female-to-male distribution and presents most commonly in the 3rd to 5th decade of life, although there is a wide range from the teens upward.[404] The most common presentation is with Raynaud's phenomenon, which occurs in some 80% to 90% of cases[151] and may precede skin changes by several years. Other early manifestations include tendinitis, arthralgia, and arthritis. Treatment has little to offer,[325] and prognosis is very variable depending on the degree of visceral involvement, particularly of the heart and kidneys and, to a much lesser extent, the lungs.[418] A 50% 5-year survival rate and a 40% 10-year survival rate were found in one series of over 300 patients.[419]

Fewer than 1% of patients present with respiratory symptoms.[471] However, in established disease respiratory symptoms are common, with dyspnea in more than 60%, pleuritic chest pain in 17%, and chronic cough in 10%.[471] Respiratory function tests are commonly abnormal in PSS, but the defects are often mild.[471] The main abnormalities are a reduced carbon monoxide diffusion and a restrictive defect with airflow obstruction in some patients.[280, 470, 471] There is a poor correlation between respiratory function tests and radiologic findings[591]; and as with other lung fibroses, the interstitial fibrosis of PSS can occur although the chest radiograph appears normal.[657]

Radiologic evidence of pulmonary involvement was first described in 1941,[387, 450] and it is now generally accepted that the chest radiograph is abnormal in about 25% of patients with established disease,[280] although the range in various series is from 10% to 80%.[607] Very occasionally, chest radiographic changes consistent with fibrosis antedate the onset of scleroderma.[37] The most common radiologic abnormality is interstitial fibrosis, which causes a symmetric, diffuse, basally predominant reticulonodular pattern (Figs 11–29 and 11–30)[254, 657] that typically starts with a very fine reticulation[220] and progresses to a coarser reticulation with nodules. Sometimes, the nodular shadowing is so fine that it has the appearance of ground glass.[12] Recognized variants of distribution include unilateral[656] and total lung involvement.[607] Cystic lesions commonly develop in the areas of fibrosis and range in size from 1 to 30 mm.[280, 656] Sometimes they are aggregated

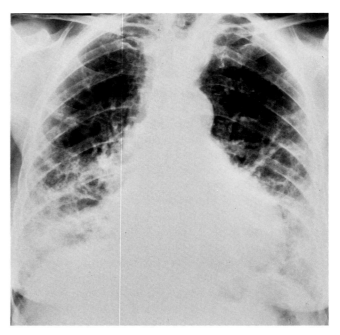

FIG 11–29.
Fibrosing alveolitis in progressive systemic sclerosis. There is bilateral middle and lower zone shadowing—partly reticulonodular and partly a ground-glass appearance with an additional coarse linear element. The findings are those of fibrosing alveolitis. (Courtesy of Dr. M.G. Britton, Chertsey, Surrey.)

and have the appearance of honeycomb shadowing. Occasionally, the cysts are quite large—more than 5 cm in diameter.[52] It is presumably the rupture of such cysts that accounts for the occasional pneumothorax seen in PSS.[254, 334] Gross fibrosis can cause airway distortion and bronchiectasis.[12] Loss of lung volume often occurs and is probably the result of the reduced compliance that is associated with fibrosis.[220] Such volume loss is manifest by elevation of the diaphragm. However, diaphragmatic muscle atrophy and replacement fibrosis have also been demonstrated, and weakness may be an additional factor contributing to elevation.[328] Pleural thickening, inflammation, adhesions, and effusion are recorded postmortem in some 50% to 80% of cases.[137, 657] Radiologically, however, pleural changes are infrequent and relatively minor.

Pulmonary arterial hypertension is common in PSS, occurring in one-third to one-half of patients, and it is unrelated to age, sex, or duration of illness (Fig 11–31).[177, 534, 639] It also occurs independently of alterations in pulmonary function,[534] and is unrelated to the degree of pulmonary fibrosis.[622, 677] Pulmonary arterial hypertension can cause enlargement of the main and proximal pulmonary arteries and lead to cor pulmonale with cardiomeg-

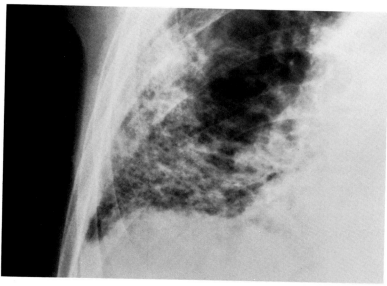

FIG 11-30.
Progressive systemic sclerosis with fibrosing alveolitis. A localized view of the right lower zone in a patient with progressive systemic sclerosis shows fine reticulonodular opacities with a basal and peripheral distribution characteristic of fibrosing alveolitis.

aly,[280] but even in cases of proved pulmonary arterial hypertension, the central pulmonary vessels can be normal in appearance.[639] It is generally accepted that there is an increased prevalence of lung carcinoma in PSS,[280] although not all studies are in agreement.[170] A particularly high prevalence of al-veolar cell carcinoma and adenocarcinoma is described.[280]

Pneumonia is a recognized complication of PSS and, in some cases, may be an aspiration pneumonia related to esophageal dysfunction.[469] Aspiration, however, is not thought to play a significant part in

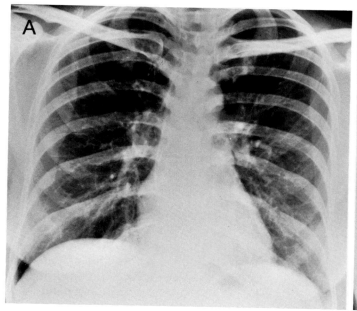
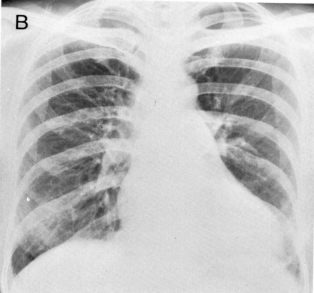

FIG 11-31.
Progressive systemic sclerosis with pulmonary arterial hypertension in a patient who developed progressive exertional dyspnea in the 5-year interval between radiographs **A** and **B**. The enlarged heart and prominent main pulmonary artery result from pulmonary arterial hypertension. Mean pulmonary artery pressure at the time of radiograph **B** was 55 mm Hg. Because pulmonary vascular changes and hypertension occur independently of alveolitis, the absence of fibrosis on the chest radiograph is not surprising.

the basal fibrotic changes.[656] Infection is a serious complication of advanced PSS,[469] and it, rather than respiratory failure, is the main cause of respiratory deaths.[471]

There are several reports of calcification of nodes (eggshell), parenchyma (micronodular), and pleura.[12, 254, 553] But there is no strong evidence that these are any more than chance associations.

Two extrapulmonary features of PSS may be seen on the chest radiograph: superior rib erosion[600] and esophageal dilatation. Superior rib erosion is not specific for PSS, being seen in rheumatoid disease, SLE,[545] and mixed connective tissue disease.[607] The resorption occurs on the upper border posterolaterally, is shallow and symmetric, with ill-defined margins. A 10% to 20% prevalence rate is reported.[279, 470]

Clinical disease of the esophagus occurs in more than one-half of cases and is present pathologically in three-quarters.[137] The esophagus becomes functionally abnormal and fibrosed, ending up as a dilated, air-filled tube that may be detected on the lateral chest radiograph.[157, 279] It does not contain an air-fluid level, as the dilatation is not associated with obstruction.[402] An air-esophagogram is found in many other conditions.[500]

An increased uptake of gallium-67 in the lung has been shown in PSS,[21, 229] but it seems unlikely that gallium scanning will find a place in routine investigation.[471]

CREST Syndrome

The CREST syndrome is a relatively benign variety of PSS that was called acrosclerosis in the older literature,[526] the terms CRST—and later CREST—being introduced more recently.[557, 669] CREST is an acronym for *c*alcinosis, *R*aynaud's phenomenon, *e*sophagus, *s*clerodactyly, and *t*elangiectasia—stressing the major features and organ involvement. Selection bias in various series makes prevalence difficult to assess, but it may well be similar to that of classic PSS.[526] The majority of patients present with Raynaud's phenomenon or swollen fingers,[526] and, CREST is, if anything, more female preponderant than PSS. It differs from PSS in that the patient's life expectancy is greater, and the disease is often mild and only slowly progressive.[526] Systemic involvement such as that of the kidney is less.[224] However, the CREST syndrome is by no means benign, and there are several reports of severe pulmonary hypertension and deaths from cor pulmonale.[224, 540, 599] In addition, although several smaller series have suggested a lower prevalence of lung disease, ranging from 0% to 11%,[224, 607, 641] in a recent large series of 88 CREST patients the prevalence of lung involvement was similar to that in PSS, with 72% having abnormal respiratory function tests and 33% having radiologic pulmonary fibrosis.[470]

Overlap-Progressive Systemic Sclerosis Syndrome

This is the other major clinical variant of PSS, constituting 10% to 27% of all cases of PSS.[404, 607, 624] Overlap occurs with one or more connective tissue disorders: SLE, rheumatoid disease, and dermatomyositis. Pleuropulmonary involvement is more common than in classic PSS, with radiologic fibrosis seen in 25% to 65%[404, 607, 624, 625] and pleural effusions in 15% to 36%.[167, 607] There is some evidence that pulmonary fibrosis is even more basally predominant than in PSS, and it has been suggested that this, possibly with pleural effusion and rib erosion should, on radiologic grounds, raise the possibility of overlap-PSS rather than classic PSS.[607]

Overlap Syndromes and Mixed Connective Tissue Disease

Some patients have an illness with the characteristic features of more than one connective tissue disorder. These patients are said to have an *overlap syndrome* or *undifferentiated connective tissue disorder*. The thoracic manifestations in these cases are those of the various connective tissue disorders that make up the overlap, and they are discussed under individual connective tissue disorders.

Mixed connective tissue disease is an overlap syndrome that is a distinct clinicopathologic entity,[568] although not everyone agrees with this view.[512] The principal characteristics are the presence of (1) features of SLE, PSS, and PM/DM occurring together or evolving sequentially during observation; and (2) antibodies to an extractable nuclear antigen.[568] These patients have a paucity of central nervous system and renal involvement. Inflammatory features (arthritis, serositis, myositis, and fever) are less frequent and, generally, the condition is more steroid-sensitive than other connective tissue disorders.[459] Those presenting with limited disease tend to show more overlap as time goes on,[601] and there is a tendency for the condition to transform eventually into PSS.[459] Eighty to ninety percent of the patients have been women.[31]

The prevalence of chest disease as assessed by pulmonary function tests together with chest radiographs is high: in the order of 80%.[148, 288, 601] In two series, the chest radiographs were abnormal in

30%[601] and 63%[288] of cases. The 30% figure represents changes on the initial chest radiograph only and undoubtedly underestimates the long-term chest involvement. The pulmonary abnormalities resemble those seen in SLE, PSS, and PM/DM.[325] Thus, pleural thickening and pleural and pericardial effusions have been described,[277, 288, 463, 575, 601] as is steroid sensitive pneumonitis, manifested as fleeting basal consolidations.[31] However, the most frequent pleuropulmonary finding has been small irregular interstitial opacities, most prevalent in the lower half of the lungs.[1, 601] Histologically, these changes are due to fibrosing alveolitis,[663] and the radiologic picture is entirely consistent with this finding. The other common finding has been pulmonary arterial hypertension,[1, 601, 663] which may produce characteristic radiographic changes but which also occurs with a normal appearance on the chest radiograph. The changes of pulmonary arterial hypertension may or may not be accompanied by a fibrosing alveolitis pattern.[31] There is a high prevalence (74%) of esophageal abnormality, which can lead to aspiration pneumonia.[601] A case has been described with mediastinal adenopathy which was nonspecific on biopsy.[277]

Although early reports suggested that the pulmonary changes responded well to steroids,[288] not all studies bear this out.[663]

Sjögren Syndrome

Sjögren syndrome (sicca syndrome, SS) is an autoimmune disorder characterized by dry eyes (keratoconjunctivitis sicca) and dry mouth (xerostomia). The syndrome is often, but not invariably, accompanied by features of one or more of the connective tissue diseases. Pathologically, the hallmark of SS is widespread tissue infiltration by immunoglobulin-producing lymphocytes. This infiltration particularly affects various exocrine glands (lacrimal, salivary, airway mucous glands) causing enlargement and later atrophy with impairment of secretion. The diagnosis is established by demonstrating reduced tear secretion (Schirmer test), a filamentary or punctate keratitis, and biopsy evidence of focal lymphocytic and plasma cell infiltration of an exocrine gland (most conveniently the labial salivary gland).[278]

The syndrome is divided into primary and secondary forms according to whether there is an associated connective tissue disorder. The connective tissue disease most commonly associated is rheumatoid arthritis, but SS may also be seen with systemic sclerosis, SLE, and polymyositis. Various autoimmune disorders occur with both primary and secondary forms and include chronic active hepatitis, primary biliary cirrhosis, Hashimoto's thyroiditis, myasthenia gravis, and celiac disease. Primary SS differs from the secondary form in that exocrine function is more severely disturbed, and extraglandular manifestations are frequent.[330] These extraglandular features include renal tubular disorders, such as renal tubular acidosis; myopathy and peripheral neuropathy and central nervous system disorders[6]; vascular disorders, including Raynaud's phenomenon, vasculitis, and purpura; and nonerosive polyarthropathy. Finally, both types of SS may develop into a lymphoproliferative disorder including pseudolymphoma and frank lymphoma.

SS is typically a disease of middle-aged women; only 10% of patients are male. The various pleuropulmonary manifestations of SS fall into three major groups (Table 11–7). These give rise to symptoms of hoarseness, cough, pleuritic pain, and exertional dyspnea. Recurrent infections, particularly bronchitis and pneumonia, are a feature.[41, 570] Factors predisposing to airway infections are complex and include mucus hyposecretion, leading to dry airways,[41] and cellular infiltration of small airway walls, causing obstruction.[458]

Obstructive, restrictive, and diffusion abnormalities are found on respiratory function testing, with different abnormalities predominating in different series.[194, 458, 472, 565] Recent evidence from a controlled study suggests that diffusion and restrictive abnormalities are more common in primary SS and that obstructive defects are more common in secondary SS.[477] Most patients have a polyclonal

TABLE 11–7.

Pleuropulmonary Manifestations of Sjögren's Syndrome

As seen in collagen vascular disease	Pleural thickening/effusion Fibrosing alveolitis* Discoid basal atelectasis Vasculitis† Diaphragm weakness†
Airway dryness/obstruction; recurrent infection	Xerotrachea* Bronchitis* Pneumonia* Bronchiectasis
Lymphoproliferative	Lymphocytic interstitial pneumonitis Pseudolymphoma Malignant lymphoma Amyloidosis†

*Common.
†Rare.

·gammopathy, especially of IgG and IgM. In 90% there is a positive rheumatoid factor, and in 70% there is a positive antinuclear antibody. Organ-specific autoantibodies are also common, and there is evidence that the presence of two precipitating antibodies to nuclear antigens (SS-A, SS-B) has diagnostic value.[278]

The prevalence of pleuropulmonary involvement is difficult to assess. Taking the symptoms and the radiologic signs together, the prevalence is probably in the order of 30%, with a range of 9% to 50%.[41, 597] When assessed by respiratory function tests, the prevalence of respiratory involvement is higher.[19, 116, 458, 472, 643] Somewhat surprisingly, the prevalence of pleuropulmonary abnormalities is about the same in primary and secondary SS.[19, 41, 477, 565, 643] Xerotrachea,[115] recurrent tracheobronchitis, recurrent pneumonia, and fibrosing alveolitis are the most common problems, each occurring in a third or more of those with chest involvement. Pleuritis with or without effusion and pleural thickening occurs in about a tenth of the patients, while other manifestations (listed in Table 11–7) have a prevalence of 5% or less.

It should be noted that a number of the manifestations, particularly fibrosing alveolitis and lymphocytic interstitial pneumonitis, give rise to basally predominant nodular or reticulonodular shadowing.[565, 597] In general the chest radiograph is not specific enough to distinguish among these processes. However, the combination of air-space shadowing[298] and an interstitial pattern suggests lymphocytic interstitial pneumonitis. It is of note that fibrosing alveolitis can occur in both primary and secondary SS.[194, 349] Enlargement of mediastinal lymph nodes or a multifocal large nodular/alveolar pattern[597] suggests the development of pseudolymphoma[194, 458, 597] or malignant lymphoma.[194, 597] In SS there is a twofold increase in malignancy in general and a 44-fold increase in malignant lymphoma. This finding applies to both primary and secondary SS.[330] The development of lymphoma is often associated with a fall in serum gammaglobulin and the disappearance of serum autoantibodies.

Relapsing Polychondritis

Relapsing polychondritis is a rare disease of unknown cause characterized by recurrent inflammatory episodes that affect various cartilaginous structures, particularly the pinna, nose, and airways. Other features include arthropathy and thoracic chondritis, medium- to large-vessel arteritis, and re-current inflammation of the eyes and inner ears.[8, 407] The mean age of onset is in the 5th decade,[407] though all age groups may be affected. The sex incidence is equal,[407] and most patients have been Caucasian.[160] About 30% of patients have an associated "autoimmune" disease, most commonly rheumatoid arthritis[407] or a systemic vasculitis.[429]

Pathologically, there is cartilage destruction with fibrous tissue replacement and surrounding inflammatory change. Cartilage antibodies have been detected[173] and are probably important in the pathogenesis.

Fifty percent of patients present with either auricular chondritis or arthropathy, and most of the remainder present with nasal chondritis, ocular inflammation, or respiratory tract involvement.[407]

Eventually just over half the patients will develop respiratory tract involvement (56%)[407] manifested by laryngeal tenderness, hoarseness, dyspnea, and stridor or wheeze. Disease of the respiratory tract is a serious development as it may be immediately life-threatening and, in the long term, is associated with a bad prognosis.[429] Airway involvement causes narrowing, primarily of the larynx or trachea, but the major bronchi can also be involved.[71, 99, 221] It seems unlikely, however, that there is significant disease beyond the main bronchi.[242] Stenoses are usually single and localized,[407] but they can be multiple.[437] Thus tracheal narrowing is typically subglottic, smooth, and from 1 cm to several centimeters long[357] but can involve the whole trachea.[99] Furthermore, stenoses may be fixed[221] when they are secondary to scarring,[160] inflammation, and edema,[407] or they may be variable. In this latter instance, increased wall compliance predisposes to dynamic collapse.[242, 455] The dynamic behavior of stenoses can be investigated by flow volume loops[437] or with fluoroscopy and cineradiography,[242] with or without contrast material. Airflow obstruction in lobar and segmental airways can lead to pulmonary oligemia and air trapping,[220] atelectasis,[437] or obstructive pneumonitis. McAdam et al., reporting that 46% of deaths were due to respiratory involvement, suggest regular assessment to detect early airway changes, particularly if there are any respiratory symptoms.[407] Such an assessment should include plain radiographs of the cervical and thoracic trachea, and tomography (either conventional or computed).[422, 437] Bronchography and laryngography are probably unnecessary and are not recommended when there are marked stenoses.[357] Cardiovascular involvement is recorded in 24% of patients,[407] and some of the described lesions such as aortic and mitral regurgitation and aortic aneurysm may produce changes on a chest radiograph. In addition, the chondritis causes nonspecific calcification of the pinna.[504, 509]

The mainstay of treatment is the use of systemic steroids, and tracheostomy may be necessary. The outcome is very variable; the course may be rapidly fatal, or may be indolent, with about a 75% 5-year survival rate.[429] The frequency of respiratory involvement as a cause of death has been 50% or more in some series,[160, 407] but was only 10% in a recent major series.[429]

DIFFUSE PULMONARY (ALVEOLAR) HEMORRHAGE

Bleeding into the lung parenchyma is common in a wide variety of disorders, but in this chapter the discussion will be limited to those conditions in which bleeding is diffuse or multifocal and contributes significantly to the radiologic changes. A triad of features suggests pulmonary parenchymal hemorrhage: hemoptysis, anemia, and air-space opacities on the chest radiograph.[53] Sometimes, the bleeding is covert and hemoptysis is absent.[581] The diagnosis is often missed, at least initially, particularly when hemoptysis is not present.[61] The *pulmonary* features of all diffuse pulmonary hemorrhage syndromes are the same, and chest radiographs are generally unhelpful in distinguishing among them.[373]

There have been a number of recent reviews,[5, 53, 373, 442, 615, 633] and the classification given in Table 11–8 has been drawn from a combination of these sources.

Causes

Antibasement Membrane Antibody Disease

Antibasement membrane antibody (ABMA) disease is the most common cause of diffuse pulmonary hemorrhage. Sixty to eighty percent of patients with ABMA disease have alveolar hemorrhage and glomerulonephritis (i.e., Goodpasture's syndrome), and most of the rest have glomerulonephritis only. A few patients with ABMA disease have alveolar hemorrhage and no kidney disease, but this is very unusual.

In 1919 Goodpasture described a patient who developed fatal pulmonary hemorrhage and glomerulonephritis 6 weeks after an attack of influenza.[257] In 1958 Stanton and Tange were the first to use the term Goodpasture's syndrome to describe the combi-

nation of pulmonary hemorrhage and glomerulonephritis.[589] With a clearer understanding of the pathogenesis, the term has taken on a restricted meaning that defines a syndrome with (1) diffuse pulmonary hemorrhage; (2) glomerulonephritis; (3) and antiglomerular basement antibodies in the serum, lung, or kidney.[615]

Goodpasture's syndrome is essentially a disease of young adult white men. In one major review the median age at onset was 21 years (range, 16 to 61 years), with 90% males and 51 of the 52 white.[32] The entity has been occasionally reported in children.[473] The clinical presentation is usually with respiratory symptoms: hemoptysis (80%), dyspnea (72%), and cough,[609] and the patients are usually found to have an iron deficient anemia (93%) and an abnormal chest radiograph (see Fig 11–32) (80%). Either at the time of presentation or in the ensuing weeks or months, urine analysis and renal function become abnormal. Occasionally, renal failure takes years to develop.[555] In one series, 55% of patients were anemic on admission, and about 80% had proteinuria or hematuria.[609] Rarely, the order of events is reversed, with pulmonary hemorrhage following a nephritic presentation.[53] Demonstration of the presence of antiglomerular basement antibodies in the serum is both a sensitive and a specific indicator of the disease and establishes the diagnosis.[373] There is, however, a general lack of correlation between the level of serum antibody and the severity of the disease.[53]

Renal biopsy shows evidence of subacute proliferative glomerulonephritis, with linear IgG deposi-

TABLE 11–8.

Causes of Diffuse Pulmonary Hemorrhage

Antibasement membrane antibody disease
  With GN* (Goodpasture's syndrome)
  Without GN
Connective tissue disorder/systemic vasculitis/
  "immune complex disease"
  With GN
    Systemic lupus erythematosus
  Without GN
    Systemic necrotizing vasculitis
    Wegener granulomatosis
    Rheumatoid disease
    Henoch-Schönlein disease
    Mixed connective tissue disease
Rapidly progressive GN
Idiopathic pulmonary hemosiderosis
Bleeding disorders
Drugs/chemicals

*GN = glomerulonephritis.

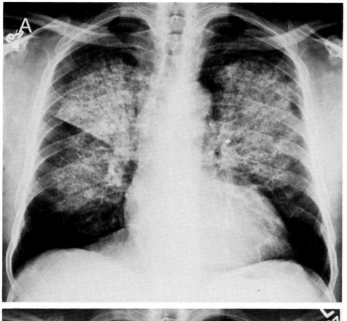

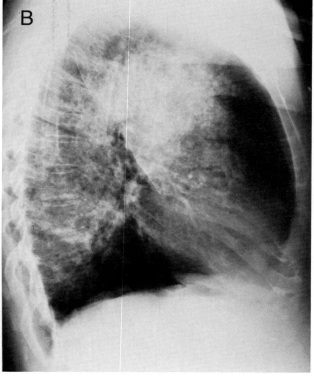

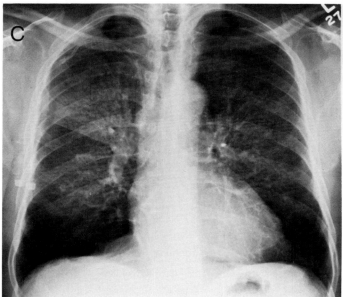

FIG 11–32.
Goodpasture's syndrome. **A,** radiograph shows bilateral perihilar consolidation, some of which is sharply marginated by the minor fissure. There is a bilateral air bronchogram. Apex and base are spared by the air-space shadowing, which is due to intra-alveolar blood. **B,** lateral view of same patient. Note hold up of consolidation by the oblique fissure and the peripheral acinar nodules. **C,** a week later there has been considerable though incomplete resolution of the consolidation. Typically pulmonary hemorrhage clears in a matter of days.

tion in the glomeruli. Lung biopsy is not usually performed, but if it were, it would show blood and hemosiderin-laden macrophages in the alveoli and hemosiderin-laden macrophages in the interstitium. In addition, there is sometimes septal thickening or fibrosis together with linear deposits of IgG on the alveolar capillary membranes.[442] Therapy, apart from supportive measures, is directed at removing ABMA by plasmapheresis and stopping its production with steroids and immunosuppressives.[511] Early on, the reported prognosis was poor, with about half the patients dying of pulmonary complications and almost all the rest dying of renal disease.[32] The occasional patient went into remission and recovered.[564] In one major series, 96% died, and there was a mean survival of 15 weeks.[32] The prognosis is better now with improved treatment and because milder cases are now included in the various series.[53]

Connective Tissue Disorders/Systemic Vasculitides/"Immune Complex Disease"

Many collagen vascular disorders and systemic vasculitides are occasionally associated with diffuse alveolar hemorrhage, with or without a glomerulonephritis. Many, and possibly all, are immune-complex mediated, though hard evidence is lacking with some of the entities. The association is most commonly seen with SLE and systemic necrotizing vasculitides of the polyarteritis nodosa type.[53]

There are 21 well-documented instances of patients with SLE who developed diffuse alveolar hemorrhage,[373] but there were only two in which the hemorrhage was a presenting feature.[73, 172] Thus, hemorrhage usually occurs with other evidence of active SLE (not necessarily renal), and it carries a bad prognosis, 70% of the patients dying within a few days.[373] Alveolar hemorrhage develops because of immune complex deposition, and there is no evidence of a pulmonary vasculitis.[373]

Alveolar hemorrhage is also well recognized in systemic necrotizing vasculitides of the polyarteritis nodosa type,[373, 480, 616] and it is usually associated with glomerulonephritis. The lung lesion is a necrotizing alveolitis, not an arteritis.[53]

Isolated case reports of alveolar hemorrhage are also reported with rheumatoid disease, progressive systemic sclerosis,[347] mixed connective tissue disease, Wegener's granulomatosis, Henoch-Schönlein syndrome (hypersensitivity vasculitis), immune complex glomerulonephritis, and essential mixed cryoglobulinemia.[53, 373] A case of microangiopathic hemolytic anemia and pulmonary vasculitis has also been recorded.[442]

Rapidly Progressive Glomerulonephritis

The rapidly progressive glomerulonephritis of Goodpasture's syndrome is associated with ABMAs and linear immunofluorescence in the renal biopsy. However, there are two types of rapidly progressive glomerulonephritis with alveolar hemorrhage, but no ABMA. One form has granular renal immunofluorescence consistent with immune complex deposition and is included in the list of diseases listed in the previous paragraph.[27] The other shows neither linear nor granular immunofluorescence[374] and, on the available evidence, does not have a demonstrable immunologic basis. In one series, 19% of patients with alveolar hemorrhage and glomerulonephritis fell into this group.[373]

Idiopathic (Primary) Pulmonary Hemosiderosis (IPH)

Idiopathic pulmonary hemosiderosis (IPH) is a disorder of unknown etiology characterized by episodic alveolar hemorrhage that eventually leads to lung fibrosis.[633] Multisystem involvement and, in particular, glomerulonephritis is not a feature. His-

tologically, the light microscopic changes are the same as those of Goodpasture's syndrome: namely, alveolar hemorrhage; hemosiderin-laden macrophages in the alveoli and, to a lesser extent, in the interstitium; and mild interstitial thickening. Late in the disease, alveolar septal fibrosis develops.[53] Some workers describe ultrastructural abnormalities of the capillary basement membranes,[162] but others view these simply as nonspecific manifestations of injury.[351]

Immunofluorescent staining for immunoglobulins and complement is negative. Unlike Goodpasture's syndrome, IPH is a disease of childhood, the onset typically occurring between 1 and 7 years of age with just one-fifth of patients presenting in the late teens and twenties.[581] It is the most common diffuse pulmonary hemorrhage syndrome in childhood.[442] The sex incidence in children is equal, but in adults, there is a twofold preponderance in men. Clinically, there is episodic cough, hemoptysis, and the signs and symptoms of anemia (tiredness, pallor, failure to gain weight). The magnitude of hemoptysis varies greatly. In some it is absent altogether, leading to diagnostic difficulties, and in others it is massive enough to cause death.[271] Bleeding into the lungs is evidenced by consolidation on the chest radiograph (Fig 11–33) and the presence of iron deficiency anemia, with low iron stores. With recurrent bleeding, pulmonary hemosiderosis and fibrosis develop, and most of those who survive several years are chronically dyspneic, anemic, and underweight.[581] Despite the fact that some patients have been followed for 20 years, it is unclear whether the disease ever permanently remits. The outcome is variable. In one series of 68 patients followed for 5 years, 29% died, 25% had active disease, 18% had inactive disease but chronic symptoms, and 28% were well.[581] Some of the deaths were due to pulmonary arterial hypertension and cor pulmonale. Treatment is supportive. Steroids and immunosuppressive drugs may be used, but there is no clear evidence that they help. Formerly splenectomy was performed, but it is no longer recommended.

Bleeding Disorders

Intrapulmonary hemorrhage is a very unusual complication of the various coagulopathies. It has been recorded with thrombocytopenia,[208, 253, 475, 576] particularly in the context of leukemia,[5, 40] anticoagulation,[207] and diffuse intravascular coagulation.[521]

Drugs/Chemicals

A number of exogenous agents are recorded as causing alveolar hemorrhage. The important ones are:

1. *d*-Penicillamine. Seven cases are recorded with the use of penicillamine for a variety of underlying disorders. The dose has been relatively high, and the drug has been used for 1 to 3 years before the onset of pulmonary hemorrhage and glomerulonephritis.[373] It is probably immune complex mediated.[442]

2. Trimellitic anhydride. This chemical, used in the plastics industry, can cause a variety of disorders, one of which is a mixed anemia with alveolar hemorrhage.[2, 307] This syndrome has an immunologic basis.[442]

3. Lymphography. There are four reported cases of diffuse pulmonary hemorrhage 2 to 10 days following lymphography.[373]

Radiology of Diffuse Pulmonary Hemorrhage

The radiographic changes of *acute* alveolar hemorrhage are the same regardless of etiology and consist of air-space consolidation. In some of the conditions under consideration, particularly primary pulmonary hemosiderosis, the bleeding tends to be recurrent over a long period of time and, in these cases, persistent interstitial changes may develop, reflecting interstitial fibrosis. When acute bleeding is superimposed on chronic changes, a mixed alveolar and interstitial pattern will be produced.

The consolidation ranges from acinar shadows (see Fig 11–32),[56, 172, 578] through patchy air-space consolidation (Fig 11–34),[32, 578] to widespread confluent consolidation with air bronchograms (see Fig 11–32).[51] At other times the consolidation may be migratory[5] or finely granular, with clustered pinpoint opacities.[51, 56] The consolidation can be widespread or show a perihilar (Fig 11–35) or mid/lower zone predominance[5, 51] and tends to be more pronounced centrally. The costophrenic angles and apices are usually spared.[247, 578] The consolidation clears quickly within about 2 to 3 days (see Fig 11–32),[51] either completely or partially, to leave a linear/reticular pattern,[603, 614] occasionally with septal (Kerley B) lines[309] or a ground-glass haziness.[51] Sometimes these two patterns are mixed.[56, 603] In any event, this interstitial shadowing is also transient and clears completely 10 to 12 days after the beginning of the episode. There are two reports of hilar adenopathy.[66, 158] Pleural effusions are not un-

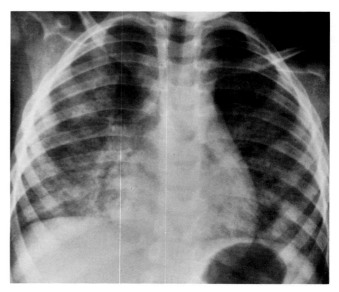

FIG 11–33.
Primary pulmonary hemosiderosis. The patient is a 2½-year-old boy who presented with a low-grade fever, cough, and hemoptysis. Chest radiograph at the time of presentation shows bilateral, coarse, partially confluent, ill-defined nodules, with air bronchograms.

common, but it seems likely that most, if not all, are secondary phenomena related to infection and fluid overload.[51]

With repeated bleeding episodes, seen typically in primary pulmonary hemosiderosis, the interstitial shadowing fails to clear completely, and the patient may be left with permanent, fine reticulonodular opacities (Figs 11–36 and 11–37)[581] that tends to increase in profusion with each acute episode. New bleeding episodes superimposed on permanent shadowing will give a mixed alveolar/interstitial pattern.

It is worthwhile noting that diffuse pulmonary bleeding can be present when the chest radiograph appears normal.[50, 193] In one series, this was found to be the case in 22% of bleeding episodes in patients with diffuse pulmonary hemorrhage[50] of Goodpasture's syndrome.

Differential Diagnosis of Alveolar Hemorrhage

Hemoptysis, iron deficient anemia, and a sudden fall in the hematocrit of more than 2 grams without bleeding elsewhere[51] are obvious pointers to the diagnosis of pulmonary hemorrhage. It is well recognized that, because alveolar hemorrhage occurs distal to the mucociliary escalator, hemoptysis may be absent. Additionally, blood brought up on the esca-

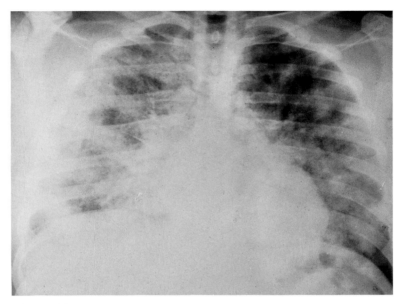

FIG 11–34.
Goodpasture's syndrome. The chest radiograph shows diffuse bilateral multifocal consolidation becoming confluent in part.

lator may be swallowed and produce a misleading positive stool blood test. Hemosiderin-laden macrophages in the sputum, gastric washings, or alveolar lavage[166] indicate bleeding within the recent past, but can also be detected with simple pulmonary edema.[51]

The most useful test for alveolar hemorrhage in clinical practice is detection of increased carbon monoxide uptake by the blood sequestered in the lungs. This can be demonstrated[193] by cyclotron produced $C^{15}O$ or, more conveniently, by the single-breath carbon monoxide uptake (Kco) test, considering a 40% rise as a positive indicator.[50]

Radionuclide scintiscans have been used in the di-

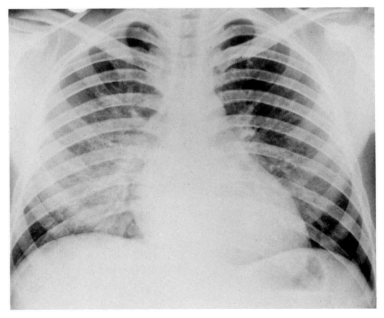

FIG 11–35.
Goodpasture's syndrome. There is homogeneous perihilar shadowing on the right which extends into the mid and lower zone. On the left there is subtle ground-glass opacification in the mid/lower zone. (Courtesy of Dr. A.N. Adam, London.)

agnosis but have not gained wide acceptance. Agents employed include ^{99m}Tc sulfur colloid, a blood pool agent useful in the diagnosis of brisk bleeding,[23] or red blood cells labeled with chromium 51,[445, 544] iron 52,[475] or ^{99m}Tc.[109] The labeled red blood cell preparations are not taken up in the lungs of healthy people, but pulmonary uptake has been detected 12 to 24 hours following administration in both Goodpasture's syndrome[445] and idiopathic pulmonary hemosiderosis.[433] However, uptake has also been reported in patients with a hemorrhagic pneumonia.[671]

Radiologic signs, unfortunately, are not particularly helpful in distinguishing between pulmonary hemorrhage and the various other causes of consolidation. The interpretation of the chest radiograph is made particularly difficult by the fact that fluid overload and infection, the two major differential diagnoses, are well recognized precipitators of alveolar hemorrhage in Goodpasture's syndrome[51] and may coexist along with hemorrhage. Bowley and coworkers found that consolidation limited by a fissure, causing loss of a major part of the diaphragmatic or cardiac silhouette or affecting the apex or costophrenic angle, suggested infection.[51] The possi-

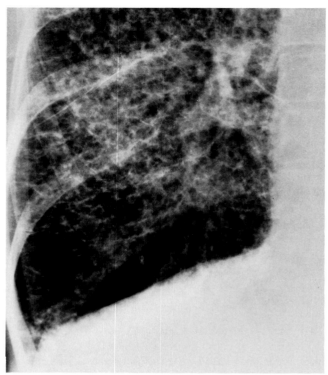

FIG 11–37.
Primary pulmonary hemosiderosis. Localized view of the right lung base. There is reticulonodular shadowing with a pronounced linear element of interstitial lines including septal (Kerley B) lines. The patient was diagnosed as having primary pulmonary hemosiderosis 30 years before the current radiograph and had been intermittently symptomatic over the intervening years. These are fixed changes due largely to fibrosis.

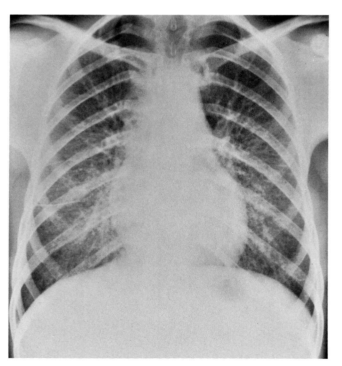

FIG 11–36.
Primary pulmonary hemosiderosis. This 17-year-old boy presented 4 months before this radiograph was obtained. In the wake of repeated bleeding episodes he has already developed indolent reticulonodular opacities about 2 mm in diameter together with interstitial lines. The minor fissure is thickened. (Courtesy of Dr. H. Massouh, Frimley, Surrey.)

bility that consolidation is the result of diffuse pulmonary (alveolar) hemorrhage should always be considered, particularly in the presence of hemoptysis, iron deficient anemia, glomerulonephritis, or a systemic vasculitis. The Kco test is probably the most useful way to confirm or exclude the diagnosis. The chest radiograph and Kco provide the best means of monitoring progress.[50] The specific etiology is usually determined by clinical assessment, serologic studies, and biopsy of the kidney or other extrapulmonary organs; lung biopsy is only needed when there are no extrapulmonary features and when anti-glomerular basement membrane antibodies are absent.[373]

EOSINOPHILIC LUNG DISEASE

The term *pulmonary eosinophilia* was introduced in 1952 to describe a group of diseases "in which pulmonary infiltration on the radiograph is accompanied by blood eosinophilia but in which pneumonia, hydatid disease of the lung, Hodgkin's disease, and sarcoidosis can be excluded."[127] Later, authors have widened this concept,[107] using the term *eosinophilic lung disease* to include all disorders associated with blood and/or tissue eosinophilia which affect major airways and/or lung parenchyma.[220] It is important to note that it is not necessary to have a blood eosinophilia to make a diagnosis of eosinophilic lung disease. The widely used term *pulmonary infiltration with eosinophilia* is synonymous with the term pulmonary eosinophilia.

Eosinophils are granulocytes that develop in the bone marrow and are carried in the blood to those epithelia that are exposed to the external environment, particularly the respiratory, gastrointestinal, and genitourinary mucosae. There is only one eosinophil in the blood compartment for every 100 in the marrow and in the tissues, and it is, therefore, not surprising that eosinophilic tissue lesions are not necessarily accompanied by blood eosinophilia.[554] Blood eosinophil counts vary between 0.05 and 0.35 $\times$ 10^9/L and show diurnal variation, with high counts in the night and low ones in the morning.[237] Eosinophilia is generally taken to mean an eosinophil count of more than 0.4 $\times$ 10^9/L, though some set the level at 0.5 $\times$ 10^9/L.[502] Eosinophils contain a range of enzymes, which accounts for their ability to damage parasitic worms, to damage cells including those of man, and to modulate mast cell–dependent reactions such as immediate hypersensitivity.

Various classifications of eosinophilic lung states have been proposed,* but none has proved entirely satisfactory. The classification used here (Table 11–9) is based on that of Schatz and co-workers.[554] The conditions considered in detail in the text are only those in which tissue and/or blood eosinophilia are a major feature. The possible causes in a patient under investigation can usually be significantly reduced by taking into account a few key historical, clinical, and laboratory findings, notably, work exposure, ethnic background, travel in endemic areas, and a history of asthma, atopy, and any medication. Useful information from first-line investigations includes the magnitude of blood eosinophilia, skin sensitivity, total serum IgE, serum *Aspergillus* precipitins, and stool examination for cysts, ova, and parasites.

Asthma

There is often a mild to moderate eosinophilia in patients with asthma.[320, 393, 430, 549] The radiology of asthma is discussed elsewhere (see Chapter 16). In

---

*References 107, 127, 237, 265, 382, 485, 554, and 584.

TABLE 11–9.

Classification of Eosinophilic Lung Disease*

Pulmonary conditions in which tissue and blood eosinophilia are pathogenically important
  Asthma
  Cryptogenic eosinophilic lung
    Acute eosinophilic pneumonia (Löffler syndrome)
    Chronic eosinophilic pneumonia
  Allergic bronchopulmonary aspergillosis
  Drug-induced disease
  Parasitic disease
    Tropical pulmonary eosinophilia
    Other worms
  Vasculitic/granulomatous disease
    Churg-Strauss syndrome
    Bronchocentric granulomatosis
  Hypereosinophilic syndrome
  Hyperimmunoglobulin E syndrome

Pulmonary conditions with occasional, or minor, tissue or blood eosinophilia
  Infections
    Bacterial *(Brucella, Mycobacterium)*
    Chlamydia
    Viral *(Adenovirus)*
    Protozoal *(Pneumocystis)*
    Fungal *(Coccidioides, Histoplasma)*
  Neoplasms[392]
    Bronchogenic carcinoma,[296] bronchial carcinoid
    Metastases
    Irradiated neoplasms
    Lymphoma (Hodgkin's and non-Hodgkin's; lymphomatoid granulomatosis)
  "Immunologic" conditions
    Wegener's granulomatosis
    Rheumatoid disease
    Extrinsic allergic alveolitis
    Sarcoidosis
  Miscellaneous
    Hemodialysis[441]

Pulmonary conditions with coincidental blood eosinophilia

*Based on Schatz M, Wasserman S, Patterson R: The eosinophil and the lung. *Arch Intern Med* 1982; 142:1515-1519.

---

addition asthma is often a prominent symptom in a number of specific eosinophilic lung states such as allergic bronchopulmonary aspergillosis and the Churg-Strauss syndrome.

Cryptogenic Eosinophilic Pneumonia

Cryptogenic eosinophilic pneumonia is commonly and usefully divided into two subgroups: acute (Löffler's syndrome) or chronic, depending on whether the condition lasts more or less than 1 month.[127] The 1-month dividing line is rather arbitrary and not universally applied, so that the acute/

chronic distinction is not always clear, particularly since steroids have been used for treatment. However, the division is useful clinically, as the majority of chronic, cryptogenic eosinophilic pneumonias (CEP) form a relatively homogeneous group.

Acute Eosinophilic Pneumonia

Synonyms for acute eosinophilic pneumonia include simple pulmonary eosinophilia and Löffler's syndrome.[391] The characteristic features of the syndrome are (1) blood eosinophilia, (2) absent or mild symptoms and signs (cough, fever, dyspnea), (3) one or more nonsegmental pulmonary consolidations that are transitory and/or migratory, and (4) spontaneous clearing of consolidations. Originally, opacities were described as disappearing within 6 to 12 days,[391] but this interval is now generally extended to a month.[127]

Löffler's syndrome may be idiopathic (cryptogenic), or it may result from a variety of inciting agents, particularly drugs (see p. 516) parasites (see p. 516) and miscellaneous agents such as nickel carbonyl.[602]

Pathologically, there is an eosinophilic pneumonia with edema and an eosinophilic infiltrate in both alveoli and interstitium.[16] Radiographically, the findings are one or more fairly homogeneous, nonsegmental consolidations that can be small or so large as to occupy much of a lobe. They are transitory and may disappear from one area while appearing in another. They have a tendency to be peripherally located. Pleural effusions, mediastinal adenopathy, and cavitation are not described.

Chronic Eosinophilic Pneumonia

By definition, CEP is of obscure etiology. This entity has a number of synonyms including prolonged eosinophilic pneumonia, prolonged pulmonary eosinophilia, and cryptogenic pulmonary eosinophilia. Pathologically, there is an eosinophil-rich exudate in alveoli and interstitium.[87, 631] Angiitis is mild, fibrosis sparse, and necrosis very rare.[87]

Since the condition was first identified in 1969,[87] several series have been published.[216, 230, 382, 411, 631] Most patients present in middle life; the mean age of onset is about 45 years (range, 7 to 77 years). Women outnumber men by 2 to 1.[216] One-third to one-half of the patients are atopic or have rhinitis, and about one-half to two-thirds have had asthma, which can antedate the condition by many years[382] or which can develop with the onset of CEP. The symptoms are often highly characteristic and range from mild to severe. Typical symptoms are dyspnea; cough with mucoid sputum; malaise; marked weight loss (8 to 12 kg); high fever, particularly in the evenings; and drenching night sweats. Occasional symptoms include chest pain and hemoptysis. It is, therefore, not surprising that patients are often believed initially to have tuberculosis—an impression that may be reinforced by the chest radiograph (Fig 11–38). Blood eosinophilia is common, but not universal, occurring in about 80% of patients[216] and ranging from mild to marked.[631] There is sputum eosinophilia in 50% to 75% of patients.[230, 631] Total white blood cell count and the ESR are raised. Serum IgE, which is normal in value or only minimally elevated,[631] is a particularly helpful finding, allowing distinction from those conditions such as allergic bronchopulmonary aspergillosis and tropical and parasitic pulmonary eosinophilias in which serum IgE levels are markedly elevated.

Most patients with chronic eosinophilic pneumonia have a characteristic radiologic pattern that is virtually pathognomonic.[91] At its most classic, the pattern consists of peripheral, nonsegmental, homogeneous opacities with radiographic features of consolidation including an ill-defined inner margin and an air bronchogram (Figs 11–38 and 11–39).[468]

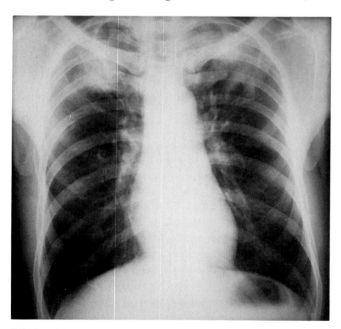

FIG 11–38.
CEP. The chest radiograph is of a 52-year-old man who presented with a 2-month fever, weight loss, and cough. He had a blood eosinophilia (2.0 × 10⁹/L) and had had nasal polypectomies in the past. The radiographic findings of bilateral apical consolidation coupled with the history was considered very suggestive of tuberculosis, and the patient was inappropriately treated for a month despite the lack of firm evidence.

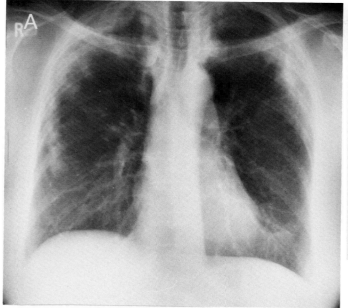

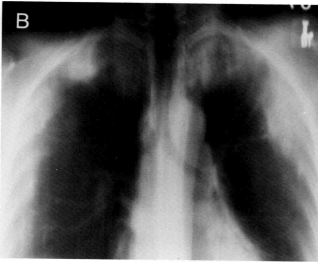

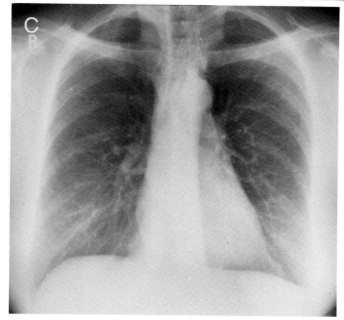

FIG 11–39.
CEP. Radiographs are of a 65-year-old woman who presented with a 1-month fever, night sweats, cough, and weight loss. The patient did not suffer from asthma but had a blood eosinophilia (1.6 × 10⁹/L). **A,** PA radiograph shows bilateral, confluent, peripheral shadowing that lines the inside of the chest wall in the mid and upper zones. It is consistent with nonsegmental consolidation. **B,** anteroposterior tomogram confirms the peripheral distribution of the shadowing, which is characteristic of CEP. **C,** radiograph 2 weeks after **A** shows complete resolution following steroid therapy.

These opacities lie against the chest wall and may surround the whole lung or just occupy the upper or lower zone. In one series the zonal distribution was 46% upper, 40% mid, and 14% lower.[411] About 50% of patients have bilateral shadowing. A variety of colorful descriptions has been applied to this striking distribution of opacities: "the photographic negative of pulmonary edema"[230] and "clouds of smoke rising after an explosion in the region of the hilum and drifting up against the chest wall peripherally."[127] Opacities may appear in one lung to be followed by others on the opposite side, or they may disappear spontaneously only to reappear elsewhere or in the same place. Although this last feature has been stressed as a characteristic finding,[230, 411] it is not unique and is also a feature of allergic bronchopulmonary aspergillosis.

Some 30% of patients with chronic eosinophilic pneumonia do not show the classic peripheral pattern described here.[216, 230, 411, 631] The consolidations may even be perihilar in distribution.[411] A common pattern is mixed peripheral and central consolidations (Fig 11–40)[411] that may even progress to opacify one lung totally.[631] Isolated lesions in the upper zone may closely mimic those of tuberculosis. Other features that are occasionally seen include a 4% prevalence of effusions,[91] possible cavitation in up to 10% of patients,[230] and the occasional case of mediastinal lymphadenopathy.[101, 468]

The disease occasionally remits spontaneously[230]; however, treatment is usually required, and it is remarkably sensitive to steroid therapy. Rapid clearing is usually seen within a few days, considerable resolution in about a week, and complete clearing by 1 month (see Fig 11–39).[87] Resolution is usually complete, but may occur by way of unusual bandlike shadows parallel to the chest wall (Fig 11–41).[230] These are highly characteristic and are particularly well seen on CT, where their platelike configuration and disregard for fissures can be easily appreciated.[468]

Relapse occurs in about one-third of patients when steroids are withdrawn,[216] and recurrent relapses and remissions are recorded as occurring for up to 26 years.[230] In such instances, chronic low-dose steroid treatment may be needed to keep the patient free of symptoms and signs. In the series of

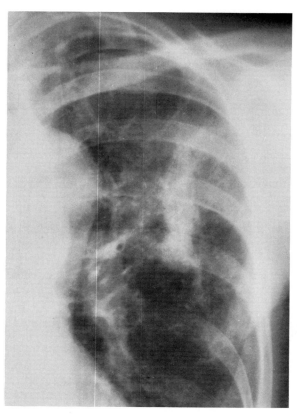

FIG 11–41.
CEP. Local view of the left mid and upper zone. Partial resolution of classic peripheral consolidation has resulted in a band opacity parallel to the chest wall. Such a finding on an interval chest radiograph is highly suggestive of CEP.

Gaensler and Carrington, in which there was a median follow-up of only 3 years, most patients were well as to their pneumonia, but four of 29 developed late-onset asthma, and one, who was untreated, died of CEP.[230] In rare instances, patients who initially have all the features of CEP go on to develop a diffuse vasculitis.[110, 230]

Allergic Bronchopulmonary Aspergillosis

Allergic bronchopulmonary aspergillosis (ABPA) is almost certainly the most common cause of eosinophilic lung disease in developed countries. It accounted for 78% of the patients in a series of 143 in the United Kingdom who were admitted to a tertiary referral center with a diagnosis of pulmonary eosinophilia.[410] First described in 1952,[315] the disease is characterized by asthma, radiographic pulmonary shadows, blood eosinophilia, and evidence of allergy to antigens of *Aspergillus* species. Its importance lies in the fact that recurrent acute episodes

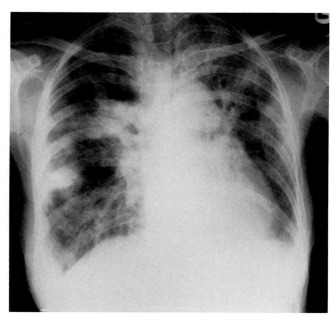

FIG 11–40.
CEP. The radiograph shows mixed peripheral and central, multifocal consolidation. This is a recognized pattern but less common than the one shown in Figure 11–39. Both costophrenic angles are blunted in this patient. On the right the blunting is almost certainly the result of peripheral consolidation, but on the left a small pleural effusion cannot be excluded. Pleural effusions are very unusual in CEP.

cause progressive lung damage that can be controlled by steroid administration.[535]

In ABPA, a hypersensitivity reaction develops to *Aspergillus* species that grow as a mycelial plug in proximal airways, usually the second or third order bronchi.[239] Tissue invasion is either absent[249] or very limited.[268] The factors that favor the initial airway colonization by *Aspergillus* are unclear[249] but are probably related in some way to the almost universal presence of asthma and atopy in affected patients. Certainly, once the fungus gets a foothold, local damage will promote further colonization. *Aspergillus* fungi are worldwide in distribution and ubiquitous. In more than 90% of patients, the species involved is *A. fumigatus,* but occasionally other species are implicated, including *A. flavus, A. niger, A. nidulans,*[249] *A. terreus,*[369] *A. oryzae,*[4] and *A. ochraceus.*[461] In addition, there are isolated case reports of an ABPA-like syndrome due to fungi other than *Aspergillus* spp, including *Candida albicans,*[3, 411] *Stemphylium lanuginosum,*[29] *Curvularia lunata,*[281] *Drechslera hawaiiensis,*[408] and *Helminthosporium* spp.[301]

Patients characteristically have evidence of both a type I and a type III Gell and Coomb's immune reactions[530] and possibly an element of a type IV reaction as well as complement activation.[267] The type I reaction is manifest by bronchospasm and is associated with a blood eosinophilia and IgE production that results in high *specific and nonspecific* serum levels. The type III reaction causes tissue damage leading to pulmonary shadowing and is associated with serum precipitins (IgG). Because antigen production is localized to the mycelial plug in the proximal airway, tissue damage tends to be greatest in this region, giving rise to the characteristic proximal bronchiectasis.

Typically, ABPA occurs in patients who are atopic and long-standing asthmatics. A few patients have been predisposed by cystic fibrosis,[372, 456] and some, particularly older ones, develop asthma concurrently with their first attack of ABPA.[410] Although unusual, the disease is well-recognized in nonasthmatics.[246, 410] Overall there is a slight preponderance of women with the condition.[239, 300, 410, 489] It may occur at any age, but 20 to 40 years of age is typical. However, patients go on presenting into their 60s[398, 489] and, at the other extreme, cases are described in children less than 2 years old.[329] The length of the interval between the onset of asthma and ABPA is inversely related to the age of onset of asthma. McCarthy and co-workers found that with asthma beginning before 10 years of age, there was an average gap of 24 years, but with late-onset asthma (30 years of age or more), the mean gap was only 3.5 years.[412] Late-onset asthma was associated with more frequent attacks of ABPA and greater lung damage.[412]

ABPA runs a relapsing and remitting course. Acute attacks are characterized by wheeze, dyspnea, and a cough that is often productive and associated with minor hemoptysis. Systemic symptoms such as fever, malaise, and weight loss are common. About 50% of patients have pleuritic pain, and about the same percentage give a history of coughing up sputum plugs.[410] These contain fungal mycelia and are important pointers to the diagnosis.[410] Plugs may be coughed up a few times a year or even monthly. They are about 1 to 2 cm long, firm, friable, and pellet-like.[410] An abnormal chest radiograph, blood eosinophilia, and an immediate skin reaction to *Aspergillus* antigens are characteristic of the acute phase. Eosinophilia is usually mild to moderate, with 74% of patients having counts between 1 and 3 $\times$ 10^9/L.[410] The eosinophil level may be depressed by steroid treatment. Serum precipitins against *Aspergillus* antigens are detected in 90% to 100% of patients in the acute phase, particularly if the serum is concentrated.[300, 410, 530] It must be remembered, however, that this test is nonspecific in that up to 25% of patients with extrinsic asthma will have a positive precipitin test.[315] Both nonspecific and *Aspergillus* antigen–specific IgE are greatly raised, perhaps 20 times normal.[530] As with the finding of positive precipitins, elevation of IgE is not diagnostic of ABPA and may be seen with atopic dermatitis, parasitic infestations, aspergilloma, and extrinsic asthma. IgE levels in asthma per se tend to be lower than in ABPA, and a level of 15,000 ng/ml is discriminatory between the two.[651]

Criteria for the diagnosis of ABPA vary from study to study. They have changed over time as knowledge about the disease has become more sophisticated; yet even now there are no universally accepted diagnostic criteria. Rosenberg and co-workers[530] have set out the following major and minor criteria and suggest that if the first six of the major criteria are satisfied, the diagnosis of ABPA can be made with reasonable certainty. The presence of central bronchiectasis makes the diagnosis certain.[530] Major criteria for ABPA are:

1. Asthma
2. Blood eosinophilia
3. Immediate skin reactivity to *Aspergillus* antigen
4. Precipitin antibodies to *Aspergillus* antigen

5. Raised levels of serum IgE
6. History of radiographic pulmonary opacities
7. Central bronchiectasis.

Minor criteria for ABPA are:

1. *A. fumigatus* in sputum
2. History of expectorating brown plugs
3. Late skin reactivity to *Aspergillus* antigen.

A great variety of radiologic changes are found in ABPA.* A consideration of the underlying disease processes makes the bewildering range of radiologic findings easier to understand and remember. In the acute stage there is mycelial plugging of segmental airways and an intense local inflammatory response that leads to bronchial wall thickening. Airway obstruction variously causes collapse, a mucoid impaction pattern, or consolidation. Judging by clinical features and response to treatment, it seems quite likely that secondary infection is an important aspect of some consolidations.[300] In the chronic phase, plugs have disappeared, leaving damaged and bronchiectatic airways, while the more distal changes have healed, often with a major fibrotic element.

The radiologic changes are best considered as acute and transient or chronic and permanent[412] (Table 11–10).

The transient changes are listed in Table 11–10. Despite some discrepancies between series, there is no doubt that consolidations are the most common type of opacity (Figs 11–42 and 11–43). They range from massive and homogeneous (occupying a whole lobe) to smaller ones that are subsegmental, to those that are even smaller (in the order of 1 cm). The smaller shadows are the more common. Consolidations show little if any zonal predilection. Larger shadows are often triangular, pointing to the hilus with a segmental or lobar configuration as might be expected of a process based on airway obstruction (see Fig 11–42). This appearance contrasts with consolidations seen in other eosinophilic states, e.g., Löffler's syndrome and cryptogenic eosinophilic pneumonia, in which nonsegmental consolidation is characteristic. Consolidations are frequently multiple. Cavitation is described in the larger consolidations with a frequency of 3% in one series[489] but rising to a surprising 14% and 21% in others.[239, 412] The cause of cavitation is largely speculative. In some cases it is undoubtedly due to bronchiectasis; in others, it may be secondary to cavitary bacterial

*References 239, 252, 300, 388, 398, 412, 436, 489, and 681.

TABLE 11–10.

Radiographic Findings in Allergic Bronchopulmonary Aspergillosis (% = Prevalence of finding)

Major	Minor
Acute (transient)	
Consolidation (80%)	Parallel line shadows
Mucoid impaction (bronchocele) (30%)	Ring shadows
	Small nodules
Atelectasis (20%)	Pleural effusion
Chronic (permanent)	
Overinflation (50%)	Pleural thickening
Tubular shadows (75%)	Mycetoma
Ring shadows (60%)	Small nodules
Vascular deficiency (30%)	Line shadows
Lobar shrinkage (40%)	

infection. Although consolidations are regarded as transient shadows, they can last for 6 weeks or more. Recently Phelan and Kerr[489] described some patients with apparently permanent consolidation. When consolidations clear, they often leave residual ring and line shadows consistent with bronchiectasis. Such bronchiectasis creates favorable conditions for fungal recolonization, a finding that accounts for the fact that 25% to 50% of consolidations recur later in the same area. It is notable that 20% to 30% of patients with radiographic consolidation are asymptomatic,[398, 535] and ABPA is one of those conditions in which gross radiographic changes may be accompanied by little in the way of symptoms.[412]

The second most common acute change is probably that of bronchocele formation (mucoid impaction). In this condition, an airway becomes obstructed and distended by retained secretions; yet, at the same time, the subtended lung remains aerated by collateral air drift allowing visualization of the impacted airway, which contrasts with the surrounding air-containing lung.[202] Bronchoceles take on a wide variety of shapes depending on the extent and degree of airway filling. The basic opacity is a linear, sharply demarcated, branched or unbranched bandlike shadow that points to the hilus (Fig 11–44)—the so-called toothpaste shadow—a band about 2- to 3-cm long and some 5- to 8-mm wide. Variants include V-shaped, inverted V-shaped, and Y-shaped opacities. Sometimes bronchoceles are more rounded than linear and can simulate a mass, if single, or a cluster of masses, if multiple ("bunch

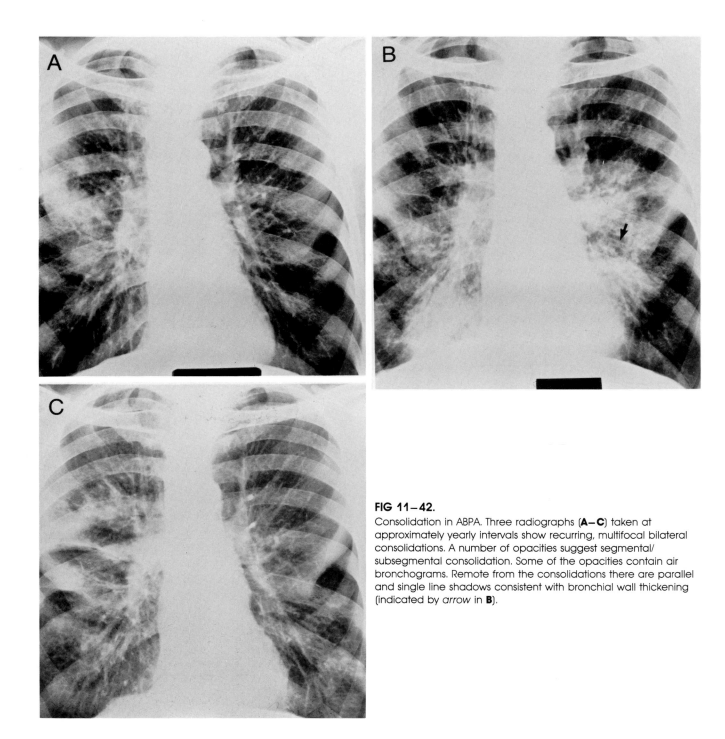

FIG 11–42.
Consolidation in ABPA. Three radiographs (**A–C**) taken at approximately yearly intervals show recurring, multifocal bilateral consolidations. A number of opacities suggest segmental/subsegmental consolidation. Some of the opacities contain air bronchograms. Remote from the consolidations there are parallel and single line shadows consistent with bronchial wall thickening (indicated by *arrow* in **B**).

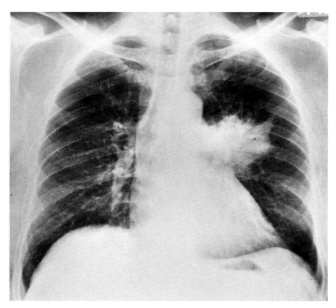

FIG 11–43.
Consolidation in ABPA simulating a mass lesion.

where wall separation is consistent with a normal airway calibre. Parallel line shadows are most commonly seen in patients less than 15 years old, an age group in which asthma alone may be associated with such shadows. Occasionally, thick-walled ring shadows (walls 3- to 5-mm wide, rings 2 to 3 cm in diameter) are seen divorced from consolidation.[412] Their pathologic basis is obscure. Small, ill-defined, rounded or irregular opacities (miliary opacities) are described as both transient and permanent shadows. It is possible that they represent granulomas formed as a result of an extrinsic allergic alveolitis. There have been a few reports of pleural effusion.[398, 449]

Permanent changes are of importance because (1) they indicate irreversible lung damage and (2) they

of grapes"). Similarly, rounded opacities will be produced by linear bronchoceles seen end-on. Impacted airways are usually proximal (typically segmental). They are often inseparable from the hilus and may simulate lymphadenopathy.[436] Another variant is produced by distal bronchiectatic airways which, when impacted, give a band shadow with a club-shaped end: the so-called "gloved finger shadow." Bronchoceles show a strong predilection for the upper zone (Fig 11–45).[398] They disappear once their contents have been coughed up, leaving ring or parallel line shadows (Fig 11–46). Like consolidations in ABPA they may recur at the same site. Occasionally they persist for many months and are recorded as remaining for at least 18 months.[239]

The third major acute manifestation of ABPA is atelectasis (Fig 11–47), which ranges in frequency from 3%[398] to 46%.[239] It may be subsegmental, segmental, lobar, or even affect a whole lung.[36, 179, 388, 489] Collapse is, of course, a complication of asthma per se.[319] Like consolidations and mucoid impaction, collapse has a tendency to recur in the same area.

A variety of other, less important, acute opacities have been described. They include parallel line shadows due to bronchial wall thickening, presumably from inflammation and edema (see Fig 11–42). McCarthy et al.[412] distinguish between two types of parallel line shadows: (1) tubular opacities, where the walls are inappropriately wide apart, consistent with bronchiectasis, and (2) tram-line opacities

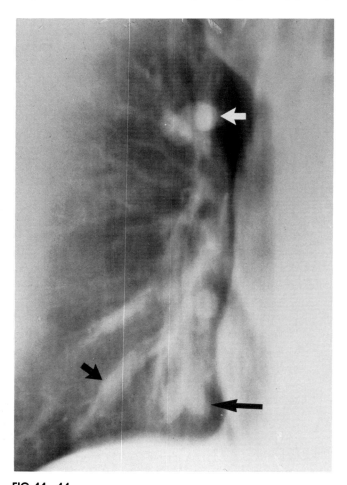

FIG 11–44.
Bronchocele in ABPA. Whole-lung tomogram demonstrates the variety of shapes adopted by bronchoceles. The most common is the bandlike opacity pointing to the hilus—the toothpaste shadow *(short black arrow)*. Other variants include Y-shaped *(long black arrow)* and rounded opacities *(white arrow)*. It is unusual to find so many bronchoceles in allergic aspergillosis, and their lower zone predominance is also unusual.

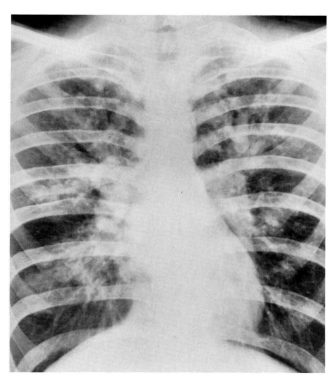

FIG 11–45.
Bronchoceles in ABPA. Bronchoceles are in the middle and upper zone, a more typical distribution than that shown in Figure 11–44. In the left upper zone there are several finger-like bronchoceles; a number on the right are clustered and rounded, overlying the hilus and giving it a lobulated appearance.

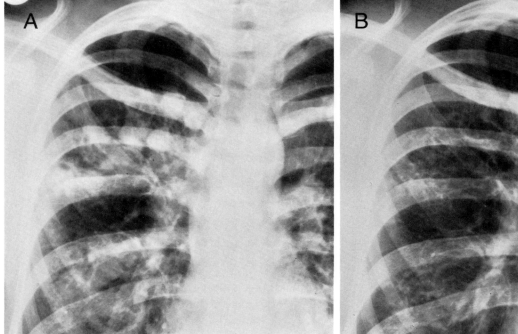

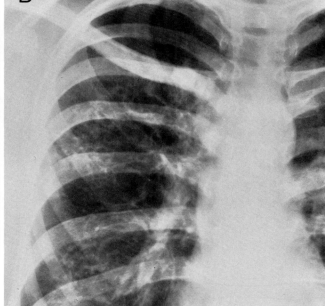

FIG 11–46.
Bronchoceles in ABPA. **A,** local view of the right upper/middle zone shows multiple rounded bronchoceles. **B,** when these clear they leave a collection of delicate curvilinear and ring opacities which are walls of bronchiectatic airways. Such opacities close to the hilus in the mid and upper zone are a characteristic interval finding in allergic aspergillosis.

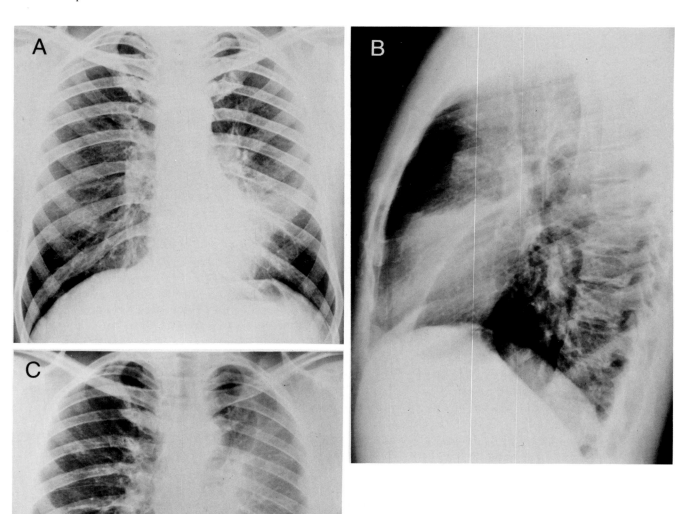

FIG 11–47.
Atelectasis in ABPA. **A** and **B,** the patient presented with lingular consolidation associated with minor volume loss, and then went on to develop complete collapse of the upper lobe (**C**).

may be the only clues that an asthmatic has ABPA when a patient is in remission.

Before discussing permanent changes, it is worthwhile considering the bronchographic findings, as these clarify the appearance seen on the plain chest radiograph (Fig 11–48). Nearly every patient with ABPA will have an abnormal bronchogram[412, 436, 530] demonstrating one or more of the following changes (see Fig 11–48):

1. Mild cylindrical bronchiectasis
2. Distal cystic bronchiectasis with occluded branches
3. Proximal bronchiectasis.

Bronchiectatic changes are a sensitive indicator of ABPA. Furthermore, proximal bronchiectasis is very specific,[422, 530] differing from other forms of bronchiectasis in that (1) it affects lobar and first and

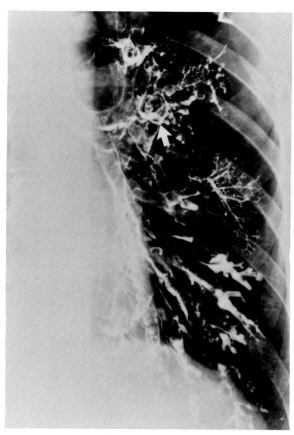

FIG 11–48.
Bronchiectasis in ABPA. In the left lower zone this bronchogram shows nonspecific cylindrical bronchiectasis. In the left upper zone, however, there is proximal cystic bronchiectasis *(arrow)* with preserved distal branches. This is a highly specific finding in ABPA.

second order segmental bronchi, and (2) normal distal airways carry on from the dilated area rather than being occluded by a bronchiolitis obliterans.[412, 547] Despite the sensitivity and specificity of proximal bronchiectasis, most workers would not consider bronchography justifiable in making or confirming a diagnosis of ABPA.[489] As an alternative approach, conventional tomography[211] and CT scanning[135] have been used. CT has been shown to be twice as sensitive as the plain chest radiograph in the detection of bronchiectasis.[135] Not all patients with ABPA will have an abnormal bronchogram,[275] and despite the generally accepted high sensitivity of this examination, some authors regard bronchiectasis as a late manifestation.[135]

Persistent radiologic changes are a direct or indirect result of bronchiectasis. Abnormally dilated airways may be visualized, particularly in perihilar regions and upper zones, as tubular and ring shadows (see Fig 11–46). Tubular shadows are parallel line

shadows in which the lines, representing bronchial walls, are more widely separated than would be expected for airways of normal caliber, implying that they must be bronchiectatic. They are bilateral and are more common in the upper zone. When filled with secretions, the dilated airways produce bronchoceles, and the transformation of bronchoceles into tubular shadows and back again is common on serial radiographs. Frequently only small segments of one wall of an airway will be seen, giving rise to single line opacities rather than tubular shadows. Thin-wall ring shadows 1 to 2 cm in diameter commonly represent bronchiectatic airways seen end-on, though some may represent bullae or some other form of abnormal air space. When filled wholly or in part with secretions, end-on bronchiectatic airways appear as nodules or ring shadows with air-fluid levels. Occasionally, aggregations of ring shadows between 0.5 and 1 cm in diameter will appear as honeycomb shadowing.

Bronchiectatic airways are also detected by their secondary effects. The reduced ventilation of lung distal to bronchiectasis is reflected in a reduction in vascularity. Parenchymal scarring commonly follows bronchiectasis and is manifest by line shadows and lobar shrinkage (Fig 11–49). Mirroring the distribu-

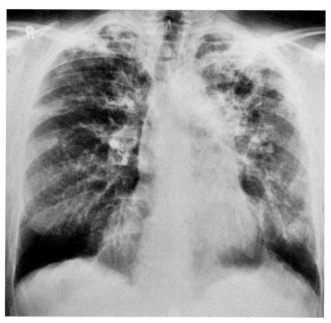

FIG 11–49.
Fibrosis in ABPA. Bilateral middle and upper zone fibrosis following multiple acute attacks of ABPA. The upper zone shadowing is a complex mixture of linear, ring, nodular, and conglomerate opacities, reflecting the diverse underlying pathology including bronchiectasis, scarring, and bulla formation.

tion of bronchiectasis, these features have a strong upper zone predilection, with 78% being so distributed in one series.[412] Such lobar shrinkage is accompanied by a variety of ring and linear shadows. Lower lobe shrinkage, though described, is very unusual.[489] Although there is often chronic lobar shrinkage, the overall lung volume is frequently increased, reflecting airflow limitation, emphysema and bulla formation. Between 30% and 40% of patients in one series showed overinflation.[489] Pleural thickening is not a major feature, having a prevalence of 18% in the same series.

Mycetomas may form in the bronchiectatic cavities. In one series of 111 patients with ABPA, eight had mycetomas, predominantly mid zonal.[412] Since mid zone mycetomas are unusual in other conditions, it has been suggested that one found in this position should raise the possibility of underlying ABPA.[412] It might be expected that patients with ABPA and mycetoma would be particularly symptomatic because of their immune status coupled with massive antigen production, but this does not appear to be so. However, it is of interest that an ABPA type of syndrome has been recorded as developing as a result of a mycetoma lodged in a tuberculous cavity.[176]

In summary, a chest radiograph of an asthmatic showing consolidation; collapse; upper zone fibrosis; or, particularly, mucoid impaction should prompt consideration of ABPA, as should the more subtle changes of perihilar and upper zone bronchiectasis.

Drug-Induced Eosinophilic Lung Disease

A large number of drugs are recorded as producing pulmonary opacities together with blood eosinophilia; these are listed in Table 11–11. Some patients develop an associated rash and pyrexia, and this can provide a helpful clue to the nature of the radiologic shadowing. A variety of chest radiographic patterns are produced:

1. Air-space consolidation (Fig 11–50), which may be localized or diffuse. In some instances the pattern is that of Löffler's syndrome. Drugs that are particularly associated with a consolidative pattern include penicillin, sulfonamides, para-aminosalicylic acid, chlorpropamide, nitrofurantoin, methotrexate, carbamazepine, mephenesin, imipramine, trimipramine, and hydrochlorothiazide.

2. Hilar lymphadenopathy. This is recorded with the anti-epileptic drugs phenytoin and trimethadione.[446]

3. Pleural effusions. These are occasionally seen with nitrofurantoin (see Chapter 14).

4. Reticulonodular shadowing. A fibrosing alveolitis type of pattern is produced in particular by nitrofurantoin and methotrexate (see Chapter 10). With nitrofurantoin the chronic interstitial pattern is associated with a blood eosinophilia in about 40% of patients.[121] Other drugs that produce an interstitial pattern include gold[446] and clofibrate.[303]

5. Other patterns. Patterns other than those described and which are not easy to classify are recorded with a number of drugs such as penicillamine.[140]

Tropical Pulmonary Eosinophilia

This is a specific systemic disease caused by hypersensitivity to microfilariae, the early larval forms of various filarial nematodes, the most important being *Brugia malayi* and *Wuchereria bancrofti*. Tropical pulmonary eosinophilia is found in all parts of the world where filariasis is endemic, particularly the Indian subcontinent, Southeast Asia, the South Pacific, North Africa, and South America. It occurs chiefly in the indigenous residents (particularly in the In-

TABLE 11–11.
Drugs Associated With Eosinophilic Lung Disease

Antibiotics
Ampicillin[121]	Penicillin[121, 446, 554, 584]
Capreomycin[584]	Rifampicin[584]
Isoniazid[121, 584]	Sulfonamides[121, 446, 554, 584]
Nitrofurantoin[121, 446, 554, 584]	Tetracycline[554]
Para-aminosalicylic acid[121, 446, 554, 584]	

Analgesics/anti-inflammatory drugs
Aspirin[554, 584]
Gold[446]
Naproxen[452]

Cytotoxics
Azathioprine[120]	Methotrexate[120, 446, 554, 584]
Bleomycin[120, 584]	Procarbazine[120]

Sulfonylureas
Chlorpropamide[121, 446, 554]
Tolazamide[48]
Tolbutamide[584]

Neuropsychiatric drugs
Carbamazepine[121, 132, 554, 584]	Mephenesin[121, 554, 584]
Chlorpromazine[554]	Phenytoin[121]
Dantrolene[121]	Trimethadione[446]
Imipramine[121, 554]	

Miscellaneous drugs
Beclomethasone[554]	Hydralazine[121]
Clofibrate[303]	Methylphenidate[121, 554]
Cromogylcate[554]	Penicillamine[140]

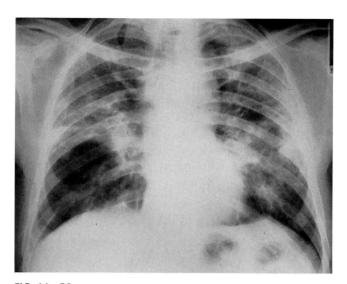

FIG 11–50.
Drug-related eosinophilic lung disease. Multifocal nonsegmental consolidations in a 66-year-old man who developed a nonproductive cough and dyspnea after starting a nonsteroidal anti-inflammatory drug (naproxen). There was a blood eosinophilia (6.4 × 10⁹/L). The opacities cleared after naproxen was discontinued and systemic steroids begun. (Courtesy of Dr. J.D. Stevenson, Poole, Dorset.)

dian subcontinent[163, 308]) and is very uncommon in visitors unless they have resided in the area for many months.[457] In nonendemic areas the disease is seen in immigrants and, because of the persistence of the parasite in the host, may present as long as 3 years after returning from an endemic area.[136] Occurrence is extremely rare in Caucasians.[356]

The disease is more common in men, in some series by as much as a 4 : 1 ratio,[585] but this is not a universal finding.[356] The usual age at presentation is between 5 and 40 years,[585] though the range can be larger; in one series of 350, age at onset varied from 1.5 years to 74 years.[308] The principal features of the illness are a systemic disturbance marked by fatigue, weight loss, and low-grade fever together with respiratory symptoms. The main respiratory symptoms are chronic cough, which is particularly troublesome at night and may be productive of mucoid or mucopurulent sputum with occasional hemoptysis, dyspnea, and wheeze. Even without treatment, disease symptoms tend to remit after several weeks or months only to recur later.[457] On auscultation of the patient's chest, there are crackles and wheezes. Hepatosplenomegaly and nodal enlargement are rarely seen except in children.[585] There is a gross eosinophilia of more than 3 × 10⁹/L, characteristically, between 5 and 60 × 10⁹/L; IgE levels are greatly elevated, usually more than

1,000 units/ml; and there is a high titer of antifilarial antibody.

Several reports have described the radiologic findings in the chest.[17, 24, 308, 356, 499] The chest radiograph has a normal appearance in 2% to 13% of cases. The most common abnormalities, seen in one-third to two-thirds of patients, of fine linear opacities distributed diffusely and symmetrically, accompanied by hilar haziness and an accentuation or blurring of vessels. Some authors[356] describe a basal preponderance, and others stress a general loss in transradiancy accompanying the diffuse shadowing.[308] Small nodules are a slightly less common finding—seen in about 30% to 50% of patients (Fig 11–51). The nodules range in size from 1 to 5 mm and may occur alone or with the linear opacities previously described.[356] Though generally bilateral and symmetric, nodulation may be asymmetric or even

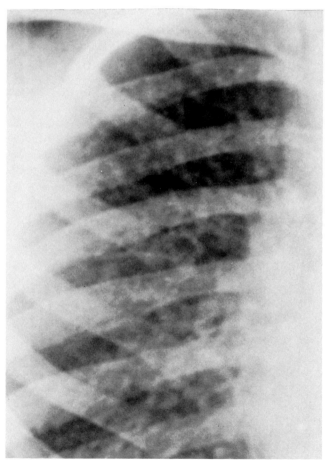

FIG 11–51.
Tropical pulmonary eosinophilia. The chief finding in this patient was 2- to 3-mm nodulation distributed throughout the lungs but more marked on the right side. (Courtesy of Professor C.J.F. Spry, London.)

unilateral.[499] Other patterns are much less common and consist of areas of consolidation that are generally small and single. They can, however, be large,[338] multifocal,[24, 356] or even cavitary.[331] Diffuse ground-glass opacification[24] and small pleural effusions[499] are also described. Many accounts describe bilateral hilar enlargement or prominence.[17, 24, 308, 499] Enlargement is almost always mild and has been ascribed to vessels rather than nodes,[308] though there was pathologic evidence of slight hilar adenopathy in one study.[658]

Eosinophilic Lung Disease From Other Worm Infestations

The larval stages of a number of worms other than filarial nematodes pass through the lung and may, in the process, induce an allergic response; these responses most commonly take the form of Löffler's syndrome with transient, migratory, nonsegmental areas of consolidation associated with a blood eosinophilia (Fig 11–52).[510] Nearly all the worms that cause this response are nematodes: *Ascaris lumbricoides*,[25, 240] *As. suum*,[490] *Strongyloides stercoralis*,[510] *Toxocara canis*,[673] *T. cati*,[510] *Ancylostoma braziliense*,[72] *An. duodenale, Necator americanus*,[221] *Trichuris trichiura*,[127] *Taenia saginata*,[127] *Echinococcus alveolaris*,[127] and *Schistosoma* spp.[145] It is possible that, in

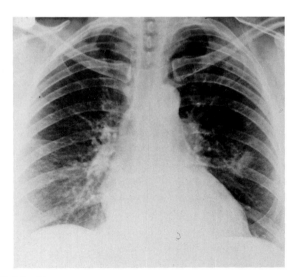

FIG 11–52.
Eosinophilic lung disease following worm infestation. This 52-year-old woman presented with a buttock rash caused by cutaneous larva migrans (due to *Ancylostoma braziliense*) acquired on vacation in the West Indies. She had a blood eosinophilia and a dry cough. The chest radiograph shows two areas of consolidation: one in the left mid-zone and the other peripherally in the left upper zone. They cleared in 2 weeks.

at least some of these infestations, the pulmonary reaction is not related to local larvae but rather is a remote response to a soluble antigen.[72] Thus in 26 patients with eosinophilic lung disease due to *An. braziliense* (see Fig 11–52), it was not possible to demonstrate larvae in the sputum.[673] Some idea of the possible frequency of eosinophilic lung disease caused by nematode infestations may be gained from the last authors, who found lung shadowing in 34% of 76 patients with cutaneous larva migrans (hookworm infestation).

Bronchocentric Granulomatosis

This form of pulmonary granulomatosis, first described by Liebow in 1973,[380] differs from other lung granulomatoses, such as Wegener's, in that it is localized to the lung and centered around airways (bronchocentric) rather than vessels (angiocentric). Pathologically, small airways and bronchioles are filled with and replaced by cellular debris and necrotic granulomas surrounded by palisaded epithelioid cells. In asthmatics the major part of the cellular infiltrate is made up of eosinophils, whereas in nonasthmatics the plasma cell is dominant.[352] Large airways may show mucoid impaction, and distal lung is often consolidated by an eosinophilic or obstructive pneumonitis. Vasculitic changes appear to be minor and incidental.

Only three series of patients with bronchocentric granulomatosis have been recorded,[352, 363, 539] representing a total of 55 cases; however, there have been many additional case reports.

Patients commonly present in their 40s, but there is a wide age range (9 to 76 years) and a tendency for asthmatics to present at a younger age (mean age, 22 years) than nonasthmatics (mean age, 50 years).[352] The incidence is equal in both sexes. In the combined series, 16 (29%) of the 55 patients have been asthmatic, and some patients have had associated disorders, though the significance of this observation is unclear. These disorders include rheumatoid disease,[33] ankylosing spondylitis,[527] glomerulonephritis,[652] and echinococcosis.[146] Symptoms may be absent or minor and, when present, are not particularly characteristic. They consist of fever, cough, chest pain, wheeze, and hemoptysis. About 50% of patients have had a blood eosinophilia, a finding that appears to be limited to asthmatics.[352, 363]

Radiologically,[352, 363, 524, 539] two major patterns are seen: consolidations, or masslike lesions. Consolidations may be lobar or sublobar and may be accompanied by volume loss (Fig 11–53,A). They are thought to represent either eosinophilic or obstructive pneumonitis.[352] They tend to be more common in the upper zones[352, 524] and are unilateral in about 75% of patients. Sublobar consolidation was the commonest finding (16/22) in one large series.[352] Masslike lesions are commonly solitary but can be multiple. They are considered to represent a mass of necrotic tissue with surrounding granulomatous or organizing pneumonitis. They vary in size from 2 to 15 cm[33] and are often not particularly well defined. Occasionally they cavitate.[33, 352] Less common radiologic patterns include mucoid impaction (Fig 11–54)[108, 352] and reticulonodular opacities. On some occasions the reticulonodular shadowing has evolved from antecedent consolidation.

There is considerable evidence that bronchocentric granulomatosis in asthmatics is different etiologically from that seen in nonasthmatics. In many asthmatics there is histologic, serologic, and microbiological evidence that bronchocentric granulomatosis is caused by *Aspergillus* and forms part of the spectrum of allergic bronchopulmonary aspergillosis.[283] It is also possible that there is sensitivity to other fungi

such as *Candida* spp.[352] In nonasthmatics the cause is obscure.

Patient prognosis is good. Lesions may clear spontaneously or with steroids and generally do not recur following surgical removal. If this should happen, recurrences can usually be controlled with steroid treatment.

Hypereosinophilic Syndrome

Hypereosinophilic syndrome is a rarely encountered, heterogeneous group of disorders characterized by (1) prolonged and marked eosinophilia (a blood count of more than 1.5×10^9/L for more than 6 months), (2) no recognizable cause for the eosinophilia such as parasitic infestation or allergy, and (3) signs or symptoms of organ dysfunction.[106] The illness varies in severity from mild to fatal, involving in particular the cardiovascular and nervous systems. In the past it has gone under a variety of other names including Löffler's syndrome with cardiac involvement, Löffler's fibroplastic endocarditis, and disseminated eosinophilic collagen disease.[189]

Pathologically there is widespread tissue infiltra-

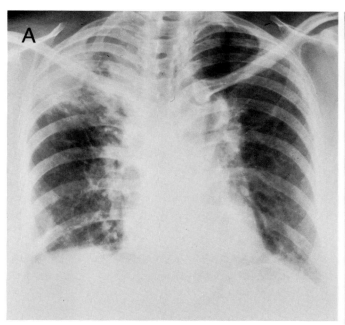

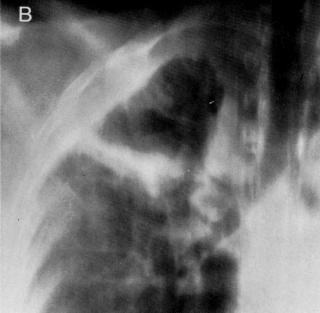

FIG 11–53.
Bronchocentric granulomatosis. This 52-year-old woman presented with weight loss and cough. **A,** the chest radiograph shows right upper zone consolidation with some volume loss and scattered linear/nodular opacities in the left upper zone, these latter changes being ascribed to old granulomatous disease. The patient was treated with antituberculous therapy without an estab-

lished diagnosis. **B,** localized tomogram of the right upper zone 1 month later. The consolidation has been replaced by a thick-walled, 5-cm-diameter cavity. Following right upper lobectomy, the patient developed asthma and blood eosinophilia. There were hyphae of *Aspergillus* in the pathologic specimen.

A
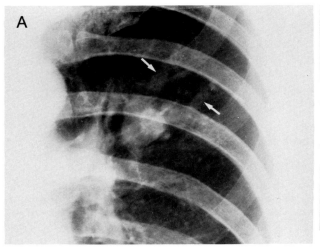

B
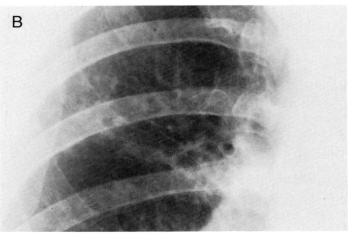

FIG 11–54.
Bronchocentric granulomatosis. **A,** localized view of the left mid zone in a 50-year-old woman shows a 2 × 3-cm lobulated well-demarcated masslike lesion with two finger-like projections *(arrows)* that strongly suggest a bronchocele. **B,** localized view of the right mid zone shows thin curvilinear and ring opacities due to bronchiectasis resulting from allergic aspergillosis. (Courtesy of Dr. J.D. Stevenson, Poole, Dorset.)

tion with mature eosinophils that cause tissue damage,[197] particularly endocardial damage leading to endocardial fibrosis, restrictive cardiomyopathy, and thrombosis.

Almost all patients have been men, typically young or middle-aged adults who present with progressive cardiopulmonary symptoms, skin rash, or myalgia together with systemic symptoms such as weight loss, weakness, fatigue, and fever. The peripheral blood shows a marked eosinophilia, often in the order of 30% to 70% of the total white blood cell count (10 to 50 × 10^9/L), some of the eosinophils being degranulated and vacuolated. Some patients have a mild increase in IgE. The organ systems most commonly affected are the nervous and cardiovascular systems and the skin. Cardiovascular involvement is usually the dominant feature and is a major cause of morbidity, with signs of restrictive cardiomyopathy and pump failure, mitral and tricuspid regurgitation, and endocardial thrombosis. This latter leads .o systemic emboli in about 5% of patients[481] or pulmonary emboli if the thrombus is right-sided.[197]

Clinical pulmonary involvement has been recorded in about 40% of patients.[106, 197] In most, these are findings related to heart failure[189] and include pulmonary edema and pleural effusions.[106] Because the cardiomyopathy is restrictive in type, any accompanying cardiomegaly is often mild.[481] Pulmonary emboli were recorded in 9% of 57 patients reviewed from the literature.[106] Other less common pulmonary manifestations include transient

consolidations, which are presumably eosinophilic pneumonias, and diffuse interstitial fibrosis.[106, 481]

Before the use of steroids and cytotoxic drugs the prognosis was poor, with a 25% 2-year survival-rate,[106] but this figure has now improved considerably, and the 3-year mortality is down to 4%.[482]

Hyperimmunoglobulin E, Recurrent-Infection (Job's) Syndrome

This rare primary immunodeficiency syndrome was first described in 1966[142] and is characterized by (1) recurrent bacterial sinopulmonary disease and recurrent skin infections dating from birth or early childhood and (2) a more than tenfold elevation of serum IgE.[161] The immunologic derangement is complex and is only partly understood.[424] Patients have a characteristically coarse facies, eczematous skin rash, and recurrent furunculosis and cutaneous cold abscesses which may be large. The lack of the usual systemic and local inflammatory findings with the abscesses is a striking feature, particularly because most are due to *Staphylococcus aureus*. Mucocutaneous candidiasis is common, as are recurrent bronchitis and pneumonia, often due to *S. aureus* or *Hemophilus influenzae*. Eosinophilia is a common feature, occurring in 77% of patients in one series[161] and in all the patients in another series,[424] but it is usually only mild or mild to moderate. Occasionally, however, eosinophilia is marked.[67] Radiologic findings in the chest have been well described[424] and consist of recurrent infective consolidations and cyst formation. Infective consolidations usually begin before 3 years of age and are commonly segmental or lobar. All the patients in the series of Merten et al.,[424] in which the average age was 18 years, had lung cysts. Some cysts disappeared after a few years, while others were recurrent or persistent. About a third of the cysts were multiple and could be very large, occupying much of a hemithorax, while their walls were usually smooth but of varying thickness. The pathogenesis of these cysts is not definitely established. Some are probably pneumatoceles and others arise in a cavitating consolidation. In a number of cases, however, their development could not be related to an infective episode.[424] One out of 11 patients had plain radiographic evidence of bronchiectasis, and 9 out of 11 had evidence of chronic sinusitis.

EXTRINSIC ALLERGIC ALVEOLITIS

Extrinsic allergic alveolitis (EAA) is a disorder in which repeated inhalation of particulate organic antigens causes a predominantly immunologic response in the air-exchange units of the lung. There are several synonyms for this condition, the most common being hypersensitivity pneumonitis.

A large number of causal antigens have already been identified, including microorganisms (bacteria, fungi, thermophilic actinomycetes, amebas), animal and plant proteins, drugs, and some small molecular weight chemicals.[542] Thermophilic actinomycetes are particularly important agents. They are widely distributed bacteria with morphologic features of fungi that thrive in the high temperatures (45° to 60° C) commonly found in decomposing vegetable matter.[516] Agents that cause EAA are all particulates of such a size (1 to 5 μm) that they can enter and be retained in the gas exchange units of the lung, particularly the alveoli. In order to induce disease, the exposure has to be heavy—either short and intense or prolonged and low grade. With one or two exceptions, for example exposure to pet birds or to agents from humidifiers, such exposures are only found in association with specific occupations or hobbies.

The most important and common disorders are listed in Table 11–12, together with the inciting

TABLE 11–12.

Major Causes of Extrinsic Allergic Alveolitis

Disease	Source of Antigen	Antigen	Reference
Farmer's lung	Moldy hay	Thermophilic actinomycetes (*Micropolyspora faeni, Thermoactinomyces vulgaris*)	Cadhan[74] Campbell[80] Dickie and Rankin[154] Emanuel et al.[182] Hapke et al.[284]
Bagassosis	Moldy sugar cane	*T. sacchari*	Hargreave et al.[286]
Mushroom worker's lung	Mushroom compost	Thermophilic actinomycetes (mushroom spores)	Bringhurst et al.[62] Sakula[537] Jackson and Welch[335]
Air conditioner/ humidifier disease	Dust or mist	*T. vulgaris, T. thalpophilus*, amebas, thermotolerant bacteria	Banaszak et al.[18] Medical Research Council[417] Stankus and Salvaggio[588] Kohler et al.[360]
Maltworker's lung	Moldy barley	*Aspergillus clavatus*	Riddle et al.[519]
Bird fancier's (breeder's) lung	Droppings and feathers	Avian protein	Reed et al.[508] Hargreave et al.[287]

agents and antigens. Many other less common disorders not included in the table are recognized, including, suberosis due to moldy cork dust,[491] maple bark disease,[183] wood pulp worker's disease,[573] sauna-taker's disease,[426] sequoiosis,[112] cheese washer's lung,[152] dry rot lung,[462] grain/wheat weevil lung,[394] animal handler's lung,[90] Pauli's reagent "alveolitis,"[192] fish meal worker's lung,[15] diisocyanate alveolitis,[97] pyrethrum alveolitis,[85] *Bacillus subtilis* alveolitis,[341] *A. fumigatus* alveolitis,[642] and coffee worker's lung.[640] More comprehensive lists are available in the literature.[219, 479, 516, 523, 577]

The immunopathogenesis is complicated and incompletely worked out. Antigen inhalation probably leads to precipitin antibody formation and T-cell sensitization in all exposed individuals, only some of whom will develop EAA. The pathologic changes are probably mediated by both type III (immune complex, Arthus type) and type IV (cell mediated, delayed type) reactions. Other mechanisms, such as complement activation by the alternative pathway, probably play a part as well. Several reviews discuss the pathogenesis in detail.[479, 516, 523, 542]

Histologic changes are conventionally classified into acute, subacute, and chronic, but it has been pointed out that the so-called acute changes are in fact occurring days or weeks into the illness.[516] Early on there is an interstitial pneumonitis that starts near terminal bronchioles and extends intraparenchymally.[351] The septa develop a mononuclear cell infiltrate with lymphocytes and histiocytes. Alveolar spaces may be filled by alveolar epithelial proliferation or fluid, which can be serous, hemorrhagic, or exudative.[22, 182, 317] Bronchiolitis is common and, in some cases, obstructive.[182, 563] Vasculitis is also described,[22] but it is not a dominant feature. These acute changes are more common in the lower zones.[563] In the subacute phase, noncaseating, loose, histiocytic granulomas appear at about 3 weeks and may last up to 1 year.[563] The interstitial pneumonitis persists, as does the alveolar inflammatory exudate.[515] With the development of the chronic phase, granulomas disappear and fibrosis ensues, affecting particularly the upper zones.[219] This results in honeycomb and cystic changes with air-containing spaces varying in size between 1 mm and several centimeters.[563] Some of these air spaces represent irregular emphysema secondary to peribronchial scarring. Eventually there may be changes of pulmonary arterial hypertension and cor pulmonale.[182, 563] Pleural fibrosis is seen in about 50% of patients[317] but is not a major feature.

The age and sex patterns in the various types of EAA simply reflect differing opportunities for exposure. Bird fancier's lung, for example, when due to budgerigars (parakeets) occurs typically in women over 65 years of age. When due to pigeons it is seen in men under 45 years.[514] Another feature of EAA is the relatively low attack rate; many people develop immune reactions to recognized antigens, yet fail to develop overt lung disease.[516] Some factors that may account for variability in the attack rates have been identified and include HLA status[213] and smoking[514] which, perversely, protects against development of the disease. Farmer's lung shows seasonal fluctuations, occurring particularly in late autumn, winter, and early spring.[479] There are also regional differences in prevalence that reflect climatic differences and differences in farming practices. For example, in the United Kingdom the prevalence rates for farmer's lung are more than ten times greater in Wales than in the drier parts of England.[479] Absolute prevalence rates are difficult to assess and compare, but it would seem that, for both farmer's lung and bird fancier's lung due to budgerigars, the prevalence rate in exposed individuals is about 2% to 4% (lying between 0.5% and 7.5%), making bird fancier's lung ten times more common than farmer's lung in the United Kingdom.[302]

Three types of illness are recognized: acute, subacute, and chronic, and each presents with a variable mixture of respiratory and constitutional symptoms.[284] The acute illness follows 4 to 8 hours after heavy exposure to the antigen and consists of dry cough, chest tightness, dyspnea, wheeze, fever, and malaise. Other symptoms include sweating, shivering, anorexia, nausea, vomiting, weakness, and prostration. These symptoms are often mistakenly diagnosed as a viral or bacterial illness unless suspicions of EAA are aroused by repeated episodes. Acute exposure and presentation occurs in the majority of those with bird fancier's lung due to pigeons, where it typically follows loft cleaning, but is only seen in about one-third of patients with farmer's lung.[486] These symptoms may be accompanied by hemoptysis and followed by weight loss. Spontaneous recovery follows removal from the agent, with substantial improvement in 1 to 2 days. Recovery is usually complete by 7 to 10 days. Leucocytosis is common during the acute illness, and respiratory function tests show restrictive and obstructive abnormalities. Physical examination of the patient in the acute phase usually reveals fine to medium basal crackles[284] and, sometimes, late inspiratory squeaks. Tachypnea and central cyanosis with restlessness and apprehension are found in the more severe cases.[479]

The subacute syndrome consists of acute episodes superimposed on a background of deteriorating respiratory function. The chronic form is dominated by progressive shortness of breath and is a common mode of presentation in farmer's lung and in bird fancier's lung related to the budgerigar.[219] It is associated with continual low-grade exposure which, if allowed to persist, causes irreversible lung damage. It may be accompanied by constitutional symptoms such as malaise and weight loss. Physical signs in the chronic form are usually not very striking.

Serum precipitins have long been regarded as the hallmark of extrinsic allergic alveolitis,[219] but it must be remembered that, like asbestos-related pleural plaques, they are only indicators of exposure and not necessarily of disease. Thus, 40% of pigeon breeders clinically free of EAA had tests positive for serum precipitin antibody.[206] Positive serum precipitin tests are also present in disease-free farmers[662] and even in the community at large. It is also possible to have the reverse situation, with definite disease, but a negative serum precipitin test, especially at the more advanced, fibrotic end of the spectrum.[266, 486, 566] Nevertheless, about 90% of patients with EAA will have positive serum precipitin values at presentation, particularly if the last exposure was in the antecedent weeks or months. In a series of patients with farmer's lung, all the acute cases and 53% of chronic cases had positive serum precipitins, the precipitins remaining positive for about 2 or 3 years.[284]

The diagnosis of EAA is usually made from the characteristic clinical symptoms and signs, together with evidence of exposure and improvement following withdrawal. Supportive evidence is provided by a late reaction to intracutaneous antigen, compatible radiologic findings and respiratory function tests, and the presence of precipitins in the blood. However, none of these tests is pathognomonic. A more specific test is bronchial provocation with the suspect antigen, though this is not commonly performed and can be dangerous.[205] Histologic changes are never diagnostic save for a few types of allergic alveolitis in which organic particles can be identified (e.g., bagassosis and maple bark disease). Histologically the principal differential diagnoses are granulomatous infections, sarcoidosis, and interstitial pneumonitis (usual and lymphocytic).[351]

It is generally considered that the chest radiographic changes are the same regardless of the provocative agent,[637] but it should be remembered that not all agents have been recorded as causing the entire spectrum of possible radiologic change. In the acute stage, the chest radiograph may occasionally be normal,[11, 285] or it may be interpreted as normal because the findings may be very subtle.[479] The radiograph may also be normal later on, even in patients with abnormal diffusing capacity[439, 627] and biopsy proved granulomata.[435, 507]

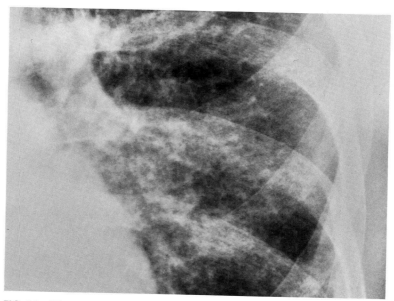

FIG 11–55.

Acute farmer's lung. A localized view of the left mid zone shows diffuse shadowing consisting predominantly of small nodules up to 2 mm in diameter.

The most common radiographic finding in the acute/subacute stage is small pulmonary nodules, usually 1 to 3 mm in diameter (Fig 11–55)[117, 435] but ranging up to 5 mm.[182, 284] These shadows may be so small and profuse that they give a ground-glass appearance (Fig 11–56).[439] The nodules may be discrete and sharply defined[284] or ill-defined.[683] They are almost always bilateral; in one series of 132 patients only 2% had unilateral nodules.[514] Opacities are most commonly found in all lung zones[285, 638] but may show a mid/lower zonal preponderance, sparing the apices,[182] or a mid/upper zone predominance, sparing the periphery at the bases.[117, 435] They appear just a few hours after exposure[49] and persist for a variable period, clearing in several weeks[435] or months.[284, 638] They can, however, persist indefinitely and become part of the chronic changes.[284] Occasionally, larger nodules in the 4-mm to 8-mm range are seen,[285] but these are far less common. Focal consolidations develop in some 10% to 25% of patients and are variously described as conglomerate shadows, fluffy opacities, and patchy clouding (Fig 11–57).[117, 182, 285, 514, 638] Sometimes the interstitial pattern takes on a more linear appearance in the acute stage, and bronchovascular markings may become accentuated.[439, 638, 683] Pleural changes are not a feature of EAA.[479] It is quite likely that when pleural changes are encountered, they are due to coincidental pleural disease, subpleural consolidation, or simple apical caps.[285] In the series of Hargreave et al.[285] there was a 15% prevalence of minor fissure thickening.[285] Septal B lines have been recorded in some series.[284, 285] Nodal enlargement has only been reported on a handful of occasions and has been described with mushroom worker's lung,[537] bird fancier's lung,[683] and farmer's lung.[22, 219]

Chronic changes reflect healing by fibrosis and may occur after one or more acute attacks[439] or may develop insidiously in relation to chronic low-grade antigen exposure as, for example, with bird fancier's lung related to budgerigars (Fig 11–58).[285] In the latter circumstances, presentation is usually by way of progressive shortness of breath. The characteristic radiological changes in the chronic stage are of a scarring process with loss of lung volume,[219] which has a marked (85%) upper lobe predominance (Figs 11–59 and 11–60)[285] and may be associated with compensatory overinflation of the lower lobes.[284, 285] The principal opacities within the lung are reticular or reticulonodular shadows, which may show a definite honeycomb pattern.[58, 285] Larger ring shadows, 1 to 4 cm in diameter, also occur and are due to bullae, blebs, cysts, or bronchiectasis. Line shadows secondary to scarring are common, particularly in the upper zones.[284] Parallel line shadows are due to bronchiectasis or simple bronchial wall thickening and, in the latter case, are often transient.[285] Other

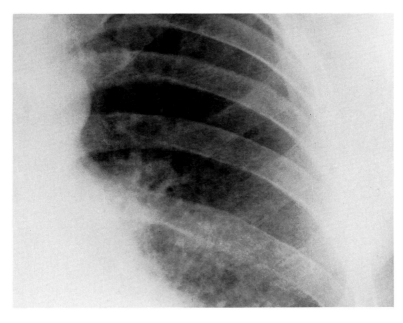

FIG 11–56.
Acute farmer's lung. A localized view of the left mid zone shows diffusely distributed micronodulation summating to give a ground-glass appearance best seen inferolaterally. (Courtesy of Dr. R.B. Pickford, Abergavenny, Gwent.)

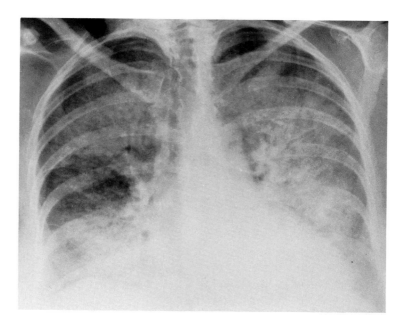

FIG 11–57.
Acute farmer's lung. Gross changes in a 55-year-old woman who was exposed during grain grinding. There is widespread, diffuse consolidation with an air bronchogram. Focal consolidation is a recognized finding in extrinsic allergic alveolitis, but such marked air-space shadowing is very unusual.

changes that are sometimes seen in the chronic stage include persisting small nodules,[284] massive opacities,[285] and evidence of cor pulmonale.[284] Pneumothorax is recorded in the fibrotic stage, but it is not common.[182]

There are a limited number of CT studies of EAA. In the subacute phase, 2- to 4-mm[454] finely granular[35] appearances are described, as well as poorly marginated opacities with air bronchograms and thickening of bronchovascular structures.[35] The distribution of changes is predominantly central.[35] In the chronic phase, linear opacities become more marked and air-space opacities become less so.[35]

The prognosis is variable. After a single attack there is usually complete recovery,[479] though there are exceptions.[22, 439] With continuing exposure, chronic changes are likely to supervene and become permanent despite cessation of exposure, the likelihood of progression being related to the number of symptomatic recurrences.[58] In a series of 143 patients with bird fancier's lung, all of whom were treated by avoidance of bird contact and 22% of whom were treated with steroids, overall only 50% showed a radiologic improvement and a significant increase in vital capacity. An age of less than 45 years and the presence of symptoms for less than 2 years correlated with improvement.[514] The death rate from farmer's lung disease in 2 series of 141 and 24 patients was 9% and 17%, respectively.[58, 182]

Pulmonary Mycotoxicosis

A small number of patients have been described who developed symptoms like those of acute EAA when exposed to moldy silage. This illness has been attributed to massive inhalation of fungi and a subsequent toxic pulmonary reaction. This condition

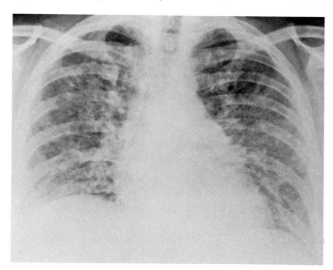

FIG 11–58.
Chronic bird fancier's lung. This patient was exposed to a budgerigar (parakeet) for many years. The basic shadowing consists of irregular 2- to 4-mm nodules with reticulation and a linear element. The appearances were essentially stable. They are unusual in that they are equally distributed in all zones.

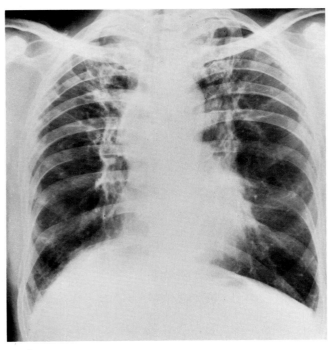

FIG 11–59.
Chronic farmer's lung. This patient had recurrent acute episodes of allergic alveolitis over a 15-year period. He then discontinued farming, and this radiograph was taken 10 years later. It shows linear scarlike shadows in both upper zones together with volume loss in the upper zones. The upper zone distribution of the scarring is typical of extrinsic allergic alveolitis. (Courtesy of Dr. R.B. Pickford, Abergavenny, Gwent.)

differs from EAA in that recurrences have been absent and hypersensitivity has not been demonstrated histologically or serologically.[184] The histologic picture is of an interstitial and intra-alveolar neutrophilic and histiocytic infiltrate with a bronchiolitis and a number of fungal elements.[351] In one series of ten patients, 50% had bilateral, basally predominant radiologic changes described as interstitial or reticulonodular.[184]

AMYLOIDOSIS AND AMYLOID DEPOSITION

The term amyloid embraces a number of abnormal proteins all of which have a characteristic configuration to their polypeptide chains (β-pleating).[248] These proteins are set down extracellularly in a number of conditions and as part of the aging process. Organ dysfunction occurs if enough amyloid material accumulates. The deposition may be generalized when it occurs as part of a systemic disease, or it may be localized to a single organ. Local deposition within an organ may itself be diffuse or focal. Localized disease never becomes generalized.

The unique structure of amyloid accounts for the histochemical findings of Congo red binding and the pathognomonic apple-green birefringence in polarized light. Two major proteins have been identified:

1. AL (amyloid light chain), which is derived from the immunoglobulin light chain. AL amyloid is manufactured by plasma cells and is found in various plasma cell dyscrasias, including primary amyloidosis, a disease now classified as an immunocyte dyscrasia with a monoclonal gammopathy.
2. AA (amyloid A), an alpha globulin that is an acute-phase reactant in inflammatory or infective conditions. As might be expected AA amyloid is found in secondary amyloidosis (reactive systemic amyloidosis).

A classification of the major clinical forms of amyloidosis and amyloid deposition together with the type of chest involvement is given in Table 11–13. It will be noted that the terms primary and secondary have been dispensed with, thus avoiding confusion over the term primary, which has been used to identify organ-limited disease, as well as what is now called AL amyloidosis with monoclonal gammopathy. Some cases of amyloidosis do not fit

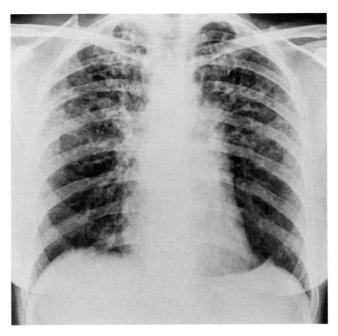

FIG 11–60.
Chronic bird fancier's lung. Alveolitis in this patient resulted from exposure to budgerigars (parakeets). There are fixed middle and upper zone changes with upper lobe volume loss. Shadowing is reticulonodular, with a predominant reticular/linear element, producing many ring shadows.

TABLE 11–13.

Major Clinical Forms of Amyloidosis and Amyloid Deposition With Type of Respiratory Involvement

Major Subdivision	Clinicopathologic Entity	Chest Involvement

Systemic amyloidosis	Immunocyte dyscrasia amyloidosis (AL amyloidosis)
	   Amyloidosis with monoclonal gammopathy
	     (formerly primary systemic amyloidosis)
	   Plasma cell myeloma
	   Waldenström's macroglobulinemia
	   Others
		Diffuse parenchymal (usually
		   subclinical) ± lymph nodes

	Reactive systemic amyloidosis (AA amyloidosis,
	   formerly secondary amyloidosis)
		Diffuse parenchymal
		   (subclinical)

	Heredofamilial amyloidosis
	   Neuropathic
	   Non-neuropathic
	     (including familial
	     Mediterranean fever)
		Diffuse parenchymal (in some)

Localized amyloidosis	Organ-limited amyloidosis
	   Lung
		Tracheobronchial
		 Parenchymal
		   Nodular
		   Diffuse
		 ± Lymph nodes

	Skin, bladder, larynx Focal amyloidosis Senile amyloidosis	

comfortably into the scheme presented in Table 11–13, and no classification is entirely satisfactory. Difficulties most commonly occur with the so-called localized disease which, although not systemic, is in many instances clearly not limited to a single organ. For example, cardiac amyloidosis is generally classified as a localized form, but is often accompanied by pathologic alveolar septal involvement of the lung.[505, 620] Thus in an autopsy series of 63 patients with cardiac amyloidosis, 49% had pulmonary amyloid infiltration, and 5% of these cases were classified as severe.[580] Another example of the difficulty in classifying every case as localized or systemic is provided by the combination of lung disease accompanied by adenopathy of the chest and cervical lymph nodes.[150, 233]

Systemic Amyloidosis

Respiratory involvement is an unimportant part of systemic amyloidosis, and clinical and radiologic findings in the chest are usually incidental or secondary to a complication such as heart failure. Should primary chest involvement occur, it takes the form of interstitial parenchymal disease or of lymphadenopathy.

AL Amyloidosis

AL amyloidosis has two main subtypes: one associated with a monoclonal gammopathy (formerly primary amyloidosis), and the other associated with

myelomatosis. They are virtually identical in their clinical manifestations, save for the fact that the prognosis of amyloidosis associated with myeloma is worse (5-month vs. 13-month mean survival).[367] In AL amyloidosis, infiltration with amyloid material affects mesenchymal tissues and, to a lesser extent, kidney, liver, and spleen. There is a 2:1 male predominance with a mean age at presentation of about 60 years.[248]

The clinical features of AL amyloidosis may be nonspecific, such as weight loss and weakness, or may be part of one or more classic disorders. The frequency of such disorders at presentation[367] is: nephrotic syndrome, 32%; carpal tunnel syndrome, 24%; restrictive cardiomyopathy, 23%; peripheral neuropathy, 17%; orthostatic hypotension, 14%; and occasionally macroglossia, purpura, papular skin rash, and arthropathy. Some 80% of patients will have proteinuria. Electrophoresis of serum shows a protein spike in 40% and, on immunoelectrophoresis, there is a monoclonal protein in 68%. When urine and blood test results are combined, 89% of patients will have a monoclonal protein.[367] The diagnosis is made by rectal biopsy, which is positive in approximately 75% of patients.[367] Bone marrow aspiration is positive in only 30% of patients, but it does allow assessment of plasma cells for the presence of possible myelomatosis. If both rectal biopsy and bone marrow aspiration are negative, then a suspect organ should be biopsied.

The median survival in a series of 229 patients

with AL amyloidosis was 12 months, with fewer than 25% alive at 3 years.[367] Renal failure is a common cause of death.[64] The presence of myeloma, heart failure and weight loss indicate a bad prognosis.

Involvement of the lungs on pathologic examination is common in AL amyloidosis, the prevalence ranging between 70% and 92%,[64, 92, 111, 580, 650] but it is not often of clinical importance. For example in a major clinical review of 229 patients with AL amyloid, there is no mention of the lung being affected.[367] Reports of significant lung involvement occur mostly in individual case reports or in small selected series.[63, 128, 348, 520, 650] In one such series, five of 12 patients with "primary" amyloidosis developed radiographic and pathologic evidence of diffuse alveolar septal amyloidosis and, in one patient, it contributed to death.[92] A further point of importance is that cardiac amyloidosis commonly accompanies lung involvement,[580] and it is well recognized that both the clinical and radiologic signs of pulmonary amyloid infiltration can be obscured by heart failure.[496, 580, 650] In the appropriate context, persistent radiologic changes despite adequate treatment of heart failure should raise the possibility of amyloid infiltration of the lungs.[312]

Reactive Systemic Amyloidosis (AA)

Reactive systemic amyloidosis (secondary/AA amyloidosis) is usually secondary to chronic infective or inflammatory processes.[366] The most common cause now is probably rheumatoid arthritis,[64] in which the prevalence of amyloidosis is usually quoted as 10%, though it seems likely that this figure is too high.[674] Other causes include tuberculosis, leprosy, osteomyelitis, bronchiectasis, chronically infected decubitus ulcers, ankylosing spondylitis, regional enteritis, and some malignancies such as Hodgkin's disease and renal cell carcinoma.[248, 366] The organs most commonly affected by amyloid deposition are the kidneys, liver, spleen, and adrenals. AA amyloidosis usually presents with renal disease (proteinuria, nephrotic syndrome, hypertension) or hepatosplenomegaly. Renal failure is the most common cause of death. The prevalence of lung involvement pathologically varies considerably in the various series. Two series give a prevalence rate of 1% to 5%,[580, 650] whereas in others the prevalence has been very high, approaching 100%.[92, 674] These discrepancies are probably unimportant as the involvement is usually diffuse within the lung and not severe enough to cause functional or radiologic changes. There are exceptions, however, and in one series of 24 patients, 16% had marked amy-

loid deposition at pathologic study.[64] There have also been a few reports of significant clinical lung involvement.[92, 440]

Radiographic Changes in Systemic Amyloidosis

The chest radiograph is normal in the majority of patients with generalized amyloidosis and lung involvement,[273] even when the lung involvement is severe enough to cause major pulmonary dysfunction.[128] When abnormalities are seen, the findings are those of an interstitial process reflecting the predominantly septal and perivascular nature of amyloid deposition.[580] The radiographic appearances in the AA and AL forms are probably similar, but descriptions in AA amyloidosis are rare. The usual findings are a diffuse micronodular or reticulonodular pattern with accentuated bronchovascular markings.[63, 348, 520, 650, 664] Parenchymal changes are usually diffuse and symmetric, but they can be segmental.[63] With progression, the nodular shadowing may become conglomerate.[650] Although the pleura may be involved pathologically in amyloidosis,[368, 559] there is no good documentation of clinically obvious disease. Pleural effusions, when they occur in the context of amyloidosis, are usually the result of heart failure secondary to myocardial infiltration.[92, 650] Cases are, however, reported with unexplained effusions that could be the result of amyloid pleural involvement.[532, 664]

Hilar and mediastinal nodal enlargement is not described in AA amyloidosis, but is occasionally seen in AL amyloidosis, either as the sole radiologic finding[63, 272, 664] or with parenchymal micronodulation.[650, 664] Both mediastinal and hilar nodes may be involved, and the enlargement is often massive. A pattern of nodal enlargement resembling sarcoidosis may be produced with symmetric bilateral hilar adenopathy or bilateral hilar and right paratracheal adenopathy.[664] Nodal calcification is common (Fig 11–61).[569, 664] The pattern of calcification is usually described as coarse or nonspecific; it may occasionally be of the eggshell type.[272] Nodal enlargement has also been described in AL amyloidosis associated with multiple myeloma[420] and Waldenström's macroglobulinemia.[92, 272]

Heart failure is common in AL amyloidosis and interstitial shadowing resulting from raised pulmonary venous pressure may obscure pulmonary lesions of amyloid infiltration.[92, 348] When AA amyloidosis is secondary to inflammatory lung disease, the chest radiograph will show major abnormalities, for example, those of cystic fibrosis or bronchiectasis.[64]

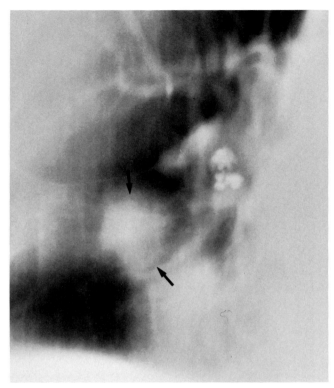

FIG 11–61.
Amyloidosis—nodular parenchymal and nodal. This patient had multiple intraparenchymal nodules, one of which is seen out of focus *(arrows)* on this right lower zone tomogram. Above and medial to this nodule there is a lobulated mass at the right hilus produced by enlarged bronchopulmonary nodes. These contain central coarse nodular calcification.

Localized Amyloidosis

Localized amyloidosis may affect either the lung parenchyma or the airways (Table 11–14). These structures are usually involved independently, but very occasionally both are affected together.[610] A few cases are recorded in which there is also amyloidosis of mediastinal nodes, and, although in these patients the disease is not strictly local (organ limited), they are usually classified as being localized in the absence of systemic involvement.

Tracheobronchial Amyloidosis

Amyloid may occur in the airways as focal or diffuse submucosal deposits[617]; both are considered together here. The mean age of patients in a large review was 53 years, with a range of 16[261] to 76 years. Twice as many men as women experience the disease.[532] Affected patients are often symptomatic[272] for several years before they finally present,[501] an indication that the disease progresses relatively slowly.

The major symptoms are cough, dyspnea, hemoptysis, stridor, and hoarseness.[501, 532] A number of patients are believed initially to have asthma,[60, 453] and recurrent pulmonary infections are common.[532]

Airway amyloid is more commonly diffuse than focal.[617] When diffuse, it can involve the trachea and main stem bronchus (Fig 11–62), and the lobar and proximal segmental bronchi, together or in part. This involvement can be demonstrated by conventional[453] or computed[235] tomography or by bronchography, all of which demonstrate multiple concentric or eccentric strictures and mural nodulation (see Fig 11–62). Although bronchography was recommended as a useful investigation in the past,[312] it has been supplanted by bronchoscopy. Bronchography was in any case poorly tolerated by some patients.[501] Local as opposed to diffuse lesions give rise to endobronchial masses that are radiologically indistinguishable from bronchial neoplasm.[123, 617] In either type of lesion, the chest radiograph may be normal in appearance[453] or show one of a number of obstructive features. The most common is collapse, which is seen in more than 50% of patients[532] (see Fig 11–62,A). Other manifestations include recurrent infective consolidations and obstructive hyperinflation.[164] A few patients have had hilar or mediastinal masses on plain chest radiography, possibly representing nodal enlargement.[416, 460, 558]

If treatment is required, the amyloid deposits may be removed, usually by intermittent bronchoscopic resection,[214] though a number of other techniques have been used, including laser photoresection.[60] Prognosis is not good, and there is a tendency for lesions to recur 6 to 12 months after treatment.[532] In one review of 39 patients, 21 were well at 4 to 6 years, but 18 were dead, 12 from respiratory causes.

TABLE 11–14.
Localized Forms of Lower Respiratory Tract Amyloidosis With Relative Percentage Prevalence*

Classification	Prevalence (%)	Form
Tracheobronchial	45	Multifocal submucosal plaques
	8	Tumor-like masses
Parenchymal	44	Nodular Solitary Multiple
	4	Diffuse alveolar septal

*After Thompson PJ, Citron KM: Amyloid and the lower respiratory tract. *Thorax* 1983; 38:84–87.

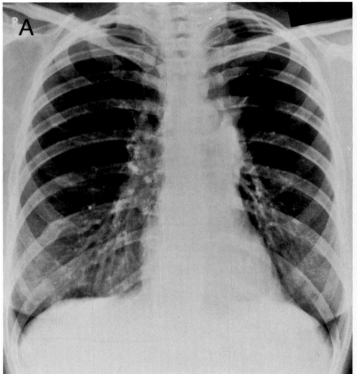

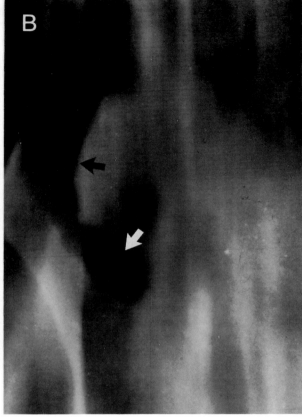

FIG 11–62.

Amyloidosis—tracheobronchial. **A,** the chest radiograph shows partial collapse of the left upper lobe due to endobronchial amyloidosis of the left main stem bronchus and upper lobar airways. **B,** a left posterior oblique (55° oblique) tomogram shows narrow-ing and irregularity of the airway at the junction of the left main stem bronchus *(white arrow)* and trachea *(black arrow)* as a result of mural amyloidosis. (Courtesy of Dr. F.J. Millard, London.)

Parenchymal Nodular Amyloidosis

This form of organ-limited amyloidosis produces one or more parenchymal nodules. Although about as common as tracheobronchial amyloid, it is still a rare condition, with only 55 reports in a recent literature review.[617] Reviews of previous cases have appeared at regular intervals.[209, 368, 532, 533, 661] The pathologic changes have been summarized by Saab and co-workers.[533] Amyloid nodules are discrete and often subpleural, puckering the adjacent pleura to which they may be adherent. They are firm, sometimes well demarcated but not encapsulated, and when sectioned they are waxy. Microscopically, lung tissue is replaced by acellular amyloid surrounded peripherally by a low-grade inflammatory infiltrate containing giant cells. Calcification, cartilage formation, and ossification within the tumor are common. Bronchioles, alveolar septa, and blood vessels in the region of the tumor often contain amyloid as well.

The mean age at presentation in several series was 68 years,[209, 368, 533] the youngest patient being 38 years old[114]; sex incidence has been equal. Unless the disease is extensive, the patients are usually asymptomatic, with only occasional reports of cough and hemoptysis.[617] The nodules may be single (Fig 11–63) or multiple (Fig 11–64). In some series, both patterns have been equally prevalent,[532] whereas in others multiple nodules have been predominant.[209] When tumors are multiple, the numbers vary from two to innumerable, with two-thirds being bilateral and one-third unilateral.[209] There is no lobar predilection.[532, 533] Characteristically, nodules are sharp and round,[272] but they may also be oval, lobulated (see Fig 11–63),[312] irregular,[123, 664] or ill-defined.[312] Generally, in any one patient, the nodules vary in size and shape. Some authors stress that a radiograph with multiple nodules of various shapes should raise the possibility of amyloidosis.

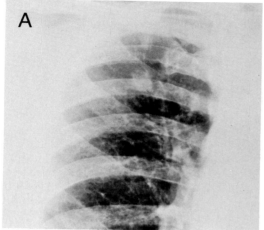

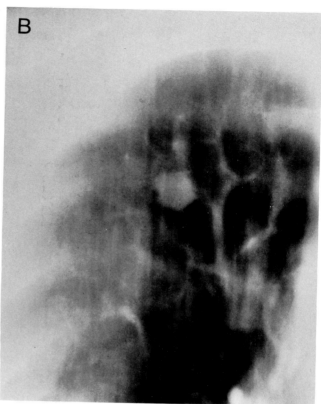

FIG 11–63.

Amyloidosis—parenchymal nodular. **A,** PA chest radiograph of this asymptomatic 72-year-old man shows an isolated 1.5-cm nodule in the right upper zone. **B,** on tomography the nodule is shown to be slightly lobulated, sharply marginated, and homogeneous.

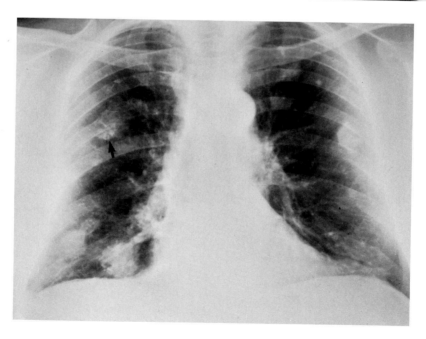

FIG 11–64.

Amyloidosis—parenchymal nodular. This 55-year-old man presented with ischemic chest pain and was found to have multiple, bilateral pulmonary nodules ranging in size from 0.5 to 3.0 cm. Several are calcified in an irregular nodular fashion best seen in the indicated nodule *(arrow).* (Courtesy of Dr. M.G. Britton, Chertsey, Surrey.)

Nodules are commonly 0.5 to 5 cm in diameter, but range from micronodular[203, 312] to massive—up to 15 cm in diameter. Calcification is quite common in both small[272, 533] and large nodules; in the latter it is variously described as irregular, cloudy, or stippled (see Fig 11–64). It may occur centrally or throughout the nodule.[209, 272, 312] Calcification is detected in approximately 30% to 50% of cases,[532, 610] depending on the method of assessment. Although calcification may be seen on the plain radiograph,[272, 661] tomography is often required for its detection.[150, 610] Calcification is clearly a very helpful finding that may suggest the nature of such lesions.[312] Although cavitation was described in 11% of cases in one review series,[532] this is probably an overestimate.[124, 661] It would seem generally to be a rare complication.[272] Occasionally, the nodules are locally confluent and mimic consolidation, an appearance which, in the upper zone, can be mistaken for tuberculosis.[438] The nodules tend to behave in a rather indolent fashion, growing slowly and sometimes remaining stable over several years.[610] In rare cases they grow rapidly, over months, behaving like a neoplasm.[209] In a few cases, additional mediastinal lymphadenopathy has been described (see Fig 11–61).[63, 368, 618]

In the absence of any systemic disorder or bronchoscopic abnormality, the diagnosis is usually established by thoracotomy, though it is possible to make the diagnosis from percutaneous needle biopsy.[38] In patients with one or a few nodules only, the prognosis is excellent, and recurrence after removal of a nodule, though recorded, is extremely rare.[171] Very occasionally, the disease is so widespread that it contributes to[203] or causes[368] death.

Parenchymal Alveolar Septal Disease

Although alveolar septal deposition of amyloid is typical of systemic amyloidosis, it is occasionally found in disease that appears to be limited to the lung.[532, 682] The radiologic pattern is of an interstitial process with fine linear or reticulonodular shadowing that can become confluent. Unlike those with the systemic alveolar septal form of the disease, these patients have had symptoms, and one died.[682] In other cases there is pathologically both septal and perivascular deposition of amyloid, often with a micronodular morphology. Radiologically these patients have a diffuse micronodular pattern that is sometimes accompanied by larger nodules, and they may be considered as one end of the spectrum of parenchymal nodular amyloidosis.[63, 203, 258, 312] These patients are often symptomatic. Alveolar septal, mi-

cronodular lung-limited amyloid and nodular parenchymal amyloidosis thus merge into one another and may be regarded as a continuum.

REFERENCES

1. Agia GA, Reddy VC, Maltby J, et al: Pulmonary involvement in mixed connective tissue disease. *Am Rev Respir Dis* 1980; 121(suppl 4):105.
2. Ahmad D, Patterson R, Morgan WKC, et al: Pulmonary haemorrhage and haemolytic anaemia due to trimellitic anhydride. *Lancet* 1979; 2:328–330.
3. Akiyama K, Mathison DA, Riker JB, et al: Allergic bronchopulmonary candidiasis. *Chest* 1984; 85:699–701.
4. Akiyama K, Takizawa H, Suzuki M, et al: Allergic bronchopulmonary aspergillosis due to *Aspergillus oryzae. Chest* 1987; 91:285–286.
5. Albelda SM, Gefter WB, Epstein DM, et al: Diffuse pulmonary hemorrhage: A review and classification. *Radiology* 1985; 154:289–297.
6. Alexander EL, Provost TT, Stevens MB, et al: Neurologic complications of primary Sjögren's syndrome. *Medicine* 1982; 61:247–257.
7. Anttila S, Sutinen S, Paakko P, et al: Rheumatoid pneumoconiosis in a dolomite worker: A light and electron microscopic, and x-ray microanalytical study. *Br J Dis Chest* 1984; 78:195–200.
8. Arkin CR, Masi AT: Relapsing polychondritis: Review of current status and case report. *Semin Arthritis Rheum* 1975; 5:41–62.
9. Armstrong JG, Steele RH: Localized pulmonary arteritis in rheumatoid disease. *Thorax* 1982; 37:313–314.
10. Aronoff A, Bywaters EGL, Fearnley GR: Lung lesions in rheumatoid arthritis. *Br Med J* 1955; 2:228–232.
11. Arshad M, Braun SR, Sunderrajan EV: Severe hypoxemia in farmer's lung disease with normal findings on chest roentgenogram. *Chest* 1987; 91:274–275.
12. Ashba JK, Ghanem MH: The lungs in systemic sclerosis. *Dis Chest* 1965; 47:52–64.
13. Asherson RA, Mackworth-Young CG, Boey ML, et al: Pulmonary hypertension in systemic lupus erythematosus. *Br Med J* 1983; 287:1024–1025.
14. Auerbach RC, Snyder NE, Bragg DG: The chest roentgenographic manifestations of pronestyl-induced lupus erythematosus. *Radiology* 1973; 109:287–290.
15. Avila R: Extrinsic allergic alveolitis in workers exposed to fish meal and poultry. *Clin Allergy* 1971; 1:343–346.
16. Baggenstoss AH, Bayley EC, Lindberg DON: Löffler's syndrome. Report of a case with pathologic examination of lungs. *Proc Mayo Clin* 1946; 21:457–465.

17. Ball JD: Tropical pulmonary eosinophilia. *Trans R Soc Trop Med Hyg* 1950; 44:237–258.

18. Banaszak EF, Thiede WH, Fink JN: Hypersensitivity pneumonitis due to contamination of an air conditioner. *N Engl J Med* 1970; 283:271–276.

19. Bariffi F, Pesci A, Bertorelli G, et al: Pulmonary involvement in Sjögren's syndrome. *Respiration* 1984; 46:82–87.

20. Barnes BE: Dermatomyositis and malignancy. A review of the literature. *Ann Intern Med* 1976; 84:68–76.

21. Baron M, Feiglin D, Hylan R, et al: [67]Gallium lung scans in progressive systemic sclerosis. *Arthritis Rheum* 1983; 26:969–974.

22. Barrowcliff DF, Arblaster PG: Farmer's lung: A study of an early acute fatal case. *Thorax* 1968; 23:490–500.

23. Barry J, Alazraki NP, Heaphy JH: Scintigraphic detection of intrapulmonary bleeding using technetium-99m sulfur colloid: Concise communication. *J Nucl Med* 1981; 22:777–780.

24. Basu SP: X-ray appearances in the lung fields in tropical eosinophilia. *Indian Med Gaz* 1954; 89:212–217.

25. Bean WJ: Recognition of ascariasis by routine chest or abdomen roentgenograms. *AJR* 1965; 94:379–384.

26. Beck ER, Hoffbrand BI: Acute lung changes in rheumatoid arthritis. *Ann Rheum Dis* 1966; 25:459–462.

27. Beirne GJ, Kopp WL, Zimmerman SW: Goodpasture's syndrome. Dissociation from antibodies to glomerular basement membrane. *Arch Intern Med* 1973; 132:261–263.

28. Bell R, Lawrence DS: Chronic pleurisy in systemic lupus erythematosus treated with pleurectomy. *Br J Dis Chest* 1979; 73:314–316.

29. Benatar SR, Allan B, Hewitson RP, et al: Allergic bronchopulmonary stemphyliosis. *Thorax* 1980; 35:515–518.

30. Benedek TG, Zawadzki ZA, Medsger TA: Serum immunoglobulins, rheumatoid factor and pneumoconiosis in coal miners with rheumatoid arthritis. *Arthritis Rheum* 1976; 19:731–736.

31. Bennett RM, O'Connell DJ: Mixed connective tissue disease: A clinicopathologic study of 20 cases. *Semin Arthritis Rheum* 1980; 10:25–51.

32. Benoit FL, Rulon DB, Theil GB, et al: Goodpasture's syndrome. *Am J Med* 1964; 37:424–444.

33. Berendsen HH, Hofstee N, Kapsenberg PD, et al: Bronchocentric granulomatosis associated with seropositive polyarthritis. *Thorax* 1985; 40:396–397.

34. Bergin CJ, Müller NL: CT in the diagnosis of interstitial lung disease. *AJR* 1985; 145:505–510.

35. Bergin CJ, Müller NL: CT of interstitial lung disease: A diagnostic approach. *AJR* 1987; 148:9–15.

36. Berkin KE, Vernon DRH, Kerr JW: Lung collapse caused by allergic bronchopulmonary aspergillosis in non-asthmatic patients. *Br Med J* 1982; 285:552–553.

37. Bettmann MA, Kantrowitz F: Rapid onset of lung involvement in progressive systemic sclerosis. *Chest* 1979; 75:509–510.

38. Bierny J-P: Multinodular primary amyloidosis of the lung: Diagnosis by needle biopsy. *AJR* 1978; 131:1082–1083.

39. Bitterman PB, Crystal RG: Is there a fibrotic gene? *Chest* 1980; 78:549–550.

40. Blank N, Castellino RA, Shah V: Radiographic aspects of pulmonary infection in patients with altered immunity. *Radiol Clin North Am* 1973; 11:175–190.

41. Bloch KJ, Buchanan WW, Wohl MJ, et al: Sjögren's syndrome. A clinical, pathological and serological study of sixty-two cases. *Medicine* 1965; 44:187–231.

42. Boey ML, Colaco CB, Gharavi AE, et al: Thrombosis in systemic lupus erythematosus: Striking association with the presence of circulating lupus anticoagulant. *Br Med J* 1983; 287:1021–1023.

43. Bohan A, Peter JB: Polymyositis and dermatomyositis. *N Engl J Med* 1975; 292:344–347; 403–407.

44. Bohan A, Peter JB, Bowman RL, et al: A computer-assisted analysis of 153 patients with polymyositis and dermatomyositis. *Medicine* 1977; 56:255–286.

45. Bombardieri S, Paoletti P, Ferri C, et al: Lung involvement in essential mixed cryoglobulinemia. *Am J Med* 1979; 66:748–756.

46. Bonafede RP, Benatar SR: Bronchocentric granulomatosis and rheumatoid arthritis. *Br J Dis Chest* 1987; 81:197–201.

47. Bonanni PP, Frymoyer JW, Jacox RF: A family study of idiopathic pulmonary fibrosis. *Am J Med* 1965; 39:411–421.

48. Bondi E, Slater S: Tolazamide-induced chronic eosinophilic pneumonia. *Chest* 1981; 80:652.

49. Bowey RR: Bird fancier's lung. *Australas Radiol* 1974; 18:292–296.

50. Bowley NB, Hughes JMB, Steiner RE: The chest x-ray in pulmonary capillary haemorrhage: Correlation with carbon monoxide uptake. *Clin Radiol* 1979; 30:413–417.

51. Bowley NB, Steiner RE, Chin WS: The chest x-ray in antiglomerular basement membrane antibody disease (Goodpasture's syndrome). *Clin Radiol* 1979; 30:419–429.

52. Boyd JA, Patrick SI, Reeves RJ: Roentgen changes observed in generalized scleroderma. *Arch Intern Med* 1954; 94:248–258.

53. Bradley JD: The pulmonary hemorrhage syndromes. *Clin Chest Med* 1982; 3:593–605.

54. Bradley JD, Pinals RS, Blumenfeld HB, et al: Giant cell arteritis with pulmonary nodules. *Am J Med* 1984; 77:135–140.

55. Brannan HM, Good CA, Divertie MB, et al: Pulmo-

nary disease associated with rheumatoid arthritis. *JAMA* 1964; 189:914–918.

56. Brannan HM, McCaughey WTE, Good CA: The roentgenographic appearance of pulmonary hemorrhage associated with glomerulonephritis. *AJR* 1963; 90:83–88.

57. Braun NMT, Arora NS, Rochester DF: Respiratory muscle and pulmonary function in polymyositis and other proximal myopathies. *Thorax* 1983; 38:616–623.

58. Braun SR, doPico GA, Tsiatis A, et al: Farmer's lung disease: Long-term clinical and physiologic outcome. *Am Rev Respir Dis* 1979; 119:185–191.

59. Brennan SR, Daly JJ: Large pleural effusions in rheumatoid arthritis. *Br J Dis Chest* 1979; 73:133–140.

60. Breuer R, Simpson GT, Rubinow A, et al: Tracheobronchial amyloidosis: Treatment by carbon dioxide laser photoresection. *Thorax* 1985; 40:870–871.

61. Briggs WA, Johnson JP, Teichman S, et al: Anti-glomerular basement membrane antibody-mediated glomerulonephritis and Goodpasture's syndrome. *Medicine* 1979; 58:348–361.

62. Bringhurst LS, Byrne RN, Gershon-Cohen J: Respiratory disease of mushroom workers. Farmer's lung. *JAMA* 1959; 171:15–18.

63. Brown J: Primary amyloidosis. *Clin Radiol* 1964; 15:358–367.

64. Browning MJ, Banks RA, Tribe CR, et al: Ten year's experience of an amyloid clinic—a clinico-pathological survey. *Q J Med* 1985; 54:213–227.

65. Brunk JR, Drash EC, Swineford O: Rheumatoid pleuritis successfully treated with decortication. Report of a case and review of the literature. *Am J Med Sci* 1966; 251:545–551.

66. Bruwer AJ, Kennedy RLJ, Edwards JE: Recurrent pulmonary hemorrhage with hemosiderosis: So-called idiopathic pulmonary hemosiderosis. *AJR* 1956; 76:98–107.

67. Buckley RH, Wray BB, Belmaker EZ: Extreme hyperimmunoglobulinemia E and undue susceptibility to infection. *Pediatrics* 1972; 49:59–70.

68. Bulgrin JG, Dubois EL, Jacobson G: Chest roentgenographic changes in systemic lupus erythematosus. *Radiology* 1960; 74:42–48.

69. Bunch TW, Tancredi RG, Lie JT: Pulmonary hypertension in polymyositis. *Chest* 1981; 79:105–107.

70. Burrows FGO: Pulmonary nodules in rheumatoid disease: A report of two cases. *Br J Radiol* 1967; 40:256–261.

71. Butcher RB, Tabb HG, Dunlap CE: Relapsing polychondritis. *South Med J* 1974; 67:1443–1449.

72. Butland RJA, Coulson IH: Pulmonary eosinophilia associated with cutaneous larva migrans. *Thorax* 1985; 40:76–77.

73. Byrd RB, Trunk G: Systemic lupus erythematosus presenting as pulmonary hemosiderosis. *Chest* 1973; 64:128–129.

74. Cadhan FT: Asthma due to grain rusts. *JAMA* 1924; 83:27.

75. Cadman EC, Lundberg WB, Mitchell MS: Pulmonary manifestations in Behçet syndrome. *Arch Intern Med* 1976; 136:944–947.

76. Callen JP: Myositis and malignancy. *Clin Rheum Dis* 1984; 10:117–130.

77. Callen JP: Dermatomyositis—an update 1985. *Semin Dermatol* 1985; 4:114–125.

78. Campbell GD, Ferrington E: Rheumatoid pleuritis with effusion. *Dis Chest* 1968; 53:521–527.

79. Campbell JA: A case of Caplan's syndrome in a boiler-scaler. *Thorax* 1958; 13:177–180.

80. Campbell JM: Acute symptoms following work with hay. *Br Med J* 1932; 2:1143–1144.

81. Caplan A: Certain unusual radiological appearances in the chest of coal-miners suffering from rheumatoid arthritis. *Thorax* 1953; 8:29–37.

82. Caplan A, Cowen EDH, Gough J: Rheumatoid pneumoconiosis in a foundry worker. *Thorax* 1958; 13:181–184.

83. Caplan A, Payne RB, Withey JL: A broader concept of Caplan's syndrome related to rheumatoid factors. *Thorax* 1962; 17:205–212.

84. Carette S, Macher AM, Nussbaum A, et al: Severe, acute pulmonary disease in patients with systemic lupus erythematosus: Ten years of experience at the National Institutes of Health. *Semin Arthritis Rheum* 1984; 14:52–59.

85. Carlson JE, Villaveces JW: Hypersensitivity pneumonitis due to pyrethrum. *JAMA* 1977; 237:1718–1719.

86. Carr DT, Mayne JG: Pleurisy with effusion in rheumatoid arthritis, with reference to the low concentration of glucose in pleural fluid. *Am Rev Respir Dis* 1962; 85:345–350.

87. Carrington CB, Addington WW, Goff AM, et al: Chronic eosinophilic pneumonia. *N Engl J Med* 1969; 280:788–798.

88. Carrington CB, Gaensler EA, Coutu RE, et al: Natural history and treated course of usual and desquamative interstitial pneumonia. *N Engl J Med* 1978; 298:801–809.

89. Carrington CB, Liebow AA: Limited forms of angiitis and granulomatosis of Wegener's type. *Am J Med* 1966; 41:497–527.

90. Carroll KB, Pepys J, Longbottom JL, et al: Extrinsic allergic alveolitis due to rat serum proteins. *Clin Allergy* 1975; 5:443–456.

91. Case record of the Massachusetts General Hospital (Case 39-1981). *N Engl J Med* 1981; 305:748–756.

92. Celli BR, Rubinow A, Cohen AS: Patterns of pulmonary involvement in systemic amyloidosis. *Chest* 1978; 74:543–547.

93. Chajek T, Fainaru M: Behçet's disease. Report of 41 cases and a review of the literature. *Medicine* 1975; 54:179–196.

94. Chamberlain MA: Behçet's syndrome in 32 patients in Yorkshire. *Ann Rheum Dis* 1977; 36:491–499.

95. Chandler PW, Shin MS, Friedman SE, et al: Radiographic manifestations of bronchiolitis obliterans with organizing pneumonia vs usual interstitial pneumonia. *AJR* 1986; 147:899–906.

96. Chang RW: Cardiac manifestations of SLE. *Clin Rheum Dis* 1982; 8:197–206.

97. Charles J, Bernstein A, Jones B, et al: Hypersensitivity pneumonitis after exposure to isocyanates. *Thorax* 1976; 31:127–136.

98. Chatgidakis CB, Theron CP: Rheumatoid pneumoconiosis (Caplan's syndrome). A discussion of the disease and a report of a case in a European Witwatersrand goldminer. *Arch Environ Health* 1961; 2:397–408.

99. Choplin RH, Wehunt WD, Theros EG: Diffuse lesions of the trachea. *Semin Roentgenol* 1983; 18:38–50.

100. Christian CL: Systemic lupus erythematosus. Clinical manifestations and prognosis. *Arthritis Rheum* 1982; 25:887–888.

101. Christoforidis AJ, Molnar W: Eosinophilic pneumonia. Report of two cases with pulmonary biopsy. *JAMA* 1960; 173:157–161.

102. Chumbley LC, Harrison EG, DeRemee RA: Allergic granulomatosis and angiitis (Churg-Strauss syndrome). Report and analysis of 30 cases. *Mayo Clin Proc* 1977; 52:477–484.

103. Churg A: Pulmonary angiitis and granulomatosis revisited. *Hum Pathol* 1983; 14:868–883.

104. Churg A, Carrington CB, Gupta R: Necrotizing sarcoid granulomatosis. *Chest* 1979; 76:406–413.

105. Churg J, Strauss L: Allergic granulomatosis, allergic angiitis and periarteritis nodosa. *Am J Pathol* 1951; 27:277–301.

106. Chusid MJ, Dale DS, West BC, et al: The hypereosinophilic syndrome: Analysis of fourteen cases with review of the literature. *Medicine* 1975; 54:1–27.

107. Citro LA, Gordon ME, Miller WT: Eosinophilic lung disease (or how to slice P.I.E.). *AJR* 1973; 117:787–797.

108. Clee MD, Lamb D, Urbaniak SJ, et al: Progressive bronchocentric granulomatosis: Case report. *Thorax* 1982; 37:947–949.

109. Coel MN, Druger G: Radionuclide detection of the site of hemoptysis. *Chest* 1982; 81:242–243.

110. Cogen FC, Mayock RL, Zweiman B: Chronic eosinophilic pneumonia followed by polyarteritis nodosa complicating the course of bronchial asthma. *J Allergy Clin Immunol* 1977; 60:377–382.

111. Cohen AS: Amyloidosis. *N Engl J Med* 1967; 277:522–530.

112. Cohen HI, Merigan TC, Kosek JC, et al: Sequoiosis. *Am J Med* 1967; 43:785–794.

113. Cohen MI, Gore RM, August CZ, et al: Tracheal and bronchial stenosis associated with mediastinal adenopathy in Wegener granulomatosis: CT findings. *J Comput Assist Tomogr* 1984; 8:327–329.

114. Condon RE, Pinkham RD, Hames GH: Primary isolated nodular pulmonary amyloidosis. Report of a case. *J Thorac Cardiovasc Surg* 1964; 48:498–505.

115. Constantopoulos SH, Drosos AA, Maddison PJ, et al: Xerotrachea and interstitial lung disease in primary Sjögren's syndrome. *Respiration* 1984; 46:310–314.

116. Constantopoulos SH, Papadimitriou CS, Moutsopoulos HM: Respiratory manifestations in primary Sjögren's syndrome. *Chest* 1985; 88:226–229.

117. Cook PG, Wells IP, McGavin CR: The distribution of pulmonary shadowing in farmer's lung. *Clin Radiol* 1988; 39:21–27.

118. Cooke NT, Bamji AN, Banks RA, et al: Rheumatoid arthritis and chronic suppurative lung disease. *Thorax* 1981; 36:229–230.

119. Cooper BJ, Bacal E, Patterson R: Allergic angiitis and granulomatosis. Prolonged remission induced by combined prednisone-azathioprine therapy. *Arch Intern Med* 1978; 138:367–371.

120. Cooper JAD, White DA, Matthay RA: Drug-induced pulmonary disease: Part 1: Cytotoxic drugs. *Am Rev Respir Dis* 1986; 133:321–340.

121. Cooper JAD, White DA, Matthay RA: Drug-induced pulmonary disease: Part 2: Noncytotoxic drugs. *Am Rev Respir Dis* 1986; 133:488–505.

122. Corrin B, Price AB: Electron microscopic studies on desquamative interstitial pneumonia associated with asbestos. *Thorax* 1972; 27:324–331.

123. Cotton RE, Jackson JW: Localized amyloid "tumours" of the lung simulating malignant neoplasms. *Thorax* 1964; 19:97–103.

124. Craver WL: Solitary amyloid tumour of the lung. *J Thorac Cardiovasc Surg* 1965; 49:860–867.

125. Cream JJ, Gumpel JM, Peachey RDG: Schönlein-Henoch purpura in the adult. *Q J Med* 1970; 39:461–484.

126. Crisp AJ, Armstrong RD, Grahame R, et al: Rheumatoid lung disease, pneumothorax, and eosinophilia. *Ann Rheum Dis* 1982; 41:137–140.

127. Crofton JW, Livingstone JL, Oswald NC, et al: Pulmonary eosinophilia. *Thorax* 1952; 7:1–35.

128. Crosbie WA, Lewis ML, Ramsay ID, et al: Pulmonary amyloidosis with impaired gas transfer. *Thorax* 1972; 27:625–630.

129. Crystal RG, Bitterman PB, Rennard SI, et al: Interstitial lung disease of unknown cause. Disorders characterized by chronic inflammation of the lower respiratory tract. *N Engl J Med* 1984; 310:154–166; 235–244.

130. Crystal RG, Fulmer JD, Roberts WC, et al: Idiopathic pulmonary fibrosis. Clinical, histologic, radiographic, physiologic, scintigraphic, cytologic and biochemical aspects. *Ann Intern Med* 1976; 85:769–788.

131. Crystal RG, Gadek JF, Ferrans VJ, et al: Interstitial lung disease: Current concepts of pathogenesis, staging and therapy. *Am J Med* 1981; 70:542–568.

132. Cullinan SA, Bower GC: Acute pulmonary hypersensitivity to carbamazepine. *Chest* 1975; 68:580–581.

133. Cunningham CDB, Hugh AE: Pneumoconiosis in women. *Clin Radiol* 1973; 24:491–493.

134. Cupps TR, Springer RM, Fauci AS: Chronic, recurrent small-vessel cutaneous vasculitis. *JAMA* 1982; 247:1994–1998.

135. Currie DC, Goldman JM, Cole PJ, et al: Comparison of narrow section computed tomography and plain chest radiography in chronic allergic bronchopulmonary aspergillosis. *Clin Radiol* 1987; 38:593–596.

136. Dalrymple W: Tropical eosinophilia. Report of two cases occurring more than a year after departure from India. *N Engl J Med* 1955; 252:585–586.

137. D'Angelo WA, Fries JF, Masi AT, et al: Pathologic observations in systemic sclerosis (scleroderma). *Am J Med* 1969; 46:428–440.

138. Davies BH, Tuddenham EGD: Familial pulmonary fibrosis associated with oculocutaneous albinism and platelet function defect. *Q J Med* 1976; 45:219–232.

139. Davies D: Pyopneumothorax in rheumatoid lung disease. *Thorax* 1966; 21:230–235.

140. Davies D, Lloyd Jones JK: Pulmonary eosinophilia caused by penicillamine. *Thorax* 1980; 35:957–958.

141. Davies JD: Behçet's syndrome with haemoptysis and pulmonary lesions. *J Pathol* 1973; 109:351–356.

142. Davis SD, Schaller J, Wedgwood RJ: Job's syndrome. Recurrent, "cold," staphylococcal abscesses. *Lancet* 1966; 1:1013–1015.

143. Davison AG, Thompson PJ, Davies J, et al: Prominent pericardial and myocardial lesions in the Churg-Strauss syndrome (allergic granulomatosis and angiitis). *Thorax* 1983; 38:793–795.

144. Degesys GE, Mintzer RA, Vrla RF: Allergic granulomatosis: Churg-Strauss syndrome. *AJR* 1980; 135:1281–1282.

145. deLeon EP, deTavera MP: Pulmonary schistosomiasis in the Phillipines. *Dis Chest* 1968; 53:154–161.

146. Den Hertog RW, Wagenaar SS, Westermann CJJ: Bronchocentric granulomatosis and pulmonary echinococcosis. *Am Rev Respir Dis* 1982; 126:344–347.

147. Dennison AR, Watkins RM, Gunning AJ: Simultaneous aortic and pulmonary artery aneurysms due to giant cell arteritis. *Thorax* 1985; 40:156–157.

148. Derderian SS, Tellis CJ, Abbrecht PH, et al: Pulmonary involvement in mixed connective tissue disease. *Chest* 1985; 88:45–48.

149. DeRemee RA, Weiland LH, McDonald TJ: Respiratory vasculitis. *Mayo Clin Proc* 1980; 55:492–498.

150. Desai RA, Mahajan VK, Benjamin S, et al: Pulmonary amyloidoma and hilar adenopathy. *Chest* 1979; 76:170–173.

151. de Takats G, Fowler EF: Raynaud's phenomenon. *JAMA* 1962; 179:1–8.

152. DeWeek AL, Gutersohn J, Butikofer E: La maladie des laveurs de fromage ("Kasenwacherkranheit"): Une forme particuliere du syndrome du poumon du fermir. *Schweiz Med Wochenschr* 1969; 99:872–876.

153. Dickey BF, Myers AR: Pulmonary disease in polymyositis/dermatomyositis. *Semin Arthritis Rheum* 1984; 14:60–76.

154. Dickie HA, Rankin J: Farmer's lung—an acute granulomatous interstitial pneumonitis occurring in agricultural workers. *JAMA* 1958; 167:1069–1076.

155. Dieppe PA: Empyema in rheumatoid arthritis. *Ann Rheum Dis* 1975; 34:181–185.

156. Dill J, Ghose T, Landrigan P, et al: Cryptogenic fibrosing alveolitis. *Chest* 1975; 67:411–416.

157. Dinsmore RE, Goodman D, Dreyfuss JR: The air esophagogram: A sign of scleroderma involving the esophagus. *Radiology* 1966; 87:348–349.

158. Ditto WR, Ognibene AJ: Idiopathic pulmonary hemosiderosis without anemia. Report of two cases. *Arch Intern Med* 1964; 114:490–493.

159. Doctor L, Snider GL: Diffuse interstitial pulmonary fibrosis associated with arthritis. *Am Rev Respir Dis* 1962; 85:413–422.

160. Dolan DL, Lemmon GB, Teitelbaum SL: Relapsing polychondritis. Analytical literature review and studies on pathogenesis. *Am J Med* 1966; 41:285–299.

161. Donabedian H, Gallin JI: The hyperimmunoglobulin E recurrent-infection (Job's) syndrome. *Medicine* 1983; 62:195–208.

162. Donald KJ, Edwards RL, McEvoy JDS: Alveolar capillary basement membrane lesions in Goodpasture's syndrome and idiopathic pulmonary hemosiderosis. *Am J Med* 1975; 59:642–649.

163. Donohugh DL: Tropical eosinophilia. An etiologic inquiry. *N Engl J Med* 1963; 269:1357–1364.

164. Dood AR, Manan JD: Primary diffuse amyloidosis of the respiratory tract. *Arch Pathol* 1959; 67:39–42.

165. Dreisin RB: Pulmonary vasculitis. *Clin Chest Med* 1982; 3:607–618.

166. Drew WL, Finley TN, Golde DW: Diagnostic lavage and occult pulmonary hemorrhage in thrombocytopenic immunocompromised patients. *Am Rev Respir Dis* 1977; 116:215–221.

167. Dubois EL, Chandor S, Friou GJ: Progressive systemic sclerosis (PSS) and localized scleroderma (morphea) with positive LE cell test and unusual systemic manifestations compatible with systemic lupus erythematosus (SLE). *Medicine* 1971; 50:199–222.

168. Dubois EL, Tuffanelli DL: Clinical manifestations of systemic lupus erythematosus. Computer analysis of 520 cases. *JAMA* 1964; 190:104–111.

169. Duncan PE, Griffin JP, Garcia A, et al: Fibrosing alveolitis in polymyositis. A review of histologically confirmed cases. *Am J Med* 1974; 57:621–626.

170. Duncan SC, Winkelmann RK: Cancer and scleroderma. *Arch Dermatol* 1979; 115:950–955.

171. Dyke PC, Demaray MJ, Delavan JW, et al: Pulmonary amyloidoma. *Am J Clin Pathol* 1974; 61:301–305.

172. Eagen JW, Memoli VA, Roberts JL, et al: Pulmonary hemorrhage in systemic lupus erythematosus. *Medicine* 1978; 57:545–560.

173. Ebringer R, Rook G, Swana GT, et al: Autoantibodies to cartilage and type II collagen in relapsing polychondritis and other rheumatic disease. *Ann Rheum Dis* 1981; 40:473–479.

174. Edwards CW: Vasculitis and granulomatosis of the respiratory tract, editorial. *Thorax* 1982; 37:81–87.

175. Efthimiou J, Johnston C, Spiro SG, et al: Pulmonary disease in Behçet's syndrome. *Q J Med* 1986; 58:259–280.

176. Ein ME, Wallace RJ, Williams TW: Allergic bronchopulmonary aspergillosis-like syndrome consequent to aspergilloma. *Am Rev Respir Dis* 1979; 119:811–820.

177. Eisenberg H: The interstitial lung diseases associated with the collagen-vascular disorders. *Clin Chest Med* 1982; 3:565–578.

178. Eisenberg H, Dubois EL, Sherwin RP, et al: Diffuse interstitial lung disease in systemic lupus erythematosus. *Ann Intern Med* 1973; 79:37–45.

179. Ellis RH: Total collapse of the lung in aspergillosis. *Thorax* 1965; 20:118–123.

180. Ellman P, Ball RE: "Rheumatoid disease" with joint and pulmonary manifestations. *Br Med J* 1948; 2:816–820.

181. Ellman P, Cudkowicz L: Pulmonary manifestations in the diffuse collagen diseases. *Thorax* 1954; 9:46–57.

182. Emanuel DA, Wenzel FJ, Bowerman CI, et al: Farmer's lung. Clinical, pathologic and immunologic study of twenty-four patients. *Am J Med* 1964; 37:392–401.

183. Emanuel DA, Wenzel FJ, Lawton BR: Pneumonitis due to cryptostroma corticale (maple bark disease). *N Engl J Med* 1966; 274:1413–1418.

184. Emanuel DA, Wenzel FJ, Lawton BR: Pulmonary mycotoxicosis. *Chest* 1975; 67:293–297.

185. England DM, Unger JM: Roentgenogram of the month. Pleural-based mass in an elderly man with arthralgias. *Chest* 1987; 91:603–604.

186. Epler GR, McLoud TC, Gaensler EA, et al: Normal chest roentgenograms in chronic diffuse infiltrative lung disease. *N Engl J Med* 1978; 298:934–939.

187. Epler GR, Snider GL, Gaensler EA, et al: Bronchiolitis and bronchitis in connective tissue disease. A possible relationship to the use of penicillamine. *JAMA* 1979; 242:528–532.

188. Epstein DM, Gefter WB, Miller WT, et al: Spontaneous pneumothorax. An uncommon manifestation of Wegener granulomatosis. *Radiology* 1980; 135:327–328.

189. Epstein DM, Taormina V, Gefter WB, et al: The hypereosinophilic syndrome. *Radiology* 1981; 140:59–62.

190. Eraut D, Evans J, Caplin M: Pulmonary necrobiotic nodules without rheumatoid arthritis. *Br J Dis Chest* 1978; 72:301–306.

191. Estes D, Christian CL: The natural history of systemic lupus erythematosus by prospective analysis. *Medicine* 1971; 50:85–95.

192. Evans WV, Seaton A: Hypersensitivity pneumonitis in a technician using Pauli's reagent. *Thorax* 1979; 34:767–770.

193. Ewan PW, Jones HA, Rhodes CG, et al: Detection of intrapulmonary hemorrhage with carbon monoxide uptake. Application in Goodpasture's syndrome. *N Engl J Med* 1976; 295:1391–1396.

194. Fairfax AJ, Haslam PL, Pavia D, et al: Pulmonary disorders associated with Sjögren's syndrome. *Q J Med* 1981; 50:279–295.

195. Farrelly C, Foster DR: Atypical presentation of Wegener's granulomatosis. *Br J Radiol* 1980; 53:721–722.

196. Farrelly CA: Wegener's granulomatosis: A radiological review of the pulmonary manifestations at initial presentation and during relapse. *Clin Radiol* 1982; 33:545–551.

197. Fauci AS, Harley JB, Roberts WC, et al: The idiopathic hypereosinophilic syndrome. Clinical, pathophysiologic, and therapeutic considerations. *Ann Intern Med* 1982; 97:78–92.

198. Fauci AS, Haynes BF, Katz P: The spectrum of vasculitis. Clinical, pathologic, immunologic, and therapeutic considerations. *Ann Intern Med* 1978; 89:660–676.

199. Fauci AS, Haynes BF, Katz P, et al: Wegener's granulomatosis: Prospective clinical and therapeutic experience with 85 patients for 21 years. *Ann Intern Med* 1983; 98:76–85.

200. Fayemi AO: Pulmonary vascular disease in systemic lupus erythematosus. *Am J Clin Pathol* 1976; 65:284–290.

201. Feigin DS, Friedman PJ: Chest radiography in desquamative interstitial pneumonitis: A review of 37 patients. *AJR* 1980; 134:91–99.

202. Felson B: Mucoid impaction (insipissated secretions) in segmental bronchial obstruction. *Radiology* 1979; 133:9–16.

203. Fenoglio C, Pascal RR: Nodular amyloidosis of the lungs. *Arch Pathol* 1970; 90:577–582.

204. Fergusson RJ, Davidson NM, Nuki G, et al: Dermatomyositis and rapidly progressive fibrosing alveolitis. *Thorax* 1983; 38:71–72.

205. Fink J: The use of bronchoprovocation in the diagnosis of hypersensitivity pneumonitis. *J Allergy Clin Immunol* 1979; 64:590–591.

206. Fink JN, Schlueter DP, Sosman AJ, et al.: Clinical survey of pigeon breeders. *Chest* 1972; 62:277–281.

207. Finley TN, Aronow A, Cosentino AM: Occult pulmonary hemorrhage in anticoagulated patients. *Am Rev Respir Dis* 1975; 112:23–29.

208. Fireman Z, Yust I, Abramov AL: Lethal occult pulmonary hemorrhage in drug-induced thrombocytopenia. *Chest* 1981; 79:358–359.

209. Firestone FN, Joison J: Amyloidosis. A cause of primary tumors of the lung. *J Thorac Cardiovasc Surg* 1966; 51:292–299.

210. Fisher MR, Christ ML, Bernstein JR: Necrotizing sarcoid-like granulomatosis: Radiologic-pathologic correlation. *J Can Assoc Radiol* 1984; 35:313–315.

211. Fisher MR, Mendelson EB, Mintzer RA, et al: Use of linear tomography to confirm the diagnosis of allergic bronchopulmonary aspergillosis. *Chest* 1985; 87:499–502.

212. Fishman AP: Chronic cor pulmonale. *Am Rev Respir Dis* 1976; 114:775–794.

213. Flatherty DK, Iha T, Chmelik F, et al: HL-A8 in farmer's lung. *Lancet* 1975; 2:507.

214. Flemming AFS, Fairfax AJ, Arnold AG, et al: Treatment of endobronchial amyloidosis by intermittent bronchoscopic resection. *Br J Dis Chest* 1980; 74:183–188.

215. Flint A: The interstitial lung diseases. A pathologist's view. *Clin Chest Med* 1982; 3:491–502.

216. Fox B, Seed WA: Chronic eosinophilic pneumonia. *Thorax* 1980; 35:570–580.

217. Fraire AE, Greenberg SD: Carcinoma and diffuse interstitial fibrosis of lung. *Cancer* 1973; 31:1078–1086.

218. Fraser RG: The radiology of interstitial lung disease. *Clin Chest Med* 1982; 3:475–484.

219. Fraser RG, Pare JAP: Extrinsic allergic alveolitis. *Semin Roentgenol* 1975; 10:31–42.

220. Fraser RG, Pare JAP: *Diagnosis of Diseases of the Chest,* ed 2. Philadelphia, WB Saunders Co, 1978, vol 2.

221. Fraser RG, Pare JAP: *Diagnosis of Diseases of the Chest,* ed 2. Philadelphia, WB Saunders Co, 1979, vol 3.

222. Frazier AR, Miller RD: Interstitial pneumonitis in association with polymyositis and dermatomyositis *Chest* 1974; 65:403–407.

223. Friedman PJ: Idiopathic and autoimmune type III-like reactions: Interstitial fibrosis, vasculitis, and granulomatosis. *Semin Roentgenol* 1975; 10:43–51.

224. Fritzler MJ, Kinsella TD: The CREST syndrome: A distinct serological entity with anticentromere antibodies. *Am J Med* 1980; 69:520–526.

225. Fromm GB, Dunn LJ, Harris JO: Desquamative interstitial pneumonitis. Characterization of free intraalveolar cells. *Chest* 1980; 77:552–554.

226. Fulmer JD: An introduction to the interstitial lung diseases. *Clin Chest Med* 1982; 3:457–473.

227. Fulmer JD, Kaltreider HB: The pulmonary vasculitides. *Chest* 1982; 82:615–624.

228. Fulmer JD, Sposovska MS, von Gal ER, et al: Distribution of HLA antigens in idiopathic pulmonary fibrosis. *Am Rev Respir Dis* 1978; 118:141–147.

229. Furst D, Davis J, Clements P, et al: Abnormalities of pulmonary vascular dynamics and inflammation in early progressive systemic sclerosis. *Arthritis Rheum* 1981; 14:1403–1408.

230. Gaensler EA, Carrington CB: Peripheral opacities in chronic eosinophilic pneumonia: The photographic negative of pulmonary edema. *AJR* 1977; 128:1–13.

231. Gaensler EA, Carrington CB: Open biopsy for chronic diffuse infiltrative lung disease: Clinical, roentgenographic, and physiological correlations in 502 patients. *Ann Thorac Surg* 1980; 30:411–426.

232. Gaensler EA, Goff AM, Prowse CM: Desquamative interstitial pneumonia. *N Engl J Med* 1966; 274:113–128.

233. Gallegos FG, Canelas JLC: Hilar enlargement in amyloidosis. *N Engl J Med* 1974; 291:531.

234. Gamsu G, Webb WR: Pulmonary hemorrhage in systemic lupus erythematosus. *J Can Assoc Radiol* 1978; 29:66–68.

235. Gamsu G, Webb WR: Computed tomography of the trachea and mainstem bronchi. *Semin Roentgenol* 1983; 18:51–60.

236. Gardner DL, Duthie JJR, Macleod J, et al: Pulmonary hypertension in rheumatoid arthritis: Report of a case with intimal sclerosis of the pulmonary and digital arteries. *Scott Med J* 1957; 2:183–188.

237. Geddes DM: Pulmonary eosinophilia. *J R Coll Physicians Lond* 1986; 20:139–145.

238. Geddes DM, Corrin B, Brewerton DA, et al: Progressive airway obliteration in adults and its association with rheumatoid disease. *Q J Med* 1977; 46:427–444.

239. Gefter WB, Epstein DM, Miller WT: Allergic bronchopulmonary aspergillosis: Less common patterns. *Radiology* 1981; 140:307–312.

240. Gelpi AP, Mustafa A: Ascaris-pneumonia. *Am J Med* 1968; 44:377–389.

241. Genereux GP: The end-stage lung. Pathogenesis, pathology and radiology. *Radiology* 1975; 116:279–289.

242. Gibson GJ, Davis P: Respiratory complications of relapsing polychondritis. *Thorax* 1974; 29:726–731.

243. Gibson GJ, Edmonds JP, Hughes GRV: Diaphragm function and lung involvement in systemic lupus erythematosus. *Am J Med* 1977; 63:926–932.

244. Gibson RN, Morgan SH, Krausz T, et al: Pulmonary artery aneurysms in Behçet's disease. *Br J Radiol* 1985; 58:79–82.

245. Gilliam JN, Smiley JD: Cutaneous necrotizing vasculitis and related disorders. *Ann Allergy* 1976; 37:328–339.

246. Glancy JJ, Elder JL, McAleer R: Allergic broncho-

pulmonary fungal disease without clinical asthma. *Thorax* 1981; 36:345–349.

247. Glay A, Rona G: The pulmonary renal syndrome of Goodpasture: Case report. *Radiology* 1964; 83:314–318.

248. Glenner GG: Amyloid deposits and amyloidosis. The β fibrilloses. *N Engl J Med* 1980; 302:1283–1292; 1333–1343.

249. Glimp RA, Bayer AS: Fungal pneumonias: Part 3. Allergic bronchopulmonary aspergillosis. *Chest* 1981; 80:85–94.

250. Gockerman JP: Drug-induced interstitial lung diseases. *Clin Chest Med* 1982; 3:521–536.

251. Gohel VK, Dalinka MK, Israel HL, et al: The radiological manifestations of Wegener's granulomatosis. *Br J Radiol* 1973; 46:427–432.

252. Goldberg B: Radiological appearances in pulmonary aspergillosis. *Clin Radiol* 1962; 13:106–114.

253. Golde DW, Drew WL, Klein HZ, et al: Occult pulmonary haemorrhage in leukaemia. *Br Med J* 1975; 2:166–168.

254. Gondos B: Roentgen manifestations in progressive systemic sclerosis (diffuse scleroderma). *AJR* 1960; 84:235–247.

255. Gonzalez L, Van Ordstrand HS: Wegener's granulomatosis. *Radiology* 1973; 107:295–300.

256. Good JT, King TE, Antony VB, et al: Lupus pleuritis. Clinical features and pleural fluid characteristics with special reference to pleural fluid antinuclear antibodies. *Chest* 1983; 84:714–718.

257. Goodpasture EW: The significance of certain pulmonary lesions in relation to the etiology of influenza. *Am J Med Sci* 1919; 158:863–870.

258. Gordonson JS, Sargent N, Jacobson G: Roentgenographic manifestations of pulmonary amyloidosis. *J Can Assoc Radiol* 1972; 23:269–272.

259. Gorevic PD, Katler EI, Agus B: Pulmonary nocardiosis. Occurrence in men with systemic lupus erythematosus. *Arch Intern Med* 1980; 140:361–363.

260. Gottlieb AJ, Spiera H, Teirstein AS, et al: Serologic factors in idiopathic diffuse interstitial pulmonary fibrosis. *Am J Med* 1965; 39:405–410.

261. Gottlieb LS, Gold WM: Primary tracheobronchial amyloidosis. *Am Rev Respir Dis* 1972; 105:425–429.

262. Gough J, Rivers D, Seal RME: Pathological studies of modified pneumoconiosis in coal-miners with rheumatoid arthritis (Caplan's syndrome). *Thorax* 1955; 10:9–18.

263. Gould DM, Daves ML: Roentgenologic findings in systemic lupus erythematosus. An analysis of 100 cases. *J Chronic Dis* 1955; 2:136–145.

264. Gould DM, Daves ML: A review of roentgen findings in systemic lupus erythematosus (SLE). *Am J Med Sci* 1958; 235:596–610.

265. Grant IWB: Bronchopulmonary eosinophilia. *Hosp Update* 1982; 8:491–501.

266. Grant IWB, Blyth W, Wardrop VE, et al: Prevalence of farmer's lung in Scotland. A pilot survey. *Br Med J* 1972; 1:530–534.

267. Greenberger PA, Patterson R: Allergic bronchopulmonary aspergillosis. *Chest* 1987; 91(suppl):165s–171s.

268. Greene R: Pulmonary aspergillosis: Three distinct entities or a spectrum of disease. *Radiology* 1981; 140:527–530.

269. Grenier P, Bletry O, Cornud F, et al: Pulmonary involvement in Behçet disease. *AJR* 1981; 137:565–569.

270. Grigor R, Edmonds J, Lewkonia R, et al: Systemic lupus erythematosus. A prospective analysis. *Ann Rheum Dis* 1978; 37:121–128.

271. Grill C, Szogi S, Bogren H: Fulminant idiopathic pulmonary haemosiderosis. *Acta Med Scand* 1962; 171:329–334.

272. Gross BH: Radiographic manifestations of lymph node involvement in amyloidosis. *Radiology* 1981; 138:11–14.

273. Gross BH, Felson B, Birnberg FA: The respiratory tract in amyloidosis and the plasma cell dyscrasias. *Semin Roentgenol* 1986; 21:113–127.

274. Gross M, Esterly JR, Earle RH: Pulmonary alterations in systemic lupus erythematosus. *Am Rev Respir Dis* 1972; 105:572–577.

275. Groves TS, Fink JN, Patterson R, et al: A familial occurrence of allergic bronchopulmonary aspergillosis. *Ann Intern Med* 1979; 91:378–382.

276. Grunebaum M, Salinger H: Radiologic findings in polymyositis-dermatomyositis involving the pharynx and upper oesophagus. *Clin Radiol* 1971; 22:97–100.

277. Guit GL, Shaw PC, Ehrlich J, et al: Mediastinal lymphadenopathy and pulmonary arterial hypertension in mixed connective tissue disease. *Radiology* 1985; 154:305–306.

278. Gumpel JM: Sjögren's syndrome. *Br Med J* 1982; 285:1598.

279. Gurtte KF, Erbe W, Kreysel HW, et al: Roentgenologic internal observations of the chest in progressive scleroderma. *Fortschr Geb Roentgenstr Nuklearmed* 1977; 126:97–101.

280. Guttadauria M, Ellman H, Kaplan D: Progressive systemic sclerosis: Pulmonary involvement. *Clin Rheum Dis* 1979; 5:151–166.

281. Halwig JM, Brueske DA, Greenberger PA, et al: Allergic bronchopulmonary curvulariosis. *Am Rev Respir Dis* 1985; 132:186–188.

282. Hamman L, Rich AR: Acute diffuse interstitial fibrosis of the lungs. *Bull Johns Hopkins Hosp* 1944; 74:177–212.

283. Hanson G, Flod N, Wells I, et al: Bronchocentric granulomatosis: A complication of allergic bronchopulmonary aspergillosis. *J Allergy Clin Immunol* 1977; 59:83–90.

284. Hapke EJ, Seal RM, Thomas GO, et al: Farmer's

lung. A clinical, radiographic, functional, and serological correlation of acute and chronic stages. *Thorax* 1968; 23:451–468.

285. Hargreave F, Hinson KF, Reid L, et al: The radiological appearances of allergic alveolitis due to bird sensitivity (bird fancier's lung). *Clin Radiol* 1972; 23:1–10.

286. Hargreave FE, Pepys J, Holford-Strevens V: Bagassosis. *Lancet* 1968; 1:619–620.

287. Hargreave FE, Pepys J, Longbottom JL, et al: Bird breeder's (fancier's) lung. *Lancet* 1966; 1:445–449.

288. Harmon C, Wolfe F, Lillard S, et al: Pulmonary involvement in mixed connective tissue disease (MCTD). *Arthritis Rheum* 1976; 19:801.

289. Harmon CE, Portanova JP: Drug-induced lupus: Clinical and serological studies. *Clin Rheum Dis* 1982; 8:121–135.

290. Hart FD: Complicated rheumatoid disease. *Br Med J* 1966; 2:131–135.

291. Harvey AM, Shulman LE, Tumulty PA, et al: Systemic lupus erythematosus: Review of the literature and clinical analysis of 138 cases. *Medicine* 1954; 33:291–437.

292. Haslam PL, Turton CWG, Lukoszek A, et al: Bronchoalveolar lavage fluid cell counts in cryptogenic fibrosing alveolitis and their relation to therapy. *Thorax* 1980; 35:328–339.

293. Haupt HM, Moore GW, Hutchins GM: The lung in systemic lupus erythematosus. Analysis of the pathologic changes in 120 patients. *Am J Med* 1981; 71:791–798.

294. Hayes DS, Posner E: A case of Caplan's syndrome in a roof tile maker. *Tubercle* 1960; 41:143–145.

295. Haynes BF, Allen NB, Fauci AS: Diagnostic and therapeutic approach to the patient with vasculitis. *Med Clin North Am* 1986; 70:355–368.

296. Healy TM: Eosinophilia in bronchogenic carcinoma. *N Engl J Med* 1974; 291:794.

297. Heitzman ER: *The Lung: Radiologic-Pathologic Correlations.* St Louis, CV Mosby Co, 1984.

298. Heitzman ER, Markarian B, DeLise CT: Lymphoproliferative disorders of the thorax. *Semin Roentgenol* 1975; 10:73–81.

299. Hellems SO, Kanner RE, Renzetti AD: Bronchocentric granulomatosis associated with rheumatoid arthritis. *Chest* 1983; 83:831–832.

300. Henderson AH: Allergic aspergillosis: Review of 32 cases. *Thorax* 1968; 23:501–512.

301. Hendrick DJ, Ellithorpe DB, Lyon F, et al: Allergic bronchopulmonary helminthosporiosis. *Am Rev Respir Dis* 1982; 126:935–938.

302. Hendrick DJ, Faux JA, Marshall R: Budgerigar-fancier's lung: The commonest variety of allergic alveolitis in Britain. *Br Med J* 1978; 2:81–84.

303. Hendrickson RM, Simpson F: Clofibrate and eosinophilic pneumonia. *JAMA* 1982; 247:3082.

304. Heng MCY: Henoch-Schönlein purpura. *Br J Dermatol* 1985; 112:235–240.

305. Hensley MJ, Feldman NT, Lazarus JM, et al: Diffuse pulmonary hemorrhage and rapidly progressive renal failure. An uncommon presentation of Wegener's granulomatosis. *Am J Med* 1979; 66:894–898.

306. Heppleston AG: The pathology of honeycomb lung. *Thorax* 1956; 11:77–93.

307. Herbert FA, Orford R: Pulmonary hemorrhage and edema due to inhalation of resins containing trimellitic anhydride. *Chest* 1979; 76:546–551.

308. Herlinger H: Pulmonary changes in tropical eosinophilia. *Br J Radiol* 1963; 36:889–901.

309. Herman PG, Balikian JP, Seltzer SE, et al: The pulmonary-renal syndrome. *AJR* 1978; 130:1141–1148.

310. Herzog CA, Miller RR, Hoidal JR: Bronchiolitis and rheumatoid arthritis. *Am Rev Respir Dis* 1981; 124:636–639.

311. Hewitt CJ, Hull D, Keeling JW: Fibrosing alveolitis in infancy and childhood. *Arch Dis Child* 1977; 52:22–37.

312. Himmelfarb E, Wells S, Rabinowitz JG: The radiologic spectrum of cardiopulmonary amyloidosis. *Chest* 1977; 72:327–332.

313. Hindle W, Yates DAH: Pyopneumothorax complicating rheumatoid lung disease. *Ann Rheum Dis* 1965; 24:57–60.

314. Hinson KFW, Moon AJ, Plummer NS: Bronchopulmonary aspergillosis. *Thorax* 1952; 7:317.

315. Hoehne JH, Reed CE, Dickie HA: Allergic bronchopulmonary aspergillosis is not rare. *Chest* 1973; 63:177–181.

316. Hoffbrand BI, Beck ER: "Unexplained" dyspnea and shrinking lungs in systemic lupus erythematosus. *Br Med J* 1965; 1:1273–1277.

317. Hogg JC: The histologic appearance of farmer's lung. *Chest* 1982; 81:133–134.

318. Holgate ST, Glass DN, Haslam P, et al: Respiratory involvement in systemic lupus erythematosus. A clinical and immunological study. *Clin Exp Immunol* 1976; 24:385–395.

319. Hopkirk JAC, Stark JE: Unilateral pulmonary collapse in asthmatics. *Thorax* 1978; 33:207–210.

320. Horn BR, Robin ED, Theodore J, et al: Total eosinophil counts in the management of bronchial asthma. *N Engl J Med* 1975; 292:1152–1155.

321. Hsu JT: Limited form of Wegener's granulomatosis. *Chest* 1976; 70:384–385.

322. Hudgson P: Polymyositis and dermatomyositis in adults. *Clin Rheum Dis* 1984; 10:85–93.

323. Hudson AR, Halprin GM, Miller JA, et al: Pulmonary interstitial fibrosis following alveolar proteinosis. *Chest* 1974; 65:700–702.

324. Hughes JP, Stovin PG: Segmental pulmonary artery aneurysms with peripheral venous thrombosis. *Br J Dis Chest* 1959; 53:19–27.

325. Hunninghake GW, Fauci AS: Pulmonary involvement in the collagen vascular diseases. *Am Rev Respir Dis* 1979; 119:471–503.

326. Hurd ER: Extraarticular manifestations of rheumatoid arthritis. *Semin Arthritis Rheum* 1979; 8:151–176.

327. Hyun BH, Diggs Cl, Toone EC: Dermatomyositis with cystic fibrosis (honeycombing) of the lung. *Dis Chest* 1962; 42:449–453.

328. Iliffe GD, Pettigrew NM: Hypoventilatory respiratory failure in generalised scleroderma. *Br Med J* 1983; 286:337–338.

329. Imbeau SA, Cohen M, Reed CE: Allergic bronchopulmonary aspergillosis in infants. *Am J Dis Child* 1977; 131:1127–1130.

330. Isenberg D, Crisp A: Sjögren's syndrome. *Hosp Update* 1985; 11:273–283.

331. Islam N, Haq AWMN: Eosinophilic lung abscess—a new entity. *Br Med J* 1962; 1:1810–1811.

332. Israel HL: The pulmonary manifestations of disseminated lupus erythematosus. *Am J Med Sci* 1953; 226:387–392.

333. Israel HL, Patchefsky AS, Saldana MJ: Wegener's granulomatosis, lymphomatoid granulomatosis and benign lymphocytic angiitis and granulomatosis of lung. *Ann Intern Med* 1977; 87:691–699.

334. Israel MS, Harley BJS: Spontaneous pneumothorax in scleroderma. *Thorax* 1956; 11:113–118.

335. Jackson E, Welch KMA: Mushroom worker's lung. *Thorax* 1970; 25:25–30.

336. Jackson LK: Idiopathic pulmonary fibrosis. *Clin Chest Med* 1982; 3:579–592.

337. Jacome AF: Pulmonary hemorrhage and death complicating anaphylactoid purpura. *South Med J* 1967; 60:1003–1004.

338. Jain VK, Beniwal OP: Unusual presentation of tropical pulmonary eosinophilia. *Thorax* 1984; 39:634–635.

339. Jaspan T, Davison AM, Walker WC: Spontaneous pneumothorax in Wegener's granulomatosis. *Thorax* 1982; 37:774–775.

340. Javaheri S, Lederer DH, Pella JA, et al: Idiopathic pulmonary fibrosis in monozygotic twins: The importance of genetic predisposition. *Chest* 1980; 78:591–594.

341. Johnson CL, Bernstein IL, Gallagher JS, et al: Familial hypersensitivity pneumonitis induced by *Bacillus subtilis*. *Am Rev Respir Dis* 1980; 122:339–348.

342. Jones FL, Blodgett RC: Empyema in rheumatoid pleuropulmonary disease. *Ann Intern Med* 1971; 74:665–671.

343. Jordan JD, Snyder CH: Rheumatoid disease of the lung and cor pulmonale. *Am J Dis Child* 1964; 108:174–180.

344. Jordan JW: Pulmonary fibrosis in a worker using an aluminum powder. *Br J Ind Med* 1961; 18:21–23.

345. Jurik AG, Davidsen D, Graudal H: Prevalence of pulmonary involvement in rheumatoid arthritis and its relationship to some characteristics of the patients. *Scand J Rheumatol* 1982; 11:217–224.

346. Jurik AG, Graudal H: Pleurisy in rheumatoid arthritis. *Scand J Rheumatol* 1983; 12:75–80.

347. Kallenbach J, Prinsloo I, Zwi S: Progressive systemic sclerosis complicated by diffuse pulmonary haemorrhage. *Thorax* 1977; 32:767–770.

348. Kanada DJ, Sharma OP: Long-term survival with diffuse interstitial pulmonary amyloidosis. *Am J Med* 1979; 67:879–882.

349. Karlish AJ: Lung changes in Sjögren's syndrome. *Proc R Soc Med* 1969; 62:1042–1043.

350. Kathuria S, Chejfec G: Fatal pulmonary Henoch-Schönlein syndrome. *Chest* 1982; 82:654–656.

351. Katzenstein A-L, Askin FB: *Surgical Pathology of Non-neoplastic Lung Disease.* Philadelphia, WB Saunders Co, 1982.

352. Katzenstein A-LA, Liebow AA, Friedman PJ: Bronchocentric granulomatosis, mucoid impaction, and hypersensitivity reactions to fungi. *Am Rev Respir Dis* 1975; 111:497–537.

353. Kaufman JM, Cuvelier CA, Van der Straeten M: Mycoplasma pneumonia with fulminant evolution into diffuse interstitial fibrosis. *Thorax* 1980; 35:140–144.

354. Kay JM, Banik S: Unexplained pulmonary hypertension with pulmonary arteritis in rheumatoid disease. *Br J Dis Chest* 1977; 71:53–59.

355. Kerr IH: Interstitial lung disease: The role of the radiologist. *Clin Radiol* 1984; 35:1–7.

356. Khoo FY, Danaraj TJ: The roentgenographic appearance of eosinophilic lung (tropical eosinophilia). *AJR* 1960; 83:251–259.

357. Kilman WJ: Narrowing of the airway in relapsing polychondritis. *Radiology* 1978; 126:373–376.

358. Kinney WW, Angelillo VA: Bronchiolitis in systemic lupus erythematosus. *Chest* 1982; 82:646–649.

359. Klein RG, Hunder GG, Stanson AW, et al: Large artery involvement in giant cell (temporal) arteritis. *Ann Intern Med* 1975; 83:806–812.

360. Kohler PF, Gross G, Salvaggio J, et al: Humidifier lung: Hypersensitivity pneumonitis related to thermotolerant bacterial aerosols. *Chest* 1976; 69:294–296.

361. Koss MN, Antonovych T, Hochholzer L: Allergic granulomatosis (Churg-Strauss syndrome). Pulmonary and renal morphologic findings. *Am J Surg Pathol* 1981; 5:21–28.

362. Koss MN, Hochholzer L, Feigin DS, et al: Necrotizing sarcoid-like granulomatosis: Clinical, pathologic, and immunopathologic findings. *Hum Pathol* 1980; 11(suppl):510–519.

363. Koss MN, Robinson RG, Hochholzer L: Bronchocentric granulomatosis. *Hum Pathol* 1981; 12:632–638.

364. Kramer N, Perez H: Pulmonary hypertension in sys-

temic lupus erythematosus: Report of four cases and review of the literature. *Semin Arthritis Rheum* 1981; 11:177–181.

365. Kus J, Bergin C, Miller R, et al: Lymphocyte sub-populations in allergic granulomatosis and angiitis (Churg-Strauss syndrome). *Chest* 1985; 87:826–827.

366. Kyle RA, Bayrd ED: Amyloidosis: Review of 236 cases. *Medicine* 1975; 54:271–299.

367. Kyle RA, Greipp PR: Amyloidosis (AL). Clinical and laboratory features in 229 cases. *Mayo Clin Proc* 1983; 58:665–683.

368. Laden SA, Cohen ML, Harley RA: Nodular pulmonary amyloidosis with extrapulmonary involvement. *Hum Pathol* 1984; 15:594–597.

369. Laham MN, Carpenter JL: *Aspergillus terreus,* a pathogen capable of causing infective endocarditis, pulmonary mycetoma, and allergic bronchopulmonary aspergillosis. *Am Rev Respir Dis* 1982; 125:769–772.

370. Landman S, Burgener F: Pulmonary manifestations in Wegener's granulomatosis. *AJR* 1974; 122:750–757.

371. Lanham JG, Elkon KB, Pusey CD, et al: Systemic vasculitis with asthma and eosinophilia: A clinical approach to the Churg-Strauss syndrome. *Medicine* 1984; 63:65–81.

372. Laufer P, Fink JN, Bruns WT, et al: Allergic bronchopulmonary aspergillosis in cystic fibrosis. *J Allergy Clin Immunol* 1984; 73:44–48.

373. Leatherman JW, Davies SF, Hoidal JR: Alveolar hemorrhage syndromes: Diffuse microvascular lung hemorrhage in immune and idiopathic disorders. *Medicine* 1984; 63:343–361.

374. Leatherman JW, Sibley RK, Davies SF: Diffuse intrapulmonary hemorrhage and glomerulonephritis unrelated to anti-glomerular basement membrane antibody. *Am J Med* 1982; 72:401–410.

375. Leavitt RY, Fauci AS: Pulmonary vasculitis. *Am Rev Respir Dis* 1986; 134:149–166.

376. Lee SL, Chase PH: Drug-induced systemic lupus erythematosus: A critical review. *Semin Arthritis Rheum* 1975; 5:83–103.

377. Levin DC: Pulmonary abnormalities in the necrotizing vasculitides and their rapid response to steroids. *Radiology* 1970; 97:521–526.

378. Levin DC: Proper interpretation of pulmonary roentgen changes in systemic lupus erythematosus. *AJR* 1971; 111:510–517.

379. Lie JT: Disseminated visceral giant cell arteritis. *Am J Clin Pathol* 1978; 69:299–305.

380. Liebow AA: The J. Burns Amberson lecture— pulmonary angiitis and granulomatosis. *Am Rev Respir Dis* 1973; 108:1–18.

381. Liebow AA, Carrington CB: The interstitial pneumonias, in Simon M, Potchen EJ, LeMay M (eds): *Frontiers of Pulmonary Radiology.* New York, Grune & Stratton 1969, pp 102–141.

382. Liebow AA, Carrington CB: The eosinophilic pneumonias. *Medicine* 1969; 48:251–285.

383. Liebow AA, Steer A, Billingsley JG: Desquamative interstitial pneumonia. *Am J Med* 1965; 39:369–404.

384. Lillington GA: Ban the boomerang. *Chest* 1981; 80:122.

385. Lindars DC, Davies D: Rheumatoid pneumoconiosis. A study in colliery populations in the East Midlands coalfield. *Thorax* 1967; 22:525–532.

386. Line BR, Fulmer JD, Reynolds HY, et al: Gallium 67 citrate scanning in the staging of idiopathic pulmonary fibrosis: Correlation with physiologic and morphological features and bronchoalveolar lavage. *Am Rev Respir Dis* 1978, 118:355–365.

387. Linenthal H, Talkov R: Pulmonary fibrosis in Raynaud's disease. *N Engl J Med* 1941; 224:682–684.

388. Lipinski JK, Wisbrod GL, Sanders DE: Unusual manifestations of pulmonary aspergillosis. *J Can Assoc Radiol* 1978; 29:216–220.

389. Livingstone JL, Lewis JG, Reid L, et al: Diffuse interstitial pulmonary fibrosis. A clinical, radiological and pathological study based on 45 patients. *Q J Med* 1964; 33:71–103.

390. Locke GB: Rheumatoid lung. *Clin Radiol* 1963; 14:43–53.

391. Löffler W: Zur Differential-Diagnose der Lungen Infiltreierunger: III. Uber fluchtige Succedan— Infiltrate (mit Eosinophilia). Beitr Klin Tuberk 1932; 79:368–392.

392. Lowe D, Jorizzo J, Hutt MSR: Tumour-associated eosinophilia: A review. *J Clin Pathol* 1981; 34:1343–1348.

393. Luksza AR, Jones DK: Comparison of whole-blood eosinophil counts in extrinsic asthmatics with acute and chronic asthma. *Br Med J* 1982; 285:1229–1231.

394. Lunn JA, Hughes DTD: Pulmonary hypersensitivity to the grain weevil. *Br J Ind Med* 1967; 24:158–161.

395. MacFarlane JD, Dieppe PA, Rigden BG, et al: Pulmonary and pleural lesions in rheumatoid disease. *Br J Dis Chest* 1978; 72:288–300.

396. MacFarlane JD, Franken CK, Van Leeuwen AWFM: Progressive cavitating pulmonary changes in rheumatoid arthritis: A case report. *Ann Rheum Dis* 1984; 43:98–101.

397. Maguire R, Fauci AS, Doppman JL, et al: Unusual radiographic features of Wegener's granulomatosis. *AJR* 1978; 130:233–238.

398. Malo JL, Pepys J, Simon G: Studies in chronic allergic bronchopulmonary aspergillosis. 2 Radiological findings. *Thorax* 1977; 32:262–268.

399. Mark EJ, Ramirez JF: Pulmonary capillaritis and hemorrhage in patients with systemic vasculitis. *Arch Pathol Lab Med* 1985; 109:413–418.

400. Martel W, Abell MR, Mikkelsen WM, et al: Pulmonary and pleural lesions in rheumatoid disease. *Radiology* 1968; 90:641–653.

401. Martens J, Demedts M, Vanmeenen MT, et al: Respiratory muscle dysfunction in systemic lupus erythematosus. *Chest* 1983; 84:170–175.

402. Martinez LO: Air in the esophagus as a sign of scleroderma. *J Can Assoc Radiol* 1974; 25:234–237.

403. Masi AT, Kaslow RA: Sex effects in systemic lupus erythematosus. *Arthritis Rheum* 1978; 21:480–484.

404. Masi AT, Rodnan GP, Medsger TA, et al: Preliminary criteria for the classification of systemic sclerosis (scleroderma). *Arthritis Rheum* 1980; 23:581–590.

405. Mason AMS, McIllmurray MB, Golding PL, et al: Fibrosing alveolitis associated with renal tubular acidosis. *Br Med J* 1970; 4:596–599.

406. Matthay RA, Schwarz MI, Petty TL, et al: Pulmonary manifestations of systemic lupus erythematosus: Review of twelve cases of acute lupus pneumonitis. *Medicine* 1974; 54:397–409.

407. McAdam LP, O'Hanlan MA, Bluestone R, et al: Relapsing polychondritis. Prospective study of 23 patients and a review of the literature. *Medicine* 1976; 55:193–215.

408. McAleer R, Kroenert DB, Elder JL, et al: Allergic bronchopulmonary disease caused by *Curvularia lunata* and *Drechslera hawaiiensis*. *Thorax* 1981; 36:338–344.

409. McCann BG, Hart GJ, Stokes TC, et al: Obliterative bronchiolitis and upper-zone pulmonary consolidation in rheumatoid arthritis. *Thorax* 1983; 38:73–74.

410. McCarthy DS, Pepys J: Allergic bronchopulmonary aspergillosis. Clinical immunology: (1) Clinical features. *Clin Allergy* 1971; 1:261–286.

411. McCarthy DS, Pepys J: Cryptogenic pulmonary eosinophilias. *Clin Allergy* 1973; 3:339–351.

412. McCarthy DS, Simon G, Hargreave FE: The radiological appearances in allergic broncho-pulmonary aspergillosis. *Clin Radiol* 1970; 21:366–375.

413. McCluskey RT, Fienberg R: Vasculitis in primary vasculitides, granulomatoses, and connective tissue diseases. *Hum Pathol* 1983; 14:305–315.

414. McDonald TJ, Neel HB, DeRemee RA: Wegener's granulomatosis of the subglottis and the upper portion of the trachea. *Ann Otol Rhinol Laryngol* 1982; 91:588–592.

415. McGregor MBB, Sandler G: Wegener's granulomatosis. A clinical and radiological survey. *Br J Radiol* 1964; 37:430–439.

416. McGurk FM: Primary bronchial amyloidosis. *Br J Radiol* 1968; 41:795–797.

417. Medical Research Council symposium. Humidifier fever. *Thorax* 1977; 32:653–663.

418. Medsger TA, Masi AT: Survival with scleroderma: II. A life-table analysis of clinical and demographic factors in 358 male US veteran patients. *J Chronic Dis* 1973; 26:647–660.

419. Medsger TA, Masi AT, Rodnan GP, et al: Survival with systemic sclerosis (scleroderma): A life-table analysis of clinical and demographic factors in 309 patients. *Ann Intern Med* 1971; 75:369–376.

420. Melato M, Antonutto G, Falconieri G, et al: Massive amyloidosis of mediastinal lymph nodes in a patient with multiple myeloma. *Thorax* 1983; 38:151–152.

421. Mendeloff J: Disseminated nodular pulmonary ossification in the Hamman-Rich lung. *Am Rev Respir Dis* 1971; 103:269–274.

422. Mendelson DS, Som PM, Crane R, et al: Relapsing polychondritis studied by computed tomography. *Radiology* 1985; 157:489–490.

423. Mendelson EB, Fisher MR, Mintzer RA, et al: Roentgenographic and clinical staging of allergic bronchopulmonary aspergillosis. *Chest* 1985; 87:334–339.

424. Merten DF, Buckley RH, Pratt PC, et al: Hyperimmunoglobulinemia E syndrome: Radiographic observations. *Radiology* 1979; 132:71–78.

425. Metheny JA: Dermatomyositis. A vocal and swallowing disease entity. *Laryngoscope* 1978; 88:147–161.

426. Metzger WJ, Patterson R, Fink J, et al: Sauna-taker's disease. *JAMA* 1976; 236:2209–2211.

427. Meyer EC, Liebow AA: Relationship of interstitial pneumonia honeycombing and atypical epithelial proliferation to cancer of the lung. *Cancer* 1965; 18:322–351.

428. Miall WE, Caplan A, Cochrane AL, et al: An epidemiological study of rheumatoid arthritis associated with characteristic chest x-ray appearances in coal workers. *Br Med J* 1953; 2:1231–1236.

429. Michet CJ, McKenna CH, Luthra HS, et al: Relapsing polychondritis. Survival and predictive role of early disease manifestations. *Ann Intern Med* 1986; 104:74–78.

430. Middleton WG, Paterson IC, Grant IWB, et al: Asthmatic pulmonary eosinophilia: A review of 65 cases. *Br J Dis Chest* 1977; 71:115–122.

431. Millar JW: Infectious mononucleosis and fibrosing alveolitis. *Br Med J* 1977; 1:612.

432. Miller LR, Greenberg SD, McLarty JW: Lupus lung. *Chest* 1985; 88:265–269.

433. Miller T, Tanaka T: Nuclear scan of pulmonary hemorrhage in idiopathic pulmonary hemosiderosis. *AJR* 1979; 132:120–121.

434. Mills ES, Mathews WH: Interstitial pneumonitis in dermatomyositis. *JAMA* 1956; 160:1467–1470.

435. Mindell HJ: Roentgen findings in farmer's lung. *Radiology* 1970; 97:341–346.

436. Mintzer RA, Rogers LF, Kruglik GD, et al: The spectrum of radiologic findings in allergic bronchopulmonary aspergillosis. *Radiology* 1978; 127:301–307.

437. Mohsenifar Z, Tashkin DP, Carson SA, et al: Pulmonary function in patients with relapsing polychondritis. *Chest* 1982; 81:711–717.

438. Moldow RE, Bearman S, Edelman MH: Pulmonary amyloidosis simulating tuberculosis. *Am Rev Respir Dis* 1972; 105:114–117.

439. Monkare S, Ikonen M, Haahtela T: Radiologic find-

ings in farmer's lung. Prognosis and correlation to lung function. *Chest* 1985; 87:460–466.

440. Monreal FA: Pulmonary amyloidosis: Ultrastructural study of early alveolar septal deposits. *Hum Pathol* 1984; 15:388–390.

441. Montoltu J, Lopez-Pedret J, Andreu L, et al: Eosinophilia in patients undergoing dialysis. *Br Med J* 1981; 282:2098.

442. Morgan PGM, Turner-Warwick M: Pulmonary haemosiderosis and pulmonary haemorrhage. *Br J Dis Chest* 1981; 75:225–242.

443. Morgan WKC: Rheumatoid pneumoconiosis in association with asbestosis. *Thorax* 1964; 19:433–435.

444. Morgan WKC, Wolfel DA: The lungs and pleura in rheumatoid arthritis. *AJR* 1966; 98:334–342.

445. Morita R, Ikekubo K, Ito H, et al: Lung scintigraphy with 51 Cr erythrocytes in Goodpasture's syndrome: Case report. *J Nucl Med* 1976; 17:702–703.

446. Morrison DA, Goldman AL: Radiographic patterns of drug-induced lung disease. *Radiology* 1979; 131:299–304.

447. Muller NL, Miller RR, Webb WR, et al: Fibrosing alveolitis: CT-pathologic correlation. *Radiology* 1986; 160:585–588.

448. Muller NL, Staples CA, Miller RR, et al: Disease activity in idiopathic pulmonary fibrosis: CT and pathologic correlation. *Radiology* 1987; 165:731–734.

449. Murphy D, Lane DJ: Pleural effusion in allergic bronchopulmonary aspergillosis: Two case reports. *Br J Dis Chest* 1981; 75:91–95.

450. Murphy JR, Krainin P, Gerson MJ: Scleroderma with pulmonary fibrosis. *JAMA* 1941; 116:499–501.

451. Murphy KC, Atkins CJ, Offer RC, et al: Obliterative bronchiolitis in two rheumatoid arthritis patients treated with penicillamine. *Arthritis Rheum* 1981; 24:557–560.

452. Nader DA, Schillaci RF: Pulmonary infiltrates with eosinophilia due to naproxen. *Chest* 1983; 83:280–282.

453. Naef AP, Savary M, Schmid de Gruneck JM, et al: Amyloid pseudotumor treated by tracheal resection. *Ann Thorac Surg* 1977; 23:578–581.

454. Nakata H, Kimoto T, Nakayama T, et al: Diffuse peripheral lung disease: Evaluation by high-resolution computed tomography. *Radiology* 1985; 157:181–185.

455. Neilly JB, Winter JH, Stevenson RD: Progressive tracheobronchial polychondritis: Need for early diagnosis. *Thorax* 1985; 40:78–79.

456. Nelson LA, Callerame ML, Schwartz RH: Aspergillosis and atrophy in cystic fibrosis. *Am Rev Respir Dis* 1979; 120:863–873.

457. Neva FA, Ottesen EA: Tropical (filarial) eosinophilia. *N Engl J Med* 1978; 298:1129–1131.

458. Newball HH, Brahim SA: Chronic obstructive airway disease in patients with Sjögren's syndrome. *Am Rev Respir Dis* 1977; 115:295–304.

459. Nimelstein SH, Brody S, McShane D, et al: Mixed connective tissue disease: A subsequent evaluation of the original 25 patients. *Medicine* 1980; 59:239–248.

460. Noring O, Paaby H: Diffuse amyloidosis in the lower air passages. *Acta Pathol Microbiol Immunol Scand* 1952; 31:470–475.

461. Novey HS, Wells ID: Allergic bronchopulmonary aspergillosis caused by *Aspergillus ochraceus*. *Am J Clin Pathol* 1978; 70:840–843.

462. O'Brien IM, Bull J, Creamer B, et al: Asthma and extrinsic allergic alveolitis due to *Merulius lacrymans*. *Clin Allergy* 1978; 8:535–542.

463. Oetgen WJ, Mutter ML, Lawless OJ, et al: Cardiac abnormalities in mixed connective tissue disease. *Chest* 1983; 83:185–188.

464. Ognibene AJ: Systemic "rheumatoid disease" with interstitial pulmonary fibrosis. *Arch Intern Med* 1960; 105:762–769.

465. O'Hara JM, Szemes G, Lowman RM: The esophageal lesions in dermatomyositis. A correlation of radiologic and pathologic findings. *Radiology* 1967; 89:27–31.

466. Olsen GN, Swenson EW: Polymyositis and interstitial lung disease. *Am Rev Respir Dis* 1972; 105:611–617.

467. O'Neill WM, Hammar SP, Bloomer HA: Giant cell arteritis with visceral angiitis. *Arch Intern Med* 1976; 136:1157–1160.

468. Onitsuka H, Onitsuka S, Yokomizo Y, et al: Computed tomography of chronic eosinophilic pneumonia. *J Comput Assist Tomogr* 1983; 7:1092–1094.

469. Opie LH: The pulmonary manifestations of generalised scleroderma (progressive systemic sclerosis). *Dis Chest* 1955; 28:665–680.

470. Owens GR, Fino GJ, Herbert DL, et al: Pulmonary function in progressive systemic sclerosis. Comparison of CREST syndrome variant with diffuse scleroderma. *Chest* 1983; 84:546–550.

471. Owens GR, Follansbee WP: Cardiopulmonary manifestations of systemic sclerosis. *Chest* 1987; 91:118–127.

472. Oxholm P, Bundgaard A, Birk Masden E, et al: Pulmonary function in patients with primary Sjögren's syndrome. *Rheumatol Int* 1982; 2:179–181.

473. Ozsoylu S, Hisconmex G, Berkel I, et al: Goodpasture's syndrome. Pulmonary haemosiderosis with nephritis. *Clin Pediatr* 1976; 15:358–360.

474. Pachman LM, Maryjowski MC: Juvenile dermatomyositis and polymyositis. *Clin Rheum Dis* 1984; 10:95–115.

475. Palmer PES, Finley TN, Drew WL, et al: Radiographic aspects of occult pulmonary haemorrhage. *Clin Radiol* 1978; 29:139–143.

476. Panettiere F, Chandler BF, Libcke JH: Pulmonary cavitation in rheumatoid disease. *Am Rev Respir Dis* 1968; 97:89–95.

477. Papathanasiou MP, Constantopoulos SH, Tsampoulas C, et al: Reappraisal of respiratory abnormalities

in primary and secondary Sjögren's syndrome. A controlled study. *Chest* 1986; 90:370–374.

478. Park S, Nyhan WL: Fatal pulmonary involvement in dermatomyositis. *Am J Dis Child* 1975; 129:723–726.

479. Parkes WR: *Occupational Lung Disorders*, ed 2. London, Butterworth, 1982.

480. Parkin TW, Rusted IE, Burchell HB, et al: Hemorrhagic and interstitial pneumonitis with nephritis. *Am J Med* 1955; 18:220–236.

481. Parrillo JE, Borer JS, Herisy WL, et al: The cardiovascular manifestations of the hypereosinophilic syndrome. Prospective study of 26 patients, with review of the literature. *Am J Med* 1979; 67:572–582.

482. Parrillo JE, Fauci AS, Wolff SM: Therapy of the hypereosinophilic syndrome. *Ann Intern Med* 1978; 89:167–172.

483. Patchefsky AS, Israel HL, Hoch WS, et al: Desquamative interstitial pneumonia: Relationship to interstitial fibrosis. *Thorax* 1973; 28:680–693.

484. Patterson CD, Harville WE, Pierce JA: Rheumatoid lung disease. *Ann Intern Med* 1965; 62:685–697.

485. Patterson R, Irons JS, Kelly JF, et al: Pulmonary infiltrates with eosinophilia. *J Allergy Clin Immunol* 1974; 53:245–255.

486. Pepys J: Pulmonary hypersensitivity disease due to inhaled organic antigens, editorial. *Ann Intern Med* 1966; 64:943–948.

487. Petrie GR, Bloomfield P, Grant IWB, et al: Upper lobe fibrosis and cavitation in rheumatoid disease. *Br J Dis Chest* 1980; 74:263–267.

488. Petty TL, Scoggin CH, Good JT: Recurrent pneumonia in Behçet's syndrome. *JAMA* 1977; 238:2529–2530.

489. Phelan MS, Kerr IH: Allergic broncho-pulmonary aspergillosis: The radiological appearance during long-term follow-up. *Clin Radiol* 1984; 35:385–392.

490. Phills JA, Harrold AJ, Whiteman GV, et al: Pulmonary infiltrates, asthma, and eosinophilia due to *Ascaris suum* infestation in man. *N Engl J Med* 1972; 286:965–970.

491. Pimentel JC, Avila R: Respiratory disease in cork workers ("suberosis"). *Thorax* 1973; 28:409–423.

492. Pinching AJ, Rees AJ, Pussell BA, et al: Relapses in Wegener's granulomatosis: The role of infection. *Br Med J* 1980; 281:836–838.

493. Pines A, Kaplinsky N, Olchovsky D, et al: Pleuropulmonary manifestations of systemic lupus erythematosus: Clinical features of its subgroups. *Chest* 1985; 88:129–135.

494. Pinsker KL, Schneyer B, Becker N, et al: Usual interstitial pneumonia following Texas A₂ influenza infection. *Chest* 1981; 80:123–126.

495. Pisetsky DS: Systemic lupus erythematosus. *Med Clin North Am* 1986; 70:337–353.

496. Poh SC, Tjia TS, Seah HC: Primary diffuse alveolar septal amyloidosis. *Thorax* 1975; 30:186–191.

497. Popper MS, Bogdonoff ML, Hughes RL: Interstitial rheumatoid lung disease. *Chest* 1972; 62:243–249.

498. Portner MM, Gracie WA: Rheumatoid lung disease with cavitary nodules, pneumothorax and eosinophilia. *N Engl J Med* 1966; 275:697–700.

499. Prasad M, Bhargava SK, Tewari SG, et al: Radiological changes in tropical pulmonary eosinophilia. *Indian J Radiol* 1979; 33:25–31.

500. Proto AV, Lane EJ: Air in the esophagus: A frequent radiographic finding. *AJR* 1977; 129:433–440.

501. Prowse CB: Amyloidosis of the lower respiratory tract. *Thorax* 1958; 13:308–320.

502. Pulmonary eosinophilia, editorial. *Br Med J* 1977; 2:480–481.

503. Purnell DC, Baggenstoss AH, Olsen AM: Pulmonary lesions in disseminated lupus erythematosus. *Ann Intern Med* 1955; 42:619–628.

504. Rabuzzi DD: Relapsing polychondritis. *Arch Otolaryngol* 1970; 91:188–194.

505. Rajan VT, Kikkawa Y: Alveolar septal amyloidosis in primary amyloidosis. *Arch Pathol* 1970; 89:521–525.

506. Ramirez-RJ, Lopez-Majano V, Schultze G: Caplan's syndrome. A clinicopathologic study. *Am J Med* 1964; 37:643–652.

507. Rankin J, Jaeschke WH, Callies QC, et al: Farmer's lung. Physiopathologic features of the acute interstitial granulomatous pneumonitis of agricultural workers. *Ann Intern Med* 1962; 57:606–626.

508. Reed CE, Sosman A, Barbee RA: Pigeon-breeders' lung. *JAMA* 1965; 193:261–265.

509. Reeder MM, Felson B: *Gamuts in Radiology.* Cincinnati, Audiovisual Radiology of Cincinnati, 1975.

510. Reeder MM, Palmer PES: Acute tropical pneumonias. *Semin Roentgenol* 1980; 15:35–49.

511. Rees AJ: Pulmonary injury caused by antibasement membrane antibodies. *Semin Respir Med* 1984; 5:264–272.

512. Reichlin M: Problems in differentiating SLE and mixed connective-tissue disease. *N Engl J Med* 1976; 295:1194–1195.

513. Reingold IM, Mizunoue GS: Idiopathic disseminated pulmonary ossification. *Dis Chest* 1961; 40:543–546.

514. Research Committee of the British Thoracic Society: A national survey of bird fanciers' lung: Including its possible association with jejunal villous atrophy. *Br J Dis Chest* 1984; 78:75–87.

515. Reyes CN, Wenzel FJ, Lawton BR, et al: The pulmonary pathology of farmer's lung disease. *Chest* 1982; 81:142–146.

516. Reynolds HY: Hypersensitivity pneumonitis. *Clin Chest Med* 1982; 3:503–519.

517. Richards RL, Milne JA: Cancer of the lung in progressive systemic sclerosis. *Thorax* 1958; 13:238–245.

518. Rickards AG, Barrett GM: Rheumatoid lung

changes associated with asbestosis. *Thorax* 1958; 13:185–193.

519. Riddle HFV, Channell S, Blyth W, et al: Allergic alveolitis in a maltworker. *Thorax* 1968; 23:271–280.

520. Road JD, Jacques J, Sparling JR: Diffuse alveolar septal amyloidosis presenting with recurrent hemoptysis and medial dissection of pulmonary arteries. *Am Rev Respir Dis* 1985; 132:1368–1370.

521. Robboy SJ, Minna JD, Colman RW, et al: Pulmonary hemorrhage syndrome as a manifestation of disseminated intravascular coagulation: Analysis of ten cases. *Chest* 1973; 63:718–721.

522. Roberts DH, Jimenez JF, Golladay ES: Multiple pulmonary artery aneurysms and peripheral venous thromboses—the Hughes-Stovin syndrome. *Pediatr Radiol* 1982; 12:214–216.

523. Roberts RC, Moore VL: Immunopathogenesis of hypersensitivity pneumonitis. *Am Rev Respir Dis* 1977; 116:1075–1090.

524. Robinson RG, Wehunt WD, Tsou E, et al: Bronchocentric granulomatosis: Roentgenographic manifestations. *Am Rev Respir Dis* 1982; 125:751–756.

525. Rodnan GP: in McCarthy DJ (ed): *Progressive Systemic Sclerosis (Scleroderma), Arthritis and Allied Conditions*, ed 9. Philadelphia, Lea & Febiger, 1979, pp 762–809.

526. Rodnan GP, Jablonska S, Medsger TA: Classification and nomenclature of progressive systemic sclerosis (scleroderma). *Clin Rheum Dis* 1979; 5:5–13.

527. Rohatgi PK, Turrisi BC: Bronchocentric granulomatosis and ankylosing spondylitis. *Thorax* 1984; 39:317–318.

528. Ropes MW, Bennett GA, Cobb S, et al: 1958 Revision of diagnostic criteria for rheumatoid arthritis. *Bull Rheum Dis* 1958; 9:175–176.

529. Rose GA, Spencer H: Polyarteritis nodosa. *Q J Med* 1957; 26:43–81.

530. Rosenberg M, Patterson R, Mintzer R, et al: Clinical and immunologic criteria for the diagnosis of allergic bronchopulmonary aspergillosis. *Ann Intern Med* 1977; 86:405–414.

531. Rosenberg TF, Medsger TA, DeCicco FA, et al: Allergic granulomatous angiitis (Churg-Strauss syndrome). *J Allergy Clin Immunol* 1975; 55:56–67.

532. Rubinow A, Celli BR, Cohen AS, et al: Localized amyloidosis of the lower respiratory tract. *Am Rev Respir Dis* 1978; 118:603–611.

533. Saab SB, Burke J, Hopeman A, et al: Primary pulmonary amyloidosis. *J Thorac Cardiovasc Surg* 1974; 67:301–307.

534. Sackner MA, Akgun N, Kimbel P, et al: The pathophysiology of scleroderma involving the heart and respiratory system. *Ann Intern Med* 1964; 60:611–630.

535. Safirstein BH, D'Souza MF, Simon G, et al: Five-year follow-up of allergic bronchopulmonary aspergillosis. *Am Rev Respir Dis* 1973; 108:450–459.

536. Sahn SA: Immunologic disease of the pleura. *Clin Chest Med* 1985; 6:83–102.

537. Sakula A: Mushroom-worker's lung. *Br Med J* 1967; 3:708–710.

538. Saldana MJ: Necrotizing sarcoid granulomatosis: Clinicopathologic observations in 24 patients. *Lab Invest* 1978; 38:364.

539. Saldana MJ: Bronchocentric granulomatosis: Clinicopathologic observations in 17 patients. *Lab Invest* 1979; 40:281–282.

540. Salerni R, Rodnan GP, Leon DF, et al: Pulmonary hypertension in the CREST syndrome variant of progressive systemic sclerosis (scleroderma). *Ann Intern Med* 1977; 86:394–399.

541. Salmeron G, Greenberg SD, Lidsky MD: Polymyositis and diffuse interstitial lung disease. A review of the pulmonary histopathologic findings. *Arch Intern Med* 1981; 141:1005–1010.

542. Salvaggio JE, Karr RM: Hypersensitivity pneumonitis: State of the art. *Chest* 1979; 75(2, suppl):270–274.

543. Sams WM, Thorne EG, Small P, et al: Leukocytoclastic vasculitis. *Arch Dermatol* 1976; 112:219–226.

544. Samuels LD, Bass TC: 51 Cr lung scan in idiopathic pulmonary hemosiderosis. *J Nucl Med* 1969; 10:106–107.

545. Sargent EN, Turner AF, Jacobson G: Superior marginal rib defects. An etiologic classification. *AJR* 1969; 106:491–505.

546. Scadding JG: Fibrosing alveolitis. *Br Med J* 1964; 2:686.

547. Scadding JG: The bronchi in allergic aspergillosis. *Scand J Respir Dis* 1967; 48:372–377.

548. Scadding JG: The lung in rheumatoid arthritis. *Proc R Soc Med* 1969; 62:227–238.

549. Scadding JG: Eosinophilic infiltration of the lungs in asthmatics. *Proc R Soc Med* 1971; 64:381–392.

550. Scadding JG: Diffuse pulmonary alveolar fibrosis. *Thorax* 1974; 29:271–281.

551. Scadding JG: Fibrosing alveolitis with autoimmune haemolytic anaemia: Two case reports. *Thorax* 1977; 32:134–139.

552. Scadding JG, Hinson KFW: Diffuse fibrosing alveolitis (diffuse interstitial fibrosis of the lungs). Correlation of histology at biopsy with prognosis. *Thorax* 1967; 22:291–304.

553. Schacherl M, Holzmann H: Eierschalenartige Verkalkung vergrosserter Hiluslymphknoten bei progressiver Sklerodermie. *Z Haut Geschlechtskr* 1968; 43:273–276.

554. Schatz M, Wasserman S, Patterson R: The eosinophil and the lung. *Arch Intern Med* 1982; 142:1515–1519.

555. Scheer RL, Grossman MA: Immune aspects of the glomerulonephritis associated with pulmonary hemorrhage. *Ann Intern Med* 1964; 60:1009–1021.

556. Schiavi EA, Roncoroni AJ, Puy RJM: Isolated bilat-

eral diaphragmatic paresis with interstitial lung disease. An unusual presentation of dermatomyositis. *Am Rev Respir Dis* 1984; 129:337–339.

557. Schimke RN, Kirkpatrick CH, Delp MH: Calcinosis, Raynaud's phenomenon, sclerodactyly, and telangiectasia. *Arch Intern Med* 1964; 119:365–370.

558. Schmidt HW, McDonald JR, Clagett OT: Amyloid tumours of the lower respiratory tract and mediastinum. *Ann Otol Rhinol Laryngol* 1953; 62:880–893.

559. Schuller H, Bolin H, Linder E, et al: Tumor-forming amyloidosis of the lower respiratory system. *Dis Chest* 1962; 42:58–67.

560. Schumacher HR, Schimmer B, Gordon GV, et al: Articular manifestations of polymyositis and dermatomyositis. *Am J Med* 1979; 67:287–292.

561. Schwartz MI, Matthay RA, Sahn SA, et al: Interstitial lung disease in polymyositis and dermatomyositis: Analysis of six cases and review of the literature. *Medicine* 1976; 55:89–104.

562. Scott DCI, Bacon PA, Tribe CR: Systemic rheumatoid vasculitis: A clinical and laboratory study of 50 cases. *Medicine* 1981; 60:288–297.

563. Seal RME, Hapke EJ, Thomas GO, et al: The pathology of the acute and chronic stages of farmer's lung. *Thorax* 1968; 23:469–489.

564. Seaton A, Meland JM, Lapp NL: Remission in Goodpasture's syndrome: Report of two patients treated by immunosuppression and review of the literature. *Thorax* 1971; 26:683–688.

565. Segal I, Fink G, Machtey I, et al: Pulmonary function abnormalities in Sjögren's syndrome and the sicca complex. *Thorax* 1981; 36:286–289.

566. Sennekamp J, Niese D, Stroehmann I, et al: Pigeon breeder's lung lacking detectable antibodies. *Clin Allergy* 1978; 8:305–310.

567. Sharma SS, Reynolds PMG: Broncho-pleural fistula complicating rheumatoid lung disease. *Postgrad Med J* 1982; 58:187–189.

568. Sharp GC, Irvin WS, Tan EM, et al: Mixed connective tissue disease—an apparently distinct rheumatic disease syndrome associated with a specific antibody to an extractable nuclear antigen [ENA]. *Am J Med* 1972; 52:148–159.

569. Shaw P, Grossman R, Fernandes BJ: Nodular mediastinal amyloidosis. *Hum Pathol* 1984; 15:1183–1185.

570. Shearn MA: Sjögren's syndrome. *Med Clin North Am* 1977; 61:271–282.

571. Shiel WC, Prete PE: Pleuropulmonary manifestations of rheumatoid arthritis. *Semin Arthritis Rheum* 1984; 13:235–243.

572. Shimizu T, Ehrlich GE, Inaba G, et al: Behçet disease (Behçet syndrome). *Semin Arthritis Rheum* 1976; 3:223–260.

573. Shlueter DP, Fink JN, Hensley GT: Wood-pulp workers' disease: A hypersensitivity pneumonitis caused by *Alternaria. Ann Intern Med* 1972; 77:907–914.

574. Sieniewicz DJ, Martin JR: Cavitating rheumatoid nodules in the lungs: Follow up report. *J Can Assoc Radiol* 1967; 18:401–403.

575. Silver TM, Farber SJ, Bole GG, et al: Radiological features of mixed connective tissue disease and scleroderma—systemic lupus erythematosus overlap. *Radiology* 1976; 120:269–275.

576. Singer C, Armstrong D, Rosen PP, et al: Diffuse pulmonary infiltrates in immunosupressed patients. Prospective study of 80 cases. *Am J Med* 1979; 66:110–120.

577. Slavin RG, Avioli LV: The Jewish Hospital of St. Louis Therapeutic Grand Rounds, No. 14. Hypersensitivity pneumonitis. *Arch Intern Med* 1976; 136:352–356.

578. Slonim L: Goodpasture's syndrome and its radiological features. *Aust J Radiol* 1969; 13:164–172.

579. Smith MJL, Benson MK, Strickland ID: Coeliac disease and diffuse interstitial lung disease. *Lancet* 1971; 1:473–475.

580. Smith RRL, Hutchins GM, Moore GW, et al: Type and distribution of pulmonary parenchymal and vascular amyloid. Correlation with cardiac amyloidosis. *Am J Med* 1979; 66:96–104.

581. Soergel KH, Sommers SC: Idiopathic pulmonary hemosiderosis and related syndromes. *Am J Med* 1962; 32:499–511.

582. Solliday NH, Williams JA, Gaensler EA, et al: Familial chronic interstitial pneumonia. *Am Rev Respir Dis* 1973; 108:193–204.

583. Songcharoen S, Raju SF, Pennebaker JB: Interstitial lung disease in polymyositis and dermatomyositis. *J Rheumatol* 1980; 7:353–360.

584. Spry CJ: Lung diseases associated with eosinophils, in Goetzl EJ, Kay AB (eds): *Current Perspectives in Allergy.* Edinburgh, Churchill Livingstone, 1983, vol 1, pp 67–77.

585. Spry CJ, Kumaraswami V: Tropical eosinophilia. *Semin Haematol* 1982; 19:107–115.

586. Stack BHR, Choo-Kang YFJ, Heard BE: The prognosis of cryptogenic fibrosing alveolitis. *Thorax* 1972; 27:535–542.

587. Stack BHR, Grant IWB, Irvine WJ, et al: Idiopathic diffuse interstitial lung disease. *Am Rev Respir Dis* 1965; 92:939–948.

588. Stankus RP, Salvaggio JE: Hypersensitivity pneumonitis. *Clin Chest Med* 1983; 4:55–62.

589. Stanton MC, Tange JD: Goodpasture's syndrome (pulmonary haemorrhage associated with glomerulonephritis). *Aust Ann Med* 1958; 7:132–144.

590. Staples CA, Müller NL, Vedal S, et al: Usual interstitial pneumonia: Correlation of CT with clinical, functional and radiologic findings. *Radiology* 1987; 162:377–381.

591. Steen VD, Owens GR, Fino GJ, et al: Pulmonary

involvement in systemic sclerosis (scleroderma). *Arthritis Rheum* 1985; 28:759–767.

592. Stein MG, Gamsu G, Webb WR, et al: Computed tomography of diffuse tracheal stenosis in Wegener granulomatosis. *J Comput Assist Tomogr* 1986; 10:868–870.

593. Steinberg DL, Webb WR: CT appearances of rheumatoid lung disease. *J Comput Assist Tomogr* 1984; 8:881–884.

594. Stephen JG, Baimbridge MV, Corrin B, et al: Necrotizing "sarcoidal" angiitis and granulomatosis of the lung. *Thorax* 1976; 31:356–360.

595. Stokes TC, McCann BG, Rees RT, et al: Acute fulminating intrapulmonary haemorrhage in Wegener's granulomatosis. *Thorax* 1982; 37:315–316.

596. Strickland B, Brennan J, Denison DM: Computed tomography in diffuse lung disease: Improving the image. *Clin Radiol* 1986; 37:335–338.

597. Strimlan CV, Rosenow EC, Divertie MB, et al: Pulmonary manifestations of Sjögren's syndrome. *Chest* 1976; 70:354–361.

598. Strohl KP, Feldman NT, Ingram RH: Apical fibrobullous disease with rheumatoid arthritis. *Chest* 1979; 75:739–741.

599. Stupi AM, Steen VD, Owens GR, et al: Pulmonary hypertension in the CREST syndrome variant of systemic sclerosis. *Arthritis Rheum* 1986; 29:515–524.

600. Subbarao K, Jacobson HG: Systemic disorders affecting the thoracic cage. *Radiol Clin North Am* 1984; 22:497–517.

601. Sullivan WD, Hurst DJ, Harmon CE, et al: A prospective evaluation emphasizing pulmonary involvement in patients with mixed connective tissue disease. *Medicine* 1984; 63:92–107.

602. Sunderman FW, Sunderman FW: Löffler's syndrome associated with nickel sensitivity. *Arch Intern Med* 1961; 107:405–408.

603. Sybers RG, Sybers JL, Dickie HA, et al: Roentgenographic aspects of haemorrhagic pulmonary-renal disease (Goodpasture's syndrome). *AJR* 1965; 94:674–680.

604. Tablan OC, Reyes MP: Chronic interstitial pulmonary fibrosis following *Mycoplasma pneumoniae* pneumonia. *Am J Med* 1985; 79:268–270.

605. Talbott JA, Calkins E: Pulmonary involvement in rheumatoid arthritis. *JAMA* 1964; 189:911–913.

606. Tan EM, Cohen AS, Fries JF, et al: The 1982 revised criteria for the classification of systemic lupus erythematosus. *Arthritis Rheum* 1982; 25:1271–1277.

607. Taormina VJ, Miller WT, Gefter WB, et al: Progressive systemic sclerosis subgroups: Variable pulmonary features. *AJR* 1981; 137:277–285.

608. Taylor TL, Ostrum H: The roentgenologic evaluation of systemic lupus erythematosus. *AJR* 1959; 82:95–107.

609. Teague CA, Doak PB, Simpson IJ, et al: Goodpasture's syndrome. An analysis of 29 cases. *Kidney Int* 1978; 13:492–504.

610. Teixidor HS, Bachman AL: Multiple amyloid tumours of the lung. *AJR* 1971; 111:525–529.

611. Tellesson WG: Rheumatoid pneumoconiosis (Caplan's syndrome) in an asbestos worker. *Thorax* 1961; 16:372–377.

612. Teplick JG, Haskin ME, Nedwich A: The Hughes-Stovin syndrome. *Radiology* 1974; 113:607–608.

613. Thadani U: Rheumatoid lung disease with pulmonary fibrosis necrobiotic nodules and pleural effusion. *Br J Dis Chest* 1973; 67:146–152.

614. Theros EG, Reeder MM, Eckert JF: An exercise in radiologic-pathologic correlation. *Radiology* 1968; 90:784–791.

615. Thomas HM, Irwin RS: Classification of diffuse intrapulmonary hemorrhage. *Chest* 1975; 68:483–484.

616. Thomashow BM, Felton CP, Navarro C: Diffuse intrapulmonary hemorrhage, renal failure and a systemic vasculitis. *Am J Med* 1980; 68:299–304.

617. Thompson PJ, Citron KM: Amyloid and the lower respiratory tract. *Thorax* 1983; 38:84–87.

618. Thompson PJ, Jewkes J, Corrin B, et al: Primary bronchopulmonary amyloid tumour with massive hilar lymphadenopathy. *Thorax* 1983; 38:153–154.

619. Thompson PL, MacKay IR: Fibrosing alveolitis and polymyositis. *Thorax* 1970; 25:504–507.

620. Thomsen OF: Primary amyloidosis in lungs and heart. *Acta Med Scand* 1968; 184:125–128.

621. Tomasi TB, Fudenberg HH, Finby N: Possible relationship of rheumatoid factors and pulmonary disease. *Am J Med* 1962; 33:243–248.

622. Trell E, Lindstrom C: Pulmonary hypertension in systemic sclerosis. *Ann Rheum Dis* 1971; 30:390–400.

623. Tubbs RR, Benjamin SP, Reich NF, et al: Desquamative interstitial pneumonitis—cellular phase of fibrosing alveolitis. *Chest* 1977; 72:159–166.

624. Tuffanelli DL, Winkelmann RK: Systemic scleroderma. *Arch Dermatol* 1961; 84:359–371.

625. Tuffanelli DL, Winkelmann RK: Scleroderma and its relationship to the "collangenoses": Dermatomyositis, lupus erythematosus, rheumatoid arthritis and Sjögren's syndrome. *Am J Med Sci* 1962; 243:133–146.

626. Tukiainen P, Taskinen E, Holsti P, et al: Prognosis of cryptogenic fibrosing alveolitis. *Thorax* 1983; 38:349–355.

627. Tukiainen P, Taskinen E, Korhola O, et al: Farmer's lung: Needle biopsy findings and pulmonary function. *Eur J Respir Dis* 1980; 61:3–11.

628. Tumulty PA: The clinical course of systemic lupus erythematosus. *JAMA* 1954; 156:947–953.

629. Turner-Stokes L, Turner-Warwick M: Intrathoracic manifestations of SLE. *Clin Rheum Dis* 1982; 8:229–242.

630. Turner-Warwick M: Fibrosing alveolitis and chronic liver disease. *Q J Med* 1968; 37:133–149.

631. Turner-Warwick M, Assem ESK, Lockwood M: Cryptogenic pulmonary eosinophilia. *Clin Allergy* 1976; 6:135–145.

632. Turner-Warwick M, Burrows B, Johnson A: Cryptogenic fibrosing alveolitis: Clinical features and their influence on survival. *Thorax* 1980; 35:171–180.

633. Turner-Warwick M, Dewar A: Pulmonary haemorrhage and pulmonary haemosiderosis. *Clin Radiol* 1982; 33:361–370.

634. Turner-Warwick M, Evans RC: Pulmonary manifestations of rheumatoid disease. *Clin Rheum Dis* 1977; 3:549–564.

635. Turner-Warwick M, Lebowitz M, Burrows B, et al: Cryptogenic fibrosing alveolitis and lung cancer. *Thorax* 1980; 35:496–499.

636. Turton CWG, Morris LM, Lawler SD, et al: HLA in cryptogenic fibrosing alveolitis. *Lancet* 1978; 1:507–508.

637. Unger GF, Scanlon GT, Fink JN, et al: A radiologic approach to hypersensitivity pneumonias. *Radiol Clin North Am* 1973; 11:339–356.

638. Unger J DeB, Fink JN, Unger GF: Pigeon breeder's disease. A review of the roentgenographic pulmonary findings. *AJR* 1968; 90:683–687.

639. Ungerer RG, Tashkin DP, Furst D, et al: Prevalence and clinical correlates of pulmonary arterial hypertension in progressive systemic sclerosis. *Am J Med* 1983; 75:65–74.

640. Van Toorn DW: Coffee worker's lung. A new example of extrinsic allergic alveolitis. *Thorax* 1970; 25:399–405.

641. Velayos EE, Masi AT, Stevens MB, et al: The "CREST" syndrome. Comparison with systemic sclerosis (scleroderma). *Arch Intern Med* 1979; 139:1240–1244.

642. Vincken W, Roels P: Hypersensitivity pneumonitis due to *Aspergillus fumigatus* in compost. *Thorax* 1984; 39:74–75.

643. Vitali C, Tavoni A, Viegi G, et al: Lung involvement in Sjögren's syndrome: A comparison between patients with primary and with secondary syndrome. *Ann Rheum Dis* 1985; 44:455–461.

644. Wade G, Ball J: Unexplained pulmonary hypertension. *Q J Med* 1957; 26:83–119.

645. Wagenaar SSC, Westermann CJJ, Corrin B: Giant cell arteritis limited to large elastic pulmonary arteries. *Thorax* 1981; 36:876–877.

646. Walker WC: Pulmonary infections and rheumatoid arthritis. *Q J Med* 1967; 36:239–251.

647. Walker WC, Wright V: Rheumatoid pleuritis. *Ann Rheum Dis* 1967; 26:467–474.

648. Walker WC, Wright V: Pulmonary lesions and rheumatoid arthritis. *Medicine* 1968; 47:501–520.

649. Wall CP, Gaensler EA, Carrington CB, et al: Comparison of transbronchial and open biopsies in chronic infiltrative lung diseases. *Am Rev Respir Dis* 1981; 123:280–285.

650. Wang CC, Robbins LL: Amyloid disease. Its roentgen manifestations. *Radiology* 1956; 66:489–501.

651. Wang JLF, Patterson R, Rosenberg M, et al: Serum IgE and IgG antibody activity against *Aspergillus fumigatus* as a diagnostic aid in allergic bronchopulmonary aspergillosis. *Am Rev Respir Dis* 1978; 117:917–927.

652. Warren J, Pitchenik AE, Saldana MJ: Bronchocentric granulomatosis with glomerulonephritis. *Chest* 1985; 87:832–834.

653. Ward R: Pleural effusion and rheumatoid disease. *Lancet* 1961; 2:1336–1338.

654. Watson AJ, Black J, Doig AT, et al: Pneumoconiosis in carbon electrode makers. *Br J Ind Med* 1959; 16:274–285.

655. Watters LC, King TE, Schwartz JA, et al: A clinical, radiographic, and physiologic scoring system for the longitudinal assessment of patients with idiopathic pulmonary fibrosis. *Am Rev Respir Dis* 1986; 133:97–103.

656. Weaver AL, Divertie MB, Titus JL: The lung in scleroderma. *Mayo Clin Proc* 1967; 42:754–766.

657. Weaver AL, Divertie MB, Titus JL: Pulmonary scleroderma. *Dis Chest* 1968; 54:490–498.

658. Webb JKG, Job CK, Gault EW: Tropical eosinophilia. Demonstration of microfilariae in lung, liver, and lymph-nodes. *Lancet* 1960; 1:835–842.

659. Webb WR, Gamsu G: Cavitary pulmonary nodules with systemic lupus erythematosus: Differential diagnosis. *AJR* 1981; 136:27–31.

660. Webb WR, Goodman PC: Fibrosing alveolitis in patients with neurofibromatosis. *Radiology* 1977; 122:289–293.

661. Weiss L: Isolated multiple nodular pulmonary amyloidosis. *Am J Clin Pathol* 1960; 33:318–329.

662. Wenzel FJ, Gray RL, Roberts RC, et al: Serologic studies in farmer's lung. *Am Rev Respir Dis* 1974; 109:464–468.

663. Wiener-Kronish JP, Solinger AM, Warnock ML, et al: Severe pulmonary involvement in mixed connective tissue disease. *Am Rev Respir Dis* 1981; 124:499–503.

664. Wilson SR, Sanders DE, Delarue NC: Intrathoracic manifestations of amyloid disease. *Radiology* 1976; 120:283–289.

665. Winchester RJ, Litwin SD, Koffler D, et al: Observations of the eosinophilia of certain patients with rheumatoid arthritis. *Arthritis Rheum* 1971; 14:650–665.

666. Winkelmann RK: Dermatomyositis in childhood. *Clin Rheum Dis* 1982; 8:353–368.

667. Winkelmann RK, Ditto WB: Cutaneous and visceral syndromes of necrotizing or "allergic" angiitis: A study of 38 cases. *Medicine* 1964; 43:59–89.

668. Winslow WA, Ploss LN, Loitman B: Pleuritis in systemic lupus erythematosus: Its importance as an

early manifestation in diagnosis. *Ann Intern Med* 1958; 49:70–88.

669. Winterbauer RH: Multiple telangiectasia, Raynaud's phenomenon, sclerodactyly, and subcutaneous calcinosis: A syndrome mimicking hereditary hemorrhagic telangiectasia. *Bull Johns Hopkins Hosp* 1964; 114:361–383.

670. Winterbauer RH, Hammar SP, Hallman KO, et al: Diffuse interstitial pneumonitis. Clinicopathologic correlations in 20 patients treated with prednisone/azothioprine. *Am J Med* 1978; 65:661–672.

671. Winzelberg GG, Laman D, Sachs M, et al: Detection of pulmonary hemorrhage with technetium-labelled red cells. *J Nucl Med* 1981; 22:884–885.

672. Wolpert SM, Kahn PC, Farbman K: The radiology of the Hughes-Stovin syndrome. *AJR* 1971; 112:383–388.

673. Wright DO, Gold EM: Loeffler's syndrome associated with creeping eruption (cutaneous helminthiasis). *Arch Intern Med* 1946; 78:303–312.

674. Wright JR, Calkins E: Clinical-pathologic differentiation of common amyloid syndromes. *Medicine* 1981; 60:429–448.

675. Wright PH, Buxton-Thomas M, Kreel L, et al: Cryptogenic fibrosing alveolitis: Pattern of disease in the lung. *Thorax* 1984; 39:857–861.

676. Wright PH, Heard BE, Steel SJ, et al: Cryptogenic fibrosing alveolitis: Assessment by graded trephine lung biopsy histology compared with clinical, radiographic and physiologic features. *Br J Dis Chest* 1981; 75:61–70.

677. Young RH, Mark GJ: Pulmonary vascular changes in scleroderma. *Am J Med* 1978; 64:998–1004.

678. Yousem SA, Colby TV, Carrington CB: Lung biopsy in rheumatoid arthritis. *Am Rev Respir Dis* 1985; 131:770–777.

679. Yue CC, Park CH, Kushner I: Apical fibrocavitary lesions of the lung in rheumatoid arthritis. Report of two cases and review of the literature. *Am J Med* 1986; 81:741–746.

680. Yum MN, Ziegler JR, Walker PD, et al: Pseudolymphoma of the lung in a patient with systemic lupus erythematosus. *Am J Med* 1979; 66:172–176.

681. Zimmerman RA, Miller WT: Pulmonary aspergillosis. *AJR* 1970; 109:505–515.

682. Zundel WE, Prior AP: An amyloid lung. *Thorax* 1971; 26:357–363.

683. Zylak CJ, Dyck DR, Warren P, et al: Hypersensitive lung disease due to avian antigens. *Radiology* 1975; 114:45–49.

Pulmonary Diseases of Unknown Origin and Miscellaneous Pulmonary Disorders

SARCOIDOSIS

Sarcoidosis is a common systemic disease characterized by widespread development of noncaseating epithelioid cell granulomas that eventually either resolve or convert into fibrous tissue. Although its etiology and pathogenesis are obscure, the disease is likely to be the result of an immunologically mediated response to one or more unidentified and possibly inhaled agents. Various agents have been suggested including *Mycobacterium* species, either alone or with viruses; pollen; and inorganic dusts,[324] but no one theory has gained widespread acceptance. There is evidence that the immunologic response is influenced by genetic factors and human lymphocyte antigen (HLA) status.[110, 303]

Pathology/Clinical Features

It is now generally accepted that granuloma formation in the lung is preceded by a mononuclear alveolitis[264] in which monocytes, macrophages, and lymphocytes all accumulate.[59] The early granulomas are loose collections of monocytes, macrophages, and lymphocytes with a few epithelioid cells; they evolve into mature granulomas that consist of a tightly packed central collection of epithelioid cells, macrophages, and multinucleate giant cells surrounded by lymphocytes, monocytes, and fibroblasts.[324] There is morphologic evidence that all three cellular elements in the center of granulomas

are secretory and that the surrounding lymphocytes are activated T cells. Necrosis is rare and, when it does occur, it is minimal and confined to the center of granulomas.[87] Granulomas remain stable for months or years and then, in about 80% of cases, they resolve completely. In the remaining 20%, the granulomas become obliterated by centripetal fibrosis, which probably originates from the fibroblasts in the periphery of the granuloma. This fibrosis may develop into extensive interstitial fibrosis, with destruction of lung architecture and the eventual production of an end-stage lung.

Sarcoid granulomas are nonspecific and resemble those in many other granulomatous processes[140] except granulomas resulting from tuberculosis, in which there is usually some caseous necrosis. Sarcoid granulomas are found in all organs and tissues—although some, like the adrenal gland, are not commonly involved.[196] The generalized nature of the sarcoid response is an important feature that distinguishes sarcoidosis from various local sarcoid-like responses associated with neoplastic conditions.[106]

Incidence rates for sarcoidosis vary greatly from country to country and depend, among other factors, on race, the sophistication of medical care, and use of screening programs. Quoted figures are in the order of 1 to 10 cases per 100,000 population per year, but this is almost certainly an underestimate because many cases remain subclinical.[177] Sarcoidosis occurs with about ten times greater frequency in blacks than in whites.[18, 76, 196, 273] About

1% to 3% of patients with sarcoidosis have a positive family history of the disease.[149, 196, 275, 293] There is no evidence that HLA type influences susceptibility, but it does have some affect on prognosis.[93] A number of conditions have been suggested as showing an association with sarcoidosis, the relationship being best established for tuberculosis.[186, 278, 305] In a series of 425 patients with sarcoidosis, tuberculosis immediately preceded sarcoidosis in 1.6%, and in 1.9%, sarcoidosis developed into overt tuberculosis.[277] In addition, *Mycobacterium* organisms were isolated from 5% of patients with typical sarcoidosis.

Presentation is commonest in patients between 20 and 40 years of age,[136, 163, 196] but the age range is wide, even including the first year of life[121] and the 8th decade.[196] In whites there is a more or less equal sex incidence or slight female preponderance, whereas in blacks there is a definite twofold to threefold excess in females.[88, 136, 163, 196, 261]

The mode of presentation varies greatly among series, depending particularly on racial mix and the use of screening radiography. In white-dominated series, presentation as an incidental radiographic finding is common and may occur in 40% to 50% of cases.[141, 261] Respiratory illness (21%), erythema nodosum (16%), ocular symptoms (7%), and other skin lesions (4%)[141] represent the other common presentations. In series with significant or dominant numbers of black patients, respiratory symptoms and systemic symptoms such as fatigue, malaise, weakness, weight loss, and fever tend to dominate.[290] A striking difference between blacks and whites at presentation is the frequency of erythema nodosum. This finding is uncommon in blacks but very common in whites, particularly in the United Kingdom, where 30% to 40% of patients present with the condition,[76, 126, 141, 210] often as part of the erythema nodosum/febrile arthralgia syndrome, with or without uveitis.[275] In general the disease in blacks is later in onset and more likely to become chronic and disseminated—with the involvement of peripheral nodes, skin, and eyes. The prognosis is worse in blacks than whites.[17, 18, 76, 126, 139, 320]

Findings on Investigation

Laboratory investigations may show an anemia, leukopenia, or a raised erythrocyte sedimentation rate. A significant blood eosinophilia is seen in up to one-quarter of patients.[196] Both hypercalcemia and hypercalciuria are recorded. The former is often transient and occurs in 10% to 20% of patients.[140, 196, 299] Hypercalcemia can cause metastatic

calcification and renal failure.[163] Hypercalciuria is two to three times more common than hypercalcemia.[208, 210] Disordered calcium homeostasis is due to synthesis of 1,25-dihydroxyvitamin D by activated sarcoid macrophages[1] and is rapidly responsive to steroids.[271]

Serum levels of angiotensin converting enzyme (ACE) are raised in about 50% to 60% of patients because of its production by activated macrophages.[182, 183] Serum ACE levels correlate with the activity of clinical disease as a whole[260] but not convincingly with the degree and activity of pulmonary disease.[282, 324] The presence of raised levels of serum ACE is not specific for sarcoidosis, and there is a false positive rate of approximately 10%.[290]

Various immunologic derangements are seen with sarcoidosis. Cutaneous anergy is well recognized. About two-thirds of patients have a negative tuberculin test, and in many of the remainder it is only weakly positive.[141, 196, 290] Cutaneous anergy is probably related to the relative abundance of suppressor T cells in the peripheral blood following sequestration of helper T cells in active sarcoid lesions. Activated helper T cells stimulate nonspecific antibody production by B cells,[324] producing a whole range of antibodies[140] and resulting in hypergammaglobulinemia in about 50% of patients, particularly blacks.[141] In the acute disease, about half the patients have circulating immune complexes, the presence of which correlates with various clinical features such as erythema nodosum.[244]

Over the last decade bronchoalveolar lavage (BAL) has provided substantial information about sarcoid alveolitis and its pathogenesis.[59] The usefulness of BAL to predict outcome and to monitor treatment is, however, still debated.[324] In patients with active sarcoidosis, the percentage of lymphocytes in lavage fluid increases above the normal 10%, and many of these are activated helper T lymphocytes.[59, 290] Some authors distinguish a high- and low-intensity alveolitis, depending on whether lymphocytes make up more or less than 28% of the total BAL cell count.[59]

Another investigation that has been used during the last decade in much the same way as BAL is gallium scintigraphy.[185] Gallium-67 citrate was introduced as a scintigraphic scanning agent in 1969,[77] and uptake in pulmonary sarcoidosis was first noted in 1972.[174] Gallium-67 is a gamma ray emitter with an 88 hour half-life and three photopeaks (92, 185, and 399 keV). Lung scanning is usually performed at 48 or 72 hours after an intravenous dose of between 100 to 300 MBq (2.6 to 8 mCi). A gamma camera with a large field of view and multiple pulse-height analyzers are used. At 48 hours, there is normally a little uptake in bone, but none in the lung or mediastinum. In sarcoidosis there is both lung and mediastinal (nodal) uptake.[120, 135, 200] It is still not clear exactly what cells take up the agent. Some studies suggest activated macrophages,[224] while other workers, on indirect evidence, suggest activated T lymphocytes.[59] Irrespective of which cell is involved, it seems possible that gallium uptake may reflect the degree of "activity" of the sarcoid process. Unfortunately, there is no consensus regarding the criteria of activity, and no clear-cut way of using gallium scanning has emerged; its clinical value, therefore, remains undefined.[16, 254]

Respiratory function tests are commonly deranged in sarcoidosis. There is a decrease in total lung capacity, a reduced diffusing capacity, a restrictive defect of ventilatory capacity, reduced compliance and, in advanced disease, abnormal airway function.[178, 278, 339] There is a loose relationship between respiratory function tests and chest radiographic changes.[339] The mean values for respiratory function tests correlate well with the radiographic stage, becoming worse from stage I to stage III.[213] However, individual exceptions to this correlation are common. For example, several studies have shown that about 50% of patients in stage I may have a diffusion defect.[127, 291, 339] Also, respiratory function tests can give results in the normal range in stage II and III disease.[127] Discrepancies between radiographs and function are most likely to arise when patients are treated with steroids, which commonly improve function in the face of an unchanging chest radiograph.[339]

Diagnosis/Prognosis

To make a firm diagnosis of sarcoidosis there must be consistent clinicoradiological findings and histologic evidence of widespread noncaseating epithelioid cell granulomas in more than one organ or a positive Kveim skin test. In clinical practice, the organs most commonly sampled are lymph nodes, liver, and lung. In sarcoidosis, even though the chest radiograph shows adenopathy with clear lungs, pathologically the lung is diffusely infiltrated with granulomas.[263] Lung biopsies are usually performed by means of a fiberoptic bronchoscope and, provided enough tissue samples are obtained,[95] positive rates for the test are in the order of 90%.[168, 218, 257, 318]

A large number of conditions can produce granulomatous lesions[140] and, if the diagnosis of sarcoidosis rests on histologic appearances, these other conditions must be excluded as far as possible by history, special histologic stains, and microbiological culture. It is also important to establish the widespread nature of the granulomatous process, as local sarcoid-like reactions can be produced by a number of primary processes, including lymphoma and carcinoma.[86, 106] In everyday clinical practice it is common to accept a diagnosis of sarcoidosis without biopsy provided clinical, laboratory, and radiologic features are typical, particularly when they correspond to a classic syndrome such as erythema nodosum, arthropathy, and bilateral hilar adenopathy. When the clinical diagnosis is less firmly based, then histologic proof, either from biopsy or a Kveim test, is mandatory.

The Kveim test is based on the fact that, in sarcoidosis, the intracutaneous injection of a saline suspension of human sarcoid tissue leads to the development of a granulomatous nodule within 4 to 6 weeks. About two-thirds to three-quarters of tests are positive in the first 2 years after patient presentation, with the positive rate falling off with time[296] and with the development of stage III disease.[26, 155, 296] There is about a 2% false positive rate, seen especially in Crohn's disease.

When death occurs due to sarcoidosis, it is most commonly related to pulmonary involvement: cor pulmonale, hemorrhage, mycetoma formation, and respiratory failure. In two series of 85 sarcoid-related deaths, 67% resulted from pulmonary involvement.[128, 146] In several large series, overall mortality ranged between 2.2% and 7.6%.*

Staging of Sarcoidosis

It is common practice to stage sarcoidosis according to its appearance on the chest radiograph. Several different classifications have been proposed. DeRemee[68] recently reviewed the subject and recommended the following:

- Stage 0—Clear chest radiograph;
- Stage I—Node enlargement only;
- Stage II—Node enlargement and parenchymal shadowing;
- Stage III—Parenchymal shadowing alone.

The objection to this particular system is that it does not permit a distinction between transient (non-

---

*References 78, 128, 141, 196, 297, and 305.

fibrotic) and fixed (fibrotic) parenchymal shadowing. Several other systems in use attempt to overcome this problem. DeRemee maintains, and we agree, that the distinction between fibrotic and nonfibrotic shadowing cannot be reliably made on radiologic criteria.[68] Another objection is that the term "stage" suggests a temporal evolution from stage 0 to a higher stage, which almost certainly does not happen in every patient. For example, stage 0 is a common late finding, and there are cases in which it seems unlikely that stage III was preceded by a stage I or II. Nevertheless, it is common for patients to pass sequentially from Stage I to III, and the term is so hallowed by use that it is unlikely to be changed.

At presentation, the percentages of patients at each stage are: stage 0, 5% to 15%; stage II, 30% to 40%; and stage III, 10% to 15%. The stage at presentation is generally considered to correlate with prognosis[296]; it therefore provides a useful method for characterizing patient groups in studies and as a guide to clinical management. In the worldwide series of 3,679 patients,[141] 65% of stage I patients showed resolution of the chest radiographic findings. The corresponding figures for stages II and III were 49% and 20%, respectively. Not all workers, however, agree that there is a correlation between outcome and stage.[132]

Chest Radiology

The chest radiograph is abnormal at some point in 90% to 95% of patients with sarcoidosis.[196] About 5% to 15% of patients have a clear chest radiograph at presentation,* but pulmonary granulomas can be demonstrated on biopsy in these patients despite the absence of radiologic change.[201, 252]

Lymph Nodes

Lymphadenopathy is the most common intrathoracic manifestation of sarcoidosis, occurring in 75% to 80% of patients at some point in their illness.[141, 164, 297] Pulmonary shadowing as a result of sarcoidosis that antedates adenopathy is extremely rare[21, 82, 186, 206] and, as a working rule, can be discounted. Possibly less rare, but still extremely unusual, is thoracic adenopathy that develops after documented involvement of extrathoracic sites such as eyes and skin.[78, 190, 221, 261]

Symmetric, bilateral hilar adenopathy and some form of paratracheal adenopathy is the classic pat-

*References 136, 140, 141, 164, 196, and 210.

tern in sarcoidosis (Fig 12–1). In one series of 150 patients with sarcoidosis and an abnormal chest radiograph, about 30% had bilateral hilar lymphadenopathy (BHL) alone, 30% had BHL with right paratracheal adenopathy, and 30% had BHL with bilateral paratracheal adenopathy.[164] This series and earlier ones probably underestimate the prevalence of left paratracheal adenopathy which is, in general, not as easy to detect as right-sided adenopathy.[22] The lowest part of the left paratracheal chain, the aortopulmonary (ductus) nodes, have only recently received attention, and these are seen to be enlarged in most patients,[343] producing a characteristic local convexity in the aortopulmonary window (Fig 12–2).[15] It is worth noting that isolated paratracheal or isolated aortopulmonary adenopathy have rarely been recorded in sarcoidosis.[15, 256]

Bilateral hilar adenopathy is common to all of these major patterns and is the most characteristic aspect of nodal enlargement in sarcoidosis. The degree of hilar node enlargement ranges from barely detectable to massive, in which case nodes may reach halfway to the chest wall (Fig 12–3). The outer margins of the hili are usually lobulated[300] and well-demarcated unless there is adjacent parenchymal shad-

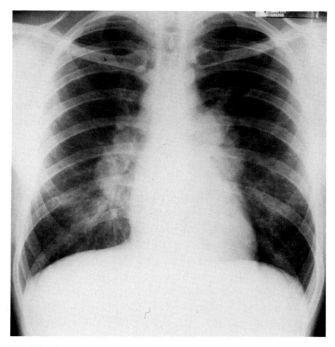

FIG 12–1.
Sarcoidosis showing characteristic lymphadenopathy. Hilar nodes are symmetrically enlarged, with involvement of both the proximal tracheobronchial and the more distal bronchopulmonary nodes. Right paratracheal and aortopulmonary nodes are mildly affected.

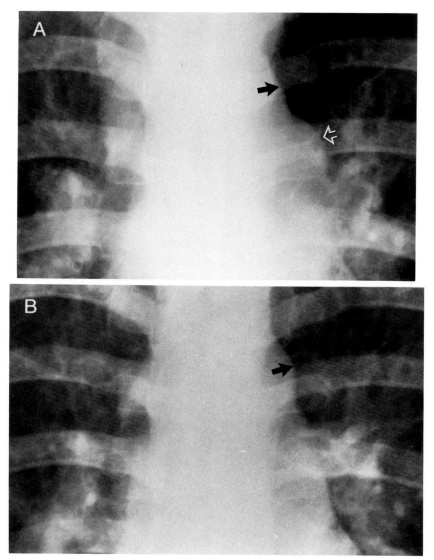

FIG 12—2.

Sarcoidosis—aortopulmonary nodes. Local view of the mid mediastinum and hilar regions. **A,** local convexity *(open arrow)* below the aortic knob *(closed arrow)* is due to aortopulmonary nodal enlargement. **B,** same patient 8 months later; the convexity below the aortic knob *(arrow)* has disappeared and has been replaced by the shadow of a normal main pulmonary artery.

owing.[245, 278] Both the more proximal tracheobronchial and the more distal bronchopulmonary nodes are involved in sarcoidosis, and enlargement of the latter is characteristic.[300] These more peripheral nodes may have lung or lower lobe bronchus on their medial aspect and, thus, when enlarged they typically have a clearly demarcated inner border[300] and the inferior aspect of the hilum takes on a rather squared off appearance (Fig 12–3).[337] Symmetry is an important diagnostic feature of the hilar adenopathy associated with sarcoidosis because symmetrical adenopathy is unusual in the major diagnostic alternatives such as lymphoma, tuberculosis and metastatic disease (Fig 12–4). Sometimes, the adenopathy will appear more marked on the right on a frontal radiograph simply because the right hilus normally stands more proud than the left,[187] and because left paratracheal nodes are more difficult to identify. Tomography can clarify this situation.[88] In about 3% of patients, the asymmetry may be real and striking, even to the extent that the adenopathy may be considered unilateral (Fig 12–5).[142, 164, 245, 261] In one series of 135 patients, an exceptionally high proportion of patients (9.6%)

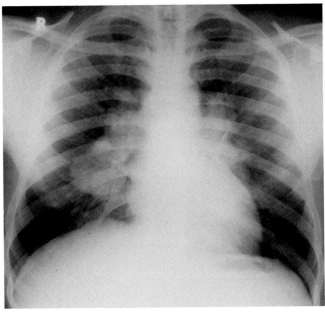

FIG 12—3.
Sarcoidosis. The hilar adenopathy is more massive than in Figure 12—1 and reaches halfway to the chest wall. The bronchopulmonary nodes are markedly enlarged and clearly demarcated medially. The lower aspect of the right hilus presents a "squared off" appearance.

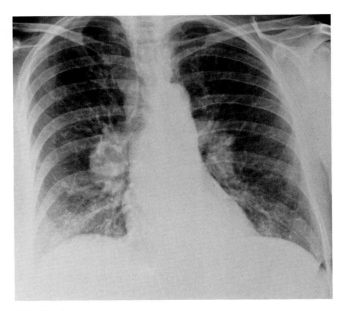

FIG 12—4.
Chronic lymphatic leukemia. Symmetric bilateral hilar and right paratracheal adenopathy simulates sarcoidosis. Adenopathy in tuberculosis, histoplasmosis, and lymphoma is usually asymmetric, but in leukemia, metastatic disease, and silicosis, symmetric nodal enlargement is well recognized.

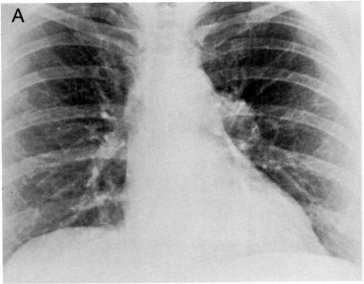

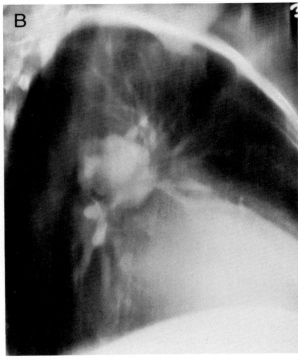

FIG 12—5.
Sarcoidosis—unilateral adenopathy. **A,** PA chest radiograph shows unilateral hilar adenopathy resulting from biopsy proved sarcoidosis. **B,** lateral tomogram in same patient.

showing true unilateral hilar adenopathy was recorded.[78] Unilateral hilar adenopathy is about twice as common on the right as on the left and can occur either alone or with right paratracheal adenopathy.[78, 307]

Other nodes in the chest may be involved with a recorded frequency that reflects the imaging modality used and the diligence with which they are sought. In general, involvement of these other nodal groups accompanies the more classic adenopathy, and the degree of enlargement is usually modest. Anterior mediastinal nodes are difficult to appreciate on plain radiographs, but CT scanning shows involvement in 25% to 66% of patients (Fig 12–6; see also Fig 12–14).[114, 304, 343] Isolated anterior mediastinal adenopathy is rare[43, 202, 245, 326] and should strongly suggest a diagnosis other than sarcoidosis, particularly lymphoma.

Subcarinal adenopathy (Fig 12–7) may occasionally be marked and can cause airway compression[21] or dysphagia.[317] The prevalence of subcarinal adenopathy in a study not using CT was 21%,[15] but with CT (Fig 12–8), the figures are in the order of 50%.[114, 343] Involvement of subcarinal nodes in the absence of hilar adenopathy is rare, but has been recorded.[154]

Posterior mediastinal adenopathy (Figs 12–9 through 12–11) is one of the least common patterns in sarcoidosis, ranging in frequency from 2% to 20%.[15, 279, 304] There is only one case report of sarcoidosis presenting with isolated posterior mediastinal adenopathy.[171]

Most mediastinal nodes are at their maximum size when first seen[300]; they decrease in size over the next 3 to 6 months so that two-thirds are no longer visible after 1 year[300] and very few are visible after 2 years.[142, 278] In one review only 6% persisted at 2 years and most of these were smaller in size than at presentation.[278] If nodes persist for 2 years, it is common for them to remain unchanged for many years[138, 300] and probably indefinitely. Therefore, given a chest radiograph with mediastinal node enlargement, it is always worth considering the possibility that adenopathy is a residuum from previous sarcoidosis.

Of those patients who present with stage I disease, about 60% will go on to complete resolution,[78, 140, 261, 275, 300] the figure being higher in those with erythema nodosum and arthropathy.[278] The remaining 30% to 40% of patients presenting with adenopathy will go on to develop parenchymal shadowing,[278, 300] usually within the 1st year, though longer intervals are not uncommon,[300] and gaps of 10 years or more are recorded.[138] The adenopathy has commonly begun to decrease in size at the time that parenchymal shadowing appears,[163, 278, 300] a feature that can be helpful in distinguishing sarcoidosis from lymphoma or carcinoma in which the

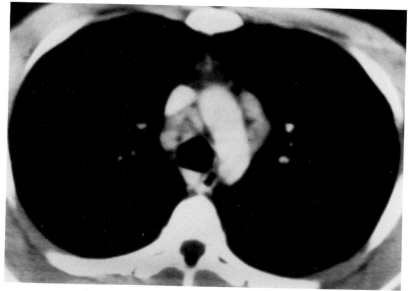

FIG 12–6.
Sarcoidosis—anterior mediastinal nodes. Contrast-enhanced CT scan shows prevascular (aortic) nodes on the left and pretracheal nodes, between superior vena cava and trachea, on the right.

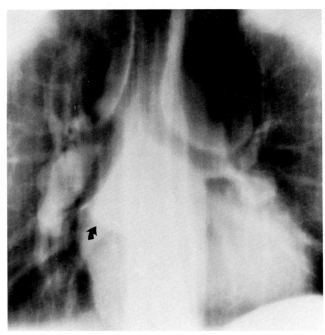

FIG 12–7.
Sarcoidosis—subcarinal nodes. AP tomogram of the mediastinum shows subcarinal adenopathy. This deviates the azygoesophageal interface *(arrow)* to the right to meet the intermediate stem bronchus distally. There is also bilateral hilar adenopathy.

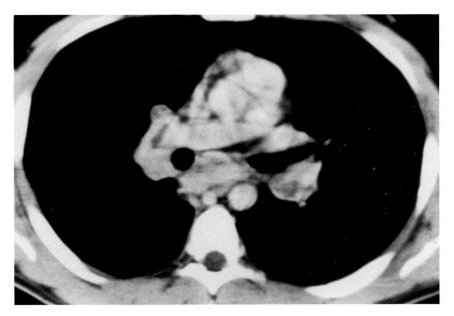

FIG 12–8.
Sarcoidosis—subcarinal nodes. Contrast-enhanced CT scan below the level of the carina reveals bilateral hilar adenopathy and enlarged subcarinal lymph nodes lying between the aorta, azygos vein, and right main stem bronchus.

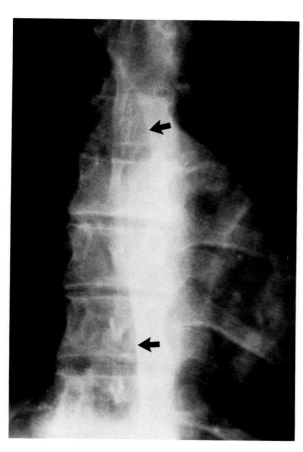

FIG 12–9.
Sarcoidosis—posterior mediastinal nodes. A penetrated PA view of the dorsal spine from D-6 to D-11 shows the middle third of the azygoesophageal interface *(arrows)* distorted and effaced by posterior mediastinal adenopathy.

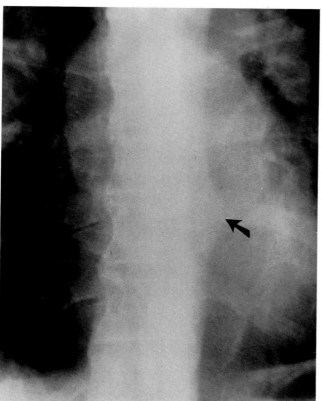

FIG 12–10.
Sarcoidosis—posterior mediastinal nodes. Localized view of lower mediastinum is taken from a high-kVp chest radiograph. There is a local convexity *(arrow)* of the para-aortic interface due to posterior mediastinal, preaortic node enlargement.

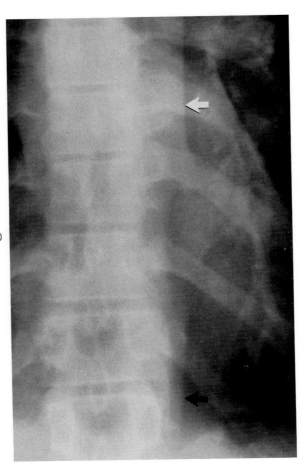

FIG 12–11.

Sarcoidosis—posterior mediastinal nodes. Localized view of lower mediastinum taken from a high-kVp chest radiograph. As in Figure 12–10 there is posterior mediastinal adenopathy, but here the loss of the para-aortic interface *(arrows)* over a 5-cm segment is the most striking finding.

nodes would be expected to remain stable or to enlarge.[78]

Fluctuation of nodal enlargement during intermittent steroid therapy is well recognized (Fig 12–12),[308] but once the nodes have completely resolved radiologically it is very unusual for them to enlarge again spontaneously. Such a train of events should raise the possibility of malignant adenopathy.[30] Only about ten cases of nodal recurrence are reported, and these spanned periods of up to 20 years.[189] Nodal recurrence developed either alone[187, 308] or with other features of sarcoidosis.[316] Recurrences may be multiple, and as many as three or four episodes have been recorded.[184, 275] Different nodal groups may be involved in separate episodes, as in one patient in whom first one hilus, then the other, was affected.[158, 245]

Sarcoid nodes may calcify (Fig 12–13); the frequency is related to duration of disease and period of observation.[256] In short-term studies, nodal calcification is seen in about 1% to 3% of cases,[137, 163, 275, 289] but in a longer term study of 111 patients observed for 10 years or more, the prevalence was 20%.[134] Calcification is thought to develop only in diseased nodes, occurring in a dystrophic fashion in fibrous tissue. Its occurrence appears unrelated to either hypercalcemia or coincident tuberculosis. Most descriptions are of paratracheal and hilar involvement, but any nodal group may be involved.[22] Radiographically the morphology of the calcification is generally variable and nonspecific. However, a number of patients develop peripheral, eggshell calcification (Fig 12–14).[22, 107, 202, 245, 275] Eggshell calcification is of diagnostic value, as its occurrence is largely limited to sarcoidosis and silicosis.[107] There is a single report of spontaneous resolution of eggshell calcification.[275]

Parenchymal Sarcoidosis

Parenchymal shadowing is seen at the time of presentation in approximately half the patients with sarcoidosis.* In addition, about a third of patients

*References 78, 136, 141, 164, 196, 201, 210, 261, and 301.

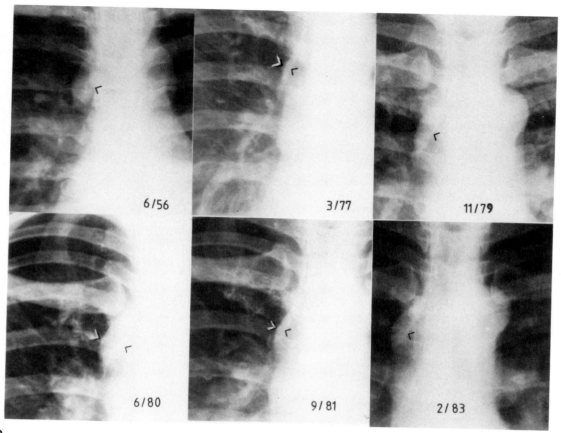

FIG 12–12.
Sarcoidosis—nodal recurrence. Localized views of the right para-tracheal region shows the azygos node *(arrowheads)*. The initial adenopathy in 1956 was a result of tuberculosis. Subsequent ade- nopathy has been associated with sarcoidosis and has fluctuated in degree in relation to steroid therapy.

presenting with stage I disease will go on to develop parenchymal shadowing with a frequency that shows a marked variation from series to series, ranging from 10% to 43%.* Such parenchymal shadowing frequently develops within the 1st year and is usually accompanied, at least to some degree, by nodal re- gression.

It has been customary to divide parenchymal shadowing in sarcoidosis into prefibrotic and fi- brotic.[275] This distinction is often not clear-cut, and a more practical division between reversible and ir- reversible shadowing will be used here.

Reversible Changes

Reversible changes consist of three patterns: re- ticulonodular opacities; ill-defined opacities with the characteristics of consolidation ("alveolar"); and large nodules. These patterns can occur either alone or in varying combinations.[164] They may resolve

*References 78, 140, 261, 278, 301, and 305.

partially or completely, or they may progress to an irreversible, fibrotic pattern. The approximate fre- quency of the various forms of parenchymal shad- owing is reticulonodular, 75% to 90%; "alveolar," 10% to 20%; and large nodular, 2%.

(Reticulo)nodular Opacities.—Small rounded or irregular opacities constitute by far the most frequent pulmonary pattern and are seen in some 75% to 90% of patients with parenchymal shadow- ing.[78, 132, 201, 275, 301] Reticulonodular opacities are more common than pure nodular shadows. In an at- tempt to characterize these opacities, a number of workers have used the pneumoconiosis classification of the ILO/UC (International Labour Office/Univer- sity of Cincinnati; see Chapter 9), extending it to in- clude x, y, and z opacities to denote small rounded opacities from which arise irregular linear tenta- cles.[41, 201] In the study by McLoud et al., 35% of opacities were classified as xyz, 33% as pqr, and 19% as stu.[201] The nodules range in size from just under

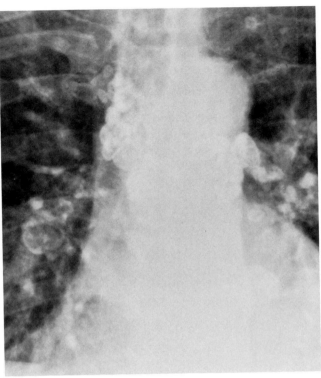

FIG 12–13.
Sarcoidosis—nodal calcification. Local view of the middle and lower mediastinum shows extensive calcification affecting hilar, paratracheal, subcarinal, posterior mediastinal, and anterior mediastinal lymph nodes.

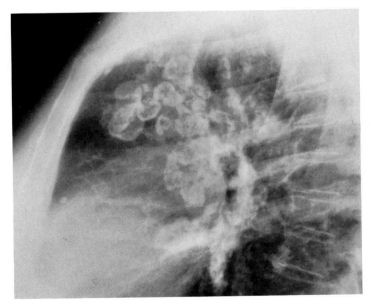

FIG 12–14.
Sarcoidosis—nodal calcification. Lateral view of the upper chest shows extensive nodal calcification, much of which has an eggshell pattern. Many of the nodes are in the anterior mediastinum.

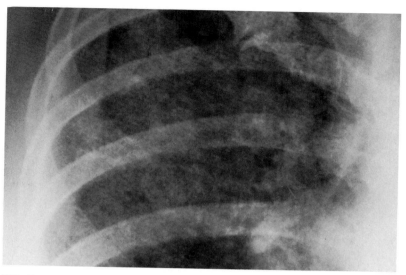

FIG 12–15.
Sarcoidosis—parenchymal. Localized view of the right upper zone shows profuse and evenly distributed multiple small nodules about 1 mm or less in diameter.

1 mm (Fig 12–15) to over 5 mm, with most being 2 to 4 mm (Fig 12–16) in diameter.[132, 164, 275, 301] Very small nodules, 1 mm or less in diameter, may take on a ground-glass appearance.[78] In addition to discrete interstitial abnormalities such as nodules, more diffuse changes occur and are seen on radiographs as bronchial wall thickening, air bronchograms, and subpleural and fissural thickening (Fig 12–17).[243] These changes can also be appreciated at CT.[243] There is a suggestion that these latter findings might give a better idea of "activity" in sarcoidosis than reticulonodular opacities, and their presence certainly correlates quite well with "disease activity" indicated by gallium scanning.[243] Sometimes parenchymal changes, which may themselves be quite mild, will silhouette the outer aspect of the hilus and blur it, giving rise to the so-called "hilar haze" sign.[245] The CT appearances of reticulonodular parenchymal disease have not been systematically studied. Reported changes include isolated small subpleural "granulomatous" nodules not seen on the chest radiograph,[114, 304] a diffuse micronodular pattern,[20, 114] peribronchial and perivascular interstitial changes,[243] and increased lung density.[94, 114]

The reticulonodular shadows are usually bilaterally symmetric (see Fig 12–17), with about 15% showing significant asymmetry.[275] In exceptional cases, parenchymal changes are strictly unilateral. In three series, this pattern was seen in fewer than 1% of the cases.[78, 136, 287] Unilateral change was, however, recorded in 8% in one recent series.[132] Unilateral parenchymal disease is usually, but not exclu-

sively,[24, 256] of the (reticulo)nodular type and may occur with or without adenopathy.[67, 112, 206, 256, 275]

Opacities tend to occur in all zones, often showing a mid zone, or mid and upper zone predominance (Fig 12–18).[275, 301] Isolated lower zone involvement is seen in less than 4% of patients.[132, 301]

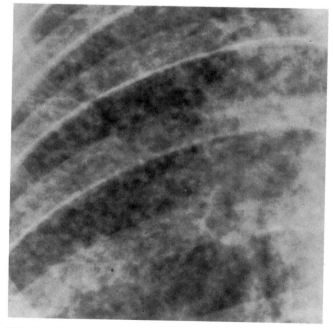

FIG 12–16.
Sarcoidosis—parenchymal. Localized view of the right middle zone shows profuse nodules, larger than in Figure 12–15. These nodules are the size more typically seen in sarcoidosis, ranging from 2 to 4 mm. Some nodules are rounded; others, irregular.

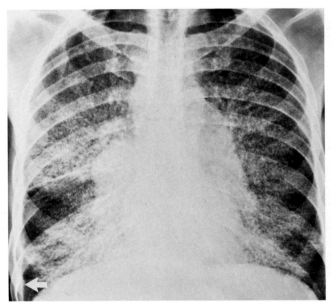

FIG 12–17.
Sarcoidosis—parenchymal and nodal. Diffuse fine reticulonodular opacities affect all zones in a symmetric fashion, sparing the apices. Minor fissure is thickened, and there is subpleural thickening ("laminar effusion") *(arrow)* in the right lower zone laterally. These latter findings are a feature of acute, active sarcoidosis.

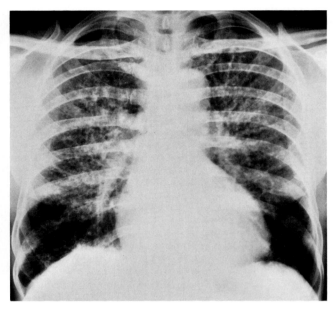

FIG 12–18.
Sarcoidosis—parenchymal. The adenopathy has subsided leaving predominantly mid and upper zone, 2- to 4-mm reticulonodular opacities.

Occasionally, there is a strictly upper zone distribution,[132] which may resemble tuberculosis.[319]

Calcification in parenchymal sarcoidosis is rarely reported. It developed in 5 out of 136 patients in one series followed for at least 5 years[274] and in 3 out of 111 cases followed for 10 or more years.[134] However, it is not possible to exclude other granulomatous causes, such as tuberculosis, in these patients.

"Alveolar" Opacities.—Some 10% to 20% of patients with sarcoidosis develop opacities that have features variously described as consolidative, alveolar, or air-space shadowing. These opacities form a spectrum ranging from ill-defined, irregular shadows of nondescript shape to those that are focal, nodular, and quite well-defined (Fig 12–19). In the past, many authors have regarded these latter nodules as a separate entity—so called large nodular sarcoidosis—and, although this is an artificial distinction,[256] it will be maintained here as it makes consideration of the literature easier. The pathologic basis for alveolar shadowing in sarcoidosis is loss of alveolar air and increase in soft tissue. This loss can be produced by a purely interstitial process if it compresses and obliterates alveoli, or it can be seen with

an alveolar process that directly replaces alveolar air by inflammatory cells. In sarcoidosis there is evidence that both interstitial compression[88, 245, 251] and alveolar filling[245] play a part. Histologically, alveoli may be filled with macrophages[269] or granulomas.[245, 295] In some cases, the pathogenesis appears to be airway occlusion by granulomas, causing obstructive pneumonitis.[251]

Alveolar sarcoidosis has a prevalence rate of about 10% to 20%, but the range is large: 4% to 27%.* The typical appearance is of bilateral, multifocal, poorly defined opacities[21, 164] ranging in size from about 1 to 10 cm (Fig 12–20).[245] These opacities can occur anywhere, but they show a predilection for the peripheral midzone,[13, 245, 295] sparing the costophrenic angles.[13] The peripheral distribution is particularly well seen at CT.[114, 343] An air bronchogram is commonly present (see Fig 12–19).[13, 21, 164] At the edge, the lesions often break up into a nodular pattern that may be very fine, creating an appearance of acinar rosettes.[347] Reticulonodular opacities are also present in about two-thirds of these patients,[13, 164] and their detection provides a helpful clue when one is faced with disseminated multifocal consolidations of obscure origin (see Fig 12–20). Another helpful pointer is me-

*References 13, 78, 164, 186, 245, 275, 287, and 295.

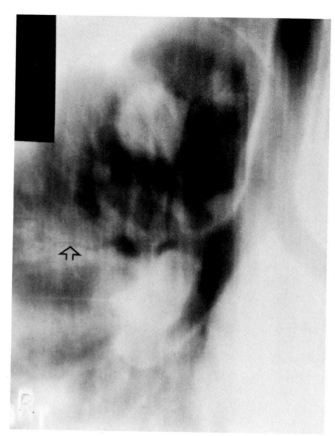

FIG 12–19.
Sarcoidosis—large nodular/alveolar. Tomogram of right mid and upper zone in a patient with coexisting large nodular and alveolar sarcoidosis. In the right upper zone there is an unusually well defined 3-cm nodule. Below it and just above the minor fissure there is an ill-defined opacity approximately 2.5 × 4 cm. This opacity has features that suggest consolidation, including an air bronchogram *(arrow)*. In addition there are right hilar nodes and thickening of the minor fissure.

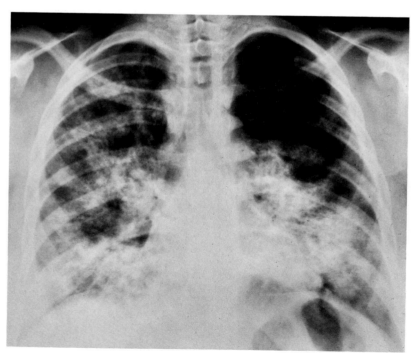

FIG 12–20.
Sarcoidosis—alveolar. There are bilateral multifocal opacities with the radiographic features of consolidation (air-space shadowing). Adenopathy usually accompanies alveolar sarcoidosis. Here there is paratracheal lymphadenopathy, and although hilar nodes are probably enlarged, they are obscured by adjacent parenchymal changes. Minor nodulation in the right mid and upper zones is of diagnostic value.

diastinal adenopathy, which is an even more common accompaniment, being present in over 80% of cases (see Fig 12–20).[13, 164] Kirks and Greenspan[164] point out that all of their patients with alveolar sarcoidosis had either mediastinal adenopathy and/or reticulonodular shadowing.

Recognized variants of the alveolar pattern include unilateral distribution,[186] upper zone distribution simulating tuberculosis (Fig. 12–21),[112] or a peripheral pattern that resembles cryptogenic eosinophilic pneumonia. In one series of 64 patients, 9% showed a pronounced peripheral distribution, some with an alveolar and some with a reticulonodular pattern.[96] Sharma describes two confusing patients in whom the peripheral alveolar pattern was accompanied by blood eosinophilia, yet lung biopsy showed noncaseating granulomas consistent with sarcoidosis.[287] Some authors have stressed the good prognosis and tendency for rapid clearing with alveolar sarcoidosis, 21 of 22 patients experiencing clearing with or without steroids in one series[13] and 66% clearing within 9 months in another.[295] Not all authors agree, and in the San Francisco series of 150 patients, clearing occurred in only 31%.[164] The rapidity of change in some cases suggests that some clearing may result from resolution of obstructive pneumonitis.[251]

Large Nodular Sarcoidosis.—Focal opacities with the radiologic features of large nodules are an uncommon, but well-recognized, finding in sarcoidosis, and when the various series are combined, there is a 2.4% prevalence rate (35 of 1,449 cases).* The nodules are usually bilateral and multiple, ranging in size from 0.5 to 5 cm (Fig 12–22).[82, 256] They can occur in any zone but, as with alveolar sarcoid, there is a slight midzone predilection.[82] The margins of the nodules are occasionally sharp,[82, 256, 287] but are much more often ill-defined and hazy.[13] Some nodules may go on to coalesce.[287] They may contain an air bronchogram,[275] a feature that is particularly well seen at CT,[114] and they develop sharp margins when they come into contact with a pleural surface.[164] Most are accompanied by mediastinal adenopathy, but there are a few cases recorded in which adenopathy was absent.[82, 232, 292]

The nodules behave unpredictably over time and may remain static for years[292] or show partial[82] or complete regression.[292] There are scattered reports of a single large sarcoid nodule,[50, 229, 237, 256, 275] and in such cases the radiologic appearances strongly suggest bronchial carcinoma.

Primary cavitation is rarely seen in either alveo-

*References 13, 164, 186, 261, 275, and 292.

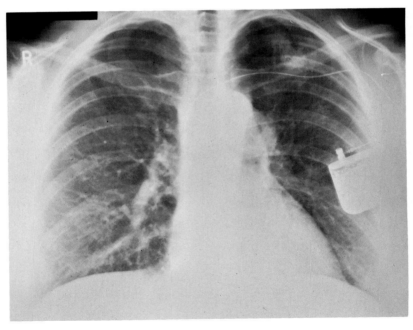

FIG 12–21.
Sarcoidosis—alveolar. Localized alveolar sarcoidosis in the left upper zone with ipsilateral hilar adenopathy. This unusual pattern raised the possibility of tuberculosis or bronchial carcinoma. The diagnosis in this case was proved at thoracotomy. The patient has a pacemaker for complete heart block, possibly the result of cardiac sarcoidosis, but unproved.

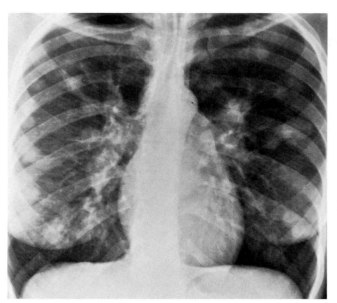

FIG 12–22.
Sarcoidosis—large nodular. There are multiple, relatively well-defined nodules ranging in size from 1 to 3 cm. In addition there is mild bilateral hilar and right paratracheal adenopathy. Nodal enlargement is an almost universal finding in large nodular sarcoidosis.

lar or large nodular sarcoidosis. It probably occurs because of ischemic necrosis in conglomerate granulomas. Only about ten cases are recorded.* Cavitation can be an early or late manifestation and may even be a presenting feature.[148] Cavities can be sin-

*References 24, 113, 148, 196, 259, and 321.

gle or multiple and may occur with or without adenopathy. The walls of the cavity have a variable appearance: thick or thin, and smooth or irregular. Sarcoid cavities may resolve either with or without steroids.[256] Although usually benign, fatal hemoptysis has been recorded.[75]

Irreversible Changes

Sarcoid granulomas may resolve completely, or they may heal by fibrosis (Fig 12–23). Such fibrosis ranges from the minor and radiologically undetectable[301] to the gross, with much scarlike shadowing and distortion on the chest radiograph. Gross fibrosis is present on the initial chest radiograph in about 5% to 25% of patients.[88, 164, 301] Additionally, gross fibrosis will develop in 10% to 15% of patients who present initially with stages 0 to II disease.[21, 78, 301] The fibrosis usually takes years to develop[21] with a range in one series of 2 to 14 years.[301]

The radiologic changes of gross fibrosis in sarcoidosis are fairly characteristic. Some authors consider that they are almost pathognomonic.[278] The findings classically consist of permanent coarse linear opacities radiating out laterally from the hilus into adjacent upper and mid zones (Fig 12–24).[245] On lateral view, this shadowing can be seen to predominate in the lower part of the upper lobes.[278] Predominant scarring remote from mid/mid-upper zones is unusual.[278] For example, in one series, only 4% of patients had fibrosis, most marked in the lower zone.[301] Coincident with the development of

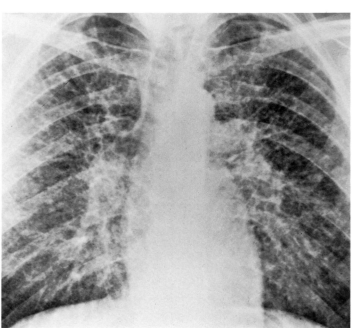

FIG 12–23.
Sarcoidosis—parenchymal. There is mild adenopathy and mild hilar elevation. Parenchymal shadowing is reticulonodular with a pronounced linear element that suggests the development of scarring. The uniformity of the changes in all zones is unusual.

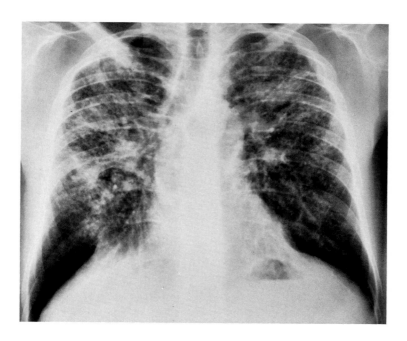

FIG 12–24.
Sarcoidosis—fibrosis. Though there is some nodular shadowing, the predominant opacities are linear. The shadowing is maximal in the mid and upper zones. Areas of confluent shadowing prob- ably represent conglomerate fibrosis. The hili are elevated, and the over-expanded lower zones are transradiant.

scarring, the extreme upper and lower zones tend to become transradiant (see Fig 12–24). In the upper zones this transradiancy is the result of cyst and bulla formation, whereas in the lower zones it is more commonly due to compensatory hyperinflation consequent upon upper zone volume loss. The hili are generally pulled upward and outward, and vessels and fissures are distorted.[78, 164] The fibrosis is occasionally so pronounced that it gives rise to massive parahilar opacities in the mid/upper zones that resemble those seen in progressive massive fibrosis.[114, 278, 301] At the other extreme there may just be minor localized linear scarring.[164] Cor pulmonale may supervene in the fibrotic stage[12, 196, 199, 275, 305] and may be radiologically recognizable.

Cystic shadows are particularly common in the upper zones in gross fibrosis.[88] Many are thin-walled and due to bronchiectasis[114, 301] or bullae (Fig 12–25).[88, 304] Ring opacities are occasionally thick-walled when due to an infected bulla, abscess, tuberculous cavity, or necrosis within a mass of conglomerate fibrosis.[88, 245, 275] A few cases are reported of "vanishing lung" with marked emphysema and bulla formation.[212, 233]

Mycetoma

Mycetoma formation (Fig 12–26) is a well-recognized complication of stage III cystic sarcoido- sis.[103, 341] Indeed, sarcoidosis is probably the second most common predisposing condition after tuberculosis.[256] This is particularly so in the United States, where the higher black population results in more cases of sarcoidosis that progress to gross fibrobullous disease.[133] In a series of mycetomas reported from Philadelphia, 45% were in patients with sarcoidosis,[180] whereas in a series of 26 patients in the United Kingdom only 15% were in sarcoidosis patients.[255] The frequency of mycetoma formation in sarcoidosis varies from series to series and ranges between 1% and 10% depending on racial mix of the patients and method of detection.* In the subset of sarcoid patients with stage III fibrocystic disease, the number of patients harboring a mycetoma can be in the order of 50%.[245, 341]

Hemoptysis is the most common and worrysome symptom and may be life-threatening.[131, 145, 153, 341] In one small series of sarcoid patients with mycetoma, major hemoptysis occurred every 5 years and minor ones every 2.5 years.[153] It has been stated that hemorrhage from mycetoma is the second most common cause of death in sarcoidosis,[133] but this is by no means a universal experience, and the 6.5% mycetoma-related deaths in one series of 46 deaths in sarcoidosis[146] is probably closer to the general ex-

*References 88, 153, 164, 245, 275, and 341.

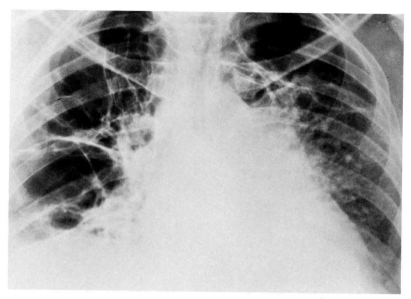

FIG 12–25.
Sarcoidosis—fibrosis. Most of the right lung and left apex are replaced by large cystic spaces.

perience. There is no evidence that steroid treatment predisposes to mycetoma formation.[341]

The radiology of mycetoma is discussed elsewhere (see Chapter 6). In sarcoidosis, mycetoma formation is worth consideration in patients with grade III fibrocystic disease who develop any sort of new shadowing, particularly masslike lesions or pleural thickening.[180] Serum precipitins against *Aspergillus* spp. are almost always positive. Conventional tomography is more sensitive than plain chest radiographs in the detection of mycetomas, but CT scanning is probably the most sensitive imaging modality.[29, 255] Mycetomas are confined virtually to the upper lobes and are commonly bilateral, 50% of cases in one series.[153]

Pulmonary and Systemic Veins

Although there is often massive mediastinal adenopathy in sarcoidosis, it is rare that compression of the great veins leads to a superior vena caval syndrome, a fact that has been ascribed to the lack of perinodal fibrosis in sarcoidosis.[256] A handful of cases are described, some of which presented with superior vena caval obstruction and others in which it punctuated the course of established disease.[27, 102, 161, 220] A single case of innominate vein obstruction which produced a large exudative effusion is recorded.[143] The rarity of the superior vena caval syndrome with sarcoidosis is such that other causes of obstruction should be sought.[43, 247]

There is a recent report of granulomatous involvement of small pulmonary veins causing obliteration and resultant pulmonary arterial hypertension. The chest radiograph showed dilated proximal pulmonary arteries and a basal "interstitial pattern" resembling veno-occlusive disease.[123]

Pulmonary Arteries

Large-vessel involvement is rare in sarcoidosis[281] and is usually the result of compression by large nodes.[80, 97, 122, 159, 335] Typically it is the lobar divisions, particularly the upper lobe vessels, that are involved, and pulmonary arterial hypertension is usually absent. Perfusion scans show corresponding large defects.[114, 335] A few cases are reported in which stenosis of major pulmonary arteries was attributed to sarcoid-induced scarring[12, 61, 283]; there is a reported case in which multiple stenoses caused pulmonary arterial hypertension.[114]

Small vessel involvement by granulomas is common pathologically and is usually accompanied by widespread parenchymal disease.[41, 265] Granulomas can lead to vessel narrowing, but not usually vascular necrosis or thrombosis. These changes probably account for patchy perfusion defects found on scintigraphy[230, 294] and for pulmonary arterial hypertension.

Pulmonary artery hypertension in sarcoidosis may be caused by granulomatous vasculitis,[42, 64, 176, 221, 302] by fibrobullous disease,[12, 314] or rarely, by large vessel disease.[114]

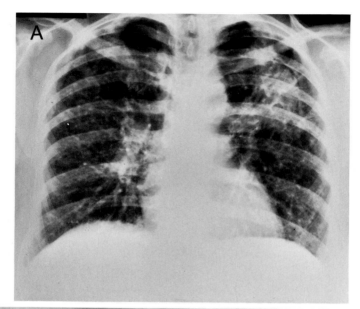

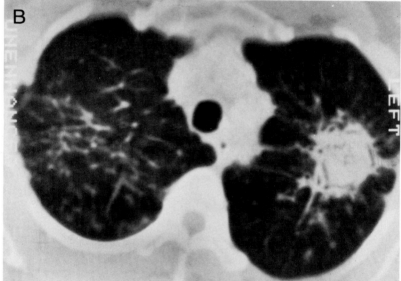

FIG 12–26.

Sarcoidosis—mycetoma. **A,** chest radiograph reveals diffusely distributed low profusion linear and small nodular densities. In the left mid-upper zone there are two masslike opacities. The lower mass has a peripheral air crescent. **B,** CT scan through lower mass demonstrates an unequivocal, inhomogeneous intracavitary body resulting from a mycetoma.

Airways

Sarcoidosis can affect the trachea, bronchi, or bronchioles. Tracheal involvement is rare[28] and, in the few reported cases, has always been associated with laryngeal involvement.[278] Both the proximal and distal trachea may be involved, and the stenosis can be smooth,[69, 118] irregular and nodular,[165] or even masslike.[334]

The bronchi may be narrowed by external nodal compression (Fig 12–27), extrinsic scarring, or by mural granulomas and fibrosis. It is generally considered that intrinsic mural disease is the most important mechanism.[256] It is a curious fact that despite the sometimes massive enlargement of nodes in sarcoidosis, lymphadenopathy on its own is a rare cause of symptomatic airway narrowing.[204, 221] Occasional examples are, however, recorded, particularly affecting the middle lobe.[70, 222, 317] The middle lo-

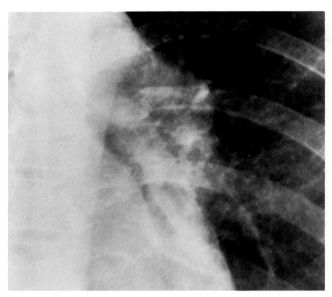

FIG 12–27.
Sarcoidosis—airways. Local view of left hilar region. There is mild narrowing of the left lower lobar airway, probably the result of extrinsic nodal compression. Such compression does not usually cause significant bronchial narrowing.

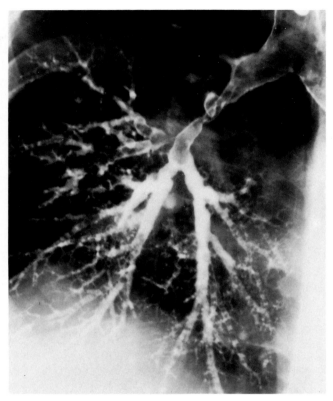

FIG 12–28.
Sarcoidosis—airways. Right bronchogram shows gross cicatricial narrowing of the right upper lobar and intermediate stem bronchi. (From Hadfield JW, Page RL, Flower CDR, et al: Localized airway narrowing in sarcoidosis. *Thorax* 1982; 37:443–447. Used by permission.)

bar airway seems to be particularly at risk because it is relatively long and narrow and is surrounded by lymph nodes.[99] The general lack of effect of sarcoid nodes on airways has been ascribed to the fact that node capsules remain intact so that scarring and fixation are rare. In addition nodes do not erode into airways.[256]

Thus, significant and symptomatic large airway narrowing is chiefly due to mural granulomas and fibrosis (Fig 12–28), and nodes play only a minor aggravating role. Bronchial wall granulomas are commonly present in all stages of sarcoidosis[89] and may be present even when the chest radiograph is normal in appearance. Although stenoses occur most commonly in well-established disease,[278] often with pulmonary fibrosis, they have been recorded early in the course of sarcoidosis and with stage 0 radiographic disease.[111, 231] The frequency of large airway narrowing is about 5% (range, 2.5% to 9%).[231, 278, 301] Patients present either with wheeze, stridor, and airflow limitation[111, 336] or with episodes of lobar or segmental collapse and consolidation.[52, 125] Collapse is a well-recognized, but uncommon, manifestation of sarcoidosis, occurring in about 1% of cases.* Any lobe may be affected, most commonly the middle (Fig 12–29),[99, 146, 256, 261] and collapse of a whole lung has been recorded.[146]

*References 78, 88, 146, 164, 245, and 261.

Although middle lobe collapse is the most common, stenoses themselves are distributed throughout the lung and show no particular lobar or segmental predilection. The stenoses may be single[231, 278] or multiple[52, 111, 125, 231] and most commonly affect main stem, lobar, or proximal segmental divisions (see Fig 12–28). They may be assessed by bronchoscopy or bronchography, and some workers consider the latter to be the more sensitive investigation.[111] Depending on the stage of the disease, the mucosa may be granular and hyperemic or even frankly inflamed and edematous.[151] Granulomas may even give rise to a local obstructing endobronchial mass.[58] Later on when there is healing by fibrosis, the mucosa may appear normal.[111] In view of the variable disease processes underlying stenoses, it is not surprising that they and their secondary effects show variable behavior, clearing spontaneously or with steroid treatment,[146, 222] or remaining unchanged.[231]

Airflow obstruction is common in sarcoido-

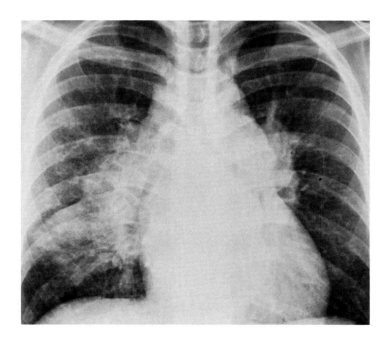

FIG 12–29.

Sarcoidosis—airways. Massive bilateral hilar and mediastinal adenopathy associated with collapse and consolidation of the right middle lobe. The middle lobe is the most frequently collapsed lobe in sarcoidosis. Low profusion, small nodular shadowing is present in the right lung as well.

sis.[25, 178, 214, 288] There is evidence that this is usually the result of small airway obstruction, presumably on the basis of granulomatous distortion,[288] and increased airflow resistance can be demonstrated even in stage I disease.[291]

Obstructive bronchiectasis as a result of endobronchial sarcoidosis is considered to be rare[256] though in the context of gross fibrobullous disease, it is often difficult to be sure of the exact pathogenesis of the bronchiectasis. Only a few cases have been described.[114, 256]

Pleural Sarcoidosis

In sarcoidosis, granulomas may be found on both the visceral and parietal pleura. These pleural granulomas commonly cause no signs or symptoms.[60] They may on rare occasions, however, be associated with a dry pleurisy[92] or a pleural effusion that is usually painless[14] but may be painful.[147] These effusions are classically lymphocyte-rich exudates that, in nearly one-fifth of cases, are sanguinous or serosanguinous.[227]

The reported frequency of pleural effusion secondary to sarcoidosis varies between 0%[196] and 7%.[338] In 1,870 cases of sarcoidosis taken from major series in the world literature, there were 55 cases with pleural effusions, giving a prevalence of 1.9%.* Effusions may occur at the time the sarcoidosis presents,[287] but more usually they develop during the course of established disease, a few months to 16 years after onset.[51] As expected, sarcoid effusions often accompany extensive pulmonary disease or multisystem involvement,[51] particularly stage II or III disease.[338] However, pleural effusions with stage I disease are recorded,[164, 286] and there are even cases in which patients had an otherwise normal chest radiograph.[147, 209] About a third of the effusions are bilateral[51] and, while they are usually small, large effusions are also described.[23, 152, 227, 330] The effusions resolve spontaneously in weeks or months and are almost invariably gone by 6 months.[186] Resolution is usually complete, but some 20% of patients are left with residual pleural thickening,[245, 338] which is occasionally marked. It appears that pleural thickening can develop without an antecedent effusion.[338]

In general, pleural effusion is a relatively minor and incidental finding in the course of sarcoidosis. However, because it is an atypical feature, it may prove a diagnostic puzzle. In addition, several authors stress the importance of excluding other

*References 51, 78, 88, 164, 196, 245, 261, 287, and 338.

causes, particularly tuberculosis, which may occur concurrently.[78, 167] Cases are also reported in which venous and possibly lymphatic obstruction by lymph node involvement may have played a part in the pathogenesis of pleural effusion.[143]

Bones

Bone involvement that is detectable on the chest radiograph is rare, and only about 20 cases are reported, the spine being the most common site and the sternum the least common. Spinal sarcoid is usually symptomatic, with multiple levels of involvement and extraspinal osseous lesions as well. The lower thoracic spine is the site of predilection[256]; lesions are typically lytic and confined to a vertebral body, which often loses height or collapses completely. A few cases have simulated infective spondylitis with narrowed disc spaces and associated paravertebral soft tissue mass.[312] Entirely sclerotic lesions of vertebral bodies are described.[344] The chest radiograph does not necessarily show changes of non-osseous sarcoidosis and, in one review, two of eight cases were of this type.[31] Rib lesions have been recorded in five cases[256] and have been lytic or permeative in most cases, one presenting as a rib fracture.[109] One patient had sclerotic lesions.[344] The one reported sternal lesion was lytic, and was part of widespread spine and rib involvement.[312]

Bone sarcoidosis, particularly of the hands, has a highly characteristic appearance, and its demonstration is of great diagnostic value in a patient with suspected chest sarcoidosis.[309] The overall prevalence of bone disease, which is largely of the extremities, is about 5% in sarcoidosis in general.[195, 225, 272] Some subgroups have a higher than average prevalence of bone disease, particularly blacks and those with chronic skin involvement. The likelihood of bone lesions at the time of presentation with sarcoidosis, which is the time when the diagnosis is most likely to be in doubt, is probably in the order of 1% to 2%.[187]

PRIMARY PULMONARY HISTIOCYTOSIS X (EOSINOPHILIC GRANULOMA OF LUNG)

Histiocytosis X is a generic term that encompasses three rare clinical disorders: eosinophilic granuloma (EG), Hand-Schüller-Christian disease, and Letterer-Siwe disease. Granulomatous infiltration by histiocytic cells with eosinophilic cytoplasm is a feature shared by all three conditions. The histiocytes in question are now thought to be Langerhans cells, which are antigen-presenting cells found especially in skin, lymph nodes, spleen, and thymus.[323] Their uncontrolled proliferation is probably related to an unidentified immunologic abnormality.[44, 81] Histiocytic proliferation may affect many or just a few organ systems. In Letterer-Siwe disease, the involvement is widespread. Typical features of this disease include skin lesions, fever, hepatosplenomegaly, anemia, thrombocytopenia, and pulmonary lesions. The condition is largely confined to neonates and infants. In EG, a disorder that affects older children or adults, histiocyte proliferation is less widespread and is confined to one or at most a few organ systems. Thus, the term EG of lung will include cases with limited extrapulmonary involvement—usually bone lesions —but excludes patients with widely disseminated disease, which, although unusual, is recorded in adults.[345] Hand-Schüller-Christian disease is a subset of EG with limited but characteristic organ system involvement that includes bone lesions (skull defects, exophthalmos) and neurologic lesions (diabetes insipidus).

Pathologically,[8, 55, 90, 156, 241] the typical pulmonary lesion is a stellate interstitial nodule that is usually a few millimeters in size, but ranges from 1 to 15 mm and lies most commonly in the walls of small airways. The nodules are granulomas containing characteristic histiocytes (histiocytosis X cells) and a variable number of eosinophils, plasma cells, and lymphocytes. Some of the histiocytes show typical ultrastructural features of the antigen-presenting Langerhans cell. The granulomas may encroach on airways and vessels and obstruct them. With the passage of time, there is fibrous replacement of the nodule from the center outward. Sometimes, the alveoli adjacent to the granulomas are filled with macrophages and desquamated alveolar lining cells. The appearances may, therefore, resemble desquamative interstitial pneumonia. Scarring, if gross, eventually leads to a picture of end-stage lung with honeycombing.

Since the first description of primary eosinophilic granuloma of lung,[79] more than 200 cases have been described in the world literature.[241] There are no good data on the prevalence of EG, but it is clearly considerably lower than that of sarcoidosis, possibly by a factor of 20.[246] EG used to be regarded as a male-predominant disease, but it is now considered equally common in both sexes.[55, 90, 172, 179, 332] The disease may be milder in women. Its prevalence in blacks is low.[90] Most patients present in their 3rd or 4th decade, but the age spread is wide, ranging from the teens to over 60 years. Patients present with pulmonary symptoms, systemic symptoms, or an asymptomatic radiographic abnormality. In one series of 100 patients, 23% were asymptomatic and were detected radiographically, 31% had systemic symptoms, and 72% had pulmonary symptoms.[90] Systemic symptoms usually coexist with pulmonary ones,[11, 90] and it is unusual for the patient to present with constitutional symptoms alone.[241] The most common symptoms are cough, dyspnea, chest pain (nonspecific, pleuritic, or bony), and fever.[90] Pneumothorax is one of the classic manifestations of pulmonary eosinophilic granuloma (Fig 12–30). The frequency of pneumothorax as a presenting feature varies from series to series and may be as high as 14%.[172] Pneumothoraces will occur in 6% to 25% of patients at some time during the course of the illness.[55, 179] They are commonly recurrent, may be bilateral, and are sometimes fatal.[90] Respiratory function tests show great variation from subject to subject. The usual pattern is restriction, reduced carbon monoxide diffusion, and evidence of airflow obstruction and small airway disease in 20% to 50%.[11, 90, 241] The diagnosis of EG can be made by transbronchial lung biopsy, but since specific lesions are focal and widespread,

they can easily be missed.[55] The diagnosis has also been made by finding the characteristic histiocytosis X cells in bronchoalveolar lavage material[11] though doubt has been cast on the specificity of this finding.[241] If these methods fail, open lung biopsy should be considered. It is of note that blood eosinophilia is rarely found in patients with EG.[241]

In many cases, pulmonary EG progresses through identifiable stages beginning with symptomatic disease, a stage of abnormal radiographic and functional findings, then a period of waning activity followed by partial or complete resolution. There is evidence that the prognosis is currently better than was suggested in early series.[90] There is a high rate of spontaneous remission and a low rate of morbidity.[241] Features that indicate a poor prognosis are extremes of age, multiple pneumothoraces, extensive multisystem disease, prolonged constitutional disturbance, extensive cysts/honeycombing on the chest radiograph, and a grossly decreased single-breath carbon monoxide uptake (Kco).[11] There is also some evidence that young adult men probably have a more severe form of the disease.[90] It is very unusual for EG presenting in adulthood to go on to disseminated disease. However, bone involvement accompanying pulmonary disease is recognized in 4% to 13% of patients.[90, 179] Diabetes insipidus occurs in approximately the same number.

As with other interstitial processes, the chest radiograph in adult patients with primary lung involvement can be normal with proved disease.[179] When findings are present, the characteristic radiographic appearance[6, 90, 172, 179, 223, 332] consists of a diffuse, symmetric, reticulonodular pattern or, less commonly, a solely nodular pattern (Fig 12–31). If anything, the shadowing has a slight mid and upper zone predominance,[90, 179] though some series show a mid/lower zone predominance.[172] At any one time all zones tend to be affected, but in a fifth of cases in one series only half the lung was radiologically involved.[172] There are also isolated reports of shadowing that is initially unilateral.[6, 179, 223] The nodules are characteristically ill-defined,[6] presumably reflecting their stellate histologic structure. They vary in size from 1 to 15 mm, generally averaging about 5 mm (see Fig 12–31).[172] The nodules are usually innumerable, but occasionally they will be sufficiently few in number to be countable.[90] Large nodules occasionally mimic metastases[223] and, in rare cases, the initial radiographic opacity shows the pattern of airspace consolidation.[223, 332] Although necrosis and cavitation in nodules is not uncommon pathologically,[11] it is very unusual radiologically, being seen

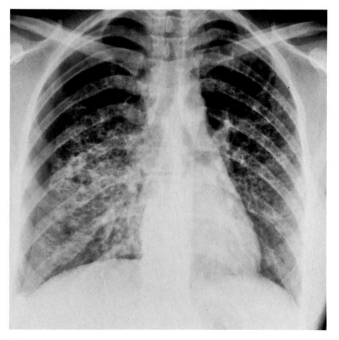

FIG 12–30.
Histiocytosis X. Chest radiograph of a 21-year-old woman who presented with a right pneumothorax. There are bilateral changes throughout both lungs, mainly ring and linear opacities.

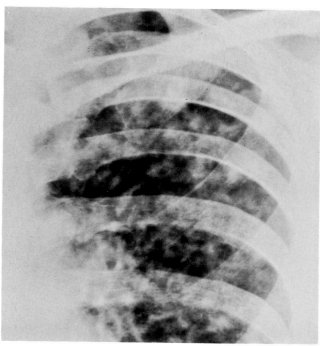

FIG 12–31.
Histiocytosis X. Localized view of the left middle and upper zone at presentation. Shadowing consists chiefly of ill-defined 3- to 8-mm nodules. There is also a minor linear element to the shadowing.

rarely in the larger nodules.[53, 228] From early on, a linear/reticular element usually accompanies the nodulation (see Fig 12–31) and was present in 94% of cases in one series.[172] With time this element tends to become dominant. Air spaces develop, and some areas show honeycomb shadows,[11] a feature which is more typical of EG than of any other disorder (Fig 12–32). In addition, larger air spaces up to 5 cm (cysts, blebs, bullae) may form (Fig 12–33).[179, 332] They have a predilection for the mid and upper zones and for the periphery.[11, 90] Probably because of the development of these abnormal air spaces, lung volume does not decrease with time. If anything the reverse occurs,[172] and in one series, a third of cases showed a definite increase in lung volume radiologically (see Fig 12–33).[90] This progression to fibrobullous disease is by no means inevitable, and in 1982, Lacronique and co-workers[172] found that, radiologically, about one-third cleared (Fig 12–34), one-third remained stable, and one-third deteriorated. In other series, the outcome has been even more favorable.[90] Late in the course of severe disease there may be evidence of pulmonary arterial hypertension.

Pleural effusion is extremely uncommon. A few cases have been reported, and in two the effusion was probably secondary to bone involvement.[108, 234] Mediastinal and hilar node enlargement is likewise uncommon; there are occasional reports, some of which have been histologically unconfirmed.[90, 194]

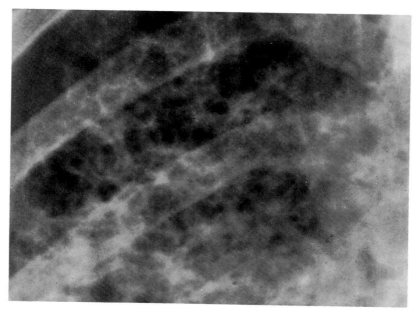

FIG 12–32.
Histiocytosis X. Localized view of the right mid zone shows multiple small ring shadows. Many of these are in the 5- to 8-mm range and could be described as honeycomb opacities. A pneumothorax was present.

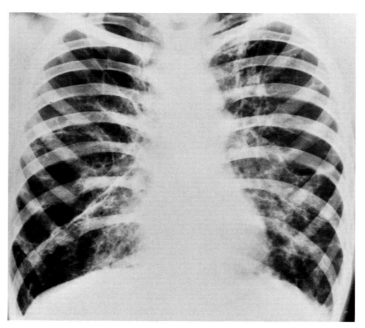

FIG 12–33.
Histiocytosis X. "Vanishing lungs." There has been progression to gross lung destruction in this patient, with much of both lungs replaced by avascular bullae and other air spaces.

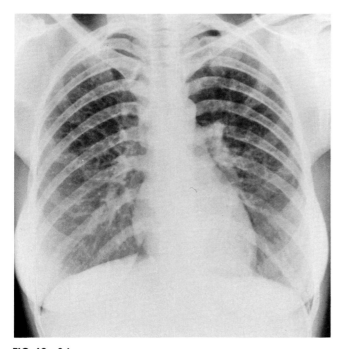

FIG 12–34.
Histiocytosis X. Same patient as in Figure 12–30. This radiograph, obtained 14 months after the image in Figure 12–30, shows almost complete resolution of parenchymal opacities.

Of the 10% or so of patients with bone involvement, possibly one-fifth will have rib involvement that will be detectable on the chest radiograph.

NEUROCUTANEOUS SYNDROMES (PHAKOMATOSES)

Five conditions are included in this group of disorders: neurofibromatosis, tuberous sclerosis, ataxia telangiectasia, Sturge-Weber syndrome, and von Hippel-Lindau syndrome. In these conditions, aberrant development of neuroectodermal tissue causes neurologic abnormalities associated with skin and/or eye lesions. In some cases, there are additional mesodermal and endodermal abnormalities.[7]

Neurofibromatosis and tuberous sclerosis are considered in this section. Pulmonary lymphangiomyomatosis is also discussed here because, although it is not a neurocutaneous disorder, it has many features in common with pulmonary tuberous sclerosis.

Neurofibromatosis

Neurofibromatosis (von Recklinghausen's disease) is an autosomal dominant neurocutaneous syndrome (neurocristopathy) that chiefly affects the ectoderm and mesoderm, though any germ cell layer can be involved. There is a prevalence rate of about one case per 3,000 births,[253] half the cases being mutants.[84] There is no sex or racial predominance. The principal features are cafe au lait spots and peripheral neural tumors (neurofibromas/schwannomas) that particularly affect the skin (fibroma molluscum). There are, however, a multitude of other features, and virtually any organ can be affected.[166]

Neurofibromatosis has a variety of manifestations in the chest (Table 12–1).

Chest Wall

Cutaneous tumors, especially if they are polypoid, will appear as nodules on the chest radiograph. If they are peripheral and unequivocally cutaneous in position, they are diagnostic of neurofibromatosis. If, however, they are projected over the lungs, they may resemble intrapulmonary nodules (Fig 12–35). It is important not to assume that because some nodules are unequivocally cutaneous that they all are[280]; otherwise, one runs the risk of missing a primary or secondary pulmonary neoplasm. The latter consideration is particularly important, as about 5% of patients with generalized neurofibromatosis develop neurofibrosarcomas (see Fig 12–35)[235] which often metastasize to the lungs.[170]

A neural tumor arising from intercostal nerves away from the spine will, if large enough, give rise to the signs of an extrapleural soft tissue mass[83] possibly combined with pressure remodeling (notching) of the adjacent ribs. This remodeling may occur on the upper or lower rib margin. The resulting well-marginated defect is usually relatively wide and shallow compared with the notches seen in coarctation of the aorta. Alternatively rib notching may be due

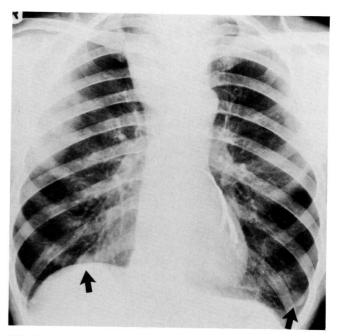

FIG 12–35.
Neurofibromatosis. Superior mediastinal mass is the result of a neurofibrosarcoma. Skin nodules (fibroma molluscum) are projected over the lungs *(arrows)* and simulate intrapulmonary nodules. Aspirated barium lies in the left bronchial tree. (Courtesy of Mr. N.L. Wright, London.)

to a primary defect in bone formation[166] unrelated to local soft tissue masses. Ribs may also be deformed in a characteristic manner that has been likened to a twisted ribbon.[46, 130] This malformation is also regarded as a primary defect. Another described pattern of rib abnormality is altered architecture with cyst formation.[266]

Kyphoscoliosis is common and, although a prevalence of about 10% is usually quoted,[130] some recent series have recorded kyphoscoliosis in up to 60% of patients.[46] Kyphosis occurs only in the presence of a scoliosis.[124] Although the appearance of the scoliosis may be nonspecific, some patterns are characteristic, in particular low thoracic, short segment, angular scolioses involving five vertebrae or fewer in the primary curve.[124, 130, 207] Vertebral lesions include the following modeling and developmental abnormalities: (1) vertebral body scalloping—posterior, lateral, or anterior[270]; (2) hypoplastic or pressure remodeled pedicles, particularly mesial flattening; (3) intervertebral foramen enlargement; and (4) transverse process hypoplasia. The most common and best-known of these abnormalities is posterior vertebral scalloping, which is typically sharply marginated and smooth, and extends over several segments.[45, 207] It is usually associated

TABLE 12–1.
Thoracic Lesions of Neurofibromatosis

Location	Lesion
Chest wall	
Skin	Cutaneous tumors (fibroma molluscum)
Nerves	Intercostal nerve tumors
Spine	Kyphoscoliosis, vertebral body modeling abnormality
Ribs	Modeling and architecture abnormality, notching
Mediastinum	
Middle	Neural tumor
Posterior	Lateral meningocele, neural tumor, pheochromocytoma
Lungs	Interstitial fibrosis, airway tumors

with, and probably causally related to, dural ectasia, though it will occasionally result from pressure by a tumor or to simple developmental hypoplasia.

Mediastinal Masses

Posterior mediastinal masses are usually due to a neural tumor (neurofibroma or neurilemmoma and their malignant counterparts) or a lateral thoracic meningocele. Lateral thoracic meningoceles are produced by gross dural ectasia, and two-thirds occur at the apex of a scoliosis on its convex aspect.[166] Right-sided lesions predominate, and about 10% are multiple.[211] They are often, but not invariably, associated with vertebral scalloping and expansion of intervertebral foramina.[211] Affected patients are commonly middle-aged (30 to 60 years old) and, more often than not, asymptomatic.[211] Some consider that lateral thoracic meningoceles are the most common posterior mediastinal mass in neurofibromatosis,[166] but this is not borne out by all series.[46] The radiology of lateral thoracic meningocele is discussed elsewhere (see Chapter 15).

Neural tumors cause well-demarcated, rounded paraspinal masses, and are discussed in detail in the section on posterior mediastinal masses. Neural tumors can become malignant. There is much doubt about the true transformation rate, but it is probably in the order of 5%[7] and is a serious complication, as neural sarcomas carry a poor prognosis. Clinically, such a transformation may be heralded by pain, the appearance of a mass, or the enlargement of a known mass.

The third type of associated posterior mediastinal mass is the pheochromocytoma. There is a 1% prevalence of pheochromocytoma in neurofibromatosis,[166] and its presence should be considered as an explanation for concomitant hypertension in neurofibromatosis.

Two types of middle mediastinal mass are recognized in neurofibromatosis: one localized; and the other diffuse. Discrete masses are the result of solitary neurofibromas, neurilemmomas, or their malignant counterparts affecting the vagus or phrenic nerves (see Fig 12–35). They are usually asymptomatic, but may cause hoarseness if the recurrent laryngeal nerve is affected.[72, 226, 311] Diffuse masses often extend down from the thoracic inlet to hilar level and may be bilateral. They are the result of plexiform neurofibromas, normal nerve elements bizarrely arranged in a network of fusiform swellings that often infiltrate and incorporate adjacent fat and muscle.[7] Though usually slow growing and asymptomatic, they can cause tracheal and bronchial compression.[49]

Lung Involvement

Parenchymal lung involvement in neurofibromatosis takes the form of a fibrosing alveolitis that was first recognized in 1963.[65] Its prevalence increases with age, the youngest patient recorded being 28 years old.[331] The prevalence rate in adults with neurofibromatosis is about 20%,[192, 331] and there is probably no sex difference. Symptoms are often mild, though some patients progress to respiratory failure and cor pulmonale.[266] Respiratory function tests show a mixed obstructive and restrictive pattern with impaired diffusion.[331]

The radiologic findings are interstitial shadowing and bullous disease. Interstitial shadowing is initially finely linear, with or without a nodular element, and is usually basally predominant. Septal (Kerley B) lines are sometimes present.[331] In time the linear element becomes more marked and widespread (Fig 12–36), and honeycomb shadows may develop.[331] The other principal findings are thin-walled bullae (see Fig 12–36),[192, 193, 331] largely mid/upper zonal, often asymmetric and sometimes large (occupying at least one lung zone). Bullae are sometimes an isolated radiologic finding,[192] but lung biopsy in these circumstances always shows an occult

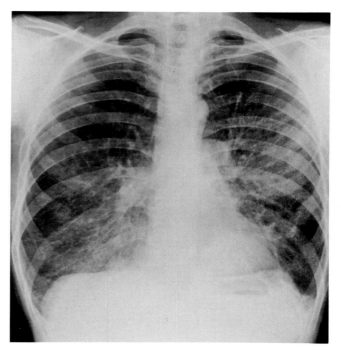

FIG 12–36.
Neurofibromatosis. There is diffuse interstitial shadowing, predominantly fine and linear. In the transradiant right upper zone, vessels are stretched and reduced in number due to bullae. The overall lung volume is increased. The combination of interstitial opacities with bullae and hyperexpanded lungs is characteristic but not pathognomonic of neurofibromatosis.

alveolitis.[331] The rather benign nature of lung involvement in neurofibromatosis contrasts with the much more sinister outcome of lung disease in tuberous sclerosis. Occasionally, there is radiographic evidence of pulmonary artery hypertension.

Rarely, a neurofibroma or neurilemmoma will produce a parenchymal mass that appears as a peripheral well-demarcated, lobulated nodule.[191] Just as rarely these lesions may arise endobronchially and cause obstructive bronchiectasis.[10, 331]

Tuberous Sclerosis

Like neurofibromatosis, tuberous sclerosis is an autosomal dominant[35] neurocutaneous syndrome with an equal sex incidence. It is, however, only half as common as neurofibromatosis. About half the cases are hereditary and the rest sporadic, arising as a result of mutation.[85] The clinical expression is variable and often incomplete, giving rise to formes frustes, which make it difficult to define the condition for diagnostic purposes. It is, for example, not clear whether a person with isolated, multiple renal angiomyolipomas should be regarded as suffering from tuberous sclerosis.[203]

The classic clinical features make up a triad of mental retardation, epilepsy, and dermal angiofibromas (adenoma sebaceum). Additional major manifestations include other skin lesions (ungual fibromas, shagreen patches, achromic patches), cerebral and paraventricular hamartomas, renal angiomyolipomas, retinal phakomas, bone lesions including calvarial sclerosis, and rhabdomyomas of the heart. The diagnostic criteria used by some workers are the presence of one or more of the following: (1) adenoma sebaceum; (2) retinal phakomas; (3) mental retardation or epilepsy, plus a close relative with adenoma sebaceum or retinal phakomas; (4) mental retardation, epilepsy and intracranial calcifications.[173] Other authors have used less stringent criteria.[85] CT scanning has proved particularly useful in the detection of the highly prevalent intracranial calcifications,[85] and the renal angiomyolipomas and cysts.[219] The prognosis is poor, 75% of patients dying by age 20.[203]

Pulmonary involvement is distinctly unusual and occurs in about 1% of cases.[74, 181] Given the low prevalence of tuberous sclerosis in the population (6 to 7 cases per million persons),[101] there can only be a handful of pulmonary tuberous sclerosis patients in either the United States or the United Kingdom at any one time. There are considerable clinical, radiologic, and pathologic similarities between pulmonary involvement in tuberous sclerosis and that found in lymphangiomyomatosis (Table 12–2), some of which will be touched on here.

Pathologically, the lungs in tuberous sclerosis show perivascular smooth muscle proliferation and small adenomatoid nodules, both of which probably contribute to the reticulonodular pattern seen radiologically. Proliferating smooth muscle spreads into the walls of airspaces, bronchioles, arterioles, and venules and causes obstruction of these structures. Venular obstruction accounts for hemoptysis, and airway obstruction causes the focal emphysema, cyst/bulla formation, and air trapping that may lead to pneumothorax. The smooth muscle proliferation in tuberous sclerosis, in general, tends to spare lymphatics[57, 310] and probably accounts for the rarity of lymphatic complications such as chylothorax. Some workers, however, have found smooth muscle proliferation in pulmonary lymphatics and in lymph nodes.[327] The adenomatoid proliferations are a few millimeters in diameter and are scattered throughout the lung.[181]

The clinical features of patients with pulmonary tuberous sclerosis[74] have been shown to be quite different from those of tuberous sclerosis in general. The patients were older, the mean age of presentation with respiratory symptoms being 34 years of age. They were predominantly women (85%), and there was a lower prevalence of mental retardation (46%) and epilepsy (20%) than has been seen in tuberous sclerosis in general. However, most had adenoma sebaceum,[117] and 60% had renal angiomyolipomas. Once respiratory symptoms had developed, they tended to dominate the clinical picture—with progressive dyspnea, recurrent pneumothoraces (in 50%), and, less seriously, cough and hemoptysis. Eighty-five percent of patients had died within 5 years from either cor pulmonale (59%) or pneumothorax (41%).

The radiologic findings in the chest consist of an interstitial process with symmetric nodular, reticular, or reticulonodular opacities. The nodules are small, in the order of 1 to 2 mm,[105, 181] and are often overshadowed by a more dominant, linear element (Fig 12–37).[181] The changes may be diffuse or basally predominant.[34, 105] With progression of the disease, the linear and reticular element becomes more marked, and honeycomb and cystic changes may develop.[105, 181, 203] The cystic shadows tend to be small, less than 1 cm. Large cysts are uncommon.[203]

Unlike most other interstitial processes the lung volume tends to be increased, because of small airway obstruction, focal emphysema, air-trapping, and cyst formation. Respiratory function tests support this observation and show airflow obstruction, in-

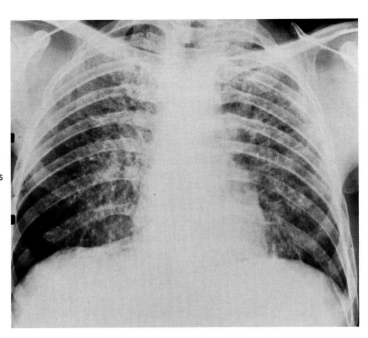

FIG 12–37.
Tuberous sclerosis. There is diffuse interstitial pulmonary shadowing consisting of small irregular and rounded opacities with a predominantly linear element. Although lung volume is commonly increased, it is not so in this patient.

creased static compliance and increased total lung volume, together with an impaired carbon monoxide diffusion.[181]

Pneumothorax is common,[66, 117] frequently recurrent, and sometimes bilateral.[105] Late in the disease, there may be evidence of pulmonary arterial hypertension and cor pulmonale. Pleural effusions are not common in tuberous sclerosis. There are, however, a few reports of chylous effusions.[188, 327] Bone changes are described and may be visible on the chest radiograph, notably an expanded dense rib resembling fibrous dysplasia or Paget's disease.[7]

Lymphangio(leio)myomatosis

Although it is not a neurocutaneous disorder, lymphangio(leio)myomatosis (LAM) shares many *pulmonary* features with pulmonary tuberous sclerosis (PTS). It differs from PTS in that it is not heredofamilial and, clinically, lacks many of the neuroectodermal features of PTS such as adenoma sebaceum, epilepsy, and mental retardation. Furthermore, some findings, such as chylothorax, that are unusual in PTS are common in LAM. The features of LAM and PTS are compared in Table 12–2.

TABLE 12–2.
Comparison of Lymphangioleiomyomatosis and Pulmonary Tuberous Sclerosis

Factor	Lymphangioleiomyomatosis	Pulmonary Tuberous Sclerosis
Familial	No	Commonly
Female sex	All	85%
Age	Reproductive	Reproductive
Adenoma sebaceum	No	85%
Epilepsy	No	20%
Intelligence (IQ)	Normal	Low (46%)
Dyspnea	Yes	Yes
Pneumothorax	Yes	Yes
Chylous pleural effusions/ascites	Yes	Rare
Hemoptysis	Yes	Yes
Chest radiograph	Interstitial opacities, cysts, pleural effusion	Interstitial opacities, cysts
Renal angiomyolipoma	Occasional	60%

There have been several major reviews of LAM[40, 57, 298] and, by 1977, there were more than 67 cases in the world literature.

The pathologic changes in the chest in LAM are similar to those in PTS insofar as both show smooth muscle proliferation. However, the muscle proliferation in LAM differs from that in PTS in two major ways: (1) it is primarily perilymphatic, with later spread to involve airways, air spaces, and vessels; and (2) it can affect pulmonary, mediastinal, and retroperitoneal lymph nodes.[169, 310] In one series of patients with LAM, 69% had mediastinal and 53% had retroperitoneal node involvement.[298] Lymphatic involvement is a major feature in LAM, but a minor one in PTS; hence chylothorax (and chyloperitoneum) are major features of LAM, but unusual in PTS. Interstitial fibrosis is typically not found in LAM.[169] Some workers view LAM and PTS as different entities on histologic and other grounds,[310] while others consider the question unresolved.[57] One of the reasons for holding the latter view is that overlap cases occur. Thus renal angiomyolipomas, a characteristic finding in tuberous sclerosis, may occur in cases which, on all other criteria, are cases of LAM.[57, 205] In addition, both chylothorax[32, 188] and lymph node involvement are recorded in PTS.[150] The issue is even more complicated because other patients have been identified who have chylothorax or chyloperitoneum and lymph node involvement (mediastinal and retroperitoneal), which are typical findings of LAM, but whose lungs are normal.[298] Such patients have been reported to develop lung disease many years later.[298]

All patients with LAM have been women, and there is no familial tendency. Presentation is usually in the 3rd or 4th decade with progressive dyspnea, pneumothorax, chylothorax, or hemoptysis. Pneumothoraces as an initial event are quite common, occurring in 21% of patients in one series,[57] and they often recur (Fig 12–38).[40] The overall prevalence of pneumothorax in the 67 cases reported up to 1977 was 39.3%.[40] Chylous pleural effusions in LAM are a recognized presenting feature, and were the initial event in 7% of patients in one series.[57] Effusions occurred at some time or other during the course of the disease in 75% of 67 cases.[40] Effusions may be unilateral or bilateral and are typically large, recurrent,[298] and chylous.[169] Hemoptysis occurs in 40% of cases[40] and is occasionally the presenting feature. Chylous ascites is not uncommon, being seen in 25% of one series,[57] and it is often accompanied by a pleural effusion.[298] Some unusual manifestations were noted in the review by Silverstein et al.[298]

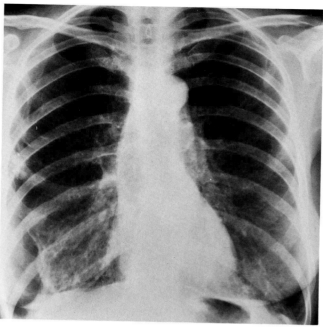

FIG 12–38.
Lymphangiomyomatosis. There is basally predominant diffuse interstitial shadowing, chiefly fine and linear. Upper zones are transradiant because of bulla formation, and lung volume is increased. There is a right pneumothorax, a common presenting feature.

These included chylopericardium, chyluria, and chyloptysis. There was also a group of seven patients who developed delayed pulmonary parenchymal changes up to 5 years after presenting with lymph node involvement or chylous effusion.[298] Respiratory function tests usually show airflow obstruction, increased total lung capacity, increased compliance, and impaired diffusion.[40]

As with other interstitial processes, the chest radiograph may appear normal despite histologically proved disease. This finding has been demonstrated in patients presenting with pneumothorax in whom a pleurectomy and lung biopsy were performed.[40] The earliest radiographic signs of lung disease consist of fine nodular, reticular, or reticulonodular shadows (Fig 12–39).[57] These changes are symmetric; they may be either generalized[216] or sometimes basally predominant, at least initially.[298] With time, there is a tendency for the reticular pattern, which may be very delicate and sharp (Fig 12–40),[57] to become coarser and more irregular. Some of the linear elements have features of septal (Kerley B) lines and may be transient.[40, 216] Cysts, bullae,[216] and honeycomb shadows can develop (Fig 12–41), the latter having thinner walls than the usual honeycomb shadows.[40] During this stage it is common for lung volumes to increase. The combination of interstitial

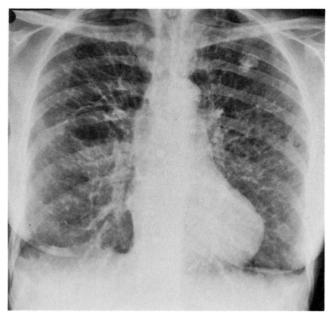

FIG 12–39.
Lymphangiomyomatosis. There is diffuse fine reticulonodular shadowing with a predominant linear pattern. Lung volume is increased, and there are thin-walled ring shadows in the right mid and upper zones. The combination of interstitial shadowing and increased lung volume is characteristic of lymphangiomyomatosis. The calcified opacity in the left upper zone is an incidental granuloma.

shadowing and increasing lung volume is very characteristic of LAM, unlike the progressive loss in volume that usually accompanies most other interstitial lung disorders (see Figs 12–38 and 12–39).[40] CT is more sensitive than the chest radiograph in demon-

strating the cystic changes that accompany increasing lung volumes.[19, 205]

Chylous pleural effusions occur in some 75% of cases (Fig 12–42).[40] They may be unilateral or bilateral[216] and are typically large and recurrent.[298] Pleural effusion and pneumothorax may coexist.[216] In advanced disease the proximal pulmonary arteries enlarge with the development of cor pulmonale (Fig 12–42).[57] Occasionally, mediastinal lymph node involvement will give rise to a radiographically visible mediastinal mass.[216] Lymphography has only occasionally been performed, since most patients have major respiratory dysfunction.[298]

The prognosis is poor once respiratory symptoms have developed, about two-thirds of the patients dying after a mean survival time of 4 years. Most patients die because of pulmonary complications.[298] Lungs that are of large volume on radiographic criteria indicate a particularly poor prognosis.[57]

Until recently, treatment has been symptomatic. However, with the demonstration of progesterone receptors on the smooth muscle of the lung, hormone therapy has been introduced with some success.[2, 197, 315] It has thus become more important to make the diagnosis as early as possible. Although LAM is a rarity, it should be considered in women of childbearing age with chylous effusion or repeat pneumothoraces, particularly if there is airflow obstruction and disproportionately poor gas exchange together with large-volume lungs and interstitial shadowing on the chest radiograph.[40]

FIG 12–40.
Lymphangiomyomatosis. Localized view of right upper zone shows interstitial shadowing, which has a characteristically predominant fine linear element.

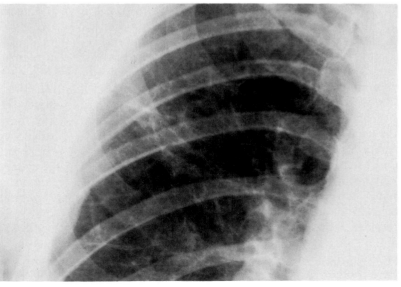

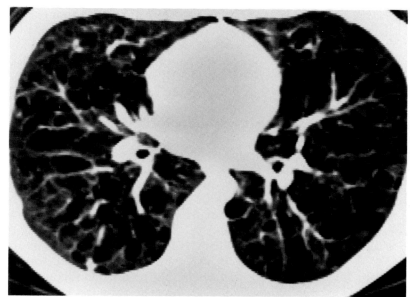

FIG 12–41.
Lymphangiomyomatosis. CT scan shows multiple thin-walled cystic lesions ranging in size from 0.5 to 2.0 cm. (Courtesy of Dr. M.K. Palmer, London.)

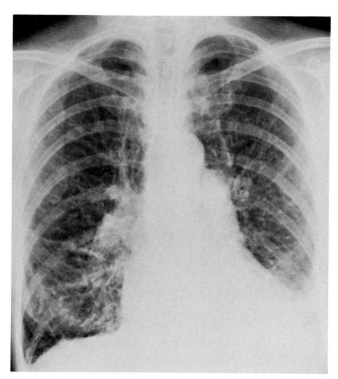

FIG 12–42.
Lymphangiomyomatosis. There is diffuse reticulonodular interstitial shadowing. The pleural effusion at the left base proved to be chylous, and there had been a right chylous effusion 4 years before. The proximal pulmonary arteries are large, indicating the presence of pulmonary artery hypertension, a recognized complication of lymphangiomyomatosis.

ANKYLOSING SPONDYLITIS

Ankylosing spondylitis (AS) is a seronegative spondyloarthritis that primarily affects the axial skeleton, causing pain and progressive stiffness of the spine. It is five to ten times more common in men than women. It has a striking familial incidence and a 90% to 95% association with HLA B27 antigen. Characteristically, AS presents in men less than 40 years of age as insidious low backache that is worse in the morning and improves with exercise. Sacroiliitis is a consistent early feature followed by synovitis and an enthesopathy which affects the axial skeleton and commonly leads to spinal fusion. The peripheral joints are involved in 35% of patients.[37] Extra-articular features may develop; these include anterior uveitis (up to 25%), aortic regurgitation (up to 10% in long-standing cases),[104] cardiac conduction defects, and constitutional symptoms. The prognosis is variable. In some patients, there is no progression beyond sacroiliitis, whereas others develop progressive, widespread disease leading in particular to complete fusion of the axial joints and the intervertebral discs of the spine.

Pleuropulmonary involvement is of two kinds: (1) chest wall restriction and (2) upper lobe fibrobullous disease.[129]

Restrictive disease is due to fusion of costovertebral and costotransverse joints. Changes in lung function are surprisingly small as the chest becomes fixed at a high resting volume, allowing the diaphragm to make a greater contribution than usual to inspiration.[129] Generally, total lung capacity and vital capacity are mildly or moderately reduced while functional residual capacity and residual volume are normal or slightly increased.[129]

Upper zone "fibrobullous" disease was first recorded in 1941,[73] but its recognition as an extra-articular manifestation of AS had to wait more than 20 years for the paper by Campbell and MacDonald in 1965.[38] The phenomenon is rare; its frequency, based on a review of 2,080 patients at the Mayo Clinic, is 1.25%.[267] Pathologically, the findings are nonspecific, and consist of fibrosis and a chronic inflammatory cell infiltrate, often lymphocytic, together with dilated bronchi, thin-walled bullae and cavities.[342]

The radiologic changes[38, 47, 63, 144, 267, 342] consist of nodular and linear shadowing or pleural thickening which begins in the lung apices. The early changes are usually symmetrical, but may be asymmetrical (one-third in one series).[63] After a while, the shadowing tends to become bilateral and symmetrical, and the nodules and pleural thickening become more pronounced and confluent (Fig 12–43). After a further interval, often of several years,[38] one or more rounded transradiancies appear in most cases.[63, 267, 342] The transradiancies are usually multi-

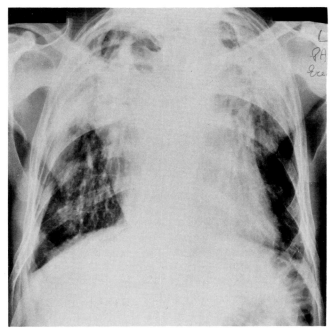

FIG 12–43.
Ankylosing spondylitis. Symmetric bilateral upper zone shadowing is largely confluent. There are transradiancies within the shadowing ranging in diameter from a few millimeters to several centimeters. There is marked volume loss of the upper lobes.

ple; they may be small or large and have thin or thick walls. These apical changes usually progress slowly,[63] but they can remain stable for many years.[267] At this stage the process is essentially one of fibrosis; the hili become elevated, producing an overall appearance that mimics tuberculosis (Fig 12–44). The changes are, however, not due to tuberculosis, nor are they due to radiation which was, at one time, used as a form of therapy for AS.[38, 47, 63] Apical fibrosis is usually seen only in patients who have marked spinal involvement[47] and long-standing ankylosing spondylitis, 15 to 20 years on average.[63, 267, 342] A few cases are recorded in which the lung changes apparently appeared within a few years of the onset of AS.[38, 267]

The cavities that develop within the fibrotic lung may be colonized by a variety of fungi and nontuberculous mycobacteria,[129, 157] most commonly *Aspergillus fumigatus*.[63] In some series, 50% to 60% of cavities have been colonized by *A. fumigatus*,[38, 63] leading to the suggestion that AS cavities are more susceptible than tuberculous cavities to mycetoma formation.[63] In other series, the colonization rate has been lower and more comparable to that expected in tuberculosis.[267] Hemoptysis is common in patients with mycetoma and may be life-threatening. Surgical removal is often attended by complications,[129] and bronchial artery embolism has therefore been used as an alternative treatment with some success.

By the time the pulmonary changes are visible, the skeletal manifestations of AS[71] are usually obvious on PA and lateral chest radiographs. The findings that are most easily seen on frontal view are ossification of costotransverse joints (particularly the first), vertebral syndesmophytes, and interspinous ossification. The diagnosis of AS is, however, generally more easily made from a lateral radiograph (see Fig 12–44,B). The principal changes are kyphosis, syndesmophytes (particularly at D-9 to D-12 level), and squared or barrel-shaped vertebral bodies. The manubriosternal joint is frequently eroded or fused.[285]

Pleural effusions and pleural thickening remote from the lung apex[160] have been seen in association with AS, but the prevalence is so low (only three of the 2,080 cases in the Mayo Clinic series[267]) that they are almost certainly chance findings. The pneumothorax rate, is, however, significantly increased, with a prevalence of about 8%.[267] The association of pulmonary fibrosis of AS and adenocarcinoma has been described.[3]

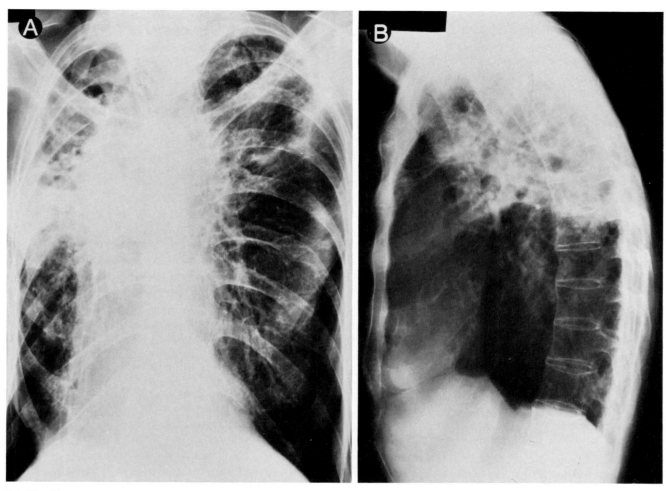

FIG 12–44.
Ankylosing spondylitis. **A,** PA chest radiograph with bilateral but grossly asymmetric apical changes. There is marked upper zone volume loss and many ring shadows. **B,** lateral radiograph of same patient demonstrating spinal fusion.

PULMONARY ALVEOLAR PROTEINOSIS

Pulmonary alveolar proteinosis (PAP) is a rare disorder characterized pathologically by filling of the alveoli with a proteinaceous material (positive to periodic acid-Schiff) while the lung interstitium remains relatively normal.[156] It probably represents a nonspecific response to some exogenous or possibly endogenous insult.[39] Although a history of exposure to dust is sometimes obtained,[62] a definite relationship has only been established for acute silicosis,[119] particularly that involving sand blasting.[268, 313, 346] Other associations that seem to be etiologically important, at least in some cases, are with hematological malignancies (lymphoma and leukemia)[39] and immunologic abnormalities, particularly in children. In one review, 30% of children with PAP had thymic alymphoplasia.[56] Also, familial cases in children have been associated with immunoglobulin abnormalities.[333] The alveolar material is partly phospholipid, resembling surfactant but lacking its surface-active properties. It is derived from type II pneumocytes. The rest of the alveolar material is protein from plasma and cellular debris. It is not clear whether phospholipid accumulation is the result of overproduction, reduced clearance, or both.[242] Alveolar filling with this material has two principal effects. First, it interferes with gas exchange and, second, it impairs pulmonary defenses against microorganisms. It is as if, by trying to clear the alveoli of proteinaceous matter, the macrophages become "lethargic and overfed" and, therefore, functionally impaired.[98]

The disease is most common in adults, though it is described in children and has even been recorded to occur at less than 1 year of age.[62] The peak age of presentation is between 30 and 50 years,[175] with 80% of patients being men.[62] Children with this disorder are usually compromised hosts, and the disease is then progressive and often fatal, whereas in adults there is generally no underlying disorder.[250] In about one-fifth of cases, the onset is acute, with fever, weight loss, and dyspnea, either with or without a super-added opportunistic infection.[62] Most of the other cases have an insidious onset of progressive dyspnea, cough, and sputum production. Occasionally, the disease is discovered by chest radiography in asymptomatic individuals.[268] The clinical signs are scattered crepitations on auscultation and, sometimes, hypoxemia and clubbing. PAP is one of those conditions in which the radiological signs are often striking even when the symptoms and clinical signs are mild.[5, 175] The diagnosis is established by bronchoalveolar lavage or transbronchial lung biopsy.

The main radiologic finding is air-space shadowing, since the pathologic changes are almost entirely the result of alveolar filling. In some cases, however, mild interstitial fibrosis and septal cellular infiltration and edema are present,[62, 215, 262, 268] and probably account for occasional "interstitial" features on the chest radiograph (Fig 12–45). The classic radiologic finding is bilateral symmetric air-space shadowing, particularly in a perihilar or hilar and basal distribution (Fig 12–46).[62, 248, 262] This shadowing often has a fine granularity (Fig 12–47), sometimes with alveolar rosettes.[248] At other times the pattern consists of rather coarse (5-mm), ill-defined

acinar nodules, perhaps in part confluent (see Fig 12–46).[198] The nodules may be particularly obvious toward the edge of confluent areas of consolidation[268] and, at times, the shadowing may even be reticulonodular.[198, 215, 268] Although usually symmetric, the consolidation can be asymmetric,[268] unilateral,[238, 262] or lobar.[39, 262] Sometimes, the consolidation is basally predominant,[39] peripheral rather than central,[5] and multifocal rather than diffuse.[238] Simultaneous evolution and regression, producing a shifting pattern similar to that found in the eosinophilic lung states, has been described.[236] Occasional features include septal (Kerley B) lines.[238, 248] Rounded transradiancies—varying in size from pinpoint[248] to several millimeters, or even a centimeter—may sometimes create a honeycomb pattern.[5, 240] Such air collections are, at least in part, thought to result from obstructive overinflation of distal respiratory units by proteinaceous material. Rupture of these respiratory units has given rise to pneumothorax.[5] Obstruction may also give rise to areas of collapse.[238, 240, 248]

Because of the functional macrophage impairment, complicating infections by pathogenic bacteria[248] or opportunistic agents are common and are a major cause of death.[62] *Nocardia* is particularly prevalent.[4, 39, 62, 116, 268] Other agents include *Candida*, *Aspergillus*, *Cryptococcus*,[39] cytomegalovirus,[39, 250] and nontuberculous *Mycobacteria*.[39] Radiologic pointers to such an opportunistic infection (particularly *Nocardia*) include the development of focal consolidation, cavitation, and pleural effusion.[62]

PAP is treated with saline lung lavage,[249] which

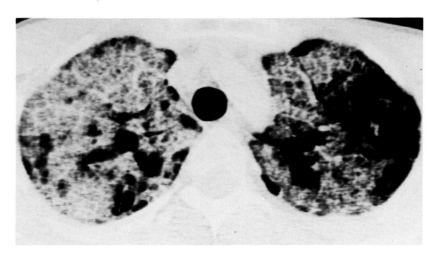

FIG 12–45.
Pulmonary alveolar proteinosis. CT scan demonstrates the geographical nature of much of the consolidation. Medially in the right lung an air bronchogram is present. The high-density reticulation is the result of septal edema. (Courtesy of Dr. C. Murch and the Royal College of Radiologists, London.)

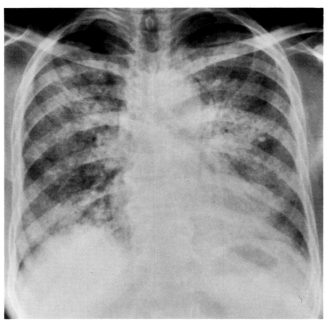

FIG 12–46.
Pulmonary alveolar proteinosis. There is bilateral air-space shadowing with elements of an air bronchogram. On the left the shadowing is in the classic perihilar distribution. Toward the edge of the parenchymal, changes are acinar nodules.

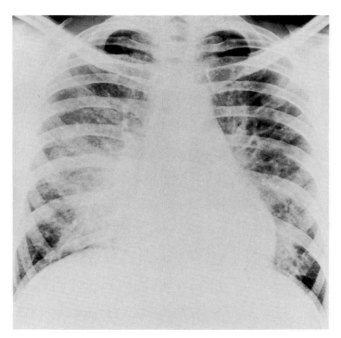

FIG 12–47.
Pulmonary alveolar proteinosis. Although the changes are bilateral, they are asymmetric. The shadowing on the right spreads out from the hilus and has a ground-glass quality.

has improved the prognosis. In a review of cases, studied chiefly before the use of therapeutic lavage, 35% of patients died, 38% continued with radiologic and symptomatic disease, and the disease cleared in 27%,[62] whereas in the more recent series mortality has been virtually eliminated.[258] When patients are treated with lavage, the chest radiograph is used to decide which side should be treated and to detect any complications.[91]

PULMONARY ALVEOLAR MICROLITHIASIS

Pulmonary alveolar microlithiasis is a rare disorder, with only about 170 cases in the world literature.[329] Its cause is unknown, and it is one of those conditions in which there may be gross radiographic changes in the face of minor clinical symptoms.

Alveolar microlithiasis is characterized pathologically by the accumulation of numerous, largely intra-alveolar calcified bodies (calcispherites or microliths). In addition, a few calcified bodies may also be found in the interstitium and airway submucosa.[284] Microliths contain calcium phosphate, and they range in size from several microns to a millimeter or more,[156] with the mean diameter about 200 μm.[48] Dystrophic ossification occasionally develops around microliths.[48] There have been rare descriptions of extrapulmonary microliths.[54, 284] Alveolar walls are commonly normal,[239] but later on in the disease, interstitial fibrosis may develop together with bullae and blebs.[284, 306]

Alveolar microlithiasis was first described in 1918.[115] About 40% of cases are sporadic while the remainder show a strong familial association,[36] for practical purposes restricted to siblings and consistent with an autosomal recessive transmission. Sex incidence is approximately equal.[239] Patients are commonly first detected in their 3rd and 4th decades,[239] but the range is large, with the disorder recorded in neonates[36] and in an 80-year-old person.[284] About 25% of patients in the literature have presented at less than 18 years of age and, in Japan, peak presentation is in childhood, a fact that has been ascribed to the greater use of screening radiography.[162]

Patients are usually asymptomatic and most commonly present with an abnormal screening or "routine" chest radiograph.[217] Later in the course of the disease, cough may appear, and a small proportion of patients will develop hemoptysis, clubbing, dyspnea, and cor pulmonale.[239, 306, 328] Respiratory function tests have been abnormal in about a third of reported cases and most commonly show a restric-

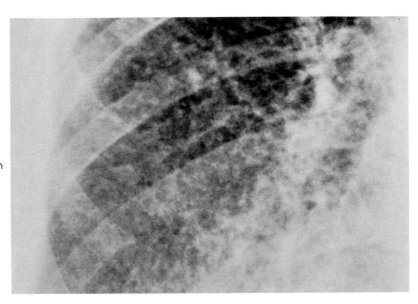

FIG 12−48.
Alveolar microlithiasis. Localized view of the right mid zone shows the basic element of the shadowing: high-density nodules less than 1 mm in diameter. (Courtesy of Dr. O. Heldaas, Konigsberg, Norway.)

tive defect or a decreased carbon monoxide diffusing capacity.[239]

The chest radiograph is quite characteristic,[306] with a diffuse distribution of innumerable, pinpoint nodules of calcific density (Fig 12−48). Nodules are less than 1 mm in diameter, but they may summate in areas to give a ground-glass or more coarsely nodular (up to 5 mm) pattern (Fig 12−49).[9] The radiographic density due to the opacities reflects local lung volume and is greatest at the bases.[306] In gross disease the radiographic opacity is so great that anatomic landmarks become completely obscured. Thus the heart may "vanish"[9] or even appear as a transra-

diant area on a penetrated radiograph (Fig 12−50). Pleural fissures can appear thickened.[9, 100, 325] A peripheral rimlike density to the lung may be seen on CT,[340] and this has been interpreted as pleural calcification. However, it seems likely that this peripheral curvilinear density is the result of (sub)pleural fibrosis rather than pleural calcification,[48] the calcification remaining strictly intrapulmonary.[306] In addition, CT scanning sometimes demonstrates striking soft tissue thickening between the chest wall and calcified lung[48] that may be seen on plain radiographs as a transradiant peel to the lung.[9] Bullae and blebs develop with late fibrosis,[239, 284, 306] and these are par-

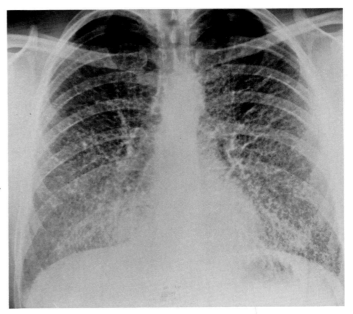

FIG 12−49.
Alveolar microlithiasis. The opacities are distributed symmetrically throughout both lungs, sparing the apices. Although the basic opacity is a high-density nodule less than 1 mm in diameter, there is a tendency, as shown here, for summation to produce larger nodules several millimeters in diameter. (Courtesy of Dr. O. Heldaas, Konigsberg, Norway.)

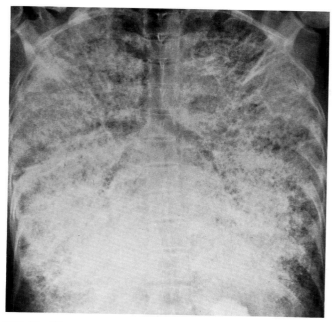

FIG 12–50.
Alveolar microlithiasis. Gross disease. The mediastinum appears less dense radiographically than the lungs.

ticularly well seen on CT.[48, 340] Such blebs and bullae probably predispose to pneumothorax and pneumomediastinum, which are recognized complications.[284, 340] Line shadows are not a feature of microlithiasis, but septal lines (Kerley B) are occasionally seen.[9, 217]

Very few patients with microlithiasis are recorded in whom a preceding normal chest radiograph has been documented.[162, 322] The micronodular opacities in microlithiasis usually appear from the beginning to be of calcific density. A few patients, however, have been described with nodulation that was initially of soft tissue density and which later became definitely calcific.[162] Bone-seeking agents such as technetium-99m diphosphonate are taken up by microliths, and this may be shown scintigraphically.[33]

Prognosis is variable. Many patients remain asymptomatic with stable chest radiographs for many years.[33] Others, sometimes after many years of stability, go on to experience pulmonary fibrosis and/or cor pulmonale, and ultimately die of the disease.[48, 284, 306, 328]

REFERENCES

1. Adams JS, Gacad MA, Singer FR, et al. Production of 1, 25-dihydroxyvitamin D3 by pulmonary alveolar macrophages in patients with sarcoidosis. *Ann NY Acad Sci* 1986; 465:587–594.

2. Adamson D, Heinrichs WL, Raybin DM, et al: Successful treatment of pulmonary lymphangiomyomatosis with oophorectomy and progesterone. *Am Rev Respir Dis* 1985; 132:916–921.

3. Ahern MJ, Maddison P, Mann S, et al: Ankylosing spondylitis and adenocarcinoma of the lung. *Ann Rheum Dis* 1982; 41:292–294.

4. Andriole VT, Ballas M, Wilson GL: The association of nocardiosis and pulmonary alveolar proteinosis. A case study. *Ann Intern Med* 1964; 60:266–275.

5. Anton HC, Gray B: Pulmonary alveolar proteinosis presenting with pneumothorax. *Clin Radiol* 1967; 18:428–431.

6. Arnett NL, Schulz DM: Primary pulmonary eosinophilic granuloma. *Radiology* 1957; 69:224–230.

7. Aughenbaugh GL: Thoracic manifestations of neurocutaneous diseases. *Radiol Clin North Am* 1984; 22:741–756.

8. Auld D: Pathology of eosinophilic granuloma of the lung. *Arch Pathol Lab Med* 1957; 63:113–131.

9. Balikian JP, Fuleihan FJD, Nucho CN: Pulmonary alveolar microlithiasis. Report of five cases with special reference to roentgen manifestations. *AJR* 1968; 103:509–518.

10. Bartlett JP, Adams WE: Solitary primary neurogenic tumor of the lung. *J Thorac Surg* 1946; 15:251–260.

11. Basset F, Corrin B, Spencer H, et al: Pulmonary histiocytosis X. *Am Rev Respir Dis* 1978; 118:811–820.

12. Battesti JP, Georges R, Basset F, et al: Chronic cor pulmonale in pulmonary sarcoidosis. *Thorax* 1978; 33:76–84.

13. Battesti JP, Saumon G, Valeyre D, et al: Pulmonary sarcoidosis with an alveolar radiographic pattern. *Thorax* 1982; 37:448–452.

14. Beekman JF, Zimmet SM, Chun BK, et al: Spectrum of pleural involvement in sarcoidosis. *Arch Intern Med* 1976; 136:323–330.

15. Bein ME, Putman CE, McLoud TC, et al: A reevaluation of intrathoracic lymphadenopathy in sarcoidosis. *AJR* 1978; 131:409–415.

16. Bekerman C, Szidon JP, Pinsky S: The role of gallium-67 in the clinical evaluation of sarcoidosis. *Semin Roentgenol* 1985; 20:400–409.

17. Benatar SR: Sarcoidosis in South Africa. A comparative study in whites, blacks and coloureds. *S Afr Med J* 1977; 52:602–606.

18. Benatar SR: A comparative study of sarcoidosis in white, black and coloured South Africans, in Williams WJ, Davies BH (eds): *Eighth International Conference on Sarcoidosis and Other Granulomatous Diseases.* Cardiff, Wales, Alpha Omega Publishing, Ltd, 1980, pp 508–513.

19. Berger JL, Shaff MJ: Pulmonary lymphangioleiomyomatosis. *J Comput Assist Tomogr* 1981; 5:565–567.

20. Bergin CJ, Muller NL: CT in the diagnosis of interstitial lung disease. *AJR* 1985; 145:505–510.

21. Berkmen YM: Radiologic aspects of intrathoracic sarcoidosis. *Semin Roentgenol* 1985; 20:356–375.

22. Berkmen YM, Javors BR: Anterior mediastinal lymphadenopathy in sarcoidosis. *AJR* 1976; 127:983–987.

23. Berte SJ, Pfotenhauer MA: Massive pleural effusion in sarcoidosis. *Am Rev Respir Dis* 1962; 86:261–264.

24. Bistrong HW, Tenney RD, Sheffer AL: Asymptomatic cavitary sarcoidosis. *JAMA* 1970; 213:1030–1032.

25. Bower JS, Dantzker DR: Airway obstruction in sarcoidosis. *Am Rev Respir Dis* 1977; 115(suppl 4):91.

26. Bradstreet CMP, Dighero MW, Mitchell DN: The Kveim test: Analysis of results of tests using K 19 materials, in Williams WJ, Davies BH (eds): *Eighth International Conference on Sarcoidosis and other Granulomatous Diseases.* Cardiff, Wales, Alpha Omega Publishing Ltd, 1980, pp 674–677.

27. Brandstetter RD, Hansen DE, Jarowski CI, et al: Superior vena cava syndrome as the initial clinical manifestation of sarcoidosis. *Heart Lung* 1981; 10:101–104.

28. Brandstetter RD, Messina MS, Sprince NL, et al: Tracheal stenosis due to sarcoidosis. *Chest* 1981; 80:656.

29. Breuer R, Baigelman W, Pugatch RD: Occult mycetoma. *J Comput Assist Tomogr* 1982; 6:166–168.

30. Brincker H, Wilbek E: The incidence of malignant tumours in patients with respiratory sarcoidosis. *Br J Cancer* 1974; 29:247–251.

31. Brodey PA, Pripstein S, Strange G, et al: Vertebral sarcoidosis. A case report and review of the literature. *AJR* 1976; 126:900–902.

32. Broughton RBK: Pulmonary tuberous sclerosis presenting with pleural effusion. *Br Med J* 1970; 1:477–478.

33. Brown ML, Swee RG, Olson RJ, et al: Pulmonary uptake of 99mTc diphosphonate in alveolar microlithiasis. *AJR* 1978; 131:703–704.

34. Bruwer AJ, Kierland RR, Schmidt HW: Pulmonary tuberous sclerosis. Report of a case. *AJR* 1956; 75:748–750.

35. Bundey S, Evans K: Tuberous sclerosis: A genetic study. *J Neurol Neurosurg Psychiatry* 1969; 32:591–603.

36. Caffrey PR, Altman RS: Pulmonary alveolar microlithiasis occurring in premature twins. *J Pediatr* 1965; 66:758–763.

37. Calin A: Ankylosing spondylitis. *Clin Rheum Dis* 1985; 11:41–60.

38. Campbell AH, MacDonald CB: Upper lobe fibrosis associated with ankylosing spondylitis. *Br J Dis Chest* 1965; 59:90–101.

39. Carnovale R, Zornoza J, Goldman AM, et al: Pulmonary alveolar proteinosis: Its association with hematologic malignancy and lymphoma. *Radiology* 1977; 122:303–306.

40. Carrington CB, Cugell DW, Gaensler EA, et al: Lymphangioleiomyomatosis. Physiologic-pathologic-radiologic correlations. *Am Rev Respir Dis* 1977; 116:977–995.

41. Carrington CB, Gaensler EA, Mikus JP, et al: Structure and function in sarcoidosis. *Ann NY Acad Sci* 1976; 278:265–283.

42. Case records of the Massachusetts General Hospital: Case 51–1974. *N Engl J Med* 1974; 291:1402–1408.

43. Case records of the Massachusetts General Hospital: Case 11–1984. *N Engl J Med* 1984; 310:708–716.

44. Case records of the Massachusetts General Hospital: Case 40–1985. *N Engl J Med* 1985; 313:874–883.

45. Casselman ES, Mandell GA: Vertebral scalloping in neurofibromatosis. *Radiology* 1979; 131:89–94.

46. Casselman ES, Miller WT, Lin SR, et al: von Recklinghausen's disease. Incidence of roentgenographic findings with a clinical review of the literature. *CRC Crit Rev Diagn Imaging* 1977; 9:387–419.

47. Chakera TMH, Howarth FH, Kendall MJ, et al: The chest radiograph in ankylosing spondylitis. *Clin Radiol* 1975; 26:455–460.

48. Chalmers AG, Wyatt J, Robinson PJ: Computed tomographic and pathological findings in pulmonary alveolar microlithiasis. *Br J Radiol* 1986; 59:408–411.

49. Chalmers AH, Armstrong P: Plexiform mediastinal neurofibromas. A report of two cases. *Br J Radiol* 1977; 50:215–217.

50. Chrisholm JC, Lang GR: Solitary circumscribed pulmonary nodule. An unusual manifestation of sarcoidosis. *Arch Intern Med* 1966; 118:376–378.

51. Chusid EL, Siltzbach LE: Sarcoidosis of the pleura. *Ann Intern Med* 1974; 81:190–194.

52. Citron KM, Scadding JG: Stenosing non-caseating tuberculosis (sarcoidosis) of the bronchi. *Thorax* 1957; 12:10–17.

53. Clark RL, Margulies SI, Mulholland JH: Histiocytosis X. A fatal case with unusual pulmonary manifestations. *Radiology* 1970; 95:631–632.

54. Coetzee T: Pulmonary alveolar microlithiasis with involvement of the sympathetic nervous system and gonads. *Thorax* 1970; 25:637–642.

55. Colby TV, Lombard C: Histiocytosis X in the lung. *Hum Pathol* 1983; 14:847–856.

56. Colon AR, Lawrence RD, Mills SD: Childhood pulmonary alveolar proteinosis (PAP). Report of a case and review of the literature. *Am J Dis Child* 1971; 121:481–485.

57. Corrin B, Liebow AA, Friedman PJ: Pulmonary lymphangiomyomatosis. *Am J Pathol* 1975; 79:348–382.

58. Corsello BF, Lohaus GH, Funahashi A: Endobronchial mass lesion due to sarcoidosis: Complete resolution with corticosteroids. *Thorax* 1983; 38:157–158.

59. Crystal RG, Roberts WC, Hunninghake GW, et al:

Pulmonary sarcoidosis: A disease characterized and perpetuated by activated lung T-lymphocytes. *Ann Intern Med* 1981; 94:73–94.

60. Da Costa JL, Chiang SC: Pleural sarcoidosis. *Singapore Med J* 1975; 6:224–226.

61. Damuth TE, Bower JS, Cho K, et al: Major pulmonary artery stenosis causing pulmonary hypertension in sarcoidosis. *Chest* 1980; 78:888–891.

62. Davidson JM, Macleod WM: Pulmonary alveolar proteinosis. *Br J Dis Chest* 1969; 63:13–28.

63. Davies D: Ankylosing spondylitis and lung fibrosis. *Q J Med* 1972; 41:395–417.

64. Davies J, Nellen M, Goodwin JF: Reversible pulmonary hypertension in sarcoidosis. *Postgrad Med J* 1982; 58:282–285.

65. Davies PDB: Diffuse pulmonary involvement in von Recklinghausen's disease. A new syndrome. *Thorax* 1963; 18:198.

66. Dawson J: Pulmonary tuberous sclerosis and its relationship to other forms of the disease. *Q J Med* 1954; 23:113–145.

67. Demicco WA, Fanburg BL: Sarcoidosis presenting as a lobar or unilateral lung infiltrate. *Clin Radiol* 1982; 33:663–669.

68. DeRemee RA: The roentgenographic staging of sarcoidosis. *Chest* 1983; 83:128–133.

69. Di Benedetto R, Lefrak S: Systemic sarcoidosis with severe involvement of the upper respiratory tract. *Am Rev Respir Dis* 1970; 102:801–807.

70. Di Benedetto RJ, Ribaudo C: Bronchopulmonary sarcoidosis. *Am Rev Respir Dis* 1966; 94:952–955.

71. Dihlmann W: Current radiodiagnostic concept of ankylosing spondylitis. *Skeletal Radiol* 1979; 4:179–188.

72. Dunbar R, Boyd W, Kijak J, et al: Mediastinal and extrapleural masses in a young adult. *Chest* 1978; 74:565–566.

73. Dunham CL, Kautz FG: Spondylarthritis ankylopoietica. Review and report of 20 cases. *Am J Med Sci* 1941; 201:232–250.

74. Dwyer JM, Hickie JB, Garvan J: Pulmonary tuberous sclerosis: Report of three patients and a review of the literature. *Q J Med* 1971; 40:115–125.

75. Edelman RR, Johnson TS, Jhaveri HS, et al: Fatal hemoptysis resulting from erosion of a pulmonary artery in cavitary sarcoidosis. *AJR* 1985; 145:37–38.

76. Edmondstone WM, Wilson AG: Sarcoidosis in caucasians, blacks and Asians in London. *Br J Dis Chest* 1985; 79:27–36.

77. Edwards CL, Hayes RL: Tumor scanning with 67Ga citrate. *J Nucl Med* 1969; 10:103–105.

78. Ellis K, Renthal G: Pulmonary sarcoidosis. Roentgenographic observations on course of disease. *AJR* 1962; 88:1070–1083.

79. Farinacci CJ, Jeffrey HC, Lackey RW: Eosinophilic granuloma of lung: Report of two cases. *US Armed Forces Med J* 1951; 2:1085–1093.

80. Faunce HF, Ramsay GC, Sy W: Protracted yet variable major pulmonary artery compression in sarcoidosis. *Radiology* 1976; 119:313–314.

81. Favara BE, McCarthy RC, Mierau GW: Histiocytosis X. *Hum Pathol* 1983; 14:663–676.

82. Felson B: Uncommon roentgen patterns of pulmonary sarcoidosis. *Dis Chest* 1958; 34:357–367.

83. Felson B: The extra pleural space. *Semin Roentgenol* 1977; 12:327–333.

84. Fienman NL, Yakovac WC: Neurofibromatosis in childhood. *J Pediatr* 1970; 76:339–346.

85. Fleury P, de Groot WP, Delleman JW, et al: Tuberous sclerosis: The incidence of sporadic cases versus familial cases. *Brain Dev* 1980; 2:107–117.

86. Fossa SD, Abeler V, Marton PF, et al: Sarcoid reaction of hilar and paratracheal lymph nodes in patients treated for testicular cancer. *Cancer* 1985; 56:2212–2216.

87. Freiman DG: The pathology of sarcoidosis. *Semin Roentgenol* 1985; 20:327–339.

88. Freundlich IM, Libshitz HI, Glassman LM, et al: Sarcoidosis. Typical and atypical thoracic manifestations and complications. *Clin Radiol* 1970; 21:376–383.

89. Friedman OH, Blaugrund SM, Siltzbach LE: Biopsy of the bronchial wall as an aid in the diagnosis of sarcoidosis. *JAMA* 1963; 183:646–650.

90. Friedman PJ, Liebow AA, Sokoloff J: Eosinophilic granuloma of lung. Clinical aspects of primary pulmonary histiocytosis in the adult. *Medicine* 1981; 60:385–396.

91. Gale ME, Karlinsky JB, Robins AG: Bronchopulmonary lavage in pulmonary alveolar proteinosis: Chest radiograph observations. *AJR* 1986; 146:981–985.

92. Gardiner IT, Uff JS: Acute pleurisy in sarcoidosis. *Thorax* 1978; 33:124–127.

93. Gardner J, Kennedy HG, Hamblin A, et al: HLA associations in sarcoidosis: A study of two ethnic groups. *Thorax* 1984; 39:19–22.

94. Gilman MJ, Laurens RG, Somogyi JW, et al: CT attenuation values of lung density in sarcoidosis. *J Comput Assist Tomogr* 1983; 7:407–410.

95. Gilman MJ, Wang KP: Transbronchial lung biopsy in sarcoidosis. An approach to determine the optimal number of biopsies. *Am Rev Respir Dis* 1980; 122:721–724.

96. Glazer HS, Levitt RG, Shackelford GD: Peripheral pulmonary infiltrates in sarcoidosis. *Chest* 1984; 86:741–744.

97. Goffman TE, Bloom RL, Dvorak VC: Acute dyspnea in a young woman taking birth control pills. *JAMA* 1984; 251:1465–1466.

98. Golde DW: Alveolar proteinosis and the overfed macrophage. *Chest* 1979; 76:119–120.

99. Goldenberg GJ, Greenspan RH: Middle-lobe atelectasis due to endobronchial sarcoidosis with hy-

percalcemia and renal impairment. *N Engl J Med* 1960; 262:1112–1116.

100. Gomez GE, Lichtemberger E, Santamaria A, et al: Familial pulmonary alveolar microlithiasis: Four cases from Colombia SA. Is microlithiasis also an environmental disease? *Radiology* 1959; 72:550–561.

101. Gomez MR: *Tuberous Sclerosis.* New York, Raven Press, 1979.

102. Gordonson J, Trachtenberg S, Sargent EN: Superior vena cava obstruction due to sarcoidosis. *Chest* 1973; 63:292–293.

103. Gorske KJ, Fleming RJ: Mycetoma formation in cavitary pulmonary sarcoidosis. *Radiology* 1970; 95:279–285.

104. Graham DC, Smythe HA: The carditis and aortitis of ankylosing spondylitis. *Bull Rheum Dis* 1958; 9:171–174.

105. Green GJ: The radiology of tuberose sclerosis. *Clin Radiol* 1968; 19:135–147.

106. Gregorie HB, Othersen HB, Moore MP: The significance of sarcoid-like lesions in association with malignant neoplasms. *Am J Surg* 1962; 104:577–586.

107. Gross BH, Schneider HJ, Proto AV: Eggshell calcification of lymph nodes: An update. *AJR* 1980; 135:1265–1268.

108. Guardia J, Pedreira JD, Esteban R, et al: Early pleural effusion in histiocytosis X. *Arch Intern Med* 1979; 139:934–936.

109. Guildford WB, Mentz WM, Kopelman HA, et al: Sarcoidosis presenting as a rib fracture. *AJR* 1982; 139:608–609.

110. Guyatt GH, Bensen WG, Stolmon LP, et al: HLA-B8 and erythema nodosum. *Can Med Assoc J* 1982; 127:1005–1006.

111. Hadfield JW, Page RL, Flower CDR, et al: Localised airway narrowing in sarcoidosis. *Thorax* 1982; 37:443–447.

112. Hafermann DR, Solomon DA, Byrd RB: Sarcoidosis initially occurring as apical infiltrate and pleural reaction. *Chest* 1978; 73:413–414.

113. Hamilton R, Petty TL, Haiby G: Cavitary sarcoidosis of the lung. *Arch Intern Med* 1965; 116:428–430.

114. Hamper UM, Fishman EK, Khouri NF, et al: Typical and atypical CT manifestations of pulmonary sarcoidosis. *J Comput Assist Tomogr* 1986; 10:928–936.

115. Harbitz F: Extensive calcification of the lungs as a distinct disease. *Arch Intern Med* 1918; 21:139–146.

116. Harris JO: Pulmonary alveolar proteinosis. Abnormal in vitro function of alveolar macrophages. *Chest* 1979; 76:156–159.

117. Harris JO, Waltuck BL, Swenson EW: The pathophysiology of the lungs in tuberous sclerosis. A case report and literature review. *Am Rev Respir Dis* 1969; 100:379–387.

118. Henry DA, Cho SR: Tracheal stenosis in sarcoidosis. *South Med J* 1983; 76:1323–1324.

119. Heppleston AG, Wright NA, Stewart JA: Experi-

mental alveolar lipo-proteinosis following the inhalation of silica. *J Pathol* 1970; 101:293–307.

120. Heshiki A, Schatz SL, McKusick KA, et al: Gallium 67 citrate scanning in patients with pulmonary sarcoidosis. *AJR* 1974; 122:744–749.

121. Hetherington S: Sarcoidosis in young children. *Am J Dis Child* 1982; 136:13–15.

122. Hietala S, Stinnett RG, Faunce HF: Pulmonary artery narrowing in sarcoidosis. *JAMA* 1977; 237:572–573.

123. Hoffstein V, Ranganathan N, Mullen JBM: Sarcoidosis simulating pulmonary veno-occlusive disease. *Am Rev Respir Dis* 1986; 134:809–811.

124. Holt JF: Neurofibromatosis in children. *AJR* 1978; 130:615–639.

125. Honey M, Jepson E: Multiple bronchostenoses due to sarcoidosis. Report of two cases. *Br Med J* 1957; 2:1330–1334.

126. Honeybourne D: Ethnic differences in the clinical features of sarcoidosis in South-East London. *Br J Dis Chest* 1980; 74:63–69.

127. Huang CT, Heurich AE, Rosen Y, et al: Pulmonary sarcoidosis: A radiographic, functional and pathological correlation, in Williams WJ, Davies BH (eds): *Eighth International Conference on Sarcoidosis and Other Granulomatous Diseases.* Cardiff, Wales, Alpha Omega Publishing, 1980, pp 368–377.

128. Huang CT, Heurich AE, Sutton AL, et al: Mortality in sarcoidosis, in Williams WJ, Davies BH (eds): *Eighth International Conference on Sarcoidosis and Other Granulomatous Diseases.* Cardiff, Wales, Alpha Omega Publishing, 1980, pp 522–526.

129. Hunninghake GW, Fauci AS: Pulmonary involvement in the collagen vascular diseases. *Am Rev Respir Dis* 1979; 119:471–503.

130. Hunt JC, Pugh DG: Skeletal lesions in neurofibromatosis. *Radiology* 1961; 76:1–20.

131. Israel HL: Experience with the treatment of aspergillosis complicating sarcoidosis, in *Proceedings of the Sixth International Conference on Sarcoidosis 1972.* Baltimore, University Park Press, 1974.

132. Israel HL, Karlin P, Menduke H, et al: Factors affecting outcome of sarcoidosis. Influence of race, extrathoracic involvement, and initial radiologic lung lesion. *Ann NY Acad Sci* 1986; 465:609–617.

133. Israel HL, Lenchner GS, Atkinson GW. Sarcoidosis and aspergilloma. The role of surgery. *Chest* 1982; 82:430–432.

134. Israel HL, Lenchner G, Steiner RM: Late development of mediastinal calcification in sarcoidosis. *Am Rev Respir Dis* 1981; 124:302–305.

135. Israel HL, Park CH, Mansfield CM: Gallium scanning in sarcoidosis. *Ann NY Acad Sci* 1976; 278:514–516.

136. Israel HL, Sones M: Sarcoidosis. Clinical observation on one hundred sixty cases. *Arch Intern Med* 1958; 102:766–776.

137. Israel HL, Sones M, Roy RL, et al: The occurrence

of intrathoracic calcification in sarcoidosis. *Am Rev Respir Dis* 1961; 84:1–11.

138. Israel HL, Sperber M, Steiner RM: Course of chronic hilar sarcoidosis in relation to markers of granulomatous activity. *Invest Radiol* 1983; 18:1–15.

139. Israel HL, Washburne JD: Characteristics of sarcoidosis in black and white patients. Analysis of 162 recent cases, in Williams WJ, Davies BH (eds): *Eighth International Conference on Sarcoidosis and Other Granulomatous Diseases.* Cardiff, Wales, Alpha Omega Publishing, 1980, pp 497–507.

140. James DG, Carstairs LS: Pulmonary sarcoidosis. *Hosp Update* 1982; 8:1022–1030.

141. James DG, Neville E, Siltzbach LE, et al: A worldwide review of sarcoidosis. *Ann NY Acad Sci* 1976; 278:321–335.

142. James DG, Williams WJ: Sarcoidosis and other granulomatous disorders. Philadelphia, W B Saunders Co, 1985.

143. Javaheri S, Hales CA: Sarcoidosis: A cause of innominate vein obstruction and massive pleural effusion. *Lung* 1980; 157:81–85.

144. Jessamine AG: Upper lung lobe fibrosis in ankylosing spondylitis. *Can Med Assoc J* 1968; 98:25–29.

145. Johns CJ: Management of hemoptysis with pulmonary fungus balls in sarcoidosis. *Chest* 1982; 82:400–401.

146. Johns CJ, MacGregor MI, Zachary JB, et al: Chronic sarcoidosis: Outcome, unusual features and complications, in Williams WJ, Davies BH (eds): *Eighth International Conference on Sarcoidosis and Other Granulomatous Diseases.* Cardiff, Wales, Alpha Omega Publishing, 1980, pp 558–566.

147. Johnson N McI, Martin NDT, McNicol MW: Sarcoidosis presenting with pleurisy and bilateral pleural effusions. *Postgrad Med J* 1980; 56:266–267.

148. Jones DK, Dent RG, Rimmer MJ, et al: Thin-walled ring shadows in early pulmonary sarcoidosis. *Clin Radiol* 1984; 35:307–310.

149. Jorgensen G: Die gewnetik der Sarkoidose. *Acta Med Scand* 1964; (suppl)425:213–215.

150. Kaku T, Toyoshima S, Enjoji M: Tuberous sclerosis with pulmonary and lymph node involvement. Relationship to lymphangiomyomatosis. *Acta Pathol Jpn* 1983; 33:395–401.

151. Kalbian VV: Bronchial involvement in pulmonary sarcoidosis. *Thorax* 1957; 12:18–23.

152. Kanada DJ, Scott D, Sharma OP: Unusual presentations of pleural sarcoidosis. *Br J Dis Chest* 1980; 74:203–205.

153. Kaplan J, Johns CJ: Mycetomas in pulmonary sarcoidosis: Nonsurgical management. *Johns Hopkins Med J* 1979; 145:157–161.

154. Karasick SR: Atypical thoracic lymphadenopathy in sarcoidosis. *AJR* 1979; 133:928–929.

155. Kataria YP, Sharma OM, Israel H, et al: Kveim antigen CRI, in Williams WJ, Davies BH (eds): *Eighth International Conference on Sarcoidosis and Other Granu-*

lomatous Diseases. Cardiff, Wales, Alpha Omega Publishing, 1980, pp 660–667.

156. Katzenstein A-LA, Askin FB: Surgical pathology of non-neoplastic lung disease. Philadelphia, WB Saunders Co, 1982.

157. Kennedy WPU, Milne LJR, Blyth W, et al: Two unusual organisms, *Aspergillus terreus* and *Metchnikowia pulcherrima,* associated with the lung disease of ankylosing spondylitis. *Thorax* 1972; 27:604–610.

158. Kent DC: Recurrent unilateral hilar adenopathy in sarcoidosis. *Am Rev Respir Dis* 1965; 91:272–276.

159. Khan MM, Gill DS, McConkey B: Myopathy and external pulmonary artery compression caused by sarcoidosis. *Thorax* 1981; 36:703–704.

160. Kinnear WJM, Shneerson JM: Acute pleural effusions in inactive ankylosing spondylitis. *Thorax* 1985; 40:150–151.

161. Kinney EL, Murthy R, Ascunce G, et al: Sarcoidosis: Rare cause of superior vena caval obstruction. *Pa Med* 1980; 83:31.

162. Kino T, Kohara Y, Tsuji S: Pulmonary alveolar microlithiasis. A report of two young sisters. *Am Rev Respir Dis* 1972; 105:105–110.

163. Kirks DR, Greenspan RH: Sarcoid. *Radiol Clin North Am* 1973; 11:279–294.

164. Kirks DR, McCormick VD, Greenspan RH: Pulmonary sarcoidosis. Roentgenologic analysis of 150 patients. *AJR* 1973; 117:777–786.

165. Kirschner BS, Hollinger PH: Laryngeal obstruction in childhood sarcoidosis. *J Pediatr* 1976; 88:263–265.

166. Klatte EC, Franken EA, Smith JA: The radiographic spectrum in neurofibromatosis. *Semin Roentgenol* 1976; 11:17–33.

167. Knox AJ, Wardman AG, Page RL: Tuberculous pleural effusion occurring during corticosteroid treatment of sarcoidosis. *Thorax* 1986; 41:651.

168. Koerner SK, Sakowitz AJ, Appelman RI, et al: Transbronchial lung biopsy for the diagnosis of sarcoidosis. *N Engl J Med* 1975; 293:268–270.

169. Kruglik GD, Reed JC, Daroca PJ: RPC from the AFIP. *Radiology* 1976; 120:583–588.

170. Kumar AJ, Kuhajda FP, Martinez CR, et al: Computed tomography of extra cranial nerve sheath tumours with pathological correlation. *J Comput Assist Tomogr* 1983; 7:857–865.

171. Kutty CPK, Varkey B: Sarcoidosis presenting with posterior mediastinal lymphadenopathy. *Postgrad Med* 1982; 71:64–66.

172. Lacronique J, Roth C, Battesti J-P, et al: Chest radiological features of pulmonary histiocytosis X: A report based on 50 adult cases. *Thorax* 1982; 37:104–109.

173. Lagos JC, Gomez MR: Tuberous sclerosis: Reappraisal of a clinical entity. *Mayo Clin Proc* 1967; 42:26–49.

174. Langhammer H, Glaubitt G, Grebe SF, et al: 67 Ga for tumor scanning. *J Nucl Med* 1972; 13:25–30.

175. Larson RK, Gordinier R: Pulmonary alveolar proteinosis. *Ann Intern Med* 1965; 62:292–312.

176. Levine BW, Saldana M, Hutter AM: Pulmonary hypertension in sarcoidosis. *Am Rev Respir Dis* 1971; 103:413–417.

177. Levinsky L, Cummiskey J, Romer FK, et al: Sarcoidosis in Europe: A cooperative study. *Ann NY Acad Sci* 1976; 278:335–346.

178. Levinson RS, Metzger LF, Stanley NN, et al: Airway function in sarcoidosis. *Am J Med* 1977; 62:51–59.

179. Lewis JG: Eosinophilic granuloma and its variants with special reference to lung involvement. *Q J Med* 1964; 33:337–359.

180. Libshitz HI, Atkinson GW, Israel HL: Pleural thickening as a manifestation of *Aspergillus* superinfection. *AJR* 1974; 120:883–886.

181. Lie JT, Miller RD, Williams DE: Cystic disease of the lungs in tuberous sclerosis. Clinicopathologic correlation, including body plethysmographic lung function tests. *Mayo Clin Proc* 1980; 55:547–553.

182. Lieberman J: Elevation of serum angiotensin converting enzyme (ACE) level in sarcoidosis. *Am J Med* 1975; 59:365–372.

183. Lieberman J, Nosal A, Schlessner LA, et al: Serum angiotensin-converting enzyme for diagnosis and therapeutic evaluation of sarcoidosis. *Am Rev Respir Dis* 1979; 120:329–335.

184. Lim KH: Four episodes of sarcoidosis after pulmonary tuberculosis. *Tubercle* 1961; 42:350–354.

185. Line BR, Hunninghake GW, Keogh BA, et al: Gallium-67 scanning to stage the alveolitis of sarcoidosis: Correlation with clinical studies, pulmonary function studies, and bronchoalveolar lavage. *Am Rev Respir Dis* 1981; 123:440–446.

186. Littner MR, Schachter EN, Putman CE, et al: The clinical assessment of roentgenographically atypical pulmonary sarcoidosis. *Am J Med* 1977; 62:361–368.

187. Lofgren S: Primary pulmonary sarcoidosis. *Acta Med Scand* 1953; 145:424–431; 465–474.

188. Luna CM, Gene R, Jolly EC, et al: Pulmonary lymphangiomyomatosis associated with tuberous sclerosis. *Chest* 1985; 88:473–475.

189. MacFarlane JT: Recurrent erythema nodosum and pulmonary sarcoidosis. *Postgrad Med J* 1981; 57:525.

190. MacPherson P: A survey of erythema nodosum in a rural community between 1954 and 1968. *Tubercle* 1970; 51:324–327.

191. Madewell JE, Feigin DS: Benign tumors of the lung. *Semin Roentgenol* 1977; 12:175–186.

192. Massaro D, Katz S: Fibrosing alveolitis: Its occurrence, roentgenographic and pathologic features in von Recklinghausen's neurofibromatosis. *Am Rev Respir Dis* 1966; 93:934–942.

193. Massaro D, Katz S, Matthews MJ, et al: Von Recklinghausen's neurofibromatosis associated with cystic lung disease. *Am J Med* 1965; 38:233–240.

194. Masson RG, Tedeschi LG: Pulmonary eosinophilic granuloma with hilar adenopathy simulating sarcoidosis. *Chest* 1978; 73:682–683.

195. Mather G: Calcium metabolism and bone changes in sarcoidosis. *Br Med J* 1957; 1:248–253.

196. Mayock RL, Bertrand P, Morrison CE, et al: Manifestations of sarcoidosis. Analysis of 145 patients, with a review of nine series selected from the literature. *Am J Med* 1963; 35:67–89.

197. McCarty KS, Mossler JA, McLelland R, et al: Pulmonary lymphangiomyomatosis responsive to progesterone. *N Engl J Med* 1980; 303:1461–1465.

198. McCook TA, Kirks DR, Merten DF, et al: Pulmonary alveolar proteinosis in children. *AJR* 1981; 137:1023–1027.

199. McCort JJ, Pare PJ: Pulmonary fibrosis and cor pulmonale in sarcoidosis. *Radiology* 1954; 62:496–504.

200. McKusick KA, Soin JS, Ghiladi A, et al: Gallium 67 accumulation in pulmonary sarcoidosis. *JAMA* 1973; 223:688.

201. McLoud TC, Epler GR, Gaensler EA, et al: A radiographic classification for sarcoidosis. Physiologic correlation. *Invest Radiol* 1982; 17:129–138.

202. McLoud TC, Putman CE, Pascual R: Eggshell calcification with systemic sarcoidosis. *Chest* 1974; 66:515–517.

203. Medley BE, McLeod RA, Houser OW: Tuberous sclerosis. *Semin Roentgenol* 1976; 11:35–54.

204. Mendelson DS, Norton K, Cohen BA, et al: Bronchial compression: An unusual manifestation of sarcoidosis. *J Comput Assist Tomogr* 1983; 7:892–894.

205. Merchant RN, Pearson MG, Rankin RN, et al: Computerized tomography in the diagnosis of lymphangioleiomyomatosis. *Am Rev Respir Dis* 1985; 131:295–297.

206. Mesbahi SJ, Davies P: Unilateral pulmonary changes in the chest x-ray in sarcoidosis. *Clin Radiol* 1981; 32:283–287.

207. Meszaros WT, Guzzo F, Schorsch H: Neurofibromatosis. *AJR* 1966; 98:557–569.

208. Meyrier A, Valeyre D, Bouillon R, et al: Resorptive versus absorptive hypercalciuria in sarcoidosis. *Q J Med* 1985; 54:269–281.

209. Mikhail JR, Lovell D, McGhee KJ, et al: Sarcoidosis presenting with a pleural effusion. *Tubercle* 1976; 57:226–228.

210. Mikhail JR, Mitchell DN, Sutherland I, et al: Sarcoidosis presenting in a district general hospital, in Williams WJ, Davies BH (eds): *Eighth International Conference on Sarcoidosis and Other Granulomatous Diseases.* Cardiff, Wales, Alpha Omega Publishing, 1980, pp 532–536.

211. Miles J, Pennybacker J, Sheldon P: Intrathoracic meningocele. Its development and association with neurofibromatosis. *J Neurol Neurosurg Psychiatry* 1969; 32:99–110.

212. Miller A: The vanishing lung syndrome associated with pulmonary sarcoidosis. *Br J Dis Chest* 1981; 75:209–214.

213. Miller A, Einstein K, Thornton J, et al: Physiologic classification and staging of intrathoracic sarcoidosis, in Williams WJ, Davies BH (eds): *Eighth International Congress on Sarcoidosis and Other Granulomatous Diseases.* Cardiff, Wales, Alpha Omega Publishing, 1980, pp 331–336.

214. Miller A, Teirstein AS, Jackler I, et al: Airway function in chronic pulmonary sarcoidosis with fibrosis. *Am Rev Respir Dis* 1974; 109:179–189.

215. Miller PA, Ravin CE, Walker Smith GJ, et al: Pulmonary alveolar proteinosis with interstitial involvement. *AJR* 1981; 137:1069–1071.

216. Miller WT, Cornog JL, Sullivan MA: Lymphangiomyomatosis. A clinical-roentgenologic-pathologic syndrome. *AJR* 1971; 111:565–572.

217. Miro JM, Moreno A, Coca A, et al: Pulmonary alveolar microlithiasis with an unusual radiological pattern. *Br J Dis Chest* 1982; 76:91–96.

218. Mitchell DM, Mitchell DN, Collins JV, et al: Transbronchial lung biopsy through fibre optic bronchoscope in diagnosis of sarcoidosis. *Br Med J* 1980; 280:679–681.

219. Mitnick JS, Bosniak MA, Hilton S, et al: Cystic renal disease in tuberous sclerosis. *Radiology* 1983; 147:85–87.

220. Morgans WE, Al-Jilahawi AN, Mbatha PB: Superior vena caval obstruction caused by sarcoidosis. *Thorax* 1980; 35:397–398.

221. Moyer JH, Ackerman AJ: Sarcoidosis. A clinical and roentgenological study of twenty-eight cases. *Am Rev Tuberc* 1950; 61:299–322.

222. Munt PW: Middle lobe atelectasis in sarcoidosis. Report of a case with prompt resolution concomitant with corticosteroid administration. *Am Rev Respir Dis* 1973; 108:357–360.

223. Nadeau PJ, Ellis FH, Harrison EG, et al: Primary pulmonary histiocytosis X. *Dis Chest* 1960; 37:325–339.

224. Nakano I, Tsuneta Y, Terai T, et al: Clinical significance of bronchoalveolar lavage, Ga scintigraphy and serum angiotensin converting enzyme activity in granulomatous lung disease. *Jpn J Thorac Dis* 1983; 21:615–621.

225. Neville E, Carstairs LS, James DG: Sarcoidosis of bone. *Q J Med* 1977; 46:215–227.

226. Newman A, So SK: Bilateral neurofibroma of the intrathoracic vagus associated with von Recklinghausen's disease. *AJR* 1971; 112:389–392.

227. Nicholls AJ, Friend JAR, Legge JS: Sarcoid pleural effusion: Three cases and review of the literature. *Thorax* 1980; 35:277–281.

228. Noble RH, Williams AJ: Multiple cavitating pulmonary nodules due to eosinophilic granuloma. *Clin Notes Resp Dis* 1982; 21:10–12.

229. Nutting S, Carr I, Cole FM, et al: Solitary pulmonary nodules due to sarcoidosis. *Can J Surg* 1979; 22:584–586.

230. O'Brien LE, Forsman PJ, Wiltse HE: Early onset sarcoidosis with pulmonary function abnormalities. *Chest* 1974; 65:472–474.

231. Olsson T, Bjornstad-Pettersen H, Stjernberg NL: Bronchostenosis due to sarcoidosis. *Chest* 1979; 75:663–666.

232. Onal E, Lopata M, Lourenco RV: Nodular pulmonary sarcoidosis. Clinical, roentgenographic, and physiologic course in five patients. *Chest* 1977; 72:296–300.

233. Packe GE, Ayres JG, Citron KM, et al: Large lung bullae in sarcoidosis. *Thorax* 1986; 41:792–797.

234. Pappas CA, Rheinlander HF, Stadecker MJ: Pleural effusion as a complication of solitary eosinophilic granuloma of the rib. *Hum Pathol* 1980; 11:675–677.

235. Patel YD, Moorhouse HT: Neurofibrosarcomas in neurofibromatosis: Role of CT scanning and angiography. *Clin Radiol* 1982; 33:555–560.

236. Phillips WJE, Constance TJ: Pulmonary alveolar proteinosis. *Med J Aust* 1963; 2:357–359.

237. Pinsker KL: Solitary pulmonary nodule in sarcoidosis. *JAMA* 1978; 240:1379–1380.

238. Prakash UBS, Barham SS, Carpenter HA, et al: Pulmonary alveolar phospholipoproteinosis: Experience with 34 cases and a review. *Mayo Clin Proc* 1987; 62:499–518.

239. Prakash UBS, Barham SS, Rosenow EC, et al: Pulmonary alveolar microlithiasis. A review including ultrastructural and pulmonary function studies. *Mayo Clin Proc* 1983; 58:290–300.

240. Preger L: Pulmonary alveolar proteinosis. *Radiology* 1969; 92:1291–1295.

241. Prophet D: Primary pulmonary histiocytosis X. *Clin Chest Med* 1982; 3:643–653.

242. Pulmonary alveolar proteinosis, editorial. *Br Med J* 1972; 395.

243. Putman CE, Hoeck B: Reassessing the standard chest radiograph for intraparenchymal activity. *Ann NY Acad Sci* 1986; 465:595–608.

244. Quismorio FP, Sharma OP, Chandor S: Immunopathological studies on the cutaneous lesions in sarcoidosis. *Br J Dermatol* 1977; 97:635–642.

245. Rabinowitz JG, Ulreich S, Soriano C: The usual unusual manifestations of sarcoidosis and the "hilar haze"—a new diagnostic aid. *AJR* 1974; 120:821–831.

246. Radenbach KL, Brandt HL, Freise CG, et al: Special diagnostic and therapeutic aspects of pulmonary histiocytosis X—twelve cases from 1969 to 1975 (author's translation). *Z Erkr Atmungsorgane* 1977; 147:26–40.

247. Radke JR, Kaplan H, Conway WA: The significance of superior vena cava syndrome developing in a patient with sarcoidosis. *Radiology* 1980; 134:311–312.

248. Ramirez RJ: Pulmonary alveolar proteinosis: A roentgenologic analysis. *AJR* 1964; 92:571–577.

249. Ramirez RJ: Bronchopulmonary lavage. New tech-

niques and observations. *Dis Chest* 1966; 50:581–
588.

250. Ranchod M, Bissell M: Pulmonary alveolar proteinosis and cytomegalovirus infection. *Arch Pathol Lab
Med* 1979; 103:139–142.

251. Reed JC, Madewell JE: The air bronchogram in interstitial disease of the lungs. *Radiology* 1975; 116:
1–9.

252. Reid L, Lorriman G: Lung biopsy in sarcoidosis. *Br
J Dis Chest* 1960; 54:321–334.

253. Riccardi VM: Von Recklinghausen neurofibromatosis. *N Engl J Med* 1981; 305:1617–1627.

254. Rizzato G, Blasi A: A European survey on the usefulness of 67Ga lung scans in assessing sarcoidosis.
Experience in 14 research centres in seven different
countries. *Ann NY Acad Sci* 1986; 465:463–478.

255. Roberts CM, Citron KM, Strickland B: Intrathoracic
aspergilloma: Role of CT in diagnosis and
treatment. *Radiology* 1987; 165:123–128.

256. Rockoff SD, Rohatgi PK: Unusual manifestations of
thoracic sarcoidosis. *AJR* 1985; 144:513–528.

257. Roethe RA, Fuller PB, Byrd RB, et al: Transbron-
choscopic lung biopsy in sarcoidosis. Optimal number and sites for diagnosis. *Chest* 1980; 77:400–402.

258. Rogers RM, Levin DC, Gray BA, et al: Physiologic
effects of bronchopulmonary lavage in alveolar proteinosis. *Am Rev Respir Dis* 1978; 118:255–264.

259. Rohatgi PK, Schwab LE: Primary acute pulmonary
cavitation in sarcoidosis. *AJR* 1980; 134:1199–1203.

260. Rohrback MS, DeRemee RA: Pulmonary sarcoidosis
and serum angiotensin-converting enzyme. *Mayo
Clin Proc* 1982; 57:64–66.

261. Romer FK: Presentation of sarcoidosis and outcome
of pulmonary changes. *Dan Med Bull* 1982; 29:27–
32.

262. Rosen SH, Castleman B, Liebow AA: Pulmonary
alveolar proteinosis. *N Engl J Med* 1958; 258:1123–
1142.

263. Rosen Y, Amorosa JK, Moon S, et al: Occurrence of
lung granulomas in patients with stage I sarcoidosis.
AJR 1977; 129:1083–1085.

264. Rosen Y, Athanassiades TJ, Moon S, et al: Nongran-
ulomatous interstitial pneumonitis in sarcoidosis.
Relationship to the development of epithelioid granulomas. *Chest* 1978; 74:122–125.

265. Rosen Y, Moon S, Huang C, et al: Granulomatous
pulmonary angiitis in sarcoidosis. *Arch Pathol Lab
Med* 1977; 101:170–174.

266. Rosenberg DM: Inherited forms of interstitial lung
disease. *Clin Chest Med* 1982; 3:635–641.

267. Rosenow EC, Strimlan CV, Muhm JR, et al: Pleuropulmonary manifestations of ankylosing spondylitis.
Mayo Clin Proc 1977; 52:641–649.

268. Rubin E, Weisbrod GL, Sanders DE: Pulmonary alveolar proteinosis. Relationship to silicosis and pulmonary infection. *Radiology* 1980; 135:35–41.

269. Sahn SA, Schwarz MI, Lakshminarayan S: Sarcoidosis: The significance of an acinar pattern on chest
roentgenogram. *Chest* 1974; 65:684–687.

270. Salerno NR, Edeiken J: Vertebral scalloping in neurofibromatosis. *Radiology* 1970; 97:509–510.

271. Sandler LM, Winearls CG, Fraher LJ, et al: Studies
of the hypercalcaemia of sarcoidosis. *Q J Med* 1984;
53:165–180.

272. Sartoris DJ, Resnick D, Resnick C, et al:
Musculoskeletal manifestations of sarcoidosis. *Semin
Roentgenol* 1985; 20:376–386.

273. Sartwell PE: Racial differences in sarcoidosis. *Ann
NY Acad Sci* 1976; 278:368–370.

274. Scadding JG: Calcification in sarcoidosis. *Tubercle*
1961; 42:121–135.

275. Scadding JG: *Sarcoidosis.* London, Eyre and Spottis-
woode, 1967.

276. Scadding JG: Further observations on calcification in
sarcoidosis. *Scand J Respir Dis* 1968; 65:235–242.

277. Scadding JG: Further observations on sarcoidosis
associated with *M tuberculosis* infection, in *Proceedings
5th International Conference on Sarcoidosis*, 1969.
Prague, 1971, pp 89–92.

278. Scadding JG, Mitchell DN: *Sarcoidosis*, ed 2. London,
Chapman and Hall, 1985.

279. Schabel SI, Foote GA, McKee KA. Posterior lymphadenopathy in sarcoidosis. *Radiology* 1978;
129:591–593.

280. Schabel SI, Schmidt GE, Vujic I: Overlooked pulmonary malignancy in neuro-fibromatosis. *J Can Assoc Radiol* 1980; 31:135–136.

281. Schermuly W, Behrend H: Die Angiographie de
Lung ensarkoidose. *Radiologie* 1968; 8:116–123.

282. Schoenberger CI, Line BR, Keogh BA, et al: Lung
inflammation in sarcoidosis: Comparison of serum
angiotensin-converting enzyme levels with bronchoalveolar lavage and gallium-67 scanning assessment
of the T lymphocyte alveolitis. *Thorax* 1982; 37:19–
25.

283. Schowengerdt CG, Suyemoto R, Main FB: Granulomatous and fibrous mediastinitis. *J Thorac Cardiovasc
Surg* 1969; 57:365–379.

284. Sears MR, Chang AR, Taylor AJ: Pulmonary alveolar microlithiasis. *Thorax* 1971; 26:704–711.

285. Sebes JI, Salazar JE: The manubriosternal joint in
rheumatoid disease. *AJR* 1983; 140:117–121.

286. Selroos O: Exudative pleurisy and sarcoidosis. *Br J
Dis Chest* 1966; 60:191–196.

287. Sharma OP: Sarcoidosis. Unusual pulmonary manifestations. *Postgrad Med* 1977; 61:67–73.

288. Sharma OP: Airway obstruction in sarcoidosis. *Chest*
1978; 73:6–7.

289. Sharma OP: Unusual manifestations of pulmonary
sarcoidosis: A radiographic panorama, in Williams
WJ, Davies BH (eds): *Eighth International Conference
on Sarcoidosis and Other Granulomatous Diseases.*
Cardiff, Wales, Alpha Omega Publishing, 1980, pp
378–385.

290. Sharma OP: Sarcoidosis: Clinical, laboratory, and immunologic aspects. *Semin Roentgenol* 1985; 20:340–355.

291. Sharma OP, Colp C, Williams MH: Pulmonary function studies in patients with bilateral sarcoidosis of hilar lymph nodes. *Arch Intern Med* 1966; 117:436–439.

292. Sharma OP, Hewlett R, Gordonson J: Nodular sarcoidosis: An unusual radiographic appearance. *Chest* 1973; 64:189–192.

293. Sharma OP, Neville E, Walker AN, et al: Familial sarcoidosis: A possible genetic influence. *Ann NY Acad Sci* 1976; 278:386–400.

294. Shibel EM, Tisi GM, Moser KM: Pulmonary photoscan-roentgenographic comparisons in sarcoidosis. *AJR* 1969; 106:770–777.

295. Shigematsu N, Emori K, Matsuba K, et al: Clinicopathologic characteristics of pulmonary acinar sarcoidosis. *Chest* 1978; 73:186–188.

296. Siltzbach LE: The Kveim test in sarcoidosis. A study of 750 patients. *JAMA* 1961; 178:476–482.

297. Siltzbach LE, James DG, Neville E, et al: Course and prognosis of sarcoidosis around the world. *Am J Med* 1974; 57:847–852.

298. Silverstein EF, Ellis K, Wolff M, et al: Pulmonary lymphangiomyomatosis. *AJR* 1974; 120:832–850.

299. Singer FR, Adams JS: Abnormal calcium homeostasis in sarcoidosis. *N Engl J Med* 1986; 315:755–757.

300. Smellie H, Hoyle C: The hilar lymph-nodes in sarcoidosis with special reference to prognosis. *Lancet* 1957; 2:66–70.

301. Smellie H, Hoyle C: The natural history of pulmonary sarcoidosis. *Q J Med* 1960; 29:539–559.

302. Smith LJ, Lawrence JB, Katzenstein AA: Vascular sarcoidosis: A rare cause of pulmonary hypertension. *Am J Med Sci* 1983; 285:38–44.

303. Smith MJ, Turton CWG, Mitchell DN, et al: Association of HLA-B8 with spontaneous resolution in sarcoidosis. *Thorax* 1981; 36:296–298.

304. Solomon A, Kreel L, McNicol M, et al: Computed tomography in pulmonary sarcoidosis. *J Comput Assist Tomogr* 1979; 3:754–758.

305. Sones M, Israel HL: Course and prognosis of sarcoidosis. *Am J Med* 1960; 29:84–93.

306. Sosman MC, Dodd, GD, Jones WD, et al: The familial occurrence of pulmonary alveolar microlithiasis. *AJR* 1957; 77:947–1012.

307. Spann RW, Rosenow EC, DeRemee RA, et al: Unilateral hilar or paratracheal adenopathy in sarcoidosis: A study of 38 cases. *Thorax* 1971; 26:296–299.

308. Steiger V, Fanburg BL: Recurrence of thoracic lymphadenopathy in sarcoidosis. *N Engl J Med* 1986; 314:1512.

309. Stein GN, Israel HL, Sones M: A roentgenographic study of skeletal lesions in sarcoidosis. *Arch Intern Med* 1956; 97:532–536.

310. Stovin PGI, Lum LC, Flower CDR, et al: The lungs in lymphangiomyomatosis and in tuberous sclerosis. *Thorax* 1975; 30:497–509.

311. Strickland B, Wolverson MK: Intrathoracic vagus nerve tumours. *Thorax* 1974; 29:215–222.

312. Stump D, Spock A, Grossman H: Vertebral sarcoidosis in adolescents. *Radiology* 1976; 121:153–155.

313. Suratt PM, Winn WC, Brody AR, et al: Acute silicosis in tombstone sandblasters. *Am Rev Respir Dis* 1977; 115:521–529.

314. Svanborg N: Studies on the cardiopulmonary function in sarcoidosis. *Acta Med Scand* [Suppl] 1961; 170:366.

315. Svendsen TL, Viskum K, Hansborg N, et al: Pulmonary lymphangioleiomyomatosis: A case of progesterone receptor positive lymphangioleiomyomatosis treated with medroxyprogesterone, oophorectomy and tamoxifen. *Br J Dis Chest* 1984; 78:264–271.

316. Symmons DPM, Woods KL: Recurrent sarcoidosis. *Thorax* 1980; 35:879.

317. Talbot FJ, Katz S, Matthews MJ: Bronchopulmonary sarcoidosis. Some unusual manifestations and the serious complications thereof. *Am J Med* 1959; 26:340–355.

318. Teirstein AS, Chuang M, Miller A, et al: Flexible-bronchoscope biopsy of lung and bronchial wall in intrathoracic sarcoidosis. *Ann NY Acad Sci* 1976; 278:522–527.

319. Teirstein AS, Siltzbach LE: Sarcoidosis of the upper lung fields simulating pulmonary tuberculosis. *Chest* 1973; 64:303–308.

320. Teirstein AS, Siltzbach LE, Berger H: Patterns of sarcoidosis in three population groups in New York City. *Ann NY Acad Sci* 1976; 278:371–376.

321. Tellis CJ, Putnam JS: Cavitation in large multinodular pulmonary disease. A rare manifestation of sarcoidosis. *Chest* 1977; 71:792–793.

322. Thind GS, Bhatia JL: Pulmonary alveolar microlithiasis. *Br J Dis Chest* 1978; 72:151–154.

323. Thomas JA, Janossy G, Chilosi M, et al: Combined immunological and histochemical analysis of skin and lymph node lesions in histiocytosis X. *J Clin Pathol* 1982; 35:327–337.

324. Thomas PD, Hunninghake GW: Current concepts of the pathogenesis of sarcoidosis. *Am Rev Respir Dis* 1987; 135:747–760.

325. Thurairajasingam S, Dharmasena BD, Kasthuriratna T: Pulmonary alveolar microlithiasis. *Australas Radiol* 1975; 19:175–180.

326. Tsou E, Romano MC, Kerwin DM, et al: Sarcoidosis of anterior mediastinal nodes, pancreas, and uterine cervix: Three unusual sites in the same patient. *Am Rev Respir Dis* 1980; 122:333–338.

327. Valensi QJ: Pulmonary lymphangiomyoma, a probable forme frust of tuberous sclerosis. *Am Rev Respir Dis* 1973; 108:1411–1415.

328. Viswanathan R: Pulmonary alveolar microlithiasis. *Thorax* 1962; 17:251–256.

329. Volle E, Kaufmann HJ: Pulmonary alveolar microlithiasis in pediatric patients—review of the world literature and two new observations. *Pediatr Radiol* 1987; 17:439–442.

330. Watts R, Thompson JR, Jasuja ML: Sarcoidosis presenting with massive pleural effusion. *IMJ* 1983; 163:57–58.

331. Webb WR, Goodman PC: Fibrosing alveolitis in patients with neurofibromatosis. *Radiology* 1977; 122:289–293.

332. Weber WN, Margolin FR, Nielsen SL: Pulmonary histiocytosis X. A review of 18 patients with reports of 6 cases. *AJR* 1969; 107:280–289.

333. Webster JR, Battifora H, Furey C, et al: Pulmonary alveolar proteinosis in two siblings with decreased immunoglobulin A. *Am J Med* 1980; 69:786–789.

334. Weisman RA, Canalis RF, Powell WJ: Laryngeal sarcoidosis with airway obstruction. *Ann Otol Rhinol Laryngol* 1980; 89:58–61.

335. Westcott JL, deGraff AC: Sarcoidosis, hilar adenopathy and pulmonary artery narrowing. *Radiology* 1973; 108:585–586.

336. Westcott JL, Noehren TH: Bronchial stenosis in chronic sarcoidosis. *Chest* 1973; 63:893–897.

337. Wigh R, Montague ED: Evaluation of intrapulmonic adenopathy in sarcoidosis. *Radiology* 1955; 64:810–817.

338. Wilen SB, Rabinowitz JG, Ulreich S, et al: Pleural involvement in sarcoidosis. *Am J Med* 1974; 57:200–209.

339. Winterbauer RH, Hutchinson JF: Use of pulmonary function tests in the management of sarcoidosis. *Chest* 1980; 78:640–647.

340. Winzelberg GG, Boller M, Sachs M, et al: CT evaluation of pulmonary alveolar microlithiasis. *J Comput Assist Tomogr* 1984; 8:1029–1031.

341. Wollschlager C, Khan F: Aspergillomas complicating sarcoidosis. A prospective study in 100 patients. *Chest* 1984; 86:585–588.

342. Wolson AH, Rohwedder JJ: Upper lobe fibrosis in ankylosing spondylitis. *AJR* 1975; 124:466–471.

343. Yotsumoto H, Hachiya J, Furuie T, et al: An estimation of computed tomography in detecting the intrathoracic changes of sarcoidosis, in Williams WJ, Davies BH (eds): *Eighth International Conference on Sarcoidosis and Other Granulomatous Diseases.* Cardiff, Wales, Alpha Omega Publishing, 1980, pp 386–393.

344. Young DA, Laman ML: Radiodense skeletal lesions in Boeck's sarcoid. *AJR* 1972; 114:553–558.

345. Zinkham WH: Multifocal eosinophilic granuloma. Natural history, etiology and management. *Am J Med* 1976; 60:457–463.

346. Ziskind M, Jones RN, Weill H: Silicosis. *Am Rev Respir Dis* 1976; 113:643–665.

347. Ziskind MM, Weill H, Payzant AR: The recognition and significance of acinus-filling processes of the lung. *Am Rev Respir Dis* 1963; 87:551–559.

13

Congenital Disorders of the Lungs and Airways

DEVELOPMENTAL LESIONS OF THE LUNGS

It is apparent from common clinical experience that congenital or developmental lesions of the lungs are neither as frequent nor, in general, as significant as their counterparts in the heart. Objective evidence from autopsy series supports this impression. For example, in a detailed analysis of over 2,000 autopsies Sotelo-Avila and Skanklin[76] showed that some form of major or minor congenital malformation occurred in 46% of cases. Of these, 30% were cardiovascular, 10% urinary, and only 3% respiratory.

Classification of congenital lesions of the lungs and airways is difficult because the embryogenesis of specific pulmonary malformations is often obscure. Classification is further complicated by associated congenital heart disease, which can lead to difficulty in deciding whether a particular malformation should be categorized as a lung lesion or as a cardiovascular anomaly. In this presentation, for example, unilateral pulmonary artery aplasia and the scimitar syndrome are included with pulmonary lesions, whereas the various forms of pulmonary atresia and anomalous pulmonary venous return are excluded.

The list presented in Table 13–1 is, therefore, just one of many arbitrary classifications. The conditions discussed in this or other chapters are given in italics, while less common or frankly rare conditions are only referenced. It must be recognized that though some of the conditions are not present at birth, they are nevertheless developmental in origin.

The fact that the lungs continue to form for an extended period of time after birth allows deleterious factors operating postnatally to affect their development, for example, in the Swyer-James syndrome and congenital bronchiectasis.

Tracheoesophageal Fistula

Most tracheoesophageal fistulas are associated with esophageal atresias and present in the neonatal period. They will not be discussed further. In rare instances, the so-called H-type tracheoesophageal fistula may not be detected until adult life even though symptoms may have been present from infancy.[77] The H-type fistula connects the adjacent trachea and esophagus, the fistula forming the transverse bar of the H (Fig 13–1). This type of fistula constitutes approximately 2% to 4% of all tracheoesophageal fistulae.[38, 87] The symptoms are recurrent aspiration, including paroxysmal coughing, feeding difficulties, and recurrent pneumonias. The pulmonary infiltrates seen on the chest radiograph reflect the extent and severity of the aspiration. Excessive quantities of air may pass through the fistula into the esophagus and on to the gut. In infants with H-type fistulas air esophagograms may be noted on the chest radiographs, and there may be unusual degrees of gaseous distention of the bowel.[83] Diagnosis of the condition by contrast studies of the esophagus can be difficult because the fistula may be relatively small, and aspiration through it may be intermit-

TABLE 13–1.

A Classification of Developmental Lesions of the Lungs*

Abnormalities of separation from foregut
Tracheoesophageal fistula
Bronchobiliary fistula[75]
Bronchogenic cyst
Tracheal diverticulum[40]
Bronchopulmonary foregut malformation[36]

Abnormal development of the branching outgrowth from foregut
Tracheal agenesis[86]
Tracheal stenosis[15]
Tracheal abnormalities in skeletal dysplasias[54]
Tracheomalacia and tracheobronchomegaly (Mounier-Kühn syndrome) (see Chapter 16)
Bronchial isomerism syndromes[53]
Tracheal bronchus, abnormal bronchial branching patterns
Bridging bronchus[33]
Bronchial atresia
Bronchial stenosis[17]
Bronchomalacia[58]
Bronchiectasis (see Chapter 16)
Congenital lobar emphysema
Absence (agenesis, aplasia) of the lungs or lobes of the lungs
Horseshoe lung[30]
Ectopia of the lungs[19]
Scimitar syndrome
Emphysema[39]
Hypoplasia of the lung
Potter syndrome (oligohydramnios tetrad)

Abnormalities of the pulmonary vasculature
Congenital pulmonary lymphangiectasis[28]
Scimitar syndrome
Pulmonary arteriovenous fistula
Tracheobronchial narrowing resulting from extrinsic vascular pressure-pulmonary sling, congenital absence of the pulmonary valves, vascular rings, etc.[57]
Pulmonary isomerism syndromes[53]
Pulmonary artery aplasia
Peripheral pulmonary stenosis[31]

Abnormalities related to a local or systemic biochemical or cellular defect
Pulmonary microlithiasis (see Chapter 12)
Immotile cilia syndrome (see Chapter 16)
Alpha₁-antitrypsin deficiency (see Chapter 16)
Fibrocystic disease (mucoviscidosis)
Chronic granulomatous disease

Abnormalities forming a component of a systemic familial or nonfamilial disease process
Hereditary telangiectasia
Pulmonary lymphangiomyomatosis (see Chapter 12)
Potter syndrome (oligohydramnios tetrad)
The yellow nail syndrome (see Chapter 14)

Familial abnormalities of the lungs
Familial primary pulmonary hypertension[73]
Familial spontaneous pneumothorax[56]
Familial fibrocystic pulmonary dysplasia[51]
Familial pulmonary fibrosis[43]

Ectopic or hamartomatous development. Hyperplasias.
Congenital cystic adenomatoid malformation
Intrapulmonary and extrapulmonary sequestration
Hamartomas of lung
Interstitial masses, hemangioma, thyroid[42]
Focal muscular hyperplasia of the trachea[6]

*Superscript numbers refer to the references listed at the conclusion of this chapter.

tent.[5] It is recommended that the patient be examined in the prone position, with lateral fluoroscopy and video recording. It is advantageous to inject the contrast material through a feeding tube as it is withdrawn along the length of the esophagus. In problem cases, thin suspensions of barium or nonionic water-soluble contrast media are useful with lateral radiography. The purpose of these measures is to encourage the contrast medium to enter the fistula.[81] In certain cases it may be necessary to repeat the contrast studies on more than one occasion in order to establish the diagnosis.[18] This clearly requires a high degree of suspicion and a dedication to proving the diagnosis.

There is a relatively high incidence of other congenital abnormalities in association with tracheoesophageal fistulae,[3] and this association may provide a clue to the presence of an H-type fistula. There is an extensive literature that describes the differing patterns of associated anomalies.[53, 54]

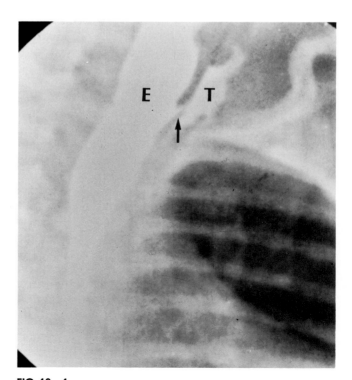

FIG 13–1.
H-type tracheoesophageal fistula in an infant. *Arrow* indicates fistula between the esophagus *(E)* and trachea *(T)*.

These patterns have been designated by a series of acronyms—the VATER complex (vertebral, anal, tracheoesophageal, and renal), the VACTEL complex (vertebral, anal, cardiac, tracheoesophageal, and limb), and the ARTICLE ± V complex (anal, renal, tracheal, intestinal, cardiac, limb, and esophageal ± vertebral). Other congenital pulmonary lesions such as pulmonary hypoplasia, tracheal stenosis, and pulmonary sequestration occur in approximately 2% of patients with these complexes.[84]

Bronchogenic Cyst

Bronchogenic cysts (synonym; bronchial cysts) are uncommon, usually isolated, lesions representing a cystic reduplication of the tracheobronchial tree. The cysts are lined with respiratory epithelium and contain mucoid material that may be remarkably viscid. Most bronchogenic cysts arise in the mediastinum or hilar regions. In one large series, over 85% of all bronchogenic cysts were found to be centrally located, with fewer than 15% being truely intraparenchymal.[69] Most bronchogenic cysts are asymptomatic and are detected on routine screening chest radiographs[49] usually before the patients' 4th decade.[72] Bronchogenic cysts may become manifest clinically as result of infection or hemorrhage into the cyst (Fig 13–2). Complications related to the bulk of

the cyst are relatively uncommon despite the central location.[72] On rare occasions, usually in infancy, a bronchogenic cyst may undergo rapid inflation with air, presumably through a check valve mechanism (Fig 13–3). In these cases the compressive effects may cause a surgical emergency.[23, 89]

On the chest radiograph a bronchogenic cyst is usually seen as a mass in the mediastinum or hilus (Fig 13–4). Those margins of the lesion that can be defined are usually well circumscribed. Bronchial cysts have a certain plasticity and mould around normal anatomic structures, a feature that may account for the paucity of pressure effects. Calcification, either rim calcification or calcification of the contents, has been described[9, 29] but is quite exceptional. Cavitation may occur, and this is frequently a complication of infection of the cyst contents. If the cyst contains air, the smooth, thin wall and the central location of the cavity should indicate its nature and should permit distinction from primary abscess formation.

In the past, barium swallow examination has been extensively used to define the size and position of mediastinal mass lesions. Computed tomography has diminished the role of esophagography, the extent to which each is used being to some extent dependent on the facilities available. The esophagogram may exclude intrinsic lesions of the esophagus

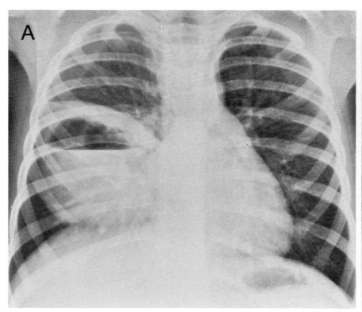

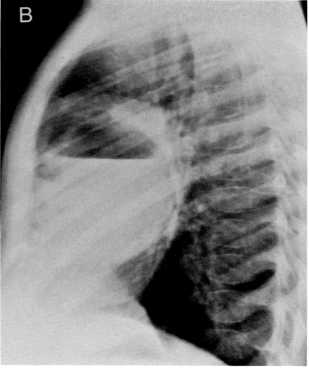

FIG 13–2.
Infected bronchogenic cyst in a child. Cyst wall is considerably thickened by inflammation. **A,** PA view. **B,** lateral view.

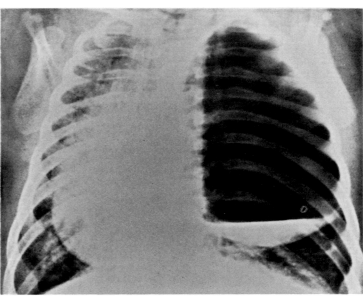

FIG 13–3.
Huge expansile bronchogenic cyst in an infant. Note the marked mediastinal shift and fluid in the bottom of the cyst (*c.f.* congenital lobar emphysema). (Courtesy of Dr. Harold Jacobson, New York.)

such as leiomyomas. Bronchogenic cysts cause the smooth displacement of the esophagus, characteristic of an extrinsic mass. CT examination is, however, much more definitive. The smooth-walled cystic nature of the lesion is readily apparent, and the position of the cyst and the way it moulds to adjacent structures can be clearly visualized (Fig 13–5). In these instances, CT scanning not only confirms the diagnosis but helps to guide the surgical removal. One might expect a "cyst" to have a CT density close to that of water (i.e., 0 Hounsfield units [HU]). In fact, the densities are usually higher, in the range of 20 to 80 HU.[62, 65] This presumably reflects the proteinaceous content of the cyst, a feature that can be accentuated by hemorrhage and infection. Up to the time of writing, there has been only one published

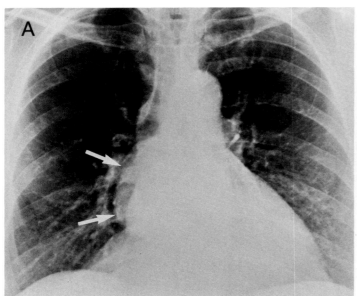

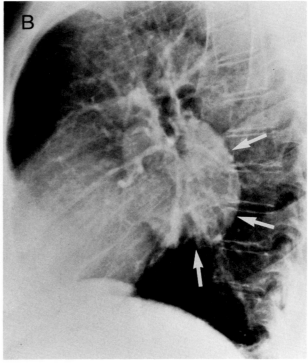

FIG 13–4.
Large central bronchogenic cyst *(arrows)* in an asymptomatic adult. **A,** PA view. **B,** lateral view.

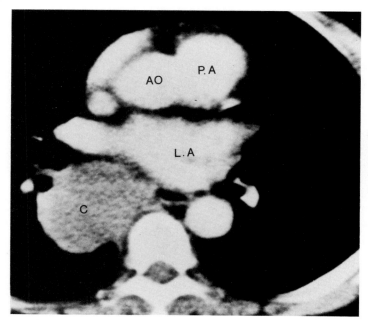

FIG 13—5.
Bronchogenic cyst demonstrated by CT scanning. *C* = cyst; *PA* = pulmonary artery; *AO* = aorta; *LA* = left atrium. Note that the cyst has a CT density comparable to that of the paraspinal muscles.

report of the diagnosis of a bronchogenic cyst using magnetic resonance imaging (MRI).[11] In this case the actual appearance of the cyst on the MR images corresponded exactly to the CT images of the same patient. However, unlike CT, MRI enabled one to distinguish mucoid bronchial plugs from vessels distal to the cyst. Real-time ultrasound has also been used in the diagnosis of mediastinal bronchogenic cysts in children (Fig 13–6). In two cases described in the literature, one lesion was clearly cystic whereas the second was an echogenic solid-appearing mass.[71]

The uncomplicated peripheral pulmonary bronchogenic cyst is an extremely well circumscribed solitary lung mass that shows little or no temporal increase in size. Complicating infection may result in communication of the cyst with the bronchial tree and the development of an air-fluid level within a smooth, thin-walled cavity. Some peripheral bronchogenic cysts have a systemic arterial supply and, therefore, may represent a form of pulmonary sequestration.[13, 14] Certainly a surgeon would be advised to consider the possibility of a systemic arterial supply in cases requiring resection.

Tracheomalacia

The term tracheomalacia implies an abnormal degree of compliance of the trachea, which tends to narrow when subjected to unusually negative intratracheal pressures during inspiration or unusually positive extratracheal pressures during expiration. Wittenborg et al.[91] have demonstrated that in most instances collapse of the trachea is a normal response to abnormal pressures (e.g., secondary to localized tracheal or laryngeal obstruction in infants or to abnormal external pressures in obstructive lung disease). True tracheomalacia secondary to defects in the supporting cartilaginous structures is rare.[54]

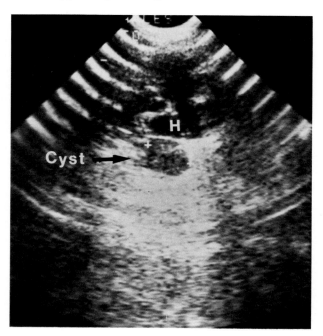

FIG 13—6.
Frame from real-time ultrasound scan of a bronchogenic cyst *(arrow).* The ribs produce the linear echoes. The heart chambers *(H)* are echolucent. The lung is echo reflective. Note that the cyst contains diffuse internal echoes.

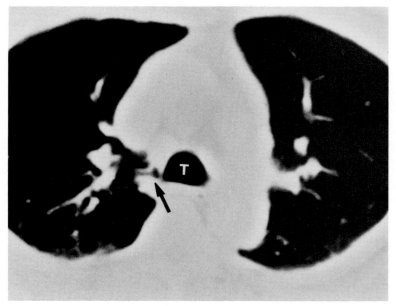

FIG 13–7.
CT demonstration of an accessory bronchus *(arrow)* to
the right upper lobe arising from the lower trachea *(T)*.

This type is usually associated with more severe congenital malformations and the tracheal abnormalities are discovered at autopsy.

Tracheal Bronchus; Abnormal Bronchial Branching Patterns

In general, the bronchial branching pattern is remarkably uniform. Major additive or subtractive bronchial anomalies are rare. Bronchography and bronchoscopy are the only methods of diagnosing such anomalies during the life of the patient. Atwell[2] analyzed 1,200 bronchograms and found only 23 with a major extra bronchial branch (Fig 13–7) and 4 with absence of a major bronchial branch. Minor bronchial branch anomalies were, however, fairly frequent, occurring in 104 cases, including 88 cases of double-stem superior-segment bronchi to the lower lobes (Fig 13–8).[2] These figures suggest that virtually 90% of the population have the standard textbook pattern of division. Most anomalous divisions have no clinical significance, though they may be confusing to the bronchoscopist searching for landmarks. Mangiulea and Stingha suggest that the accessory cardiac bronchus increases liability to infection (Fig 13–9),[61] and Remy et al.[70] found focal emphysema, presumably secondary to pulmonary artery compression, in left apicoposterior segments which arose more proximally from the left main bronchus.

Bronchial Atresia

This rare and benign condition produces a characteristic triad of radiographic findings:

1. A localized central mass density representing mucoid impaction in the bronchus distal to the focal atresia of the segmental bronchus.

2. Emphysema of the affected segment of lung—because the central bronchus is atretic, the aeration of the lung presumably occurs through collateral air drift.

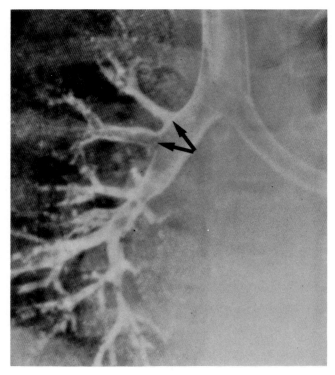

FIG 13–8.
Bronchographic demonstration of a double-stem right upper lobe bronchus *(arrows)* in an infant.

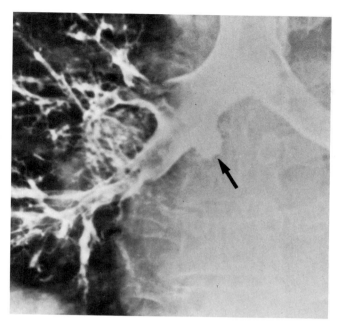

FIG 13—9.
Bronchographic demonstration of an accessory cardiac bronchus *(arrow)* largely occluded by secretions.

3. Hypoperfusion of the affected segment as indicated by a paucity of vessels in that segment (Fig 13–10).

Meng et al.[63] reviewed 36 cases of bronchial atresia and found 24 with involvement of the left upper lobe and 7 with involvement of the right upper lobe. In the affected upper lobes it is almost invariably the apical or apicoposterior segments that are involved. The clinical significance of the condition is minimal. Its importance lies in the fact that the dilated mucus-filled bronchus distal to the atresia may be misdiagnosed as a neoplasm or other significant lesion.

Congenital Lobar Emphysema

Some form of aplasia, hypoplasia, or dysplasia of bronchial supporting structures is postulated as the primary cause of congenital lobar emphysema,[80] although it has proved difficult to determine the precise cause of the obstruction in resected specimens. The congenital nature of the condition has never been unequivocally established despite the fact that the circumstantial evidence is strong. There is a definite association with congenital heart disease.[37] There is also an interesting infrequent fluid-filled form of the condition thought to be the result of amniotic fluid trapped behind an obstructed bronchus.[24]

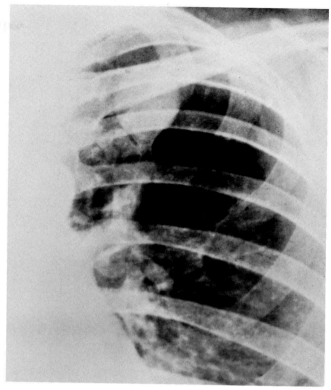

FIG 13—10.
Bronchial atresia producing an ovoid upper lobe mass representing a mucocele. Note hyperlucent lung surrounding the mucocele and paucity of lung vessels in this region.

Most cases of congenital lobar emphysema present in the neonatal period with respiratory distress, which may be life-threatening. In as many as 25% of cases, however, presentation is delayed until after the 1st month of life.

The classic, and by far the most common, radiographic appearance is hyperexpansion of an isolated lobe in one lung, usually an upper or middle lobe (Figs 13–11 and 13–12). Remarkably, the lower lobes are involved only in some 2% of all cases. Involvement of more than one lobe is equally exceptional.[37] The expanded lobe may cause compression atelectasis of the rest of the lung, accompanied by displacement of the heart, mediastinum, and diaphragm. The main differential diagnoses include localized pneumothorax and an expanding lung cyst. Careful study of the images should reveal the presence of blood vessels within the expanded lobes in cases of lobar emphysema. Pulmonary interstitial emphysema, an acquired condition, most commonly seen in babies receiving positive pressure ventilation, may affect a single lobe and closely resemble congenital lobar emphysema radiographically. Clinically, the conditions are different in that interstitial

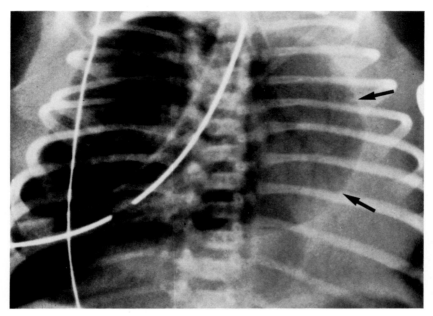

FIG 13–11.
Congenital lobar emphysema involving right upper lobe. Note the marked mediastinal shift and the mediastinal herniation *(arrows)* of the hyperexpanded lobe.

emphysema usually occurs in children who are already on ventilators because of previously known diffuse lung disease. Mucus obstruction of a bronchus occasionally leads to obstructive overinflation, which can be radiographically identical to congenital lobar emphysema. Bronchoscopy to exclude a mucus plug is, therefore, performed prior to surgical resection of any overexpanded lobe. Acute inflation of a bronchogenic cyst has already been discussed.

Congenital lobar emphysema may present initially as a fluid-filled form with the same tendency to expand.[24] Radiographically this form presents as an expansile mass of soft tissue density. Compression of the remainder of the lung and displacement of the mediastinum may occur exactly as with the more usual hyperinflated form. The entrapped fluid may drain, and conversion to the more conventional form of lobar emphysema ensues. On rare occasions, a transitional phase between the fluid-filled and the air-filled forms may be encountered.[1] In the transitional form there are linear interstitial markings resembling septal lines in the hyperexpanded lobe. These gradually clear—presumably as fluid drains or is absorbed. Resection of the affected lobe may be necessary; otherwise, a policy of nonintervention is adopted with close radiographic control in the hope that the condition will resolve.[74]

Absence (Agenesis, Aplasia) of the Lungs or Lobes of the Lungs

Unilateral absence of a lung or a lobe is a rare congenital abnormality, which in itself may cause surprisingly few clinical problems.[47, 60] Indeed, absence of a lung may be encountered de novo in an adult without that individual experiencing symptoms referable to the chest (Fig 13–13). The condition frequently occurs, however, in association with other congenital abnormalities, particularly those complexes associated with tracheoesophageal fistulas. Nearly 10% of patients with tracheobronchial malformations have unilateral pulmonary agenesis. Interestingly, there appears to be a strong association between agenesis of the right lung and esophageal atresia,[8, 12] whereas in cases of isolated tracheoesophageal fistulas without esophageal atresia the left lung is predominantly affected.[60] Absence of a lobe of a lung is less common and simulates pulmonary hypoplasia.

As one might expect, the findings in absence of a lung are absence of aeration of the lung on that side. Volume loss is manifested by elevation of the ipsilateral hemidiaphragm and shift of the mediastinum toward that side, with herniation of the opposite lung anteriorly (Fig 13–14). The principal differential diagnosis is acquired total lung collapse; further investigation with tomography, bronchography, or

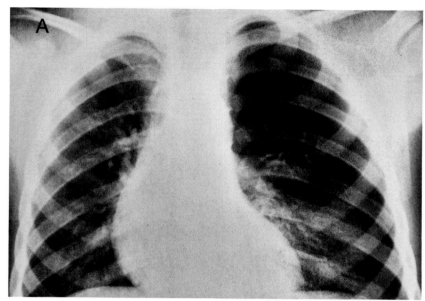

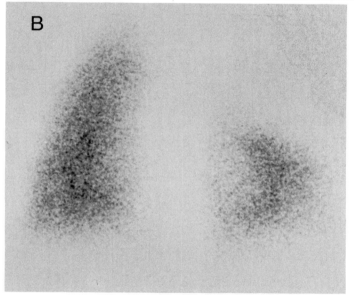

FIG 13–12.
A, PA radiograph. **B,** radionuclide ventilation scan in a 4-year-old boy with surgically proven congenital lobar emphysema of the left upper lobe.

angiography may be required in order to make the distinction. The ipsilateral pulmonary artery will be completely absent, and the bronchus to the affected lung or lobe will be either totally absent (agenesis) or rudimentary (aplasia).[26] In isolated absence of a lobe there is compensatory expansion of the remaining lobe or lobes with consequent distortion of the bronchovascular structures. The compensatory expansion is never complete, and lung volume is reduced on the affected side. As in diffuse pulmonary hypoplasia, areolar tissue and fat may occupy the anterior part of the affected hemithorax and may serve to compensate for the volume loss in the underlying lung. The chest radiographic findings in the absence

of a lobe are indistinguishable from those of generalized pulmonary hypoplasia and are dealt with under that heading. Bronchography will identify absence of a lobe by demonstrating agenesis or aplasia of the lobar bronchus with an otherwise normal bronchial tree.[26] In pulmonary hypoplasia, on the other hand, there should be an appropriate number of lobes, but the bronchial tree will be stunted and deformed.

In the infant with associated congenital abnormalities, the diagnosis of absence of a lung may be more readily apparent than in the adult, but the clinical significance of the lesion is likely to be overshadowed by the other abnormalities.

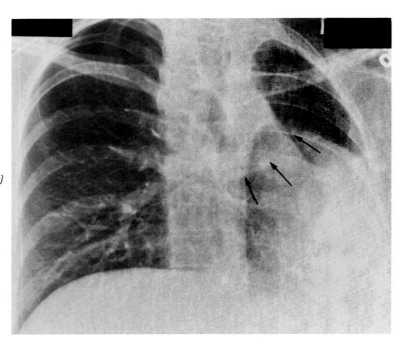

FIG 13-13.
Routine radiograph in an asymptomatic man reveals aplasia of the left lung. Right upper lobe vessels *(arrows)* course to the left apex, with the heart positioned in the left posterior portion of the chest.

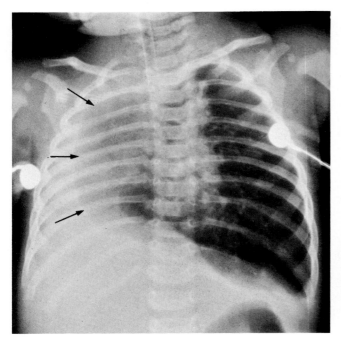

FIG 13-14.
Agenesis of the right lung in an infant showing shift of the heart into the right chest, elevation of the right hemidiaphragm, and herniation of the left lung *(arrows).*

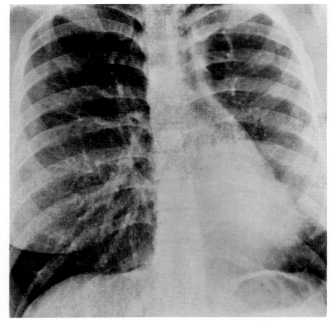

FIG 13-15.
Routine chest radiograph in an asymptomatic man with aplasia of the left pulmonary artery. The aortic arch is right sided.

Isolated aplasia of a pulmonary artery produces few, if any, clinical problems other than potential difficulties in interpreting the chest radiograph. The affected lung is of normal volume, but the pulmonary vasculature is remarkably diminished (Figs 13–15 and 13–16). The vasculature in the normal lung may appear correspondingly plethoric because the entire cardiac output is shunted through that lung. The abnormal perfusion of the lungs presumably contributes to a relative hyperlucency of the affected lung. Radioisotope ventilation/perfusion scanning will readily demonstrate the total absence of perfusion and the normal ventilation of the lung. Acquired conditions may, however, closely mimic aplasia of a pulmonary artery. Patients with the Swyer-James syndrome (see Chapter 16) should have demonstrably abnormal ventilation of the affected lung. Fibrosing mediastinitis may, on occasion, be indistinguishable radiographically from unilateral pulmonary artery aplasia. There may, however, be strong clinical pointers in favor of fibrosing mediastinitis, including a tendency for the patient's condition to worsen. Further studies such as angiography or ventilation/perfusion scanning will usually indicate bilateral pulmonary vascular abnormalities.

The Scimitar Syndrome

The alternative designation for this condition, namely, "hypogenetic lung syndrome," emphasizes that this anomaly is not simply a variant of partial anomalous pulmonary venous return but a more widespread malformation. The condition is confined to the right lung. The lung is hypoplastic, both the bronchial tree and the vascular structures in the lung being underdeveloped.[25, 66] The bronchial tree on the involved side is stunted, and the pulmonary arterial supply may derive in much greater proportion than normal from systemic arteries. The pulmonary arteries are correspondingly hypoplastic. The syndrome derives its name from the anomalous pulmonary vein that descends vertically in the lung before curving medially to enter the upper inferior vena cava. The vein broadens as it curves downward, resulting in a configuration resembling a scimitar (Fig 13–17).

The anomalously draining vein is readily visible on chest radiographs both in the frontal and lateral projections. One should also observe the associated features of reduced lung volume together with dextroposition of the heart and the abnormal bronchovascular pattern in the right hilus. If these features are present, the diagnosis of hypogenetic lung syndrome may be made with total confidence. Partial anomalous pulmonary venous return to the inferior vena cava, right atrium, or coronary sinus may occur without pulmonary hypoplasia, particularly in association with intracardiac lesions such as an atrial septal defect. The key distinguishing feature in these cases is the absence of radiographic evidence of pulmonary hypoplasia.

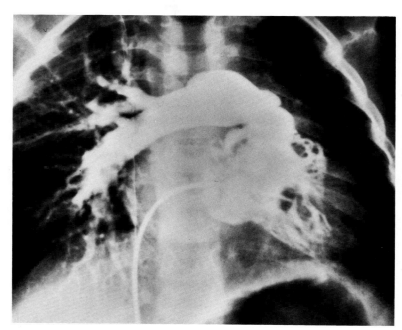

FIG 13–16.
Right ventricular angiogram in infant with aplasia of the left pulmonary artery. Left lung was normally ventilated.

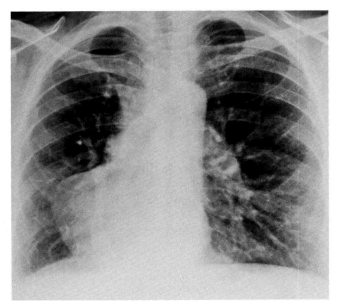

FIG 13—17.
Scimitar syndrome. Note dextropositioned heart, stunted pulmonary vascular pattern in the right lung, and scimitar-shaped vein coursing behind the heart toward the inferior vena cava.

Pulmonary Hypoplasia and the Potter Syndrome

Unilateral primary hypoplasia without accompanying scimitar syndrome is rare. Associated anomalies may be present in other body systems, and these may ultimately determine the prognosis. The patients may be asymptomatic or have recurrent episodes of wheezing and pneumonia.

More commonly pulmonary hypoplasia is secondary to any condition that stunts the growth of the lung or lungs in utero. A classic example is the pulmonary hypoplasia that may result from a congenital diaphragmatic hernia. The underlying lung exhibits varying degrees of hypoplasia depending on the size of the hernia and the period over which pressure effects on the lung were operative. The basic problem in these cases is lack of space for growth and development of the lung. The extent of the hypoplasia may be a critical determinant of survival following repair of the hernia.

The fetal lung communicates freely with the amniotic sac, and the fetus is known to exhibit respiratory movement in utero. The developing lung, therefore, contains amniotic fluid. The fact that this fluid exerts an important influence on pulmonary embryogenesis is evidenced by infants with Potter's syndrome[67] (oligohydramnios tetrad). The oligohydramnios in these infants is the result of an abnormality in the development of the urinary tract, most

commonly renal agenesis. The full tetrad consists of (1) the underlying renal abnormality that causes the oligohydramnios, (2) abnormal facies resulting from pressure effects in utero, (3) abnormal laxity of the skin, and (4) pulmonary hypoplasia.[27] There is debate as to whether the pulmonary hypoplasia results from a reduction in the amount of amniotic fluid actually within the developing lung or whether it is secondary to external pressure effects on the developing thorax. Clearly both factors could operate together.

Primary unilateral pulmonary hypoplasia may be encountered in a child or an adult. The affected lung is small, and the mediastinum is displaced toward that side. The pulmonary vascular pattern may be seen to be deformed and stunted. The lateral chest film often shows a sharply marginated opacity behind and parallel to the sternum, an appearance similar to that seen in left upper lobe collapse or combined right upper and middle lobe collapse. There is, however, no wedge or fan of tissue connected to the hilus. This retrosternal density represents extra pleural areolar tissue occupying the space that should have been occupied by lung. The presence of this tissue adjacent to the heart and mediastinum frequently results in lack of definition of these borders on the affected side (Fig 13—18).

Although the extent of secondary pulmonary hypoplasia may be a critical factor in determining survival, for example, after the repair of a diaphragmatic hernia, the radiograph does not give a reliable indication of the possible outcome. It is clearly ominous if the lung fails to expand following relief of the pressure effects.

Chronic Granulomatous Disease

In chronic granulomatous disease a hereditary leucocyte defect results in recurrent infections with catalase-positive low-grade pyogenic organisms. Host defense against these organisms devolves upon the macrophages, with a resultant granulomatous response. The leucocyte defect, which is inherited in the majority of cases as an X-linked recessive trait, appears to be an inability to produce the hydrogen peroxide necessary for the destruction of certain organisms (e.g., coagulase-positive staphylococci, *Escherichia coli* and *Serratia marcescens*.).[46] The defective leucocytes are capable of phagocytosing but not killing these organisms, which may indeed be protected from circulating antibiotics by their intracellular position.[41]

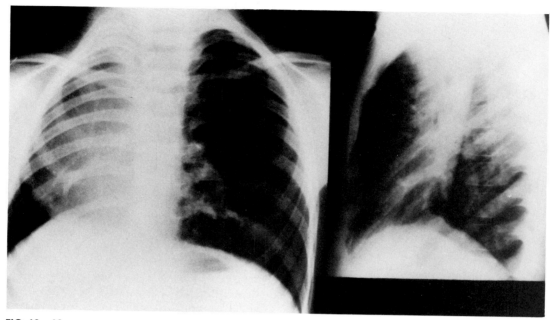

FIG 13–18.
Frontal and lateral chest radiographs in infant with hypoplasia of the left lung. Note the volume reduction and the retrosternal soft-tissue density.

Clinically, patients have recurrent skin infections, osteomyelitis, lymphadenopathy, hepatosplenomegaly, persistent rhinitis, and recurrent pneumonia.

The pneumonias are randomly distributed and

recurrent. Response to antibiotic therapy is slow and often incomplete, with residual chronic scarring in the lungs (Fig 13–19). Hilar adenopathy is often a prominent feature.[91] Chronic granulomatous disease, however, has ordinarily been diagnosed clini-

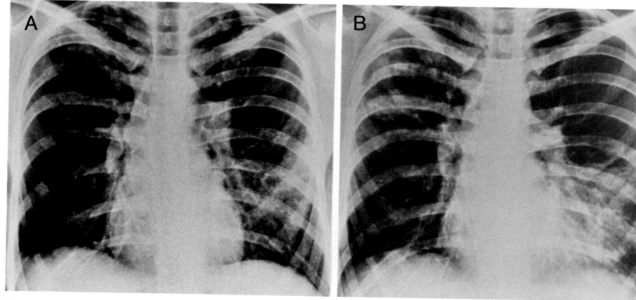

FIG 13–19.
Chronic granulomatous disease over a 5-year period of observation in a young adult man. **A,** some patchy infiltrates are in right upper lobe; there is lingular pneumonia. **B,** 5 years later, there is patchy pulmonary infiltration and scarring, notably in the apices and left base.

TABLE 13–2.

Differentiation of Extralobar and Intralobar Pulmonary Sequestration*

Parameter	Extralobar Sequestration	Intralobar Sequestration
Relation to normal lung	Separate with own pleural covering	Within the normal lung and its pleural cover
Venous drainage	Systemic	Pulmonary
Side affected	Left 90%	Left 60% to 70%
Associated congenital anomalies	Frequent	Uncommon
Age at diagnosis	60%, 1 yr	50%, 20 yr
Sex ratio	M:F = 4:1	M = F
Infection and/or communication with normal lung	Rare	Common

*Modified from De Parades CG, Pierce WS, Johnson DG, et al: Pulmonary sequestration in infants and children: A 20 year experience and review of the literature. *Pediatr Surg* 1970; 5:136–147.

cally and by specialized leucocyte studies. The role of chest radiography is primarily to diagnose and follow the recurrent pneumonias.

Pulmonary Sequestration

Pulmonary sequestration is defined as the presence of an abnormal mass of pulmonary tissue that does not communicate with the tracheobronchial tree through a normal bronchial connection and which receives its blood supply via an anomalous systemic artery. The arterial supply may arise from the descending thoracic aorta or from the abdominal aorta or one of its branches. Pulmonary sequestrations are often divided into intralobar and extralobar types,[79] the intralobar variety being much more common. However, it is important to realize that one may encounter variants that do not fit neatly into these two categories.[10] The differentiating features are best summarized in tabular form (Table 13–2).[21]

Intralobar sequestrations produce symptoms only when they become infected, usually in adolescence or in early adult life. Extralobar sequestrations are usually asymptomatic and are often discovered

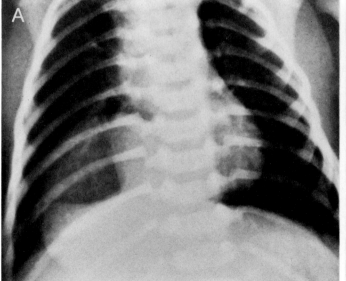
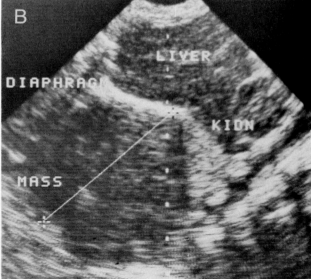

FIG 13–20.

A and **B,** extralobar sequestration in infant. Well-circumscribed right posterior basal mass lesion (**A**) is shown by ultrasound (**B**) to be a solid mass.

incidentally during surgical repair of a congenital diaphragmatic hernia, with which they are frequently associated.

The appearances on plain chest radiograph are typically those of an opacity situated at one or other base posteromedially (Fig 13–20). There is a distinct affinity for the left side. In the uncomplicated lesion, the mass is uniformly dense. With the extralobar variety, the lateral margin is well-defined because of the pleural envelope, whereas medially the lesion abuts the mediastinum so closely that it is usually confused with a mediastinal mass. The intralobar variety often has more ill-defined margins and resembles an area of pneumonia, though it may have rounded or lobulated contours and resemble an intrapulmonary mass (Fig 13–21). On occasion, one or more air-fluid levels will be seen within sequestrated segments. Such air-fluid levels are a consequence of infection with fistula formation to the adjacent lung.

The demonstration of a systemic artery supplying the lesion is the critical diagnostic feature. This can be readily demonstrated by aortography and particularly by selective angiography which will also demonstrate the venous drainage (Figs 13–22 and 13–23). Arteriography is particularly important if surgical treatment is being considered, because inadvertent damage to the artery during surgery can

cause significant hemorrhage.[16] The systemic artery can also be demonstrated by CT using intravenous contrast enhancement[64] or, on occasion, by ultrasound.[48, 82] The systemic vascular perfusion of pulmonary sequestrations has also been demonstrated by comparison of the pulmonary and systemic phases at radionuclide angiography.[34, 50]

A cystic form of pulmonary sequestration may be encountered. This may be caused by infection of a previously solid mass with subsequent communication to the adjacent lung (Fig 13–24). Reference has already been made to a possible overlap with peripheral bronchogenic cysts.[20] The presence or absence of a systemic arterial supply is the critical feature in such instances. The infected communicating pulmonary sequestration may contain fluid levels and lack definition because of inflammatory changes in adjacent lung. Indeed, the appearances may exactly mimic a simple lung abscess, and only the position of the lesion and the clinical circumstances may lead one to suspect an infected pulmonary sequestration. On the other hand, many cavitated sequestrations are sterile at the time of presentation or surgical removal. Communication with the bronchial tree may be demonstrated by bronchography but, in practice, bronchography is of limited value in evaluating bronchopulmonary sequestration. On rare occasions,

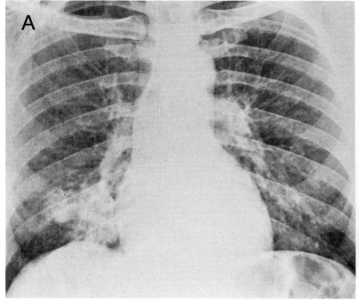
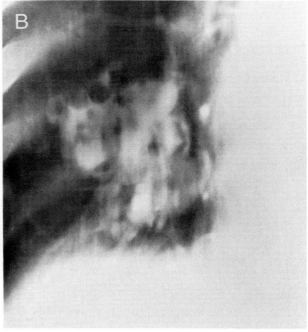

FIG 13–21.
A and **B,** intralobar sequestration in right lower lobe. The lobulated mass contains some air spaces indicating communication with the bronchial tree.

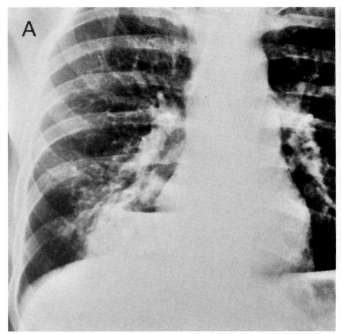

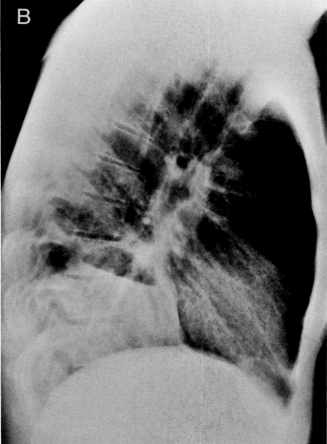

FIG 13–22.
PA (**A**) and lateral (**B**) radiographs of a young man who presented with sudden onset of fever and cough (see Fig 13–23).

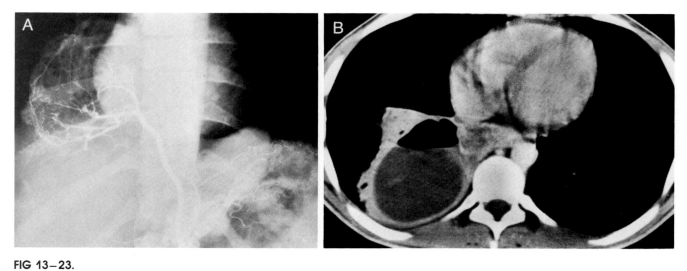

FIG 13–23.
A, same patient as in Figure 13–22. Large feeding vessel arising from abdominal aorta supplies an intralobar sequestration. **B,** this vessel was not visualized on the CT examination.

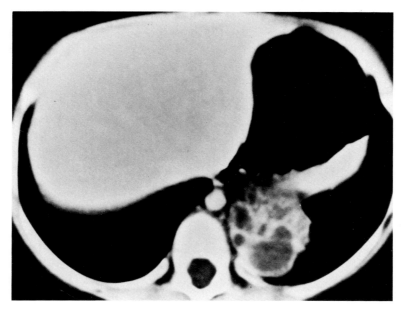

FIG 13–24.
A cystic form of intralobar sequestration demonstrated by CT scanning.

calcifications may occur in pulmonary sequestration and are readily detected by CT.[85] The differential diagnosis of lower paravertebral masses would include neurogenic tumors and lateral meningoceles. In these lesions pressure erosions of the vertebrae and the proximal ribs may be observed, a finding not seen with pulmonary sequestration. Other paravertebral masses such as extramedullary hematopoiesis or pleural tumors may be indistinguishable from pulmonary sequestration. In essence, the diagnosis of pulmonary sequestration depends as much on the position of the lesion and the clinical features as on the radiographic appearances alone.

Pulmonary Hamartomata

A hamartoma is a benign tumor composed of an agglomeration of tissues normally encountered in the organ in which it is found. Pathologically, pulmonary hamartomas are effectively benign pulmonary chondromas.[4] The cartilage content of these tumors allows definite diagnosis by percutaneous needle biopsy[35] and also results on occasion in a characteristic pattern of calcification (Fig 13–25). According to this definition of a hamartoma, cystic adenomatoid malformation of the lung is a hamartomatous lesion. However, it is clinically, radiologically, and pathologically distinct from the classic pulmonary hamartoma and is considered separately.

The pulmonary hamartoma is assumed to be a congenital lesion, although it virtually never mani-

fests itself during childhood.[44] This lesion is usually asymptomatic and is discovered by chance on radiographs. Some 8% to 12% may be central and endobronchial in position[52] and may cause problems comparable to those caused by bronchial adenomas. Most are isolated peripheral lung tumors with well-

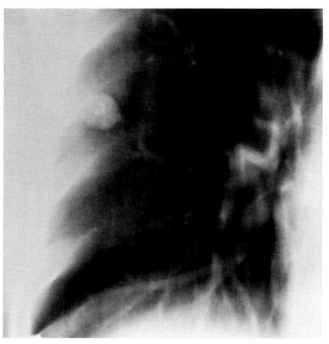

FIG 13–25.
Pulmonary hamartoma showing a central nidus of calcification.

circumscribed often lobulated margins. Only in exceptional cases is more than one hamartoma encountered.[7] Chondroid calcification has a characteristic pattern described as a series of rings and whorls. In the pulmonary hamartoma a central focus of popcorn-like calcification is highly characteristic and diagnostic. However, calcification is stated to occur in no more than 5% of hamartomas.[55] Thus, in many cases, no specific diagnostic features are apparent on the chest radiograph. Ledor et al. studied the CT characteristics in one surgically proven case of pulmonary hamartoma and found that the lesion had attenuation characteristics indicating a high fat content,[55] a previously described histologic feature of hamartomas.[4] These authors suggest that a fatty lung tumor probably represents either a pleural lipoma or a hamartoma, in both instances benign lesions. It is important to realize that growth occurs in these lesions as, indeed, it must, if they are to become visible in the first place. Growth is usually very slow but on occasion may be unexpectedly rapid, and a hamartoma may overlap slow-growing malignancies.[45] Pulmonary hamartomas are frequently removed surgically as a precaution, thereby grouping them with granulomas and infarcts as benign lesions that may be removed for perfectly valid reasons. However, percutaneous biopsy can obviate the need for surgical removal.[35] Central endobronchial hamartomas causing significant pressure effects may be identified by the presence of atelectasis or postobstructive pneumonia. In theory at least calcification in the tumor might allow identification; however, confusion with the far more common nodal calcification of granulomatous disease seems likely.

Pulmonary Arteriovenous Fistulae

Pulmonary arteriovenous fistulas may be single or multiple as part of Rendu-Osler-Weber disease (hereditary telangiectasia). They may be associated with other congenital abnormalities, notably cardiac malformations. In infants and children the lesions may be large enough to cause a detectable bruit and enough right to left shunting to produce cyanosis (Fig 13–26). More usually, however, pulmonary arteriovenous fistulae are occult and are discovered by chance or during investigation of a patient with known Rendu-Osler-Weber disease. On occasion, the patient may present with systemic abscesses or infarction, notably of the brain, because the right-to-left shunting of blood bypasses the lung filter[32] (Fig 13–27).

On plain chest radiographs an arteriovenous malformation is seen as a pulmonary nodule that usually has a lobulated outline. In peripheral lesions, the vessels feeding and draining the fistula can usually be seen on plain films—and this feature may be confirmed, if necessary, by conventional tomography

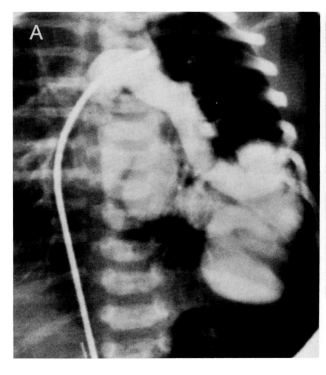
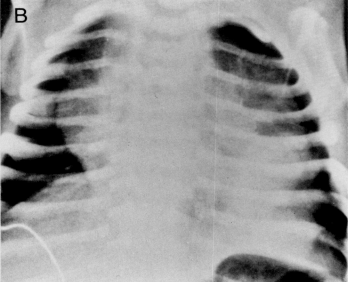

FIG 13–26.
Lateral (**A**) and PA (**B**) views of pulmonary arteriovenous fistula demonstrated by pulmonary arteriography in a cyanotic infant.

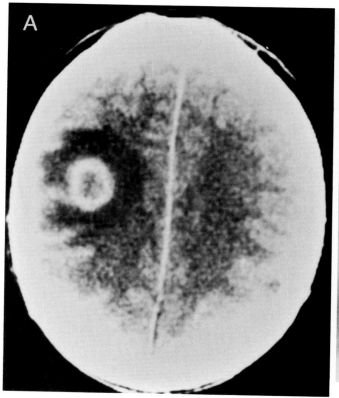

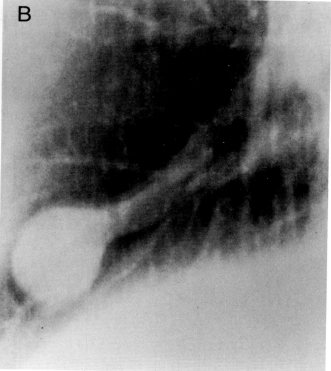

FIG 13–27.
A, brain abscess demonstrated by CT scan in a previously healthy young man. **B,** tomogram of same individual shows a large arteriovenous malformation in the right lung. (Courtesy Dr. Bech-Olsen, Tonsberg, Norway.)

or CT scanning. Contrast-enhanced CT[68] or pulmonary angiography can be used not only to opacify the malformation in order to confirm the diagnosis but also to search for additional lesions elsewhere in the lungs, particularly in those cases where surgical excision is contemplated (Fig 13–28). Selective vascular occlusion using, for example, detachable balloons is an alternative method of treatment, and this requires pulmonary arteriography prior to occlusive therapy.

Multiple lesions may be confused with metastases if the enlarged feeding vessels are overlooked[22] (Fig 13–29).

Congenital Cystic Adenomatoid Malformation of the Lung

This rare life-threatening condition almost invariably manifests itself in the neonatal period. The basic lesion is a hamartomatous mass of fibrous tissue and smooth muscle usually containing numerous cystic spaces lined with bronchial or cuboidal epithelium.[78] Unlike the classic pulmonary hamartoma, cartilage is notably absent from the lesion. The process usually involves just one lobe. Involvement of more than one lobe or bilaterality is exceedingly rare. It is the expansile nature of the lesion that is life-threatening, a feature frequently compounded by secondary hypoplasia of the uninvolved lung.

Radiographically, one observes a marked expansion of what appears to be one entire lung with a shift of the mediastinum and compression of the contralateral lung. The involved lung is composed of opaque tissue interspersed with cystic, air-containing spaces of varying size which may contain fluid levels (Fig 13–30). Occasionally a single cyst predominates.[59] The lesion may initially appear solid if the radiograph is obtained before the fetal lung fluid has drained; it will appear cystic only where air replaces the fluid. The similarity to a congenital diaphragmatic hernia can on occasion be quite striking. In diaphragmatic hernia the abdomen tends to be scaphoid with a paucity of gas shadows in the abdomen. In congenital cystic adenomatoid malformation of the lung, both the abdominal gas pattern and the shape of the abdomen are normal. Immediate diag-

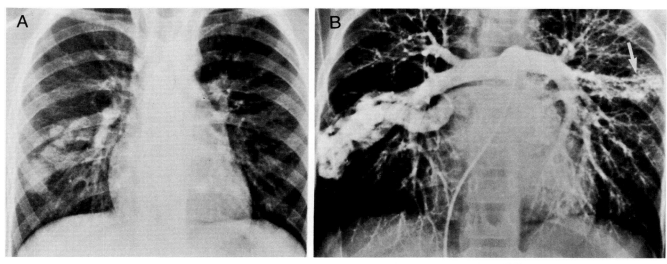

FIG 13–28.
A, large arteriovenous malformation in the right lung. No other lesion could be identified with certainty. **B,** pulmonary arteriography reveals a second arteriovenous malformation in the left midzone *(arrow).*

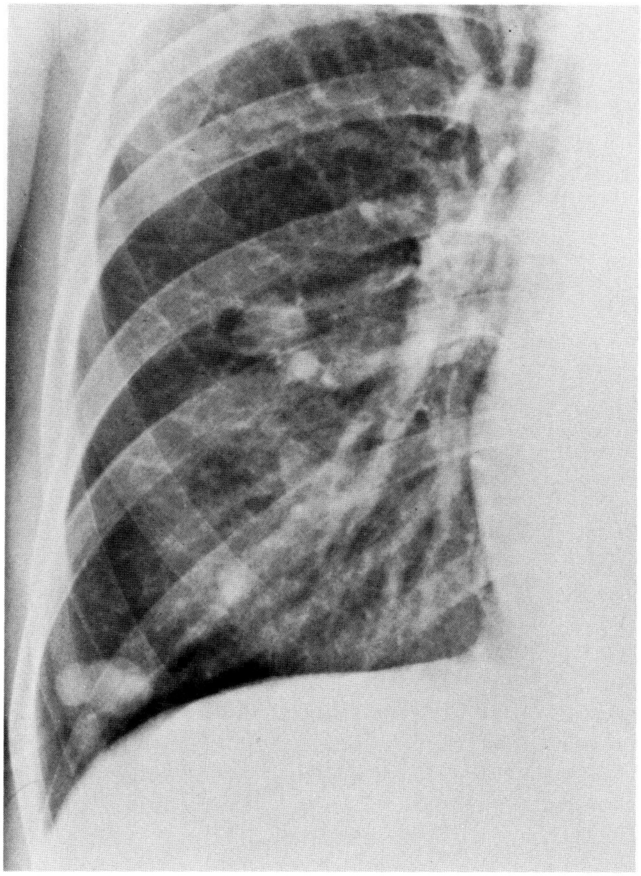

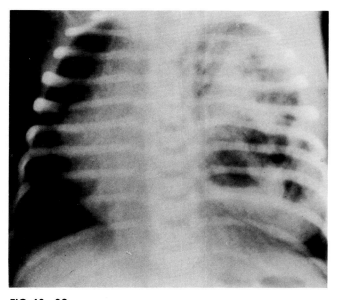

FIG 13–29.
Multiple small arteriovenous malformations in a middle-aged woman presenting with severe gastrointestinal bleeding. These lesions were initially suspected to be metastases from a neoplasm of the gastrointestinal tract.

nosis is essential in both conditions, and treatment for both is surgical. As indicated, the extent of any underlying pulmonary hypoplasia will probably play a significant role in determining the outcome.

Cystic Fibrosis of the Pancreas (Mucoviscidosis)

This relatively common congenital disorder is variously termed cystic fibrosis of the pancreas, fibrocystic disease, and mucoviscidosis. The term mucoviscidosis will be used in this presentation because

FIG 13–30.
Radiograph of neonate with congenital cystic adenomatoid malformation of the left lung.

it underlines the primary feature of this condition, the presence of excessively viscid mucous secretions in a wide systemic distribution. Nevertheless, the term is not encompassing because it does not cover the associated abnormalities in the exocrine glands. A summary of mucoviscidosis and its diverse effects is given in Table 13–3. The pulmonary manifestations are the most significant, causing the greatest morbidity and mortality.

The pulmonary manifestations of mucoviscidosis are progressive from birth but do not become radiologically apparent for months or years (Fig 13–31). The earliest changes are variable and may include focal atelectasis, recurrent pneumonias, diffuse peribronchial infiltration, emphysema, and hilar adenopathy. Clinical features, rather than chest radiographic findings alone, usually point to the diagnosis. The role of chest radiography is to follow the course of the pulmonary infections. Deterioration is inexorable in spite of treatment, but the rate of deterioration varies among individual patients. Patients with early manifestations of the disease tend to deteriorate the most rapidly. In the fully developed form of the disease, the radiographic findings are remarkably uniform. These findings include:

1. Emphysema. The widespread parenchymal changes may obscure the lung changes of emphysema, but the chest is usually barrel-shaped with an increased sagittal diameter and low, flat diaphragms.

2. Enlarged hilar shadows and diffuse increase in the perihilar shadows (Fig 13–32). The increase in size of the hili is probably caused by hilar adenopathy, dilatation of the pulmonary arteries with pulmonary hypertension, and inflammatory changes adjacent to the hili. The widespread peribronchial and bronchial infiltration causes the diffuse perihilar densities.

3. Bronchiectasis. This may be both tubular and cystic. The cystic changes are perhaps a hallmark of the disease (Fig 13–33). The cysts may be as much as 1 to 2 cm in diameter and often have relatively thin walls. Walls may be thickened by associated infection, and the cysts may contain variable quantities of fluid.

4. Atelectasis and focal infiltration. Patchy focal parenchymal densities are common and may be observed to wax and wane in association with intercurrent infections.

Taken as a whole, the pulmonary shadows in mucoviscidosis are often predominant in the upper zones, a reverse of the usual situation with bronchiectasis. Pulmonary complications include pneumothorax as a result of rupture of an emphysematous bleb and massive hemoptysis. Arteriography may be required to determine the site of bleeding. The hemoptysis can be abated by the interventional techniques of selective vascular occlusion. Lung abscess and empyema are surprisingly rare, probably because of a hyperimmune state resulting from prolonged chronic infection.

Chest radiographs over the years will reflect the patient's deteriorating status, but short-term clinical fluctuations are not necessarily accompanied by any readily detectable radiographic changes. In part, this must result from obscuration of minor changes by preexisting major chronic abnormalities. Eventually the patient will probably succumb to respiratory failure, possibly precipitated by a major complication such as massive hemoptysis or cor pulmonale, in which case increasing heart size may be apparent.

TABLE 13–3.
Effects of Mucoviscidosis

Incidence: 1 in 1,600 live births
Inheritance: Mendelian recessive
Carrier state: 1 in 20 are heterozygotes
Race: High incidence in whites
Effects:
  Related to the viscid secretions
    Pancreas
      Antenatal: Meconium ileus
      Postnatal: Pancreatitis, pancreatic insufficiency, diabetes mellitus
    Liver
      Focal biliary cirrhosis
      Cirrhosis leading to portal hypertension, varices, hypersplenism
    Gallbladder
      Thick-walled with viscid secretions
    Intestines
      Meconium ileus
      Atresia
      Constipation leading to rectal prolapse and inguinal hernias
    Upper respiratory tract
      Abnormal salivary secretions
      Nasal polyps
      Sinusitis
    Lower respiratory tract
      Bronchiectasis, bronchitis, bronchopneumonia, atelectasis, emphysema, hilar adenopathy, pulmonary hypertension, cor pulmonale, hemoptysis, respiratory failure
    Female genital tract
      Reduced fertility
  Eccrine gland abnormality
    Salt depletion due to increased salt content of sweat
    Heat stroke
  Secondary aplasia in male genitalia (vas deferens, epididymis, seminal vesicles) leading to sterility

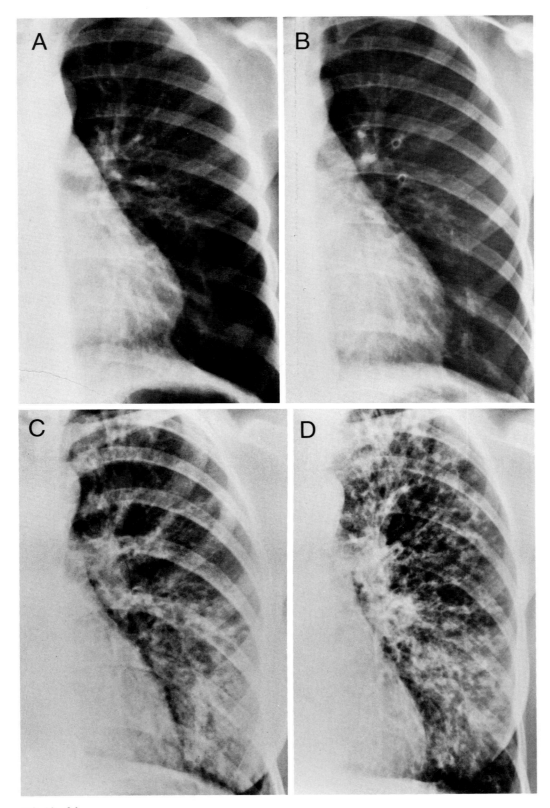

FIG 13–31.
A series of radiographs obtained over a 13-year period in an individual with mucoviscidosis. **A,** age 6 years. **B,** age 10 years. **C,** age 16 years. **D,** age 19 years.

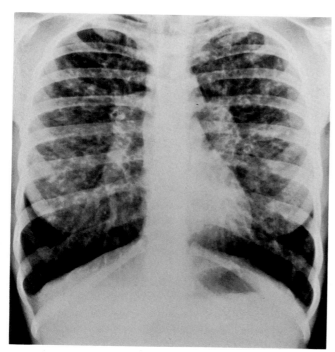

FIG 13–32.
Mucoviscidosis. Enlarged hilar shadows and diffuse perihilar infiltration are seen.

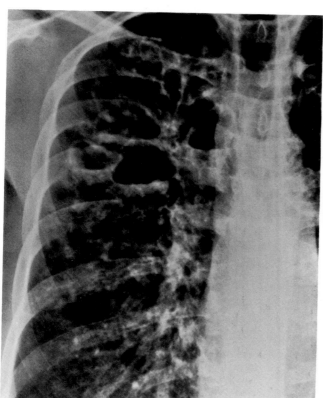

FIG 13–33.
Mucoviscidosis. There is cystic bronchiectasis in the upper lobe and diffuse peribronchial infiltration with upper zone predominance.

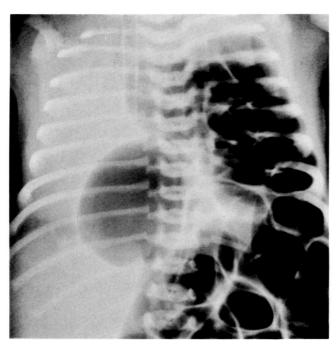

FIG 13—34.
Congenital diaphragmatic hernia in neonate with severe respiratory distress.

CONGENITAL DIAPHRAGMATIC ABNORMALITIES

Congenital Diaphragmatic Hernia

The exact embryologic basis for these hernias is disputed. Some at least may be acquired and relate to phrenic nerve trauma at birth. Wayne et al.[88] reported that 10 out of 60 cases of diaphragmatic eventration they reviewed resulted from birth trauma. Nevertheless, 48 were truly congenital, and of these, 3 had coincident pulmonary hypoplasia. The most common congenital diaphragmatic hernia consists of a relatively central defect in one hemidiaphragm.

Classically congenital diaphragmatic hernias present as an emergency in the neonatal period. A major portion of the abdominal viscera may be in one hemithorax with compressive effects on the lungs and mediastinum. Swallowed air enters the stomach and the bowel fairly quickly, and the diagnosis is not ordinarily very difficult (Fig 13–34). The chief differential diagnosis is cystic adenomatoid malformation of the lung (see earlier section). If a nasogastric tube is inserted, this may either be impeded up in the region of the esophagogastric junction or it may turn up into the chest cavity (Fig 13–35). The abdomen is likely to be scaphoid instead of showing the normal protuberance of the in-

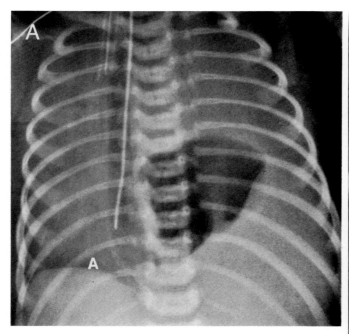

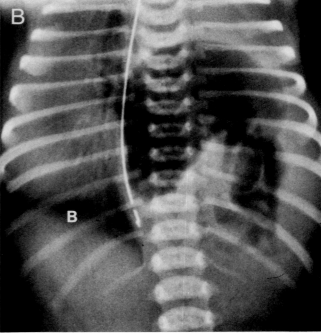

FIG 13—35.
Congenital diaphragmatic hernia in neonate with respiratory distress. The nasogastric tube could not be advanced into the stomach. Early image (**A**) shows gas in stomach but not in herniated small bowel. Later (**B**), gas appears in the small bowel.

fant. Aeration of the lungs may be severely re-stricted and, additionally, there may be underlying pulmonary hypoplasia, the extent of which cannot be determined on the initial radiographs.

Accessory Diaphragm

This rare anomaly consists of an accessory fibro-muscular diaphragmatic sheet within the oblique fis-sure. The hemithorax is thereby separated into two compartments. In an uncomplicated case, the only inkling of the presence of an accessory diaphragm is the visualization of an unusually thick oblique fissure on that side. An accessory diaphragm may be associ-ated with and be incidental to more significant pul-monary anomalies such as lobar hypoplasia or the scimitar syndrome.

The Morgagni Hernia

The Morgagni hernia may be encountered in patients of any age and represents a herniation of abdominal contents through the diaphragm between its costal and sternal attachments. The heart hinders herniation on the left, and the hernia normally pre-sents in the right cardiophrenic sulcus. Morgagni hernias are normally small and often contain only liver or omentum—in which case they are of homo-geneous density on plain radiographs. The margins are smooth and rounded, and the chief differential diagnoses include pericardial cysts, prominent car-diac fat pads and focal pleural or pulmonary paren-chymal masses (Fig 13–36). CT scanning may be helpful in determining the high fat content of con-tained omentum or cardiac fat pads or in confirming the presence of a pericardial cyst. Ultrasound scan-ning may also be useful in showing herniation of liver into the chest. When the hernia contains bowel—usually transverse colon—the diagnosis is simplified. Morgagni hernias are more often a dif-ferential diagnostic problem on chest radiography than a clinical problem.

Bochdalek Hernias

Bochdalek hernias represent herniations through a posterior diaphragmatic defect close to the crura. The defect is a relic of the pleuroperitoneal canal of the embryo. Bochdalek mistakenly believed that the herniation occurred under the lateral arcuate liga-ment of the diaphragm; nevertheless, his name is consistently applied to herniations through posterior diaphragmatic defects.[90] Bochdalek hernias may be

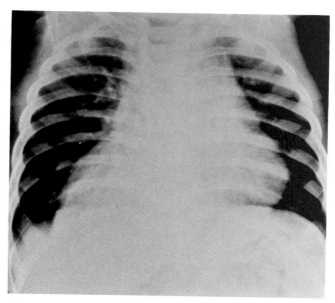

FIG 13–36.
Morgagni hernia in the right cardiophrenic angle in a child. The hernia contained liver and omentum and was isodense with the heart.

bilateral and symmetric, minor degrees of herniation being fairly common and inconsequential (Fig 13–37). In these instances, one may observe sym-metric hemispherical bulges on the diaphragmatic contours posteriorly slightly medial to the midlines of each lung. These small herniations contain only

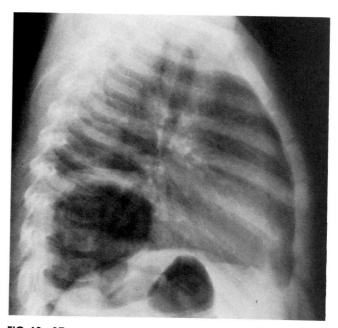

FIG 13–37.
Bochdalek hernia in a child, which contained herniated stomach.

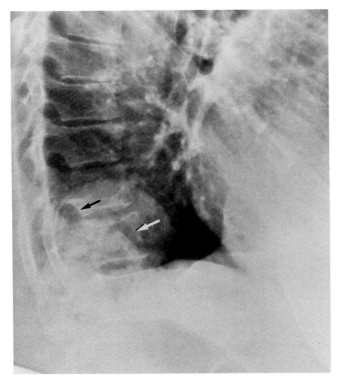

FIG 13–38.
Bochdalek hernia in an adult, which contained a small knuckle of gas-filled bowel *(arrows)*.

perinephric fat. Rarely Bochdalek hernias may be larger and contain portions of the kidney and even viscera, such as the stomach and small bowel (Fig 13–38). Ordinarily the presence of the liver prevents visceral herniation on the right.

REFERENCES

1. Allen RP, Taylor RL, Reiquam CW: Congenital lobar emphysema with dilated septal lymphatics. *Radiology* 1966; 86:929–931.
2. Atwell SW: Major anomalies of the tracheobronchial tree with a list of the minor anomalies. *Dis Chest* 1967; 52:611–615.
3. Barnes JC, Smith WL: The Vater association. *Radiology* 1978; 126:445–449.
4. Bateson EM: Relationship between intrapulmonary and endobronchial cartilage containing tumors (so called hamartomata). *Thorax* 1965; 20:447–461.
5. Bedard P, Girvan DP, Shandling B: Congenital H type tracheoesophageal fistula. *J Pediatr Surg* 1974; 9:663–668.
6. Benisch BM, Wood WG, Kroeger GB, et al: Focal muscular hyperplasia of the trachea. *Arch Otolaryngol* 1974; 99:226–227.
7. Bennett LL, Lesar MSL, Tellis CJ: Multiple calcified chondrohamartomas of the lung: CT appearance. *J Comput Assist Tomogr* 1985; 9:180–182.
8. Benson JE, Olsen MM, Fletcher BD: A spectrum of bronchopulmonary anomalies associated with tracheoesophageal malformations. *Pediatr Radiol* 1985; 15:377–380.
9. Bergstrom JF, Yost RV, Ford KT, et al: Unusual roentgen manifestations of bronchogenic cysts. *Radiology* 1973; 107:49–54.
10. Blesovsky A: Pulmonary sequestration: A report of an unusual case and a review of the literature. *Thorax* 1967; 22:351–357.
11. Brasch RC, Gooding CA, Lallemond DP, et al: Magnetic resonance imaging of the thorax in childhood: Work in progress. *Radiology* 1984; 150:463–467.
12. Brereton RJ, Rickwood AM: Esophageal atresia with pulmonary agenesis. *J Pediatr Surg* 1983; 18:618–620.
13. Bressler S, Wiener D: Bronchogenic cyst associated with an anomalous pulmonary artery arising from the thoracic aorta. *Surgery* 1954; 35:815–819.
14. Bruwer A, Clagett OT, McDonald JR: Anomalous arteries to the lung associated with congenital pulmonary abnormality. *J Thorac Surg* 1950; 19:957–972.
15. Cantrell JR, Guild HG: Congenital stenosis of the trachea. *Am J Surg* 1964; 108:297–305.
16. Carter R: Pulmonary sequestrations. *Ann Thorac Surg* 1969; 7:68–88.
17. Chang N, Hertzler JH, Gregg RH, et al: Congenital stenosis of the right main stem bronchus: A case report. *Pediatrics* 1968; 41:739–742.
18. Cumming WA: Esophageal atresia and tracheoesophageal fistula. *Radiol Clin North Am* 1975; 13:277–295.
19. Cunningham MD, Peter ER: Cervical hernia of the lung associated with cri du chat syndrome. *Am J Dis Child* 1969; 118:769–771.
20. Demos NJ, Teresi A: Congenital lung malformations: A unified concept and case report. *J Thorac Cardiovasc Surg* 1975; 70:260–264.
21. De Parades CG, Pierce WS, Johnson DG, et al: Pulmonary sequestration in infants and children: A 20 year experience and review of the literature. *J Pediatr Surg* 1970; 5:136–147.
22. Dines DE, Seward JB, Bernatz PE: Pulmonary arteriovenous fistulas. *Mayo Clin Proc* 1983; 58:176–181.
23. Eraklis AJ, Griscom NT, McGovern JB: Bronchogenic cysts of the mediastinum in infancy. *New Engl J Med* 1969; 281:1150–1155.
24. Fagan CJ, Swischuk LE: The opaque lung in lobar emphysema. *AJR* 1972; 114:300–304.
25. Farnsworth AE, Ankeney JL: The spectrum of the scimitar syndrome. *J Thorac Cardiovasc Surg* 1974; 68:673–674.
26. Felson B: Pulmonary agenesis and related anomalies. *Semin Roentgenol* 1972; 7:17–30.
27. Fraga JR, Mirza AM, Reichelderfer TE: Association of pulmonary hypoplasia, renal anomalies and Potter's facies. *Clin Pediatr* 1973; 12:150–153.

28. France NE, Brown RJK: Congenital pulmonary lymph-angiectasis: Report of 11 examples with special reference to cardiovascular findings. *Arch Dis Child* 1971; 46:528–532.

29. Fraser RG, Pare JAP: in *Diagnosis of Diseases of the Chest*. Philadelphia, WB Saunders Co, 1977, pp 612–622.

30. Freedom RM, Burrows PE, Moes CA: "Horseshoe" lung: Report of five new cases. *AJR* 1986; 146:211–215.

31. Freedom RM, Culham JAG, Moes CAF: Anomalies of pulmonary arteries, in *Angiocardiography of Congenital Heart Disease*. New York, Macmillan Publishing Co, 1984, pp 254–273.

32. Gibbons JR, McIlrath TE, Bailey IC: Pulmonary arteriovenous fistula in association with recurrent cerebral abscess. *Thorac Cardiovasc Surg* 1985; 33:319–321.

33. Gonzalez-Crussi F, Padilla LM, Miller JK, et al: "Bridging bronchus" a previously undescribed airway anomaly. *Am J Dis Child* 1976; 130:1015–1018.

34. Gooneratne N, Conway JJ: Radionuclide angiographic diagnosis of bronchopulmonary sequestration. *J Nucl Med* 1976; 17:1035–1037.

35. Hamper VM, Khouri NF, Stitik FP, et al: Pulmonary hamartoma: Diagnosis by transthoracic needle aspiration biopsy. *Radiology* 1985; 155:150–158.

36. Heithoff KB, Sane SM, Williams HJ, et al: Bronchopulmonary foregut malformations. A unifying etiologic concept. *AJR* 1976; 126:46–55.

37. Hendren W, McKee DM: Lobar emphysema of infancy. *J Pediatr Surg* 1966; 1:24–39.

38. Holder TM, Cloud DT, Lewis JE, et al: Esophageal atresia and tracheoesophageal fistula. *Pediatrics* 1964; 34:542–549.

39. Hole BV, Wasserman K: Familial emphysema. *Ann Intern Med* 1965; 63:1009–1017.

40. Holinger PH, Johnstone KC, Schild JA: Congenital anomalies of the tracheobronchial tree and of the esophagus. *Pediatr Clin North Am* 1962; 9:1113–1124.

41. Holmes B, Quie PG, Windhorst DB: Protection of phagocytosed bacteria from the killing action of antibiotics. *Nature* (London) 1966B; 210:1131–1132.

42. Hudson HL, McAlister WH: Obstructing tracheal hemangioma in infancy. *AJR* 1965; 93:428–431.

43. Hughes EW: Familial interstitial pulmonary fibrosis. *Thorax* 1964; 19:515–525.

44. Izzo C, Rickham PP: Neonatal pulmonary hamartoma. *J Pediatr Surg* 1968; 3:77–83.

45. Jensen KG, Schiodt T: Growth considerations of hamartoma of the lung. *Thorax* 1958; 13:233–237.

46. Johnston RB, Baehner RL: Chronic granulomatous disease—correlation between pathogenesis and clinical findings. *Pediatrics* 1971; 48:730–739.

47. Jones HE, Howells CHL: Pulmonary agenesis. *Br Med J* 1961; 2:1187–1189.

48. Kaude JV, Laurin S: Ultrasonographic demonstration of systemic artery feeding extrapulmonary sequestration. *Pediatr Radiol* 1984; 14:226–227.

49. Kirwan WO, Walbaum PR, McCormack RJM: Cystic intrathoracic derivatives of the foregut and their complications. *Thorax* 1973; 28:424–432.

50. Kobayashi Y, Abe T, Sato A, et al: Radionuclide angiography in pulmonary sequestration. *J Nucl Med* 1985; 26:1035–1038.

51. Koch B: Familial fibrocystic pulmonary dysplasia: Observations in one family. *Can Med Assoc J* 1965; 92:801–808.

52. Koutras P, Urschel HC Jr, Paulson DL: Hamartoma of the lung. *J Thorac Cardiovasc Surg* 1971; 61:768–776.

53. Landing BH: Syndromes of congenital heart disease with tracheobronchial anomalies. *AJR* 123:679–686.

54. Landing BH, Wells TR: Tracheobronchial anomalies in children. *Perspect Pediatr Pathol* 1973; 1:1–32.

55. Ledor K, Fish B, Chaise L, et al: CT diagnosis of pulmonary hamartomas. *J Comput Assist Tomogr* 1981; 5:343–344.

56. Leites V, Tannerbaum E: Familial spontaneous pneumothorax. *Am Rev Respir Dis* 1960; 82:240–241.

57. Lincoln JCR, Deverall PB, Stark J, et al: Vascular anomalies compressing the esophagus and trachea. *Thorax* 1969; 24:295–306.

58. MacMahon HE, Ruggieri J: Congenital segmental bronchomalacia. *Am J Dis Child* 1969; 118:923–926.

59. Madewell JE, Stoacker JT, Korsower JM: Cystic adenomatoid malformation of the lung: Morphologic analysis. *AJR* 1975; 124:436–448.

60. Maltz DL, Nadas AS: Agenesis of the lung. Presentation of eight new cases and review of the literature. *Pediatrics* 1968; 42:175–188.

61. Mangiulea VG, Stinghe RV: The accessory cardiac bronchus: Bronchologic aspect and review of the literature. *Dis Chest* 1968; 54:433–436.

62. Mendelson DS, Rose JS, Efremedis SC, et al: Bronchogenic cysts with high CT numbers. 1983; 140:463–465.

63. Meng RL, Jensik RJ, Faber LP, et al: Bronchial atresia. *Ann Thorac Surg* 1978; 25:184–192.

64. Miller PA, Williamson BRJ, Minor GR, et al: Pulmonary sequestration: Visualization of the feeding artery by CT. *J Comput Assist Tomogr* 1982; 6:828–830.

65. Nakata H, Nakayama C, Komoto T, et al: Computed tomography of mediastinal bronchogenic cysts. *J Comput Assist Tomogr* 1982; 6:733–738.

66. Neill CA, Ferencz C, Sabiston DC, et al: The familial occurence of hypoplastic right lung with systemic arterial supply and venous drainage: Scimitar syndrome. *Bull Johns Hopkins Hosp* 1960; 107:1–21.

67. Potter EL: Bilateral renal agenesis. *J Pediatr* 1946; 29:68.

68. Rankin S, Faling LJ, Pugatch RD: CT diagnosis of pulmonary arteriovenous malformations. *J Comput Assist Tomogr* 1982; 6:746–749.

69. Reed JC, Sobonya RE: Morphologic analysis of foregut cysts in the thorax. *AJR* 1974; 120:851–860.

70. Remy J, Smith M, Marache P, et al: La bronche "trachéale" gauche pathogene: Revue de la literature á propos de 4 observations. *Radiol Electrol Med Nucl* 1977; 58:621–630.

71. Ries T, Currarino G, Nikaido H, et al: Real-time ultrasonography of subcarinal bronchogenic cysts. *Radiology* 1982; 145:121–122.

72. Rogers LF, Osmer JC: Bronchogenic cyst: A review of 46 cases. *AJR* 1964; 91:273–283.

73. Rogge JD, Mishkin ME, Genovese PD: The familial occurrence of primary pulmonary hypertension. *Ann Intern Med* 1966; 65:672–684.

74. Roghair GD: Non operative management of lobar emphysema. Long-term follow-up. *Radiology* 1972; 102:125–127.

75. Sane SM, Sieber WK, Girdany BR: Congenital bronchobiliary fistula. *Surgery* 1971; 69:599–608.

76. Sotelo-Avila C, Skanklin DR: Congenital malformations in an autopsy series. *Arch Pathol* 1967; 84:272–279.

77. Stephens RW, Lingeman RE, Lawson LJ: Congenital tracheoesophageal fistulas in adults. *Ann Otol Rhinol Laryngol* 1976; 85:613–617.

78. Stocker A: Congenital cystic adenomatoid malformation. *Hum Pathol* 1977; 8:155–171.

79. Stocker JT, Drake RM, Madewell JE: Cystic and congenital lung disease in the newborn, in Rosenberg H, Bolande R (eds): *Perspectives in Pediatric Pathology*. Chicago, Year Book Medical Publishers, 1978, vol 4, pp 93–154.

80. Stovin PGI: Congenital lobar emphysema. *Thorax* 1959; 14:254–261.

81. Stringer DA, Ein SH: Recurrent tracheoesophageal fistula: A protocol for investigation. *Radiology* 1984; 151:637–641.

82. Thind CR, Pilling DW: Case Report: Pulmonary sequestration: The value of ultrasound. *Clin Radiol* 1985; 36:437–439.

83. Thomas PS, Chrispin AR: Congenital tracheoesophageal fistula without esophageal atresia. *Clin Radiol* 1969; 20:371–374.

84. Toyama WM: Esophageal atresia and tracheoesophageal fistula in association with bronchial and pulmonary anomalies. *J Pediatr Surg* 1972; 7:302–307.

85. Van Dyke JA, Sagel SS: Calcified pulmonary sequestration: CT demonstrations. *J Comput Assist Tomogr* 1985; 9:372–374.

86. Warfel KA, Schulz DM: Agenesis of the trachea: Report of a case and review of the literature. *Arch Pathol Lab Med* 1976; 100:357–359.

87. Waterston DJ, Carter REB, Aberdeen E: Oesophageal atresia, tracheo-oesophageal fistula. A study of survival in 218 infants. *Lancet* 1962; 1:819–822.

88. Wayne ER, Campbell JB, Burrington JD, et al: Eventration of the diaphragm. *J Pediatr Surg* 1974; 9:643–651.

89. Weichert RF, Lindsey ES, Pearce CW, et al: Bronchogenic cyst with unilateral obstructive emphysema. *J Thorac Cardiovasc Surg* 1970; 59:287–291.

90. White JJ, Suzuki H: Hernia through the foramen of Bochdalek: A misnomer. *J Pediatr Surg* 1972; 7:60–61.

91. Wittenborg MH, Gyepes MT, Crocker D: Tracheal dynamics in infants with respiratory distress, stridor and collapsing trachea. *Radiology* 1967; 88:653–662.

92. Wolfson J, Quie PG, Laxdol SD, et al: Roentgenologic manifestations in children with a genetic defect of polymorphonuclear leucocyte function. *Radiology* 1968; 91:37–48.

14

The Pleura and Pleural Disorders

PLEURAL ANATOMY

The pleural space is lined by a smooth serosal membrane and is lubricated by a small amount of fluid, which allows the lungs to change shape easily and provides low-friction mechanical coupling between the lungs and the chest wall. The visceral and parietal pleura are lined by a single layer of flat mesothelial cells. In the parietal pleura, these mesothelial cells lie directly on connective tissue in continuity with the endothoracic fascia. In the visceral pleura, however, there are five layers[284, 566]: (1) a mesothelial layer; (2) a thin layer of connective tissue; (3) a strong layer of connective tissue—the chief layer; (4) a vascular layer; and (5) the limiting lung membrane, which is connected by collagen and elastic fibers to the chief layer.[284] The blood supply of the parietal pleura is from systemic vessels, while the visceral pleura is supplied largely by the pulmonary circulation with some bronchial contribution.[284] Both the parietal and the visceral pleura are supplied by lymphatics, but only parietal lymphatics communicate with the pleural space.

The Pleural Cavity

The parietal and visceral pleura, which enclose the pleural cavity, are continuous with one another at the hilus of the lung and along the (inferior) pulmonary ligament. Inferiorly the parietal pleura is tucked into the costophrenic sulcus. The disposition of the sulcus helps to explain some of the radiologic

findings in pleural disease and is important in upper abdominal interventional procedures. On the surface of the body, the inferior edge of the sulcus crosses the xiphoid and eighth costochondral junction to reach the mid-axillary line at the level of the tenth rib,[364, 368] and then passes horizontally across the 11th and 12th ribs to reach the first lumbar vertebral body. The cephalad part of the sulcus is occupied to a variable extent by lung, whereas caudally the sulcus is empty and the diaphragm and chest wall are separated only by the two layers of the visceral pleura. The distance between the lowest part of the sulcus and the lung edge depends on the phase of respiration and the segment of sulcus being considered. The right intercostal midaxillary approach is often used for percutaneous introduction of needles into the upper abdomen and, because the pleural reflection reaches the tenth rib in this region, it would be usual for the parietal pleura to be punctured, for example, during percutaneous transhepatic cholangiography or biliary drainage.[364, 368] Somewhat surprisingly, the complication rate of these procedures is low. In fine-needle transhepatic cholangiography, for example, only two pneumothoraces were recorded in 2,005 procedures.[191] This low complication rate undoubtedly reflects the fact that the lung rarely occupies the depth of the sulcus, except possibly in young patients taking a maximum inspiration. The complications are more serious and frequent when drainage catheters pass through the pleural cavity because abdominal fluid collections/pus may then flow into the pleural space.[368]

Fissures and Junctional Lines

On a plain chest radiograph the pleura cannot be seen as such, except where the visceral pleura invaginates into the lung to form the fissures and where the two lungs contact one another at junctional lines (see Chapter 3). Fissures are of two sorts: standard and accessory.

Standard Fissures

Standard fissures consist of a double layer of infolded visceral pleura. They are normally very thin and are only seen on plain radiographs when they are tangential to the x-ray beam, appearing as a hairline of soft tissue density. Many fissures are incomplete and fail to extend all the way to the hilus. They are often partially hidden by ribs. As a result, it is uncommon to see complete fissures either on frontal or lateral radiographs. There are two standard fissures: the major and the minor.

The Major Fissure.—This fissure, also called the oblique or greater fissure, separates the upper lobe from the lower lobe on the left, and the upper and middle lobes from the lower lobe on the right. On plain chest radiographs, the major fissures are best seen on lateral projection (Fig 14–1). In Proto and Speckman's study of plain lateral radiographs, a part of the right fissure was seen in 22% of the images, part of the left fissure was seen in 14%, and part of a major fissure of indeterminate size was seen in 62%; in only 2% of radiographs was a complete major fissure identified.[404] When the major fissure is incom-

pletely seen, it is almost always the lower portion that is detected (see Fig 14–1).

Anatomically the right fissure is wider and shorter than the left and has a greater overall area.[411] Both fissures face forward and pass obliquely downward, parallel to the fifth rib, from about the body of the fifth thoracic vertebra, to meet the diaphragm several centimeters behind the sternum (see Fig 14–1).[124] Neither fissure is flat, both being mildly twisted in the middle, a configuration that has been likened to a propeller. The twist is such that the upper half, which is concave forward (Fig 14–2), faces outward while the lower half, which is convex forward, faces medially (Fig 14–3).[400, 404] On the radiograph the fissure is detected where it becomes tangential to the x-ray beam. This means that in a lateral chest radiograph, the caudad portion of the oblique fissure tends to lie along the anterior edge of the lower lobe, whereas the cephalad portion is projected over the body of the lower lobe (Fig 14–4). Normal undulations in the oblique fissure can lead to the following misinterpretations on the lateral chest radiograph[404]:

1. Because the lateral aspect of the minor fissure extends more posteriorly than the medial aspect of the right major fissure, the two can appear to cross in lateral view. This appearance can lead to problems in identifying the right major fissure and can also lead to mistaken identification of the posterior aspect of the minor fissure as a superior accessory fissure. Confusion between minor fissure and superior accessory fissure can be avoided if it is realized

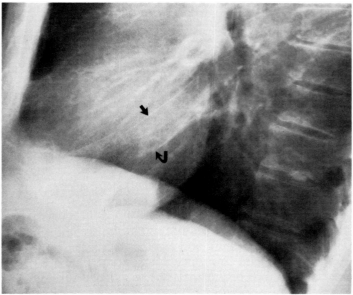

FIG 14–1.
Major fissures. As is often the case only the lower halves of these major fissures are detectable. The right fissure *(straight arrow)* is anterior to the left *(curved arrow)*, and both make contact with their ipsilateral hemidiaphragms 5 to 7 cm behind the sternum.

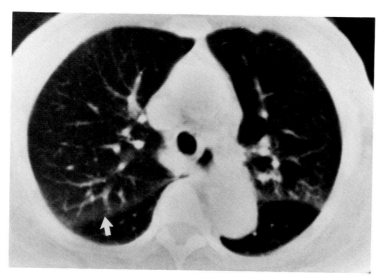

FIG 14–2.
The upper part of the major fissures shown as band opacities on computed tomography (CT). That on the right *(arrow)* is concave forward, the usual configuration at this level; the left is atypical and convex forward.

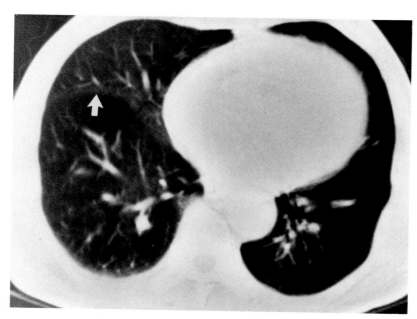

FIG 14–3.
The inferior part of the right oblique fissure. This is demonstrated on a CT scan as a band opacity which is convex forward *(arrow)*.

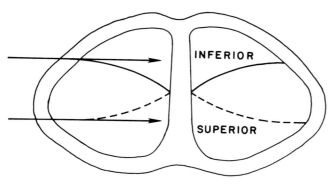

FIG 14–4.
The major fissure. Diagram of a CT scan, oriented in the conventional way, shows the configuration of the major fissure in its upper half ("superior") and lower half ("inferior"). The upper segment is concave, facing forward and laterally, and the lower is convex facing forward and medially. The lateral x-ray beam *(long arrows)* is tangential to the anterior aspect of the lower part of the fissure and to the posterior aspect of the upper part of the fissure.

that the minor fissure often ends before the vertebral bodies. Furthermore, the superior accessory fissure cannot appear to be continuous with the minor fissure because the fissures have to straddle the origins of the middle lobe and apical lower bronchi,[404] both of which arise at essentially the same level.

2. If, because of undulations, the medial aspect of the major fissure is visualized in the lower zone rather than the more usual lateral aspect, the apparent backward shift of the fissure may be interpreted as indicating volume loss of the lower lobe.

3. If parenchymal lesions are close to but do not abut a major fissure, it is not possible to localize them with certainty to a particular lobe. Tomography will usually resolve this type of problem.

Fissures are commonly incomplete, failing to extend to the hilus or mediastinum,[194] and in these regions there is parenchymal fusion between lobes, often over quite a large area. The frequency of incomplete fissures in different series has ranged from 12.5% to 73% for the major fissure[411] and from 60% to 90% for the minor fissure.[194, 238, 327, 602] An incomplete fissure allows pathologic processes such as pneumonia to spread easily from one lobe to another and also allows collateral air drift so that, even with complete obstruction of the large airway, there may be no atelectasis.[209, 473]

It is sometimes useful to be able to distinguish the left and right major fissures on a lateral chest radiograph (see Fig 14–1). The most helpful points are that the right fissure (1) is more oblique, (2) ends farther forward inferiorly, (3) merges with the right hemidiaphragm, and (4) joins with the minor fissure.

The major fissure is not usually seen on a frontal radiograph, but there are three circumstances under which it may be detected. First, the upper edge, where it contacts the posterior chest wall, may become visible when extrapleural fat enters the lips of the fissure.[401] This generates the "superolateral major fissure" (Fig 14–5), a curved line or edge that starts medially above the hilus and curves downward and laterally, concave to the mediastinum.[401] Second, the upper aspect of the major fissure can become tangential to the frontal x-ray beam, generating a hairline opacity that runs obliquely across the midzone (Fig 14–6). Medially this fissure line often crosses the hilus to end up against the spine, allowing it to be distinguished from the minor fissure, which never crosses hilar vessels. This part of the major fissure becomes tangential to the frontal x-ray beam with lordotic projections and because of undulations in the fissure or volume loss of the lower

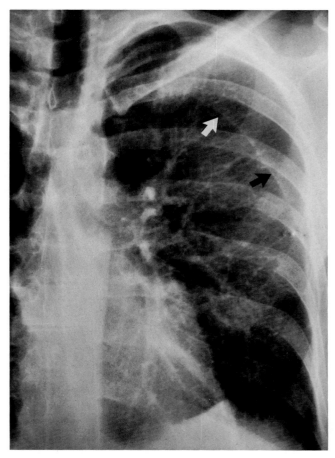

FIG 14–5.
Superolateral major fissure. This curvilinear opacity *(arrows)* marks the line along which the major fissure contacts the posterior chest wall.

lobe,[132] particularly the apical segment. Third, reorientation of the lateral aspect of the lower part of the oblique fissure probably accounts for the vertical fissure,[83, 146, 573] a vertical hairline seen particularly on the right, low down and toward the chest wall. It is most often described in babies with lower lobe volume loss and cardiomegaly.[83]

The major fissure can be appreciated on standard computed tomographic (CT) sections in some 80% to 95% of patients.[400] The most common appearance, present in some 80% of cases, is a curvilinear avascular band (Fig 14–7) extending from the hilus to the chest wall, reflecting the lack of vessels in the subcortical zone of the lung.[149, 174, 311] In some 10% of cases the major fissure, particularly in the upper third, is seen as a curvilinear line or band density (see Fig 14–2).[400] It is of interest that the upper part of the fissure is more easily detected with CT scanning, whereas the reverse is true of plain ra-

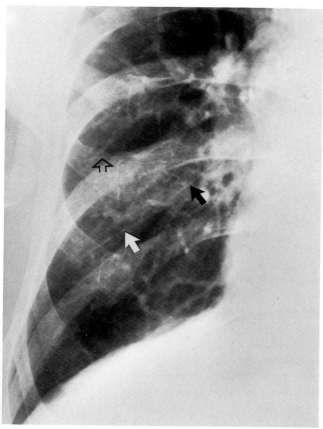

FIG 14–6.
The major fissure on a frontal radiograph. A reoriented major fissure *(closed arrows)* is visible on a frontal radiograph as an oblique line. It can be distinguished from the minor fissure *(open arrow)* because it passes more medially, overlying the right hilus and ending at the spine.

diography. The left fissure is the longer; it is seen one or two sections higher than the right.[400] In about a fifth of patients, supradiaphragmatic fat invaginates into the lower end of the major fissure and is detectable at CT scanning.[152]

The Minor Fissure.—The minor fissure separates the anterior segment of the right upper lobe from the right middle lobe, and because of its orientation it is seen on both frontal and lateral chest radiographs. It lies approximately horizontally on the right side at the level of the anterior fourth rib or interspace (Fig 14–8).[124, 140] On frontal chest radiographs, some or all of the fissure is seen in about 50% to 60% of patients.[124] The whole fissure is seen in only 7% of individuals, and when just a segment is seen, it is much more commonly the lateral portion than the medial. Felson pointed out that on a frontal chest radiograph the fissure ends medially at the interlobar pulmonary artery within about a centimeter of the point where the superior vein crosses (see Fig 14–8).[124] This observation can be helpful in finding and identifying the fissure. On lateral view, the fissure is seen in about half of the radiographs: in part in 44% and in toto in 6%.[404]

The upper surface of the middle lobe is either flat or convex, and it is common for the anterior and lateral aspects of the minor fissure to curve downward in a caudad direction (see Fig 14–8). Because of undulations, the minor fissure may appear sigmoid or double.

Felson has related the position of the minor fissure to the anterior ribs in order to assess pathologic

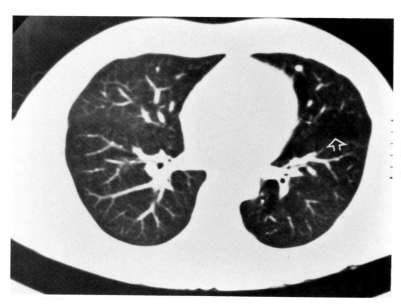

FIG 14–7.
The inferior part of the left oblique fissure on CT demonstrated as a broad avascular zone *(arrow).*

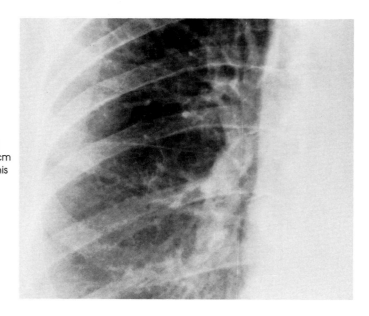

FIG 14–8.
The minor fissure. The minor fissure stops medially at the lateral margin of the interlobar pulmonary artery at a point about 1 cm beyond the Y-point of the hilus where artery and vein cross. This is a useful identifying feature of the minor fissure.

displacement.[124] He found 67% of minor fissures were on a level with the fourth anterior interspace, with 15% above and 18% below. Two percent were above the anterior third rib, and 3% were below the anterior sixth rib. He believed the variation was so great that, to diagnose pathologic shift, displacement had to be striking or the shape and direction of the fissure had to be altered.

On CT, the minor fissure is seen as an avascular zone extending from the major fissure to the chest wall (Fig 14–9). The avascular area has a triangular or occasionally rounded or oval configuration. It is usually best seen on a single section midway between

the origins of the upper and middle lobe bronchi. The overall detection rate in one series was 52%.[400]

Accessory Fissures

Accessory fissures are clefts of varying depth in the outer surface of the lung that delineate accessory lobes. Six important accessory fissures are recognized, and one or more of these is commonly present.[140] In a CT study of 50 patients, 22% had some form of accessory fissure.[169] It is important to recognize accessory fissures for the following reasons: (1) to avoid their misinterpretation as pathologic structures such as bullae, scars, or pneumotho-

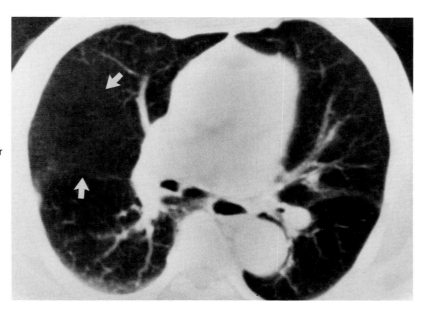

FIG 14–9.
The minor fissure. On CT scans, the minor fissure produces an approximately triangular, avascular area *(arrows)* in front of the major fissure on sections midway between the upper and lower lobar bronchi.

rax[169]; (2) to avoid incorrect localization of an intrapulmonary lesion; (3) because they give consolidation a sharp margin, and the resulting opacity may be misinterpreted as atelectasis, consolidation of a whole lobe, or mediastinal mass[169]; and (4) because of the atypical appearance of a pneumothorax in the presence of an azygos fissure.

The Azygos Fissure.—This is the best known accessory fissure, with a prevalence of 0.4% to 1% in various clinical and postmortem series.[508] There is some evidence of a male predominance,[133] and a familial occurrence has been described.[399] The azygos fissure produces a hairline curvilinear opacity, concave to the mediastinum, that extends obliquely across the right upper zone (Fig 14–10). It originates peripherally, where there may be a little triangle of soft tissue density, and it ends medially in the tear drop of the displaced azygos vein above and to the right of its normal location in the angle between trachea and right main stem bronchus.

The azygos fissure supports the azygos vein in a sling and is therefore sometimes called the mesoazygos. Unlike all other fissures, it consists of four layers of pleura: two visceral and two parietal. These four layers are present because the precursor of the

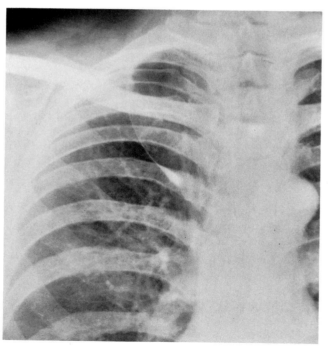

FIG 14–10.
Azygos fissure. Plain radiograph, right upper zone, demonstrating hairline azygos fissure ending medially in the teardrop of the azygos vein.

azygos vein, the right posterior cardinal vein, initially lies lateral to the lung and instead of migrating over the lung apex, it pushes through the upper lobe taking both the visceral and the parietal pleura with it.[508] On CT (Fig 14–11), the azygos vein lies 2 to 4 cm higher than usual, forming a C-shaped band coursing through the lung.[508] The azygos arch ends anteriorly at the right brachiocephalic vein/superior vena cava junction. The cephalic part of the azygos vein as it runs upward in a paravertebral position courses more laterally than usual and can be mistaken for a lung nodule or subpleural mass (see Fig 14–11).[403] Below the carina, the azygos vein returns to its usual prevertebral position.[508]

A left "azygos" fissure is rare[273, 581] and most likely involves the hemiazygos vein in an analogous way to the azygos vein on the right.[124]

The Inferior Accessory Fissure.—The inferior accessory fissure usually incompletely separates the medial basal segment from the rest of the lower lobe. Because this segment lies anteromedially in the lower lobe, the accessory fissure will have components that are oriented both sagittally and coronally. As a result, parts of the fissure are tangential to frontal and lateral x-ray beams. Despite this it is rarely seen on lateral radiographs. The frequency of occurrence is difficult to ascertain as the fissure varies greatly in depth and in its prominence from one examination to the next.[169] The prevalence also depends critically on the method of detection. It is present in 30% to 50% of anatomic specimens,[124, 140] in 16% of CT scans,[169] and in 5% to 10% of plain radiographs.[124, 169, 433]

On the frontal radiograph the fissure is a hairline that arises from the medial aspect of the hemidiaphragm and ascends obliquely toward the hilus (Fig 14–12). Sometimes there is a little triangular peak of the diaphragm at its lower end and this, together with a very short fissure line, may be all that is seen.[169] At the other extreme, the fissure may be long, reaching all the way to the hilus.[124] Although the left lower lobe lacks a separate medial basal segment, the anteromedial basal bronchus divides early into two components analogous to the medial and anterior segmental bronchi on the right,[169] and anatomically an inferior accessory fissure is about as common on the left as the right. Radiologically, however, it is not detected with equal frequency, and in one series of 500 radiographs 80% of inferior accessory fissures were right-sided, 12% left-sided, and 7% bilateral.[433] On the lateral radiograph the inferior accessory fissure is occasionally seen as a vertical

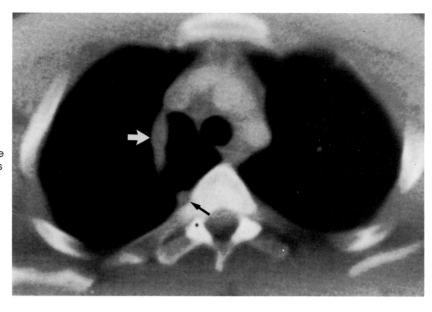

FIG 14–11.
Azygos fissure. A CT scan at the level of the lower trachea shows the C-shaped band of the displaced azygos venous arch *(white arrow).* Note the lateral displacement of the ascending azygos vein *(black arrow),* which must be distinguished from a lung or pleural nodule.

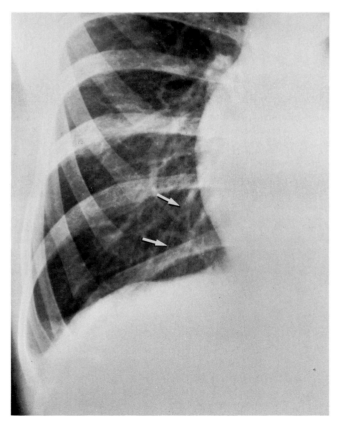

FIG 14–12.
Inferior accessory fissure *(arrows).* This fissure separates the medial basal segment from the rest of the lower lobe.

line, often associated with a diaphragmatic peak in the region of the esophagus.[169] The pulmonary ligament is very close to the medial portion of the inferior accessory fissure, and it is quite possible that diaphragmatic peaks on the lateral radiograph in this region are really the result of the inferior pulmonary ligament and its septum. On CT scans the fissure appears on sections near the diaphragm as an arc, concave to the mediastinum, extending from the major fissure back to the mediastinum near the esophagus. It is best demonstrated with thin, 5.0-mm or 1.5-mm sections.[169]

Should the inferior accessory fissure marginate a pneumonia in the medial basal segment, it will give a sharp outer border to the triangular opacity (Fig 14–13),[544] which may mimic a collapsed lower lobe. Other lesions such as pleural effusion, mediastinal mass, hernia, or fat pad may be simulated.[169] Occasionally the appearance is reversed (Fig 14–14).

The Superior Accessory Fissure.—The superior accessory fissure separates the apical segment of a lower lobe from the basal segments and superficially resembles a minor fissure on a frontal radiograph. It was identified on 6% of lateral radiographs in one series,[404] a percentage that seems very high when judged by general experience. The minor fissure lies above the middle lobe bronchus and the superior accessory fissure below the apical lower bronchus. Because both of these airways arise at approximately the same level, the superior accessory fissure is projected below the minor fissure on frontal radiographs (Fig 14–15). On the lateral view it

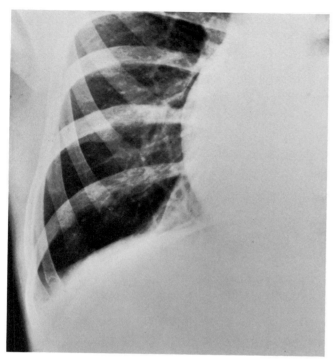

FIG 14—13.
Inferior accessory fissure. Same patient as in Figure 14—12. Consolidation in the medial basal segment of the right lower lobe is sharply demarcated laterally by the inferior accessory fissure. (Courtesy Dr. C.J. Dow, London.)

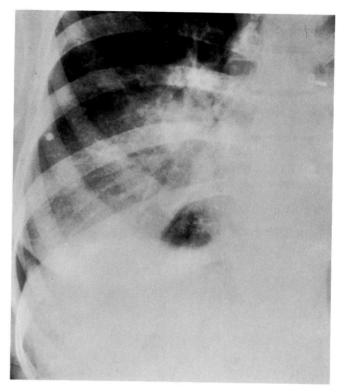

FIG 14—14.
Inferior accessory fissure. The exudate of a right lower lobe consolidation has been excluded from the medial basal segment by an inferior accessory fissure. (Courtesy Dr. C.J. Dow, London.)

differs from the minor fissure in that it extends backward across the vertebral bodies (Fig 14—16).[404] On CT, like the minor fissure, it appears as an avascular area that needs to be distinguished from downward angulation of the upper end of the major fissure, a distinction which depends on the identification of the apical lower bronchus.[169]

The Left Minor Fissure.—The left minor fissure is present anatomically in 8% to 18% of people, but is only rarely detected on PA and lateral radiographs, with a quoted frequency of 1.6%.[13] It separates the lingula from the rest of the left upper lobe and is analogous to the minor fissure. It is usually arched and located more cephalad than the minor fissure. It slopes medially and downward (Fig 14—17).

The (Inferior) Pulmonary Ligament

The pulmonary ligament is a double sheet of pleura that hangs down from the hilus like a curtain and joins the lung to the mediastinum and to the medial part of the diaphragm.[413] The two layers of pleura contact each other below the inferior pulmonary vein and end in a free border which usually lies over the inner third of the hemidiaphragm but which is sometimes displaced towards the hilus. The right ligament is short and wide-based and related on its mediastinal aspect to the inferior vena cava and azygos vein. On the left, the ligament is longer and it attaches to the mediastinum close to the esophagus anterior to the aorta (Fig 14—18).[413] The ligament overlies a septum within the lung that separates posterior and medial basal segments,[170] and it is probably the septum, rather than the ligament itself, which is radiographically detectable. The bare area of the ligament contains connective tissue, bronchial veins, lymphatics, and nodes.[142]

The ligament is not visible on chest radiographs but may occasionally be seen in posterior oblique tomograms.[142] On CT, it is visible in about 50% to 75% of patients.[69, 170, 450] It is best detected just above the diaphragm[450] as a thin curvilinear line passing outward and slightly backward from the mediastinum. At the mediastinal base of the ligament there is often a triangular elevation. The ligament may appear thickened with asbestos exposure and with fat or fluid infiltration.[413]

The ligament and variations in its degree of de-

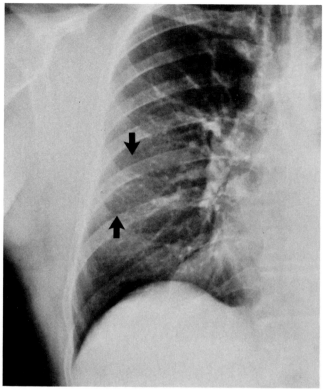

FIG 14–15.
Posteroanterior (PA) chest radiograph demonstrating the relationship of the minor fissure *(upper arrow)* and the superior accessory fissure *(lower arrow).*

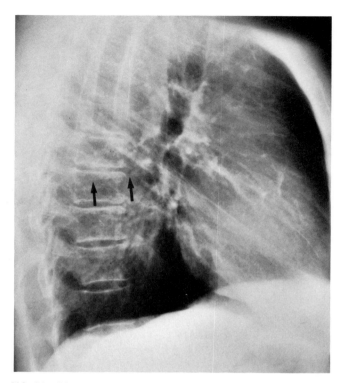

FIG 14–16.
Superior accessory fissure. Lateral radiograph demonstrates the posterior location of the fissure, which overlies the vertebral bodies.

velopment have been considered to be important for the following reasons:

1. It determines the shape of a collapsed lower lobe,[414] because the lobe, as it loses volume, folds backward—hinged along the line of the fixed mediastinal attachment of the ligament. In frontal view, the characteristic triangular shape of lower lobe collapse results because the inferior part of the lobe is being held away from the mediastinum by the diaphragmatic part of the ligament. If the ligament is not well developed and it lacks a diaphragmatic attachment, the whole lower lobe collapses against the mediastinum, giving an oval-shaped paravertebral opacity (Fig 14–19).[413] This can usually be distinguished from a mediastinal mass by looking for an air bronchogram or following the course of the left lower bronchus.

2. It determines the ultimate shape of the collapsed lung in a pneumothorax.[414]

3. Pleural effusion collecting posterior to the ligament tends to produce a triangular opacity, not unlike a lower lobe collapse.[413]

4. The juxtaphrenic peak sign described with

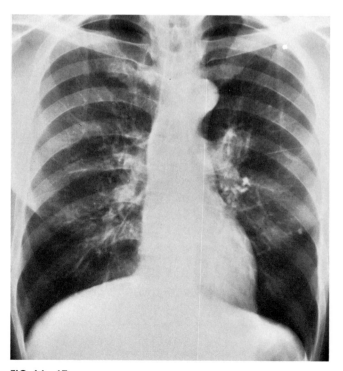

FIG 14–17.
Left minor fissure. This separates the lingula from the rest of the left upper lobe. It characteristically slopes downward and medially.

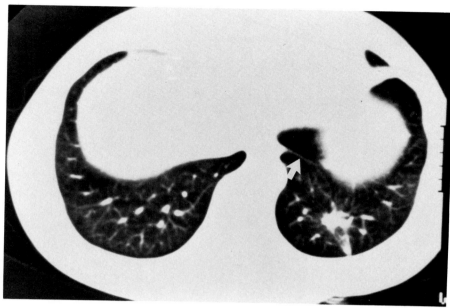

FIG 14–18.
Left pulmonary ligament. CT scan at the level of the left hemidiaphragm shows the left pulmonary ligament and associated septum *(arrow)*. The medial end of the ligament is marked by a small triangular elevation that lies in relation to the esophagus, just anterior to the aorta.

volume loss of an upper lobe[234] (see Chapter 5) may be due to reorientation and hyperexpansion of the lower lobe, causing diaphragmatic traction by way of the ligament and septum.

5. The ligament provides a pathway from lung to mediastinum and allows pathologic processes to spread in either direction. It may contain lung tumors, esophageal varices, the vascular supply to sequestered segments, and lymph nodes.[450] Posttraumatic paramediastinal air cysts (see Fig 14–64) were at one time considered to result from air collections within the inferior pulmonary ligament. There is now evidence that they represent loculated pneumothoraces or pneumomediastinum (see the section "Loculated/Localized Pneumothorax" on p. 683).

PLEURAL PHYSIOLOGY

The outward pull of the chest wall and the inward recoil of the lung tend to separate the parietal and visceral pleura. These membranes are permeable both to gases and liquid, and they are kept in apposition only because there are mechanisms for maintaining the pleural space essentially gas and liquid free.[5] Gas is removed by the venous blood because the total gas pressure in venous blood is about 70 cm H_2O subatmospheric, and this provides a steep absorption gradient.

The formation and absorption of pleural fluid is more complex and follows Starling's law, depending on (1) the hydrostatic pressure of systemic and pulmonary capillaries, (2) the oncotic pressure of pleural fluid and blood, and (3) the pleural surface pressure. There is a vertical gradient of pleural surface pressure of about -0.2 cm H_2O per centimeter with a mean value for the pleural space of about -5 cm H_2O. Plasma oncotic pressure is taken as 34 cm H_2O. The interplay of the various forces is illustrated in Fig 14–20.

The distribution of these forces is such that there is a net flow of fluid from the parietal to the visceral pleura, the rate depending on the net pressure gradient and on the permeability of the vessels and pleural membranes. An overall pressure gradient arises across the pleura simply because of differences in capillary pressure between the high-pressure systemic vessels of the parietal pleura and the low-pressure pulmonary circulation. About 2.5 L of fluid pass through the pleural space per day.[284] While most of this is absorbed by the visceral pleura, a small amount (250 to 500 ml) leaves the pleural space every day by way of the lymphatics.[270, 522] Lymphatic drainage from the pleural space occurs by way of 2- to 6-μm diameter stomata that communicate with lymphatic channels. Stomata are distributed only on the parietal pleura low down on the chest wall and mediastinum.[284, 566] The importance of lymphatic drainage is that it is the only way that

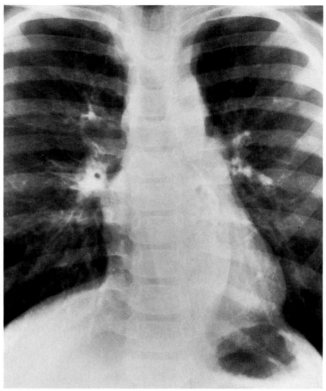

FIG 14–19.
A convex paravertebral opacity is the result of collapse of the left lower lobe. This atypical appearance probably results from underdevelopment of the pulmonary ligament, with resultant lack of tethering of the lower lobe to the diaphragm. The disposition of the left main stem bronchus and the air bronchogram within the opacity indicate the correct diagnosis.

proteins, particulates, and cells can leave the pleural space. This is particularly important in pathologic states, but even under normal conditions, a certain amount of protein leaks into the pleural space, possibly up to 4 gm/day,[284] and were this not removed

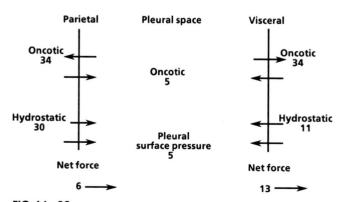

FIG 14–20.
Forces acting across the pleura (given in cm H$_2$O). (Adapted from Wang N-S: Anatomy and physiology of the pleural space. *Clin Chest Med* 1985; 6:3–16.)

the subsequent rise in oncotic pressure in the pleural fluid would lead to progressive pleural fluid accumulation. In pathologic states, once the protein content of pleural fluid reaches 4 g/dl, capillary absorption ceases and clearance is entirely by way of the lymphatics. While these mechanisms explain many aspects of pleural fluid dynamics, inexplicable findings are not uncommon. For example, the pleural space may be dry in cor pulmonale despite a right atrial pressure of 30 cm H$_2$O.[284] In addition, in pathologic states, critical factors affecting secretion and absorption may change (e.g., pleural thickening reduces permeability, and lymphatic stomata become blocked with cells and debris). Although the pleural space is completely gas-free, it is normally lubricated by a small amount of pleural fluid. This liquid coupling provides instantaneous transmission of perpendicular forces between pleural surfaces and allows the pleural membranes to slide in response to shear forces.[4] The film of liquid is thin, in the order of only 10 to 30 μm.[6] Normally, the volume of pleural fluid is approximately 1 to 5 ml, but in some subjects there may be up to 15 ml, particularly in pregnancy or during exercise.[357, 601] In one study small pleural effusions, usually bilateral, occurred in two-thirds of post-partum patients within 24 hours of delivery.[214] Using lateral decubitus chest radiographs to detect pleural fluid, a technique that has a threshold sensitivity of about 5 ml,[353] Hessen found a 10% prevalence of definite or probable pleural fluid in healthy adults.[198] This was sometimes unilateral and sometimes bilateral, and varied in the same individual from time to time. Normal pleural fluid has a protein concentration of 1 to 2 gm/dl, a cell count of 1,500 to 4,500/μl (60% to 70% monocytes), and less than half the serum concentration of large protein molecules like lactic acid dehydrogenase (LDH).[566]

PLEURAL EFFUSION

A variety of liquids may accumulate in the pleural space—transudate, exudate, blood, chyle, and occasionally more exotic liquids such as bile, cerebrospinal fluid, peritoneal dialysate, and intravenous infusions. By convention, and often in ignorance of the true contents of the pleural space, liquid in the pleural space is usually called pleural effusion. Alternative and more specific terms such as hemothorax, pyothorax, and chylothorax may be used as appropriate.

In clinical practice, the majority of effusions are either transudates or exudates. This distinction is based on the specific gravity, protein, and LDH content of the fluid. Transudates classically have a specific gravity of 1.016 or less and a protein content of 3 gm/dl or less. Recently, more sophisticated and specific criteria have been introduced to define a transudate: (1) a ratio of pleural fluid protein to serum protein of <0.5; (2) an LDH ratio of <0.6; and (3) an absolute pleural LDH of <200 IU/L.[284]

Transudates develop because of a change in the physical factors that affect the rate of pleural fluid formation and resorption: capillary pressure; plasma oncotic pressure; and, occasionally, pleural surface pressure. Once the altered factor or factors have been identified, attention can be directed away from the pleura, which is itself normal, to the underlying systemic abnormality. The important causes of transudative pleural effusions are listed in Table 14–1.

An exudative effusion, on the other hand, indicates that the pleural surface is pathologically altered, with an accompanying increase in permeability and/or a decrease in lymph flow. The list of possible causes for an exudative effusion is much longer than that for a transudate, and is presented in Table 14–2. The table gives a combined list of transudative and exudative effusions because there is some degree of overlap. The list is rather daunting; however, in practice, more than 90% of effusions result from heart failure, cirrhosis, ascites, pleuropulmonary infection, malignancy, and pulmonary embolism.[227] Very large effusions are seen especially in malignant disease as a result of metastases, notably lung and breast, but these may also occur in heart failure, cirrhosis, tuberculosis, empyema, and hemothorax.[304] Bilateral effusions tend to be transudates, though there are notable exceptions, particularly with metastatic disease, lymphoma, pulmonary embolism, and systemic lupus erythematosus.[412]

Once the presence and location of a pleural effusion have been established by an imaging investigation, the next step is to establish its cause.[205] This

TABLE 14–1.

Causes of Pleural Transudates

Raised venous pressure	Heart failure Constrictive pericarditis
Reduced plasma oncotic pressure	Hepatic cirrhosis Nephrotic syndrome Hypoalbuminemia (other causes)
Reduced pleural surface pressure	Atelectasis
Various other causes	Nephrogenic effusion Myxedema Pulmonary embolism

TABLE 14–2.

Causes of Pleural Effusion (Excluding Chylothorax and Hemothorax)

Physiologic	Normal (exceptionally), post-partum
Infectious	Bacteria (including *Mycobacterium*) Viruses, *chlamydia* Fungi Protozoa, metazoa Adjacent-subphrenic abscess, hepatic abscess (including amoebic)
Neoplastic	Bronchial carcinoma, metastases (lung/pleura) Lymphoma, leukemia, macroglobulinemia Pleural tumor (mesothelioma-diffuse, localized) Chest wall neoplasm
Cardiovascular	Heart failure, constrictive pericarditis Postcardiac injury syndrome Superior vena caval obstruction Pulmonary thromboembolism
Hepatic	Cirrhosis
Pancreatic	Pancreatitis
Renal	Nephrotic syndrome, acute nephritic syndrome, renal tract obstruction
Ascitic	Meigs' syndrome, peritoneal dialysis Ascites (benign, malignant)
Traumatic	Open/closed chest trauma, including esophageal rupture Iatrogenic, including abdominal surgery, radiation
Inhalational	Asbestos
Inflammatory	Rheumatoid disease, systemic lupus erythematosus, Wegener's granulomatosis
Drug-induced	Methotrexate and other drugs
Miscellaneous	Sarcoidosis Myxedema Yellow nail syndrome Familial Mediterranean fever

will depend on patient history, the examination, and a hierarchy of investigations which, depending on possible diagnoses, include blood and urine tests; thoracocentesis, with an examination of the pleural fluid; and pleural biopsy. Exudates should be examined, in particular, for microorganisms, malignant cells, and autoantibodies. Other investigations that may be used include thoracoscopy, bronchoscopy, and open biopsy. Imaging procedures play an early and important part in this work-up and may disclose abnormalities both inside and outside the chest that can establish or suggest a probable cause for the effusion. In addition, imaging techniques are used to direct biopsy or interventional therapy.

Several large series indicate that about a fifth of pleural effusions that come to thoracocentesis are of indeterminate cause despite extensive investigation.[205, 274, 523] Nearly half of such patients have a definite diagnosis made on follow-up, most commonly of a malignant disorder.[182, 461]

Imaging of Pleural Effusion

Conventional radiography, CT, and ultrasound are all specific and sensitive ways of demonstrating pleural fluid. The appearance of an effusion depends critically on the position of the patient at the time of the examination and the mobility of the effusion, which may be free or constrained to a variable extent.

With a moderate sized pleural effusion, fluid collects around and under the lung and it takes on a characteristic configuration. This shape is determined by the interplay of the hydrostatic pressure in the effusion, the pleural liquid pressure, and the pleural surface pressure in the various zones from apex to base. In the erect subject, fluid collects mainly in the lower zone. Here the hydrostatic pressure is positive and the lung is compressed, so that it floats away from the chest wall and diaphragm.[4, 6] Homeostatic mechanisms, particularly tissue interdependence, prevent the lower lung zones from collapsing as much as might be predicted from the local pleural liquid pressure.[161] In contrast, in the highest zone, normal conditions obtain and pleural liquid pressure is much lower than pleural surface pressure. In this zone the thickness of fluid is essentially normal and radiologically undetectable. In the middle zone, the visceral-parietal pleural contact is lost, and pleural liquid and surface pressures become identical. Descending in this zone, pleural liquid pressure remains subatmospheric but becomes more positive because of the increasing head of effusion, and thus the recoil of the lung has to become less to allow the pleural surface pressure to rise (become less negative). This is achieved by lung volume decreasing since at smaller lung volumes recoil is less. Because lung volume decreases, the thickness of pleural fluid increases progressively. The end result of the interactions between these forces is that the lung eventually sits in the pleural fluid rather like an egg in an egg cup, and the upper surface of the effusion takes on a meniscus-like shape (Fig 14–21). The three-dimensional shape of effusions has been illustrated with casts.[84, 136]

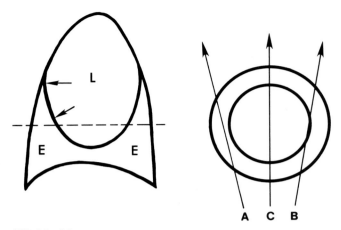

FIG 14–21.
Left, diagramatic vertical section through the lung *(L)* and a pleural effusion *(E)* to illustrate the disposition of pleural fluid. *Arrows* mark the lung/pleural fluid interface, which has a meniscus-like shape. *Right,* a transaxial section at the level indicated in the diagram at *left.* The letters A, B, and C represent x-ray beams. See text for explanation. (From Wilson AG: The interpretation of shadows on the adult chest radiograph. *Br J Hosp Med;* 37:526–534. Used by permission.)

The classic plain radiographic changes in a patient with a moderate pleural effusion are of a homogeneous lower zone opacity with a curvilinear upper border, quite sharply marginated and concave to the lung (Fig 14–22). A consideration of Figure 14–21 explains how this type of shadow is produced. In transaxial view it can be seen that the x-ray beam will be more attenuated laterally than centrally because the marginal beam passes through a greater thickness of fluid. A pleural effusion is therefore dense laterally, and because it presents a tangential fluid/air interface, it will have a sharp inner margin, with the classic meniscus shape produced by the inner fluid envelope. More centrally, the x-ray beam is less attenuated and the effusion just produces a general haziness, the upper edge of which cannot be seen because it has wedge-shaped geometry (see Fig 14–22). The meniscus is often higher laterally than medially because lung attachments (hilus and pulmonary ligament) alter the distribution of forces (see Fig 14–22).

Sometimes other types of shadow will be seen with a moderate effusion. Most of these result from free pleural fluid within fissures—and the radiographic appearance will depend on the shape and orientation of the fissure, the location of the fluid within it, and the direction of the x-ray beam.[410] A common appearance is a curvilinear interface on a frontal chest radiograph (see Fig 14–53). Such an opacity may be faint; typically, it is relatively transra-

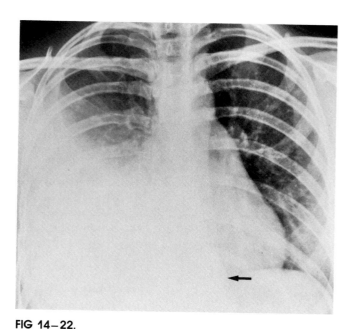

FIG 14–22.
Pleural effusion. The right-sided opacity has the classic features of a free pleural effusion in an erect patient. The opacity is homogeneous, occupies the inferior part of the chest, and has a concave upper margin that extends higher laterally than medially. Medial to the lateral limb of the meniscus there is a characteristic haziness without a clear upper border. At first glance the shadow low and to the left *(arrow)* resembles a displaced azygoesophageal recess, as sometimes occurs with pleural effusion. Its configuration is, however, not quite as expected, and it was found to result from a tuberculous paravertebral abscess—the cause of the effusion.

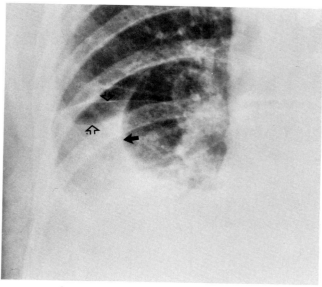

FIG 14–23.
The "middle lobe step." There is a steplike intrusion of pleural fluid into the fissures below the minor fissure. Features due to the minor fissure *(open arrows)* and major fissure *(closed arrow)* are indicated.

diant medially and more dense laterally and superiorly.[410] The medial curvilinear interface marks the limit of fluid intrusion into the fissure which may or may not be at the point of fissural fusion.[80] A somewhat similar shadow but higher and more peripheral may be produced by fluid accumulations between chest wall and the lips of contact of the major fissure[194] (see Fig 14–26). Such tongue-like intrusions of fluid into the margins of fissures are common and may be seen quite early on in the development of a pleural effusion, an observation that has been confirmed in studies with animals.[5] It gives rise to the thorn sign when a small amount of fluid accumulates laterally in the minor fissure on frontal view.[377]

A rather more complex shadow also now attributed to fissural intrusion is the middle lobe step (Fig 14–23). It consists of a steplike accumulation of fluid laterally below the minor fissure. When originally described it was thought to indicate a diseased middle lobe with reduced compliance.[136] This is no longer accepted, and it is now explained on the basis of overlapping fluid intrusion into incomplete major and minor fissures.[194, 410]

Other unusual appearances that may be seen with moderate sized effusions include encapsulation of a lobe, particularly the lower lobe, simulating consolidation.[126, 136, 194] Sometimes fluid collects preferentially against the mediastinum, particularly on the left, and gives a triangular retrocardiac density simulating lower lobe collapse, from which it can be differentiated by analyzing the position of the lower lobe bronchus. This distribution of fluid has been attributed to the modifying influence of the pulmonary ligament.[344, 414]

Early in their development pleural effusions are small, and it is now generally accepted that such effusions collect initially between the lower lobes and the diaphragm (Fig 14–24).[6, 198, 432] After a variable amount of fluid has accumulated, it spills into the posterior and then into the lateral costophrenic angles[136] and may cause subtle changes in the contour of the inferior aspect of the lower lobe. The only study to assess the amount of pleural fluid needed to blunt the costophrenic angles on PA radiographs is a postmortem study in erect cadavers at which it was found that, on average, the required volume was 175 ml (range, 25 to 525 ml).[66]

When effusions are too small to be detected on conventional PA and lateral chest radiographs, they may be demonstrated with special radiographic views or by ultrasound or CT. The most widely used special radiographic view is the lateral decubi-

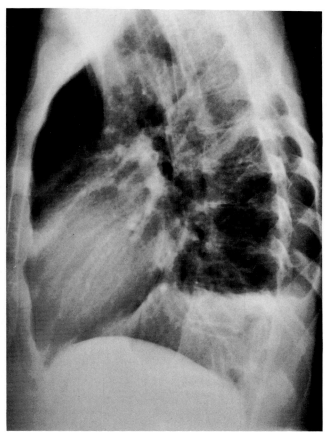

FIG 14–24.
Pleural effusion—subpulmonic. Lateral radiograph with patient erect demonstrates the characteristic horizontal upper border to the effusion and the abrupt angulation anteriorly against the oblique fissure.

tus view (see Fig 14–26),[198, 357, 555] with which it may be possible to detect 3 to 10 ml of fluid.[353, 357, 555] A variant on this technique, which can be performed in relatively immobile patients and by the bedside if necessary, is the oblique semisupine view.[349] The sensitivity of ultrasound and CT has not been formally assessed, but it is probably in the same sort of order as that of decubitus radiographs.

Subpulmonic Effusion

Occasionally, for reasons that are obscure, large quantities of pleural fluid accumulate in a subpulmonic location rather than escaping into the general pleural cavity. Attempts to attribute this distribution to an underlying abnormality in the lower lobe with subsequent distortion of pleural forces have not been convincing.[136, 432] Pleural adhesions are not a factor either, as most subpulmonic effusions prove completely mobile with postural changes.[198] Also,

for no clear reason, subpulmonic effusions are often transudates and are associated with renal failure, liver cirrhosis, congestive heart failure, and nephrotic syndrome.[100, 556] There are, however, many exceptions.[140] These effusions may be unilateral or bilateral; when unilateral they are more commonly right-sided,[394] and when bilateral they can easily be missed on the chest radiograph.[556]

The upper edge of the fluid mimics the contour of the diaphragm on the chest radiograph, so that the principal sign is an apparent elevation of the hemidiaphragm,[555] with the minor fissure appearing to be closer to the apparent diaphragm than usual. The "elevated hemidiaphragm" may have one or more of the following features, which should suggest the correct diagnosis:

1. The "hemidiaphragm" peaks more laterally than usual (Fig 14–25), and the contour on either side of the peak is straighter. The medial slope tends to be gradual; the lateral one, steep.[46, 136, 394]

2. These appearances, particularly the lateral peaking, are accentuated on expiration,[46] a phenomenon that has been attributed to the presence of the pulmonary ligament.[456]

3. The costophrenic angle is usually ill-defined, blunted (Figs 14–24 and 14–26), or shallow,[198, 556] but, exceptionally, both the lateral and the posterior angles can be clear.[140]

4. In the lateral radiograph the posterior aspect of the "hemidiaphragm" tends to be flat beneath the lower lobe (see Fig 14–24). On reaching the major fissure, the silhouette usually slopes steeply downward (Figs 14–24, and 14–26), and there may be a tail of fluid passing up into the fissure itself.[124, 394, 556] The perceived lack of fluid under the lung anteriorly may be more apparent than real.[410]

5. The rather flat upper surface of the fluid means that on the frontal view there is not the usual wedge of lung passing down below the silhouette of the diaphragm. Thus, on frontal view vessels are not seen below the superior surface of the diaphragm.[480]

6. On the left side there will be a greater than usual separation of gastric air bubble and the upper surface of the "hemidiaphragm." Unfortunately, this distance is very variable in healthy patients. Comparison with previous radiographs may help assessment. Some authors suggest that a distance of more than 2 cm is suggestive.[198]

7. On the frontal radiograph there will, occasionally, be a diaphragmatic spur associated with fluid entering the inferior accessory fissure[556] or a

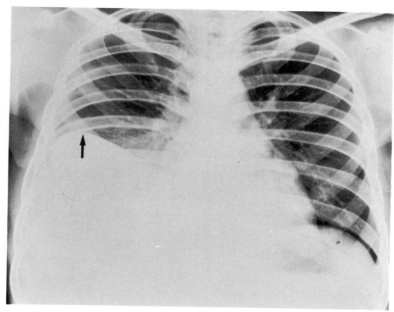

FIG 14–25.
Pleural effusion—subpulmonic. Appearances on the right superficially resemble those of an elevated hemidiaphragm. The configuration is, however, unusual—with a lateral peak that is characteristic of a subpulmonic effusion.

more substantial triangular retrocardiac shadow. This latter opacity—which effaces the medial "hemidiaphragmatic" contour and the left paravertebral interface—results from paramediastinal extension of the subpulmonic fluid.[100]

Subpulmonic pleural fluid is rarely loculated, and the diagnosis may, therefore, be confirmed by obtaining a decubitus radiograph (Fig 14–26).[198] Alternatively, its presence may be confirmed by ultrasound or CT.

Large pleural effusions obscure the border of the heart and displace the mediastinum, the airways, and the diaphragm. Visualization of the pericardial fat as a curvilinear transradiancy sometimes allows assessment of heart size even when the heart border is completely obscured by pleural fluid.[150] Large pleural effusions should lead to contralateral displacement of the mediastinum (see Fig 14–27), and right-sided effusions may give a mediastinally based retrocardiac density convex to the left as a result of herniation of the fluid-filled azygoesophageal recess[387] (see Fig 14–45). A central mediastinum in the face of a large pleural effusion suggests that either the mediastinum is fixed (most commonly the result of malignant infiltration by carcinoma or mesothelioma) or there is obstructive collapse, usually because of bronchial carcinoma of the underlying lung.[278, 556] In contrast, relaxation collapse of the

lung, which normally accompanies a large pleural effusion, is not usually so great that it makes up for the volume of the effusion. On lateral views posterior pleural collections cause anterior displacement of central airways, a helpful feature in differentiating effusion from collapse or consolidation.[402]

Inversion of the hemidiaphragm is an occasional but well-recognized finding.[124, 358, 528] It is seen with large or moderate effusions, more commonly on the left than on the right,[556] a difference ascribed to the lack of liver support on the left.[605] On plain chest radiography, diaphragmatic inversion is easier to recognize on the left, where displacement of gastric and colonic gas indicates the shape and position of the left hemidiaphragm (Fig 14–28). On the right side it is most easily diagnosable by ultrasound (Fig 14–29; see also Fig 14–45).[296, 525, 606] It has been brought to light by liver scintigraphy, which demonstrates deformity of the dome of the liver.[89, 235] An inverted right hemidiaphragm on CT examination superficially resembles a cystlike lesion of the liver (Fig 14–30).[235, 276] Other lesions that may invert the hemidiaphragm include pneumothorax, lobar emphysema, diaphragmatic neoplasm, pericardial cyst, and myocardial aneurysm.[440] Diaphragm inversion is generally unimportant clinically. However, the following effects have been described: (1) it may cause or simulate an upper abdominal mass[78, 89]; (2) it leads to paradoxic diaphragmatic movement[525] that

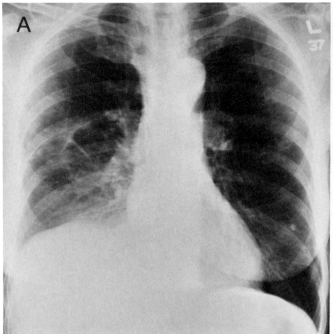

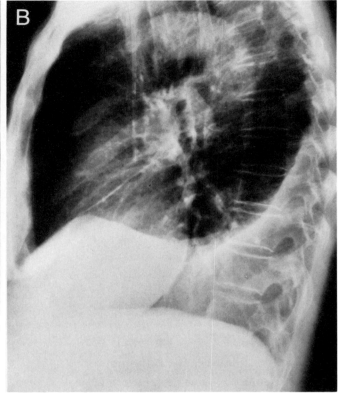

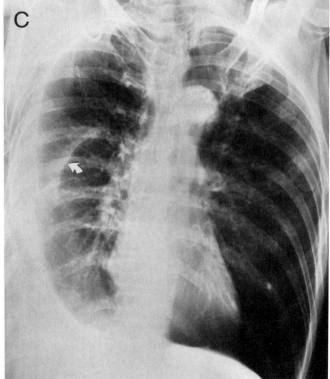

FIG 14–26.

Pleural effusion—subpulmonic. **A,** the right hemidiaphragm is elevated, and although it does not have the classic contour associated with a subpulmonic effusion, it does have a longer horizontal medial segment than is usual on the right. The costophrenic angle is clear, but there is haziness in the cardiophrenic angle region. **B,** lateral view of the same patient. There is pleural fluid underneath the right lower lobe but it is not entirely subpulmonic, as the posterior costophrenic angle is obscured and fluid extends up against the posterior chest wall. The rather flat lower margin to the lower lobe and the steep down slope at the major fissure are characteristic of subpulmonic fluid. **C,** right lateral decubitus view. The subdiaphragmatic fluid has run up the lateral chest wall, giving a band of soft tissue density. The curvilinear shadow medially *(arrow)* indicates intrusion of fluid into the lips of the major fissure.

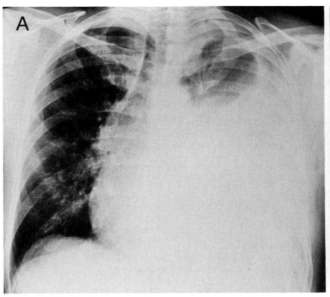

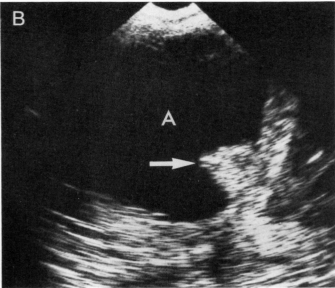

FIG 14-27.
Pleural effusion—large. **A,** mesothelioma is a recognized cause for a large pleural effusion unaccompanied by mediastinal shift. Exceptions to this finding are, however, not uncommon, as in this patient. **B,** ultrasound examination demonstrates echo-free pleu-ral fluid *(A)* and one of several areas of nodular pleural thickening *(arrow).* Diagnosis was made by biopsy study of a local pleural mass under ultrasound control. (Courtesy of Dr. A.E.A. Joseph, London.)

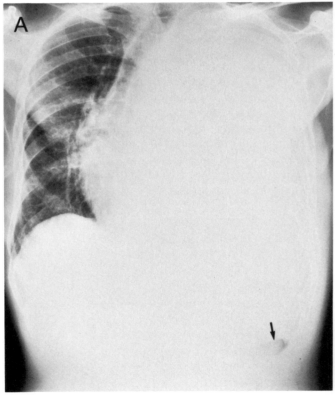

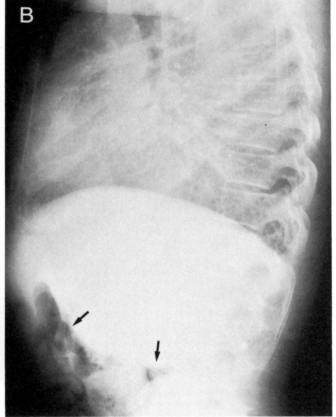

FIG 14-28.
Pleural effusion—hemidiaphragm inversion. **A,** PA chest radio-graph shows a large left pleural effusion displacing the mediasti-num to the right and colonic gas inferiorly *(arrow).* **B,** lateral radio-graph on the same patient shows more clearly the position of the left hemidiaphragm, indicated by displaced bowel gas *(arrows).*

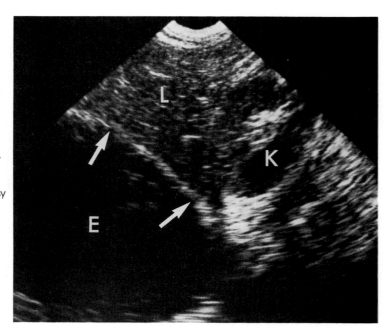

FIG 14–29.
Pleural effusion—inverted hemidiaphragm. Ultrasound examination of the right upper quadrant of the abdomen. Liver *(L)* and kidney *(K)* to the right are separated from an essentially echo-free pleural effusion *(E)* by the hemidiaphragm *(arrows)*, which is convex to liver. (Courtesy of Dr. A.E.A. Joseph, London.)

could lead to dyspnea because of pendulum breathing (expired air from the ipsilateral lung being inspired contralaterally)[358]; and (3) should the inversion disappear following thoracocentesis, the apparent size of the pleural effusion on a chest radiograph may not change significantly.

Loculated Pleural Effusion

Pleural fluid may loculate (encyst) within the fissures, or between parietal and visceral pleura when there is partial fusion of the pleural layers.

Loculations against the chest wall are the most frequent. They take on a variety of configurations, the most common being a dome-shaped projection into the lung (Fig 14–31). The appearances of this on plain radiographs depends on the projection. If the loculation is seen *en face* or obliquely, it produces a rounded opacity with part of the margin sharp and part ill-defined. On a frontal radiograph the clear margin is usually medial and the hazy one lateral (Fig 14–32). This appearance is the same as that illustrated with a (sub)pleural lipoma (see Fig 14–51). When viewed tangentially a loculation is classically convex to lung and sharply demarcated on its pulmonary aspect because of its pleural covering, just as it appears on CT (see Fig 14–31). These lesions tend to have greater length than height, and because of the weight of contained fluid the greatest height is

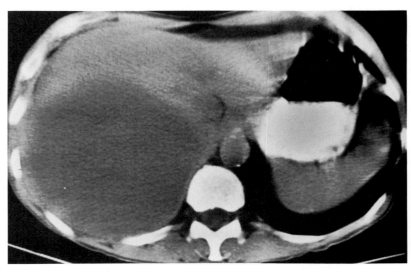

FIG 14–30.
Pleural effusion—inverted hemidiaphragm. A CT examination of the upper abdomen shows a large, rounded, low-density area apparently lying posteriorly in the liver caused by a right pleural effusion inverting the right hemidiaphragm.

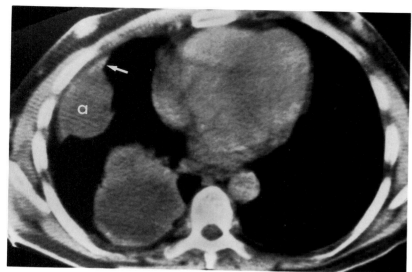

FIG 14–31.
Pleural effusion—loculated. The opacities on the right are loculated hematomas, in part clotted. The upper one is against the chest wall, and the lower is a dome-shaped collection resting on the hemidiaphragm. Opacity *a* has the classic shape of a loculated pleural collection; it is sharply marginated and convex to lung, and it lifts off a tail of pleura *(arrow),* giving its margin an obtuse angle with the chest wall.

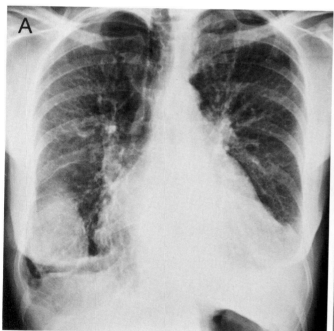

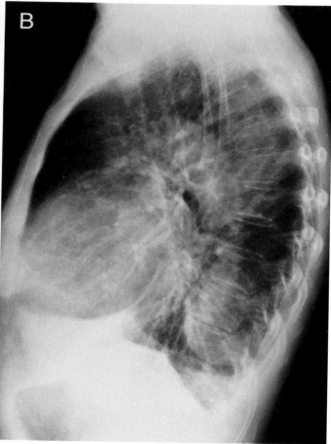

FIG 14–32.
Pleural effusion—loculated. This 68-year-old woman was in heart failure due to mixed mitral valve disease. There is bilateral pleural fluid, which on the right is loculated against the chest wall. **A,** PA radiograph shows an oval right lower zone opacity with the characteristics of a chest wall or pleural lesion; it is homogeneous, the margin in part sharp and in part ill-defined. Much of the sharp margin is on the medial aspect of the opacity, as is usually the case with localized pleural/chest wall lesions. **B,** lateral view of the same patient confirms the radiographic features of the pleural loculation and shows blunting of the posterior costophrenic angle and fluid entering the major fissure on the right.

not necessarily over the center of the lesion. The margins of the loculus make an obtuse angle with the chest wall, elevating a "tail" of pleura (see Fig 14–31). Radiologically these lesions share many features with chest wall or (extra)pleural masses[125] and they are often indistinguishable. Extrapleural chest wall lesions, however, tend to stand more proud, to be as high as they are long, to have their greatest depth opposite the center of attachment, and—most important of all—they may show rib involvement.[125] A pleural lesion may well show evidence of pleural disease elsewhere in the pleural cavity (see Fig 14–32).

Pleural fluid may also loculate within fissures, particularly in heart failure.[122, 200, 578] Because these collections tend to come and go, they have been called vanishing/phantom tumors and pseudotumors.[200] Such loculations are seen more commonly on the right[120] and in the minor rather than the major fissures despite the greater area of the latter (Fig 14–33). In the minor fissure on a lateral radiograph loculated fluid has a characteristic lenticular shape, often with a pathognomonic tail extending along the fissure for a short distance. In frontal view it usually appears rounded or oval and sharply demarcated. Usually there is no problem in making the diagnosis if account is taken of the distinctive shape and posi-

tion of the lesion, particularly in the presence of heart failure.

Loculated collections in the major fissure have the expected distinctive appearance in lateral views (Fig 14–34), but in frontal projection they commonly do not have the masslike features of those in the minor fissure. This is because the long axis of these lesions is tilted relative to the frontal x-ray beam, and the shadow generated is either hazy and veil-like or more discrete—with margins that are in part ill-defined and in part distinct (Fig 14–34). Loculations in the caudad part of the major fissure (Fig 14–35) may resemble middle lobe collapse/ consolidation (Fig 14–36). Points in this situation that favor loculated fluid rather than collapse are: (1) identification of a separate minor fissure; (2) one or more convex margins in lateral projection (with collapse, usually at least one border is concave or straight); (3) right border of the heart not effaced on frontal view; and (4) both ends of the opacity taper in lateral view (with collapse, the anterior end is usually broad).[124] Two findings that favor collapse are: (1) contact between the anterior end of the shadow and the chest wall; and (2) an air bronchogram[124, 140] (Fig 14–37).

Other peripheral fluid loculations (against diaphragm and mediastinum) are not so common as

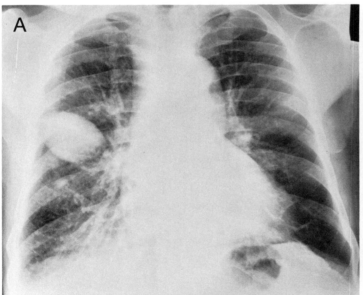
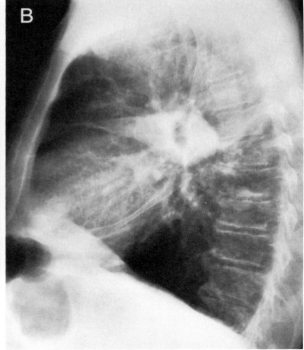

FIG 14–33.
Pleural effusion—loculated. This 77-year-old man is in heart failure. The PA chest radiograph **(A)** shows a 7 × 4-cm well-demarcated oval opacity in the right mid-zone projected in the region of the minor fissure. The lateral radiograph **(B)** shows a lenticular opacity occupying the minor fissure, with a characteristic tail anteriorly.

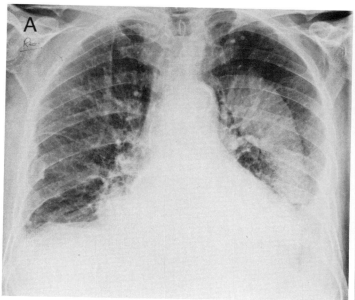

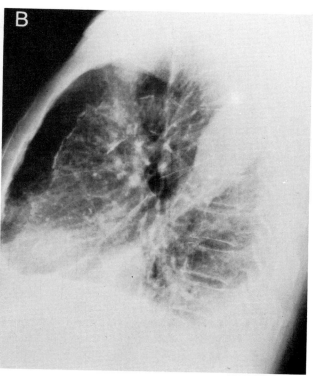

FIG 14–34.
Pleural effusion—loculated. **A,** anteroposterior (AP) and **B,** lateral views of fluid encysted in the major fissure. This effusion is unusual in that most of its margin is sharp in AP view. As with many loculated collections there is also free fluid in the pleural space.

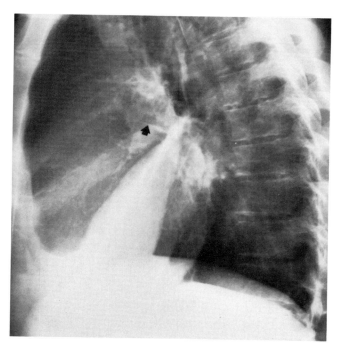

FIG 14–35.
Pleural effusion—loculated. There is a homogeneous triangular opacity in this lateral view projected over the lower end of the major fissure. Features that suggest it results from loculated fluid rather than middle lobe collapse are: (1) contact with diaphragm rather than sternum anteriorly and (2) convex borders. Identification of a separate minor fissure *(arrow)* confirms the diagnosis.

those against the chest wall, but they do occur and they are being increasingly recognized with CT. The plain radiographic features of these lesions are predictable.

So-called lamellar pleural effusions are, in fact, fluid collections in the loose connective tissue beneath the visceral pleura (Fig 14–38). They are seen with an edematous pulmonary interstitium, particularly in heart failure, and are discussed in Chapter 8.

Pleural Effusion in the Supine Patient.—When a patient is supine, free pleural fluid layers out posteriorly, and although there is a meniscus effect at the lung/fluid interface, it is not appreciated on a frontal projection because it is orientated at right-angles to the x-ray beam. It is generally accepted that the supine chest radiograph is not particularly sensitive or specific in the diagnosis of pleural effusion,[459] although in one study 90% of effusions between 200 and 500 ml were detected.[599] Sensitivity of detection falls when effusions are bilateral, and the volume of the effusion is generally underestimated.[459]

The signs produced by pleural effusions on supine radiographs are as follows:

1. Hazy, veil-like opacity of a hemithorax with preserved vascular shadows[136, 198] (Fig 14–39).

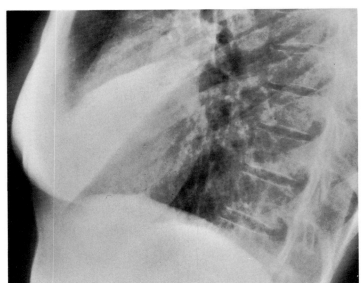

FIG 14−36.
Right middle lobe collapse. In lateral view features that suggest this is a collapsed/consolidated lobe rather than encysted fluid are: (1) anterior contact of the wedge-shaped opacity with the sternum; (2) anterior end broader than the posterior; (3) one straight border; and (4) absence of a separate minor fissure. The convexity of the upper border is atypical and a feature of encysted fluid.

When effusions are small this veiling may just occupy the lower chest, making the lower half of the hemithorax more opaque than the upper, which is the reverse of the normal situation.[599]

2. Loss of the sharp silhouette of the ipsilateral hemidiaphragm (see Fig 14−39).[349, 599]

3. Blunting of the costophrenic angle.[455, 574] Though a common sign, it is often a false positive finding.[459]

4. Capping of the lung apex with a pleural shadow (see Fig 14−39).[410] Some regard this as a relatively early sign explicable because the chest apex has a small capacity and is the most dependent part of the pleural space tangential to a frontal x-ray beam in a supine patient.[410] Other workers, however, find that effusions have to be at least moderate (more than 500 ml) before they collect at the apex.[599] With the accumulation of more fluid a bandlike opac-

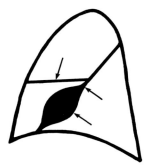
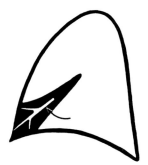

FIG 14−37.
Diagram of collapse vs. encysted fluid. The differential diagnosis of encysted fluid in the oblique fissure *(left)* vs. collapse/consolidation *(right)* of the middle lobe are illustrated. For discussion see text.

ity develops and separates the lateral lung margin from the chest wall (see Fig 14-39).

5. Thickening of the minor fissure.[410]

6. Widening of the paraspinal soft tissues.[542]

7. Apparent elevation of the hemidiaphragm and reduced visibility of lower lobe vessels behind the diaphragm.[455]

The modifying effect of additional air in the pleural space on the signs of a supine effusion are discussed by Onik and co-workers.[384]

CT of Free Pleural Fluid

Although comparative studies have not been performed, CT is undoubtedly a more sensitive modality in the detection of pleural fluid than an erect PA chest radiograph. Pleural effusion gives a homogeneous crescentic opacity in the most dependent part of the pleural cavity. The lower attenuation coefficients of pleural fluid usually allow distinction from pleural thickening and masses,[302] but the attenuation coefficient does not allow a differentiation to be made between exudate, transudate, and malignant effusion.[248, 557] It may, however, be possible to identify a hemothorax with CT as a nonhomogeneous collection with attenuation coefficients considerably higher than that of water.[591] Pleural fluid deep in the posterior and lateral costophrenic sulci may be confused with ascites, and a variety of signs have been described to differentiate pleural and ascitic fluid:

1. Displaced crus sign. Pleural fluid collects between the crus and the spine and displaces the crus

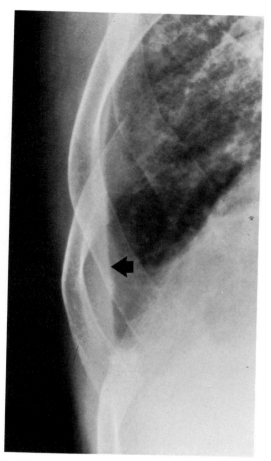

FIG 14–38.
Effusion—laminar. Localized view of the right costophrenic angle shows a band of soft tissue density parallel to the chest wall with edge enhancement due to a Mach effect *(arrow)*. This is not free pleural fluid but rather subvisceral pleural fluid, and it is seen when the lung interstitium is waterlogged—as in this patient with heart failure. Note the septal lines.

anterolaterally, whereas ascitic fluid collects anterolaterally to the crus and causes the opposite displacement (Fig 14-43).[101]

2. The interface sign. The interface between pleural fluid and liver or spleen is hazy (Fig 14–40),[535] probably because of a partial volume effect from the obliquely sectioned diaphragm. This sign must be assessed away from the dome of the diaphragm and it becomes less discriminating with thin slices (1.5–5 mm).[535]

3. The diaphragm sign. If the diaphragm can be identified, fluid inside the dome must be ascites, and fluid on the outside must be pleural, provided that the diaphragm is not inverted.[9] It is often surprisingly difficult to identify the diaphragm because the diaphragm and liver have similar attenuation values. Sometimes the curvilinear opacity produced by at-

electatic lung can mimic the appearance of the diaphragm. In general, atelectatic lung is thicker than the diaphragm, tapers laterally, and may be interrupted.[121] In addition, contiguous cuts will usually show continuity with air-containing lung or lung that contains an air bronchogram.[121]

4. Bare area sign. Because the posterior portion of the diaphragm is difficult to identify in many individuals, a knowledge of the shape of the various spaces in which peridiaphragmatic fluid may collect is helpful in assessing whether fluid is pleural or ascitic on CT.[361] Pleural fluid is free to collect along the full width of the costophrenic recess behind the liver, whereas ascitic fluid is excluded from the large bare area over the posteromedial surface of the right lobe of the liver (see Fig 14–40). This bare area, which lies between the upper and lower layers of the coronary ligament, is extraperitoneal and not accessible to ascitic fluid.[181] Therefore, fluid posteromedial to liver suggests a pleural location. Some care in interpreting this sign is needed, as ascitic fluid can lie above and below the coronary ligament. It is important, therefore, to assess multiple scan levels.[189]

Ultrasound and Pleural Fluid

Ultrasound can be used to image pleural fluid provided that there is no intervening lung. This situation obtains for pleural fluid against the chest wall and less commonly for fluid in other situations where there may be sonic access through a lung-free window such as liver. The main contributions made by ultrasound examination in the evaluation and management of pleural fluid are: (1) it is helpful in distinguishing solid from fluid pleural lesions (see Fig 14–27)[289]; (2) it enables differentiation of peripheral lung lesions from pleural fluid[96] (Fig 14–41); (3) it enables identification of pleural fluid in unusual sites such as in a subpulmonic location; (4) it pinpoints localized fluid collections for aspiration; (5) it may demonstrate solid components of a large effusion, which will enable biopsy (see Fig 14–27); and (6) it is helpful in identifying the causes of some effusions, such as those due to subphrenic or hepatic abscess.[366]

Pleural fluid is commonly echo-poor, with posterior echo enhancement just like fluid collections elsewhere in the body.[406] Posterior echo enhancement is, however, of limited diagnostic value because any interface with air-containing lung has high acoustic impedence. In addition, while solid lesions are usually echogenic and reliably identified,[289] there are exceptions. This is particularly recognized when im-

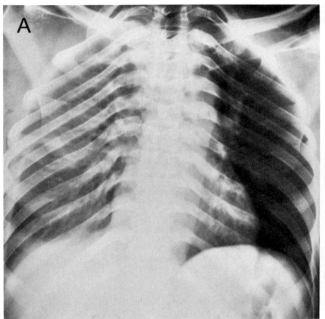

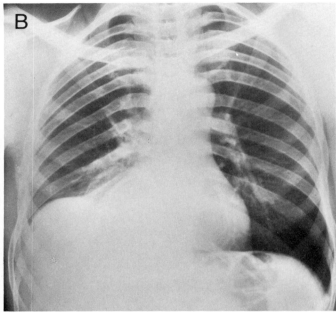

FIG 14—39.
Effusion—supine. **A,** supine view in a patient with a right-sided pleural effusion. There is hazy opacification of the whole right hemithorax with preserved vascular markings. The diaphragm silhouette is hazy. The right costophrenic angle is, unfortunately, ex-

cluded from the image, but with a lateral band of fluid against the chest wall it would almost certainly have been blunted. The lung is capped with apical fluid. **B,** radiograph on the same day with patient erect; the effusion is largely in a subpulmonic location.

aging clotted blood.[259] Conversely, fluid lesions may contain echoes, especially those indicative of debris and septa (Fig 14—42),[206] which are particularly common in empyema. Septation and change in shape of pleural lesions during the examination are

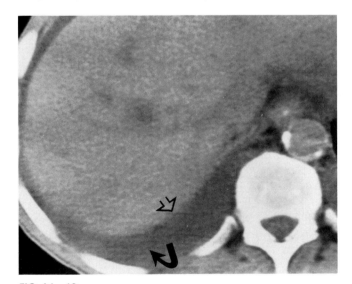

FIG 14—40.
Pleural effusion—CT. CT scan at the level of the liver and posterior costophrenic sulcus. The homogeneous opacity behind the liver is pleural fluid and not ascites. The hazy liver margin *(open arrow)* and the absence of a bare area *(curved arrow)* are supporting evidence.

indications that fluid is present and that a pleural aspiration will be successful.[311, 443]

Magnetic Resonance Imaging and Pleural Fluid

Preliminary in vitro studies have suggested that magnetic resonance imaging has the potential for differentiation among pleural effusions of different chemical composition.[558] In vivo results have not been so encouraging,[546] although they have shown that old hemorrhage can be differentiated from other effusions.

Specific Pleural Effusions

In the following sections, specific causes of pleural effusion are considered in detail. Effusions caused by pleuropulmonary infection, neoplasm, trauma, exposure to asbestos, and collagen vascular diseases are considered elsewhere. The major causes of pleural effusion other than chylothorax and hemothorax are listed in Table 14—2.

Adjacent Infection

Infectious processes in the upper abdomen commonly cause pleural effusions, which are usually sterile transudates. This happens particularly with subphrenic (and hepatic) abscesses, but also occurs

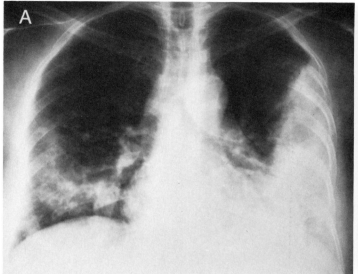
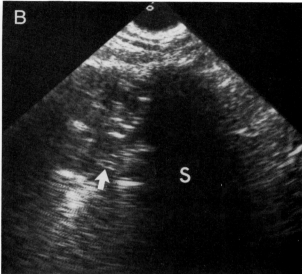

FIG 14–41.
A, PA chest radiograph of a patient with pneumonia. It was questioned whether or not the opacity against the left chest wall was a loculated pleural effusion. Its overall shape was suggestive but the irregular inner margin was atypical. **B,** ultrasound examination shows acoustic shadowings because of rib. The lesion itself is echogenic and contains parallel linear reflections *(arrow)* that could either be airways or vessels. In either case this offers definite evidence that the opacity is the result of consolidated lung. The distinction between vessels and airways is academic but can be made by assessing pulsation. (Courtesy of Dr. A.E.A. Joseph, London.)

with other forms of upper abdominal suppuration such as perinephric abscess.[463]

Subphrenic Abscess.— This most commonly follows upper abdominal surgery, particularly involving the stomach and spleen.[467] A significant proportion of cases, between 10% and 20%,[86, 467, 488] are not directly related to surgery but follow perforation of a hollow viscus, pancreatitis, or trauma, and a small number are cryptogenic. When a subphrenic abscess follows surgery, there is commonly a delay of about 1 to 3 weeks, but this may be prolonged to many months.[284] With abscesses in contact with the diaphragm there are nearly always changes on the plain chest radiograph (Fig 14–43).[86] About 80% of patients have a pleural effusion,[86, 340, 467, 582] which is usually small to moderate in size. Additional radiographic findings commonly include an elevated hemi-

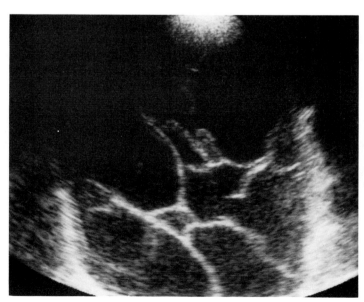

FIG 14–42.
Ultrasound examination of an empyema demonstrates multiple septa and echo-rich spaces in between. Empyema fluid is commonly echogenic because of its content of cells and debris.

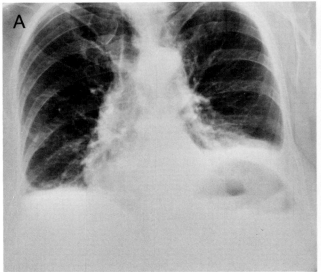

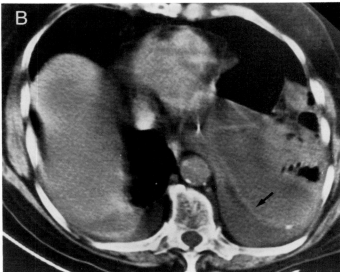

FIG 14–43.
Pleural effusion—subphrenic abscess. **A,** PA chest radiograph shows a raised left hemidiaphragm, pleural fluid, two air-fluid levels underneath the left hemidiaphragm, and collapse/consolidation of the left lower lobe. **B,** CT of the same patient shows a slightly thickened diaphragm *(arrow)* between posterior pleural fluid and the more anterior subdiaphragmatic fluid which contains gas, at least some of which is in bowel.

diaphragm, basal collapse and consolidation, and an air-fluid level below the diaphragm (Fig 14–43). The diagnosis may be virtually established by ultrasound or CT scanning[184] (Fig 14–43).

Hepatic Abscess.—In a series of 53 patients with pyogenic liver abscesses the chest radiograph was abnormal in 53%.[453] The changes most commonly noted were basilar atelectasis/pneumonitis (44%), hemidiaphragm elevation (31%), and pleural effusion (20%). There was an air-fluid level below the hemidiaphragm in 7% of these patients. The possibility of a hepatic abscess (amebic or pyogenic) should be considered in all patients with an obscure right-sided exudative pleural effusion,[285] particularly if there is fever, anorexia, and abdominal pain. Investigation by ultrasound and CT plays a pivotal role in diagnosis and management, but their consideration is beyond the scope of this discussion.

Cardiovascular

Heart Failure.—In clinical practice heart failure is probably the most common cause of a transudative pleural effusion; the volume ranges from barely detectable to considerable.[304] It is generally taught that pleural effusions in heart failure are more common and larger on the right, but a review of autopsy and clinical series shows that the excess of right-sided effusions over left is not very marked: 26% right-sided, 16% left-sided, 59% bilateral.* Some authors consider that isolated left pleural effusion in heart failure indicates an additional disease process, such as pulmonary embolism.[292] Again, this view receives some, but not strong, support from the autopsy series in which a fifth of those with right-sided and a third of those with left-sided effusions had pulmonary infarcts.[415, 584] Two unusually distributed forms of fluid collection occur particularly in heart failure: (1) encysted effusion[120, 122] and (2) lamellar "effusion" (see Chapter 8).

There is still debate about the mechanism responsible for the development of pleural effusion in heart failure. Most authors have suggested that a mixture of left and right heart failure is necessary.[141] A much-quoted experiment conducted in dogs[333] showed that elevation of right-sided pressures caused a greater accumulation of pleural fluid than elevation of left-sided pressures, but that an increase of both right- and left-sided pressures together was the most effective maneuver. On the other hand, a recent study on humans in heart failure following myocardial infarction showed that the presence of an effusion correlated much better with elevated left atrial pressure than it did with elevated right-sided pressures,[587] an observation that fits bet-

---

*References 24, 274, 325, 392, 415, 577, and 584.

ter with the generally low prevalence of pleural effusions in cor pulmonale.[586, 587]

Pericardial Disease.—Pericardial disease, both inflammatory and noninflammatory, may be associated with pleural effusions. Weiss and Spodick[576] assessed a series of 35 patients with pleural effusions and a variety of pericardial diseases and found that effusions were solely left-sided in 60% and predominantly left-sided in 71% (Fig 14−44) (9% were right predominant and 20% were equal bilaterally).

Post−Cardiac Injury Syndrome.—Post−cardiac injury syndrome follows a variety of myocardial and/or pericardial injuries and is most commonly seen after myocardial infarction (Dressler's syndrome)[98] or cardiac surgery (postpericardiotomy syndrome).[110] It is characterized by fever, pleuritis, pneumonitis, and pericarditis days or weeks after the precipitating event and often runs an intermittent course. Study of the condition has been hampered by lack of a diagnostic test and by clinical similarities with pneumonia, extension of myocardial infarction, heart failure, and pulmonary embolism. The prevalence rate following myocardial infarction is probably in the order of a few percent[98, 283] and

somewhat higher after cardiac surgery.[462] In one series,[519] the syndrome developed on average 20 days after cardiac injury (range, 2 to 86 days). The most common symptoms and signs were pleuritic chest pain (91%), fever, pericardial rub, dyspnea, and pleural rub. Nearly all the patients had a high erythrocyte sedimentation rate, and 50% had a leukocytosis. None had hemoptysis.

The post−cardiac injury syndrome is usually self-limiting. Should treatment be required, the usual drugs used are aspirin, nonsteroidal anti-inflammatory agents, or steroids. Relapse may occur following drug withdrawal.[462]

The chest radiograph is abnormal in more than 90% of patients, the chief findings being pleural effusion, consolidation, and a large heart. Pleural effusions were present in 81% of patients in four combined series,[98, 275, 519, 531] unilateral and bilateral effusions being equally common. When unilateral, effusions are more common on the left than on the right.[519] About half of the patients have consolidation, which is usually unilateral, and about half have a large cardiac silhouette. In the appropriate clinical setting the diagnosis should be suspected on radiologic grounds if pleural effusion(s) and consolidation develop with concomitant rapid enlargement of

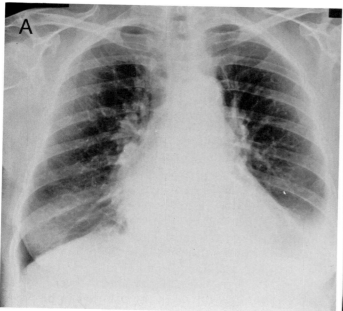

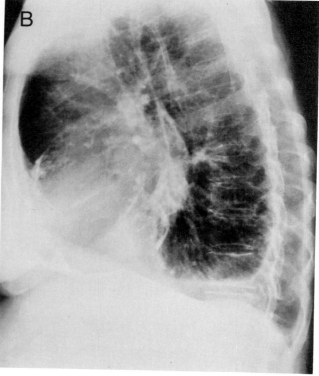

FIG 14−44.

Pleural effusion—pericarditis. **A,** PA chest radiograph in constrictive pericarditis. There is a left-sided pleural effusion. **B,** lateral chest radiograph of the same patient shows that the pleural fluid is confined to the left side. There is heavy pericardial calcification.

the cardiac silhouette without evidence of heart failure.[506] Echocardiography will establish the pericardial nature of the cardiac enlargement. The pleural fluid is a serosanguinous or bloody exudate.[519] It is important to identify the postcardiac injury syndrome if only to avoid iatrogenic complications from unnecessary therapy for incorrect diagnoses such as pulmonary embolism.

Superior Vena Caval Syndrome.—Occlusion of the superior vena cava might be expected to predispose to the formation of pleural effusion[333] because (1) it increases the parietal pleural hydrostatic pressure, thereby increasing fluid filtration from parietal pleural capillaries; and (2) it reduces lymphatic flow from the thoracic duct and right bronchomediastinal trunk.[529] However, pleural effusion secondary to vena caval obstruction is not common. In a series of 35 patients with superior vena caval syndrome, eight had effusions but in only two did obstruction of the superior vena cava seem a reasonable explanation for its development.[217] In a larger series of 84 patients with superior vena caval obstruction, all four effusions were the result of malignancy.[391] Apart from these series there are isolated case reports of pleural effusion associated with innominate vein[226] and superior vena caval obstruction.[173] In the last case the effusion followed iatrogenic thrombosis and was a transudate, but in other case reports it has been chylous.[91, 481]

Pulmonary Embolism.—Pleural effusion is common in pulmonary embolism occurring in a quarter to a half of the cases.* Effusions are more likely to occur with infarction but can be seen without it; in some series, effusion without infarction was considered to be very unusual.[52, 71]

The characteristics of pleural effusions in pulmonary embolism have been well described in a prospective study of 155 patients with pulmonary embolism.[52] Effusion was the only chest radiographic sign in 18% of the patients; more commonly, it was associated with other signs of pulmonary embolism. Effusions tended to be small, occupying 15% of a hemithorax on average, and none occupied more than a third of the hemithorax. The vast majority (98%) were unilateral with no side predilection. This observation is somewhat at variance with other series in which a higher prevalence of bilateral effusions was found.[77, 135, 532] The effusions were nearly always painful and tended to be at a maximum within

the first 3 days of clinical illness. Only 3% enlarged after this time, an event that should suggest recurrent embolism, infection, or possibly anticoagulant-induced hemorrhage.[494] The effusions tended to disappear within about a week (72% disappearing by 7 days), but effusions accompanied by pulmonary consolidation usually took longer to clear.

Cirrhosis of the Liver

Pleural effusion is a recognized finding in patients with hepatic cirrhosis. A prevalence varying between 0.4%[351] and 12%[221] has been recorded in various series, a range that reflects the differing severity of the underlying liver disease. Effusions may be small to massive,[232, 320] and they show a predilection for the right side (Fig 14–45). Thus, in 55 cases from six series, 60% were right-sided, 22% left-sided, and 18% bilateral.† In one series that looked at cirrhosis with isolated left pleural effusion, 18% of effusions were found to be tuberculous.[346] These authors concluded that isolated left-sided effusions in the context of cirrhosis should be fully investigated and not assumed to be the result of the liver disease per se.[346]

Although raised lymphatic pressure, azygos vein hypertension, and hypoalbuminemia play a part in generating cirrhotic effusions,[32] there is considerable evidence indicating that transdiaphragmatic passage of fluid is the most important mechanism.[282] Under these circumstances the development of pleural effusions depends on the presence of ascites, and this is indeed an almost universal finding in cirrhotic pleural effusion (Fig 14–45),[221, 232, 320] with only a few exceptions having been reported.[55, 143] The corollary, that all patients with cirrhotic ascites have pleural effusions, is by no means true. In one series of 330 patients with hepatic ascites, only 5.5% had pleural effusions on plain chest radiography.[281] Early workers theorized that fluid crossed the diaphragm by way of the lymphatics,[232, 330] but today's consensus opinion is that it passes through defects in the diaphragm. Transfer of fluid from the peritoneal cavity to the chest has been clearly demonstrated by studies in which blue dye, Indian ink, and labeled albumin have been introduced into ascitic fluid.[232, 281] It is also well recognized that air in the peritoneal cavity can enter the pleural cavity, usually on the right.‡ Furthermore, defects have been identified in the diaphragm at postmortem examination,[109, 281, 500] at thoracotomy, and at thoracoscopy.[134, 281, 363] Fluid and air have been seen to pass

---

*References 52, 352, 490, 516, 532, and 551.

†References 221, 232, 281, 282, 320, and 589.
‡References 39, 72, 233, 281, 282, 447, and 589.

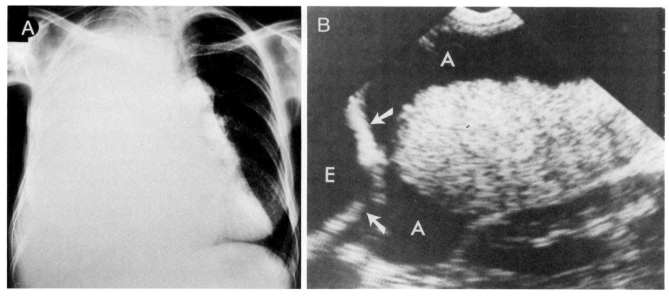

FIG 14–45.
Pleural effusion—hepatic cirrhosis. **A,** PA radiograph shows a massive right pleural effusion with mediastinal displacement to the left. The right-sided location of the effusion is characteristic. **B,** longitudinal ultrasound scan of the right upper quadrant shows the diaphragm *(arrows)* between pleural effusion *(E)* and ascites *(A)*. The diaphragm is convex to liver and inverted. The cirrhotic liver has a nodular surface. (Courtesy of Dr. A.E.A. Joseph, London.)

through these defects.[281] The defects are usually found in the tendinous part of the diaphragm and are probably tears produced by the stretching that occurs in the presence of ascites.[282] Localized muscle thinning where vessels pass through the diaphragm may be another predisposing factor. The pathology of these lesions has been elegantly demonstrated by Lieberman and Peters.[282] Some of the defects were still closed by peritoneum and appear as fluid-filled blebs on the pleural side of the diaphragm, whereas in others the peritoneal membrane had ruptured, leaving a hole. The structure of the blebs, their possible sudden rupture, and their later occlusion by adhesions probably accounts for the fact that many people with ascites have no pleural effusion[281] and that effusions may develop or resolve suddenly.[281, 282, 589] The right-sided predilection of effusions in ascites may be related to the greater exposure of the tendinous diaphragm on the right, where it is not covered by the heart.

Pancreatic Disease

Pleural effusion occurs in both acute and chronic pancreatitis.[285]

The prevalence in *acute pancreatitis* is about 10% to 20%, with figures ranging between 4%[130] and 38%.[360] The presence of an effusion suggests severe pancreatitis.[341] Because of the close relationship of the pancreas, particularly the tail, to the left hemi-

diaphragm, effusions are usually left-sided (70%) or bilateral (15%).[130, 237, 341, 360] There may be additional elevation of the hemidiaphragm together with basal consolidation.[442] The clinical picture is usually dominated by abdominal symptoms, though occasionally there is dyspnea or pleuritic chest pain.[285]

The effusions are exudates and often hemorrhagic. The amylase levels of the pleural fluid are high and may exceed those in the serum. Pleural amylase values remain elevated even after serum levels have returned to normal values.[321] An elevated amylase level in pleural fluid is not, however, a specific indicator of pancreatitis and may be seen with esophageal perforation and occasionally with pleural malignancy.[285] The effusions usually resolve completely, but pleural calcification has been described as a possible sequel in three patients[51]; curiously, these were bilateral in all three cases.

Effusions associated with *chronic pancreatitis* are often large and recurrent,[10, 345] and in contrast to acute pancreatitis, chest symptoms usually dominate the clinical picture.[285] Indeed, patients may present with effusions. Such effusions are frequently associated with pancreatic pseudocysts[237] which, having dissected into the mediastinum by way of the aortic or esophageal hiatus,[242, 295] burst into the pleural space. Communication between the pleural space and the pancreatic pseudocyst may be demonstrated by endoscopic retrograde cholangiopancreatography (ERCP) or operative pancreatography,[54, 90] by CT,[118, 295] or by introducing contrast material into the pleural effusion itself.[541] Excision of the pancreaticopleural fistulous track is the treatment of choice. Pleural effusions resulting from chronic pancreatitis may cause gross pleural thickening, requiring decortication.[285]

Renal Disease

Nephrogenic effusions are associated with the following six conditions and treatments[166, 463].

1. *Uremic pleurisy and hemodialysis.* A fibrinous pleuritis is common in uremia.[213] It may develop despite hemodialysis[30] and is often accompanied by pericarditis. Patients may be asymptomatic or have chest pain and fever.[30, 369] The effusions are exudates[369] and are commonly bloody.[153] In one series, 79% were unilateral.[30] The effusions may be small or large. In patients who continue on hemodialysis, they quite often subside over weeks. Sometimes, however, fibrous pleural thickening ensues and decortication may be required.[160, 437]

2. *Urinothorax.* Urinothorax is an unusual condition; only 22 cases had been reported up to 1986.[464] It is usually an aftermath of obstruction and rupture of the urinary tract with urinoma formation.[21, 22] It may also follow blunt[258] or penetrating trauma, particularly iatrogenic, such as renal biopsy[464] or nephrostomy.[424] A few cases have been described that are a result of hydronephrosis in which no urinoma was demonstrable.[71, 257, 376] It seems likely that a urinothorax develops when retroperitoneal urine dissects upward into the mediastinum, which then ruptures, allowing urine to escape into the pleural space.[464] The mediastinal widening that accompanies this process may be detectable radiographically.[22]

The effusions are usually unilateral and on the same side as the obstructed or traumatized kidney.[463] The presence of urine can be established by comparing the urea and/or creatinine levels of the pleural fluid with those in the blood.[22, 145, 513] Urinothorax has also been identified through scintigraphy with [99mTc] DTPA (diethylenetriaminepentaacetic acid).[417] The pleural collections subside following drainage of the urinomas and relief of the hydronephrosis.

3. *Nephrotic syndrome.* Transudative effusions develop in about 20% of patients with nephrotic syndrome because of the associated hypoalbuminemia.[463] The effusions tend to be bilateral and are

commonly subpulmonic[100] and recurrent.[229] If the effusion is an exudate and/or bloody, pulmonary embolism should be suspected.[291]

4. *Acute glomerulonephritis.* Effusions are also common in acute glomerulonephritis, occurring in some 50% of cases.[212, 243] The effusions are often multifactorial in origin, with disturbed fluid balance playing an important role.

5. *Peritoneal dialysis.* Acute hydrothorax can develop during peritoneal dialysis.[104, 457] The effusions most commonly develop within hours of initiation of dialysis.[129] Like ascites-related pleural effusions, those resulting from dialysis are usually on the right[463] though a few have been left-sided.[362] Elevated levels of glucose will confirm the presence of dialysate in the pleural effusion.[293] In some and possibly all cases, the mechanism is believed to be direct transfer of fluid from the peritoneal cavity into the pleural space through diaphragmatic defects. There have, however, been several unsuccessful attempts at demonstrating such communications in patients on peritoneal dialysis with pleural effusions.[252, 293, 362] It is therefore possible that other mechanisms play a part in the development of dialysis-related effusion. Their appearance is a contraindication to peritoneal dialysis, as they usually recur when interrupted dialysis is begun again.[457]

6. *Renal infection*[398]/*perinephric abscess.*[463]

Ascitic Effusion

Ascitic fluid of any cause may be associated with a pleural effusion. The mechanism of pleural effusion formation in the majority of these patients would seem to be transdiaphragmatic passage of fluid. The association of ascitic and pleural fluid is well-recognized in hepatic cirrhosis, peritoneal dialysis, ovarian hyperstimulation syndrome,[475] and Meigs' syndrome. The first two conditions are considered elsewhere, and the pathogenesis of ascites-related effusions is discussed in some detail in the section on cirrhosis.

Meigs' Syndrome.—The earliest descriptions of this syndrome are those of Salmon in 1934[331] and Meigs and Cass in 1937.[465] The syndrome has four components: (1) ascites; (2) pleural effusion; (3) ovarian fibroma; and (4) resolution of ascites and hydrothorax with removal of the tumor. The definition was later extended[305, 328] to include other ovarian tumors—theca cell, granulosa cell, and Brenner tumors. More recently there has been a tendency to include all female pelvic neoplasms, both ovarian and uterine.[506] Some authors call this extended syndrome the atypical (pseudo) Meigs' syndrome.[190,378] Majzlin and Stevens[305] reviewed 128 cases of the more limited syndrome and found ovarian fibroma in 82%, theca cell tumor in 9.4%, granulosa cell tumor in 4.7% and Brenner tumor in 1.6%. The fluid in the chest and abdomen were the same—usually clear, amber-colored transudates. However, various appearances of the effusions are described, including hemorrhagic.[329] Pleural effusions are more commonly right-sided, with a frequency of 65% on the right, 10% on the left, and 22% bilaterally (Fig 14–46).[305] Meigs' syndrome is not common; in one series of 283 patients with ovarian fibromas, 51 had ascites but only 2 had pleural effusions as well.[94] The source of the ascites is not clearly established, but there is some evidence that it is produced by transudation from the surface of the larger tumors, possibly on the basis of vascular compromise.[94] Once formed, ascitic fluid almost certainly enters the chest through diaphragmatic defects (see earlier discussion in the section "Cirrhosis of the Liver" on p. 656).

The importance of Meigs' syndrome lies in the fact that neither ascites nor pleural effusion can be

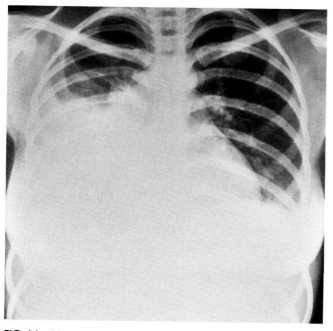

FIG 14–46.
Pleural effusion—Meigs' syndrome. This 17-year-old presented with lower abdominal pain and irregular menstrual periods. There was a large pleural effusion, which did not contain malignant cells, and also ascites with an ovarian mass. Removal of the mass (a granulosa cell tumor) was followed by resolution of both ascites and pleural effusion. Three years later the patient remained well.

taken as necessarily indicative that a pelvic mass is malignant and has metastasized. Furthermore, Meigs'-type syndromes have been described with malignant tumors.[348]

Traumatic

Abdominal Surgery.—Half the patients in a series of 200 investigated 2 to 3 days after abdominal surgery with bilateral decubitus chest radiographs had a pleural effusion.[286] Factors that predisposed included upper rather than lower abdominal surgery and postoperative atelectasis. All but one of these effusions settled without complications.

Such small early effusions need to be distinguished from the larger ones that develop later as these are more commonly of clinical significance, suggesting a complication such as subphrenic abscess (see p. 653).[467]

Radiation.—Pleural changes following radiation are recognized, but unusual.[280,583] In one series of 11 patients, pleural effusions were usually small, gradually reducing and sometimes disappearing in a rather indolent fashion over many months or years.[17] Suggested criteria for the diagnosis of radiation pleuritis are: (1) effusion within 6 months of completing radiation therapy; (2) coexisting radiation pneumonitis; and (3) spontaneous resolution.[17] Reaccumulation or rapid increase in the pleural effusion suggests metastasis.

Drugs and the Pleura

A number of drugs may cause pleural effusions or pleural thickening. Relevant drugs are listed in Table 14–3; all are considered in this section apart from those associated with systemic lupus erythematosus. Drug-induced pleural disease has been recently and comprehensively reviewed.[456]

Cytotoxic Drugs.—Pleural changes are described with all types of *methotrexate* regimens: intermittent high dose,[550] intermittent low dose,[560] and maintenance.[115] Urban and colleagues[550] described a 9% prevalence of pleuritis with a high-dose regimen which produced thickening of fissures on the radiograph but no free fluid. An intermittent low-dose regimen gave a 4% prevalence of pleuritis, but only about 1% had radiographic evidence of pleural effusion.[550] Maintenance therapy may be associated with pulmonary eosinophilia in which parenchymal shadowing may occasionally be accompanied by a small pleural effusion.[115] *Procarbazine* may cause bi-

TABLE 14–3.

Drugs Causing Pleural Changes

Drugs causing systemic lupus erythematosus	Hydralazine Isoniazid Phenytoin Procainamide Others (rarely)
Cytotoxic drugs	Bleomycin Busulfan Methotrexate Mitomycin Procarbazine
Antibacterial drugs	Nitrofurantoin
Antimigraine drugs	Ergotamine Methysergide
Antiarrhythmic drugs	Amiodarone
Skeletal muscle relaxants	Dantrolene
Vasodilator antihypertensives	Minoxidil
Dopaminergic receptor stimulants	Bromocriptine
Beta-adrenergic blockers	Acebutolol Practolol Propanolol

lateral interstitial shadowing accompanied by blood eosinophilia and pleural effusions,[103] and pleural effusions have also been described with *mitomycin,*[385] *busulfan,*[499] and *bleomycin.*[388]

Antibacterial Drugs.—Two syndromes are recognized with *nitrofurantoin* toxicity: (1) an acute syndrome that comes on after hours or days and is probably immunologically based, because there is usually previous nitrofurantoin exposure and eosinophilia; and (2) a chronic syndrome less commonly associated with eosinophilia that appears months or years after therapy begins.[462] In one large series, 35% of acute reactions were accompanied by interstitial lung shadowing and pleural effusions, while isolated pleural effusions developed in a further 8%. In the chronic syndrome there was a 7% prevalence of effusions, which were never the sole manifestation.[211]

Antimigraine Drugs.—There are now more than 30 cases of *methysergide*-induced pleuropulmonary disease in the literature following the first re-

port in 1966.[177] The syndrome may appear between 1 month and 6 years after initiation of therapy.[462] Radiographically there are unilateral or bilateral pleural thickening and effusions.[176, 204, 247] Pleural effusions sometimes appear to be loculated.[157] Localized pleural and subpleural fibrosis can simulate a mass lesion.[176] *Ergotamine* has been implicated in causing unilateral pleural thickening with effusion,[530] and it is possible that *ergonovine* has the same effect.[157]

Antiarrhythmic Drugs.—*Amiodarone* may produce a variety of changes on the chest radiograph, most commonly parenchymal opacities with either acinar or interstitial characteristics.[70] Pleural thickening and effusions are occasionally present.[172, 416, 607] On average the onset is 6 months after start of treatment, but this ranges from 1 month to several years and it is rarely seen if the dose is less than 400 mg/day. The prevalence rate varies between 1% and 6%.[70] All patients with pleural abnormality have had parenchymal involvement.[172]

Skeletal Muscle Relaxants.—*Dantrolene* may cause pleural effusion, which can be unilateral and eosinophil-rich.[395]

Vasodilator Antihypertensives.—There is one case report of *minoxidil* administration being associated with bilateral pleural and pericardial exudative effusions.[570]

Dopaminergic Receptor Stimulants.—There are two reports of *bromocriptine* being associated with pleural effusion and thickening and, in both, there was additional interstitial pulmonary shadowing.[277, 434] Of the eight patients in these reports, five were also on levodopa. Thus, some workers consider that a cause-and-effect relationship between effusion and bromocriptine therapy is not clearly established.

Beta-adrenergic blockers.—*Practolol,* which was withdrawn in 1976, caused a variety of side effects including pleural thickening and effusion.[112, 137, 186, 315] There is one case report of patchy visceral pleural thickening associated with lung fibrosis due to *acebutolol* which resembles practolol chemically. The radiologic changes were subtle and could be demonstrated only with CT.[597] *Propanolol* has been implicated in causing a pleural effusion in a patient with sclerosing peritonitis, but the effusion developed after surgery, and a clear cause and effect was not established.[7] A single case report of pleural thickening thought to be due to the related *oxprenolol* was in fact found later to be due to mesothelioma.[386]

Miscellaneous Causes of Pleural Effusion

Myxedema.—Pleural effusions are described in myxedema,[45] but it is not clear whether they are more commonly transudates or exudates.[58, 284] In one series of patients with myxedema about half had a pleural effusion,[312] and these were usually accompanied by pericardial effusions, though isolated pleural effusion is recorded.[478] Effusions disappear with treatment of the myxedema.[478]

Pleural Effusion With Yellow Nails and Primary Lymphedema.

—The association between yellow nails and primary lymphedema was first described in 1964,[466] and in the same year the association between pleural effusion and primary lymphedema was recorded.[216] Two years after these accounts, the triad of yellow nails, pleural effusion, and primary lymphedema was reported,[108] and by 1986 nearly 100 cases were on record.[371] The nails are not only yellow but are also dystrophic[25] and subject to both onycholysis and infection. Lymphedema typically affects the lower legs and is mild.[605] The pleural effusions may be unilateral or bilateral, small or large[25, 201] and are characteristically chronic

and persistent (Fig 14–47).[371] The exudates are rich in protein and lymphocytes but, since there is no reflux from the thoracic duct into the lungs, they are not chylous. Other respiratory manifestations are common and include recurrent bronchitis, pneumonia, pleurisy, bronchiectasis, and sinusitis. Bronchiectasis was present in 25% of patients in two series totaling 32 cases.[25, 201] Other less common features include erysipelas and hypogammaglobulinemia.[371]

In a review of 97 patients the male:female ratio was 1:1.6 and median age at presentation was 40 years.[371] There is, however, a wide range in the age at presentation and in the severity of the manifestations. At presentation, only about half of the patients will have the classic triad. All elements of the triad are thought to be explicable on the basis of defective lymphatics. In the visceral pleura there are dilated lymphatics consistent with downstream obstruction,[504] and there is reduced lymphatic drainage from the pleural space.[458] The exact mechanism of changes of the nails is, however, not clear.[605] Neither is the pathogenesis of recurrent sinusitis and bronchiectasis; in some it may be related to hypogammaglobulinemia.

The effusions may require pleurectomy or chemical pleurodesis.[216, 371]

Familial Mediterranean Fever.—This rare, genetically determined, disorder is characterized by recurrent attacks of abdominal pain, arthralgia, and pleuritic pain accompanied by fever. It has several synonyms including periodic disease, periodic fever, recurrent polyserositis, and familial paroxysmal polyserositis.[68] It occurs almost exclusively in non-Ashkenazic Jews, Armenians, Turks, and Arabs, with disease occurring in 50% of those affected in their 1st decade and occurring in 75% before the age of 20 years (range, 1 to 40 years). Men outnumber women 2:1.[20] The most common presentation is with paroxysmal, recurrent peritonitis and fever lasting 1 to 4 days, which often leads to unnecessary laparotomy. The peritonitis is commonly accompanied by a pleurisy, which is often overlooked. At presentation, between 13% and 40% of patients have pleuritis.[20, 195, 374, 492, 503] Isolated pleurisy, however, as a presenting feature is uncommon.[20, 309, 374] Febrile arthropathy, usually of large joints, is the second most frequent presentation. Colchicine prevents attacks and to some extent suppresses symptoms once an attack has begun.[68] The prognosis is good unless renal amyloidosis develops.

Radiologic manifestations in the chest are un-

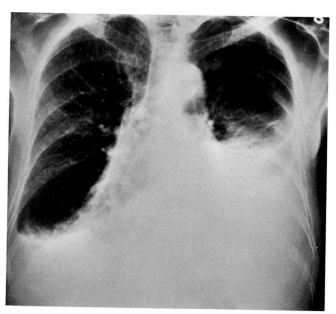

FIG 14–47.
Pleural effusion—yellow nail syndrome. Bilateral pleural effusions in a 74-year-old man. These had been present for several years, and this persistence is characteristic. Effusions are not chylous.

common and include diaphragmatic elevation, small pleural effusions, diaphragmatic haziness, and discoid atelectasis.*

CHYLOTHORAX

A chylothorax contains fluid that is largely chyle (lymph of intestinal origin) and, because chyle usually contains suspended fat in the form of chylomicrons, chylothorax fluid is milky. A chylothorax needs to be distinguished from other milky effusions, particularly empyema and pseudochylothorax, which are discussed later. Before considering the causes of chylothorax the anatomy of the thoracic duct and its tributaries and the physiology of chyle will be briefly reviewed.

Anatomy of the Thoracic Duct and its Tributaries*

The thoracic duct connects the cisterna chyli to the great veins in the root of the neck and transports all of the body lymph except that from most of the lungs and the right upper quadrant of the body (Fig 14–48).

The cisterna chyli is formed by the fusion of the two lumbar lymphatic trunks[446] and lies in front of the D-12 to L-2 vertebral bodies. The thoracic duct arises from the cisterna chyli. It is 2 to 8 mm in diameter[375] and is valved, particularly in its upper half,[236, 375, 446] effectively preventing retrograde flow.[236] Although the thoracic duct is thought of as a single structure, it is commonly multiple in part of its course[552] and may consist of up to eight separate channels.[446] Indeed, in one study, entirely single ducts were less common than multiple ones, and at the level of the diaphragm where the duct is commonly ligated therapeutically, about one-third were double.[236] The duct or ducts pass up from the cisterna behind the median arcuate ligament and ascend on the anterior aspect of the vertebral bodies and right intercostal arteries between the azygos vein and aorta. At the level of D-6, the thoracic duct crosses to the left of the spine[326] and ascends along the lateral aspect of the esophagus behind the aorta and left subclavian artery. Having reached the neck, it arches forward across the subclavian artery and inserts into a large central vein within 1 cm of the junction of the left internal jugular and subclavian veins. The number of channels and the site of inser-

*References 20, 106, 107, 309, 337, and 503.
*References 31, 76, 236, 446, 470, 479, and 524.

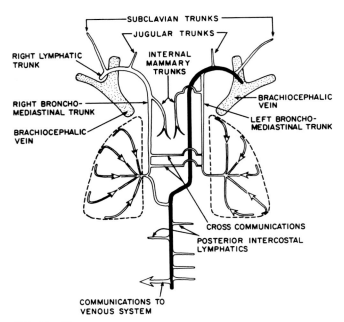

FIG 14–48.
Lymphatics of the thorax. The thoracic duct is shown in black. A major feature is the extensive lymphatic anastomoses between both lungs, right bronchomediastinal trunk, and the thoracic duct. Another important feature is lymphatic-venous connections remote from the brachiocephalic vein. The richness of these anastomoses and connections is such that simply obstructing the thoracic duct does not produce a chylothorax.

tion of the terminal thoracic duct vary.[298] Near its termination, the thoracic duct receives the left bronchomediastinal trunk, which drains the left lung, the left jugular trunk, and the left subclavian trunk (see Fig 14–48). Any or all of these vessels may end separately in the great veins.

On the right side, there is a right lymphatic duct which receives the right jugular, right subclavian, right internal mammary, and right bronchomediastinal trunks. The right bronchomediastinal trunk also receives communications from the left trunk (through which it commonly drains the caudad half of the left lung) and from the thoracic duct by way of the right posterior intercostal lymphatics (see Fig 14–48).

The thoracic duct anatomy is clinically important for the following reasons:

1. Immediately after thoracic duct rupture, chyle commonly collects in the mediastinum and may cause a mediastinal swelling.[537] Eventually, however, it bursts through into the pleural space—after a delay that varies from days to months.

2. Because the thoracic duct crosses from right to left in the mid-dorsal region, chylothorax tends to

be right-sided with low chest trauma and left-sided with trauma high in the chest.

3. The thoracic duct is closely related to the aortic arch and mid esophagus, and surgery to these structures is more likely to cause chylothorax than other types of cardiothoracic operations.

4. Obstruction to the thoracic duct per se does not result in a chylothorax because of the duct's extensive lymphatic and venous communications.[43, 367] This means that it can be tied off therapeutically without adverse consequences[261] and also implies that neoplastic blockade, as with lymphoma, must lead to rupture if it is to cause chylothorax.[236, 326] As might be expected, obstruction of the superior vena cava or of both brachiocephalic veins may produce a chylothorax, as this maneuver compromises the drainage of both the thoracic duct and potential anastomotic channels.[33, 91, 250, 481, 538]

Mechanisms of Chylothorax Formation

Three main mechanisms account for chyle collections in the pleural space: first, leakage from a discrete rupture of the thoracic duct or a large lymphatic vessel; second, a general oozing from pleural lymphatics; and third, passage of chylous ascites through the diaphragm.[240, 521]

Direct drainage from the duct occurs with disruption resulting from trauma or neoplastic involvement. There may be a phase of accumulation within the mediastinum before the mediastinal pleura becomes breached and chyle spills over into the pleural cavity.

Blockage of the thoracic duct can cause extensive collateral formation in the parietal pleura and these may rupture, allowing seepage of chyle from the *parietal pleura* (Fig 14–49). The degree and type of collateral formation with thoracic duct block may vary depending on the richness of an individual's lymphatic-lymphatic and lymphatic-venous connections. Another factor that promotes pleural seepage is reflux of chyle into the lungs. Normally, with a few exceptions,[179] chyle does not gain access to the lungs or visceral pleura because both the intrapulmonary lymphatics and the thoracic duct are valved.[543] Valvular incompetence, however, allows chyle to reflux into the lungs and to ooze from the *visceral pleura* over the lung surface (see Fig 14–49). The development of a "lymphangitic" radiologic pattern in the lungs and a chylothorax after obstruction of the thoracic duct and the right bronchomediastinal trunk have been described.[27, 481] The "lymphangitic" pattern in these cases almost certainly represented di-

lated lung lymphatics distended by chylous reflux (see Fig 14–49). Factors that promote reflux are lymphatic vessel dilation; increased thoracic duct and lymphatic vessel pressure; and maldevelopment of valves and lymphatic vessel walls.[575] Seepage of chyle from fragile lymphatic vessels and collaterals is possibly the mechanism for chylothorax formation associated with lymphangiomatous malformations.[99]

The third mechanism of chylous effusion formation is transdiaphragmatic passage of chylous ascites. This is a recognized but rare occurrence.[240] The mechanism is the same as that involved with transdiaphragmatic passage of cirrhotic ascites (see "Cirrhosis of the Liver" earlier in this chapter).

Physiology of Chyle*

Lymph flowing up the thoracic duct is derived principally from the gut (60%) and to a lesser extent from the liver (35%) and the peripheral lymphatics (5%). About 1.5 to 2.5 L is produced per day.[375, 569] It flows upward because of contractions of the duct wall, adjacent arterial pulsations, gut contractions, the pressure gradient from the abdomen to the thorax, and vis a tergo.[31] Flow is increased by increased fluid intake and, particularly, by fat ingestion, an effect that may increase flow tenfold for several hours. Sixty to seventy percent of the fat absorbed by the gut passes by way of the thoracic duct. Chyle contains about 0.5 to 6.0 gm/dl fat, 3.0 gm/dl protein, and electrolytes as in serum. There are 2,000 to 20,000 white blood cells per ml chyle,[297] mostly T lymphocytes. Loss of chyle from the body—as occurs with drainage of a chylothorax—has serious consequences, leading to inanition, lymphopenia, and immune compromise.

Most of the fat in chyle is carried as triglycerides in the form of chylomicrons, which gives chyle its characteristic milky appearance. Two other types of pleural fluid may appear milky and need to be distinguished: (1) empyema, in which the milkiness is due to leukocytes which, unlike chylomicrons, settle out on standing or centrifugation; and (2) pseudochylous effusions, in which the milkiness is due to cholesterol and/or lecithin-globulin complexes. Pseudochylous effusions may be distinguished from true chylous effusions by their high cholesterol content and the fact that they usually occur in characteristic clinical settings in which there has been long-standing disease with much pleural thickening. It is important to note that not all chylous effusions are

*References 284, 297, 314, 448, and 470.

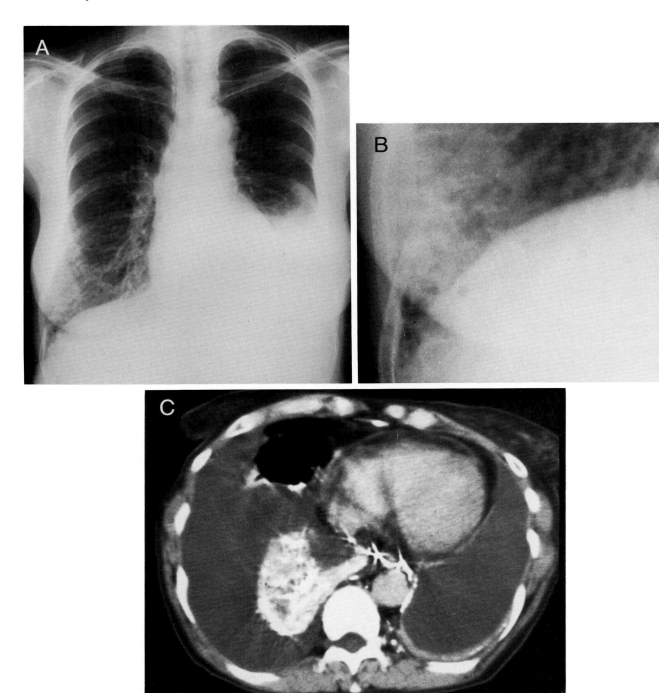

FIG 14–49.

Chylothorax—cryptogenic. **A,** PA chest radiograph of a 64-year-old woman who presented with dyspnea and was found to have a left chylothorax. At the right lung base there are thick septal lines. The patient had had a right chylothorax 7 years previously. **B,** localized view of septal lines. **C,** CT following lymphangiogram shows multiple lymphatic channels in the posterior mediastinum, lymphatic collaterals in the left parietal pleura, and gross reflux of contrast into the collapsed right lung. There are bilateral effusions (chylothoraces) at this stage with a CT (Hounsfield) number of about 20. Lymphatic channels in the mediastinum could not be traced above D-3. The cause was obscure. Chylothorax presumably was formed by reflux into the lung and seepage from the visceral pleura. A contribution from parietal pleura seems likely as well.

milky, and in one series 53% of 38 chylous effusions were initially undiagnosed because they were turbid or bloody.[512] Furthermore, during starvation, as may occur following surgery, flow is reduced and the characteristic milkiness may disappear.[38, 448] The diagnosis of a chylous effusion is made by measuring the triglyceride levels of the effusion.[512] Levels above 110 mg/dl are taken as positive; levels below 50 mg/dl, as negative. In patients with intermediate values, lipoprotein electrophoresis[482] should be performed. It should not be assumed with bilateral effusions that if one is chylous both are.[269] Chyle is bacteriostatic and does not irritate the pleura, giving neither pain nor pleuritis or fibrosis.

Causes of Chylothorax

Chylothoraces can be conveniently classified (Table 14–4) as neoplastic, traumatic, idiopathic, and of miscellaneous origins.[470] In most series, about 50% have been neoplastic,[38, 301, 452] with some 25% traumatic and 15% idiopathic[470]:

1. *Neoplastic causes.* Lymphomas make up about 75% of the neoplastic lesions,[38, 301, 452, 512] and chylothorax can be the presenting feature of lympho-

TABLE 14–4.
Causes of Chylothorax

Neoplastic
  Lymphoma
  Metastatic carcinoma
Traumatic
  Operative
    Cardiac
    Esophageal
    Thoracic
    Cervical
  Penetrating injuries
  Closed injuries
    Major
    Minor
Miscellaneous
  Systemic venous hypertension
  Obstruction of central systemic veins
  Scarring processes
    Mediastinal
    Nodal (filariasis)
  Developmental anomalies
    Thoracic duct atresia
    Lymphangioma
    Lymphangiectasia
    Lymphangioleiomyomatosis/tuberous sclerosis
  Cryptogenic

mas.[284] When chylothorax is associated with carcinoma it suggests mediastinal metastasis.[448]

2. *Trauma.* The most common form of trauma is surgery, particularly cardiac surgery. The frequency of chylothorax with cardiothoracic surgery is between 0.2% and 0.56%[38, 56, 307] and the condition is most commonly seen with surgery for Fallot's tetralogy, patent ductus arteriosus, and coarctation of the aorta. Chylothorax is also described with coronary artery surgery,[251, 574] thoracoplasty and pneumonectomy (Fig 14–50), esophagoscopy and esophageal resection,[470] thoracic sympathectomy, and block dissection of the neck.[470] Chylothorax may follow penetrating injuries such as stab and bullet wounds.

Closed chest trauma—ranging from major trauma with crush injuries and spinal fractures[297] to very minor injuries—are recognized as causing chylothorax. Minor injuries include vomiting and weight lifting,[470] coughing,[261] and the hyperextension and stretching that accompanies yawning.[425] It has been suggested that, for such trivial trauma to cause duct rupture, there must be a duct that is distended by a high postprandial lymphatic flow.[31]

3. *Idiopathic.* A significant number of cases of chylothorax are cryptogenic (see Fig 14–49), and in the neonatal period this variety is the most common cause of a pleural effusion. Many adult cases may arise following trauma that is so minor it is not recalled or recorded.

4. *Miscellaneous.* The remaining 10% of chylothoraces result from a great variety of causes, many of which fall into one of three subgroups. (1) Impaired venous drainage. This has been recorded with raised venous pressure due to heart disease[42, 301] and with central venous thrombosis that affects subclavian and brachiocephalic veins and superior vena cava.* Despite a number of case reports, chylothorax remains a rare complication of central venous thrombosis, and in one series of 25 cases, no examples of chylothorax were encountered.[3] (2) Scarring processes. This is probably the common mechanism in chronic pancreatitis,[255] fibrosing mediastinitis, radiation exposure, tuberculosis,[553] and filariasis.[144] (3) Developmental anomalies. Under this broad heading it is possible to include thoracic duct atresia,[452] tuberous sclerosis and lymphangioleiomyomatosis, pulmonary lymphangiectasia—either per se or as part of Noonan's syndrome[156, 479]—and lymphangioma-

*References 91, 105, 203, 250, 358, and 481.

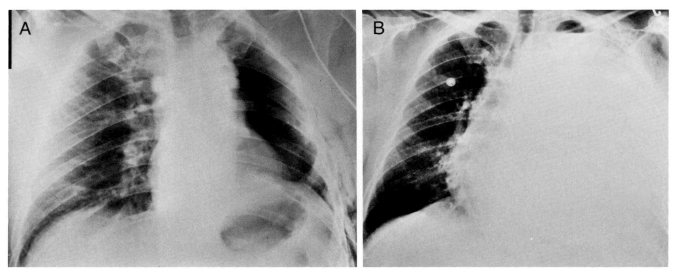

FIG 14–50.
Chylothorax—traumatic. **A,** AP chest radiograph immediately following left pneumonectomy for carcinoma of lung. **B,** just over 1 week later a pleural effusion developed rapidly and proved to be a chylothorax. This complication of cardiothoracic surgery is seen especially following operations for Fallot's tetralogy, patent ductus arteriosus, and coarctation of the aorta.

tous anomalies, which are often associated with massive osteolysis.[18, 44, 99, 389, 517]

Radiology of Chylothorax

The changes with chylothorax on plain radiographs cannot be distinguished from other effusions. Chylothoraces vary from small to massive, can be unilateral or bilateral, and are slightly more frequent on the right side in large series.[297] Reference has already been made to the mass-like accumulation in the mediastinum that may precede the effusion[117, 298, 537] and the delay—which can vary from days to months—between trauma and the eventual development of chylothorax.† CT may demonstrate a causal mediastinal lymphoma that is covert on the chest radiograph. The CT attenuation density of chyle, despite the fat content, is usually indistinguishable from that of other effusions because it is protein-rich (see Fig 14–49), though there is one report in which the CT density was significantly reduced.[269]

Lymphography has been commonly performed in assessments of chylothorax.‡ Lymphography can show leakage of contrast material into the pleural space[479] and may also demonstrate the exact site of thoracic duct rupture,[193] which will help in direct-

ing surgical repair. It will also demonstrate lymphoma,[144] duct blockage with accompanying collaterals (see Fig 14–49),[144, 553] and lymphatic malformations, including lymphangiectasia.[18] The exact place of lymphography in the investigation of chylothorax is not firmly established. CT scanning is probably the best approach in screening for lymphoma, and once neoplasia is excluded, details about the exact mechanism and point of leakage often play little part in treatment, because if medical management fails, the usual approach is to tie the thoracic duct at the diaphragm and/or perform a pleurodesis.

Pseudochylothorax

Pseudochylothorax is also a milky effusion, but the milky appearance is the result of cholesterol and/or lecithin-globulin complexes rather than chylomicrons. There have been several reviews of the condition.[64, 202, 284, 470] Pseudochylothorax characteristically occurs in pleural disease of many years' duration, with chronic encysted effusion, pleural thickening, and sometimes calcification. It most commonly follows, or is associated with, tuberculosis[202] and rheumatoid disease.[64, 127] Unusual causes have been described,[470] including paragonimiasis.[231] The clinical context in which the effusion occurs is so characteristic that pseudochylothorax rarely causes any diagnostic confusion with a true chylothorax.

---

†References 199, 301, 422, 437, 448, and 476.
‡References 57, 91, 144, 193, 343, 479, 553, 575, and 585.

HEMOTHORAX

Hemothorax usually results from trauma but it may, on occasion, occur in other conditions (Table 14–5). The natural history of hemothorax depends in part on the source of the bleeding. Low-pressure bleeding from the lung tends to stop spontaneously because the pleural fluid compresses and collapses the lung. High-pressure bleeding from systemic vessels is less susceptible to the tamponade effect of pleural fluid,[429] and the bleeding may be rapid and persistent, with the formation of a tension hemothorax.[19] In the context of trauma, other causes of rapidly accumulating pleural fluid should be considered; these include ruptured esophagus, ruptured thoracic duct, traumatic subarachnoid-pleural fistula,[409] and iatrogenic causes, particularly those related to venous lines.

In the acute state there is nothing on the plain chest radiograph that distinguishes hemothorax from other collections of pleural fluid. However, on CT, a hemothorax may show areas of hyperdensity.[596] With clotting of the blood there is a tendency for loculation to occur, and fibrin bodies may form.[124, 592] Hemothorax may eventually organize

TABLE 14–5.

Causes of Hemothorax

Cause	Reference
Trauma	
Open	—
Closed (with or without fracture)	—
Iatrogenic	Milner et al.[342]
Infection	
Varicella	Rodriguez et al.[439]
Coagulopathy	
Hemophillia	Rasaretnam et al.[418]
Anticoagulants	Banks et al.,[19] Millard[338]
Vascular abnormality	
Arteriovenous malformation	Spear et al.[507]
Dissecting aortic aneurysm	—
Atherosclerotic aneurysm	Defrance et al.[87]
Pulmonary neoplasm	Defrance et al.[87]
Extramedullary hemopoiesis	Sulis and Floris[527]
Pneumothorax	Calvert and Smith,[53] Willson et al.[592]
Catamenial hemothorax (endometriosis)	Yeh[603]
Idiopathic	Deaton and Johnston,[85] Slind and Rodarte[498]

and cause massive pleural thickening (fibrothorax), necessitating decortication, a complication that can be avoided by early evacuation of the pleural space.

PLEURAL MASS

Pleural mass lesions are uncommon. Radiographically they may resemble pleural fluid collections loculated against the chest wall, chest wall masses, or pleurally based parenchymal lung masses. An important feature of these lesions on plain radiographs is that they look entirely different when viewed *en face* and tangentially.

En face, chest wall and localized pleural lesions characteristically appear as homogeneous, often partly rounded opacities with a sharp medial edge and an ill-defined lateral margin (Fig 14–51). This typical appearance is produced because the medial border is usually aligned in a tangential fashion to the x-ray beam, thereby generating a sharp marginal image. The lateral beam, on the other hand, is angled away from the tangent of the lung/soft tissue interface and passes through a wedge-shaped mass of soft tissue, which will, therefore, have no clearly defined lateral margin (Fig 14–52). Tangentially both chest wall and localized pleural lesions are convex to lung and are sharply marginated, as they are both covered on the lung aspect by pleura. At their periphery these lesions often lift off a tail of pleura, creating an obtuse angle of contact with the chest wall (Fig 14–51). Plain radiographs frequently do not allow a distinction to be made between localized lesions of the chest wall and pleura unless there is rib remodeling or destruction. These signs are characteristic of a chest wall lesion, and apart from the occasional neoplastic or infective lesion (actinomycosis, tuberculosis), they are rarely seen with pleural or lung processes. Rarely, a chest wall lesion will have a detectable layer of extrapleural fat on its inner aspect, allowing it to be unequivocally localized to the chest wall on a plain radiograph—the pleural coif sign.[426]

Intrapulmonary lesions differ from pleural lesions in that they tend to have a less clearly defined lung interface (see Fig 14–41), and they may show characteristic inhomogeneities, such as an air bronchogram. Classically, they make an acute angle of contact with the visceral pleura, but with local infiltration, as may occur with a neoplasm, this can become obtuse.[591]

Ultrasound examination is helpful in establish-

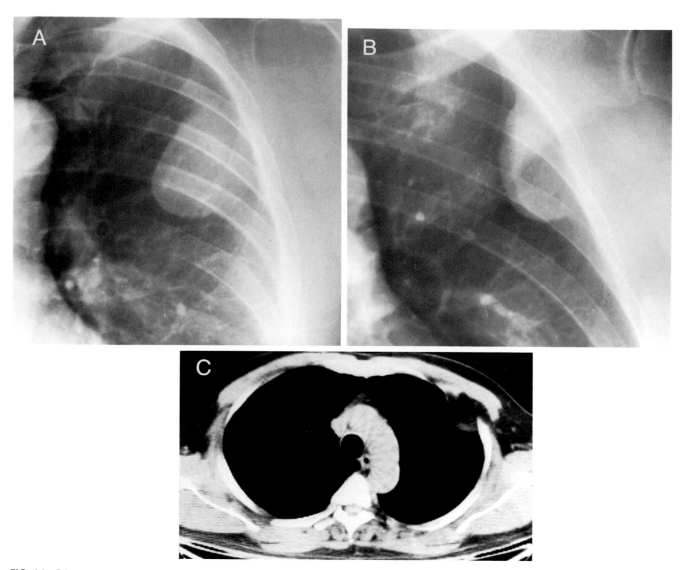

FIG 14–51.
Pleural mass—lipoma. **A,** localized view of left upper zone shows a 3 × 5-cm homogeneous mass lesion. It is pleurally based and has a sharp inner border, but its outer margin fades off into the soft tissues of the chest wall. The ribs are unaffected. The opacity could be pleural or extrapleural. **B,** a tangential view adds little information. The lesion makes an obtuse angle where it contacts the chest wall superiorly. The inferior angle cannot be analyzed. The inner margin of the lesion is clear and sharp. **C,** CT shows a low-density lesion that has the attenuation of fat. A component of the lesion lies in the chest wall. The exact site of origin, although it could be pleural, is indeterminate.

ing the solid nature of a pleural mass lesion.[289] Mass lesions are typically homogeneous and echogenic but may be echo-free.[259, 406] The presence of septation and change in shape with respiration are reliable indicators that a collection is fluid.[313]

CT provides a more sensitive way of detecting the signs that are assessed on plain radiographs and in placing a lesion in an anatomic compartment.[591] CT is particularly helpful in detecting invasion of the chest wall with disruption of soft tissue planes and the formation of a mass.[406] In one study comparing the abilities of plain radiography and CT in a variety of peripheral abnormalities (lung, pleura, and chest wall), CT provided information that was not readily available on the plain radiograph in two-thirds of patients.[405]

Conditions that produce local pleural masses are listed in Table 14–6.

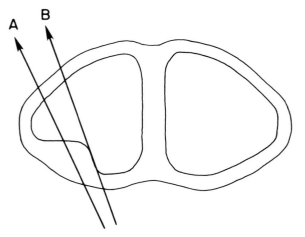

FIG 14–52.
Diagramatic cross-section of the chest shows the relationship between a pleural mass lesion and two x-ray beams. The medial beam *(B)* is oriented tangentially to the medial margin of the mass, which will therefore have a well-defined edge on the radiograph. The lateral aspect of the mass does not have a tangential interaction with *(A)* and will not produce a well-marginated image. Similar considerations will apply to chest wall lesions and loculated pleural collections. (From Wilson AG: The interpretation of shadows on the adult chest radiograph. *Br J Hosp Med* 1987; 37:526–534. Used by permission.)

Lipoma

Lipomas are the most common benign soft tissue tumor of the chest wall.[382] Their exact origin is not always clear, but they can arise from subpleural adipose tissue and present as a local pleural mass. They can extend into the chest wall, taking on an hourglass configuration (see Fig 14–51)[444] and remodeling adjacent ribs.[533] Because they are soft lesions they may change shape with respiration.[178] Although they are of soft tissue density on plain radiographs, they have a diagnostically low fat density on CT (Fig 14–51).[111, 406]

TABLE 14–6.

Causes of Localized Pleural Masses

Cause	Reference
Metastasis	—
Localized mesothelioma	—
Lymphoma	Bramson et al.,[40] Shuman and Libshitz[491]
Lipoma	—
Fibrin body	—
Thoracic splenosis	—
Others	
Endometriosis	Im et al.,[219] Yeh[603]
Multiple benign fibromas	Scattini and Orsi[474]
Amyloid	Lundin et al.[299]

Fibrin Body

Fibrin bodies develop in the pleural cavity from fibrin-rich fluid[48] particularly, but not necessarily, when there is air as well as fluid in the pleural space. They were common when therapeutic pneumothorax was used to treat tuberculosis and, in one series, were present in 21% of cases,[435] though the usual figure was more in the order of 1%.[113] Fibrin bodies are usually single, homogeneous, well-demarcated, spherical or ovoid mass lesions lying near the diaphragm (Fig 14–53).[48] They may be mobile or fixed[113] and are uncommonly more than 4 cm in diameter.[536] They may spontaneously and rapidly decrease in size and disappear, or may remain stable for many years.[48] Their only importance lies in possible confusion with a fungal or neoplastic mass.[155] They should always be considered in the differential diagnosis when a pleural mass or nodule develops after a pleural effusion or thoracotomy (Fig 14–53).[124]

Thoracic Splenosis

Thoracic splenosis is a rare condition[79] in which tissue from a traumatized spleen crosses an injured diaphragm and proliferates within the left thorax.[472] The resulting pleural nodules are often multiple; they are usually less than 3 cm in diameter, but they may be up to 7 cm.[472] The nodules are implanted on parietal or visceral pleura, including fissures.[350] Radiologically, they usually appear as pleural mass lesions of water density, but some may show intraparenchymal features both on conventional radiographs and at CT.[472] It seems likely that the majority of these apparently intrapulmonary lesions have pleural contact, though it is possible that some have been implanted in a lung laceration rather than on the pleural surface. The combination of left-sided subpleural or pleural nodules in a patient with a history of splenic and diaphragmatic injury is very suggestive of thoracic splenosis.[472] Should the spleen have been removed at the time of trauma, the absence of Howell-Jolly bodies in a blood smear would suggest persisting ectopic splenic activity.

The diagnosis, when suspected, may be confirmed with scintiscans using ^{99m}Tc sulfur colloid, ^{99m}Tc labeled heat-damaged erythrocytes or indium-111 labeled platelets, all of which will be taken up by the ectopic splenic tissue.[82, 472]

The main importance of these lesions is that they may be misinterpreted as resulting from a neoplastic disorder.

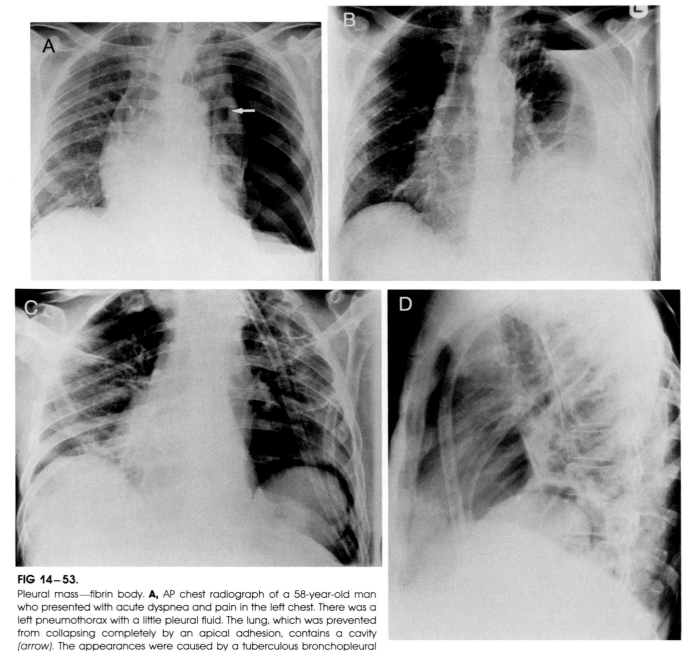

FIG 14—53.
Pleural mass—fibrin body. **A,** AP chest radiograph of a 58-year-old man who presented with acute dyspnea and pain in the left chest. There was a left pneumothorax with a little pleural fluid. The lung, which was prevented from collapsing completely by an apical adhesion, contains a cavity *(arrow).* The appearances were caused by a tuberculous bronchopleural fistula. **B,** 2 months later there is a persisting hydropneumothorax with much protein-rich fluid despite repeated thoracocentesis. **C** and **D,** 1 month later left chest drains have been inserted, draining the fluid and revealing a 10-cm rounded mobile mass lesion in the pleural space. This is homogeneous and has a smooth, sharp margin. There was no evidence of a fungal infection of the pleural space, and the mass was assumed to be a fibrin body despite its unusually large size.

PLEURAL THICKENING

Pleural thickening can be localized or generalized and usually represents the organized end-stage of a variety of active processes, particularly infective and noninfective inflammation, hemothorax, and absestos- and drug-related disease. It is virtually always present after thoracotomy and pleurodesis[323] and may follow exposure to radiation. Particularly gross examples are seen following tuberculosis. If it is very extensive, pleural thickening is termed a fibrothorax, in which case it may be associated with significant ipsilateral volume loss and ventilatory impairment.

Changes on the plain radiograph in this condition are more commonly unilateral than bilateral and consist of soft tissue shadowing—characteristically in the more dependent, lateral, and posterior parts of the chest. Blunting of the costophrenic angle is common and is often angular, distinguishing it from the more smoothly curvilinear pleural fluid. Decubitus radiographs and ultrasound scans are particularly helpful in making this distinction. En face, extensive pleural thickening gives a veillike opacity that has no clear margins and crosses known pulmonary boundaries. Tangentially, it appears as a soft tissue density immediately inside and parallel to the chest wall, sharply marginated on its inner aspect, and fading into the soft tissues of the chest wall laterally. Such pleural thickening can extend into and thicken fissures.

On ultrasound, pleural thickening produces a homogeneously echo-dense layer subjacent to the chest wall. There is no posterior echo enhancement, but this is often difficult to assess because the soft tissue/lung interface is normally so reflective. CT shows a layer of soft tissue attenuation lining the chest wall.

A number of normal findings originating from the chest wall can closely resemble local or generalized pleural thickening:

1. *Apical pleural cap.* An apical pleural cap is an irregular, usually homogeneous, soft tissue density that may be found at the extreme lung apex (Fig 14–54).[428] The lower border is usually sharply marginated and it may be smoothly curvilinear, tented, or undulating.[427] A cap is usually less than 5 mm thick, but its width is variable. In two series, it was about as common unilaterally (11% and 7%) as it was bilaterally (11% and 12%).[223, 427] When bilateral, it was usually asymmetric. The frequency of occur-

rence increased with age being 6.2% in patients up to 45 years of age, and 15.9% in those over 45 years of age.[428] Pathologically, the opacity is formed by an apical subpleural scar that is nonspecific and not related to tuberculosis.[50] The idiopathic apical cap is significant because it must be distinguished from other lesions (Fig 14–55), particularly a Pancoast tumor.[324]

2. *Rib companion shadows.* Rib companion shadows are bands of soft tissue density lying inside ribs. They have smooth margins and are almost parallel to the ribs.[428] Occasionally they appear as a line of soft tissue density separated from the rib by a less attenuating layer. This sandwich appearance could be the result of subpleural fat but is more likely to be a Mach effect.[75, 265] Companion shadows are best developed posterolaterally inside the second and third ribs and are also present lower down against the chest wall in relation to the sixth to ninth ribs.

3. *Serratus anterior shadowing.* Serratus anterior shadowing can produce a variety of soft tissue densities,[67, 162] mostly low down and laterally, overlying the anterolateral ends of the ribs. Here the digitations of the serratus create repeating triangular shadows with sharp inner margins that fade laterally. The other common pattern is a convex, low-profile shadow that projects inward from the lateral chest wall and closely resembles asbestos-related pleural plaques. It is usually possible to make this distinction between muscle slips and plaques on plain radiographs.[469] CT allows unequivocal differentiation should there be any doubt.

4. *Extrapleural fat.* Extrapleural fat may generate confusing shadows that can resemble generalized pleural thickening or plaques.[114, 468, 554] The distribution varies from patient to patient. Sometimes the fat is widely distributed in the form of a peel; more commonly it is localized, and develops particularly

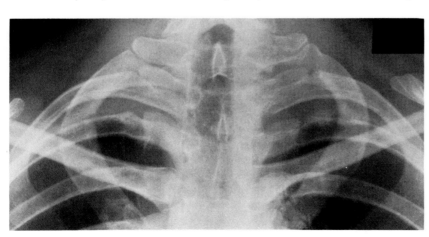

FIG 14–54.
Apical pleural caps. Symmetric soft tissue opacities are projected under both second ribs. They are slightly atypical for pleural caps, being thicker (1 cm) than usual, with some irregularity of their lower margins. The appearance of pleural caps is quite variable.

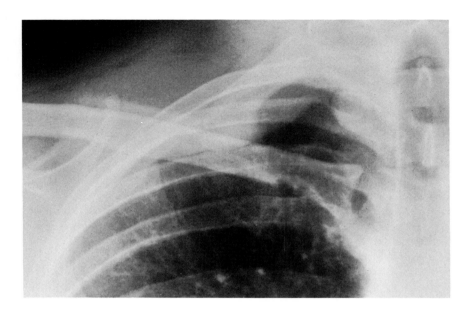

FIG 14–55.
Pleural thickening—pseudoapical cap. A localized apical view in a 27-year-old asymptomatic man shows a lenticular soft tissue density projected under the posterior aspect of the second rib. Its maximum width is 2 cm, and it is sharply demarcated from lung. It has the appearances of an apical pleural cap, although some features are unusual: its particularly sharp demarcation from lung, its lateral offset from the true apex, and its thickness. The ribs appear normal. The findings could indicate either a pleural or extrapleural lesion, and the final diagnosis was neurofibroma. There is a rhomboid fossa in the clavicle.

over the fourth to eighth ribs between the anterior axillary line and the rib angles.[468] Excess thoracic fat often occurs in obese patients, but there are exceptions. The more localized forms of fat deposition can be difficult to distinguish from plaques on plain radiographs because both are of soft tissue density. Change over time on repeated radiographs may provide discriminative information but, if there is still doubt, CT becomes the examination of choice, with its ability to identify fat.[468]

Pleural thickening, particularly when generalized, is often correctly dismissed as an inactive residuum. Care, however, must be taken to distinguish it from various active processes, some of which are neoplastic. While a number of these conditions tend to give plaquelike, nodular or irregular shadowing (Fig 14–56), they can on occasions closely resemble simple inactive pleural thickening. Disorders to consider include (1) mycetoma-related pleural thickening, (2) diffuse pleural mesothelioma, (3) diffuse pleural metastases, (4) leukemia, (5) lymphoma, and (6) Wegener's granulomatosis.

PLEURAL CALCIFICATION

Virtually any process that can cause pleural thickening can go on to calcify,[556] but, in practice, most cases of pleural calcification are the result of infection, hemorrhage, or exposure to asbestos. The recognized causes are listed in Table 14–7.

Calcification in asbestos inhalation and related conditions is very characteristic morphologically,[469] and is considered elsewhere in this volume (see Chapter 9). Calcification following infection and hemorrhage generally cannot be distinguished. Such calcification is usually unilateral and varies from barely detectable to massive (Fig 14–57). In the latter circumstance it becomes sheetlike and, reflecting the gravitationally determined distribution of the

TABLE 14–7.
Causes of Pleural Calcification

Infection
    Tuberculous empyema
    Nontuberculous empyema

Hemothorax

Mineral inhalation
    Asbestos (including tremolite talc)
    Mica
    Zeolites

Miscellaneous
    Chronic pancreatitis[51]
    Chronic hemodialysis[568]
    Calcified metastasis

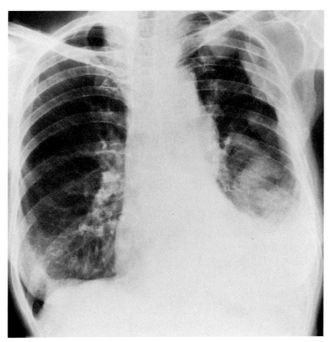

FIG 14–56.
Pleural thickening—diffuse. In the left hemithorax there is diffuse pleural thickening. It is irregular and coarsely nodular and is accompanied by a pleural effusion. Pleural thickening also affects the mediastinal pleura and distorts the mediastinal silhouette. The combination of findings is very suggestive of a malignant process, in this case metastatic adenocarcinoma. A mesothelioma could have an identical appearance.

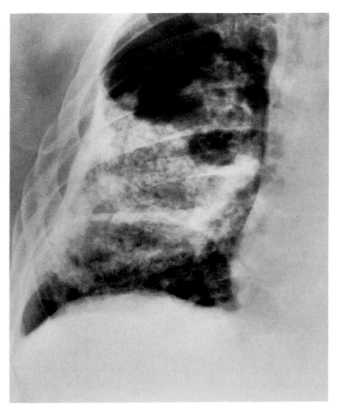

FIG 14–57.
Pleural calcification. Localized view of the right mid and lower zone shows sheetlike calcification. Laterally, where the calcification is tangential to the x-ray beam, it is dense and homogeneous, but medially—where it is seen en face—it is more broken-up and nodular. On the outside of the axillary calcification there is a 1-cm soft tissue band as a result of pleural thickening. The appearances occurring low down and unilaterally are characteristic of post-empyema (tuberculous) pleural calcification. The calcification occurs in thickened pleura, both parietal and visceral.

preceding pleural fluid, is often best developed posterolaterally.[556] En face, it appears as a hazy veil-like opacity, but in profile it is dense and linear, often parallel to the inner chest wall. The calcification in old empyemas is in both visceral and parietal pleura.[477, 484] Sometimes these calcified layers are separated, an observation that can be made on plain radiographs or, more easily, on CT scans.[477] In a series of 140 calcified fibrothoraces, 15.7% of cases had a persistent effusion sandwiched between layers of thickened calcified pleura demonstrable on CT by virtue of its attenuation, location, homogeneity, and failure to enhance.[477] This can be suspected on the plain radiograph with pleural thickening of more than 2 cm and a double layer of calcification.[477] Active infection of these encysted collections is manifested by expansion of the pleural opacity and the development of an air-fluid level signifying the presence of a bronchopleural fistula.[484]

PNEUMOTHORAX

Traditionally, pneumothorax is divided into spontaneous and traumatic types. The more common causes in the adult are listed (Table 14–8). Only spontaneous pneumothorax will be discussed in this chapter, apart from a brief consideration of pneumothorax associated with mechanical ventilation.

Primary Spontaneous Pneumothorax

A pneumothorax occurring without an obvious precipitating traumatic event is spontaneous; if the individual is apparently healthy, it is, in addition, primary. Primary spontaneous pneumothorax is typically a disease of young adult men. The peak prevalence is between the ages of 20 and 40 years, during which time two-thirds of the patients will present.[239] The male:female ratio is approximately 5:1.[220, 239, 334] There is a slight predominance of right-sided over left-sided pneumothorax, a predominance thought simply to reflect the slightly

TABLE 14–8.
Causes and Varieties of Pneumothorax in Adults

Spontaneous
  Primary
  Secondary
    Primary spontaneous pneumothorax*
    Familial pneumothorax*
    Airflow obstruction
      Asthma, chronic irreversible
    Infection
      Cavitary pneumonias
      Pneumatocele
      Tuberculous, fungal, hydatid disease
    Infarction*
      Septic, aseptic
    Neoplasm
      Primary, secondary, radiation
    Diffuse lung disease
      Eosinophilic granuloma, lymphangiomyomatosis,
        tuberous sclerosis, fibrosing alveolitis, sarcoidosis, cystic
        fibrosis
    Catamenial pneumothorax*
    Hereditable disorders of fibrous connective tissue*

Traumatic:
  Iatrogenic
    Thoracotomy, thoracocentesis
    Percutaneous biopsy (lung, kidney, etc.)
    Tracheostomy
    Central venous punctures
    Artificial ventilation
    Feeding tube perforation
  Noniatrogenic
    Closed
      Ruptured esophagus
      Ruptured trachea
      Perse ± rib fracture
    Penetrating.

*Discussed in this section.

larger volume of the right lung.[239] Bilateral pneumothoraces occur but are unusual,[180] and are more likely to occur metachronously than simultaneously. Thus, in one series of 242 cases, 10% were bilateral, but only 2.5% were simultaneous.[454] The incidence is about ten per hundred thousand of population per year.[334] Primary spontaneous pneumothorax is nearly always the result of rupture of an apical pleural bleb.[244] Blebs are said to be detectable on chest radiographs in 15% of cases in the presence of pneumothorax; they are seen in 54% of patients at thoracoscopy and in 92% at thoracotomy.[239] They are rarely seen, however, on the interval chest radiograph. The formation and/or rupture of blebs is probably encouraged by the greater mechanical stresses that occur at the lung apex[580] where the pleural surface pressure is much more negative than at the base. The transpulmonary pressure, which is

the force distending the lungs, is therefore greater at the apex than at the base, causing apical alveoli to be more distended.[165, 210] These stresses are magnified in subjects with long lungs, possibly explaining why pneumothoraces are more common in tall, thin individuals.[138, 595] Interestingly, if the prevalence of spontaneous pneumothorax is compared in male and female groups of the same height, then any sex difference in prevalence disappears.[335] Other predisposing factors are smoking[225] and, in familial spontaneous pneumothorax, human lymphocyte antigen (HLA) type.[485] There is some difference of opinion regarding the importance of stressful activity in precipitating the actual event. Some authors suggest that this happens only occasionally,[180] but in other series, about a quarter of patients were engaged in stressful activity, coughing, or sneezing.[239]

The clinical presentation is with chest pain (92%) and/or dyspnea (79%).[239] A few patients are asymptomatic. The pathophysiologic effect is usually mild, but there is a restrictive ventilatory defect[163] and sometimes transient hypoxemia and widening of the $(A-a)O_2$ gradient.[372] The pneumothorax will resorb once the causal pleural break seals. Absorption is slow and occurs at a rate of about 1.25% of the hemithoracic volume per day.[241] Thus, even a 15% pneumothorax will take 10 days to resolve. In one large series, the average time for resorption was 25 days.[239] Breathing 100% oxygen increases resorption rate.[373] Without definitive treatment, the likelihood of having another pneumothorax is about 40%, and this is three times more likely on the ipsilateral as the contralateral side.[239] The chance of recurrence rises with each episode from about 25% with the first to about 50% after several episodes, at which point the risk flattens off.[239] More than 60% of recurrences occur within 2 years, though they have been reported up to 12 years after the initial pneumothorax.[239]

Primary spontaneous pneumothorax may be treated conservatively with chest tube drainage, or with chemical or surgical pleurodesis, the latter usually being combined with bullectomy.[230, 239]

Familial pneumothorax has been occasionally reported since its first description in 1921.[485] The subject was reviewed in 1960[272] and again in 1979.[593] These last authors found reports of 61 pneumothoraces in 22 families. The male:female ratio was 1.8:1. The reported cases did not allow the mode of inheritance to be determined. Familial pneumothorax does not seem to be definitely related to stature, although in some reports patients have been marfanoid[526] Other workers have raised the possibility of a relationship to HLA haplotype (A2,B40) and α_1-antitrypsin phenotype.[485] There is a recent report of concurrent spontaneous pneumothoraces in 71-year-old identical twins.[419] There is also a report of pneumothoraces associated with large bullae in sisters.[159]

Secondary Spontaneous Pneumothorax

A pneumothorax developing without a precipitating traumatic event in a patient with predisposing lung disease is said to be a spontaneous secondary pneumothorax. These are generally considered to be less common than primary spontaneous pneumothoraces. Important causes are listed in Table 14–8. They include the following:

Airflow Obstruction.— Pneumothorax is a serious complication of chronic obstructive lung disease. It can lead to significant morbidity and possibly to death.[92, 158] The incidence in patients with chronic obstructive pulmonary disease has been estimated to be 0.4% per year,[239] and the mortality is 3% or higher.[92, 239]

Pneumothorax is an unusual complication of asthma in adults. The frequency of occurrence in patients with asthma severe enough to warrant hospitalization varies from 0.26%[423] to 2.5%,[49, 271] the lower figure probably being the more reliable, as it is based on two very large series. The association is seen more often in children (see Chapter 16), but even so is not very common.[128]

Pulmonary Infarction.— Pulmonary infarcts due to aseptic emboli are occasionally associated with a pneumothorax, 25 cases having been reported up to 1977.[187] At the time the pneumothorax develops, the infarct may be sterile,[35, 187, 421] or it may have become secondarily infected.[319] Such infarcts are usually large. Only about one-third have had obvious cavities in the consolidation on the chest radiograph.[187] Half of the patients go on to develop a large or persistent bronchopleural fistula. Septic pulmonary emboli may also cause pneumothorax.[222]

Primary Neoplasm.— The association of primary bronchial neoplasm and pneumothorax has recently been reviewed.[267, 518] The prevalence of this association is low, well under 1% of pneumothoraces being due to primary carcinoma of the lung.[93, 518] Looked at the other way around, 0.5% of lung carci-

nomas present with pneumothorax.[518] The suggested mechanisms include:

1. Coincidental occurrence, possibly associated with chronic obstructive pulmonary disease[180, 518].
2. Tumor wall necrosis with direct pleural invasion and rupture; unexpectedly, only a few of the carcinomas associated with pneumothorax have been cavitary.[267]
3. Rupture of lung that is overexpanded to compensate for adjacent carcinoma-induced collapse.[518]
4. Endobronchial obstruction with a check-valve effect.[15, 518]

The suspicion of an underlying bronchial carcinoma is usually raised by the finding of a mass or cavitary lesion in the reexpanded lung. Sometimes, however, the reexpanded lung appears radiographically normal.[62]

Secondary Neoplasms.— In a large series from the Mayo Clinic, about 0.5% of pneumothoraces were associated with lung metastases.[93] Of 45 cases in a literature review, 89% resulted from sarcomas (Fig 14–58) and only 11% from carcinoma.[600] Osteogenic sarcoma is by far the most common sarcoma.[224, 509] Other tumors reported to cause pneumothorax include Wilm's tumor,[493] germ cell tumors,[495, 496] and lymphoma.[397, 604] Many of these patients have been on chemotherapy, and the role that such therapy plays is not clear.[294] It is important to remember that pneumothoraces associated with metastases can occur before the deposits are radiologically detectable on the plain radiograph.[600]

Radiation.— The association of radiation and pneumothorax was first reported in 1974.[279] It is very unusual, only 11 cases in the English literature being found in a review in 1985.[451] It was reported in 1% of lymphoma patients receiving mantle irradiation.[451] Usually there is no malignancy in the chest at the time the pneumothorax develops. Typically, the pneumothoraces occur 4 to 16 weeks after the end of the radiation therapy, and radiographically visible radiation pneumonitis is common. Patients without associated radiation changes in the lung have also been recorded.[34] Pneumothoraces tend to be small or moderate in size and heal spontaneously, though some may be recurrent and bilateral.[549]

Endometriosis and Catamenial Pneumothorax

Chest involvement in endometriosis is rare. The most common manifestation is catamenial pneumothorax. This disorder, together with other aspects

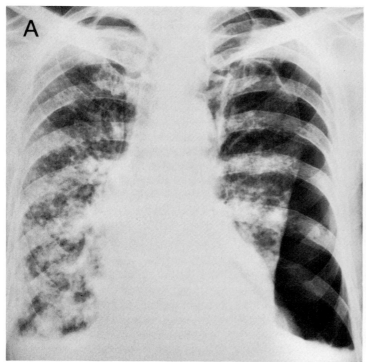

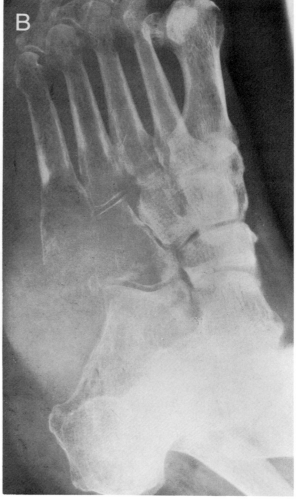

FIG 14–58.
Secondary spontaneous pneumothorax. **A,** a left pneumothorax with multiple bilateral nodular shadows, more easily appreciated in the right lung, due to metastases from a fibrosarcoma of the foot (**B**).

of endometriosis, are discussed in this section. There are two distinct forms of chest endometriosis: pleurodiaphragmatic and bronchopulmonary.[603] Each has distinct demographic, pathogenetic, and clinical features.

Pleurodiaphragmatic Endometriosis.—This presents clinically either as catamenial pneumothorax or, less commonly, as catamenial hemothorax.

Catamenial Pneumothorax.—Catamenial pneumothorax was first described by Maurer and coworkers in 1958.[316] It usually occurs in parous patients who are slightly older than patients with primary spontaneous pneumothorax.[449] Pneumothorax occurs only in relation to the menses—appearing 1 day before or up to 3 days after the periods. The pneumothorax is usually small and self-resolving.[497] It is nearly always right-sided (Fig 14–59), but left-sided[449] and bilateral instances [268, 588] have been re-

corded. Recurrence is a characteristic feature; indeed, without repeated episodes, a clear relationship to the menses cannot be established. Ten or 20 recurrences are not uncommon, and some authors have reported 30 or more.[81, 594] The other characteristic is that recurrence is prevented by pregnancy or drugs that suppress ovulation.[449]

Although 63 cases had been reported by 1982,[497] there is still some argument about the pathogenesis. No single concept can explain the occurrence of catamenial pneumothorax in all patients.[497] The most plausible theory is that air enters the peritoneal cavity by way of the genital tract during the menses, this being the only time that the cervix is not occluded by a mucus plug.[356] Having entered the peritoneal cavity, the air then passes into the pleural cavity through diaphragmatic holes that may be either simple defects (see p. 656)* or defects associated with

*References 73, 151, 316, 487, 497, and 520.

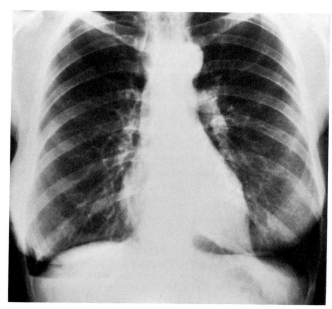

FIG 14—59.
Catamenial pneumothorax in a 34-year-old woman. This was the third episode, and all had been right-sided, as is usually the case. The air-fluid level in the costophrenic angle draws attention to the pneumothorax, which is otherwise easy to miss.

necrotic endometrial implants.[497, 502, 579] Some, but not all, of these latter patients have pelvic endometriosis. In the review by Slasky and co-workers[497] a third of catamenial pneumothoraces were associated with simple diaphragmatic defects and a fifth with diaphragmatic endometrial implants. Further support for the genital/transdiaphragmatic theory is afforded when cure follows either hormonal suppression of ovulation[288, 603] or tubal ligation.[379]

However, these mechanisms cannot account for all cases. In some patients pulmonary blebs seem to have been responsible just as in primary spontaneous pneumothorax.[288, 318] In other cases, endometriosis of the lung itself appears to have caused a direct air leak from the lung.[249, 603] The role of diaphragmatic defects and endometriosis has been comprehensively reviewed in a recent article.[497]

Catamenial Hemothorax.— A less common manifestation of pleurodiaphragmatic endometriosis in the chest is recurrent hemothorax occurring with the menses. All patients have had right-sided hemothoraces, pleural endometriosis, and pelvic endometriosis with demonstrated diaphragmatic holes in some,[603] and it seems likely that pleural implantation has occurred after transdiaphragmatic spread.

Bronchopulmonary Endometriosis.— This is a disorder of parous women aged 30 to 50 years. Gen-

erally, postmenopausal patients have been symptomless while younger ones have had recurrent hemoptysis at the time of the menses (catamenial hemoptysis). Pathologically there is usually a single focus of endometrial tissue in the lung parenchyma[228, 249, 266, 347] and occasionally in an airway,[438] together with a variable amount of parenchymal hemorrhage.[438]

Radiologically, lesions have appeared either as solitary, rounded nodules, several centimeters in diameter[266, 347] or as thin-walled cavitary lesions with septation and focal mural irregularity.[228] Sometimes the associated parenchymal bleeding is the dominant radiologic finding—appearing as consolidation that comes and goes in phase with the menses and hemoptyses.[197, 438] The chest radiograph can be normal in appearance.[445]

Catamenial hemoptysis has been successfully treated with the antigonadotropin *danazol.*[445] Patients with bronchopulmonary involvement usually give a past medical history of pregnancy and/or obstetric or gynecologic surgery (cesarean section, dilatation and curettage, abortion, hysterectomy), and it seems quite likely that pulmonary lesions are metastatic. There is experimental evidence in rabbits that this is a realistic possibility,[207] and the finding of decidua in the lungs at postmortem is well recognized.[228]

Heritable Disorders of Fibrous Connective Tissue

Five heritable disorders of fibrous connective tissue are associated with chest abnormalities. They may be classified as in Table 14—9.[407] These disorders are discussed here because pneumothorax is one of their more important respiratory manifestations.

Marfan's Syndrome.— This autosomal dominant disorder has a variable expression—involving particularly the eyes (myopia, ectopia lentis), aorta and heart (aortic aneurysm, aortic regurgitation, mitral valve disease), and musculoskeletal system (relatively long limbs in relationship to the trunk, arachnodactyly, pectus deformities, kyphoscoliosis, and joint laxity). The diagnosis is based on the clinical features, since a definite biochemical defect has yet to be identified.[408] New mutations probably account for 15% of cases.[408] Life expectancy is greatly reduced, most deaths being caused by cardiovascular complications.[359]

The chief respiratory abnormalities in Marfan's syndrome are pneumothorax, bullae, cysts, and emphysema. These findings are present in some 5% to

TABLE 14–9.
Heritable Disorders of Connective Tissue

Disorder	Major Clinical Features	Associated Chest Abnormality	
		Major	Minor
Marfan's syndrome	Myopia, ectopia lentis, aortic aneurysm, mitral valve disease, arachnodactyly, pectus deformity, lax joints	Emphysema, bullae/cysts, pneumothorax, skeletal deformity	Cor pulmonale, recurrent infection, bronchiectasis, mycetoma, pulmonary fibrosis, lobar hypoplasia
Ehlers-Danlos syndromes	Hyperextensible but elastic skin, lax joints, tissue fragility (bruising and bleeding)	Hemoptysis, bullae, pneumothorax, skeletal deformity	Recurrent infection, bronchiectasis, tracheobronchomegaly, pulmonary fibrosis
Cutis laxa	Loose inelastic skin, doleful facies	Emphysema, cor pulmonale	Recurrent infection, bronchiectasis, tracheobronchomegaly, laryngeal obstruction, pulmonary artery tortuous and stenotic, hernia, eventration of diaphragm
Pseudoxanthoma elasticum	Yellow skin papules	None	Small parenchymal nodules*

*Reported by Mamtora and Cope.[308]

10% of patients. Kyphoscoliosis may be gross and can lead to cor pulmonale and death.[565]

Pneumothorax is 30 to several hundred times more likely to occur in patients with Marfan's syndrome than in unaffected individuals.[188, 598] In such patients the frequency of pneumothorax ranges between 5% and 10%.[188, 598] Pneumothoraces are commonly bilateral and recurrent. There is an underlying chest radiographic abnormality in about two-thirds of the affected patients, either bullae or apical fibrosis.[188, 598]

A particularly striking manifestation of Marfan's syndrome is bullae occurring in young patients.[598] These may be apical in position[547] or widely distributed.[598] The bullae can become occupied by an aspergilloma.[598] Other manifestations include emphysema, congenital pulmonary malformations, apical fibrosis, bronchiectasis, and an increased frequency of lower respiratory tract infections.[598] Emphysema has been recorded at all ages from neonates to adults.[36, 102] It may cause cor pulmonale and death in the pediatric age group.[36, 95] Upper zone fibrosis is rare; only six cases have been reported in the world literature.[290] Associated congenital pulmonary malformations consist mainly of "rudimentary" middle lobes, which do not contribute to mortality or morbidity.[102] Bronchiectasis has been reported in

Marfan's syndrome,[139, 534, 598] but it is not clear if this is any more than a chance association.

The marfanoid hypermobility syndrome is classed as a separate entity that shares some of the features of both Marfan's and the Ehlers-Danlos syndromes.[561] Respiratory abnormalities consist of cysts, pneumothorax, bronchomegaly, and hemoptysis.[355]

The Ehlers-Danlos Syndromes.—These embrace a group of disorders characterized by hyperextensible skin and joints and abnormal tissue fragility that leads to bleeding and bruising.[402] The prevalence of respiratory abnormality is difficult to assess, and much of the literature has been confined to case reports.

The common clinical respiratory findings are hemoptysis, pneumothorax, and bullae. In one series of 20 patients, about 50% had respiratory symptoms or abnormal lungs on the chest radiograph,[16] and 25% had hemoptysis, probably related to vascular fragility rather than a bleeding or clotting abnormality. Bullae can occur without pneumothorax[16] and on one occasion have been both transient and fluid-filled.[23] Unlike cutis laxa, emphysema is not a feature, though exceptional cases have been reported.[74]

Pneumothorax is well-described, but appears to be less common in Ehlers-Danlos syndromes than in Marfan's syndrome.[16] It may be encountered with[63, 501] or without visible bullae on the plain chest radiograph.[16, 383]

Other findings that have been noted include recurrent sinusitis and pneumonia,[16] and, rarely, bronchiectasis,[436] tracheobronchomegaly,[1, 16] and upper zone fibrosis.[16] Skeletal abnormalities are common on the chest radiograph. In 20 cases in one series, 33% of patients had pectus excavatum, 22% had scoliosis, 17% had straight back, and 17% had thin ribs.[16]

Cutis Laxa (Generalized Elastolysis).—This condition may be acquired or congenital. Loose, inelastic skin is its characteristic feature. This results in a typical doleful facies with large earlobes, periorbital bagginess, and hook nose. Both forms demonstrate fragile, fragmented elastic tissue which shows normal collagen on histologic study. In the acquired form, the abnormality is confined to the skin. Several congenital varieties are recognized. The autosomal recessive form is characterized by neonatal onset of respiratory disease with air flow obstruction, pneumonia, emphysema, and cor pulmonale, resulting in the patient's death in childhood.[61, 171, 185, 317] The dominant form has predominant skin involvement, although other organ systems are sometimes involved.[26]

The most important respiratory abnormality accompanying this condition is emphysema, which usually develops shortly after birth[61, 185] but may be delayed until the teens[336, 548] or adulthood.[192, 260] Emphysema may be accompanied by bullae or by pulmonary arterial hypertension.[548] It commonly leads to death from cor pulmonale or respiratory failure. Other features described in children include repeated pulmonary infections,[185, 317] airflow obstruction due to large floppy cords, tracheobronchomegaly,[564] and bronchiectasis.[26] The pulmonary arteries may become tortuous and develop stenoses,[332, 336] causing abnormalities that appear on the plain chest radiograph. Hernias are a feature of cutis laxa and in the chest are manifest as hiatus hernias. In addition, the diaphragm may appear eventrated.[260, 332]

Traumatic Iatrogenic Pneumothorax

Only one of the varieties of traumatic pneumothorax is discussed here.

Mechanical Ventilation.—Pneumothorax is common in patients undergoing ventilation. Because there are so many modifying factors, it is both difficult and meaningless to give a prevalence rate. The likelihood of pneumothorax is increased by high airway pressures, long ventilation times, and abnormal lungs, and is particularly associated with infection,[88] infarction, and chronic obstructive pulmonary disease.[180, 441] Many factors cause high airway pressures: stiff lungs, volume cycling, unregulated manual inflation, large tidal volumes, endotracheal tube obstruction, right main stem bronchus intubation, atelectasis, and positive end-expired pressure.[322, 441] The development of a pneumothorax may be anticipated by the development of interstitial air, particularly in the form of "cysts."[8, 441] These appear as rounded, thin-walled transradiancies, 2 to 9 cm in diameter; they occur anywhere in the lungs but particularly at the bases, medially, or along the diaphragm. These cysts almost invariably go on to produce a tension pneumothorax. Not only are pneumothoraces common with mechanical ventilation, they are also more likely to be bilateral[180] and under tension—68% being so in one series.[441] It is therefore not surprising that pneumothorax occurring with mechanical ventilation may be rapidly fatal.[253] Immediate tube drainage is required.[515, 611]

Radiographic Signs of Pneumothorax

As with other pleural processes, the radiologic appearance of a pneumothorax depends critically on the radiographic projection, the position of the patient, and the presence or absence of loculation.

Free Pneumothorax

In the erect patient, air rises in the pleural space and separates the lung from the chest wall, allowing the visceral pleural line to become visible as a thin curvilinear opacity between vessel-containing lung and the avascular pneumothorax space (Fig 14–60). The pleural line remains approximately parallel to the chest wall. It may be difficult to identify in shallow pneumothoraces, when hidden by ribs and other bony structures. In this circumstance a radiograph taken in expiration may make the line easier to detect as it alters its orientation relative to ribs and also increases the volume of the pneumothorax space relative to the lung volume.[124] A lateral decubitus chest radiograph obtained with the suspect side uppermost may similarly be of help.[300]

Curvilinear shadows projected over the lung apex may mimic the visible visceral pleural line of a pneumothorax and cause difficulty in interpretation. Such opacities include those resulting from vascular

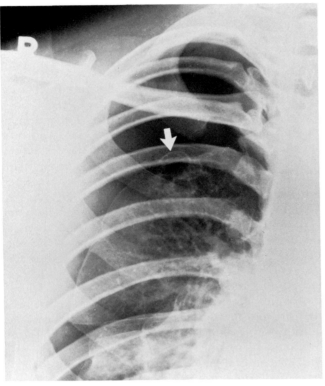

FIG 14-60.
Primary spontaneous pneumothorax. The visceral pleural line is clearly demonstrated together with the lateral avascular space. There is a pleural bleb at the apex of the lung *(arrow)*, a common finding. Such blebs are usually not detectable when the lung re-expands.

lines, tubes, clothing, hair, scapulae, skinfolds, and the walls of bullae and cavities. Careful analysis of the structure and shape of these shadows—noting whether or not they extend beyond the inner margin of the chest wall—will often allow correct identification. In practice, skinfolds and bullae are the most troublesome. Skinfold artefacts are seen on AP radiographs of very young or old, seriously ill patients and are produced when subjects with loose skin slump against a cassette. Sometimes, it will be clear that the skinfold shadow does not represent a pneumothorax when, for instance, vessels are seen beyond it, when it extends outside the margin of the chest cavity, or when it is located or oriented such that it could not possibly represent the edge of a slightly collapsed lung. A helpful feature is that a skinfold generates a broad, bandlike opacity with a sharp outer edge that fades off medially and may have a very transradiant lateral margin, whereas visceral pleura tends to produce a much thinner linear opacity.[131] The thin marginal transradiancy with a skinfold artifact is a Mach effect.[75, 265] A somewhat

similar shadow to that generated by a skinfold may be produced by the scapular companion shadow.[263]

Cysts, bullae, and cavities are probably the most troublesome mimics of pneumothorax because they produce both transradiancy and thin curvilinear shadows. These structures, however, have inner margins that are concave to the chest wall rather than convex.[180] They do not conform to the shape of the costophrenic angle when they are at the lung base,[29] and they may be demonstrably limited to a lobe.[124] Not only may a bulla mimic a pneumothorax, but the reverse sometimes occurs when synechiae cross the pleural space. Synechiae, however, are generally straight, allowing a distinction from the curved linear margins of a cyst or bulla.[180] CT may be used to differentiate bullae and pneumothorax.[37]

With a pneumothorax, the transradiancy of the ipsilateral hemithorax is variable and is related to the degree of collapse, the presence or absence of disease in the lung itself, and the degree to which perfusion is reduced because of hypoventilation.[97] With a small pneumothorax, transradiancy is unchanged or occasionally slightly increased, but with progressive collapse the opacity of the lobe increases until it eventually becomes a fistlike mass of soft tissue density at the hilus. An air bronchogram is often but not invariably present, and its absence does not necessarily mean obstruction of large airways, as has been suggested.[365] As the lung loses volume, the small apical blebs that are almost invariably associated with primary spontaneous pneumothorax frequently become clearly visible (see Fig 14-60). Searching the partially collapsed lung for other predisposing conditions (see Fig 14-53) such as bullae, interstitial disease, or metastases is also worthwhile, taking care not to misinterpret shadows that simply result from the collapse itself.[124]

Many patients, such as those who have sustained trauma and those in intensive care units, undergo radiography while *supine.* Chest radiographs of a supine patient are not very sensitive in the detection of pneumothoraces; recent series suggest a sensitivity of 50% to 70%,[539, 540, 562] but clearly such figures depend critically on the size of the pneumothorax. Failure to diagnose pneumothorax under these circumstances may have serious consequences because, if untreated, tension will develop in many of these patients.[441]

In the supine patient, the highest part of the chest cavity lies anteriorly or anteromedially at the base, and free pleural air rises to this region. If the pneumothorax is small to moderate in size, there will be no separation of the lung from the chest wall laterally or at the apex. In the absence of a displaced visceral pleural line in these regions the detection of pneumothorax depends on identification of one or more of the following signs:

1. Relative transradiancy in the hypochondrial region (Fig 14–61)[431, 539, 610] and even of the whole hemithorax.

2. Increased sharpness of the adjacent mediastinal margin (Fig 14–61) and diaphragm, which may become bordered by a band of relative transradiancy. This effect is particularly well seen in infants and neonates.[354]

3. A deep and sometimes rather tonguelike costophrenic sulcus.[175]

4. Visualization of the anterior costophrenic sulcus (Fig 14–61). This recess runs obliquely across the hypochondrium and is sigmoid shaped, with its most cephalad point medially.[246] It may be seen as an interface or, if the under surface is bordered by gastric or colonic gas, as a line.[431, 610] The term "the

double diaphragm sign" has been applied to the simultaneous visualization of the anterior sulcus and the dome of the true hemidiaphragm.[610]

5. Increased sharpness of the cardiac borders (Fig 14–61), particularly the apex and a lobulated, rounded, and often masslike appearance to the pericardial fat pads (Fig 14–62)[610] because they are no longer flattened against the heart.

6. Occasionally, anterior pleural air allows the middle lobe to retract medially away from the lateral chest wall while the lower and upper lobes still maintain chest wall contact. Under these circumstances the lateral border of the middle lobe becomes visible as a fine, linear opacity passing caudally from the lateral aspect of the minor fissure, parallel to the chest wall toward the diaphragm.[256]

7. Pleural air may also collect in the minor fissure giving a characteristic transradiancy bounded by two visceral pleural lines.[164, 510]

8. Visualization of the inferior edge of the collapsed lung[610] above the diaphragm. This must be distinguished from extrapleural extension of air

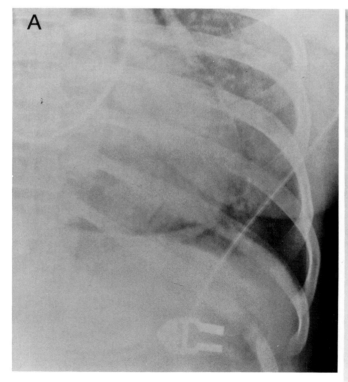

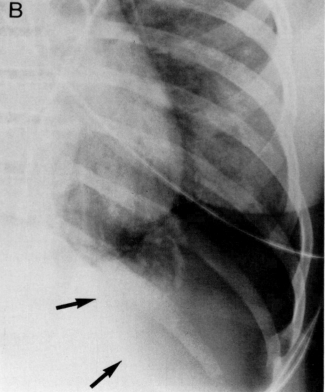

FIG 14–61.
Pneumothorax in a supine patient. **A,** pre-pneumothorax radiograph for comparison. **B,** following the development of a pneumothorax, there is a general basal transradiancy and a deep costophrenic sulcus; the left border of the heart is more distinct, and the anterior costophrenic sulcus *(arrows)* has become visible.

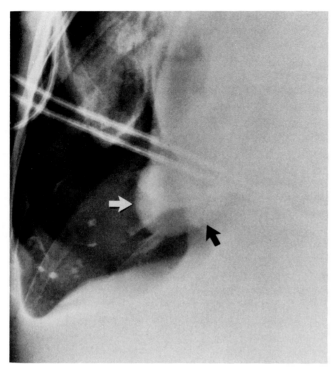

FIG 14–62.
Pneumothorax in a supine patient. Localized view of right lung base demonstrates a fat pad in the right cardiophrenic angle that has become rounded and masslike.

above the diaphragm, described in pneumomediastinum.[379]

9. Depression of the ipsilateral hemidiaphragm.[610]

If a pneumothorax is suspected in a radiograph of a supine patient it can be confirmed or excluded by other views, several of which were first described in infants and neonates. The cross-table lateral view[208] is probably the least satisfactory because of overlap of the other hemithorax. An alternative is to place a cassette 45 degrees dorsolaterally and angle the x-ray tube so that the central ray is perpendicular to the cassette. However, if the patient can be turned, the best image will result from a lateral decubitus view with the suspect side uppermost.[300] There is no doubt that CT is more sensitive than conventional radiography in the detection of pneumothorax in supine subjects.[539, 540, 562] Some authors recommend that a limited CT examination of the lung bases should be performed in all patients with severe trauma to the head at the time of cranial CT[540] to exclude unsuspected pneumothorax.

Loculated/Localized Pneumothorax

Sometimes a pneumothorax is truly loculated because of adhesions. On other occasions a free pneumothorax shows an atypical distribution (Fig 14–63). Several patterns are recognized:

1. *Subpulmonic pneumothorax.* Several authors have described subpulmonic pneumothorax with the visceral pleural line visible just above the diaphragm. This unusual location has been ascribed to preferential collection around diseased basal lobes[254] or to scarring of the rest of the pleural space, for example, following tuberculosis.[60] In another series of patients with the adult respiratory distress syndrome, subtle degrees of mediastinal shift and contour changes of the heart and hemidiaphragm suggested that these localized pneumothoraces were under tension.[167] Intrapleural air in this situation must be distinguished from extrapleural air that has dissected

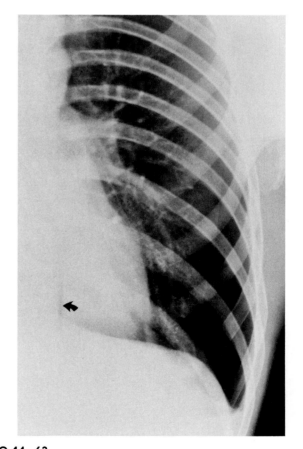

FIG 14–63.
Left pneumothorax, erect patient. There is an obvious pneumothorax. Pleural air is seen to collect in a linear manner along the left border of the heart and behind the heart *(arrow)* and must not be misinterpreted as a pneumomediastinum.

outward along the diaphragm from a pneumomediastinum[245, 287, 379] or from barotraumatic cysts.[8, 441]

2. *Encysted pneumothorax.* This may occur in the oblique fissure, giving a cystic opacity in the right mid-zone[370] or an air-fluid collection with a hemopneumothorax.[12] It may also occur in the inferior accessory fissure.[310]

3. *"Pulmonary ligament pneumatocoele."* Following trauma, particularly in children or young adults, a triangular collection of air sometimes develops against the mediastinum with its apex near the hilus (Fig 14-64). These air collections are more common on the left and may contain an air-fluid level.[116] An obvious ipsilateral pneumothorax may or may not be present, and the air collection generally clears in days or weeks.[168] In the past, these transradiancies have been ascribed to an air collection in the inferior pulmonary ligament.[123, 218, 420, 559] Recent CT evaluation, which allows more accurate localization, indicates that such transradiancies are either localized posteromedial pneumothoraces (see Fig 14-64) or air collections within the mediastinum.[147, 168]

4. *Pneumothorax adjacent to collapse.* Pleural surface pressure would be expected to be more negative over collapsed lung and thus might favor the localization of pneumothorax to that region. Pneumothorax adjacent to collapsed lobes has been recognized in adults[264] and children.[28]

Complications of Pneumothorax

About 20% of pneumothoraces are accompanied by *pleural fluid* (see Fig 14-59), which is usually small in amount and of no consequence.[239] The fluid may be clear, serosanguinous, or sanguinous. On an erect frontal radiograph a small amount of fluid appears as a C-shaped shadow in the costophrenic angle because its horizontal upper border is below the central ray and its anterior and posterior margins are projected separately. If the pneumothorax is very small and pleural separation is present only at the apex, then pleural fluid at the base will take on the classic meniscus form. In 3% or fewer of patients, a *hemothorax* develops that is large enough to warrant treatment in its own right.[2, 239] Hemothorax is much more frequent in primary than in secondary pneumothorax.[239] In keeping with this observation, 93% of patients with hemothorax in one review were men, and 92% were under 39 years of age.[563] Torn adhesions between the parietal and visceral pleura are common sources of bleeding.[85] Blood can clot in the pleural space and cause a mass, which may mimic a pleural tumor.[592] Pleural thickening is common following hemopneumothorax and, in one series, 22% of patients needed subsequent decortication.[239]

Uncommonly, purulent fluid accompanies a pneumothorax giving a *pyopneumothorax*. This is seen

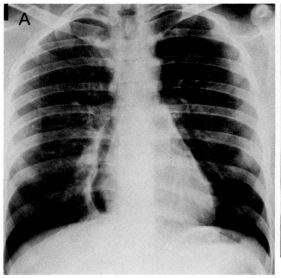
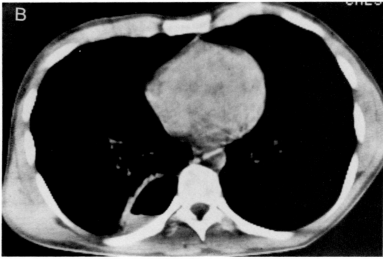

FIG 14-64.
"Pulmonary ligament pneumatocoele." **A,** following closed chest trauma, a triangular collection of air developed against the lower right mediastinum, with its apex at the hilus. **B,** CT of the same patient shows that the appearance in **A** is the result of a loculated posteromedial pneumothorax. It contains fluid that was infected, accounting for the thick pleural wall. (Courtesy of Dr. T. Bloomberg, Guildford, Surrey.)

with esophageal perforation or necrotizing pneumonia due most commonly to infection with *Staphlococcus aureus, Pseudomonas* spp., *Klebsiella* spp., or anaerobes.[230]

Tension pneumothorax is a life-threatening complication. It occurs when intrapleural pressure becomes positive for a significant part of the respiratory cycle, compressing the normal lung and causing a restrictive ventilatory defect, an increase in the work of breathing, and a ventilation/perfusion imbalance.[180] The cardiovascular effects are probably the result of respiratory failure rather than directly due to the increased pleural pressure.[183, 460] The condition must be treated by immediate decompression of the pleural space. It is usually diagnosed clinically by virtue of tachypnea, tachycardia, cyanosis, sweating, and hypotension. However, it will sometimes first be detected on radiographic examination, and the most important signs are mediastinal shift and diaphragmatic depression (Fig 14–65). Contralateral mediastinal shift must be interpreted with caution, as some movement toward the normal side is a frequent finding in a nontension pneumothorax, reflecting the fact that the pressure in the pneumothorax

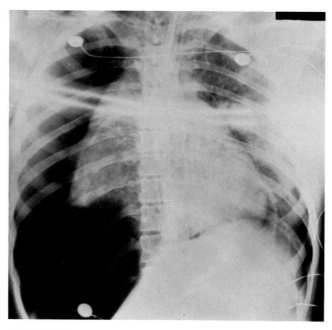

FIG 14–65.
Right tension pneumothorax. There is marked depression of the right hemidiaphragm and shift of the mediastinum to the left, indicated by the position of the heart and an endotracheal tube. The patient was being mechanically ventilated, which may account for the relative mildness of mediastinal shift compared with the gross diaphragmatic depression. Complete collapse of the right lung is prevented by consolidation. There is a small left pneumothorax as well.

space is usually not as negative as on the normal side. Should this shift be any more than mild or mild to moderate, then true tension should be considered. Unfortunately, no way of quantitating such shift has been worked out, and it seems unlikely that it ever will because mediastinal compliance varies so much from person to person. The degree of depression of the ipsilateral hemidiaphragm is a more useful observation than the extent of mediastinal shift, and the hemidiaphragm is invariably depressed, with significant tension. In patients on mechanical ventilation, diaphragmatic depression is the major sign. In such patients mediastinal shift is not a particularly marked feature of tension because airway pressure remains positive.[180] It is important to remember that significant tension can occur with little lung collapse if the underlying lung is abnormal (e.g., consolidated).[180] Tension pneumothorax occurs when the leak is through a tear, which behaves like a valve. Tension is unusual in primary pneumothorax and is seen more commonly with trauma or mechanical ventilation[441] particularly if positive end-expiratory pressure is employed.[515]

Following drainage of a pneumothorax acute *pulmonary edema* may develop in the reexpanded lung (Fig 14–66). A similar sequence of events can follow drainage of a pleural effusion. Its mechanism is obscure—some authors suggesting it is related to depletion of surfactant[339, 390, 483, 545] and others that it is due to anoxic capillary damage that leads to increased capillary permeability. There is quite a lot of evidence that supports the latter view.[47, 390, 483, 511] The edema usually develops within 2 hours of reexpansion and can progress for 1 or 2 days, resolving within 5 to 7 days. Reexpansion edema usually causes little morbidity, but patients can become hypotensive and hypoxic,[196, 230] and at least one death has been recorded.[471] It is generally held that predisposing factors are complete pneumothoraces with gross lung collapse, chronicity of the pneumothorax, and high negative aspiration pressures. Most pneumothoraces have been complete and present for at least 3 days,[303, 339, 545] but there are exceptions of shorter duration.[489] In many patients expansion has been rapid because negative aspiration pressure was used,[59, 471, 609] but again this has by no means been universal.[41, 215, 545, 567] The radiograph shows ipsilateral air-space shadowing. Exceptional cases are reported with contralateral edema[196, 514] and recurrent edema with recurrent pneumothorax.[486]

Pneumothoraces may be *recurrent*, and conditions that predispose to recurrence also predispose

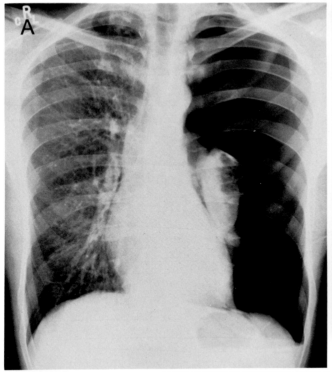

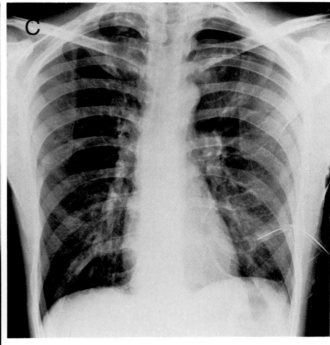

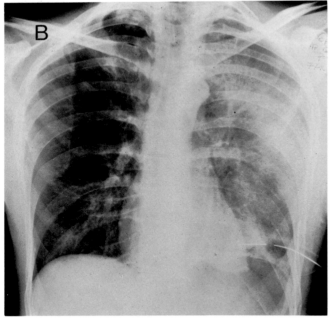

FIG 14–66.
Reexpansion pulmonary edema. **A,** complete collapse of the left lung following a primary spontaneous pneumothorax that had occurred 7 days previously. **B,** diffuse consolidation of the left lung 2 hours after insertion of a left pleural drain attached to an underwater seal drain. **C,** 24 hours after radiograph **B,** the air-space shadowing has cleared.

to *bilateral pneumothoraces.* Bilateral pneumothoraces may be synchronous or metachronous, the latter being much more common. Conditions particularly associated with bilateral pneumothoraces have been reviewed.[65] They include primary spontaneous pneumothorax and a variety of secondary pneumothoraces, in particular those associated with malig-

nant lung deposits, histiocytosis X, sarcoidosis, lymphangioleiomyomatosis, and exposure to radiation. Catamenial pneumothorax is almost invariably recurrent.

Pneumomediastinum is an unusual association of pneumothorax seen most commonly in neonates. In adults the combination may be seen in patients being mechanically ventilated, and with rupture of the esophagus,[396] trachea, or bronchi.[141] It is rare in primary spontaneous pneumothorax.

Pneumoperitoneum is an extremely rare complication of pneumothorax. Diaphragmatic defects may allow pleural air to pass into the peritoneal cavity, giving a pneumoperitoneum.[119] Presumably because of the pressure gradient across the diaphragm, the development of pneumothorax after pneumoperitoneum is much more common.

Following Progress and Management

Changes in the size of a pneumothorax can be followed on serial radiographs by measuring the interpleural distance at the apex or along a specified rib. Numerical estimates of the size of a pneumothorax can be expressed as a percentage of hemithorax volume by making simple measurements.[14, 430]

The causes to consider for failure of lung expansion include (1) tube malplacement; (2) large-airway occlusion by blood, mucus, or foreign body; (3) persistent air leak because of underlying lung disease, airway rupture, or pleural adhesions (see Fig 14–53,A); (4) visceral pleural thickening; and, possibly, (5) acute depletion of surfactant.[154] A number of these conditions may be detected radiographically. Tube malposition may be obvious, but in some cases the radiographic signs are subtle. Malposition in the oblique fissure may be suspected on an AP radiograph if the chest tube follows a gently curved or straight course upward and medially from its entry point, rather than deviating soon after entry, where it is deflected in front of or behind the lung.[572] The outer margin of pleural drainage tubes is seen by virtue of their contrast with surrounding air. Should such a tube become entirely displaced into the soft tissue of the chest wall then the outer margin of the tube will be no longer detectable. This is a useful sign of displacement.[571] Provided the degree of collapse is mild, it should be possible to detect any underlying lung diseases that may be responsible for persistent leakage, particularly diffuse interstitial fibrosis, cysts, bullae, or emphysema. Pleural adhesions that may hold open a visceral pleural tear will be seen as band shadows joining visceral to parietal pleura, distorting the lung envelope (see Fig 14–53,A).

With failure to completely reexpand the lungs, the pneumothorax becomes chronic and persistent, and this is an indication for surgery.

BRONCHOPLEURAL FISTULA

Bronchopleural fistula is an important cause of air in the pleural space (Table 14–10). It is similar to a pneumothorax except that the pleural communication is with an airway rather than with distal gas-exchange units. Although there are a number of causes, the bulk of cases are due either to surgical lung resection or necrotizing infections. Causes are listed in Table 14–11.

Bronchopleural fistulae complicating infections are considered under empyema (see Chapter 6). Postsurgical fistulae are considered here. They occur with a frequency of about 2.5% to 3%[306, 590] and usually occur within 2 weeks of surgery. They should be suspected clinically with the postoperative development of fever, hemoptysis, cough—especially if productive of a large amount of brown sputum, and a persistent large air leak from the pleural drains.

With bronchopleural fistula following recent pneumonectomy the chest radiographic signs differ from normal because there is: (1) an increased amount of air in the operated hemithorax; (2) a decreased amount of fluid; (3) loss of the normal mediastinal shift toward the operated side; and (4) sometimes an aspiration pneumonitis. Following lobectomy, or more than 6 months after a pneumonectomy, the pleural space is free of air and the development of a bronchopleural fistula is then signaled by the appearance of air in the pleural space. Occasionally, unchanged persistence of an air space following pneumonectomy indicates a fistula. This happens when the residual space is surrounded by pleural fibrosis and scarring such that it cannot change shape.[306] Extensive scarring may also prevent the mediastinal shift sign from being manifest.[262] It is not uncommon for plain radiographic signs (increasing pleural air) of bronchopleural fistula to appear in otherwise well patients who go on without complication or interference to show suc-

TABLE 14–10.

Causes of Air in the Pleural Space

Pneumothorax
Iatrogenic causes
Infection with gas-forming organism (rare)
Fistulae
    Bronchopleural
    Esophagopleural
    Via diaphragm or chest wall

TABLE 14–11.
Causes of Bronchopleural Fistula*

Trauma	Thoracic surgery/lobectomy/ pneumonectomy
	Other iatrogenic causes (chest tubes, lung biopsy, thoracocentesis, nasogastric tube misplacement, oleothorax)
Infection	Necrotizing pneumonia/empyema (especially anaerobic, tuberculous, pyogenic)
	Fungal infection
Pulmonary infarction	Sterile/septic
Miscellaneous	Neoplasms, radiation, rheumatoid nodules

*Data from Friedman PJ, Hellekant CAG: Radiological recognition of bronchopleural fistula. *Radiology* 1977, 124:289–295, and Peters ME, Gould HR, McCarthy TM: Identification of a bronchopleural fistula by computerized tomography—a case report. *J Comput Tomogr* 1983; 7:267–270.

cessful obliteration of the pleural cavity.[381] This is ascribed to a flap valve type of fistula that is self healing.

A fistula may be detected using scintigraphy and may for example be shown with xenon-133 lung scintigraphy in the washout phase.[608] Bronchography, sinography,[11] and even CT can be used to demonstrate anatomic details.

REFERENCES

1. Aaby GV, Blake HA: Tracheobronchiomegaly. *Ann Thorac Surg* 1966; 2:64–70.
2. Abyholm FE, Storen G: Spontaneous haemopneumothorax. *Thorax* 1973; 28:376–378.
3. Adams JT, McEvoy RK, DeWeese JA: Primary deep venous thrombosis of upper extremity. *Arch Surg* 1965; 91:29–42.
4. Agostoni E: Mechanics of the pleural space. *Physiol Rev* 1972; 52:57–128.
5. Agostoni E: Mechanics of the pleural space, in Geiger SR (ed): *The Handbook of Physiology;* section 3, The respiratory system, vol III, *Mechanics of Breathing,* part 2. Bethesda, Md, American Physiological Society, 1986.
6. Agostoni E, D'Angelo E: Thickness and pressure of the pleural liquid at various heights and with various hydrothoraces. *Respir Physiol* 1969; 6:330–342.
7. Ahmad S: Sclerosing peritonitis and propanolol. *Chest* 1981; 79:361–362.
8. Albelda SM, Gefter WB, Kelley MA, et al: Ventilator-induced subpleural air cysts: Clinical, radiographic and pathologic significance. *Am Rev Respir Dis* 1983; 127:360–365.
9. Alexander ES, Proto AV, Clark RA: CT differentiation of subphrenic abscess and pleural effusion. *AJR* 1983; 140:47–51.
10. Anderson WJ, Skinner DB, Zuidema GD, et al: Chronic pancreatic pleural effusions. *Surg Gynecol Obstet* 1973; 137:827–830.
11. Andrews NC, VerMeulen VR, Christoforidis AJ: Injection of contrast media in postresection pleural spaces: Diagnostic, prognostic and therapeutic value. *Dis Chest* 1967; 52:656–661.
12. Aronberg DJ, Brinkley AB, Levitt RG, et al: Traumatic fissural hemopneumothorax. *Radiology* 1980; 135:318.
13. Austin JHM: The left minor fissure. *Radiology* 1986; 161:433–436.
14. Axel L: A simple way to estimate the size of a pneumothorax. *Invest Radiol* 1981; 16:165–166.
15. Ayres JG, Pitcher DW, Rees PJ: Pneumothorax associated with primary bronchial carcinoma. *Br J Dis Chest* 1980; 74:180–182.
16. Ayres JG, Pope FM, Reidy JF, et al: Abnormalities of the lungs and thoracic cage in the Ehlers-Danlos syndrome. *Thorax* 1985; 40:300–305.
17. Bachman AL, Macken K: Pleural effusions following supervoltage radiation for breast carcinoma. *Radiology* 1959; 72:699–709.
18. Baltaxe HA, Lee JG, Ehlers KH, et al: Pulmonary lymphangiectasia demonstrated by lymphangiography in two patients with Noonan's syndrome. *Radiology* 1975; 115:149–153.
19. Banks J, Cassidy D, Campbell IA, et al: Unusual clinical signs complicating tension haemothorax. *Br J Dis Chest* 1984; 78:272–274.
20. Barakat MH, Karnik AM, Majeed HWA, et al: Familial Mediterranean fever (recurrent hereditary polyserositis) in Arabs—a study of 175 patients and review of the literature. *Q J Med* 1986; 60:837–847.
21. Barek LB, Cigtay OS: Urinothorax—an unusual pleural effusion. *Br J Radiol* 1975; 48:685–686.
22. Baron RL, Stark DD, McClennan BL, et al: Intrathoracic extension of retroperitoneal urine collections. *AJR* 1981; 137:37–41.
23. Baumer JH, Hankey S: Transient pulmonary cysts in an infant with the Ehler-Danlos syndrome. *Br J Radiol* 1980; 53:598–599.
24. Bedford DE, Lovibond JL: Hydrothorax in heart failure. *Br Heart J* 1941; 3:93–111.
25. Beer DJ, Pereira W, Snider GL: Pleural effusion associated with primary lymphedema: A perspective on the yellow nail syndrome. *Am Rev Respir Dis* 1978; 117:595–599.
26. Beighton P: Cutis laxa—a heterogeneous disorder. *Birth Defects* 1974; 10:126–131.
27. Benninghoff D, Camiel M, Takashima T: Clinical and experimental studies of chylous reflux. *Prog Lymphol* 1970; 2:269–271.
28. Berdon WE, Dee GJ, Abramson SJ, et al: Localized

pneumothorax adjacent to a collapsed lobe: A sign of bronchial obstruction. *Radiology* 1984; 150:691–694.

29. Berg RA: Giant congenital bronchogenic cyst, "Pseudopneumothorax." *Postgrad Med* 1970; 48:121–126.

30. Berger HW, Rammohan G, Neff MS, et al: Uremic pleural effusion. A study in 14 patients on chronic dialysis. *Ann Intern Med* 1975; 82:362–364.

31. Bessone LN, Ferguson TB, Burford TH: Chylothorax. *Ann Thorac Surg* 1971; 12:527–550.

32. Black LF: The pleural space and pleural fluid. *Mayo Clin Proc* 1972; 47:493–506.

33. Blalock A, Cunningham RS, Robinson CS: Experimental production of chylothorax by occlusion of the superior vena cava. *Ann Surg* 1936; 104:359–364.

34. Blane CE, Silberstein RJ, Sue JY: Radiation therapy and spontaneous pneumothorax. *J Can Assoc Radiol* 1981; 32:153–154.

35. Blundell JE: Pneumothorax complicating pulmonary infarction. *Br J Radiol* 1967; 40:226–227.

36. Bolande RP, Tucker AS: Pulmonary emphysema and other cardiorespiratory lesions as part of the Marfan abiotrophy. *Pediatrics* 1964; 33:356–366.

37. Bourgouin P, Cousineau G, Lemire P, et al: Computed tomography used to exclude pneumothorax in bullous lung disease. *J Can Assoc Radiol* 1985; 36:341–342.

38. Bower GC: Chylothorax. Observations in 20 cases. *Dis Chest* 1964; 46:464–468.

39. Bradley JWP, Fielding LP: Hydropneumothorax complicating perforated peptic ulcer. *Br J Surg* 1972; 59:72–73.

40. Bramson RT, Mikhael MA, Sagel SS, et al: Recurrent Hodgkin's disease manifesting roentgenographically as a pleural mass. *Chest* 1974; 66:89–91.

41. Brennan NJ, Fitzgerald MX: Hydropneumothorax complicating perforated peptic ulcer. *Br J Surg* 1972; 59:72–73.

42. Brenner WI, Boal BH, Reed GE: Chylothorax as a manifestation of rheumatic mitral stenosis. Its post operative management with a diet of medium-chain triglycerides. *Chest* 1978; 73:672–673.

43. Bron KM, Baum S, Abrams HL: Oil embolism in lymphangiography. Incidence, manifestations, and mechanism. *Radiology* 1963; 80:194–202.

44. Brown LR, Reiman HM, Rosenow EC, et al: Intrathoracic lymphangioma. *Mayo Clin Proc* 1986; 61:882–892.

45. Brown SD, Brashear E, Schnute RB: Pleural effusion in a young woman with myxedema. *Arch Intern Med* 1983; 143:1458–1460.

46. Bryk D: Infrapulmonary effusion. Effect of expiration on the pseudodiaphragmatic contour. *Radiology* 1976; 120:33–36.

47. Buczko GB, Grossman RF, Goldberg M: Re-

48. Bumgarner JR, Gahwyler M, Ward DE: Persistent fibrin bodies presenting as coin lesions. *Am Rev Tuberc* 1955; 72:659–662.

49. Burke GJ: Pneumothorax complicating acute asthma. *S Afr Med J* 1979; 55:508–510.

50. Butler C, Kleinerman J: The pulmonary apical cap. *Am J Pathol* 1970; 60:205–216.

51. Bydder GM, Kreel L: Pleural calcification in pancreatitis demonstrated by computed tomography. *J Comput Assist Tomogr* 1981; 5:161–163.

52. Bynum LJ, Wilson JE: Radiographic features of pleural effusions in pulmonary embolism. *Am Rev Respir Dis* 1978; 117:829–834.

53. Calvert RJ, Smith E: An analytical review of spontaneous haemopneumothorax. *Thorax* 1955; 10:64–72.

54. Cameron JL: Chronic pancreatic ascites and pancreatic pleural effusions. *Gastroenterology* 1978; 74:134–140.

55. Case records of the Massachusetts General Hospital (case 10, 1963). *N Engl J Med* 1963; 268:320–325.

56. Cevese PG, Vecchioni R, D'Amico DF, et al: Postoperative chylothorax. *J Thorac Cardiovasc Surg* 1975; 69:966–971.

57. Chavez CM, Conn JH: Thoracic duct laceration. Closure under conservative management based on lymphangiography evaluation. *J Thorac Cardiovasc Surg* 1966; 51:724–728.

58. Chetty KG: Transudative pleural effusions. *Clin Chest Med* 1985; 6:49–54.

59. Childress ME, Moy G, Mottram M: Unilateral pulmonary edema resulting from treatment of spontaneous pneumothorax. *Am Rev Respir Dis* 1971; 104:119–121.

60. Christensen EE, Dietz GW: Subpulmonic pneumothorax in patients with chronic obstructive pulmonary disease. *Radiology* 1976; 121:33–37.

61. Christiaens L, Marchand-Alphant A, Favet A: Emphyseme congenital et cutix laxa. *Presse Med* 1954; 62:1799–1801.

62. Citron KM: Spontaneous pneumothorax complicating bronchial carcinoma. *Tubercle* 1959; 40:384–386.

63. Clark JG, Kuhn C, Uitto J: Lung collagen in type IV Ehlers-Danlos syndrome: Ultrastructural and biochemical studies. *Am Rev Respir Dis* 1980; 122:971–978.

64. Coe JE, Aikawa JK: Cholesterol pleural effusion. *Arch Intern Med* 1961; 108:763–774.

65. Cohen HL, Cohen SW: Spontaneous bilateral pneumothorax in drug addicts. *Chest* 1984; 86:645–647.

66. Collins JD, Burwell D, Furmanski S, et al: Minimal detectable pleural effusions. A roentgen pathology model. *Radiology* 1972; 105:51–53.

67. Collins JS, Pagani JJ: Extrathoracic musculature mimicking pleural lesions. *Radiology* 1978; 129:21–22.

68. Cook GC: Periodic disease, recurrent polyserositis, familial Mediterranean fever, or simply "FMF." *Q J Med* 1986; 60:819–823.

69. Cooper C, Moss AA, Buy JN, et al: CT appearance of the normal inferior pulmonary ligament. *AJR* 1983; 141:237–240.

70. Cooper JAD, White DA, Matthay RA: Drug-induced pulmonary disease: Part 2. Noncytotoxic drugs. *Am Rev Respir Dis* 1986; 133:488–505.

71. Corriere JN, Miller WT, Murphy JJ: Hydronephrosis as a cause of pleural effusion. *Radiology* 1968; 90:79–84.

72. Crofts NF: Pneumothorax complicating therapeutic pneumoperitoneum. *Thorax* 1954; 9:226–228.

73. Crutcher RR, Waltuch TL, Blue ME: Recurring spontaneous pneumothorax associated with menstruation. *J Thorac Cardiovasc Surg* 1967; 54:599–602.

74. Cupo LN, Pyeritz RE, Olson JL, et al: Ehlers-Danlos syndrome with abnormal collagen fibrils, sinus of Valsalva aneurysms, myocardial infarction, panacinar emphysema and cerebral heterotopias. *Am J Med* 1981; 71:1051–1058.

75. Daffner RH: Visual illusions affecting perception of the roentgen image. *CRC Crit Rev Diagn Imaging* 1983/4; 20:79–119.

76. Dahlgren S: Anatomy of the thoracic duct from the standpoint of surgery for chylothorax. *Acta Chir Scand* 1963; 125:201–206.

77. Dalen JE, Haffajee CI, Alpert JS, et al: Pulmonary embolism, pulmonary hemorrhage and pulmonary infarction. *N Engl J Med* 1977; 296:1431–1435.

78. Dallemand S, Twersky J, Gordon DH: Pseudomass of the left upper quadrant from inversion of the left hemidiaphragm: CT diagnosis. *Gastrointest Radiol* 1982; 7:57–59.

79. Dalton ML, Strange WH, Downs EA: Intrathoracic splenosis. Case report and review of the literature. *Am Rev Respir Dis* 1971; 103:827–830.

80. Dandy WE: Incomplete pulmonary interlobar fissure sign. *Radiology* 1978; 128:21–25.

81. Davies R: Recurring spontaneous pneumothorax concomitant with menstruation. *Thorax* 1968; 23:370–373.

82. Davis HH, Varki A, Heaton WA, et al: Detection of accessory spleens with indium III-labeled autologous platelets. *Am J Hematol* 1980; 8:81–86.

83. Davis LA: The vertical fissure line. *AJR* 1960; 84:451–453.

84. Davis S, Gardner F, Qvist G: The shape of a pleural effusion. *Br Med J* 1963; 1:436–437.

85. Deaton WR, Johnston FR: Spontaneous hemopneumothorax. *J Thorac Cardiovasc Surg* 1962; 43:413–415.

86. DeCosse JJ, Poulin TL, Fox PS, et al: Subphrenic abscess. *Surg Gynecol Obstet* 1974; 138:841–846.

87. DeFrance JH, Blewett JH, Ricci JA, et al: Massive hemothorax: Two unusual cases. *Chest* 1974; 66:82–84.

88. de Lattore FJ, Tomasa A, Klamburg J, et al: Incidence of pneumothorax and pneumomediastinum in patients with aspiration pneumonia requiring ventilatory support. *Chest* 1977; 72:141–144.

89. Demos TC, Pieters C: Abdominal pseudotumor due to inverted hemidiaphragm. *Chest* 1984; 86:466–468.

90. Dewan NA, Kinney WW, O'Donohue WJ: Chronic massive pancreatic pleural effusion. *Chest* 1984; 85:497–501.

91. Diaconis JN, Weiner CI, White DW: Primary subclavian vein thrombosis and bilateral chylothorax documented by lymphography and venography. *Radiology* 1976; 119:557–558.

92. Dines DE, Clagett OT, Payne WS: Spontaneous pneumothorax in emphysema. *Mayo Clin Proc* 1970; 45:481–487.

93. Dines DE, Cortese DA, Brennan MD, et al: Malignant pulmonary neoplasms predisposing to spontaneous pneumothorax. *Mayo Clin Proc* 1973; 48:541–544.

94. Dockerty MB, Masson JC: Ovarian fibromas: A clinical and pathologic study of 283 cases. *Am J Obstet Gynecol* 1944; 47:741–752.

95. Dominguez R, Weisgrau RA, Santamaria M: Pulmonary hyperinflation and emphysema in infants with the Marfan syndrome. *Pediatr Radiol* 1987; 17:365–369.

96. Dorne HL: Differentiation of pulmonary parenchymal consolidation from pleural disease using the sonographic fluid bronchogram. *Radiology* 1986; 158:41–42.

97. Dornhorst AC, Pierce JW: Pulmonary collapse and consolidation. The role of collapse in the production of lung field shadows and the significance of segments in inflammatory lung disease. *J Fac Radiol* 1954; 5:276–281.

98. Dressler W: The post-myocardial-infarction syndrome. A report on 44 cases. *Arch Intern Med* 1959; 103:28–42.

99. Ducharme J-C, Belanger R, Simard P, et al: Chylothorax, chylopericardium with multiple lymphangioma of bone. *J Pediatr Surg* 1982; 17:365–367.

100. Dunbar JS, Favreau M: Infrapulmonary pleural effusions with particular reference to its occurrence in nephrosis. *J Can Assoc Radiol* 1959; 10:24.

101. Dwyer A: The displaced crus: A sign for distinguishing between pleural fluid and ascites on computed tomography. *J Comput Assist Tomogr* 1978; 2:598–599.

102. Dwyer EM, Troncale F: Spontaneous pneumothorax

and pulmonary disease in the Marfan syndrome. *Ann Intern Med* 1965; 62:1285–1292.

103. Ecker MD, Jay B, Keohane MF: Procarbazine lung. *AJR* 1978; 131:527–528.

104. Edwards SR, Unger AM: Acute hydrothorax—a new complication of peritoneal dialysis. *JAMA* 1967; 199:853–855.

105. Effmann EL, Ablow RC, Touloukian RJ, et al: Radiographic aspects of total parenteral nutrition during infancy. *Radiology* 1978; 127:195–201.

106. Ehrenfeld EN, Eliakim M, Rachmilewitz M: Recurrent polyserositis (familial Mediterranean fever, periodic disease). A report of fifty-five cases. *Am J Med* 1961; 31:107–123.

107. El-Kassimi FA: Roentgenogram of the month. Acute pleuritic chest pain with pleural effusion and plate atelectasis. *Chest* 1987; 91:265–266.

108. Emerson PA: Yellow nails, lymphoedema, and pleural effusions. *Thorax* 1966; 21:247–253.

109. Emerson PA, Davies JH: Hydrothorax complicating ascites. *Lancet* 1955; 1:487–488.

110. Engle MA, Ito T: The postpericardiotomy syndrome. *Am J Cardiol* 1961; 7:73–82.

111. Epler GR, McLoud TC, Munn CS, et al: Pleural lipoma. Diagnosis by computed tomography. *Chest* 1986; 90:265–268.

112. Erwteman TM, Braat MCP, Van Aken WG: Interstitial pulmonary fibrosis: A new side effect of practolol. *Br Med J* 1977; 2:297–298.

113. Euphrat EJ, Beck E: Fibrin body following traumatic pneumothorax. *AJR* 1955; 74:86–89.

114. Evander LC: Pleural fat pads: A cause of thoracic shadows. *Am Rev Tuberc* 1948; 57:495–503.

115. Everts CS, Westcott JL, Bragg DG: Methotrexate therapy and pulmonary disease. *Radiology* 1973; 107:539–543.

116. Fagan CJ, Swischuk LE: Traumatic lung and paramediastinal pneumatoceles. *Radiology* 1976; 120:11–18.

117. Fairfax AJ, McNabb WR, Spiro SG: Chylothorax: A review of 18 cases. *Thorax* 1986; 41:880–885.

118. Faling LJ, Gerzof SG, Daly BDT, et al: Treatment of chronic pancreatitic pleural effusion by percutaneous catheter drainage of abdominal pseudocyst. *Am J Med* 1984; 76:329–333.

119. Fataar S, Morton P, Schulman A: Recurrent nonsurgical pneumoperitoneum due to spontaneous pneumothorax. *Br J Radiol* 1981; 54:1100–1102.

120. Feder BH, Wilk SP: Localized interlobar effusion in heart failure: Phantom lung tumor. *Dis Chest* 1956; 30:289–297.

121. Federle MP, Mark AS, Guillaumin ES: CT of subpulmonic pleural effusions and atelectasis: Criteria for differentiation from subphrenic fluid. *AJR* 1986; 146:685–689.

122. Feldman DJ: Localized interlobar pleural effusion in heart failure. *JAMA* 1951; 146:1408–1409.

123. Felman AH, Rodgers BM, Talbert JL: Traumatic

124. Felson B: *Chest Roentgenology.* Philadelphia, WB Saunders Co, 1973.

125. Felson B: The extrapleural space. *Semin Roentgenol* 1977; 12:327–333.

126. Felson B, Fleischner FG, McDonald JR, et al: Some basic principles in the diagnosis of chest diseases. *Radiology* 1959; 73:740–748.

127. Ferguson GC: Cholesterol pleural effusion in rheumatoid lung disease. *Thorax* 1966; 21:577–582.

128. Findley LJ, Sahn SA: The value of chest roentgenograms in acute asthma in adults. *Chest* 1981; 80:535–536.

129. Finn R, Jowett EW: Acute hydrothorax complicating peritoneal dialysis. *Br Med J* 1970; 2:94.

130. Fishbein R, Murphy GP, Wilder RJ: The pleuropulmonary manifestations of pancreatitis. *Dis Chest* 1962; 41:392–397.

131. Fisher JK: Skin fold versus pneumothorax. *AJR* 1978; 130:791–792.

132. Fisher MS: Significance of a visible major fissure on the frontal chest radiograph. *AJR* 1981; 137:577–580.

133. Fisher MS: Adam's lobe, letters to the editor. *Radiology* 1985; 154:547.

134. Fitzgerald TB, Johnstone MW: Diaphragmatic defects and laparoscopy. *Br Med J* 1970; 2:604.

135. Fleischner FG: Pulmonary embolism. *Clin Radiol* 1962; 13:169–182.

136. Fleischner FG: Atypical arrangement of free pleural effusion. *Radiol Clin North Am* 1963; 1:347–362.

137. Fleming HA, Hickling P: Pleural effusions after practolol. *Lancet* 1975; 2:1202.

138. Forgacs P: Stature in simple pneumothorax. *Guys Hosp Rep* 1969; 118:199–204.

139. Foster ME, Foster DR: Bronchiectasis and Marfan's syndrome. *Postgrad Med J* 1980; 56:718–719.

140. Fraser RG, Pare JAP: *Diagnosis of Diseases of the Chest,* ed 2. Philadelphia, WB Saunders Co, 1977, vol 1.

141. Fraser RG, Pare JAP: *Diagnosis of Diseases of the Chest,* ed 2. Philadelphia, WB Saunders Co, 1979, vol 3.

142. Fraser RG, Pare JAP, Pare PD, et al: *Diagnosis of Diseases of the Chest,* ed 3. Philadelphia, WB Saunders Co, 1988, vol 1.

143. Frazer IH, Lichtenstein M, Andrews JT: Pleuroperitoneal effusion without ascites. *Med J Aust* 1983; 2:520–521.

144. Freundlich IM: The role of lymphangiography in chylothorax. A report of six nontraumatic cases. *AJR* 1975; 125:617–627.

145. Friedland GW, Axman MM, Love T: Neonatal "urinothorax" associated with posterior urethral valves. *Br J Radiol* 1971; 44:471–474.

146. Friedman E: Further observations on the vertical fissure line. *AJR* 1966; 97:171–173.

147. Friedman PJ: Adult pulmonary ligament pneumatocele: A loculated pneumothorax. *Radiology* 1985; 155:575–576.

148. Friedman PJ, Hellekant CAG: Radiological recognition of bronchopleural fistula. *Radiology* 1977; 124:289–295.

149. Frija J, Schmit P, Katz M, et al: Computed tomography of the pulmonary fissures: Normal anatomy. *J Comput Assist Tomogr* 1982; 6:1069–1074.

150. Frolich DJ, Clements JL, Weens HS: Epicardial fat line in left pleural effusion. *AJR* 1975; 124:394–396.

151. Furman WR, Wang KP, Summer WR, et al: Catamenial pneumothorax: Evaluation by fiberoptic pleuroscopy. *Am Rev Respir Dis* 1980; 121:137–140.

152. Gale ME, Greif WL: Intrafissural fat: CT correlation with chest radiography. *Radiology* 1986; 160:333–336.

153. Galen MA, Steinberg SM, Lowrie EG, et al: Hemorrhagic pleural effusion in patients undergoing chronic hemodialysis. *Ann Intern Med* 1975; 82:359–361.

154. Galvis AG, Bowen AD, Oh KS: Nonexpandable lung after drainage of pneumothorax. *AJR* 1981; 136:1224–1226.

155. Gannon WE, Greenfield H: Fibrin body in an old abscess cavity, simulating a new growth. *Radiology* 1956; 66:564–566.

156. Gardner TW, Domm AC, Brock CE, et al: Congenital pulmonary lymphangiectasis. A case complicated by chylothorax. *Clin Pediatr* 1983; 22:75–78.

157. Gefter WB, Epstein DM, Bonavita JA, et al: Pleural thickening caused by Sansert and Ergotrate in the treatment of migraine. *AJR* 1980; 135:375–377.

158. George RB, Herbert SJ, Shames JM, et al: Pneumothorax complicating pulmonary emphysema. *JAMA* 1975; 234:389–393.

159. Gibson GJ: Familial pneumothoraces and bullae. *Thorax* 1977; 32:88–90.

160. Gilbert L, Ribot S, Frankel H, et al: Fibrinous uremic pleuritis: A surgical entity. *Chest* 1975; 67:53–56.

161. Gillett D, Ford GT, Anthonisen NR: Shape and regional volume in immersed lung lobes. *J Appl Physiol* 1981; 51:1457–1462.

162. Gilmartin D: The serratus anterior muscle on chest radiographs. *Radiology* 1979; 131:629–635.

163. Gilmartin JJ, Wright AJ, Gibson GJ: Effects of pneumothorax or pleural effusion on pulmonary function. *Thorax* 1985; 40:60–65.

164. Giuffre B: Supine pneumothoraces in adults. *Australas Radiol* 1984; 28:335–338.

165. Glazier JB, Hughes JMB, Maloney JE, et al: Vertical gradient of alveolar size in lungs of dogs frozen intact. *J Appl Physiol* 1967; 23:694–705.

166. Glorioso LW, Lang EK: Pulmonary manifestations of renal disease. *Radiol Clin North Am* 1984; 22:647–658.

167. Gobien RP, Reines HD, Schabel SI: Localized tension pneumothorax: Unrecognized form of barotrauma in adult respiratory distress syndrome. *Radiology* 1982; 142:15–19.

168. Godwin JD, Merten DF, Baker ME: Paramediastinal pneumatocele: Alternative explanations to gas in the pulmonary ligament. *AJR* 1985; 145:525–530.

169. Godwin JD, Tarver RD: Accessory fissures of the lung. *AJR* 1985; 144:39–47.

170. Godwin JD, Vock P, Osborne DR: CT of the pulmonary ligament. *AJR* 1983; 141:231–236.

171. Goltz RW, Hult A-M, Goldfarb M, et al: Cutis laxa. A manifestation of generalized elastolysis. *Arch Dermatol* 1965; 92:373–387.

172. Gonzales-Rothi RJ, Hannan SE, Hood CI, et al: Amiodarone pulmonary toxicity presenting as bilateral exudative pleural effusions. *Chest* 1987; 92:179–182.

173. Good JT, Moore JB, Fowler AA, et al: Superior vena cava syndrome as a cause of pleural effusion. *Am Rev Respir Dis* 1982; 125:246–247.

174. Goodman LR, Golkow RS, Steiner RM, et al: The right mid-lung window. *Radiology* 1982; 143:135–138.

175. Gordon R: The deep sulcus sign. *Radiology* 1980; 136:25–27.

176. Graham JR: Cardiac and pulmonary fibrosis during methysergide therapy for headache. *Am J Med Sci* 1967; 254:1–12.

177. Graham JR, Suby HI, LeCompte PR, et al: Fibrotic disorders associated with methysergide therapy for headache. *N Engl J Med* 1966; 274:359–368.

178. Gramiak R, Koerner HJ: A roentgen diagnostic observation in subpleural lipoma. *AJR* 1966; 98:465–467.

179. Grant T, Levin B: Lymphangiographic visualization of pleural and pulmonary lymphatics in a patient without chylothorax. *Radiology* 1974; 113:49–50.

180. Greene R, McLoud TC, Stark P: Pneumothorax. *Semin Roentgenol* 1977; 12:313–325.

181. Griffin DJ, Gross BH, McCracken S, et al: Observations on CT differentiation of pleural and peritoneal fluid. *J Comput Assist Tomogr* 1984; 8:24–28.

182. Gunnels JJ: Perplexing pleural effusion. *Chest* 1978; 74:390–393.

183. Gustman P, Yerger L, Wanner A: Immediate cardiovascular effects of tension pneumothorax. *Am Rev Respir Dis* 1983; 127:171–174.

184. Haaga JR, Weinstein AJ: CT-guided percutaneous aspiration and drainage of abscesses. *AJR* 1980; 135:1187–1194.

185. Hajjar BA, Joyner EN: Congenital cutis laxa with advanced cardiopulmonary disease. *J Pediatr* 1968; 73:116–119.

186. Hall DR, Morrison JB, Edwards FR: Pleural fibrosis after practolol therapy. *Thorax* 1978; 33:822–824.

187. Hall FM, Salzman EW, Ellis BI, et al: Pneumothorax

complicating aseptic cavitating pulmonary infarction. *Chest* 1977; 72:232–234.

188. Hall JR, Pyeritz RE, Dudgeon DL, et al: Pneumothorax in the Marfan syndrome: Prevalence and therapy. *Ann Thorac Surg* 1984; 37:500–504.

189. Halvorsen RA, Fedyshin PJ, Korobkin M, et al: CT differentiation of pleural effusion from ascites. An evaluation of four signs using blinded analysis of 52 cases. *Invest Radiol* 1986; 21:391–395.

190. Handler CE, Fray RE, Snashall PD: Atypical Meigs' syndrome. *Thorax* 1982; 37:396–397.

191. Harbin WP, Mueller PR, Ferrucci JT: Transhepatic cholangiography: Complications and use patterns of the fine-needle technique. *Radiology* 1980; 135:15–22.

192. Harris RB, Heaphy MR, Perry HO: Generalized elastolysis (cutis laxa). *Am J Med* 1978; 65:815–822.

193. Heilman RD, Collins VP: Identification of laceration of the thoracic duct by lymphangiography. Preoperative radiography of the traumatized thoracic duct. *Radiology* 1963; 81:470–472.

194. Heitzman ER: *The lung. Radiologic-pathologic correlations,* ed 2. St Louis, CV Mosby Co, 1984.

195. Heller H, Sohar E, Sherf L: Familial Mediterranean fever. *Arch Intern Med* 1958; 102:50–71.

196. Henderson AF, Banham SW, Moran F: Re-expansion pulmonary oedema: A potentially serious complication of delayed diagnosis of pneumothorax. *Br Med J* 1985; 291:593–594.

197. Hertzanu Y, Heimer D, Hirsch M: Computed tomography of pulmonary endometriosis. *Comput Radiol* 1987; 11:81–84.

198. Hessen I: Roentgen examination of pleural fluid. A study of the localization of free effusions, the potentialities of diagnosing minimal quantities of fluid and its existence under physiological conditions. *Acta Radiol* 1951; [Suppl] (Stockh) 86:7–80.

199. Higgins CB, Mulder DG: Mediastinal chyloma. A roentgenographic sign of chylous fistula. *JAMA* 1970; 211:1188.

200. Higgins JA, Juergens JL, Bruwer AJ, et al: Loculated interlobar pleural effusion due to congestive heart failure. *Arch Intern Med* 1955; 96:180–187.

201. Hiller E, Rosenow EC, Olsen AM: Pulmonary manifestations of the yellow nail syndrome. *Chest* 1972; 61:452–458.

202. Hillerdal G: Chyliform (cholesterol) pleural effusion. *Chest* 1985; 88:426–428.

203. Hinckley ME: Thoracic-duct thrombosis with fatal chylothorax caused by a long venous catheter. *N Engl J Med* 1969; 280:95–96.

204. Hindle W, Posner E, Sweetnam MT, et al: Pleural effusion and fibrosis during treatment with methysergide. *Br Med J* 1970; 1:605–606.

205. Hirsch A, Ruffie P, Nebut M, et al: Pleural effusion: Laboratory tests in 300 cases. *Thorax* 1979; 34:106–112.

206. Hirsch JH, Rogers JV, Mack LA: Real-time sonography of pleural opacities. *AJR* 1981; 136:297–301.

207. Hobbs JE, Bortnick AR: Endometriosis of the lungs. An experimental and clinical study. *Am J Obst Gynecol* 1940; 40:832–843.

208. Hoffer FA, Ablow RC: The cross-table lateral view in neonatal pneumothorax. *AJR* 1984; 142:1283–1286.

209. Hogg JC, Macklem PT, Thurlbeck WM: The resistance of collateral channels in excised human lungs. *J Clin Invest* 1969; 48:421–431.

210. Hogg JC, Nepszy S: Regional lung volume and pleural pressure gradient estimated from the lung density in dogs. *J Appl Physiol* 1969; 27:198–203.

211. Holmberg L, Boman G: Pulmonary reactions to nitrofurantoin. 447 cases reported to the Swedish adverse drug reaction committee 1966–1976. *Eur J Respir Dis* 1981; 62:180–189.

212. Holzel A, Fawcitt J: Pulmonary changes in acute glomerulonephritis in childhood. *J Pediatr* 1960; 57:695–703.

213. Hopps HC, Wissler RW: Uremic pneumonitis. *Am J Pathol* 1955; 31:261–274.

214. Hughson WG, Friedman PJ, Feigin DS, et al: Postpartum pleural effusion: A common radiologic finding. *Ann Intern Med* 1982; 97:856–858.

215. Humphreys RL, Berne AS: Rapid re-expansion of pneumothorax. A cause of unilateral pulmonary edema. *Radiology* 1970; 96:509–512.

216. Hurwitz PA, Pinals DJ: Pleural effusion in chronic hereditary lymphedema (Nonne, Milroy, Meige's disease). *Radiology* 1964; 82:246–248.

217. Hussey HH, Katz S, Yater WM: The superior vena caval syndrome: Report of thirty-five cases. *Am Heart J* 1946; 31:1–26.

218. Hyde I: Traumatic para-mediastinal air cysts. *Br J Radiol* 1971; 44:380–383.

219. Im J-G, Kang HS, Choi BI, et al: Pleural endometriosis: CT and sonographic findings. *AJR* 1987; 148:523–524.

220. Inouye WY, Berggren RB, Johnson J: Spontaneous pneumothorax: Treatment and mortality. *Dis Chest* 1967; 51:67–73.

221. Islam N, Ali S, Kabir H: Hepatic hydrothorax. *Br J Dis Chest* 1965; 59:222–227.

222. Jaffe RB, Koschmann FB: Septic pulmonary emboli. *Radiology* 1970; 96:527–532.

223. Jamison HW: Anatomic-roentgenographic study of pleural domes and pulmonary apices, with special reference to apical subpleural scars. *Radiology* 1941; 36:302–314.

224. Janetos GP, Ochsner SF: Bilateral pneumothorax in metastatic osteogenic sarcoma. *Am Rev Respir Dis* 1963; 88:73–76.

225. Jansveld CAF, Dijkman JH: Primary spontaneous pneumothorax and smoking. *Br Med J* 1975; 4:559–560.

226. Javaheri S, Hales CA: Sarcoidosis: A cause of innominate vein obstruction and massive pleural effusion. *Lung* 1980; 157:81–85.

227. Jay SJ: Diagnostic procedures for pleural disease. *Clin Chest Med* 1985; 6:33–48.

228. Jelihovsky T, Grant AF: Endometriosis of the lung. A case report and brief review of the literature. *Thorax* 1968; 23:434–437.

229. Jenkins PG, Shelp WD: Recurrent pleural transudate in the nephrotic syndrome: A new approach to treatment. *JAMA* 1974; 230:587–588.

230. Jenkinson SG: Pneumothorax. *Clin Chest Med* 1985; 6:153–161.

231. Johnson JR, Falk A, Iber C, et al: Paragonimiasis in the United States. A report of nine cases in the Hmong immigrants. *Chest* 1982; 82:168–171.

232. Johnston RF, Loo RV: Hepatic hydrothorax. Studies to determine the source of the fluid and report of thirteen cases. *Ann Intern Med* 1964; 61:385–401.

233. Jones JS, Yuill KB: Spontaneous pneumothorax resulting from pneumoperitoneum therapy. *Br J Tuberc* 1952; 46:30–36.

234. Kattan KR, Eyler WR, Felson B: The juxtaphrenic peak in upper lobe collapse. *Semin Roentgenol* 1980; 15:187–193.

235. Katzen BT, Choi WS, Friedman MH, et al: Pseudomass of the liver due to pleural effusion and inversion of the diaphragm. *AJR* 1978; 131:1077–1078.

236. Kausel HW, Reeve TS, Stein AA, et al: Anatomic and pathologic studies of the thoracic duct. *J Thorac Surg* 1957; 34:631–642.

237. Kaye MD: Pleuropulmonary complications of pancreatitis. *Thorax* 1968; 23:297–306.

238. Kent EM, Blades B: Surgical anatomy of pulmonary lobes. *J Thorac Surg* 1942; 12:18–30.

239. Killen DA, Gobbel WG: *Spontaneous Pneumothorax.* Boston, Little, Brown & Co, 1968.

240. Kinmonth JB: *The lymphatics. Diseases, Lymphography and Surgery.* London, Edward Arnold, 1972.

241. Kircher LT, Swartzel RL: Spontaneous pneumothorax and its treatment. *JAMA* 1954; 155:24–29.

242. Kirchner SG, Heller RM, Smith CW: Pancreatic pseudocyst of the mediastinum. *Radiology* 1977; 123:37–42.

243. Kirkpatrick JA, Fleisher DS: The roentgen appearance of the chest in acute glomerulonephritis in children. *J Pediatr* 1964; 64:492–498.

244. Kjaergaard H: Spontaneous pneumothorax in the apparently healthy. *Acta Med Scand* [Suppl] 1932; 43:1–159.

245. Kleinman PK, Brill PW, Whalen JP: Anterior pathway for transdiaphragmatic extension of pneumomediastinum. *AJR* 1978; 131:271–275.

246. Kleinman PK, Raptopoulos V: The anterior diaphragmatic attachments: An anatomic and radiologic study with clinical correlates. *Radiology* 1985; 155:289–293.

247. Kok-Jensen A, Lindeneg O: Pleurisy and fibrosis of the pleura during methysergide treatment of hemicrania. *Scand J Respir Dis* 1970; 51:218–222.

248. Kollins SA: Computed tomography of the pulmonary parenchyma and chest wall. *Radiol Clin North Am* 1977; 15:297–308.

249. Kovarik JL, Toll GD: Thoracic endometriosis with recurrent spontaneous pneumothorax. *JAMA* 1966; 196:595–597.

250. Kramer SS, Taylor GA, Garfinkel DJ, et al: Lethal chylothoraces due to superior vena caval thrombosis in infants. *AJR* 1981; 137:559–563.

251. Kshettry VR, Rebello R: Chylothorax after coronary artery bypass grafting. *Thorax* 1982; 37:954.

252. Kuehnel E: Massive pleural effusion secondary to CAPD. *Kidney Int* 1981; 19:152.

253. Kumar A, Pontoppidan H, Falke KJ, et al: Pulmonary barotrauma during mechanical ventilation. *Crit Care Med* 1973; 1:181–186.

254. Kurlander GJ, Helmen CH: Subpulmonary pneumothorax. *AJR* 1966; 96:1019–1021.

255. Kutty CPK: Cause of chylous pleural effusion. *Chest* 1980; 78:357–358.

256. Lacombe P, Cornud F, Grenier PH, et al: A new sign of right anterior pneumothorax in the supine adult. Three case reports. *Ann Radiol* 1982; 25:231–236.

257. Laforet EG, Kornitzer GD: Nephrogenic pleural effusion. *J Urol* 1977; 117:118–119.

258. Lahiry SK, Alkhafaji AH, Brown AL: Urinothorax following blunt trauma to the kidney. *J Trauma* 1978; 18:608–610.

259. Laing FC, Filly RA: Problems in the application of ultrasonography for the evaluation of pleural opacities. *Radiology* 1978; 126:211–214.

260. Lally JF, Gohel VK, Dalinka MK, et al: The roentgenographic manifestations of cutis laxa (generalized elastolysis). *Radiology* 1974; 113:605–606.

261. Lampson RS: Traumatic chylothorax. A review of the literature and report of a case treated by mediastinal ligation of the thoracic duct. *J Thorac Surg* 1948; 17:778–791.

262. Lams P: Radiographic signs in post-pneumonectomy bronchopleural fistula. *J Can Assoc Radiol* 1980; 31:178–180.

263. Lams PM, Jolles H: The scapula companion shadow. *Radiology* 1981; 138:19–23.

264. Lams PM, Jolles H: The effect of lobar collapse on the distribution of free intrapleural air. *Radiology* 1982; 142:309–312.

265. Lane EJ, Proto AV, Phillips TW: Mach bands and density perception. *Radiology* 1976; 121:9–17.

266. Lattes R, Shepard F, Tovell H, et al: A clinical and pathologic study of endometriosis of the lung. *Surg Gynecol Obstet* 1956; 103:552–558.

267. Laurens RG, Pine JR, Honig EG: Spontaneous

pneumothorax in primary cavitating lung carcinoma. *Radiology* 1983; 146:295–297.

268. Laws HL, Fox LS, Younger JB: Bilateral catamenial pneumothorax. *Arch Surg* 1977; 112:627–628.

269. Lawton F, Blackledge G, Johnson R: Co-existent chylous and serous pleural effusions associated with ovarian cancer: A case report of Contarinis syndrome. *Eur J Surg Oncol* 1985; 11:177–178.

270. Leckie WJH, Tothill P: Albumin turnover in pleural effusions. *Clin Sci* 1965; 29:339–352.

271. Legge DA, Tiede JJ, Peters GA, et al: Death from tension pneumothorax and chlorpromazine cardio-respiratory collapse as separate complications of asthma. *Ann Allergy* 1969; 27:23–29.

272. Leites V, Tannenbaum E: Familial spontaneous pneumothorax. *Am Rev Respir Dis* 1960; 82:240–241.

273. Lesser MB: Left azygos lobe. Report of a case. *Dis Chest* 1964; 46:95–96.

274. Leuallen EC, Carr DT: Pleural effusion. A statistical study of 436 patients. *N Engl J Med* 1955; 252:79–83.

275. Levin EJ, Bryk D: Dressler syndrome (postmyocardial infarction syndrome). *Radiology* 1966; 87:731–736.

276. Levitt RG, Sagel SS, Stanley RJ, et al: Accuracy of computed tomography of the liver and biliary tract. *Radiology* 1977; 124:123–128.

277. LeWitt PA, Calne DB: Pleuropulmonary changes during long-term bromocriptine treatment for Parkinson's disease. *Lancet* 1981; 1:44–45.

278. Liberson M: Diagnostic significance of the mediastinal profile in massive unilateral pleural effusions. *Am Rev Respir Dis* 1963; 88:176–180.

279. Libshitz HI, Banner MP: Spontaneous pneumothorax as a complication of radiation therapy to the thorax. *Radiology* 1974; 112:199–201.

280. Libshitz HI, Southard ME: Complications of radiation therapy: The thorax. *Semin Roentgenol* 1974; 9:41–49.

281. Lieberman FL, Hidemura R, Peters RL, et al: Pathogenesis and treatment of hydrothorax complicating cirrhosis with ascites. *Ann Intern Med* 1966; 64:341–351.

282. Lieberman FL, Peters RL: Cirrhotic hydrothorax. Further evidence that an acquired diaphragmatic defect is at fault. *Arch Intern Med* 1970; 125:114–117.

283. Liem K: Incidence and significance of heart muscle antibodies in patients with acute myocardial infarction and unstable angina. *Acta Med Scand* 1979; 206:473–475.

284. Light RW: *Pleural Diseases.* Philadelphia, Lea & Febiger, 1983.

285. Light RW: Exudative pleural effusions secondary to gastrointestinal diseases. *Clin Chest Med* 1985; 6:103–111.

286. Light RW, George RB: Incidence and significance of pleural effusion after abdominal surgery. *Chest* 1976; 69:621–625.

287. Lillard RL, Allen RP: The extrapleural air sign in pneumomediastinum. *Radiology* 1965; 85:1093–1098.

288. Lillington GA, Mitchell SP, Wood GA: Catamenial pneumothorax. *JAMA* 1972; 219:1328–1332.

289. Lipscomb DJ, Flower CDR, Hadfield JW: Ultrasound of the pleura: An assessment of its clinical value. *Clin Radiol* 1981; 32:289–290.

290. Lipton RA, Greenwald RA, Seriff NS: Pneumothorax and bilateral honeycombed lung in Marfan syndrome. Report of a case and review of the pulmonary abnormalities in this disorder. *Am Rev Respir Dis* 1971; 104:924–928.

291. Llach F, Arieff AI, Massry SG: Renal vein thrombosis and nephrotic syndrome. A prospective study of 36 adult patients. *Ann Intern Med* 1975; 83:8–14.

292. Logue RB, Rogers JV, Gay BB: Subtle roentgenographic signs of left heart failure. *Am Heart J* 1963; 65:464–473.

293. Lorentz WB: Acute hydrothorax during peritoneal dialysis. *J Pediatr* 1979; 94:417–419.

294. Lote K, Dahl O, Vigander T: Pneumothorax during combination chemotherapy. *Cancer* 1981; 47:1743–1745.

295. Louie S, McGahan JP, Frey C, et al: Pancreatic pleuropericardial effusions. Fistulous tracts demonstrated by computed tomography. *Arch Intern Med* 1985; 145:1231–1234.

296. Lowe SH, Cosgrove DO, Joseph AEA: Inversion of the right hemidiaphragm shown on ultrasound examination. *Br J Radiol* 1981; 54:754–757.

297. Lowell JR: *Pleural Effusions. A Comprehensive Review.* Baltimore, University Park Press, 1977.

298. Lowman RM, Hoogerhyde J, Waters LL, et al: Traumatic chylothorax. The roentgen aspects of this problem. *AJR* 1951; 65:529–546.

299. Lundin P, Simonsson B, Winberg T: Pneumonopleural amyloid tumour. *Acta Radiol* 1961; 55:139–144.

300. MacEwan DW, Dunbar JS, Smith RD, et al: Pneumothorax in young infants—recognition and evaluation. *J Can Assoc Radiol* 1971; 22:264–269.

301. MacFarlane JR, Holman CW: Chylothorax. *Am Rev Respir Dis* 1972; 105:287–291.

302. Maffessanti M, Tommasi M, Pellegrini P: Computed tomography of free pleural effusions. *Eur J Radiol* 1987; 7:87–90.

303. Mahafan VK, Simon M, Huber GL: Re-expansion pulmonary edema. *Chest* 1979; 75:192–194.

304. Maher GG, Berger HW: Massive pleural effusion. Malignant and nonmalignant causes in 46 patients. *Am Rev Respir Dis* 1972; 105:458–460.

305. Majzlin G, Stevens FL: Meigs' syndrome. Case report and review of literature. *J Int Coll Surg* 1964; 42:625–630.

306. Malave G, Foster ED, Wilson JA, et al: Bronchopleural fistula—present-day study of an old problem. *Ann Thorac Surg* 1971; 11:1–10.

307. Maloney JV, Spencer FC: The nonoperative treatment of traumatic chylothorax. *Surgery* 1956; 40:121–128.

308. Mamtora H, Cope V: Pulmonary opacities in pseudoxanthoma elasticum: Report of two cases. *Br J Radiol* 1981; 54:65–67.

309. Mancini JL: Familial paroxysmal polyserositis, phenotype I (familial Mediterranean fever). *Am Rev Respir Dis* 1973; 107:461–463.

310. Mandell GA, Pizzica AL: Air in the inferior accessory fissure of a neonate. *J Can Assoc Radiol* 1981; 32:249–250.

311. Marks BW, Kuhns LR: Identification of the pleural fissures with computed tomography. *Radiology* 1982; 143:139–141.

312. Marks PA, Roof BS: Pericardial effusion associated with myxedema. *Ann Intern Med* 1953; 39:230–240.

313. Marks WM, Filly RA, Callen PW: Real-time evaluation of pleural lesions: New observations regarding the probability of obtaining free fluid. *Radiology* 1982; 142:163–164.

314. Marsac JH, Huchon GJ, Bismuth V: Pleural chylous effusion in Chretien J, Bignon J, Hirsch A (eds): *The Pleura in Health and Disease.* New York, Marcel Dekker, 1985.

315. Marshall AJ, Eltringham WK, Barritt DW, et al: Respiratory disease associated with practolol therapy. *Lancet* 1977; 2:1254–1257.

316. Maurer ER, Schaal JA, Mendez FL: Chronic recurring spontaneous pneumothorax due to endometriosis of the diaphragm. *JAMA* 1958; 168:2013–2014.

317. Maxwell E, Esterly NB: Cutis laxa. *Am J Dis Child* 1969; 117:479–482.

318. Mayo P: Recurrent spontaneous pneumothorax concomitant with menstruation. *J Thorac Cardiovasc Surg* 1963; 46:415–416.

319. McFadden ER, Luparello F: Bronchopleural fistula complicating massive pulmonary infarction. *Thorax* 1969; 24:500–505.

320. McKay DG, Sparling HJ, Robbins SL: Cirrhosis of the liver with massive hydrothorax. *Arch Intern Med* 1947; 79:501–509.

321. McKenna JM, Chandrasekhar AJ, Skorton D, et al: The pleuropulmonary complications of pancreatitis. *Chest* 1977; 71:197–204.

322. McLoud TC, Barash PG, Ravin CE: PEEP: Radiographic features and associated complications. *AJR* 1977; 129:209–213.

323. McLoud TC, Isler R, Head J: The radiologic appearance of chemical pleurodesis. *Radiology* 1980; 135:313–317.

324. McLoud TC, Isler RJ, Novelline RA, et al: The apical cap, review. *AJR* 1981; 137:299–306.

325. McPeak EM, Levine SA: The preponderance of right hydrothorax in congestive heart failure. *Ann Intern Med* 1946; 25:916–927.

326. Meade RH, Head JR, Moen CW: The management of chylothorax. *J Thorac Surg* 1950; 19:709–723.

327. Medlar EM: Variations in interlobar fissures. *AJR* 1947; 57:723–725.

328. Meigs JV: Fibroma of the ovary with ascites and hydrothorax—Meigs' syndrome. *Am J Obstet Gynecol* 1954; 67:962–987.

329. Meigs JV: Pelvic tumours other than fibromas of the ovary with ascites and hydrothorax. *Obstet Gynecol* 1954; 3:471–485.

330. Meigs JV, Armstrong SH, Hamilton HH: A further contribution to the syndrome of fibroma of the ovary with fluid in the abdomen and chest, Meigs' syndrome. *Am J Obstet Gynecol* 1943; 46:19–37.

331. Meigs JV, Cass JW: Fibroma of the ovary with ascites and hydrothorax. With a report of seven cases. *Am J Obstet Gynecol* 1937; 33:249–267.

332. Meine F, Grossman H, Forman W, et al: The radiographic findings in congenital cutis laxa. *Radiology* 1974; 113:687–690.

333. Mellins RB, Levine OR, Fishman AP: Effect of systemic and pulmonary venous hypertension on pleural and pericardial fluid accumulation. *J Appl Physiol* 1970; 29:564–569.

334. Melton LJ, Hepper NGG, Offord KP: Incidence of spontaneous pneumothorax in Olmsted County, Minnesota: 1950–1974. *Am Rev Respir Dis* 1979; 120:1379–1382.

335. Melton LJ, Hepper NGG, Offord KP: Influence of height on the risk of spontaneous pneumothorax. *Mayo Clin Proc* 1981; 56:678–682.

336. Merten DF, Rooney R: Progressive pulmonary emphysema associated with congenital generalized elastolysis (cutis laxa). *Radiology* 1974; 113:691–692.

337. Meyerhoff J: Familial Mediterranean fever: Report of a large family, review of the literature, and discussion of the frequency of amyloidosis. *Medicine* 1980; 59:66–77.

338. Millard CE: Massive hemothorax complicating heparin therapy for pulmonary infarction. *Chest* 1971; 59:235–237.

339. Miller WC, Toon R, Palat H, et al: Experimental pulmonary edema following re-expansion of pneumothorax. *Am Rev Respir Dis* 1973; 108:664–666.

340. Miller WT, Talman EA: Subphrenic abscess. *AJR* 1967; 101:961–969.

341. Millward SF, Breatnach E, Simpkins KC, et al: Do plain films of the chest and abdomen have a role in the diagnosis of acute pancreatitis? *Clin Radiol* 1983; 34:133–137.

342. Milner LB, Ryan K, Gullo J: Fatal intrathoracic hemorrhage after percutaneous aspiration lung biopsy. *AJR* 1979; 132:280–281.

343. Mine H, Tamura K, Tanegashima K, et al: Nontraumatic chylothorax associated with diffuse lymphatic dysplasia. *Lymphology* 1984; 17:111–112.

344. Mintzer RA, Hendrix RW, Johnson CS, et al: The radiologic significance of the left pulmonary ligament. *Chest* 1979; 76:401–405.

345. Miridjanian A, Ambruoso VN, Derby BM, et al: Massive bilateral hemorrhagic pleural effusions in chronic relapsing pancreatitis. *Arch Surg* 1969; 98:62–66.

346. Mirouze D, Juttner H-U, Reynolds TB: Left pleural effusion in patients with chronic liver disease and ascites. Prospective study of 22 cases. *Dig Dis Sci* 1981; 26:984–988.

347. Mobbs GA, Pfanner DW: Endometriosis of the lung. *Lancet* 1963; 1:472–474.

348. Mokrohisky JF: So-called "Meigs syndrome" associated with benign and malignant ovarian tumors. *Radiology* 1958; 70:578–581.

349. Moller A: Pleural effusion. Use of the semi-supine position for radiographic detection. *Radiology* 1984; 150:245–249.

350. Moncada R, Williams V, Fareed J, et al: Thoracic splenosis. *AJR* 1985; 144:705–706.

351. Morrow CS, Kantor M, Armen RN: Hepatic hydrothorax. *Ann Intern Med* 1958; 49:193–203.

352. Moses DC, Silver TM, Bookstein JJ: The complementary roles of chest radiography, lung scanning, and selective pulmonary angiography in the diagnosis of pulmonary embolism. *Circulation* 1974; 49:179–188.

353. Moskowitz H, Platt RT, Schachar R, et al: Roentgen visualization of minute pleural effusion. An experimental study to determine the minimum amount of pleural fluid visible on a radiograph. *Radiology* 1973; 109:33–35.

354. Moskowitz PS, Griscom NT: The medial pneumothorax. *Radiology* 1976; 120:143–147.

355. Motoyoshi K, Momoi H, Mikomi R, et al: Pulmonary lesions seen in a family with marfanoid hypermobility syndrome. *Jpn J Thorac Dis* 1973; 11:138–143.

356. Muller NL, Nelems B: Postcoital catamenial pneumothorax. *Am Rev Respir Dis* 1986; 134:803–804.

357. Muller R, Lofstedt S: The reaction of the pleura in primary tuberculosis of the lungs. *Acta Med Scand* 1945; 122:105–133.

358. Mulvey RB: The effect of pleural fluid on the diaphragm. *AJR* 1965; 84:1080–1085.

359. Murdoch JL, Walker BA, Halpern BL, et al: Life expectancy and causes of death in the Marfan syndrome. *N Engl J Med* 1972; 286:804–808.

360. Murphy D, Duncan JG, Imrie CW: The "negative chest radiograph" in acute pancreatitis. *Br J Radiol* 1977; 50:264–265.

361. Naidich DP, Megibow AJ, Hilton S, et al: Computed tomography of the diaphragm: Peridiaphragmatic fluid localization. *J Comput Assist Tomogr* 1983; 7:641–649.

362. Nassberger L: Left-sided pleural effusion secondary to continuous ambulatory peritoneal dialysis. *Acta Med Scand* 1982; 211:219–220.

363. Nayak IN, Lawrence D: Tension pneumothorax from a perforated gastric ulcer. *Br J Surg* 1976; 63:245–247.

364. Neff CC, Mueller PR, Ferrucci JT, et al: Serious complications following transgression of the pleural space in drainage procedures. *Radiology* 1984; 152:335–341.

365. Nelson SW: Large pneumothorax and associated massive collapse of the homolateral lung due to intrabronchial obstruction: A case report. *Radiology* 1957; 68:411–414.

366. Newlin N, Silver TM, Stuck KJ, et al: Ultrasonic features of pyogenic liver abscess. *Radiology* 1981; 139:155–159.

367. Neyazaki T, Kupic EA, Marshall WH, et al: Collateral lymphatico-venous communication after experimental obstruction of the thoracic duct. *Radiology* 1965; 85:423–432.

368. Nichols DM, Cooperberg PL, Golding RH, et al: The safe intercostal approach? Pleural complications in abdominal interventional radiology. *AJR* 1984; 142:1013–1018.

369. Nidus BD, Matalon R, Cantacuzino D, et al: Uremic pleuritis—a clinicopathological entity. *N Engl J Med* 1969; 281:255–256.

370. Nightingale RC, Flower CDR: Encysted pneumothorax, a complication of asthma. *Br J Dis Chest* 1984; 78:98–100.

371. Nordkild P, Kromann-Andersen H, Struve-Christensen E: Yellow nail syndrome—the triad of yellow nails, lymphedema and pleural effusions. *Acta Med Scand* 1986; 219:221–227.

372. Norris RM, Jones JG, Bishop JM: Respiratory gas exchange in patients with spontaneous pneumothorax. *Thorax* 1968; 23:427–433.

373. Northfield TC: Oxygen therapy for spontaneous pneumothorax. *Br Med J* 1971; 4:86–88.

374. Nugent FW, Burns JR: Periodic disease. *Med Clin North Am* 1966; 50:371–378.

375. Nusbaum M, Baum S, Hedges RC, et al: Roentgenographic and direct visualization of thoracic duct. *Arch Surg* 1964; 88:105–113.

376. Nusser RA, Culhane RH: Roentgenogram of the month. Recurrent transudative effusion with an abdominal mass. *Chest* 1986; 90:263–264.

377. Oestreich AE, Haley C: Pleural effusion: The thorn sign. *Chest* 1981; 79:365–366.

378. O'Flanagan SJ, Tighe BE, Egan TJ, et al: Meigs' syndrome and pseudo-Meigs' syndrome. *J R Soc Med* 1987; 80:252–253.

379. O'Gorman LD, Cottingham RA, Sargent EN, et al: Mediastinal emphysema in the newborn: A review and description of the new extra pleural gas sign. *Dis Chest* 1968; 53:301–308.

380. Okuda T, Tanikawa K, Shimokawa Y: Hydrothorax complicating ascites. *Jpn Med J* 1967; 2261:15–21.

381. O'Meara JB, Slade PR: Disappearance of fluid from the post-pneumonectomy space. *J Thorac Cardiovasc Surg* 1974; 67:621–628.

382. Omell GH, Anderson LS, Bramson RT: Chest wall tumors. *Radiol Clin North Am* 1973; 11:197–214.

383. O'Neill S, Sweeney J, Walker F, et al: Pneumothorax in the Ehlers-Danlos syndrome. *Ir J Med Sci* 1981; 150:43–44.

384. Onik G, Goodman PC, Webb WR, et al: Hydro-pneumothorax: Detection on supine radiographs. *Radiology* 1984; 152:31–34.

385. Orwoll ES, Kiessling PJ, Patterson JR: Interstitial pneumonia from mitomycin. *Ann Intern Med* 1978; 89:352–355.

386. Page RL: Pleural thickening—oxprenolol exonerated. *Br J Dis Chest* 1979; 73:319.

387. Pantoja E, Kattan KR, Thomas HA: Some uncommon lower mediastinal densities: A pictorial essay. *Radiol Clin North Am* 1984; 22:633–646.

388. Pascual RS, Mosher MB, Sikand RS, et al: Effects of bleomycin on pulmonary function in man. *Am Rev Respir Dis* 1973; 108:211–217.

389. Patrick JH: Massive osteolysis complicated by chylothorax successfully treated by pleurodesis. *J Bone Joint Surg* [Br] 1976; 58B:347–349.

390. Pavlin J, Cheney FW: Unilateral pulmonary edema in rabbits after re-expansion of collapsed lung. *J Appl Physiol* 1979; 46:31–35.

391. Perez CA, Presant CA, Van Amburg AL: Management of superior vena cava syndrome. *Semin Oncol* 1978; 5:123–143.

392. Peterman TA, Brothers SK: Pleural effusions in congestive heart failure and in pericardial disease. *N Engl J Med* 1983; 309:313.

393. Peters ME, Gould HR, McCarthy TM: Identification of a bronchopleural fistula by computerized tomography—a case report. *J Comput Tomogr* 1983; 7:267–270.

394. Petersen JA: Recognition of infrapulmonary pleural effusion. *Radiology* 1960; 74:34–41.

395. Petusevsky ML, Faling LJ, Rocklin RE, et al: Pleuro-pericardial reaction to treatment with dantrolene. *JAMA* 1979; 242:2772–2774.

396. Phillips LG, Cunningham J: Esophageal perforation. *Radiol Clin North Am* 1984; 22:607–613.

397. Plowman PN, Stableforth DE, Citron KM: Spontaneous pneumothorax in Hodgkin's disease. *Br J Dis Chest* 1980; 74:411–414.

398. Polsky MS, Weber CH, Ball TP: Infected pyelocaliceal diverticulum and sympathetic pleural effusion. *J Urol* 1975; 114:301–303.

399. Postmus PE, Kerstjens JM, Breed A, et al: A family with lobus venae azygos. *Chest* 1986; 90:298–299.

400. Proto AV, Ball JB: Computed tomography of the major and minor fissures. *AJR* 1983; 140:439–448.

401. Proto AV, Ball JB: The superolateral major fissures. *AJR* 1983; 140:431–437.

402. Proto AV, Merhar GL: Central bronchial displacement with large posterior pleural collections. Findings on the lateral chest radiograph and CT scans. *J Can Assoc Radiol* 1984; 35:128–132.

403. Proto AV, Rost RC: CT of the thorax: Pitfalls in interpretation. *RadioGraphics* 1985; 5:693–812.

404. Proto AV, Speckman JM: The left lateral radiograph of the chest. *Med Radiogr Photogr* 1979; 55:30–74.

405. Pugatch RD, Faling LJ, Robbins AH, et al: Differentiation of pleural and pulmonary lesions using computed tomography. *J Comput Assist Tomogr* 1978; 2:601–606.

406. Pugatch RD, Spirn PW: Radiology of the pleura. *Clin Chest Med* 1985; 6:17–32.

407. Pyeritz RE: Cardiovascular manifestations of heritable disorders of connective tissue, in Steinberg AG, Bearn AG, Motulsky AG, et al (eds): *Progress in Medical Genetics* (new series). Philadelphia, WB Saunders Co, 1983, vol 5.

408. Pyeritz RE, McKusick VA: The Marfan syndrome: Diagnosis and management. *N Engl J Med* 1979; 300:772–777.

409. Qureshi MM, Roble DC, Gindin A, et al: Subarachnoid-pleural fistula. *J Thorac Cardiovasc Surg* 1986; 91:238–241.

410. Raasch BN, Carsky EW, Lane EJ, et al: Pictorial essay. Pleural effusion: Explanation of some typical appearances. *AJR* 1982; 139:899–904.

411. Raasch BN, Carsky EW, Lane EJ, et al: Radiographic anatomy of the interlobar fissures. *AJR* 1982; 138:1043–1049.

412. Rabin CB, Blackman NS: Bilateral pleural effusion. Its significance in association with a heart of normal size. *Mt Sinai J Med (NY)* 1957; 24:45–53.

413. Rabinowitz JG, Cohen BA, Mendleson DS: The pulmonary ligament. *Radiol Clin North Am* 1984; 22:659–672.

414. Rabinowitz JG, Wolf BS: Roentgen significance of the pulmonary ligament. *Radiology* 1966; 87:1013–1020.

415. Race GA, Scheifley CH, Edwards JE: Hydrothorax in congestive heart failure. *Am J Med* 1957; 22:83–89.

416. Rakita L, Sobol SM, Mostow N, et al: Amiodarone pulmonary toxicity. *Am Heart J* 1983; 106:906–916.

417. Ralston MD, Wilkinson RH: Bilateral urinothorax identified by technetium-99m DPTA renal imaging. *J Nucl Med* 1986; 27:56–59.

418. Rasaretnam R, Chanmugam D, Sivathasan C: Spontaneous haemothorax in a mild haemophiliac. *Thorax* 1976; 31:601–604.

419. Rashid A, Sendi A, Al-Kadhimi A, et al: Concurrent spontaneous pneumothorax in identical twins. *Thorax* 1986; 41:971.

420. Ravin CE, Smith GW, Lester PD, et al: Post-traumatic pneumatocele in the inferior pulmonary ligament. *Radiology* 1976; 121:39–41.

421. Rawson AJ, Cocke JA: Infarction of an entire pulmonary lobe with subsequent aseptic softening causing sterile hemopneumothorax. *Am J Med Sci* 1947; 214:520–524.

422. Rea D: Traumatic chylothorax in a closed chest in-

jury. Report of a case. *Br J Dis Chest* 1960; 54:
82–85.

423. Rebuck AS: Radiological aspects of severe asthma. *Australas Radiol* 1970; 14:264–268.

424. Redman JF, Arnold WC, Smith PL, et al: Hypertension and urino-thorax following an attempted percutaneous nephrostomy. *J Urol* 1982; 128: 1307–1308.

425. Reilly KM, Tsou E: Bilateral chylothorax: A case report following episodes of stretching. *JAMA* 1975; 233:536–537.

426. Remy J, Mabille JP: La coiffe pleurale de le lésions parietales. Un nouveau signe du syndrome extrapleural. *Ann Radiol* 1977; 20:161–164.

427. Renner RR, Makarian B, Pernice NJ, et al: The apical cap. *Radiology* 1974; 110:569–573.

428. Renner RR, Pernice NJ: The apical cap. *Semin Roentgenol* 1977; 12:299–302.

429. Reynolds J, Davis JT: Injuries of the chest wall, pleura, pericardium, lungs, bronchi and esophagus. *Radiol Clin North Am* 1966; 4:383–401.

430. Rhea JT, DeLuca SA, Greene RE: Determining the size of pneumothorax in the upright patient. *Radiology* 1982; 144:733–736.

431. Rhea JT, vanSonnenberg E, McLoud TC: Basilar pneumothorax in the supine adult. *Radiology* 1979; 133:593–595.

432. Rigby M, Zylak CJ, Wood LDH: The effect of lobar atelectasis on pleural fluid distribution in dogs. *Radiology* 1980; 136:603–607.

433. Rigler LG, Ericksen LG: The inferior accessory lobe of the lung. *AJR* 1933; 29:384–392.

434. Rinne UK: Pleuropulmonary changes during long-term bromocriptine treatment for Parkinson's disease. *Lancet* 1981; 1:44.

435. Robins SA, Joress MH: Intrapleural fibrin bodies. *Am Rev Tuberc* 1938; 37:81–87.

436. Robitaille GA: Ehlers-Danlos syndrome and recurrent hemoptysis. *Ann Intern Med* 1964; 61:716–721.

437. Rodelas R, Rakowski TA, Argy WP, et al: Fibrosing uremic pleuritis during hemodialysis. *JAMA* 1980; 243:2424–2425.

438. Rodman MH, Jones CW: Catamenial hemoptysis due to bronchial endometriosis. *New Engl J Med* 1962; 266:805–808.

439. Rodriguez E, Martinez J, Javaloyas M, et al: Haemothorax in the course of chickenpox. *Thorax* 1986; 41:491.

440. Rogers CI, Meredith HC: Osler revisited: An unusual cause of inversion of the diaphragm. *Radiology* 1977; 125:596.

441. Rohlfing BM, Webb WR, Schlobohm RM: Ventilator-related extra-alveolar air in adults. *Radiology* 1976; 121:25–31.

442. Roseman DM, Kowlessar OD, Sleisenger MH: Pulmonary manifestations of pancreatitis. *N Engl J Med* 1960; 263:294–296.

443. Rosenberg ER: Ultrasound in the assessment of pleural densities. *Chest* 1983; 84:283–285.

444. Rosenberg RF, Rubinstein BM, Messinger NH: Intrathoracic lipomas. *Chest* 1971; 60:507–509.

445. Rosenberg SM, Riddick DH: Successful treatment of catamenial hemoptysis with danazol. *Obstet Gynecol* 1981; 57:130–131.

446. Rosenberger A, Abrams HL: Radiology of the thoracic duct. *AJR* 1971; 111:807–820.

447. Ross J, Farber JE: Right sided spontaneous pneumothorax complicating therapeutic pneumoperitoneum. *Am Rev Tuberc* 1951; 63:67–75.

448. Ross JK: A review of the surgery of the thoracic duct. *Thorax* 1961; 16:12–21.

449. Rossi NP, Goplerud CP: Recurrent catamenial pneumothorax. *Arch Surg* 1974; 109:173–176.

450. Rost RC, Proto AV: Inferior pulmonary ligament: Computed tomographic appearance. *Radiology* 1983; 148:479–483.

451. Rowinsky EK, Abeloff MD, Wharam MD: Spontaneous pneumothorax following thoracic irradiation. *Chest* 1985; 88:703–708.

452. Roy PH, Carr DT, Payne WS: The problem of chylothorax. *Mayo Clin Proc* 1967; 42:457–467.

453. Rubin RH, Swartz MN, Malt R: Hepatic abscess: Changes in clinical, bacteriologic and therapeutic aspects. *Am J Med* 1974; 57:601–610.

454. Ruckley CV, McCormack RJM: The management of spontaneous pneumothorax. *Thorax* 1966; 21:139–144.

455. Rudikoff JC: Early detection of pleural fluid. *Chest* 1980; 77:109–111.

456. Rudikoff JC: The pulmonary ligament and subpulmonic effusion. *Chest* 1981; 80:505–507.

457. Rudnick MR, Coyle JF, Beck LH, et al: Acute massive hydrothorax complicating peritoneal dialysis, report of two cases and a review of the literature. *Clin Nephrol* 1979; 12:38–44.

458. Runyon BA, Forker EL, Sopko JA: Pleural-fluid kinetics in a patient with primary lymphedema, pleural effusions, and yellow nails. *Am Rev Respir Dis* 1979; 119:821–825.

459. Ruskin JA, Gurney JW, Thorsen MK, et al: Detection of pleural effusions on supine chest radiographs. *AJR* 1987; 148:681–683.

460. Rutherford RB, Hurt HH, Brickman RD, et al: The pathophysiology of progressive tension pneumothorax. *J Trauma* 1968; 8:212–227.

461. Ryan CJ, Rodgers RF, Unni KK, et al: The outcome of patients with pleural effusion of indeterminate cause at thoracotomy. *Mayo Clin Proc* 1981; 56:145–149.

462. Sahn SA: Immunologic diseases of the pleura. *Clin Chest Med* 1985; 6:83–102.

463. Sahn SA, Miller KS: Obscure pleural effusion. Look to the kidney. *Chest* 1986; 90:631.

464. Salcedo JR: Urinothorax: Report of 4 cases and review of the literature. *J Urol* 1986; 135:805–808.

465. Salmon VJ: Benign pelvic tumours associated with ascites and pleural effusion. *J Mt Sinai Hosp* 1934; 1:169–172.

466. Samman PD, White WF: The "yellow nail" syndrome. *Br J Dermatol* 1964; 76:153–157.

467. Sanders RC: Post-operative pleural effusion and subphrenic abscess. *Clin Radiol* 1970; 21:308–312.

468. Sargent EN, Boswell WD, Ralls PW, et al: Subpleural fat pads in patients exposed to asbestos: Distinction from non-calcified pleural plaques. *Radiology* 1984; 152:273–277.

469. Sargent EN, Jacobson G, Gordonson JS: Pleural plaques: A signpost of asbestos dust inhalation. *Semin Roentgenol* 1977; 12:287–297.

470. Sassoon CS, Light RW: Chylothorax and pseudochylothorax. *Clin Chest Med* 1985; 6:163–171.

471. Sautter RD, Dreber WH, MacIndoe JH, et al: Fatal pulmonary edema and pneumonitis after reexpansion of chronic pneumothorax. *Chest* 1971; 60:399–401.

472. Scales FE, Lee ME: Nonoperative diagnosis of intrathoracic splenosis. *AJR* 1983; 141:1273–1274.

473. Scanlon TS, Benumof JL: Demonstration of interlobar collateral ventilation. *J Appl Physiol* 1979; 46:658–661.

474. Scattini CM, Orsi A: Multiple bilateral fibromas of the pleura. *Thorax* 1973; 28:782–787.

475. Schenker JG, Weinstein D: Ovarian hyperstimulation syndrome: A current survey. *Fertil Steril* 1978; 30:255–268.

476. Schmidt A: Chylothorax. Review of 5 years' cases in the literature and report of a case. *Acta Chir Scand* 1959; 118:5–12.

477. Schmitt WGH, Hubener KH, Rucker HC: Pleural calcification with persistent effusion. *Radiology* 1983; 149:633–638.

478. Schneierson SJ, Katz M: Solitary pleural effusion due to myxedema. *JAMA* 1958; 168:1003–1005.

479. Schulman A, Fataar S, Dalrymple R, et al: The lymphographic anatomy of chylothorax. *Br J Radiol* 1978; 51:420–427.

480. Schwarz MI, Marmorstein BL: A new radiologic sign of subpulmonic effusion. *Chest* 1975; 67:176–178.

481. Seibert JJ, Golladay ES, Keller C: Chylothorax secondary to superior vena caval obstruction. *Pediatr Radiol* 1982; 12:252–254.

482. Seriff NS, Cohen ML, Samuel P, et al: Chylothorax: Diagnosis by lipoprotein electrophoresis of serum and pleural fluid. *Thorax* 1977; 32:98–100.

483. Sewell RW, Fewel JG, Grover FL, et al: Experimental evaluation of reexpansion pulmonary edema. *Ann Thorac Surg* 1978; 26:126–132.

484. Shapir J, Lisbona A, Palayew MJ: Chronic calcified empyema. *J Can Assoc Radiol* 1981; 31:24–27.

485. Sharpe IK, Ahmad M, Braun W: Familial spontaneous pneumothorax and HLA antigens. *Chest* 1980; 78:264–268.

486. Shaw TJ, Caterine JM: Recurrent re-expansion pulmonary edema. *Chest* 1984; 86:784–786.

487. Shearin RPN, Hepper NGG, Payne WS: Recurrent spontaneous pneumothorax concurrent with menses. *Mayo Clin Proc* 1974; 49:98–101.

488. Sherman NJ, Davis JR, Jesseph JE: Subphrenic abscess: A continuing hazard. *Am J Surg* 1969; 117:117–123.

489. Sherman S, Ravikrishran KP: Unilateral pulmonary edema following reexpansion of pneumothorax of brief duration. *Chest* 1980; 77:714.

490. Short DS: A radiological study of pulmonary infarction. *Q J Med* 1951; 20:233–245.

491. Shuman LS, Libshitz HI: Solid pleural manifestations of lymphoma. *AJR* 1984; 142:269–273.

492. Siegal S: Familial paroxysmal polyserositis. Analysis of fifty cases. *Am J Med* 1964; 36:893–918.

493. Siegel MJ, McAlister WH: Unusual intrathoracic complications in Wilms tumor. *AJR* 1980; 134:1231–1234.

494. Simon HB, Daggett WM, DeSanctis RW: Hemothorax as a complication of anticoagulant therapy in the presence of pulmonary infarction. *JAMA* 1969; 208:1830–1834.

495. Singh A, Sethi RS, Singh G: Pneumothorax: An unusual complication of teratoma chest. *Chest* 1973; 63:1034–1036.

496. Slasky BS, Deutsch M: Germ cell tumors complicated by pneumothorax. *Urology* 1983; 22:39–42.

497. Slasky BS, Siewers RD, Lecky JW, et al: Catamenial pneumothorax: The roles of diaphragmatic defects and endometriosis. *AJR* 1982; 138:639–643.

498. Slind RO, Rodarte JR: Spontaneous hemothorax in an otherwise healthy young man. *Chest* 1974; 66:81.

499. Smalley RV, Wall RL: Two cases of busulfan toxicity. *Ann Intern Med* 1966; 64:154–164.

500. Smith CN: Induced pneumoperitoneum: A fatal case. *Br Med J* 1943; 2:404.

501. Smith J, Alberts C, Balk AG: Pneumothorax in the Ehlers-Danlos syndrome. Consequences or coincidence? *Scand J Respir Dis* 1978; 59:239–242.

502. Soderberg CH, Dahlquist EH: Catamenial pneumothorax. *Surgery* 1976; 79:236–239.

503. Sohar E, Gafni J, Pras M, et al: Familial Mediterranean fever. *Am J Med* 1967; 43:227–253.

504. Solal-Celigny P, Cormier Y, Fournier M: The yellow nail syndrome. *Arch Pathol Lab Med* 1983; 107:183–185.

505. Solomon S, Farber SJ, Caruso LJ: Fibromyomata of the uterus with hemothorax—Meig's syndrome? *Arch Intern Med* 1971; 127:307–309.

506. Soulen RL, Freeman E: Radiologic evaluation of myocardial infarction. *Radiol Clin North Am* 1971; 9:567–582.

507. Spear BS, Sully L, Lewis CT: Pulmonary arteriovenous fistula presenting as spontaneous haemothorax. *Thorax* 1975; 30:355–356.

508. Speckman JM, Gamsu G, Webb WR: Alterations in CT mediastinal anatomy produced by an azygos lobe. *AJR* 1981; 137:47–50.

509. Spittle MF, Heal J, Harmer C, et al: The association of spontaneous pneumothorax with pulmonary me-

tastases in bone tumours of children. *Clin Radiol* 1968; 19:400–403.

510. Spizarny DL, Goodman LR: Air in the minor fissure: A sign of right-sided pneumothorax. *Radiology* 1986; 160:329–331.

511. Sprung CL, Loewenherz JW, Baier H, et al: Evidence of increased permeability in reexpansion pulmonary edema. *Am J Med* 1981; 71:497–500.

512. Staats BA, Ellefson RD, Budahn LL, et al: Lipoprotein profile of chylous and nonchylous pleural effusions. *Mayo Clin Proc* 1980; 55:700–704.

513. Stark DD, Shanes JG, Baron RL, et al: Biochemical features of urinothorax. *Arch Intern Med* 1982; 142:1509–1511.

514. Steckel RJ: Unilateral pulmonary edema after pneumothorax. *N Engl J Med* 1973; 289:621–622.

515. Steier M, Ching N, Roberts EB, et al: Pneumothorax complicating continuous ventilatory support. *J Thorac Cardiovasc Surg* 1974; 67:17–23.

516. Stein GN, Chen JT, Goldstein F, et al: The importance of chest roentgenography in the diagnosis of pulmonary embolism. *AJR* 1959; 81:255–263.

517. Steiner GM, Farman J, Lawson JP: Lymphangiomatosis of bone. *Radiology* 1969; 93:1093–1098.

518. Steinhauslin CA, Cuttat JF: Spontaneous pneumothorax. A complication of lung cancer. *Chest* 1985; 88:709–713.

519. Stelzner TJ, King TE, Antony VB, et al: The pleuropulmonary manifestations of the postcardiac injury syndrome. *Chest* 1983; 84:383–387.

520. Stern H, Toole AL, Merino M: Catamenial pneumothorax. *Chest* 1980; 78:480–482.

521. Stewart CA, Linner HP: Chylothorax in the newborn infant. *Am J Dis Child* 1926; 31:654–656.

522. Stewart PB: The rate of formation and lymphatic removal of fluid in pleural effusions. *J Clin Invest* 1963; 42:258–262.

523. Storey DD, Dines DE, Coles DT: Pleural effusion. A diagnostic dilemma. *JAMA* 1976; 236:2183–2186.

524. Stranahan A, Alley RD, Kausel HW, et al: Operative thoracic ductography. *J Thorac Surg* 1956; 31:183–198.

525. Subramanyam BR, Raghavendra BN, Lefleur RS: Sonography of the inverted right hemidiaphragm. *AJR* 1981; 136:1004–1006.

526. Sugiyama Y, Maeda H, Yotsumoto H, et al: Short reports. Familial spontaneous pneumothorax. *Thorax* 1986; 41:969–970.

527. Sulis E, Floris C: Haemothorax due to thoracic extramedullary erythropoiesis in thalassaemia intermedia. *Br Med J* 1985; 291:1094.

528. Swingle JD, Logan R, Juhl JH: Inversion of the left hemidiaphragm. *JAMA* 1969; 208:863–864.

529. Szabo G, Magyar Z: Effect of increased systemic venous pressure on lymph pressure and flow. *Am J Physiol* 1967; 212:1469–1474.

530. Taal BG, Spierings ELH, Hilvering C: Pleuropulmonary fibrosis associated with chronic and excessive intake of ergotamine. *Thorax* 1983; 38:396–398.

531. Tabatznik B, Isaacs JP: Postpericardiotomy syndrome following traumatic hemopericardium. *Am J Cardiol* 1961; 7:83–96.

532. Talbot S, Worthington BS, Roebuck EJ: Radiographic signs of pulmonary embolism and pulmonary infarction. *Thorax* 1973; 28:198–203.

533. Ten Eyck EA: Subpleural lipoma. *Radiology* 1960; 74:295–297.

534. Teoh PC: Bronchiectasis and spontaneous pneumothorax in Marfan's syndrome. *Chest* 1977; 72:672–673.

535. Teplick JG, Teplick SK, Goodman L, et al: The interface sign: A computed tomographic sign for distinguishing pleural and intra-abdominal fluid. *Radiology* 1982; 144:359–362.

536. Theros EG, Feigin DS: Pleural tumors and pulmonary tumors: Differential diagnosis. *Semin Roentgenol* 1977; 12:239–247.

537. Thorne PS: Traumatic chylothorax. *Tubercle* 1958; 39:29–34.

538. Thurer RJ: Chylothorax: A complication of subclavian vein catheterization and parenteral hyperalimentation. *J Thorac Cardiovasc Surg* 1976; 71:465–468.

539. Tocino IM, Miller MH, Fairfax WR: Distribution of pneumothorax in the supine and semirecumbent critically ill adult. *AJR* 1985; 144:901–905.

540. Tocino IM, Miller MH, Frederick PR, et al: CT detection of occult pneumothorax in head trauma. *AJR* 1984; 143:987–990.

541. Tombroff M, Loicq A, De Koster J-P, et al: Pleural effusion with pancreaticopleural fistula. *Br Med J* 1973; 1:330–331.

542. Trackler RT, Brinker RA: Widening of the left paravertebral pleural line on supine chest roentgenograms in free pleural effusions. *AJR* 1966; 96:1027–1034.

543. Trapnell DH: The peripheral lymphatics of the lung. *Br J Radiol* 1963; 36:660–672.

544. Trapnell DH: The differential diagnosis of linear shadows in chest radiographs. *Radiol Clin North Am* 1973; 11:77–92.

545. Trapnell DH, Thurston JGB: Unilateral pulmonary oedema after pleural aspiration. *Lancet* 1970; 1:1367–1369.

546. Tscholakoff D, Sechtem U, de Geer G, et al: Evaluation of pleural and pericardial effusions by magnetic resonance imaging. *Eur J Radiol* 1987; 7:169–174.

547. Turner JAMcM, Stanley NN: Fragile lung in the Marfan syndrome. *Thorax* 1976; 31:771–775.

548. Turner-Stokes L, Turton C, Pope FM, et al: Emphysema and cutis laxa. *Thorax* 1983; 38:790–792.

549. Twiford TW, Zornoza J, Libshitz HI: Recurrent spontaneous pneumothorax after radiation therapy to the thorax. *Chest* 1978; 73:387–388.

550. Urban C, Nirenberg A, Caparros B, et al: Chemical pleuritis as the cause of acute chest pain following high-dose methotrexate treatment. *Cancer* 1983; 51:34–37.

551. Urokinase pulmonary embolism trial: A national cooperative study. Chapter B. Associated clinical and laboratory findings. *Circulation* 1973; 47(suppl II): II-81–II-85.

552. Van Pernis PA: Variations of thoracic duct. *Surgery* 1949; 26:806–809.

553. Vennera MC, Moreno R, Cot J, et al: Chylothorax and tuberculosis. *Thorax* 1983; 38:694–695.

554. Vix VA: Extrapleural costal fat. *Radiology* 1974; 112:563–565.

555. Vix VA: Roentgenographic recognition of pleural effusion. *JAMA* 1974; 229:695–698.

556. Vix VA: Roentgenographic manifestations of pleural disease. *Semin Roentgenol* 1977; 12:277–286.

557. Vock P, Effmann EL, Hedlund LW, et al: Analysis of the density of pleural fluid analogs by computed tomography. *Invest Radiol* 1984; 19:10–15.

558. Vock P, Hedlund LW, Herfkens RJ, et al: Work in progress: In vitro analysis of pleural fluid analogs by proton magnetic resonance. Preliminary studies at I.S.T. *Invest Radiol* 1987; 22:382–387.

559. Volberg FM, Everett CJ, Brill PW: Radiologic features of inferior pulmonary ligament air collections in neonates with respiratory distress. *Radiology* 1979; 130:357–360.

560. Walden PAM, Mitchell-Heggs PF, Coppin C, et al: Pleurisy and methotrexate treatment. *Br Med J* 1977; 2:867.

561. Walker BA, Beighton PH, Murdoch JL: The marfanoid hypermobility syndrome. *Ann Intern Med* 1969; 71:349–352.

562. Wall SD, Federle MP, Jeffrey RB, et al: CT diagnosis of unsuspected pneumothorax after blunt abdominal trauma. *AJR* 1983; 141:919–921.

563. Walsh JJ: Spontaneous pneumohemothorax. *Dis Chest* 1956; 29:329–335.

564. Wanderer AA, Ellis EF, Goltz RW, et al: Tracheobronchiomegaly and acquired cutis laxa in a child. Physiologic and immunologic studies. *Pediatrics* 1969; 44:709–715.

565. Wanderman KL, Goldstein MS, Faber J: Cor pulmonale secondary to severe kyphoscoliosis in Marfan's syndrome. *Chest* 1975; 67:250–251.

566. Wang N-S: Anatomy and physiology of the pleural space. *Clin Chest Med* 1985; 6:3–16.

567. Waqarrudin M, Bernstein A: Re-expansion pulmonary oedema. *Thorax* 1975; 30:54–60.

568. Watanabe T, Kobayashi T: Pleural calcification: A type of "metastatic calcification" in chronic renal failure. *Br J Radiol* 1983; 56:93–98.

569. Watne AL, Hatiboglu I, Moore GE: A clinical and autopsy study of tumor cells in the thoracic duct lymph. *Surg Gynecol Obstet* 1960; 110:339–345.

570. Webb DB, Whale RJ: Pleuropericardial effusion associated with minoxidil administration. *Postgrad Med J* 1982; 58:319–320.

571. Webb WR, Godwin JD: The obscured outer edge: A sign of improperly placed pleural drainage tubes. *AJR* 1980; 134:1062–1064.

572. Webb WR, LaBerge JM: Radiographic recognition of chest tube malposition in the major fissure. *Chest* 1984; 85:81–83.

573. Webber MM, O'Loughlin BJ: Variations of the pleural vertical fissure line. *Radiology* 1964; 82:461–462.

574. Weber DO, Del Mastro P, Yarnoz MD: Chylothorax after myocardial revascularization with internal mammary graft. *Ann Thorac Surg* 1981; 32:499–502.

575. Weidner WA, Steiner RM: Roentgenographic demonstration of intrapulmonary and pleural lymphatics during lymphangiography. *Radiology* 1971; 100:533–539.

576. Weiss JM, Spodick DH: Association of left pleural effusion with pericardial disease. *N Engl J Med* 1983; 308:696–697.

577. Weiss JM, Spodick DH: Laterality of pleural effusions in chronic congestive heart failure. *Am J Cardiol* 1984; 53:951.

578. Weiss W, Boucot KR, Gefter WI: Localized interlobar effusion in congestive heart failure. *Ann Intern Med* 1953; 38:1177–1186.

579. Weldon CS, Tumulty PA: Topics in clinical medicine. Recurrent pneumothorax associated with menstruation. *Johns Hopkins Med J* 1968; 123:259–263.

580. West JB: Distribution of mechanical stress in the lung, a possible factor in the localization of pulmonary disease. *Lancet* 1971; 1:839–841.

581. Weston WJ: Left-sided lobe of the azygos vein. *J Fac Radiol* 1954; 5:286–288.

582. Wetterform J: Subphrenic abscess, a clinical study of 101 cases. *Acta Chir Scand* 1959; 117:388–408.

583. Whitcomb ME, Schwartz MI: Pleural effusion complicating intensive mediastinal radiation therapy. *Am Rev Respir Dis* 1971; 103:100–107.

584. White PD, August S, Michie CR: Hydrothorax in congestive heart failure. *Am J Med Sci* 1947; 214:243–247.

585. White WF, Urquhart W: The demonstration of pulmonary lymphatics by lymphography in a patient with chylothorax. *Clin Radiol* 1966; 17:92–94.

586. Wiener-Kronish JP, Goldstein R, Matthay RA, et al: Lack of association of pleural effusion with chronic pulmonary arterial and right atrial hypertension. *Chest* 1987; 92:967–970.

587. Wiener-Kronish JP, Matthay MA, Callen PW, et al: Relationship of pleural effusions to pulmonary hemodynamics in patients with congestive heart failure. *Am Rev Respir Dis* 1985; 132:1253–1256.

588. Wilhelm JL, Scommegna A: Catamenial pneumothorax. Bilateral occurrence while on suppressive therapy. *Obstet Gynaecol* 1977; 50:227–231.

589. Williams MH: Pleural effusion produced by abdomino-pleural communication in a patient with Laennec's cirrhosis of the liver and ascites. *Ann Intern Med* 1950; 33:216–221.

590. Williams NS, Lewis CT: Bronchopleural fistula: A review of 86 cases. *Br J Surg* 1976; 63:520–522.

591. Williford ME, Hidalgo H, Putman CE, et al: Com-

puted tomography of pleural disease. *AJR* 1983; 140:909–914.

592. Willson SA, Sawicka EH, Mitchell IC: Spontaneous pneumothorax: An unusual radiological appearance. *Br J Radiol* 1985; 58:173–175.

593. Wilson WG, Aylsworth AS: Familial spontaneous pneumothorax. *Pediatrics* 1979; 64:172–175.

594. Wingfield RC: Chronic recurring spontaneous pneumothoraces associated with menstruation. *Md State Med J* 1961; 10:344–345.

595. Withers JN, Fishback ME, Kiehl PV, et al: Spontaneous pneumothorax. Suggested etiology and comparison of treatment methods. *Am J Surg* 1964; 108:772–776.

596. Wolverson MK, Crepps LF, Sundaram M, et al: Hyperdensity of recurrent hemorrhage at body computed tomography: Incidence and morphologic variation. *Radiology* 1983; 148:779–784.

597. Wood GM, Bolton RP, Muers MF, et al: Pleurisy and pulmonary granulomas after treatment with acebutolol. *Br Med J* 1982; 285:936.

598. Wood JR, Bellamy D, Child AH, et al: Pulmonary disease in patients with Marfan syndrome. *Thorax* 1984; 39:780–784.

599. Woodring JH: Recognition of pleural effusion on supine radiographs: How much fluid is required. *AJR* 1984; 142:59–64.

600. Wright FW: Spontaneous pneumothorax and pulmonary malignant disease—a syndrome sometimes associated with cavitating tumours. *Clin Radiol* 1976; 27:211–222.

601. Yamada S: Uber die serose Flussigkeit in der Pleurahohle der gesunden menschen. *Z Gesamte Exp Med* 1933; 90:342–348.

602. Yamashita H: *Roentgenologic Anatomy of the Lung.* Tokyo, Igaku-Shoin, 1978.

603. Yeh TJ: Endometriosis within the thorax: Metaplasia, implantation, or metastasis? *J Cardiovasc Surg* 1967; 53:201–205.

604. Yellin A, Benfield JR: Pneumothorax associated with lymphoma. *Am Rev Respir Dis* 1986; 134:590–592.

605. Yellow nails and oedema, editorial. *Br Med J* 1972; 4:130.

606. Yousef MMA: Case of the fall season. *Semin Roentgenol* 1980; 15:269–271.

607. Zaher C, Hamer A, Peter T, et al: Low-dose steroid therapy for prophylaxis of amiodarone-induced pulmonary infiltrates. *N Engl J Med* 1983; 308:779.

608. Zelefsky MN, Freeman LM, Stern H: A simple approach to the diagnosis of bronchopleural fistula. *Radiology* 1977; 124:843–844.

609. Ziskind MM, Weill H, George RA: Acute pulmonary edema following the treatment of spontaneous pneumothorax with negative intrapleural pressure. *Am Rev Respir Dis* 1965; 92:632–636

610. Ziter FMH, Westcott JL: Supine subpulmonary pneumothorax. *AJR* 1981; 137:699–701.

611. Zwillich CW, Pierson DJ, Creagh CE, et al: Complications of assisted ventilation. *Am J Med* 1974; 57:161–170.

Mediastinal Disorders

The standard techniques for imaging the mediastinum are plain chest radiography, barium swallow studies, and computed tomography (CT). The introduction of CT radically altered the radiologic approach to the mediastinum: CT scanning has totally replaced conventional tomography, and aortography has been relegated to the investigation of vascular disease. CT scanning is advantageous because it enables one to readily distinguish lymph nodes and masses from surrounding fat, demonstrate the larger blood vessels and accurately locate abnormalities. The problem of superimposition of structures, which often leads to confusion on plain films, is eliminated with the cross-sectional technique of CT. Fluoroscopy, ultrasound,[319] and radionuclide examinations are still used, but only in special circumstances. Early reports suggest that magnetic resonance imaging (MRI), in general, provides information comparable, though not identical, to that derived from CT scanning, the difference in intensity between a mass and the surrounding mediastinal fat being greater with MRI, but the delineation of any tumor mass being clearer with CT.[7, 105]

TECHNIQUES

High kV techniques (greater than 120 kV) have significant advantages over low kV (approximately 70 to 90 kV) in the demonstration of the mediastinum on plain chest radiography. The coefficients of x-ray absorption are closer together with higher kV techniques and, therefore, the visibility of the mediastinal interfaces is less degraded by overlying bone. When this advantage is combined with the better penetration of high kV techniques, the information content for structures within the mediastinum is significantly greater. Several specially designed wedge filters have been constructed to achieve adequate exposure of the mediastinum without over-exposing the lung.[304, 323] These filters are trough-shaped so that they are thicker over the lungs and gradually taper over the mediastinum.

A standard chest CT consists of images of the entire thorax from lung apices to costophrenic angles. Typically, the scan slice thickness is 8 to 10 mm, and the sections are usually contiguous. All modern machines can collect the necessary data within 5 seconds and thus, for most patients, it is possible to obtain each section during a single breath hold. The use of intravenous contrast media to opacify the cardiac chambers and the vessels in the mediastinum varies significantly from center to center. Because it is usually possible to identify the vascular structures without additional opacification, intravenous contrast material can be withheld as a routine and used only to clarify specific problems. Dynamic contrast-enhanced scanning can then be performed at selected levels. For dynamic scans, 40 to 50 ml of iodinated contrast are injected intravenously, and scans are obtained at a single level during the passage of the bolus. In some centers, intravenous contrast material is used routinely, unless specifically contraindicated. Contrast material is required for optimal evaluation of the hili; an appropriate technique is to scan contiguous 8- to 10-mm sections, ensuring maximum contrast opacification by injecting 50 ml of contrast material and imaging as soon as half the bolus has been injected. The sections should be exposed as rapidly as possible from the level of the plane of the right upper lobe bronchus or from the level of the inferior pulmonary veins, depending on the direction of travel of the table top.[112] In those cases where there is still difficulty in deciding whether a density is or is not a normal vessel, the level in question can be examined using contrast-enhanced dynamic scanning.

MRI examinations are usually confined to a specific portion of the mediastinum because the time taken to scan the whole mediastinum would in many instances be too long to be justifiable. For the standard spin-echo sequences, the total time taken for a multislice examination depends on the repetition time (TR) and the number of signal averages. Seven to nine sections can usually be completed for each signal average. For routine examinations, the section thickness is approximately 1 cm. In order to cover enough volume, sections are often taken with 1- to 2-cm intervals. Electrocardiographic (ECG) gating improves the quality of the images, particularly those of the hili and the aorta, and is essential for examination of the lower mediastinum.[320] There is, however, a cost to such gating in terms of extending the time needed to obtain the images. Respiratory gating is not currently in routine use. If an effective respiratory gate were to be manufactured, it too would probably extend the imaging time.

Poor spatial resolution is the chief limitation of MRI in evaluating mediastinal disease, the primary reason being the long imaging times during which respiratory and cardiac movements degrade the image. Currently, the total study time for standard mediastinal examinations by MRI is 30 to 60 minutes, depending on the number of sequences and the views chosen. T1-weighted sequences, usually spin-echo technique, (e.g., a TR of 300 to 500 msec and a TE of 30 msec or less) have been found to provide the best contrast between mediastinal tumor and mediastinal fat (Fig 15–1).[84, 178, 275] With these sequences, fat is of very high intensity, whereas tumors are, in general, of appreciably lower intensity.[310] Images with a longer TR (1,000 to 2,000 msec) have a better signal-to-noise (S/N) ratio and improved spatial resolution, but the contrast between mediastinal fat and mediastinal masses is decreased.[310] T2-weighted images (e.g., TR of 2,000 msec or more and TE of 56 msec or more) are good for showing the fluid content of mediastinal cysts but have disadvantages—notably, poor S/N ratio, poor fat/nonfat soft tissue contrast differences, and long imaging times. The diagnostic usefulness of T2-weighted sequences is, therefore, limited.

MR images are potentially capable of providing better tissue characterization than CT. Lymph node masses due to bronchial carcinoma tend to have long T1 and T2 relaxation values, while chronic inflammatory processes have intermediate T1 and T2 values.[264] Also, the long T1/long T2 characteristics of

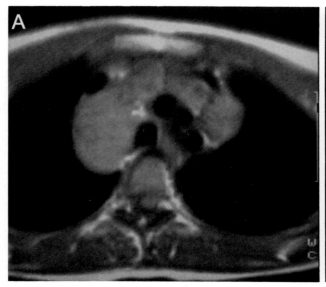

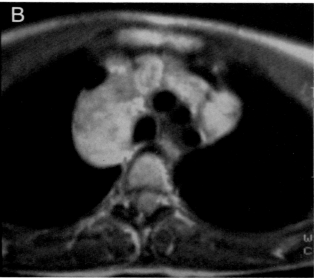

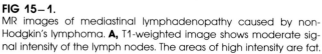

FIG 15–1.
MR images of mediastinal lymphadenopathy caused by non-Hodgkin's lymphoma. **A,** T1-weighted image shows moderate signal intensity of the lymph nodes. The areas of high intensity are fat. **B,** T2-weighted image at the same level. The signal intensity of the lymph nodes is higher and is now closer to the signal seen in fat. (Courtesy of Dr. Janet Husband, London.)

fluid can be helpful in confirming the CT impression that a mass is cystic,[240] thus limiting the differential diagnosis. Another potential advantage is that MR images show greater structural detail of mediastinal masses.[264] What remains to be seen is how useful all this information proves to be. Thus far, the hopes for improved tissue characterization have not been realized to any great extent.[7, 84, 240, 255]

Unlike CT, MRI can provide nontransaxial images of the mediastinum with the same resolution as those obtained in the transaxial plane. Coronal, sagittal, and various angled planes are readily viewed. These projections can be useful in evaluating the aortopulmonary window, imaging the aorta and its branches, defining the relationship of a mass to the spinal canal and visualizing laterally placed hilar masses.[7, 313] Intraspinal extension of mediastinal masses is well evaluated with MRI, regardless of projection, because the subarachnoid space and spinal cord are so clearly visualized.[275] Since rapidly flowing blood produces no signal, contrast media are not required to distinguish between masses and the larger blood vessels. Thus, MRI can be used to examine patients who might be endangered by iodinated contrast media. Owing to the lack of signal from fast-flowing blood in the hilar vessels, hilar lymphadenopathy and other hilar masses are particularly easy to identify[8, 53, 311] and invasion or narrowing of the large arteries and veins of the mediastinum is easy to demonstrate.[197, 240, 264, 317]

The lack of ionizing radiation with MRI, which could prove a significant advantage elsewhere in the body, is of less importance in the mediastinum since most subjects are adults, and mediastinal CT scanning does not, in any event, pose much of a radiation risk.

The place of MR imaging of the mediastinum is not yet clear. The obvious comparison is with CT, but CT is a well established modality, whereas MRI is still evolving. Rapid sequences and surface coils may significantly alter the current recommendations, but at present, the chief limitations center on the long imaging times and the resulting inevitable degradation of spatial resolution. Apart from evaluating cardiac and great vessel disorders and, possibly, hilar adenopathy, the use of MRI in diagnosing mediastinal disease is currently limited to answering questions unresolved by CT.

MEDIASTINAL MASSES

Most mediastinal disorders present as localized masses. The relative incidence of these masses is dif-

ficult to ascertain as published surgical series are biased toward patients whose lesions are being considered for biopsy or resection and there are several common causes of mediastinal mass which are not referred to the surgeon, notably, thyroid masses, aortic aneurysms, and lymphadenopathy in patients with previously established diagnoses such as malignant lymphoma or sarcoidosis. Such cases do not appear in the surgical reviews. The relative incidence of masses in two large series is listed in Table 15–1; these masses were visible on plain chest radiographs and came to surgery.[23, 331] In the series from the Mayo Clinic,[331] more than 75% of mediastinal masses in both adults and children were benign and surgically resectable. Twenty-five percent were malignant and, apart from patients with malignant lymphoma, almost all had a poor prognosis. There were significant differences between the masses encountered in children and in adults. Neurogenic tumors, teratomas, and foregut cysts accounted for almost 80% of the masses seen in children, whereas thymic neoplasms (only 1 case encountered), pericardial cysts, and thoracic goiters were rare.

The classification of mediastinal masses according to their location in the anterior, middle, or posterior mediastinal compartments is a matter of descriptive convenience because there are no anatomic boundaries that limit growth between these various compartments. Indeed, many radiologists do not even use these anatomic terms in the manner defined by textbooks of anatomy. As Heitzman[140] has pointed out, aside from being useful as a means of remembering that thymic, thyroid, and teratomatous

TABLE 15–1.

Incidence (%) of Mediastinal Masses in Two Series

Masses	Wychulis et al.* (1,064 cases)	Benjamin et al.† (214 cases)
Neural tumors	19.9	22.9
Thymic tumors	19.4	20.6
Lymphoma	10.1	14.9
Teratoma	9.3	12.6
Benign cysts (foregut cysts)	18.4	7
Thyroid masses	5.3	11.2
Granuloma	6.3	‡
Mesenchymal tumors	5.6	3.7
Primary carcinoma	2.3	‡
Vascular tumor/ malformation	‡	7.5
Miscellaneous	3.4	‡

*Data from Wychulis AR, Payne WS, Clagett OT, et al: Surgical treatment of mediastinal tumors: A 40-year experience. *J Thorac Cardiovasc Surg* 1971; 62:379–392.
†Data from Benjamin SP, McCormack LJ, Effler DB, et al: Primary tumors of the mediastinum. *Chest* 1972; 62:297–303.
‡Not listed as a separate category.

masses are found in the anterior mediastinum and that most neurogenic tumors are posteriorly situated this simple classification ". . . tends to constrict thinking and minimizes more detailed anatomic analysis." What is needed is the most accurate assessment of the position of any mass, together with a description of its size, shape, and density characteristics. This information will limit the number of possible diagnoses offered and, on occasion, will even permit a specific diagnosis to be made. The differential diagnosis of mediastinal masses is discussed on p. 696.

Thyroid Masses

Intrathoracic thyroid masses are usually colloid or adenomatous goiters; on occasion they may be due to carcinoma. They are almost invariably a downward extension of a thyroid mass that originated in the neck and descended into the mediastinum, carrying with it a vascular pedicle.[331] Development of a primary intrathoracic goiter from heterotopic thyroid tissue is extremely rare.[87, 260, 288, 331] Consequently, the continuity between the mediastinal mass and the thyroid gland in the neck is an important diagnostic feature both on conventional films and at CT.

On plain films, intrathoracic thyroid masses have a well-defined outline which may be spherical or lobular (Figs 15–2 and 15–3). Many masses displace

and narrow the trachea; occasionally the narrowing is substantial and may result in cough, or even stridor, and shortness of breath. The pattern of displacement of the trachea depends on the location of the mass, which is usually predominantly anterior or lateral to the trachea, but may be posterior to it in as many as a quarter of cases (Figs 15–3; 15–4). Posteriorly placed thyroid masses separate the trachea and the esophagus, a pattern that is shared with bronchogenic cysts and anteriorly placed leiomyomas of the esophagus, but is almost never seen with other mediastinal masses. Occasionally, intrathoracic goiter will compress the brachiocephalic veins, a process that may result in the superior vena caval syndrome.[38]

Calcifications within a goiter are common and are largely the result of benign conditions (Figs 15–5; 15–6; 15–7), the usual appearance being dense, amorphous, well-defined calcification, with a nodular, curvilinear or circular configuration. The longer the goiter has been present, the more frequently the calcifications are seen.[170] However, calcification may also be seen in carcinoma of the thyroid[147, 170, 195, 232, 306] (see Fig 15–6). In general, malignant calcification is made up of fine dots grouped in a cloudlike formation that corresponds to the psammoma bodies found pathologically in papillary and follicular carcinoma. The closest resemblance to "benign calcifications" occurs with medullary carcinoma, where the conglomerate dots

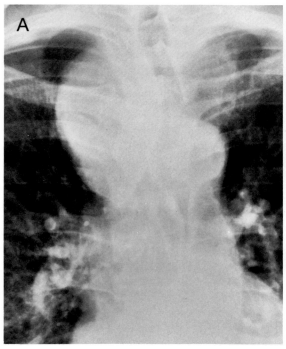

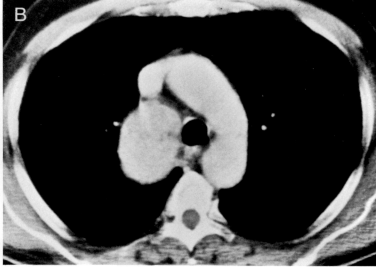

FIG 15–2.
A, Plain radiograph of benign intrathoracic goiter showing well-defined outline and tracheal deviation. **B,** CT scan shows, additionally, contrast enhancement of the thyroid tissue in the mass.

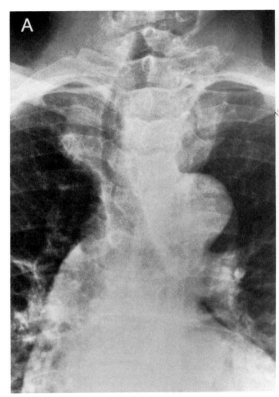

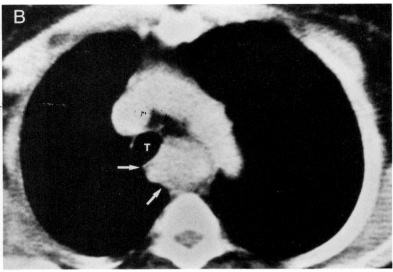

FIG 15–3.
Plain film **(A)** and CT scan **(B)** of benign intrathoracic goiter *(arrows)* lying predominantly posterior to the trachea *(T)*, displacing the trachea anteriorly and to the right. In this case, the mass caused recurrent laryngeal nerve palsy. The CT scan also shows contrast enhancement of the mass.

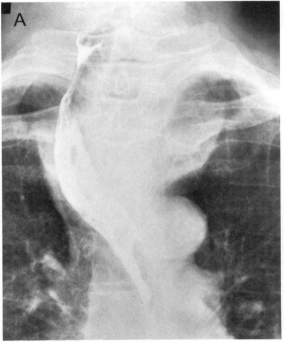

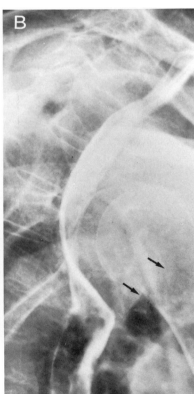

FIG 15–4.
Films from barium swallow study show a benign intrathoracic goiter splitting the esophagus from the trachea. **A,** PA view. **B,** Lateral projection. *Arrows* point to back of trachea.

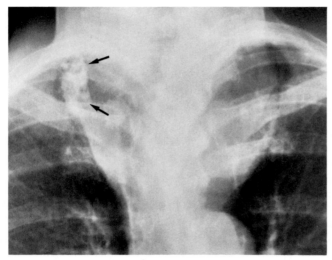

FIG 15-5.
Benign calcification *(arrows)* in an intrathoracic goiter seen on plain film.

are very dense and can be remarkably well-defined, even, on occasion, being arranged in a ring.

CT scanning[18, 27, 111, 210] demonstrates the shape, size, and position of the mass (see Figs 15-2; 15-3; 15-7; 15-8). It is usually possible to diagnose a thyroid origin by noting a well-defined mass in the paratracheal or retrotracheal region cradled by the brachiocephalic veins and lying partly or wholly behind the arteries to the head and neck. The mass will usually be continuous with the thyroid gland in the neck (see Fig 15-7). There are rare occasions, however, when the only connection is a narrow fibrous or vascular pedicle, which is not visible

at CT.[18] Another useful sign at CT is the relatively high attenuation value of the thyroid tissue compared to that of the adjacent muscles on both precontrast and postcontrast images (see Fig 15-7). In the cases published to date, there were at least some areas of increased attenuation in all the examples of intrathoracic goiter.[18, 27, 111, 210]

Calcification is better seen at CT than on plain film, the pattern being similar to that described for plain films. As expected, it is a common finding that further aids differential diagnosis.[18] Rounded, focal, low-density areas are equally common (see Fig 15-8). These low-density areas are more easily visible on the postcontrast films[18] because they do not enhance, whereas the surrounding normal thyroid shows substantial enhancement.

Early reports of MRI examinations of intrathoracic goiter[105, 264] indicate that, like CT, MRI can demonstrate cystic and solid components, but that MRI does not demonstrate calcification. T2-weighted images show very high signal intensity in what are presumed to be the cystic portions of the goiter.

Radionuclide imaging of the thyroid will show some functioning thyroid tissue in almost all intrathoracic goiters[151] (see Fig 15-8). The appropriate agents are[131]I or[127]I, partly because they have a higher energy radiation which can penetrate the sternum, but more particularly because they can be seen on delayed images thus avoiding appreciable background blood pool activity. Technetium-99m images are degraded by the background blood pool activity, and[125]I energy levels are too low to ade-

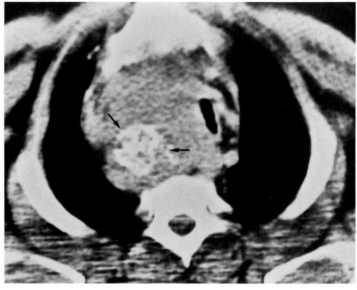

FIG 15-6.
Calcification *(arrows)* in a mucoepidermoid carcinoma of the thyroid shown at contrast-enhanced CT.

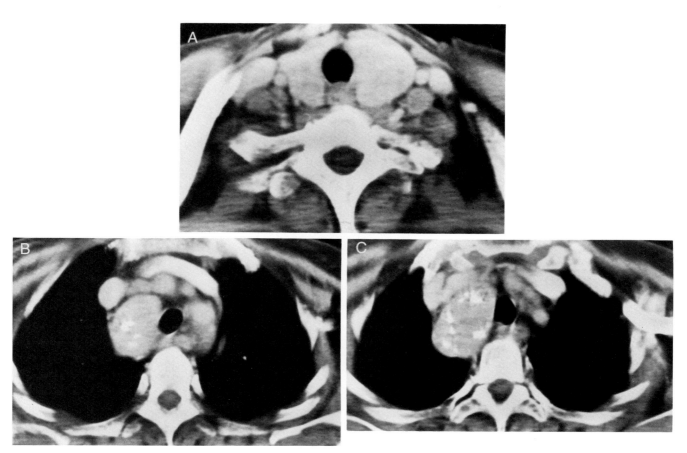

FIG 15—7.
Benign intrathoracic goiter. Three levels **(A—C)** from a contrast-enhanced CT scan illustrate the contiguity of the mass with the thyroid in the neck. Note enhancement of both mass and normal thyroid tissue. Also shown are multiple benign calcifications within the mass.

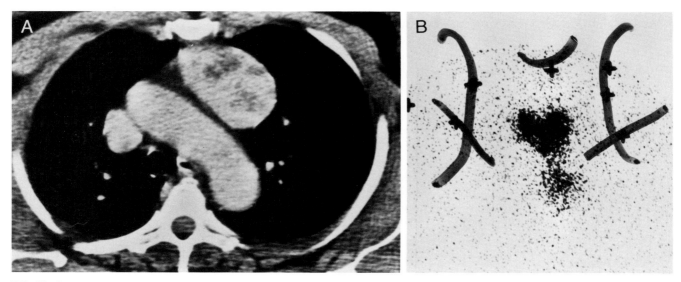

FIG 15—8.
Benign intrathoracic goiter showing **(A)** multiple, focal, rounded low-density areas on contrast-enhanced CT scan and **(B)** activity on an iodine-131 radionuclide study. (The lines indicate the neck, clavicles, and mandible.)

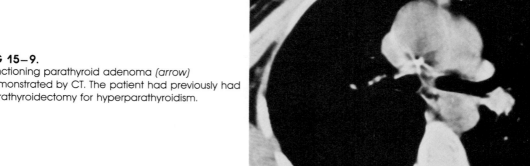

FIG 15–9.
Functioning parathyroid adenoma *(arrow)* demonstrated by CT. The patient had previously had parathyroidectomy for hyperparathyroidism.

quately penetrate the sternum.[151] The very high sensitivity and specificity of radionuclide imaging in goiters makes it a good initial diagnostic test when the diagnosis is suspected on plain film evidence.

Parathyroid Masses

Hyperparathyroidism may be caused by parathyroid adenomas that arise in ectopic parathyroid glands in the mediastinum, usually in or near the thymus.[258] These adenomas vary greatly in size, often being less than 2 cm in diameter (Fig 15–9). When larger than 3 cm they can usually be seen at CT,[171, 258] and even those between 2 and 3 cm stand a reasonable chance of detection. Just what proportion of mediastinal parathyroid adenomas less than 2 cm in diameter can be identified with modern CT equipment remains to be seen. With second generation equipment, relatively few are found.[171]

Because the smaller adenomas are the same size as normal mediastinal lymph nodes or normal thymic remnants, differential diagnosis can be difficult. Here, CT-directed needle aspiration of the suspected adenoma has proved helpful in making the diagnosis, as aspirates from adenomas contain significantly higher levels of parathormone than aspirates from lymph nodes or thymus.[70]

Thymic Masses

CT has effectively replaced conventional tomography and pneumomediastinography as the best means of evaluating the thymus. Enlargement of the thymus is usually caused by a tumor; occasionally it is caused by a cyst and, rarely, by hyperplasia.

Thymic Tumors

The most common cause of a thymic mass is thymoma. Other tumors that may occur in the thymus[176] include thymolipoma; malignant lymphoma, notably Hodgkin's disease (Fig 15–10); thymic carci-

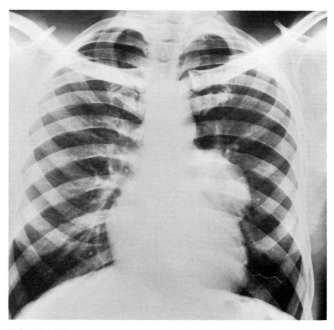

FIG 15–10.
Hodgkin's disease of the thymus. The asymptomatic mass, which was discovered on routine chest radiography, was the only focus of disease in this 33-year-old man.

noid, which may secrete adrenocorticotrophic hormone (ACTH) and consequently may be responsible for Cushing's syndrome[34] (Fig 15–11); germ cell tumors or teratomas; and thymic carcinoma.[12]

Thymomas are very unusual in patients under the age of 20.[80] They are epithelial tumors with variable lymphocytic infiltration. They may be contained within a capsule or may penetrate the capsule, eventually invading the mediastinum. It is the presence or absence of spread beyond the capsule rather than the histologic appearance within the thymus that determines whether the tumor is labeled benign or malignant by the pathologist. For this reason Zerhouni et al.[339] use the term "invasive thymoma" to describe any tumor that has spread beyond the capsule.

Approximately 30% to 40% of patients with thymoma have myasthenia gravis,[281] and the incidence of thymoma in patients with myasthenia gravis is around 10% to 17%.[80] Some 15% to 40% of thymomas turn out to be invasive tumors.[80, 120, 276] The interrelationship between thymoma and myasthenia gravis is not clearly understood. Thymectomy undoubtedly improves the myasthenia in some patients, but those who have a thymoma are no more likely to be improved by surgery than those who are tumor free.[228] Other associations in patients with thymoma include hypogammaglobulinemia, hematologic cytopenias, and nonthymic cancers.[281]

Most thymic masses arise in the upper anterior mediastinum (Fig 15–12), but may project into the adjacent middle mediastinum. They are usually found anterior to the ascending aorta above the right ventricular outflow tract and the main pulmo-

nary artery. A few are situated more inferiorly adjacent to the left or right borders of the heart (Fig 15–13), and occasionally even as low as the cardiophrenic angles. Large thymic masses may lie partly in the neck and partly in the thorax.[127]

Thymomas are usually spherical or have lobulated borders. Only the larger tumors are visible on plain film. Sometimes the mass can be recognized only in one or other plain film projection, the opacity frequently being indefinite in the lateral view. Another problem on plain chest radiographs is overdiagnosis in obese patients in whom mediastinal fat can closely resemble a thymic swelling. CT is very helpful in such cases because it readily enables one to distinguish fat from tumor.

Punctate or curvilinear calcification is seen in both benign and invasive thymomas. In thymomas large enough to be seen on plain films or conventional tomography, calcification is seen in 6% to 28% of cases.[81, 137]

All signs of thymic tumor seen on plain radiographs are best seen with CT (Figs 15–11 and 15–14),* which is the most sensitive examination for the detection of thymoma in patients with myasthenia gravis. The accuracy of diagnosis varies with the age of the patient. After 40, the normal gland is sufficiently small to permit masses to be readily distinguished. In patients over 40 they can be diagnosed even when smaller than 2 cm in diameter. Before age 40, and particularly before 30, it may be difficult to distinguish small thymomas from the normal

*References 12, 34, 35, 80, 98, 160, 207, 208, and 276.

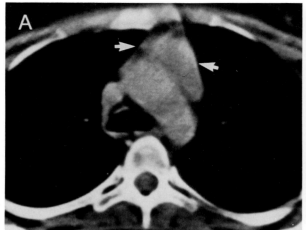
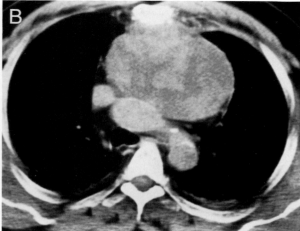

FIG 15–11.
Thymic carcinoid. **A,** contrast-enhanced CT scan shows a thymic tumor *(arrows)* in a young woman with ectopic ACTH production by the tumor. The tumor in this instance was invasive and recurred following surgery. **B,** CT scan in another patient with a large carcinoid tumor of the thymus who presented with chest pain. The mass showed areas of low density because of necrosis.

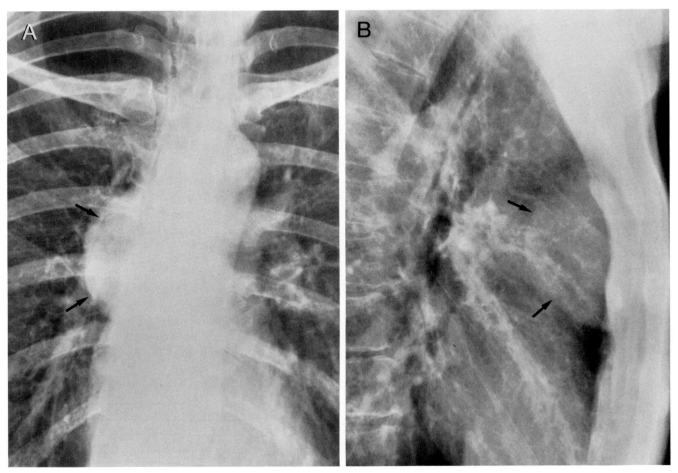

FIG 15–12.
A and **B,** thymoma. Plain films show a thymoma in the anterior mediastinum lying anterior to the ascending aorta above the right ventricular outflow tract. The lesion presented as an asymptomatic mass *(arrows).*

gland. The diagnosis depends on recognizing a focal swelling rather than applying a specific measurement. Fortunately thymoma is so rare in children that the potentially difficult problem of finding a thymoma in a child with myasthenia gravis does not arise. Care must be taken not to confuse a high main or left pulmonary artery with a thymoma (Fig 15–15).

Invasive thymomas invade the mediastinal fat and eventually spread to the pericardium and pleura, at which time transpleural spread and "drop metastases" may be noted radiographically (Fig 15–16). All of these features are best diagnosed with CT[276, 339] (Fig 15–17). Until mediastinal invasion has occurred, it is not possible to distinguish benign from invasive thymoma.

Early experience with MRI suggests that, though MRI is more accurate than plain film techniques in determining the size of the thymus, CT remains the superior technique because of its better spatial resolution and its ability to demonstrate calcification.[17] As always, MRI can more readily enable one to distinguish between mediastinal masses and the blood vessels traversing the mediastinum, a possible advantage in selected cases where CT interpretation proves difficult. With current technology, there is no evidence that MRI provides better tissue characterization of thymic masses than is available with CT. Thymomas have a signal intensity similar to muscle on T1-weighted images. T1-weighted sequences are,

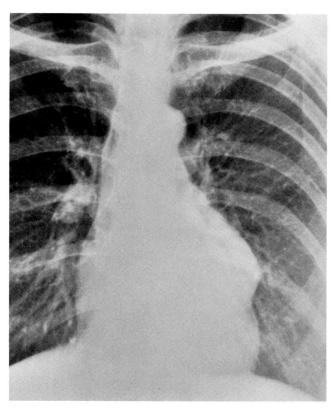

FIG 15–13.
Thymoma situated predominantly adjacent to the mid left heart border.

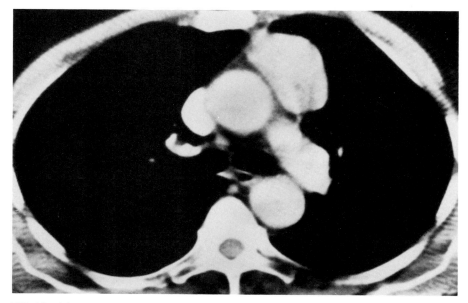

FIG 15–14.
Contrast-enhanced CT scan of benign thymoma. The patient did not have clinical or electromyographic evidence of myasthenia gravis. The mass was initially discovered on plain chest films.

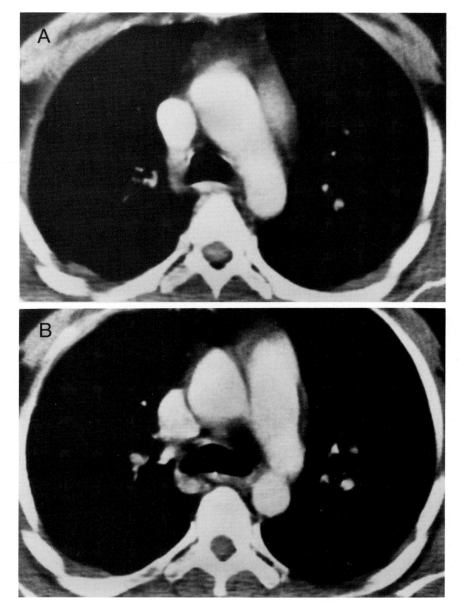

FIG 15–15.
A, high proximal left pulmonary artery mimicking a thymic mass. Its true nature was proved with contrast-enhanced scans. **B,** adjacent section showed that the apparent mass is a partial volume effect due to the left pulmonary artery.

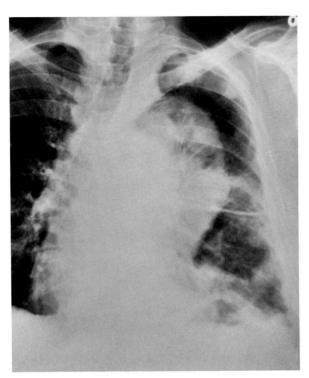

FIG 15–16.
Invasive thymoma showing contiguous spread to pleura in the left chest. Patient also had pure red cell aplasia.

therefore, the best choice for detecting thymic disease. On T2-weighted images the signal intensity increases and approaches that of fat, making distinction of thymic masses from surrounding mediastinal fat more difficult.

Thymolipomas (Fig 15–18) are rare tumors composed of a mixture of mature fat and normal-looking or involuted thymic tissue. As thymolipomas are virtually asymptomatic, they can grow to a very large size before discovery. Being soft, they mold themselves to the adjacent mediastinum and diaphragm and may mimic cardiomegaly.[295] In one reported case, CT showed the fat density of the mass and ultrasound showed the high echoreflectivity expected of fat, thereby excluding cardiac disease.[337] CT scanning shows the fatty density of the mass.

Thymic Cysts

Thymic cysts are usually simple cysts within an otherwise normal or hyperplastic gland.[266] They may, however, be found within thymomas or thymic germ cell tumors.[73, 127] Cysts have also been reported in Hodgkin's disease involving the thymus[89, 183]; even when radiation therapy eradicates the Hodgkin's disease, the size of the cysts may remain unchanged.[183] In some cases, the cysts first develop after irradiation of the mediastinum.[13, 302] At least some post-treatment cysts are benign in nature. Their pathogenesis is debated. They may be due to cystic degeneration following chemotherapy or radiation therapy or they may be due to cystic change within a focus of Hodgkin's disease and unrelated to therapy. The important point to note is that if a thymic mass develops in a patient with Hodgkin's disease following radiation therapy, the possibility of a benign cyst should be considered before further treatment for Hodgkin's disease is given.[164]

On plain film, thymic cysts are indistinguishable from other nonlobulated thymic masses, notably thymoma. CT may demonstrate the water density of the cyst.[126]

Thymic Hyperplasia

In follicular hyperplasia of the thymus, the gland may be of normal size and weight, but it may be enlarged, sometimes greatly. The most common association of thymic hyperplasia is with myasthenia gravis, but it is seen in other conditions, notably thyrotoxicosis (Fig 15–19). CT and MRI may show enlargement of both lobes of an otherwise normally shaped gland, but usually the size of the thymus is within the normal range[80] even though at surgery the thymus may be large and hyperplastic.[12, 17, 156] Thymic hyperplasia may occasionally cause a focal swelling that mimics a thymic mass.[12, 98]

Rebound Thymic Hyperplasia

The thymus gland may atrophy rapidly in response to stress or therapy with steroids and antineoplastic drugs. The gland will grow back to its original size upon recovery or cessation of treatment. Such atrophy is very common. It was seen in 90% of one group of patients who were receiving chemotherapy for extrathoracic malignancies.[49] In the phenomenon known as rebound thymic hyperplasia, the gland may grow back to an even larger size than normal (Fig 15–20). Histologically, the gland shows hyperplasia of the cortex and medulla. Rebound thymic hyperplasia has been reported after recovery from a wide variety of stresses including burns, surgery, and tuberculosis; after cessation of steroid therapy or treatment of Cushing's syndrome; and during or after antineoplastic chemotherapy.* The phenomenon is most frequent in children and young adults, in whom the incidence is approximately 25%.[49] When rebound thymic hyperplasia is seen in patients previously treated for a malignant

*References 40, 54, 71, 106, 166, 251, and 328.

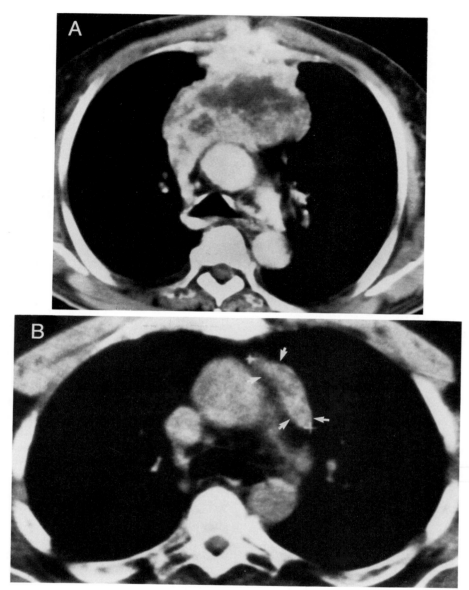

FIG 15–17.
Invasive thymoma. **A,** contrast-enhanced CT scan shows thymic mass of variable density invading adjacent mediastinum and sternum. **B,** CT scan in another patient with an invasive thymoma *(arrows)* illustrates the impossibility of distinguishing invasive from non-invasive thymoma prior to mediastinal or pleural invasion. Capsular invasion was present histologically, and the tumor recurred locally following thymectomy.

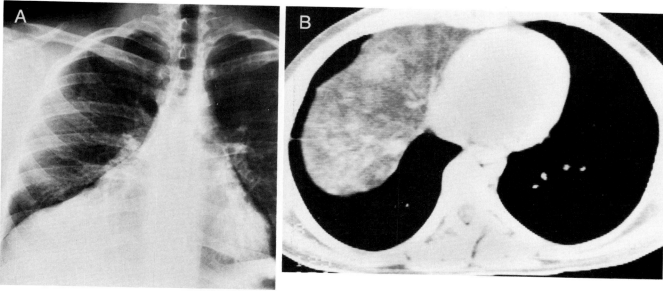

FIG 15–18.
Thymolipoma. **A,** plain film shows large low-lying thymic mass, the shape of which conforms more to the adjacent diaphragm and mediastinum than it would if it were a thymoma or other thymic mass. **B,** contrast-enhanced CT scan indicates the tumor is largely composed of fat, but has strands of soft tissue density scattered throughout.

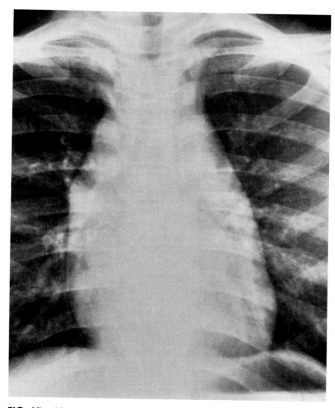

FIG 15–19.
Substantial enlargement of the thymus resulting from thymic hyperplasia in a 16-year-old girl with thyrotoxicosis.

neoplasm that could involve the thymus, there may be difficulty in distinguishing thymic involvement by neoplasm from thymic rebound. The diagnosis depends on the absence of clinical or other features indicating recurrence of tumor in a patient with a reason for thymic rebound.[54] A normal thymus will shrink on steroid therapy and, in those instances where the diagnosis is uncertain, a trial of steroids can be used to attempt to confirm thymic hyperplasia. Lymphomas and leukemias may, however, be equally responsive to steroid administration.[54] A helpful feature is that on CT scanning the gland, though enlarged, may retain a normal shape.

Teratoma and Germ Cell Tumors of the Mediastinum

A teratoma is a neoplasm derived from more than one embryonic germ layer. The term mediastinal teratoma is used in a variety of ways. Some use it to cover the entire spectrum of germinal tumors, both benign and malignant.[331] Others divide such tumors into benign teratoma and a number of malignant forms,[59] chiefly the malignant germinal tumors found in the testes: teratocarcinoma, seminoma, embryonal carcinoma, choriocarcinoma, and mixtures of these cell types.

Mediastinal teratomas are believed to develop in

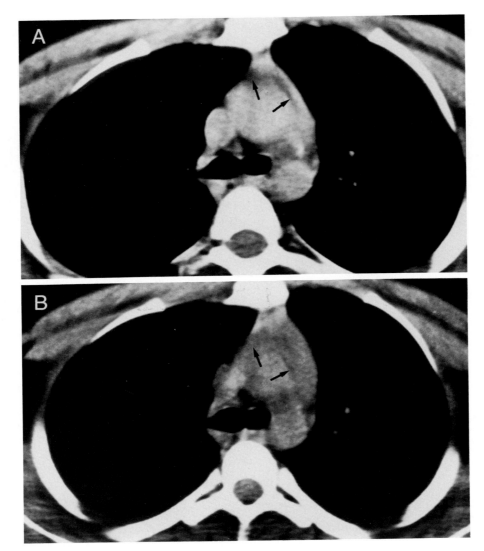

FIG 15–20.
Rebound hyperplasia of the thymus in a 13-year-old girl with osteosarcoma. **A,** the thymus *(arrows)* is normal in size prior to chemotherapy. **B,** enlarged thymus *(arrows)* after completion of chemotherapy.

aberrant cell rests. Almost all arise in the anterior mediastinum within, or in intimate contact with, the thymus.[176] Dermoid cysts, a term that is going out of use, are now usually regarded as benign or mature cystic teratomas. Benign teratomas are more common than the malignant forms[188, 331]; they are found in patients of all ages but particularly in adolescents and in young adults, with women slightly outnumbering men.

The malignant germ cell tumors are usually seen in young adults and are much more common in men than in women. In a review of 103 cases of primary mediastinal seminoma by Polansky et al., only five patients were women.[239] Even mediastinal choriocarcinoma is more common in men than in women.

Benign cystic teratoma may be asymptomatic and diagnosed incidentally on chest radiography or CT. The most common symptoms are chest pain, cough (usually productive), dyspnea, and fever. An occasional patient presents with hemoptysis.[331] Most of these lesions consist of one large cyst, though a few are made up of multiple cysts, some of which have intervening solid portions.[331] They are frequently large and may be huge, occupying much of one hemithorax.

Benign cystic teratomas usually produce a well-defined, rounded or lobulated mass in the mediastinum (Figs 15–21 and 15–22). Being benign, these lesions grow slowly, but rapid increases in size may occur due to hemorrhage. Alternatively, the cyst

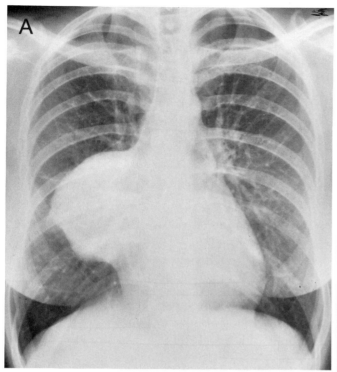

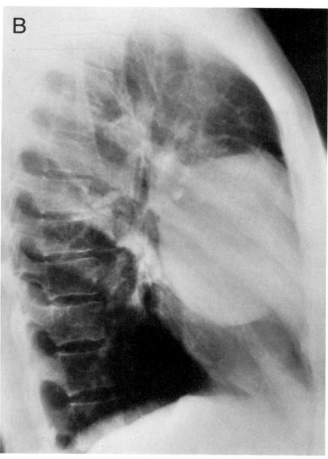

FIG 15–21.
Benign cystic teratoma in an asymptomatic 26-year-old woman. The round, well-defined anterior mediastinal mass projecting predominantly to one side is typical of the condition. **A,** PA radiograph. **B,** lateral radiograph.

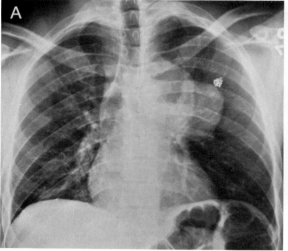

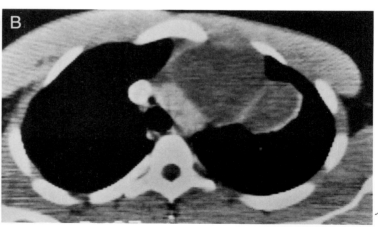

FIG 15–22.
Benign cystic teratoma showing lobular anterior mediastinal mass projecting to left side discovered on routine chest radiographs in a 27-year-old man **(A). B,** contrast-enhanced CT scan shows fluid density and septations within the mass. (Courtesy of Dr. Chuck Hubbard, Columbia, S.C.)

may rupture into the bronchial tree. Almost all cystic teratomas are in the anterior mediastinum in front of the roots of the great vessels, but a few are found in the posterior mediastinum.[69, 315, 331] Most teratomas project mainly to one side of the midline,[331] sometimes markedly so (see Figs 15—20 and 15—21). Peripheral calcification and even teeth may be visible on plain chest radiograph and, occasionally, sufficient fat is present to be detectable. CT is more sensitive than plain films in the detection of both calcification and fat.[315] The findings at CT are variable[150, 289] (Figs 15—22 and 15—23). Water density in the cystic component is common, and fat density is seen in one quarter to one half of the patients. A definite cyst wall, which occasionally shows calcification, is often visible.

Ultrasound examination of mediastinal teratomas may reveal useful information regarding the cystic components of the mass.[150] Cystic teratomas may appear cystic, solid, or complex, and when the cystic content is serous fluid, the tumor is anechoic. When the cystic component is nonserous, the tumor tends to exhibit a complex or solid echo pattern.

Mediastinal malignant germ cell tumors give rise to symptoms that are similar to those of benign cystic teratoma: namely cough, dyspnea, and chest pain.[239] Superior venal caval obstruction is not uncommon[146]; it was found in 10% of patients in a review of over 100 cases.[239] Weight loss may also be noted. About 30% are asymptomatic and are first discovered as an anterior mediastinal mass on routine radiography.[239] The plain film findings (Figs 15—24 and 15—25) of the mass itself are similar to benign teratoma except that the mass is often lobular in outline, fat density is not noted, and calcification is a rare finding. Unlike benign teratoma, the malignant forms grow rapidly, and metastases may be seen in the lungs, bones, or pleura. CT shows a lobular, asymmetric mass[179, 270] (see Figs 15—24 and 15—25). The adjacent mediastinal fat planes may be obliterated, and the tumors are either of homogeneous soft tissue density or show multiple areas of contrast enhancement interspersed with rounded areas of decreased attenuation due to necrosis and hemorrhage (see Fig 15—25). Mediastinal adenopathy may be seen. Coarse tumor calcification was reported in one patient.[179] Though suggestive, the CT features are not specific. CT cannot distinguish malignant germ cell tumor from thymoma, and in the absence of calcification, the differential diagnosis includes lymphoma of the thymus, metastatic carcinoma, and other primary malignant tumors arising in the anterior mediastinum.

Mediastinal Cysts

Most mediastinal cysts are developmental in origin. The usual entities included in this category are bronchogenic cysts, esophageal cysts, neurenteric cysts, and pericardial cysts. The distinction between

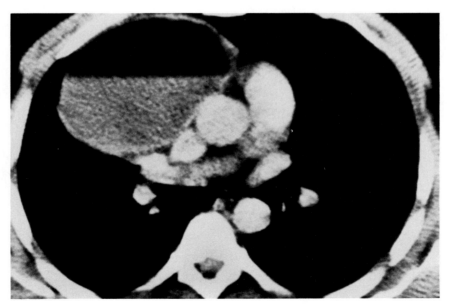

FIG 15—23.
Benign cystic teratoma showing thin wall and fat/fluid level on contrast-enhanced CT scan.

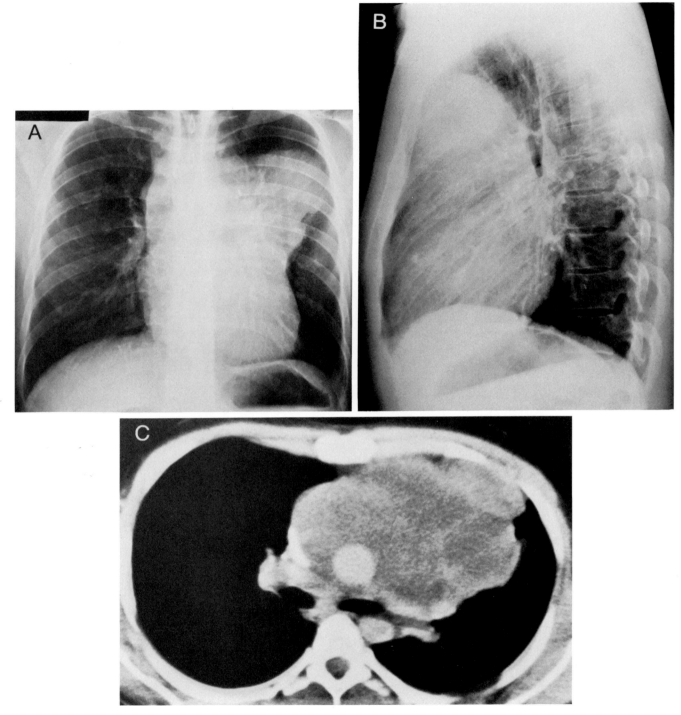

FIG 15–24.
Malignant germ cell tumor (choriocarcinoma) of mediastinum. **A** and **B,** PA and lateral chest radiographs show the lobular asymmetric mediastinal mass and small metastases in both lungs. **C,** contrast-enhanced CT scan shows variable density in the mass.

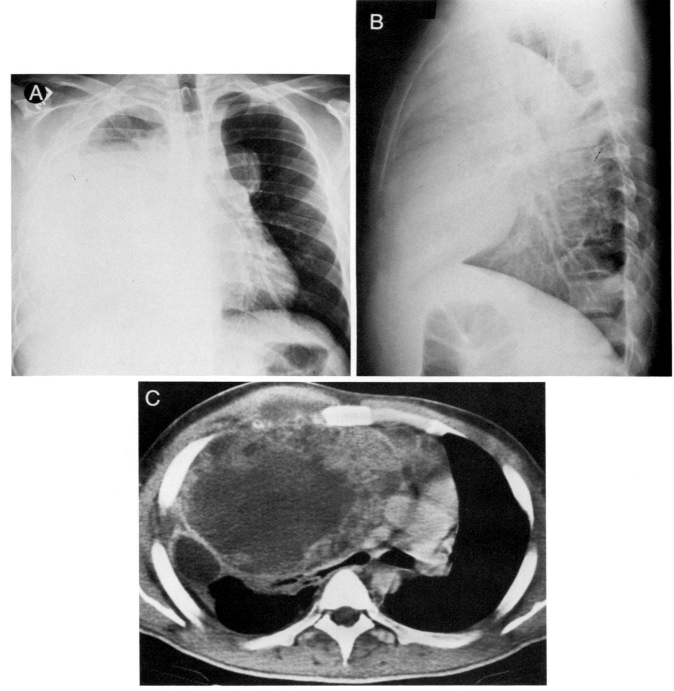

FIG 15–25.
Malignant germ cell tumor. **A** and **B**, PA and lateral chest radiographs show a huge asymmetric anterior mediastinal mass and large right pleural effusion. **C**, contrast-enhanced CT scan shows fluid density in the widespread necrotic areas within the tumor.

these cysts is not always clear-cut. For example, a cyst deep in the wall in the esophagus, and unquestionably by all anatomic criteria an esophageal cyst, may contain respiratory epithelium. It is for this reason that bronchogenic, esophageal, and neurenteric cysts are frequently classified as foregut cysts in order to emphasize their origin from the embryological foregut.[142, 221, 249] Mediastinal cysts containing cartilage are classified as definitely bronchogenic and those with gastric epithelium are classified as definitely enteric. Those with seromucinous glands are considered as probably, although not definitely, respiratory in origin. Most congenital mediastinal cysts are lined by respiratory epithelium, and these are usually labeled as bronchial cysts even though their precise origin can only be conjectured.[249]

Bronchogenic Cysts

Bronchogenic cysts are discussed in Chapter 13. The discussion in this chapter is confined to their radiographic appearances.

These lesions are almost invariably single. They are usually, but not always, found in close proximity to the major airways—typically in the paratracheal, carinal, subcarinal, or perihilar areas. The single most frequent site is immediately adjacent to the lower trachea or proximal main-stem bronchi. Anterior and posterior mediastinal cysts remote from the airways are occasionally encountered.[32, 221] As the cysts grow they displace the adjacent lung and often also displace the esophagus. The central airways are more rigid and are usually displaced little, if at all. Airway compression, though rare, is well documented; in young children it may be life-threatening. Hemorrhage into the cyst or infection of the contents may, on very rare occasions, lead to rapid expansion and serious airway compromise even in adults. Superior vena caval obstruction, though reported, is very rare.[9, 202]

On plain chest radiographs,[249] bronchogenic cysts are seen as smoothly marginated rounded or oval masses in the mediastinum or hilus with one of the surfaces of the cyst adjacent to the trachea or central bronchi (Fig 15–26). Approximately 10% show a lobular outline (Fig 15–27).[249] In most cases, the lesion is stable in size over many years. Rapid enlargement is seen with hemorrhage or infection, both of which are unusual. Calcification of the wall is seen on rare occasions,[249] and the odd case will show milk of calcium within the cyst.[24, 58] Air or air-fluid levels are seen within the cyst in a few cases.[24, 249]

Barium swallow examination shows smooth extrinsic displacement of the esophagus by the cyst in at least half the cases (Fig 15–28). Typically, the cyst invaginates between the airway and the esophagus. (Fig 15–29).

CT is now the standard technique for evaluating bronchogenic cysts[142, 218] (see Figs 15–26, 15–27, 15–29, 15–30, 15–31). The characteristic features are a smooth spherical or oval mass in contact with a major airway, with well-defined margins and no infiltration of the adjacent mediastinum. The cyst may show a CT density close to that of water, but a significant proportion show uniform soft-tissue density, presumably due to the high protein content of the cyst fluid.[218] Some show surprisingly high CT numbers, well above soft tissue; cysts with numbers as high as 120 Hounsfield units have been reported (see Fig 15–31).[199] These high densities are probably the result of previous hemorrhage. Since milk of calcium has been seen on plain film examinations, it is not surprising that, in some cysts, high density as a result of calcium crystals can be demonstrated at CT scanning.[338] Calcification of the wall of the cyst is well shown by CT.

Ultrasound can be used to demonstrate the cystic nature of the mass if the lesion can be approached without the beam traversing the lung. It has been used primarily in children. MRI shows the same anatomic features as CT, the cyst content showing the signal characteristics of fluid.

The diagnosis can be confirmed nonoperatively by needle aspiration of the contents and the subsequent injection of contrast medium to demonstrate the smoothness and thickness of the wall of the cyst. Transthoracic placement under CT control[97] is the simplest technique, but it may prove more effective to pass the needle transbronchoscopically or through an esophagoscope.[172] The cyst fluid can be examined to exclude malignant cells, and a confident diagnosis of bronchogenic cyst can obviate the need for operative removal. Needle aspiration has also been advocated for the treatment of pressure effects.[172]

Pericardial Cysts

Pericardial cysts are the result of anomalous outpouchings of the parietal pericardium, but only rarely do they have any visible communication with the pericardial sac. (Pericardial diverticula are related anomalies of the visceral pericardium that communicate with the pericardial space.[226]) The cysts contain clear yellow fluid. The interior is usually unilocular but is often trabeculated. In one series, 20% of cases examined pathologically were multilocular,[91] though in another large series of 72

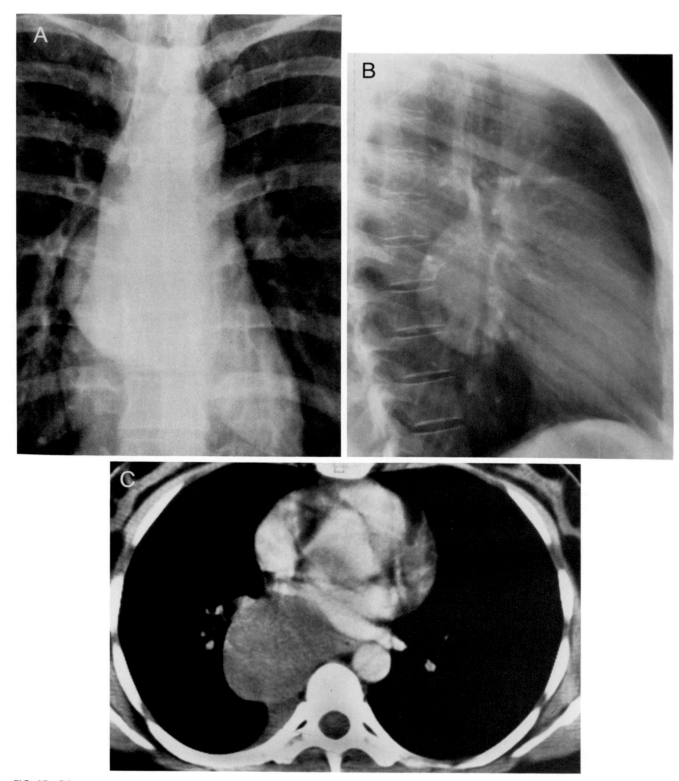

FIG 15—26.
Bronchogenic cyst in a 33-year-old woman. **A** and **B,** PA and lateral plain chest radiographs show well-defined, oval subcarinal mass which on contrast-enhanced CT scanning **(C)** demonstrates an imperceptible wall and uniform near-water density. The patient complained of dysphagia and of dyspnea relieved by lying on the right side.

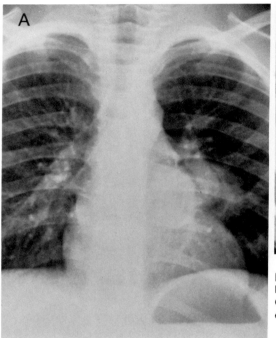

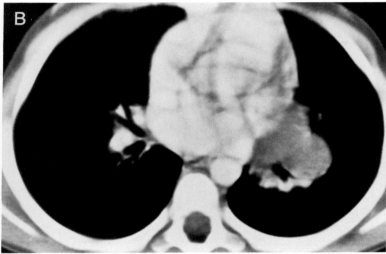

FIG 15–27.
Multilocular bronchogenic cyst in a 7-year-old boy showing uniform density on CT except for septations within the cyst. **A,** PA radiograph. **B,** contrast-enhanced CT scan.

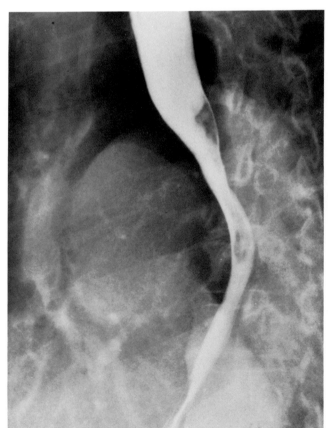

FIG 15–28.
Bronchogenic cyst interposing between airway and esophagus shows typical smooth displacement of the esophagus at barium swallow.

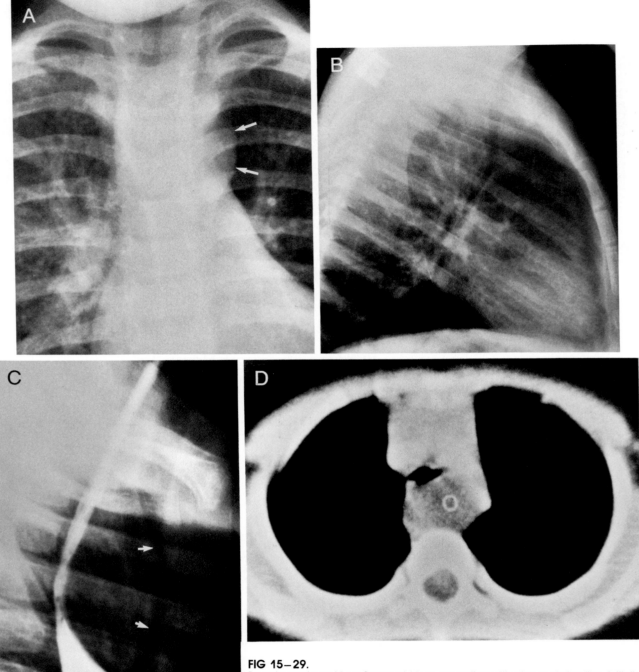

FIG 15–29.
Bronchogenic cyst in a 2-year-old boy presenting with airway obstruction, initially believed to be asthma. Note the relatively subtle findings on plain films. **A,** the cyst *(arrows)* projects to the left of the aortic knob on PA radiograph and bows the trachea forward on the lateral projection **(B). C,** the esophagogram demonstrates separation of the trachea *(arrows)* and esophagus by the mass. **D,** contrast-enhanced CT scan shows the airway displacement and the typical uniform water density of the mass.

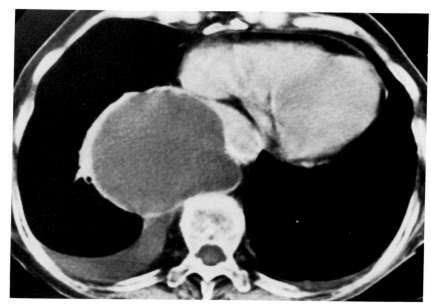

FIG 15–30.
Bronchogenic cyst in an 83-year-old woman shows pathognomonic features of a benign cyst on contrast-enhanced CT, namely the smooth wall with uniform water density to the cyst. There is an incidental right pleural effusion.

patients, only one pericardial cyst was truly loculated.[330] The wall of the cyst is composed of collagen and scattered elastic fibers lined by a single layer of mesothelial cells.[91] The great majority are asymptomatic, but in surgical series symptoms such as chest pain, cough, and dyspnea may be present in up to one-third of patients.[91, 221, 330]

There is a strong predilection for the anterior cardiophrenic angles, and the cysts typically contact the heart, the diaphragm, and the anterior chest wall. They are seen more frequently on the right than on the left. In the Mayo Clinic series,[330] 37 of 72 pericardial cysts were in the right cardiophrenic angle, and 17 were in the left cardiophrenic angle. The remaining 18 arose higher in the mediastinum, and 11 extended into the superior mediastinum. In a review of radiographs of 41 cases at the Armed Forces Institute of Pathology, the right left ratio was 4:3.[91]

On all imaging studies, the cysts are seen as smooth, round, or oval well-defined masses in contact with the heart (Fig 15–32). An oval shape coming to a point has been observed in some cases.[37, 91] Calcification is exceptional. On CT (see Fig 15–32), the cyst contents may be close to water density[244] or may be in the soft tissue range.[37] The

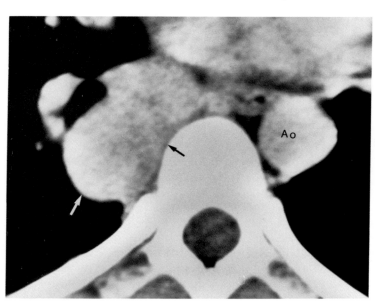

FIG 15–31.
Bronchogenic cyst *(arrows)* showing uniform high density. The cyst has the same density as the contrast-enhanced descending aorta *(Ao)*. Following resection, the cyst was found to contain thick proteinaceous fluid.

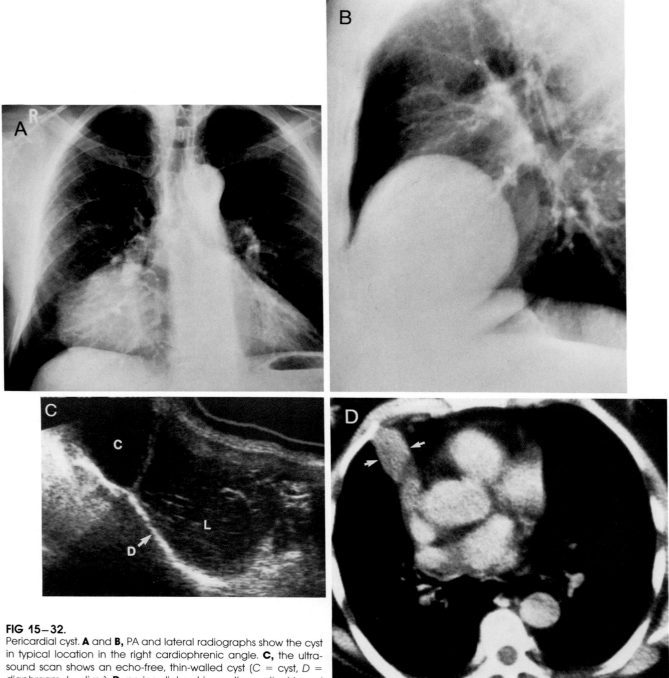

FIG 15–32.
Pericardial cyst. **A** and **B,** PA and lateral radiographs show the cyst in typical location in the right cardiophrenic angle. **C,** the ultrasound scan shows an echo-free, thin-walled cyst (C = cyst, D = diaphragm, L = liver). **D,** pericardial cyst in another patient is oval and is in contact with the pericardium on contrast-enhanced CT scan. In this case there was uniform soft-tissue density, so the lesion was removed surgically.

cysts may be of almost any size, diameters up to 16 cm having been recorded.[91, 330] Rapid change in size, particularly a decrease in size, suggests a pericardial diverticulum rather than a pericardial cyst.[167] Ultrasound can be used to demonstrate the cystic na

ture of these lesions (see Fig 15–32). The place of MRI has yet to be ascertained, but clearly the fluid characteristics of the lesion should be very helpful in establishing the diagnosis. Cyst puncture with instillation of contrast medium to establish the diagnosis of a benign cyst has been performed with pericardial cysts just as it has with other benign mediastinal cysts.[169]

Neurenteric Cysts

Neurenteric cysts are foregut cysts in which there are associated anomalies of the vertebral column. In early embryogenesis the notochord lies against the embryonic foregut, and it is believed that incomplete separation of the notochord from the alimentary tract explains the various anomalies of the vertebrae that are seen in conjunction with neurenteric cysts.[221] The vertebral anomalies include hemivertebrae and sagittal clefts in the vertebral body (including butterfly vertebra and spina bifida). The vertebral anomaly may be located above the level of the cyst itself. Neurenteric cysts are relatively rare, forming either a small minority of mediastinal cysts, or not being encountered at all in the larger surgical series.[32, 221, 331] Radiographically[191, 326] (Fig 15–33), neurenteric cysts are round, oval, or lobulated masses of water density situated in the posterior mediastinum or paravertebral region. The vertebral anomalies described earlier need to be searched for carefully, as they are difficult to see but are an important clue to the diagnosis. These cysts sometimes communicate with the subarachnoid space, a com-munication that can be demonstrated by myelography.

Mediastinal Pancreatic Pseudocyst

On very rare occasions, a pancreatic pseudocyst will extend into the mediastinum.[165, 327] Most patients are adults and have clinical features of chronic pancreatitis but they only occasionally have a palpable abdominal mass. In children, the usual cause of the pseudocyst is trauma.[165] Radiographically, most patients have pleural effusion on the left or bilaterally. The mediastinal component of the pseudocyst is almost always in the posterior mediastinum, having gained access to the chest by way of the esophageal or aortic hiatus. The esophagus is, therefore, deformed by the pseudocyst in many instances.

Lymphangioma/Hemangioma

Lymphangiomas (cystic hygromas) are tumor-like congenital malformations of the lymphatic system[26, 268] consisting of lymph channels or cystic lymph spaces lined by endothelium and containing clear or straw-colored fluid. The walls are formed by fibrous tissue and smooth muscle. These lesions do not undergo malignant change. They grow slowly and may envelop the adjacent structures. This char-

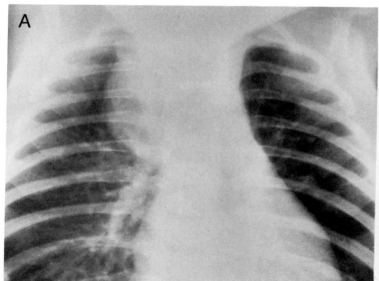
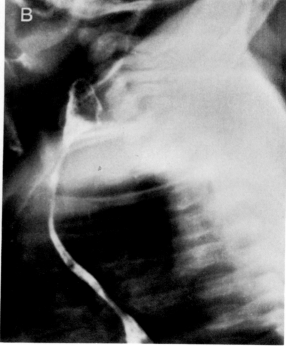

FIG 15–33.
Neurenteric cyst. **A,** plain film showing oval soft mass arising from the mediastinum. A segmentation anomaly was present in the lower cervical spine. **B,** barium swallow study shows displacement of the esophagus by the mass, placing the lesion between the spine and the esophagus. (Courtesy of Dr. Helen Carty, Liverpool.)

acteristic can make them difficult to resect, and recurrence rates are high. The most common location for lymphangiomas is the neck. Mediastinal lymphangiomas may be wholly confined to the mediastinum or may be an extension from the neck. The cervicomediastinal form is the more common of the two. It is practically always discovered in infancy, presenting as a mass in the neck. The form confined to the mediastinum is rare. It is usually asymptomatic and is first discovered on chest radiographs in older children or adults.[36, 94, 235] Lymphangiomas may, on rare occasions, compress the surrounding structures such as the esophagus,[333] airway,[193] great veins,[63] or heart.[36] Lymphangiomas vary greatly in size and histologic characteristics. Some show a capillary or cavernous structure; others take the form of unilocular or multilocular cysts.

On plain chest radiograph,[36, 193] they form well-defined, round, lobular masses, usually in the anterior or superior mediastinum (Fig 15–34). Fewer than 10% occur in the posterior mediastinum.[268] Calcification does not appear to be a feature. Unilateral or bilateral pleural effusions may be present, in which case the fluid is often chylous.

CT (Fig 15–35) shows a mass which may mould to or envelope the adjacent mediastinal structures. The CT attenuation value falls in the low soft tissue or water density range. It is sometimes possible to

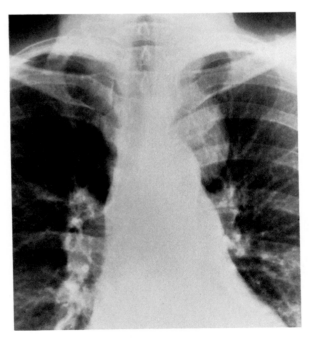

FIG 15–34.
Lymphangioma (cystic hygroma) of superior mediastinum in an asymptomatic patient. Note the contiguity with the anterior neck and the lack of tracheal displacement.

recognize that the lesion consists of serpiginous, vessel-like structures but, regardless of shape, there is no enhancement of the lesion with administration of intravenous contrast material.[36, 238, 269, 293]

The differential diagnosis from other cystic masses is based chiefly on location, lymphangiomas being situated high in the superior mediastinum in contact with, or extending into, the neck. Occasionally, lymphangiomas may invade the chest wall, leading to radiologically recognizable thinning of the ribs.[238] (Massive bone destruction in lymphangiomas is discussed below.)

Blood vessel tumors in the mediastinum occur only rarely. The benign lesions are usually capillary or cavernous hemangiomas.[64] Mixed lymphatic and blood vessel lesions such as lymphangiohemangioma,[3] hemangioendothelioma,[20, 292] and hemangiosarcoma are also occasionally encountered. Hemangiomas may be encountered in patients of any age, most often in the first decade. They usually arise in the anterior mediastinum (Fig 15–36); the next most common site is the posterior mediastinum.[51] Isolated involvement of the middle mediastinum was not encountered in an extensive review of the literature.[64] These lesions may extend into the neck. The lesions are almost always solitary, though multiple tumors have been reported. They are recognized radiologically as masses within the mediastinum. Phleboliths are an important diagnostic finding. They are seen in 10% of cases, or perhaps even more frequently if looked for carefully. Contrast opacification is another useful diagnostic feature.

Mixed lymphangioma/hemangioendothelioma is a variant of these disorders. The condition may be widespread in the body. When encountered in the chest, the malformation may involve the mediastinum, pleura, and chest wall as a single continuous lesion causing widespread lobular soft tissue swelling, bone destruction, and chylous pleural effusion. This destructive form of the disease is known as Gorham's disease. Cystic angiomatosis is another, probably separate, form of widespread lymphangiomatosis[36] in which lymphangiomas and hemangiomas may coexist. Many different sites in the body are involved, including the mediastinum, pericardium, and pleura. Multiple lytic lesions may be seen in the bones.[136] The condition is most frequently seen in children and young adults.

Traumatic lymphoceles, also known as chylous pseudocysts, are rare lesions that may follow trauma, particularly surgery.[189] Radiographically, they present as an enlarging mediastinal mass. CT scanning demonstrates a low density cystic mass.[189, 287]

FIG 15–35.
Lymphangioma (cystic hygroma) of mediastinum. This lesion is so large that, unusually, it displaces the great vessels and the trachea backward. The CT scan shows mixed density with large water density areas. The patient, a newborn child, presented with respiratory distress. **A,** PA radiograph. **B,** lateral radiograph. **C,** contrast-enhanced CT scan.

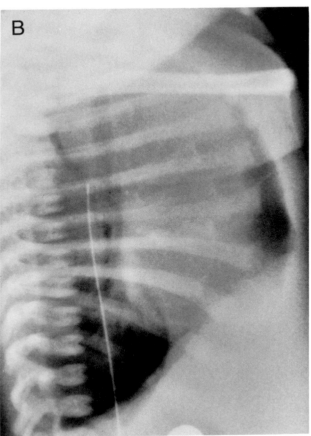

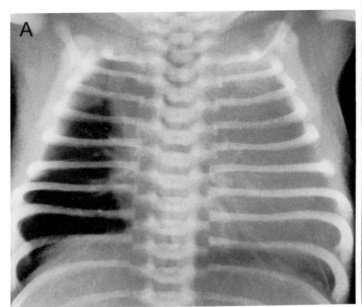

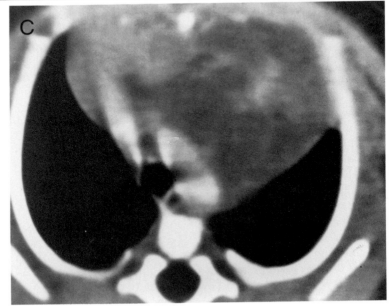

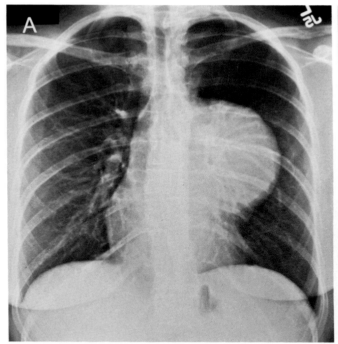

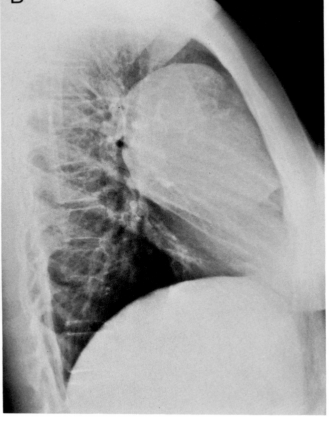

FIG 15–36.
Hemangioma of the anterior mediastinum in an asymptomatic 25-year-old woman. The mass has no specific radiologic features. **A,** PA radiograph. **B,** lateral radiograph.

Mediastinal Lipomatosis

Excessive deposition of fat may give rise to mediastinal widening, a condition sometimes known as mediastinal lipomatosis.[140, 148] When part of generalized obesity, the widening is fairly uniform and does not pose a diagnostic problem. However, in patients on steroid therapy and in those with Cushing's disease, focal collections of fat occur in many sites in the body, including the mediastinum.[241, 294] A similar phenomenon may occasionally be encountered as an incidental finding in patients with normal steroid hormone levels.[116] The usual appearance is a smooth widening of the superior mediastinum, without tracheal deformity. It may not be possible to say with certainty that the widening is of fat density from plain radiographs, but at CT the low density of fat is obvious (Fig 15–37).[22, 116, 286] If the fat deposition is symmetrical and, particularly, if it is widespread in the mediastinum, there is no diagnostic difficulty even if the only available examinations are plain radiographs. The fact that the fat pads in the costophrenic angles are also often enlarged is a helpful diagnostic feature. In those cases where the process is focal, CT scanning is indicated to distinguish

fat from neoplasm.[245] This diagnostic problem arises most often in patients with lymphoma who are being treated with steroids.

There is a rare condition called multiple symmetrical lipomatosis that resembles mediastinal lipomatosis, but is linked to a specific biochemical abnormality in which multiple masses of benign fat may compress mediastinal structures, notably the trachea.[83]

Fatty Tumors

True mediastinal tumors of fatty origin are uncommon, forming less than 1% of the series of 1,064 surgically proved cases of mediastinal masses.[331] On plain film, they present as well-defined round or oval mediastinal masses. The benign lipoma is soft and will not, therefore, compress surrounding structures unless it is very large. The moulding to the mediastinal contour may be so extreme that a large mediastinal lipoma may mimic cardiomegaly.[273] CT will show uniform fat density apart from a few strands of soft tissue.[200] Lipoblastoma, a benign tumor of childhood, may show a few more soft tissue

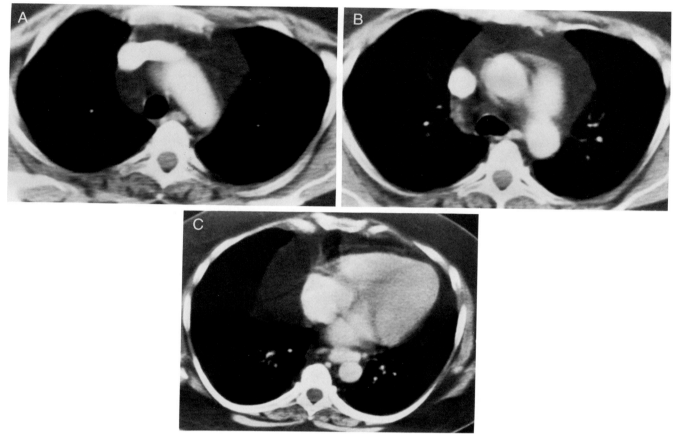

FIG 15–37.
A–C, mediastinal lipomatosis in a 47-year-old woman with Cushing's disease. Note the masslike accumulations of fat on three representative sections of the mediastinum in this typical example. Contrast-enhanced CT scans.

strands.[29, 257] In virtually every case, liposarcomas show inhomogeneity of the fat and often contain large areas of soft tissue density (Fig 15–38). Other fat-containing mediastinal tumors are teratomas (see p. 718) and thymolipomas (see p. 715).

Herniation of Abdominal Fat

Herniation of omental and perigastric fat is the most common cause of localized fatty masses in the mediastinum. The fat may herniate through the esophageal hiatus, the foramen of Morgagni, or the foramen of Bochdalek. Such herniations are usually readily diagnosed on plain films because of their characteristic locations. At CT, a CT density in the fat range eliminates confusion with other mediastinal masses.

Aggressive Fibromatosis

Aggressive fibromatosis is a locally invasive, nonmetastasizing tumor of fibrous origin that primarily

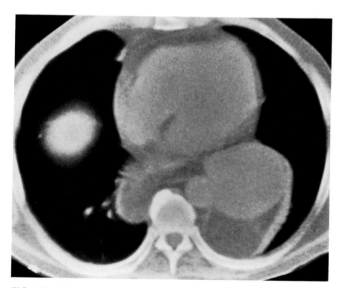

FIG 15–38.
Liposarcoma of the mediastinum. The fat density component indicates the fatty origin of the tumor; the soft tissue component within the tumor indicates its malignant nature. Contrast-enhanced CT scans.

involves the soft tissues of the extremities, neck, and trunk.[1] This tumor may, very rarely, be found in the mediastinum (Fig 15–39).[28] Plain radiographs show a soft tissue mass and may show periosteal reaction or cortical erosion of adjacent bone. CT scanning shows a mass which is isodense with skeletal muscle on precontrast images and is slightly hyperdense compared with muscle after the administration of intravenous contrast material. These masses are very vascular at angiography.[149]

Mediastinal and Hilar Adenopathy

Conventional imaging, CT, MRI, and radionuclide imaging are all capable of demonstrating intrathoracic lymphadenopathy, but plain radiography and CT scanning have become the standard techniques. With these modalities the two basic signs of intrathoracic lymphadenopathy are calcification and/or enlargement. CT is more sensitive than plain radiography in the detection of both signs and may on occasion show additional features, such as areas of decreased density within enlarged lymph nodes or evidence of invasion of the adjacent mediastinal fat. The place of MRI in the detection and diagnosis of intrathoracic lymphadenopathy is not yet clear (see p. 749). Conventional tomography is now rarely used for the evaluation of mediastinal and hilar lymph node enlargement. Although it is comparable with CT in demonstrating hilar adenopathy, CT is still the preferable technique because the state of the mediastinal nodes is so often of equal, if not greater importance, in making management decisions.[112]

To date, the best radionuclide agent is gallium 67, which localizes primarily in neoplastic or inflammatory tissue. But radionuclide imaging is rarely used nowadays in the detection of intrathoracic lymphadenopathy because, compared with CT, its sensitivity is low.

Intrathoracic Lymph Node Calcification

Intrathoracic lymph node calcification is common following tuberculous and certain fungal infections (Fig 15–40), and is also seen in other benign

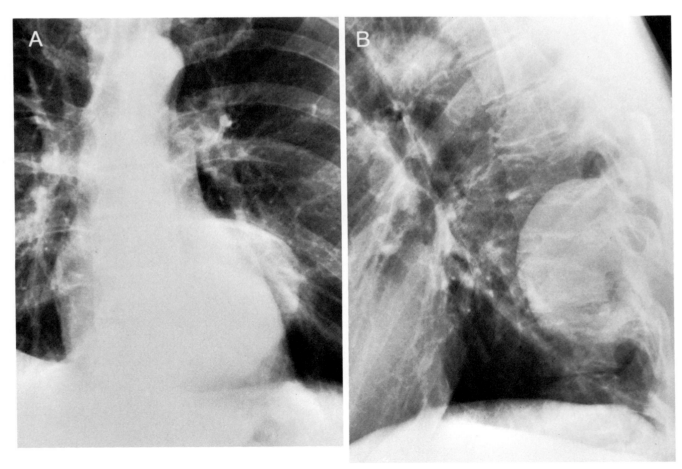

FIG 15–39.
Aggressive fibromatosis in a 34-year-old man. **A,** PA radiograph. **B,** lateral radiograph.

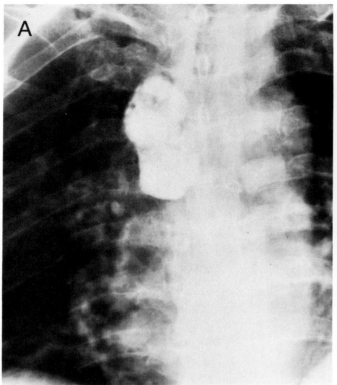 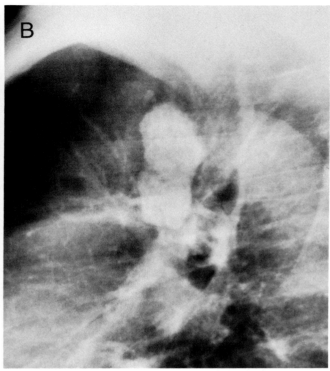

FIG 15–40.
Lymph node calcification following histoplasmosis. The large size of the nodal mass illustrates just how large infectious granulom- atous lymph nodes can be. **A,** PA radiograph. **B,** lateral radiograph.

conditions such as sarcoidosis, silicosis, and amyloidosis. Calcification, which may be the eggshell type of calcification, is not infrequent in the later stages of sarcoidosis. In one series, 17% of 111 patients eventually developed calcified intrathoracic lymph nodes.[152]

Lymph node calcification is very rarely the result of neoplastic disease. There are single case reports of calcification in metastatic bronchioloalveolar carcinoma of the lung[194] and untreated Hodgkin's disease,[332] but these cases are clearly isolated exceptions to a useful general rule that lymph node calcification is not a feature of either primary or secondary lymph node neoplasms. Tumor-bearing nodes may, however, calcify following radiation therapy. This unusual phenomenon occurs most frequently in patients treated for lymphoma.

CT will demonstrate more calcification than plain film techniques. Because calcification is not visible at MRI, an important sign of benign lymph node disease is not available with MR imaging.[178]

The two common patterns of calcification are coarse, irregularly distributed clumps within the node and homogeneous calcification of the whole node. Sometimes there is a ring of calcification at the periphery of the node—the so-called eggshell calcification (Fig 15–41). Eggshell calcification is a particular feature of prolonged exposure to dust in coal and metal mines and of sarcoidosis.[152, 153] It was seen in 3% of those who had worked in the coal industry for more than 30 years.[153] Eggshell calcification is rare in other conditions but has been reported in amyloidosis, histoplasmosis, blastomycosis, and treated Hodgkin's disease.[129]

Causes of Intrathoracic Lymph Node Enlargement

There are many causes of mediastinal and hilar lymph node enlargement—notably neoplasms, infection, sarcoidosis, and reactive hyperplasia. The infective group consists predominantly of tuberculosis and fungal disease, particularly histoplasmosis and coccidioidomycosis, each of which may cause intrathoracic adenopathy without visible pneumonia. Hilar adenopathy may also be seen in the late stages of cystic fibrosis. Hilar/mediastinal adenopathy is rare in other infections, especially in the absence of visible consolidation in the lungs. It may be seen in

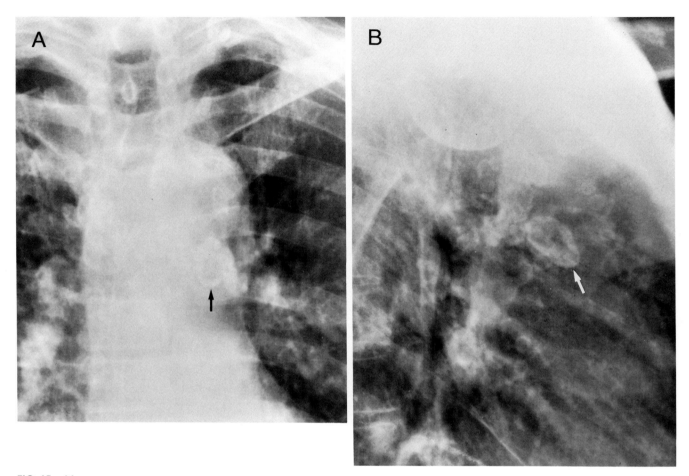

FIG 15–41.
Eggshell calcification *(arrow)* in mediastinal lymph nodes in a patient with long-standing amyloidosis. **A,** PA radiograph. **B,** lateral radiograph.

tularemia, whooping cough, anthrax and plague, and in mycoplasmal and viral infections. The neoplastic group includes malignant lymphoma, leukemia, and metastatic carcinoma—carcinoma of the bronchus, esophagus, and breast being the usual primary sites. If the primary tumor is extrathoracic, then kidney, testis, and head and neck tumors are the most likely origins.[196]

Intrathoracic lymphadenopathy may occasionally result from a variety of other disorders, including silicosis, Castleman's disease, angioimmunoblastic lymphadenopathy, amyloidosis, multiple myeloma,[157] chronic berylliosis, histiocytosis X, and mixed connective tissue disease.[131] The differential diagnosis of mediastinal and hilar node enlargement is, therefore, wide.

The associated features may point to one or other diagnosis (e.g., a known neoplasm in the lung or elsewhere) or to a previously established diagnosis of a systemic disease known to cause intrathoracic adenopathy. In many instances, however, biopsy is required to establish the specific diagnosis. Sarcoidosis is a particularly frequent cause of intrathoracic lymphadenopathy, particularly in young adults. It becomes much the most likely diagnosis when multiple node groups are involved and the adenopathy is symmetrically distributed in the hili and mediastinum in a young patient who either has no symptoms or has clinical features consistent with sarcoidosis. Lymphoma is often a major concern in such patients, but lymphoma is rarely so symmetrically distributed with equal involvement of the hili and the mediastinal lymph node groups. When doubt exists, biopsy is essential.

Only reactive hyperplasia, Castleman's disease, and angioimmunoblastic lymphadenopathy will be discussed further; the other diseases that cause lymphadenopathy are dealt with elsewhere in this book.

Reactive hyperplasia is a term which covers an acute or chronic, nonspecific inflammatory response in which both inflammation and hyperplasia are present. Lymph nodes undergo reactive changes whenever challenged by infection, cell debris, or foreign substances. Thus reactive hyperplasia is seen in nodes draining areas of pulmonary infection, in a variety of other inflammatory diseases, and also in nodes draining neoplasms. Generalized acute reactive inflammation is seen with virus infections and bacteremia.

Castleman's disease[46] (synonyms: giant lymph node hyperplasia, angiofollicular lymph node hyperplasia, angiomatous lymphoid hamartoma) is a variety of lymph node hyperplasia of particular interest to chest radiologists because the usual hyaline vascular type presents most frequently as an asymptomatic mass of mediastinal lymph nodes that may be as much as 20 cm in diameter. The mass may press on mediastinal structures, causing pressure symptoms. The less frequent plasma cell variety has been associated with fever, fatigue, anemia, gammaglobulin abnormalities, and elevated levels of lactic dehydrogenase.[163] Castleman's disease may occur in patients of any age but frequently strikes young adults. It may be multifocal and can involve extrathoracic lymph nodes. Its cause is uncertain, but it may be a chronic inflammatory response to as yet undefined antigens. Recently, a multicentric form with a high association with Kaposi's sarcoma of the skin has been reported.[48, 101] Acquired immune deficiency syndrome may be the underlying factor in these cases. Histologically, the hyaline form shows a follicular structure, the nodules consisting predominantly of small lymphocytes with large numbers of blood vessels in the interfollicular areas, whereas the plasma cell type shows sheets of interfollicular cells and fewer blood vessels.[163] The entity can be confused histologically with malignant lymphoma or with thymoma. Surgical excision is curative if the lesion is completely removed.[222]

Radiologically,[158, 222] the disorder presents as lobulated, well-defined, large masses of lymph nodes in the mediastinum or proximal hilus (Fig 15–42). Calcification has been reported.[237] The masses may extend into the neck or retroperitoneum and are very vascular at angiography.[222, 307]

The few cases examined by CT[96, 108, 224] showed soft tissue density with marked uniform contrast enhancement of the mass, a feature that could help in the differential diagnosis from cyst, thymoma, and lymphoma (Fig 15–43).

Angioimmunoblastic lymphadenopathy (immuno-blastic lymphadenopathy) is another variety of lymph node hyperplasia that may also be confused with lymphoma.[182] It is a systemic disorder with a high mortality, seen chiefly in individuals over 50 years of age and characterized by fever, weight loss and generalized lymphadenopathy, hepatosplenomegaly, a maculopapular rash, hypergammaglobulinemia, and a Coomb's positive hemolytic anemia.[243] It sometimes appears to be related to drug ingestion. On histologic examination, there is a combination of chronic inflammatory cellular infiltrate, hyperplasia of small blood vessels, and deposit of amorphous interstitial debris. The classification and nature of the condition are debated.[243] It may be caused by chronic antigenic stimulation inducing non-neoplastic proliferation of β lymphocytes. Immunoblastic sarcoma/lymphoma develops in approximately one-third of cases of angioimmunoblastic lymphadenopathy.[182, 219]

Paratracheal, anterior mediastinal, or hilar adenopathy are the most common radiologic manifestations[180, 182] (Fig 15–44). Widespread parenchymal shadows are frequent, and a reticulonodular pattern with septal lines may be seen.[340] Pulmonary nodules are also encountered, and pleural effusions are not uncommon.

Recognition of Mediastinal and Hilar Lymph Node Enlargement

The ease with which intrathoracic lymph node enlargement can be diagnosed depends on the particular location[141] and the imaging technique being used.

Conventional Techniques.— Few studies have specifically addressed how large the lymph nodes need to be in order to be visible on plain film. (The discussion here focuses on the plain chest radiograph; plain film tomography provides essentially similar information, but with greater clarity.) It would appear that most nodes with a short-axis diameter greater than 2 cm give rise to visible mediastinal widening if they lie in the right paratracheal area, the aortopulmonary window, the hilar regions, or the paravertebral areas. Pretracheal, left paratracheal, and subcarinal nodes may be larger than 2 cm without being visible on plain chest radiograph.[212]

Enlargement of the right upper paratracheal nodes[213] (Fig 15–45) (station 2R of the American Thoracic Society nomenclature[298]; see Chapter 3) causes uniform or lobular widening of the right tracheal stripe. The density of the superior vena cava increases and may equal that of the aortic knob.

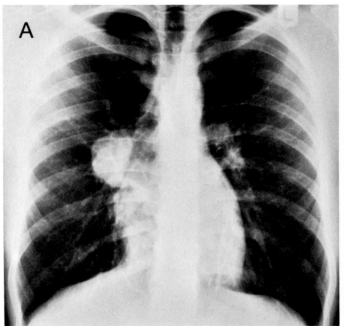

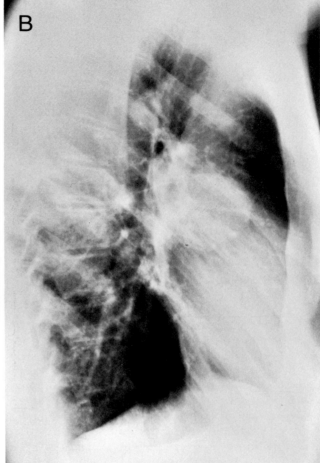

FIG 15–42.
Castleman's disease causing massive right hilar adenopathy. **A,** PA radiograph. **B,** lateral radiograph.

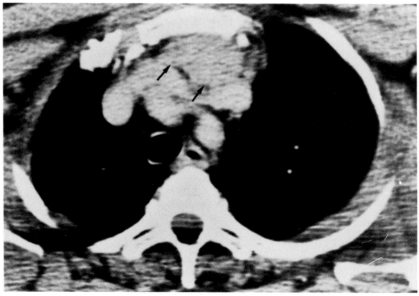

FIG 15–43.
Castleman's disease. Contrast-enhanced CT scan illustrates the enlarged anterior mediastinal lymph nodes *(arrows)* that enhanced with administration of intravenous contrast material.

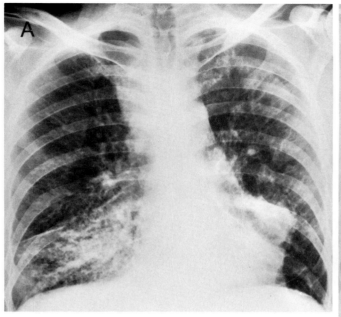

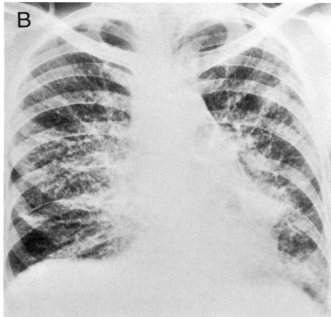

FIG 15—44.
Angioimmunoblastic lymphadenopathy in a 42-year-old man with generalized lymphadenopathy and hepatosplenomegaly. **A,** there is obvious enlargement of right and left paratracheal lymph nodes as well as the paracardiac nodes. The parenchymal reticu-

lonodular shadowing is chiefly confined to the right base. **B,** 6 months later, after an initial dramatic response to steroid therapy, the reticulonodular shadowing is seen in all lung zones. (Courtesy of Dr. Keith Simpkins, Leeds, England.)

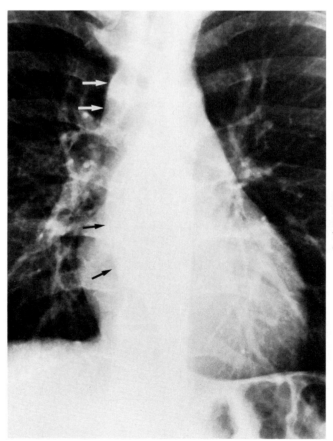

FIG 15—45.
Right paratracheal adenopathy *(white arrows)* resulting from Hodgkin's disease. The right paratracheal stripe is widened, and the right paratracheal area is as dense as the aortic knob. There is also massive subcarinal adenopathy *(black arrows).*

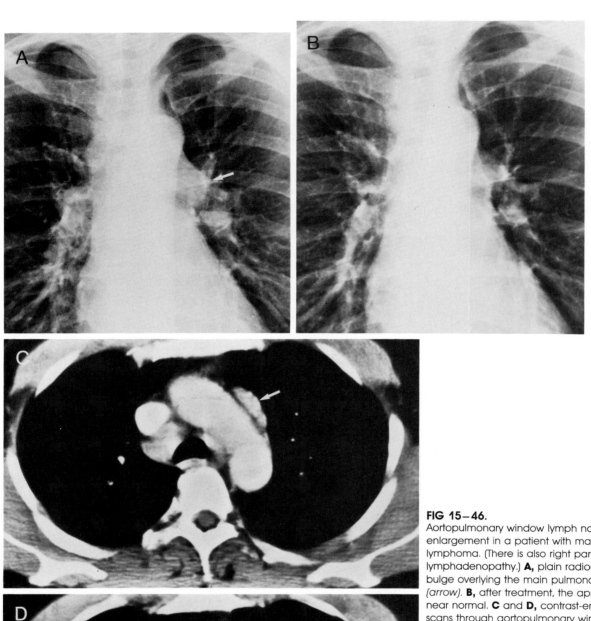

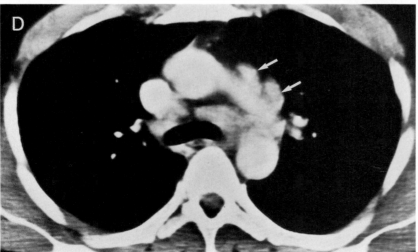

FIG 15–46.
Aortopulmonary window lymph node enlargement in a patient with malignant lymphoma. (There is also right paratracheal lymphadenopathy.) **A,** plain radiograph shows a bulge overlying the main pulmonary artery *(arrow).* **B,** after treatment, the appearance is near normal. **C** and **D,** contrast-enhanced CT scans through aortopulmonary window and aortic arch show the many enlarged nodes *(arrows).* (The right paratracheal adenopathy is also demonstrated.)

Normally, the density of the superior vena cava in the right paratracheal area is significantly less than that of the aortic arch. With substantial paratracheal adenopathy, the border of the superior vena cava may be convex, rather than flat or concave as in the normal. When the right lower paratracheal (azygos) nodes (Station 4R) enlarge, they push the azygos vein laterally so that the diameter of the combined shadows of the node and the vein enlarges proportionately (the diameter of the normal vein on an upright chest film should be 7 mm or less).[161]

If the aortopulmonary nodes (Station 5) project beyond the aortopulmonary window, they cause a bulge in the angle between the aortic arch and the main pulmonary artery[30] (Fig 15–46). Nodes beside the aortic arch will be visible as bulges even when relatively small (Fig 15–47). The left upper paratracheal (Station 2L) nodes have to be substantially enlarged if they are to cause mediastinal widening on plain chest radiograph since, to be visible, they have to project beyond the left carotid and left subclavian arteries. Those nodes anterior to the trachea (Stations 2 and 4) will have to be even larger before they cause visible deformity.

The most useful sign of subcarinal node (Station 7) enlargement on plain film is displacement of the azygoesophageal line (see Fig 15–45). This interface is normally concave towards the lung. Subcarinal lymph node masses change the contour from concave to convex. Alteration of the contour of the azygoesophageal recess is, unfortunately, a relatively insensitive sign of subcarinal adenopathy. It occurred in only 23% of the cases with subcarinal adenopathy reported by Muller et al.[212] Two other plain film signs of subcarinal adenopathy are described: increased opacity, and lack of visibility of the external surface of the medial wall of the right main-stem bronchus and the bronchus intermedius.[212] Though more sensitive, these signs are difficult to use because they are so nonspecific. Because the esophagus passes immediately behind the carina, subcarinal node enlargement will cause posterior displacement of the esophagus. If the nodes are very large, the esophagus will slip laterally. The hallmark of adenopathy, namely lobulation, is not always evident and, if the borders of the lymph node mass are smooth, the appearance may resemble left atrial enlargement both on plain films and at barium swallow examination.

To be recognizable on plain chest radiograph, enlargement of the anterior mediastinal nodes—that is, nodes anterior to the aorta, innominate artery, and trachea—must be substantial (Fig 15–48).

With enlargement of these nodes, mediastinal widening is frequently bilateral and lobulated in outline. Sometimes the only sign of enlargement is increased opacity of the retrosternal area on the lateral view, a sign that is difficult to evaluate because it is also seen in some healthy people with abundant mediastinal fat. Enlargement of the anterior intercostal nodes is easiest to recognize on the lateral chest radiograph as extrapleural soft tissue swelling along the course of the internal mammary arteries.

Enlarged paraesophageal nodes and posterior mediastinal nodes (Stations 8 and 9) produce displacement of the azygoesophageal and paraspinal lines (Fig 15–49). The plain chest radiograph is relatively insensitive in detecting enlarged nodes to the left of, or posterior to, the esophagus. Such nodes may be recognized at the barium swallow study by the appearance of localized indentations on the esophagus.

Recognizing hilar lymph node enlargement on plain chest radiographs and conventional tomography requires an understanding of the normal hilar anatomy (see Chapter 3). The basic signs are hilar enlargement, lobulation of outline, or the presence of a rounded mass of tissue in a portion of the hili that does not contain major vascular trunks[211] (Fig 15–50). In those portions of the hili that contain the major blood vessels (e.g., the crossover point of the right superior pulmonary vein and the descending limb of the right pulmonary artery) hilar node enlargement has to be substantial if it is to be recognized. Similarly the inferior poles of both hili, where the inferior pulmonary veins intermingle with the segmental divisions of the lower lobe arteries, are another particularly difficult region to interpret. By contrast, even mild nodal enlargement can be recognized, at least on lateral tomography, when the enlarged nodes lie posterior to the right main bronchus and the bronchus intermedius (see Fig 15–50), because in this region, the lung normally contacts the posterior wall of the airway. Another sensitive site to search for hilar adenopathy on lateral projection is in the angles formed by the middle lobe or lingula bronchus and the lower lobe bronchi (Fig 15–51). It is often possible to measure the transverse diameter of the lower lobe arteries, which should be no greater than 16 mm. Lymphadenopathy adjacent to these vessels will increase the diameter of the hilus and create a lobular as opposed to a tubular configuration (Fig 15–52). Lymphadenopathy in the upper portions of the hili is often easy to recognize because the vessels in these regions are normally small and the nodes therefore stand out.

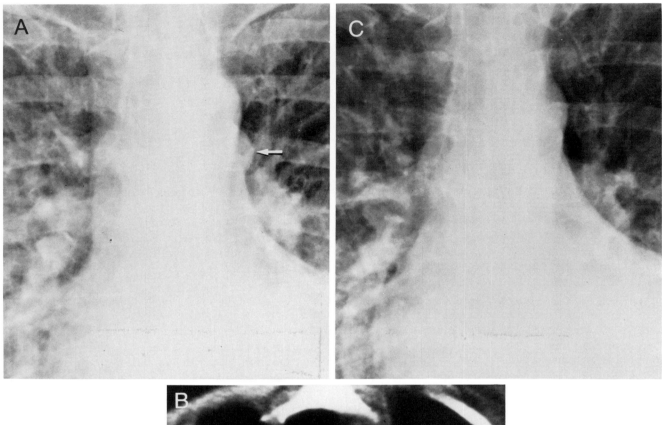

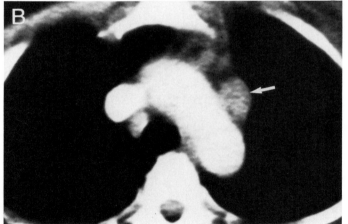

FIG 15–47.
Aortopulmonary window lymph node enlargement as a result of metastatic breast carcinoma. **A,** plain radiograph demonstrates a small bulge *(arrow)* just beneath aortic knob. **B,** in the contrast-enhanced CT scan there is an enlarged node *(arrow)* projecting to the left of the aortic arch. **C,** following treatment, the appearance of the aortopulmonary window region has returned to normal.

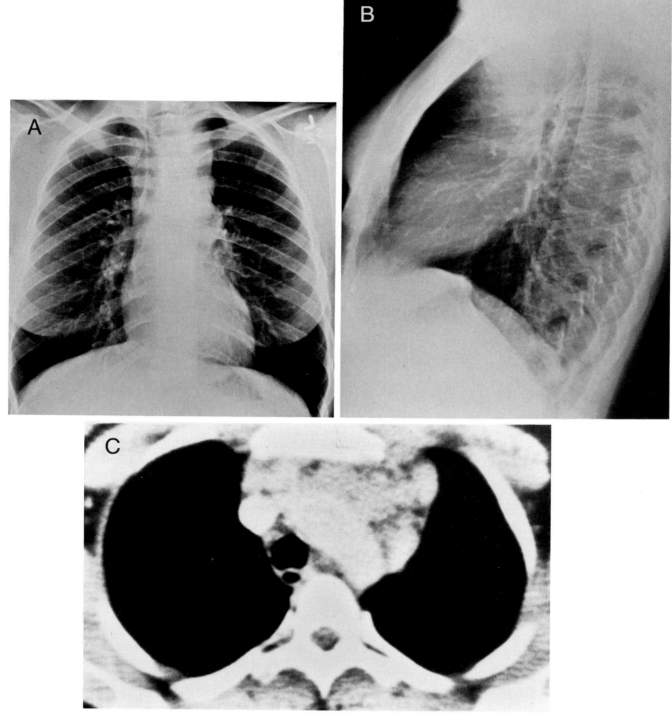

FIG 15–48.
Anterior (prevascular) mediastinal lymph node enlargement due to lymphoma. **A,** PA radiograph shows lobular left-sided widening of the upper mediastinum and aortopulmonary window. **B,** lateral radiograph shows ill-defined increase in density in the anterior mediastinum. **C,** contrast-enhanced CT scan shows massive lymphadenopathy, predominantly anterior to and to the left of the aortic arch.

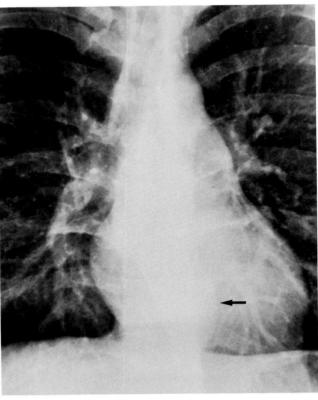

FIG 15–49.
Enlarged paraesophageal and posterior mediastinal lymph nodes
(arrow) in a patient with Hodgkin's disease.

It may, at times, be very difficult to distinguish enlarged hilar lymph nodes from the enlargement of the hilar arteries resulting from pulmonary hypertension (Fig 15–53). The analysis should center on determining whether the enlargement is truly centered on the pulmonary arteries (any mass in a site that is normally devoid of vessels would clearly favor the diagnosis of lymphadenopathy) and on evaluating the degree of lobulation, because the central pulmonary arteries, even when large, should retain their basically tubular configuration.

Computed Tomography.—The CT signs of lymphadenopathy are an increase in size of the nodes, focal bulges or lobulations of the mediastinum-lung interface, recognizable invasion of surrounding mediastinal fat, coalescence of enlarged nodes to form larger masses, and diffuse soft tissue density throughout the mediastinum obliterating the mediastinal fat. In general, the detection of lymph node enlargement depends on recognizing round or oval soft-tissue densities in the mediastinum or hili that are not the result of vascular structures (Fig 15–54). This distinction requires a secure knowledge of the normal arrangement of blood vessels and an understanding of the various anomalies and variations in the arrangement of the mediastinal vessels. Enhancement with intravenous contrast material may be needed to help distinguish vessels from lymph nodes in selected cases.

To date, three series have measured normal lymph node size at CT scanning.[107, 110, 262] In summary, they showed that nodes less than 10 mm in short-axis diameter lie within the 95th percentile and should be considered normal. Nodes between 10 and 15 mm in short-axis diameter occur in certain sites, notably the subcarinal and tracheobronchial regions, in 5% to 7% of healthy subjects. Short-axis diameter is the standard measurement because it shows the best correlation with lymph node volume at autopsy.[247]

It is easier to identify and measure right-sided mediastinal lymph nodes than to evaluate the left-sided nodes, because of the more abundant mediastinal fat and less complex vascular anatomy on the right side.[247] Two regions that are frequently difficult to analyze are the subcarinal and hilar areas.

The cardinal signs of subcarinal lymph node enlargement at CT (Fig 15–55) are (1) a soft tissue mass between the esophagus and either the left atrium or the intramediastinal portions of the right or left pulmonary arteries, and (2) a soft tissue den-

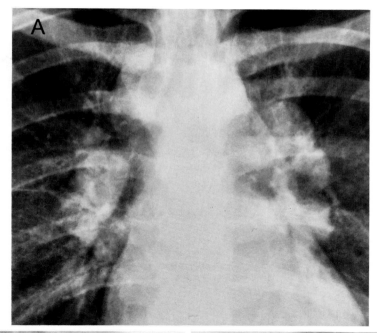

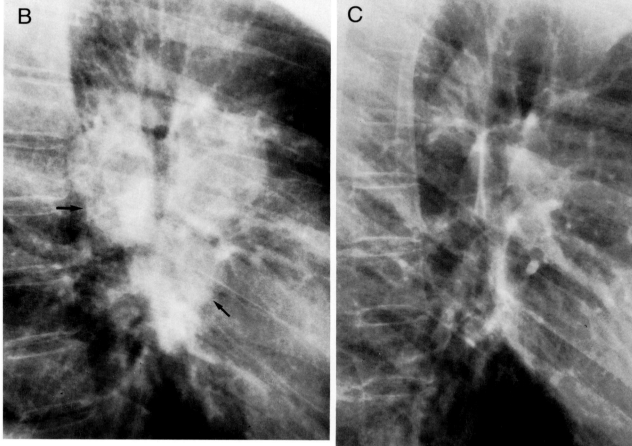

FIG 15–50.
Lobular enlargement of the hili owing to enlarged lymph nodes in a patient with sarcoidosis. **A,** PA radiograph. **B,** lateral radiograph. Recognizing the adenopathy in this example is easy, but when there is doubt it is useful to examine the lateral projection for rounded densities in areas that are devoid of vessels. *Arrows* point to two such areas: namely, posterior to the bronchus intermedius, and anterior to the lower lobe bronchus below the level of the middle lobe bronchus. **C,** a comparison lateral radiograph in another patient shows the normal anatomy.

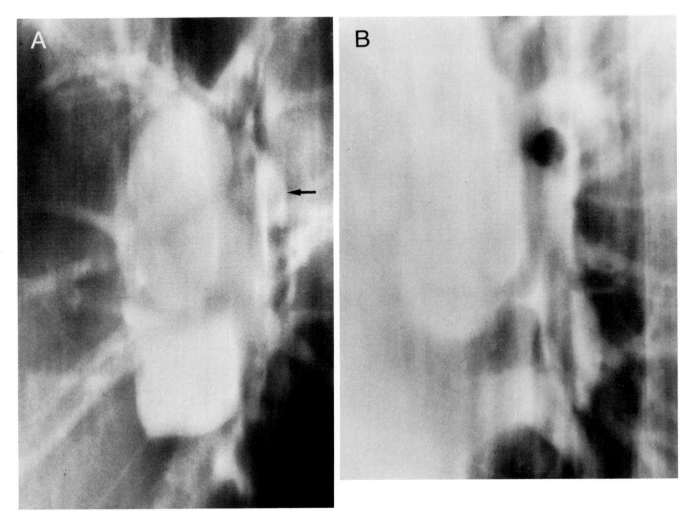

FIG 15–51.
A, lateral tomogram of a patient with sarcoidosis demonstrates a small node posterior to the bronchus intermedius *(arrow)*. Note also the very large nodes in the angle between the lower and middle lobe bronchi. **B,** lateral tomogram of right hilus in a patient with normal anatomy.

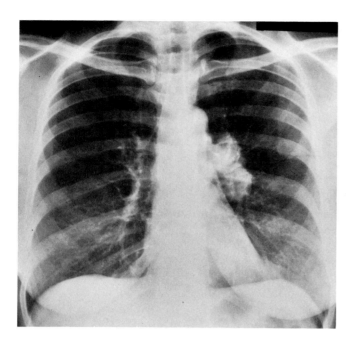

FIG 15–52.
Left hilar lymph node enlargement due to metastases from a bronchial carcinoma in the left lower lobe; typical lobular enlargement of the left hilus is seen.

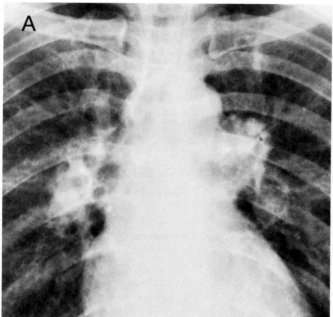

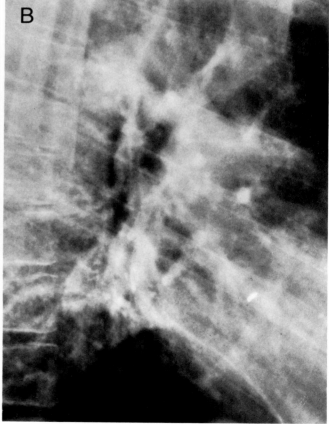

FIG 15–53.
Enlarged hilar arteries in a patient with pulmonary hypertension resulting from chronic pulmonary thromboembolism. The differentiation from hilar lymphadenopathy is best made by noting that the hilar enlargement is not lobular and is centered on those portions of the hili occupied by the lobar divisions of the pulmonary arteries. **A,** PA radiograph. **B,** lateral radiograph.

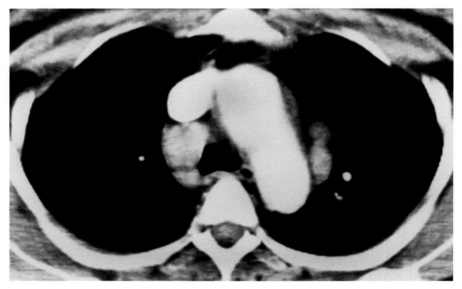

FIG 15–54.
Mediastinal lymphadenopathy demonstrated by CT (contrast enhanced). There is substantial enlargement of the right paratra-cheal lymph nodes and moderate enlargement of the prevascular nodes to the left of the aortic arch.

sity bulging into the azygoesophageal recess posterior to the bronchus intermedius and the left lower lobe bronchus.

The recognition of hilar node enlargement at CT is greatly facilitated by opacification of the hilar vessels with intravenous contrast material.[113] In general, lymph nodes do not enhance to any recognizable degree, whereas with good technique (see p. 703), the blood vessels enhance brightly. Any nonenhancing hilar tissue larger than 5 mm in short-axis diameter is considered abnormal.[114] If enhancement is uncertain or if the examination is performed without contrast material, then the recognition of nodal enlargement depends on demonstrating rounded soft tissue densities that are too large to be blood vessels (Fig 15–56).[6, 215, 216, 309] The required size will vary according to location. Some portions of the hilus are normally devoid of vessels greater than 5 mm in diameter; in others, the vessel diameters may be 15 mm, or even greater if there is increased pulmonary blood flow or pulmonary arterial hypertension. The most sensitive site to examine for lymph node enlargement is the region immediately behind the right main-stem bronchus and its divisions (the right upper lobe bronchus and the bronchus intermedius) because in these regions, the lung contacts the posterior wall of the bronchial tree[312] (Fig 15–56). The equivalent area on the left is partially occupied by the descending aorta and the descending left pulmonary artery and, therefore, only a small tongue of lung can contact the posterior wall of the left main bronchus.[308] The most difficult and, therefore, least sensitive area to evaluate is the central portion of the right hilus, where the right superior pulmonary vein passes directly anterior to the right pulmonary artery and its major divisions. Additionally, there are fat pads at the bifurcation of the

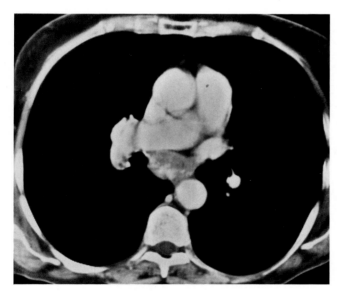

FIG 15–55.
Subcarinal mediastinal adenopathy resulting from metastatic bronchial carcinoma. The mass of nodes interposes between the descending aorta and esophagus (not seen as a separate structure) posteriorly, and the right pulmonary artery anteriorly. Note also that the lymph node mass causes a convex bulge into the azygoesophageal recess of lung. Contrast-enhanced CT scan.

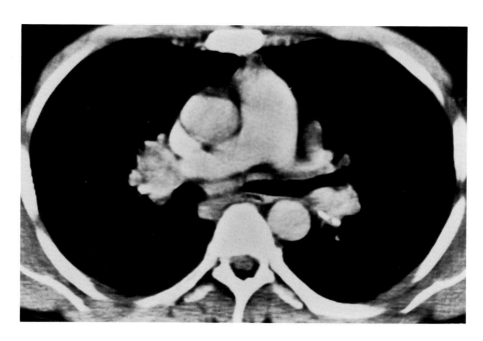

FIG 15–56.
Bilateral hilar adenopathy as a result of lymphoma. The right hilus shows lobular swelling that cannot be accounted for by the normal vascular structures (right pulmonary artery and right superior pulmonary vein). Similarly, the bulk of tissue posterior to the left bronchial tree is too great to be accounted for by the descending branch of the left pulmonary artery. (There is also subcarinal and aortopulmonary window adenopathy.) Contrast-enhanced CT scan.

right pulmonary artery that can resemble lymph node enlargement. It is usually impossible to recognize the fatty nature of these pads because of partial volume averaging with the adjacent arteries and lung.

Magnetic Resonance Imaging.— Hilar adenopathy is easier to recognize at MRI than at CT scanning[8, 178, 311] because in the healthy person the signal arises from the walls of the blood vessels and bronchi and from the small amount of fat and connective tissue that surrounds the hilar structures. No signal is generated by fast-flowing blood within the hilar blood vessels, nor is any signal generated from air within the bronchi. Hilar adenopathy, therefore, stands out as a relatively high signal of rounded or oval configuration against a background of low signal (Fig 15–57).

With current machines, MRI and CT scans provide comparable information regarding mediastinal lymphadenopathy (Fig 15–58). With standard MRI sequences the imaging times are long and motion, therefore, degrades the image. It is frequently difficult to measure the diameter of lymph nodes, and it may be impossible to distinguish a cluster of small normal nodes from a single enlarged node.[7, 178] An advantage of MRI is that

fast-flowing blood in the larger arteries and veins can be recognized as signal void, and consequently blood vessels are often easily distinguished from lymph nodes. But sometimes the averaging of low signal from flowing blood and high signal from fat may mean that a blood vessel partially in the volume is imaged as a rounded area with a signal similar to that of a soft tissue mass; it may thus closely resemble lymph node enlargement. This pitfall can be avoided by repeating the study, using a long repetition time (e.g., TR = 2,000 msec), so that the signal intensity of flowing blood remains very low, whereas the signal intensity of a soft tissue mass increases to approach that of mediastinal fat.[314] Another pitfall is that, with ECG gating of data acquisition, some images of the blood vessels will be obtained during periods of slow blood flow. Slow-flowing blood generates a signal that can be misinterpreted as a soft tissue mass.[320]

Pitfalls in the Diagnosis of Intrathoracic Lymph Node Enlargement

A variety of anatomic structures can be confused with mediastinal lymphadenopathy.[39, 115, 242] Some of these are illustrated in Figures 15–59 through 15–68.

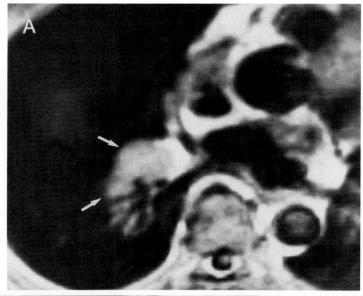

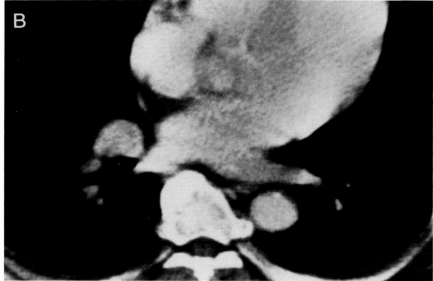

FIG 15–57.
MR image of right hilar *(arrows)* adenopathy. The high signal from the solid tissues stands out clearly against the signal void of air in the bronchi and lungs and the signal void of flowing blood in the left atrium and hilar blood vessels. **B,** Contrast-enhanced CT scan for comparison.

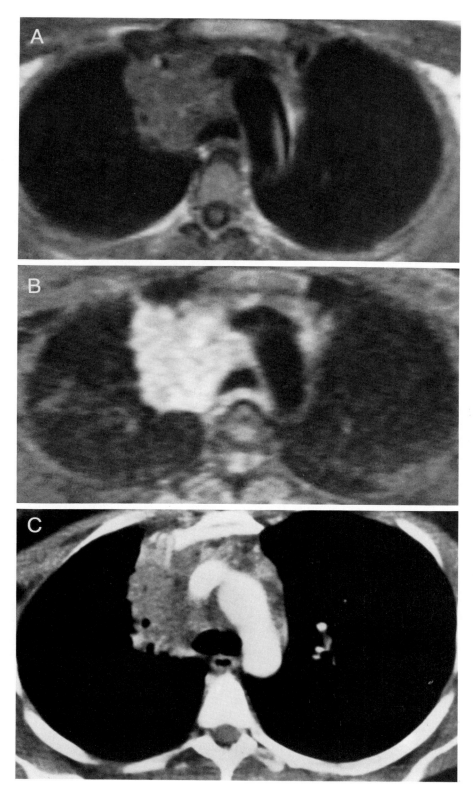

FIG 15–58.
Comparison of MRI and CT (contrast-enhanced) images of mediastinal adenopathy in a patient with Hodgkin's disease. On these axial images the information is comparable, but the compression of the right and left brachiocephalic veins is shown well without the need for intravenous contrast medium in the MR images. All images are at the same level. **A,** T1-weighted axial MR image. **B,** T2-weighted axial MR image. **C,** contrast-enhanced CT scan. (Courtesy of Dr. William C. Black, Washington, D.C.)

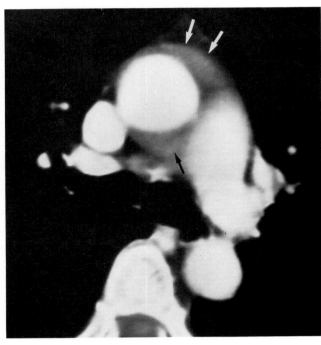

FIG 15–59.
Superior pericardial recesses anterior *(white arrows)* and posterior *(black arrow)* to the proximal descending aorta mimicking lymphadenopathy. Contrast-enhanced CT scan.

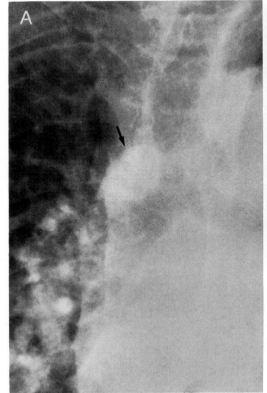

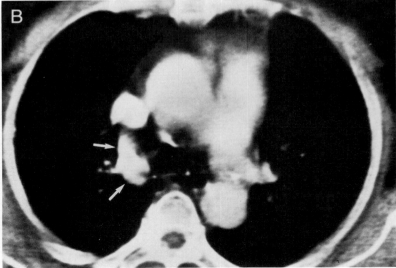

FIG 15–60.
A, the azygos vein in right tracheobronchial angle *(arrow)* is difficult to distinguish from an enlarged azygos node. **B,** contrast-enhanced CT scan of same patient demonstrates the large azygos vein *(arrows)*. No adenopathy was present on any of the sections.

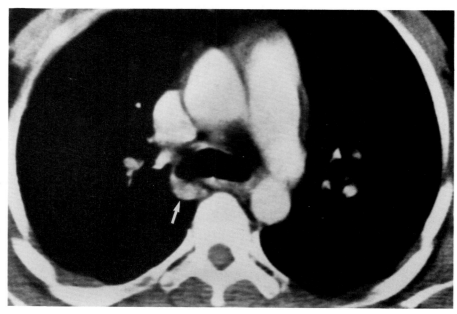

FIG 15–61.
Azygos vein lying posterior to the right main stem bronchus *(arrow)*, mimicking lymphadenopathy on CT scan. Note that even though good contrast opacification of the aorta, pulmonary ar-tery, and superior vena cava has been achieved, the azygos vein is poorly opacified.

Neural Tumors

Neural tumors can be divided into nerve sheath tumors and ganglion cell tumors. (Tumors of the paraganglionic cells are considered separately on p. 765).

The *nerve sheath tumors* comprise schwannomas (neurilemmoma), neurofibromas, and their malignant counterparts, the schwannoma being by far the most common intrathoracic nerve sheath tumor.[41, 248] All these tumors are more common in patients with neurofibromatosis. Though histologically distinct, both schwannomas and neurofibromas are derived from Schwann cells. In its classic form, the schwannoma is eccentric and encapsulated and has no nerve fibers passing through it, whereas the neurofibroma is unencapsulated and has nerve fibers scattered through the tumor. Patients with neurofibromatosis may develop large plexiform masses of neurofibromatous tissue in the mediastinum (Fig 15–69).[41, 47]

Almost all the intrathoracic nerve sheath tumors arise either from the intercostal (Fig 15–70) or the sympathetic nerves, the rare exceptions being neurofibromas or schwannomas of the phrenic or vagus nerves.[220] Many arise close to the spine and may extend through the neural exit foramina into the spinal canal (the so-called "dumbbell tu-mor"). Though dumbbell tumors are a much talked about phenomenon, they occur in less than 5% of cases.[102, 331]

Most nerve sheath tumors of the mediastinum (Fig 15–71) are benign and asymptomatic, usually being discovered incidentally on chest imaging. In contrast to ganglion cell tumors, they are rare in patients below age 20 and virtually nonexistent in patients who are less than 10 years old. The few cases that are encountered below this age are likely to be associated with neurofibromatosis. Malignant nerve sheath tumors are infrequent. They may cause pain and are usually associated with neurofibromatosis.

The *ganglion cell tumors* form a spectrum—with neuroblastoma at the malignant end and ganglioneuroma at the benign end, ganglioneuroblastoma being an intermediate form (Figs 15–72; 15–73 and 15–74). Neuroblastoma and ganglioneuroblastoma may occasionally mature into a more benign form.[2, 74] The mediastinum is the second most common primary site within the body for this spectrum of tumors, the adrenal gland being the most common. Approximately one-third to one-half of mediastinal neuroblastomas arise primarily in the mediastinum.[16, 79] The remainder are secondary to either lymph node metastases or to thoracic spread from a tumor arising primarily in the adrenal gland. Primary mediastinal neuroblastomas appear to have a

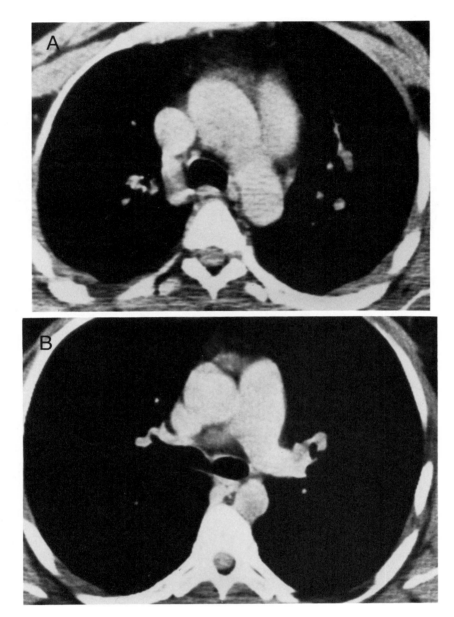

FIG 15–62.
A, high arching main and left pulmonary artery mimicking aorto-pulmonary lymphadenopathy. **B,** section 1 cm lower, illustrating the main and the left pulmonary arteries. Contrast-enhanced CT scans.

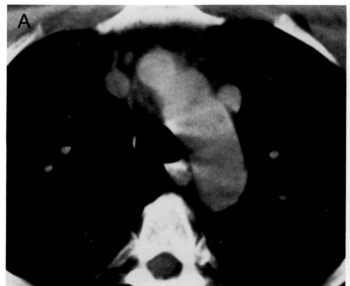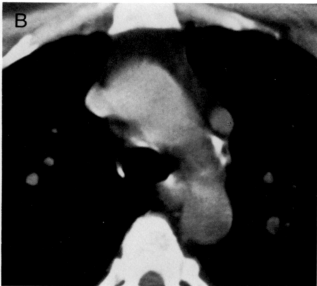

FIG 15–63.
A and **B,** persistent left superior vena cava mimicking anterior mediastinal/aortopulmonary lymphadenopathy. Confusion with lymphadenopathy is avoided once the tubular nature of the density is appreciated. The vein could be traced from the left brachiocephalic vein to the upper posterior margin of the left atrium. Non-contrast-enhanced images are illustrated since the confusion with lymphadenopathy is greatest prior to administration of contrast material.

better prognosis than those that arise primarily in the abdomen.[79, 95]

Neuroblastoma and ganglioneuroblastoma are essentially tumors of childhood,[234] fewer than 10% being seen in patients older than 20 years of age.[93, 248] In children below 1 year of age, a neural tumor is virtually certain to be one of these two types. Ganglioneuroma shows a wider and more even age distribution, which ranges from 1 to 50 years.[248]

Radiologic Features of Neurogenic Tumors

The common feature of all neurogenic tumors on plain films and CT scans[14, 93, 248] is a well-defined mass with a lobulated or smooth outline. These tumors may be almost any size; some are very large, occupying most of a hemithorax. Except for vagal and phrenic nerve tumors, and the occasional neuroblastoma, neural tumors are situated in the posterior mediastinum. Those that arise adjacent to the upper thoracic spine occupying the lung apex press down on the lung from above (see Figs 15–72 and 15–76).

Most neurogenic tumors are approximately spherical, but some ganglion cell tumors are elongated, the axis following the vertical orientation of the sympathetic chain. It may be possible to distinguish between a ganglion cell tumor and a nerve sheath tumor by observing the shape of the tumor mass, since the base of ganglion cell tumors may show a tapered interface with the adjacent chest wall or mediastinum, whereas nerve sheath tumors tend to show a sulcus at their margins.[296]

Calcification may be seen in all types of neural tumors (see Figs 15–73 and 15–74). Approximately 10% of primary mediastinal neuroblastomas are visibly calcified on plain chest radiograph,[79, 248] a figure considerably lower than that encountered with neuroblastoma arising in the adrenal gland. The incidence of calcification detectable at CT is substantially higher. In neuroblastoma the calcification is usually finely stippled, whereas in ganglioneuroblastoma and ganglioneuroma, it is denser and coarser, occurring most frequently in the larger, more benign lesions. Nerve sheath tumors calcify only occasionally. In the series of Reed et al.,[248] of 65 cases examined by plain chest radiography, only two examples were encountered, both of which were neurofibromas. In the 67 cases reported by Carey et al.,[41] calcification was seen 7 times; all 7 were schwannomas. In these cases, the calcification was curvilinear and lay in the walls of the larger masses; it can, however, be more widely distributed.[41]

An important diagnostic feature of neurogenic tumors is pressure erosion and displacement of the adjacent ribs and vertebrae (Figs 15–70; 15–72;

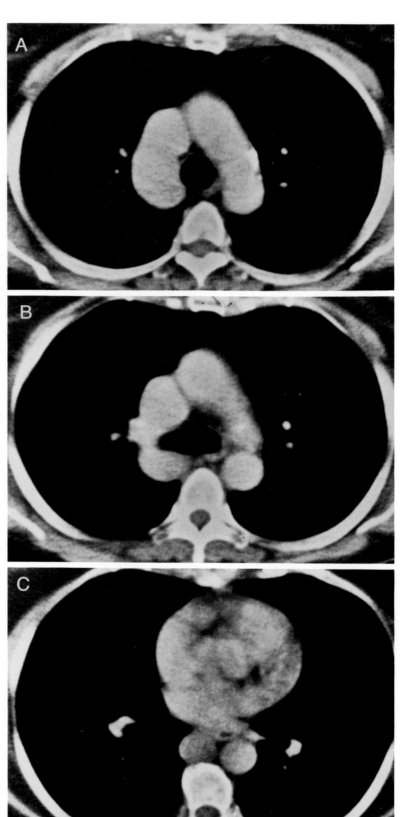

FIG 15–64.
A–C, azygos continuation of the inferior vena cava
(non-enhanced CT scans). The appearances on each
image viewed separately could be confused with a
mass or lymphadenopathy. Taken together, the
tubular nature and conformity to the anatomy of the
azygos vein are diagnostic of the condition.

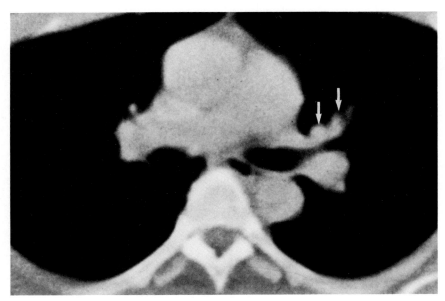

FIG 15–65.
Tributaries of the left superior pulmonary vein *(arrows)* mimicking lymph nodes anterior to the left upper lobe bronchus. Contrast-enhanced CT scan.

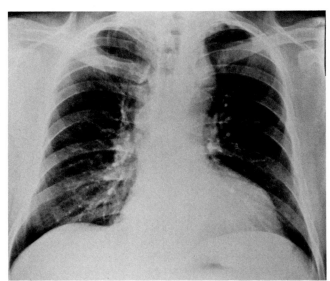

FIG 15–66.
Pseudocoarctation of the aorta mimicking a left-sided superior mediastinal mass. The angiogram and CT scan of this patient are shown in Figure 15–112.

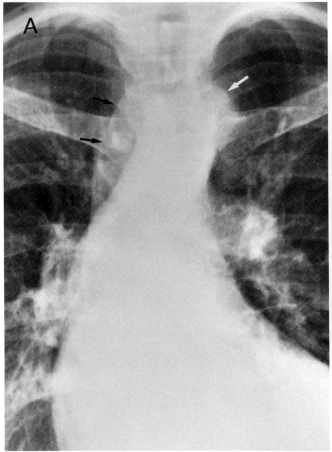

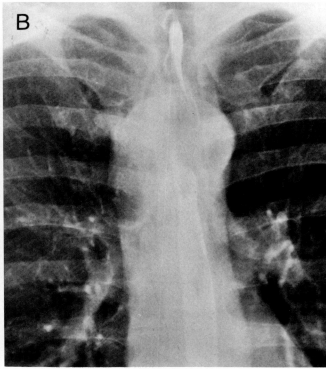

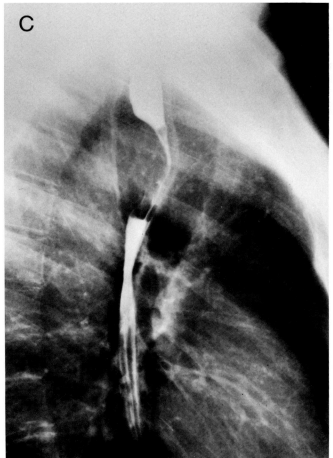

FIG 15–67.
Right aortic arch mimicking lymphadenopathy (two separate examples). **A,** PA radiograph shows the aortic arch *(black arrows)* to the right of the trachea. The density to the left of the trachea *(white arrow)* is the diverticulum from which the left subclavian artery takes origin. **B** and **C,** PA and lateral radiographs taken during the passage of a bolus of barium. The confusion with lymphadenopathy is particularly great in this case because, unusually, the descending aorta is on the left. Note the characteristic forward displacement of the esophagus and trachea on the lateral view.

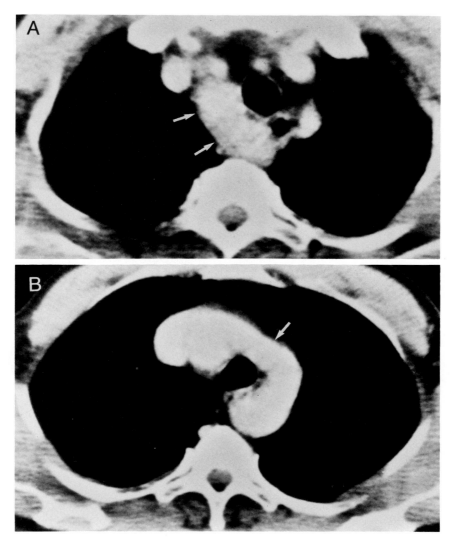

FIG 15–68.
Double aortic arch. **A,** CT section at the level of the left brachio-cephalic vein illustrates the high right-sided aortic arch *(arrows)*, mimicking right paratracheal adenopathy. **B,** CT section 3 cm lower illustrates the left-sided aortic arch *(arrow)*. Contrast-enhanced scans.

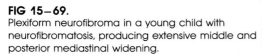

FIG 15–69.
Plexiform neurofibroma in a young child with neurofibromatosis, producing extensive middle and posterior mediastinal widening.

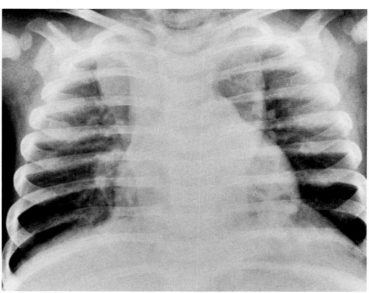

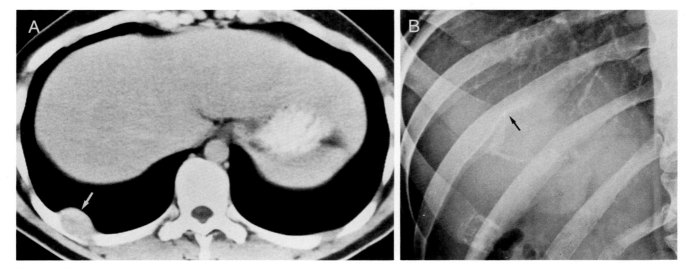

FIG 15–70.
A, Contrast-enhanced CT scan shows schwannoma *(arrow)* arising from an intercostal nerve. **B,** plain radiographs of ribs showing smooth, corticated pressure erosion of the adjacent rib *(arrow)*.

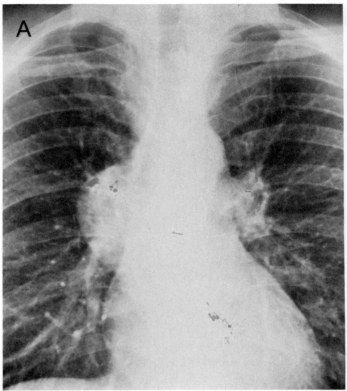

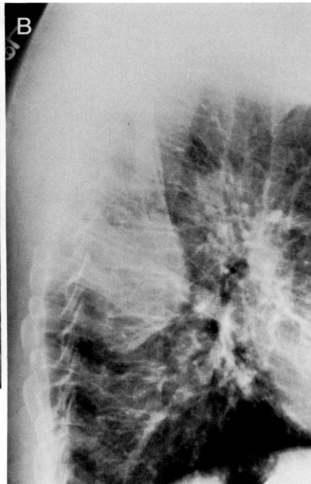

FIG 15–71.
Schwannoma arising in the posterior mediastinum in an
asymptomatic young man. **A,** PA radiograph. **B,** lateral radiograph.

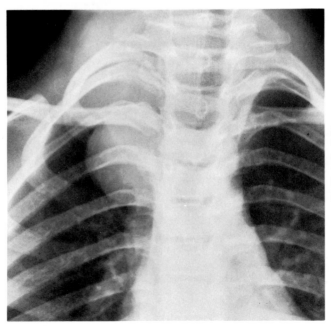

FIG 15–72.
Ganglioneuroma arising from the upper sympathetic chain in an
older child. Note the smooth, lobulated outline and the deformity of
the adjacent ribs. The second interspace is widened and the first
interspace is correspondingly narrow. The adjacent ribs show
pressure resorption but retain a corticated margin.

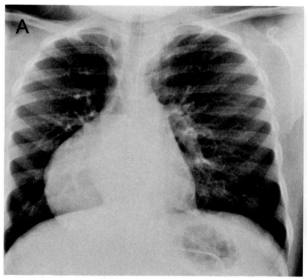
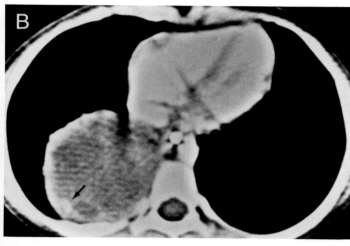

FIG 15–73.
A and **B**, ganglioneuroblastoma in a 7-year-old child. The mass is rounded and well defined. A small area of calcification *(arrow)* is noted on the contrast-enhanced CT scan.

15–75; 15–76). The bone in immediate contact with the tumor shows a scalloped edge; usually the bony cortex is preserved, and frequently it is thickened. The ribs may be thinned and splayed apart, and the intervertebral foramina may appear widened. With larger lesions, the absence of changes in the adjacent bones is a pointer against the diagnosis of a neurogenic tumor. Bone changes are most frequently encountered with the neuroblastoma/ganglioneuroma range of tumors, perhaps because such tumors are frequently large when they first present and the growing skeleton is able to react relatively quickly. Frank destruction of bone appears to be a sign of malignant invasion.[41, 55, 248] The larger tumors may be associated with scoliosis.[41]

At CT scanning many neural tumors have a low attenuation number,[55, 93] presumably because of the lipid elements in the nerve sheaths (Fig 15–77). Being vascular lesions, they enhance on images taken after the administration of intravascular contrast medium (Fig 15–78).[336]

One great advantage of CT is the superior demonstration of spinal and intraspinal involvement compared to that of plain films,[5, 86, 217] particularly if water-soluble contrast medium has previously been injected intrathecally. MRI (see Fig 15–75) is even better than CT at demonstrating intraspinal involvement. Predictably, CT is superior to conventional techniques in detecting calcification,[5] whereas MRI is far inferior. At MRI, the high signal intensity of both T1- and T2-weighted images[264] is presum-

ably related to the high lipid content. This finding is likely to prove a useful diagnostic sign of neurogenic tumors.

Lateral Intrathoracic Meningocele

Intrathoracic meningocele is a protrusion of the spinal meninges through an intervertebral foramen. It is usually detected in patients between 30 and 60 years of age.[201] Most are asymptomatic, but occasionally they are associated with pain or neurological abnormality.[201] Approximately two-thirds of cases occur in association with neurofibromatosis.[201] On rare occasions, multiple or bilateral intrathoracic meningoceles are encountered.[31, 76, 274]

On plain chest radiograph[76] there is a well-defined paravertebral mass, usually with scalloping and deformity of the adjacent ribs, pedicle, or vertebral body. Enlargement of the adjacent intervertebral foramina is an important diagnostic feature. Kyphoscoliosis is often present. These signs are identical to those seen with dumbbell nerve sheath tumors—a diagnostic problem complicated by the fact that both conditions are so frequently associated with neurofibromatosis.

CT scanning[316] documents the features listed previously and also shows the expected low attenuation value of the mass, since much of its bulk consists of cerebrospinal fluid. If the examination is performed with intrathecal contrast medium, the contrast material will enter the meningocele, thereby

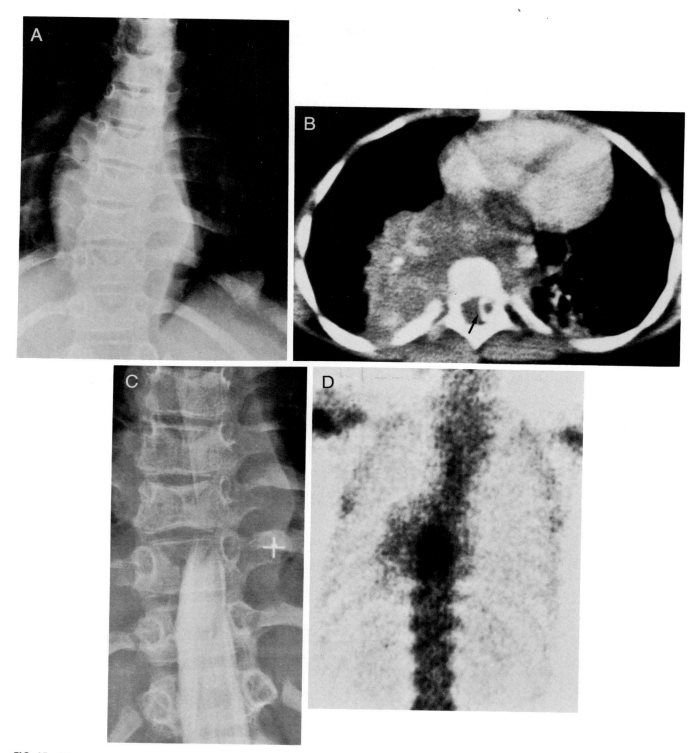

FIG 15–74.
Neuroblastoma in a 5-year-old child. The tumor straddles the midline. **A,** on the PA chest radiograph the tumor shows a smooth outline but on the CT scan (contrast enhanced) **(B),** the irregularity of the margin can be seen. The tumor is partially calcified and extends into the spinal canal, displacing the dural sac *(arrow),* which in this illustration contains contrast medium. **C,** the myelogram illustrates the extradural mass displacing the theca and narrowing the subarachnoid space. Collapse of the adjacent vertebral body is also seen. **D,** radionuclide bone scan shows intense activity in the neuroblastoma mass.

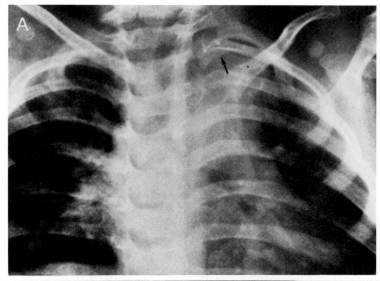

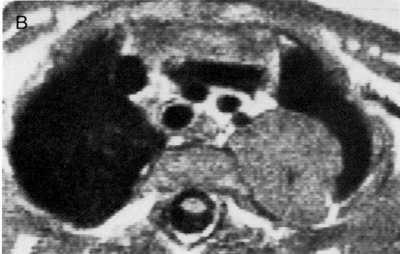

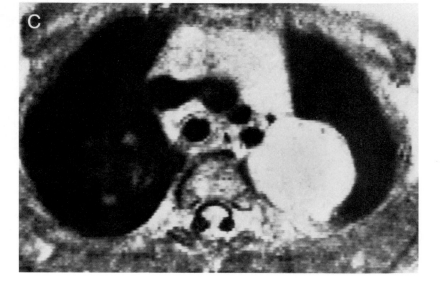

FIG 15–75.
Neuroblastoma in a 2-year-old child. **A,** PA
radiograph shows soft tissue mass plus splaying and
deformity of adjacent ribs *(arrow).* **B,** T1-weighted
and **(C)** T2-weighted MR images show the extent of
the mass between the ribs but no evidence of
extension into the spinal canal.

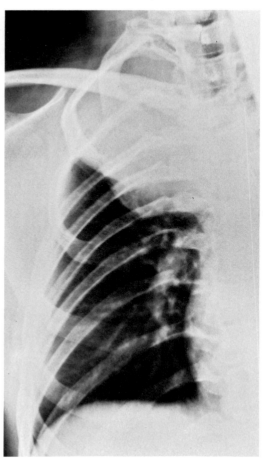

FIG 15–76.
Neurofibrosarcoma in a young woman with neurofibromatosis. Note resemblance of mass to a benign neurogenic tumor. The ribs are splayed and show corticated pressure erosion.

confirming the diagnosis. Prior to CT, such opacification was obtained with conventional myelography.

Mediastinal Paragangliomas

Paragangliomas are tumors of the paraganglionic cells; they may be benign or malignant.[223, 248, 303] In the chest, paragangliomas may be chemodectomas or pheochromocytomas (functioning paragangliomas). Almost all the chemodectomas are aortic body tumors. Mediastinal paragangliomas are rare; they formed only 2% of the large series of neural tumors of the thorax reported by Reed et al.[248] In a review of 51 cases of nonfunctioning paragangliomas, 39 were in the area of the aortic arch and were, therefore, classified as aortic body tumors, whereas 12 were located near the sympathetic chain in the paravertebral area.[223] The aortic body may be situated in one of four locations: lateral to the brachiocephalic artery; anterolateral to the aortic arch; at the angle of the ductus arteriosus; or above and to the right of the right pulmonary artery.[223] Multicentric cases are also reported.[135] In the review by Olson and Salyer,[223] eight of 41 patients with aortic body tumor had died, either from metastasis or from local invasion.

Fewer than 2% of pheochromocytomas occur in the chest.[300] Most are found in the posterior mediastinum[198] or adjacent to the heart and pericardium, particularly in the wall of the left atrium or the interatrial septum.[267, 272] The left atrial lesions indent the left atrium from the pericardial surface, rather than growing into the lumen of the atrium.[267] Ap-

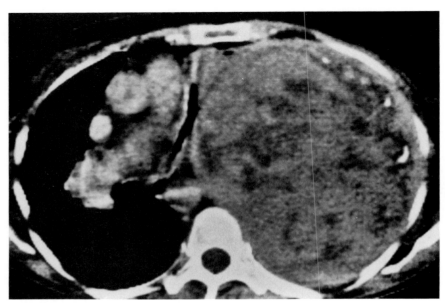

FIG 15–77.
Malignant schwannoma. This huge mass shows both low-density areas corresponding to lipid elements in the tumor and high-density areas due to calcification. Contrast-enhanced CT scan.

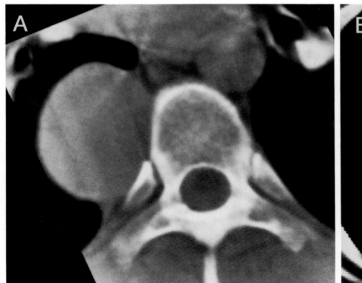

FIG 15–78.
Benign schwannoma. **A,** CT scan before administration of contrast material. **B,** following contrast material, the CT scan shows intense enhancement of the tumor. Note the schwannoma is as dense as the opacified left atrium.

proximately one-third of mediastinal pheochromocytomas are nonfunctioning and asymptomatic; the remainder present with symptoms, signs, and laboratory findings of overproduction of catecholamines.[198]

The various paragangliomas appear similar on plain chest radiography, CT, and angiography (Fig 15–79). They form rounded soft tissue masses which are extremely vascular and, therefore, enhance brightly at CT after administration of intravenous contrast material.[282] Arteriography will demonstrate enlarged feeding vessels, pathologic vessels within the tumor, and an intense tumor blush. Radionuclide ^{131}I MIBG (metaiodobenzylguanidine) images show increased activity in functioning pheochromocytomas and are an excellent method of identifying extra-adrenal tumors.[99]

Mediastinal Hemorrhage

Trauma (either penetrating or blunt) to the aorta or one of its major branches is a frequent cause of mediastinal hemorrhage. The usual spontaneous causes are dissecting hematoma, rupture of an aneurysm, and bleeding disorders or anticoagulant therapy. Other causes of spontaneous mediastinal hemorrhage are extremely unusual. They include chronic hemodialysis[82]; bleeding into pre-existing mediastinal tumors, such as thymic masses and goiter; radiation vasculitis[25]; and severe vomiting.[285]

Mediastinal hemorrhage can be asymptomatic or

can give rise to varying degrees of substernal chest pain, which often radiates to the back. Its investigation depends on the probable cause. When further tests are indicated, aortography, rather than CT or MRI, is frequently undertaken, because CT and MRI, though they would confirm or exclude hemorrhage, might not show the underlying cause with sufficient detail.

On plain chest radiography, mediastinal hemorrhage causes widening of the mediastinal shadow and widening of the right paratracheal stripe (Fig 15–80).[329] The widening may be focal or general, depending on how freely the blood tracks through the mediastinum. The blood may also track extrapleurally over the lung apices giving rise to the important sign of apical capping (Fig 15–80).[277] When the hemorrhage is severe, it may rupture into the pleural cavity and may track into the lung along perivascular and peribronchial sheaths, giving rise to pulmonary shadowing that may resemble pulmonary edema.[227] Generalized widening is often difficult to diagnose unless comparison can be made with previous examinations, whereas focal hematoma around a bleeding site causes a homogeneous mass that is far easier to recognize. Rapid widening on serial films is a useful clue to the diagnosis.

The appearance of mediastinal hemorrhage on CT scanning is fairly characteristic (Fig 15–81). Streaky soft tissue densities are seen interspersed through the mediastinal fat. On occasion, it is possible to appreciate the high density associated with

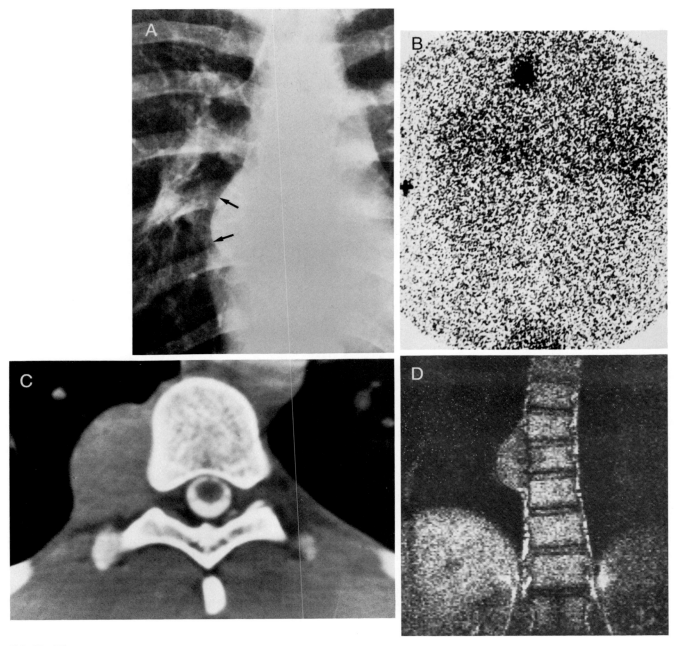

FIG 15–79.

Mediastinal pheochromocytoma in an asymptomatic patient who was screened because of a strong family history of the condition and found to have high levels of urinary catecholamines. The mass *(arrows)*, which proved to be a solitary pheochromocytoma, was first discovered on **(A)** the plain film. **B,** MIBG scan shows increased activity in the mediastinal mass but no other site of tumor.

C, CT scan (following myelogram) shows posterior mediastinal mass centered on the sympathetic chain growing toward the adjacent neural exit foramen but no displacement of the dural sac. **D,** T1-weighted (TR-500, TE-17) MR image shows an oval mass with a flat base against the thoracic spine. Signal intensity is similar to that of muscle.

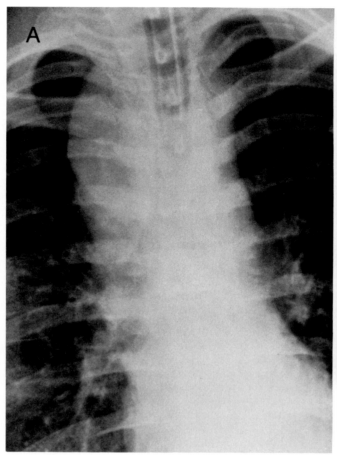

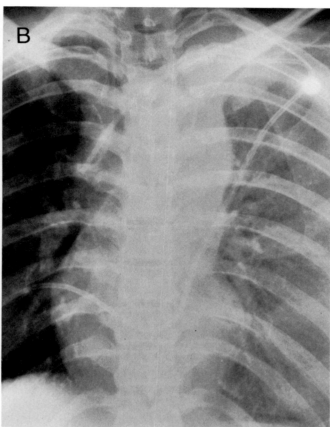

FIG 15–80.
Two examples of mediastinal hemorrhage following inadvertent arterial puncture during placement of an intravenous line. **A,** right paratracheal hemorrhage. **B,** left superior mediastinal hemorrhage tracking extrapleurally over left lung apex.

fresh thrombus. A focal hematoma may be difficult to distinguish from a solid mediastinal mass on CT findings alone (Fig 15–81), but usually the clinical situation is sufficiently different to prevent real confusion.

The appearance of hemorrhage with MRI varies with the location and the age of the hemorrhage, the degree of T1 and T2 weighting, the field strength, and the technique used. Relatively specific patterns have been described for hematomas in the brain and muscle.[122, 290] Whether the patterns for mediastinal hematoma and infiltrating hemorrhage will be as specific remains to be seen. In the acute phase, T1-weighted spin-echo images of hematomas and infiltrating hemorrhage tend to have low signal intensity compared with that of muscle. As the blood ages, the signal intensity increases significantly. On T2-weighted spin-echo images in the acute phase, the signal intensity of both hematoma and infiltrating hemorrhage is, in general, higher than that of muscle; with the passage of time, the signal intensity of

hematoma decreases to some extent, whereas the signal intensity of infiltrating hemorrhage tends to remain high. The explanations for these changing patterns include the amount of water in the area of hemorrhage and the degree of conversion from oxyhemoglobin to deoxyhemoglobin and methemoglobin.[122, 290]

Pneumomediastinum

The presence of a pneumomediastinum indicates perforation of some portion of either the respiratory or alimentary tracts. Gas-forming infection may increase the quantity of gas present. The perforation need not be within the mediastinum; indeed, it often lies beyond the confines of the mediastinum itself. The causes[128] can be divided into:

1. Alveolar rupture:
   a. Spontaneous.
   b. In patients on mechanical ventilation.

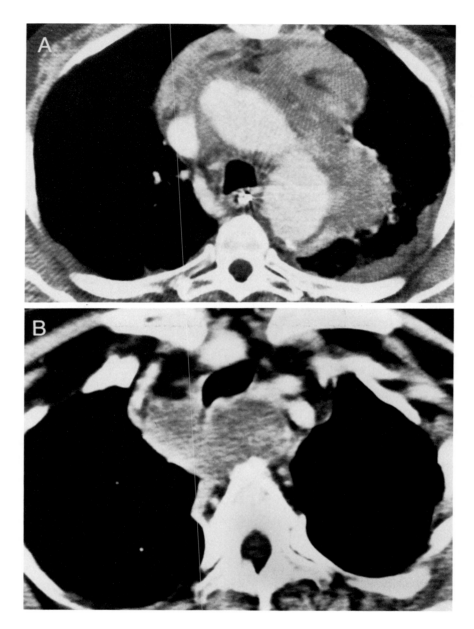

FIG 15–81.
Mediastinal hemorrhage on CT: **(A)** in a case of aortic dissection, showing blood with islands of mediastinal fat; **(B)** following a spinal fracture. Note that from this image alone it would not be possible to distinguish the hematoma from a solid mediastinal mass. Contrast-enhanced CT scans.

c. Following compressive trauma to thorax.
d. Following rupture of lung by rib fracture with tracking of air into mediastinum by way of the chest wall and neck.
2. Traumatic laceration of trachea or a central bronchus.
3. Perforation of the esophagus:
   a. Spontaneous.
   b. Following instrumentation.
4. Perforation of pharynx,[261, 299] duodenum,[283] colon, or rectum,[21] with tracking of air into mediastinum.

Alveolar Rupture

In *spontaneous alveolar rupture,* the patients are usually healthy young men or women with a history of a bout of asthma or of severe coughing, vomiting, or some other cause of sudden rise of intrathoracic pressure.[214] The conditions that have been reported to be associated with spontaneous pneumomediastinum[61, 128, 214] include asthma, strenuous exercise, marijuana smoking, nitrous oxide inhalation,[184] pneumonia, diabetic ketoacidosis,[109, 259] and childbirth. The air leak from alveolar rupture tracks through the interstitial tissues of the lung to accumulate in the mediastinum,[190] but the interstitial air is only visible if the adjacent lung is opaque, as for example, in hyaline membrane disease or adult respiratory distress syndrome. Associated rupture of air into the pleural space to produce pneumothorax is fairly common.

The patient may complain of chest pain aggravated by deep breathing and dyspnea. Fever and leukocytosis without apparent infection are frequently encountered[214] and may cause confusion with acute mediastinitis. In those cases where the air has tracked into the neck there may be palpable crepitus in the supraclavicular areas. The equivalent of crepitus may be heard as a crackling sound through a stethoscope. Hammond's sign, a crunching sound synchronous with the heartbeat which may be heard in half the patients, was at one time thought to be diagnostic of pneumomediastinum, but a similar clicking sound is heard with small pneumothoraces.[128] Spontaneous pneumomediastinum resulting from alveolar rupture, though it may cause symptoms and signs, does not in itself affect patient outcome, and it is therefore not treated.[109, 128]

Alveolar rupture is common in patients who are on mechanical ventilation, particularly those with small airway obstruction or noncompliant lungs.[254] This combination is frequent in patients in intensive care units, particularly neonatal units. Hyaline membrane disease, meconum aspiration, and neonatal pneumonia are among the many neonatal pulmonary disorders that require mechanical ventilation and produce stiff lungs. In adults, the pneumomediastinum itself rarely affects the outcome of the disease and therefore does not require treatment, though reduction of ventilatory pressure to the minimum needed is advisable.

Air in the chest wall following rib fracture or placement of a chest tube may track into the mediastinum, usually by way of the neck. This is a particularly common occurrence in patients on mechanical ventilation. Usually the chest wall emphysema is severe, and the cause of the pneumomediastinum is not in doubt.

Radiographic Findings in Pneumomediastinum

Air in the mediastinum is seen on plain chest radiograph as streaks, bubbles, or larger collections of air outlining the mediastinal blood vessels, the major airways, or the esophagus (Fig 15–82).[61, 253] The dissection of air along tissue planes may be more obvious in the lateral projection than on the frontal view. The air may dissect under the parietal layer of the mediastinal pleura so that a line shadow representing the combined parietal and visceral pleura will be seen separate from the heart and great vessels. The air is usually greatest in amount anteriorly. When limited in quantity, the only sign of pneumomediastinum on plain chest radiography may be a line or band of transradiancy in the retrosternal area.

An important plain film sign of pneumomediastinum is air dissecting under and medial to the thymus. The outlining of the thymus by air is quite specific for pneumomediastinum and may be the most striking sign of the condition (see Fig 15–82). Air may also track extrapleurally along the upper surface of the diaphragm. Air between the heart and diaphragm gives rise to the "continuous diaphragm sign,"[175] so called because air beneath the heart may form a visible line of transradiancy that permits the diaphragm to be seen even within the confines of the mediastinum (Fig 15–83).

It may, on occasion, be difficult to distinguish pneumomediastinum from pneumothorax or pneumopericardium on plain chest radiograph (see Fig 15–83). The distinction depends on the anatomic extent of the air.[61] Pneumothorax is rarely confined solely to the mediastinal border. It can usually be traced out over the lung apex to the lateral portion of the thoracic cavity. A lateral decubitus view will confirm the pleural location, though it is rarely needed. Pneumopericardium may extend from the diaphragm to just below the aortic knob, but will not extend around the aortic knob or into the superior mediastinum. Pneumopericardium can mimic the continuous diaphragm sign and can lift the thymus away from the great vessels, but the bilaterality and anatomic conformity to the pericardium is usually evident. A thin line of apparent radiolucency is frequently seen against the heart borders and aortic knob in healthy individuals due to the "Mach band" phenomenon. The Mach band may have an identical degree of radiolucency to a small pneumomediastinum. The distinction from pneumomediastinum[100] depends on analyzing both the anatomic extent and the border of the radiolucent line. A Mach band will be adjacent to a normally visualized contour, and its lateral boundary will either be unrecognizable or will be formed by a pulmonary blood vessel. The outer margin of a pneumomediastinum, on the other

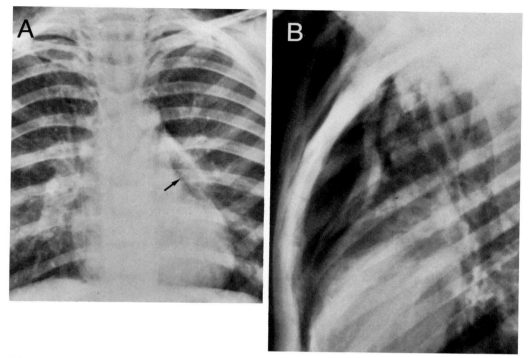

FIG 15–82.
Pneumomediastinum in asthmatic child showing air in mediastinal tissue planes. Note the air deep to the thymus *(arrow)*. **A,** PA radiograph. **B,** lateral radiograph.

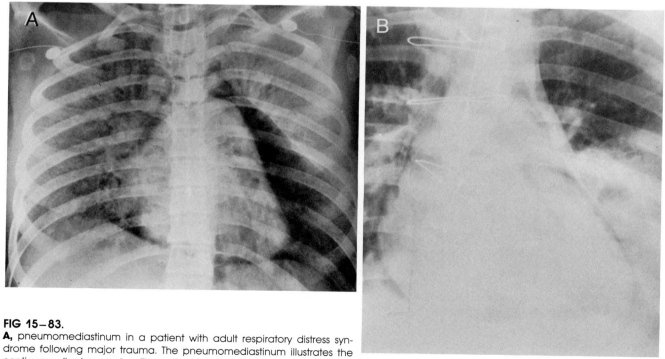

FIG 15–83.
A, pneumomediastinum in a patient with adult respiratory distress syndrome following major trauma. The pneumomediastinum illustrates the continuous diaphragm sign. The patient required high-pressure mechanical ventilation. Compare the extent of the pneumomediastinum in **A** with that in **B,** a patient with pneumopericardium following pericardiocentesis.

hand, will be the displaced mediastinal pleura.

The diagnosis of mediastinal emphysema is easy at CT (Fig 15–84), as the anatomic location of the air is self-evident on cross-sectional display. CT scanning is both more sensitive and specific than the plain chest radiograph and can be used to make the diagnosis in clinically suspected cases when the plain chest radiograph is normal or equivocal. This is usually only necessary in patients with suspected rupture of the trachea or central bronchi or in cases of suspected esophageal perforation.

Acute Mediastinitis

Acute infection of the mediastinum is relatively rare. The most common causes are esophageal perforation[233] or postoperative infection, for example, following median sternotomy.[155] Esophageal perforation is usually due to penetrating trauma, particularly from surgery, endoscopy, or swallowing sharp objects such as chicken bones. Spontaneous perforation may occur, as in Boerhaave's syndrome, where forceful vomiting causes a tear in the esophageal wall. The tear in the esophagus is almost invariably just above the gastroesophageal junction. The tear may be of any depth. Usually it is confined to the mucosa, in which case bleeding may occur, but there is no immediate danger of mediastinitis. If the tear is complete, air, alimentary juices, and food will leak into the mediastinum.

Other causes of acute mediastinal infection are leakage from the esophagus into the mediastinum through necrotic neoplasm and extension of infection from adjacent structures, particularly the neck, pharynx (Fig 15–85), or teeth,[177, 206, 280] but occasionally from the retroperitoneum, lungs, pleura, or spine. Mediastinitis may be associated with empyema or subphrenic abscess.

Clinically, the patients are often very ill with chills, high fever, tachycardia, and chest pain. Circulatory shock is frequent.[155] Dysphagia is common in those patients in whom the mediastinitis is caused by perforation of the esophagus.[233] Diffuse mediastinitis has a particularly high mortality.

The major radiologic features of acute mediastinitis are mediastinal widening, pneumomediastinum, obliteration of fat planes, localized fluid collections, and abscess formation (Figs 15–86 and 15–87). Accompanying pleural effusions in one or both pleural cavities are common. In cases of Boerhaave's syndrome, the effusion is particularly striking on the left and is often accompanied by consolidation of the left lower lobe.[253] All these features are better demonstrated on CT scans than on plain radiographs.[33, 43] CT may also show important associated abnormalities such as jugular vein thrombosis, pericardial effusion, or rupture of the hypopharynx or esophagus.

The widening of the mediastinum is the result of inflammatory swelling or abscess formation; therefore, the size and shape of the widening is determined by the cause of the infection. Because so many acute mediastinal infections are secondary to esophageal perforation, one of the important clues to the diagnosis is air within the mediastinum, a feature that may be difficult to see on plain films. The

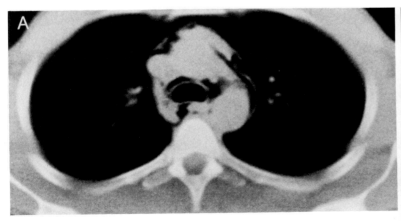
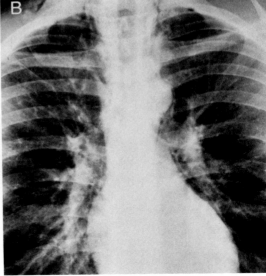

FIG 15–84.
A, CT scan of pneumomediastinum in a young man following a bout of marijuana inhalation with subsequent retching and coughing. **B,** plain chest radiograph at same time for comparison.
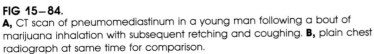

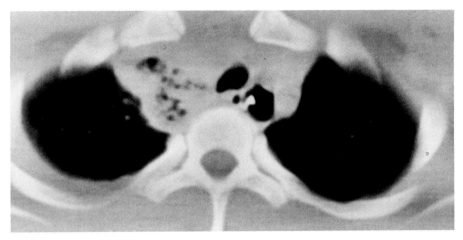

FIG 15–85.
Acute mediastinitis from a peritonsillar abscess that had tracked into the mediastinum. The mediastinal infection required surgical drainage. CT scan shows mediastinal widening due to fluid containing numerous air bubbles.

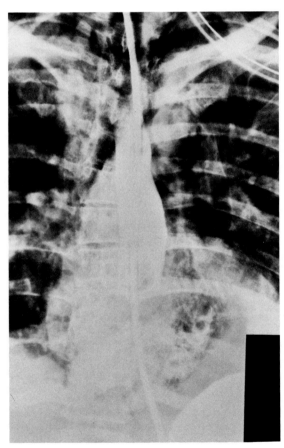

FIG 15–86.
Acute mediastinitis resulting from spontaneous perforation of the esophagus during severe vomiting (Boerhaave's syndrome). This image, taken during an esophagogram, shows pneumomediastinum and contrast material leaking into the mediastinum through a perforation of the left lower wall of the esophagus.

air may be bubbly or streaky and may be localized or widespread in distribution. As with all types of pneumomediastinum, the air may extend into the neck or retroperitoneum. In cases of diffuse mediastinitis without discrete abscess formation, CT shows widespread infiltration of the mediastinum with obliteration of the normal fat planes. Gas bubbles may be scattered through the mediastinum (see Fig 15–87). Where walled-off abscesses occur, the gas may be seen in more discrete rounded collections, together with air-fluid levels. Abscesses may be single but are frequently multiple. Discrete fluid collections within the mediastinum on CT may serve as an invaluable guide should percutaneous drainage be indicated.[33, 117]

Barium swallow examination can be critical in determining the presence and precise location of esophageal perforation or underlying tumor.[253]

The radiologic evaluation of possible complications of median sternotomy is a separate subject.[33, 123, 159] When acute mediastinitis is suspected clinically following sternotomy, CT will show the extent of inflammation, and any drainable mediastinal or pericardial fluid collections.[33, 159] With chronically draining wounds, the role of CT is uncertain.[133] Distinguishing retrosternal hematomas from reactive granulation tissues or cellulitis is difficult, as is distinguishing osteomyelitis from the direct effects of the surgical incision. Minor degrees of sternal separation and step-off are common in asymptomatic uncomplicated operations.[123, 159] It should be remembered that substernal fluid collections and dots of air are normal in the first 20 days following

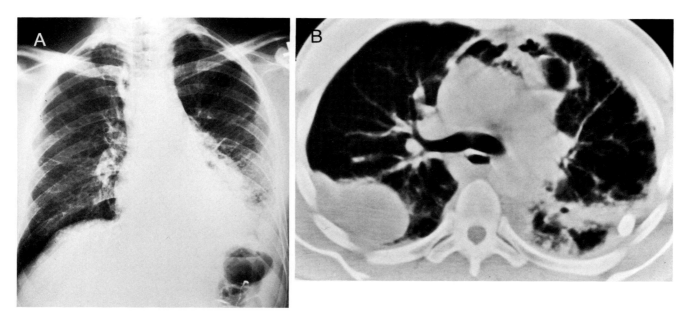

FIG 15–87.
Acute mediastinitis following perforation of the pharynx by a chicken bone. The patient, a 30-year-old man, had swallowed a chicken bone 3 weeks earlier. **A,** plain chest radiograph shows the features typical of pneumomediastinum: left lower lobe con-

solidation and left pleural effusion. **B,** CT scan following placement of tube in the left side of the chest shows an extensive air-fluid collection in the mediastinum and a right pleural empyema.

sternotomy and, therefore, the anterior mediastinum may not appear normal until 2 months have passed. Similarly, air trapped in the presternal or retrosternal soft tissues, though it usually dissipates within a few weeks, may be visible for up to 50 days on plain chest radiographs. Therefore, before gas-forming infections can be diagnosed, the air collections must appear *de novo* or must progressively increase without other explanation.[44]

Superior Vena Caval Obstruction

The most common cause of superior vena caval obstruction is compression and invasion by bronchogenic carcinoma either because the primary tumor is invading the mediastinum or because of lymph node metastases.[231] Other causes include mediastinal malignant neoplasms, notably metastatic breast and testicular neoplasm, and lymphoma; mediastinal fibrosis (see the following topic); and thrombosis, usually around a transvenous catheter.[231] In one large review, 78% of cases were due to the result of malignant neoplasm (two-thirds of which were lung carcinoma) and 22% were due to benign causes.[231]

Clinically, the features of superior vena caval obstruction are edema and visible distention of the veins of the face, neck, arms, and anterior chest wall.

Dyspnea, choking, dysphagia, and a feeling of congestion are common symptoms. Cerebral edema may occur. The severity of the symptoms and signs depends on the degree of venous collateral formation.[192] There may be no symptoms at all even with total obstruction, particularly if the obstruction is slow in developing.

A variety of imaging techniques have been used to document superior vena caval syndrome. Plain films rarely provide useful information about the venous obstruction itself. On occasion, the dilated collaterals may be visible, particularly enlargement of the azygos vein or enlargement of the superior intercostal vein (aortic nipple) draining the hemiazygos system.[45] Venography shows the obstruction, demonstrates collateral pathways, and is an excellent technique for demonstrating intraluminal thrombus. In general, however, it provides relatively little information about the cause of the obstruction. Radionuclide venography is a simple technique that can readily confirm or exclude superior vena caval obstruction,[56] but it contributes little information regarding the cause. CT with intravenous contrast material enhancement is an excellent all-purpose test that will show caval narrowing or filling defects in the superior vena cava and demonstrate the responsible pathologic process (Figs 15–88 and 15–89).[10, 19, 205] MRI (see Fig 15–89) can show the same features[197, 317]

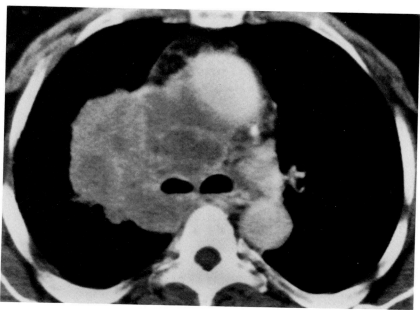

FIG 15–88.
Superior vena caval syndrome. Contrast-enhanced CT scan shows obstruction of the superior vena caval as a result of small cell carcinoma of the lung involving the mediastinum. Note that the superior vena cava has been obliterated.

and has the advantages of sagittal and coronal imaging and also the ability to distinguish rapidly flowing blood from both slowly flowing blood and thrombus.[197] The disadvantage of MRI is that it will not demonstrate calcification—an important feature in the diagnosis of granulomatous mediastinal fibrosis.

Fibrosing Mediastinitis

The most common cause of fibrosing mediastinitis is histoplasmosis, but fibrosing mediastinitis is rare, even in individuals who come from areas in which histoplasmosis is endemic. Other causes of mediastinal fibrosis include tuberculosis and drug or radiation therapy. An idiopathic variety, which may be autoimmune in origin and is sometimes combined with retroperitoneal fibrosis, has also been described.[168, 181]

When due to histoplasmosis, the fibrosis is thought to result from an idiosyncratic tendency to develop excessive fibrosis in response to a fungal antigen escaping from adjacent lymph nodes. The condition may be similar to the layers of fibrosis that form within an enlarging histoplasmoma of the lung.[124, 125] The fact that histoplasma organisms are rarely isolated is believed to be related to the inactivity of the infection at the time of nodal biopsy.

Clinically, the disorder presents in adult life with symptoms or signs related to obstruction of the various structures that traverse the mediastinum, most notably the superior vena cava. These symptoms and signs include swelling of the face, distention of the veins in the neck, cough, pulmonary infections, wheezing, hemoptysis, dyspnea, and a hoarse voice.[68, 124, 125, 263]

The radiologic features[50, 57, 68, 90, 324, 325] vary according to the bulk of the adenopathy and the severity of the obstructive phenomena. Plain films of the chest may be normal in appearance but, in cases due to histoplasmosis, almost always demonstrate enlargement and/or calcification of at least some of the mediastinal or hilar lymph nodes (Fig 15–90). The adenopathy may be unilateral or bilateral, but is most often asymmetric. It is maximal in the superior mediastinum. Narrowing of the lower trachea or major bronchi may be detectable and, if there is severe obstruction to a pulmonary artery, the resulting pulmonary oligemia may be identified, even on plain films. Pulmonary consolidation/atelectasis resulting from bronchial, venous, or lymphatic obstruction or due to pleuropulmonary scarring may be seen. Mediastinal venography and pulmonary arteriography will show smooth, tapered narrowing of the superior vena cava and brachiocephalic veins, together with numerous dilated collateral veins, and may also show narrowing of the central pulmonary arteries (Fig 15–91).[325] Barium swallow study may show narrow-

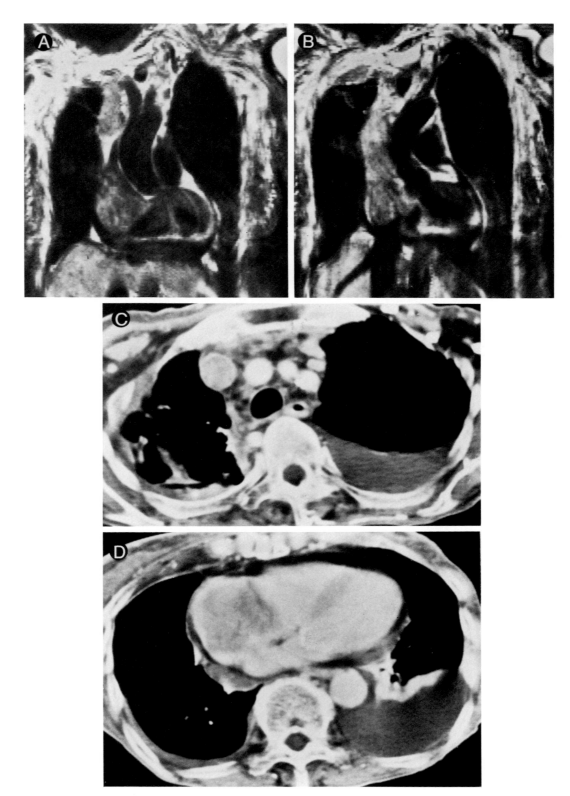

FIG 15–89.
Superior vena caval syndrome. **A** and **B,** MR images of intraluminal thyroid carcinoma growing in the superior vena cava and
right atrium. **C** and **D,** contrast-enhanced CT scans at level of right
brachiocephalic vein and right atrium show intraluminal filling defect.

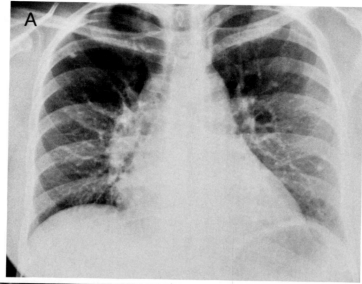

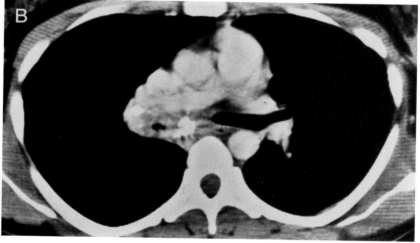

FIG 15–90.
Mediastinal fibrosis resulting from histoplasmosis. **A,** plain chest radiograph shows enlarged right hilar and paratracheal nodes as well as subcarinal lymph node enlargement. Note small calcified granulomas in lungs. **B,** contrast-enhanced CT scan through subcarinal region shows enlarged, partially calcified nodes and severe narrowing of the bronchus intermedius.

ing of the esophagus and, in rare instances, may show varices resulting from esophageal venous collaterals, the so-called downhill varices.

CT is now the best single technique for diagnosing and assessing the severity of mediastinal fibrosis (Figs 15–90; 15–92).[15, 250, 271, 318] CT shows the enlarged calcified nodes to advantage. Lymph node calcification is present in almost all patients in whom the process is the result of histoplasmosis. CT scanning also demonstrates any airway narrowing, any pulmonary or systemic vein compression, collateral venous pathways, any arterial compressions, and any pulmonary shadows resulting from the central obstructive processes. The noncalcified fibrotic tissue may be difficult to identify; there may simply be obliteration of fat planes, which makes it difficult to identify the normal vascular landmarks.

MRI[88, 250, 317] can demonstrate the vascular narrowings as well as, if not better than, CT scanning and has the additional advantage of not requiring contrast media. The major disadvantage of MRI is that it cannot reliably show calcification; consequently, an important diagnostic sign of histoplasmosis or tuberculosis is not available. But on T2-weighted spin-echo sequences, the adenopathy seen in fibrosing mediastinitis may be lower in signal intensity than that generally seen with malignancy, probably because of the presence of calcification.[250]

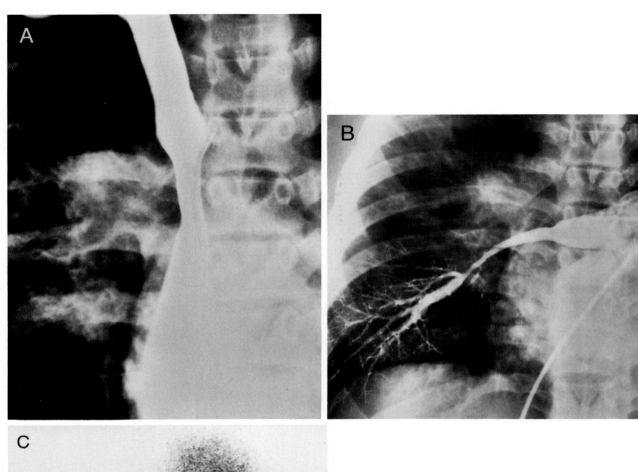

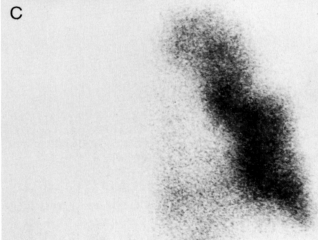

FIG 15–91.
Mediastinal fibrosis resulting from histoplasmosis. **A,** superior vena cavogram shows smooth focal narrowing. **B,** pulmonary arteriogram shows long, smooth stricture through right lower lobe artery and occlusion of the truncus anterior. **C,** ^{99m}Tc pulmonary perfusion radionuclide scan indicates substantial reduction in flow to right lung.

Radionuclide ventilation-perfusion scanning can be used to demonstrate the pulmonary arterial flow and to show which areas are underventilated.[209]

Extramedullary Hematopoiesis

Extramedullary hematopoiesis in potential blood-forming organs such as the liver, spleen, and lymph nodes is a common condition in various anemias, but only rarely does extramedullary hematopoiesis cause masslike collections within the chest. Usually the anemia is one of the congenital hemolytic anemias, notably thalassemia and sickle cell disease, though the condition may be seen in other anemias and may even occur in patients without anemia.[256] The masses themselves are usually asymptomatic, though paraplegia from cord compression may occur.[185, 229]

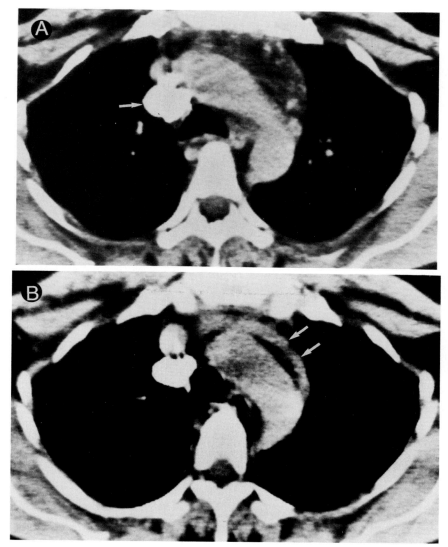

FIG 15–92.
Mediastinal fibrosis resulting from histoplasmosis. **A,** contrast-enhanced CT scan shows enlarged calcified nodes *(arrow)* adjacent to the narrowed right brachiocephalic vein. **B,** adjacent level shows collateral venous channels *(arrows).* Note that noncalcified fibrous tissue in the mediastinum is not visualized in these or other sections.

Radiologically[132, 145, 229, 256] these masses are found in the paravertebral regions, usually in the lower chest (Fig 15–93). They may be unilateral but are usually bilateral and symmetric. They are smoothly marginated, because they are covered by mediastinal pleura, and are of soft tissue density on plain chest radiographs. Calcification does not appear to be a feature. Sometimes the masses occur at multiple levels, in which case the symmetric lobular arrangement conforming to the segmental divisions of the body produces a striking and characteristic appearance.[229] Further foci of extramedullary hematopoiesis may be seen adjacent to ribs. The intervening or adjacent bone may be normal or may show marrow expansion. The extramedullary hemopoietic tissue apparently spreads from marrow within the bone.

The appearance at CT[132, 185] is that of a homogeneous mass of soft tissue or slightly higher-density matter (see Fig 15–93). In one reported case there was a large fatty component to the mass.[334] A radionuclide bone marrow scan may demonstrate activity in the mass.[132, 284]

The condition should be considered in the differential diagnosis of any paravertebral mass in a patient with severe chronic anemia. Unlike neurogenic

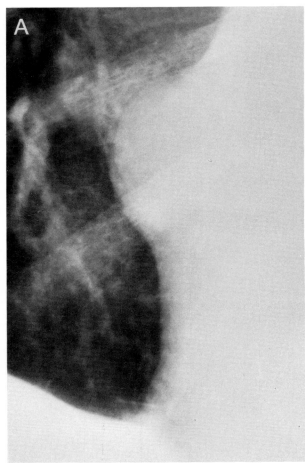

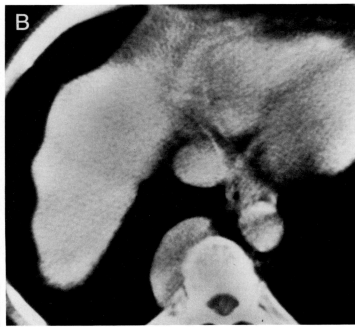

FIG 15–93.
Extramedullary hematopoiesis in the right paravertebral region. **A,** plain film. **B,** contrast-enhanced CT scan.

tumors, the major differential diagnosis, extramedullary hematopoiesis does not appear to cause pressure erosion of the adjacent spine or ribs.[256]

Aortic Aneurysm

The causes of aortic aneurysm are given in Table 15–2. A full discussion of aortic aneurysm is beyond the scope of this book. Our remarks are confined to plain film and CT findings, concentrating on the diagnostic and differential diagnostic points.

Atherosclerotic Aortic Aneurysms

Atherosclerotic aneurysms, along with generalized ectasia, are both extremely common aging/degenerative phenomena and may be fusiform or saccular in shape. Degenerative aneurysms are often first discovered on imaging studies when still asymptomatic. Chest pain and compression effects are the most common symptoms. A hoarse voice may occur because of pressure on the recurrent laryngeal nerve

TABLE 15–2.
Aortic Aneurysms

Saccular aneurysm
  True aneurysms*
    Atherosclerotic
    Congenital
    Aortitis
  False aneurysms†
    Traumatic
    Mycotic
Fusiform aneurysms
  Aging
  Atherosclerosis
  Medionecrosis
  Aortitis
Dissecting hematoma

*True aneurysms are defined as outpouchings of the aortic wall containing all three layers of the arterial wall with no disruption in continuity of the intima or media.
†False aneurysms are secondary to a break in the intima and media of the aortic wall, the wall of the aneurysm being formed by adventitia or adjacent extra-vascular tissues.

as it passes around and under the aortic arch. Compression of the left main or lower lobe bronchus may lead to atelectasis of the left lung (Fig 15–94), and compression of the esophagus may cause dysphagia with extrinsic deformity on barium swallow. Compression of the right and left pulmonary arteries has also been reported.[60, 72] Rupture is the most feared complication. Fusiform aneurysms do not pose a diagnostic problem because their anatomic conformity to the aorta is obvious.

Saccular aneurysms usually arise from the descending aorta, or very occasionally from the aortic arch, but are extremely unusual in the ascending aorta. Occasionally, they can be misdiagnosed on plain films as a neoplastic mediastinal mass.[279] They can usually be differentiated from the majority of neoplastic or cystic masses by their conformity to the aorta and by noting the presence of curvilinear calcification in the wall of the aneurysm (Fig 15–95). Such calcification is usually present, though it may be difficult to see on plain chest radiographs. At CT, the aorta is dilated; to diagnose aneurysm forma-

tion, the diameter of the aorta has to substantially exceed the normal figures of 40 mm for the ascending aorta and 30 mm for the descending aorta.[134] Peripheral calcification of the wall of the aneurysm is well demonstrated at CT, particularly prior to administration of contrast material. After intravenous opacification, the widened lumen in the region of the aneurysm is demonstrated (Fig 15–96). Most degenerative aneurysms show significant amounts of lining thrombus, which may show flecks of calcification on the inner margin of the thrombus[139] (see Fig 15–95). The thrombus is usually shaped like a crescent wedged against the outer wall of the aorta, so that some luminal dilatation at the level of the aneurysm is almost invariable. There are only a few reported occasions in which the lumen of the aneurysm was totally occupied by thrombus.[279] There may be a rim of soft tissue adjacent to the aneurysm, the result of either thickening of the aortic wall, adjacent hematoma, or reaction in the adjacent lung or pleura. This rim should not be confused with aortic dissection (Fig 15–96).

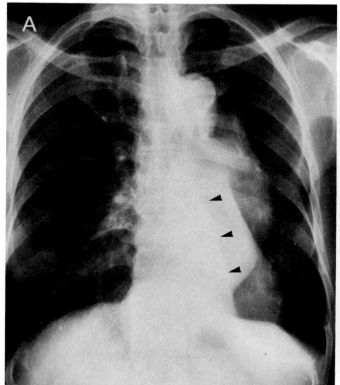

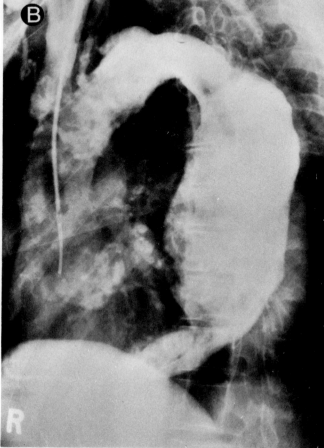

FIG 15–94.
Fusiform atherosclerotic aneurysm of the descending aorta causing left lower lobe collapse *(arrowheads)*. **A,** plain film. **B,** aortogram.

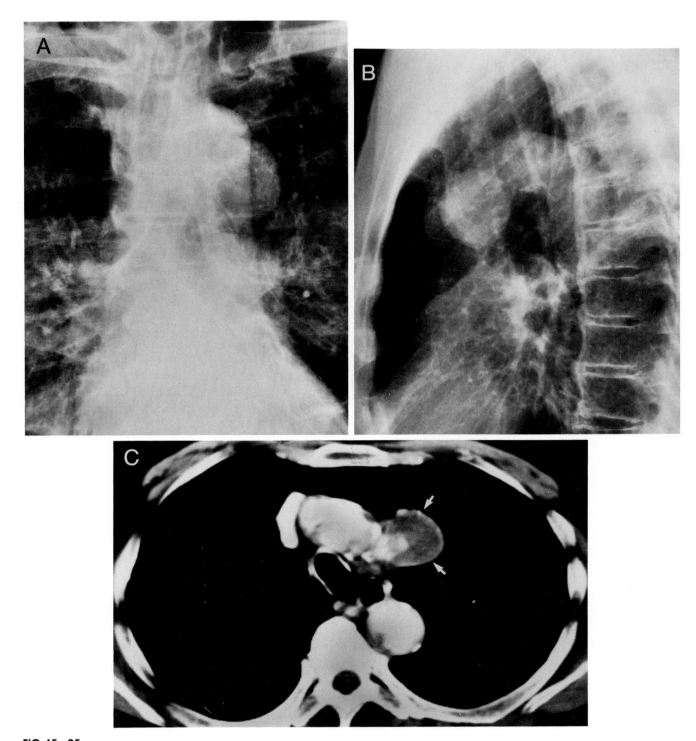

FIG 15–95.
Saccular aneurysm of the aortic arch resembling mediastinal mass in a patient with recurrent laryngeal nerve paralysis. **A** and **B,** plain chest radiographs showing a round mass in contact with the upper ascending aorta. Curvilinear calcification is visible in the wall of the aneurysm but is only seen with difficulty. **C,** CT scan shows contiguity of the mass *(arrows)* with the ascending aorta, crescentic lining thrombus, opacified central lumen, and calcification of the wall.

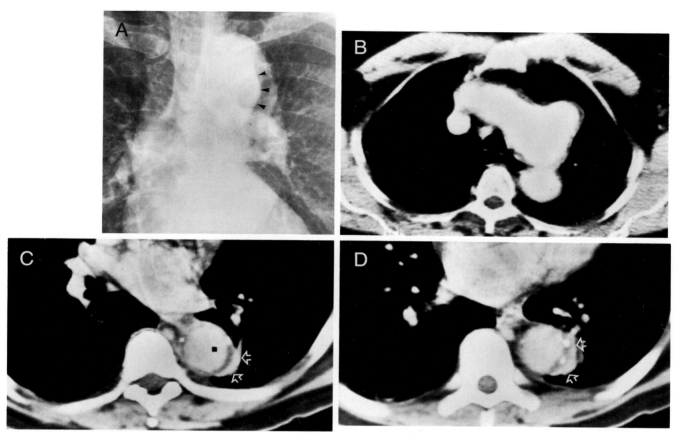

FIG 15–96.
Atheromatous disease of the aorta. **A** and **B,** saccular aneurysm. The contrast-enhanced CT scan **(B)** shows widening of the lumen of the aorta. **C** and **D,** adjacent contrast-enhanced CT sections showing atheromatous disease of descending aorta in another patient with atelectasis of lung adjacent to the aorta *(arrows)* closely mimicking an aortic dissection.

Traumatic Aneurysm

Traumatic laceration of the aorta is discussed in Chapter 17. Traumatic tears of the aorta are usually fatal if not treated surgically. In those patients who do not receive surgery soon after the trauma, a chronic false aneurysm may develop.[133, 143] These aneurysms develop in characteristic sites. With few exceptions,[144] all arise from the anteromedial wall of the distal arch or upper descending aorta close to the ligamentum arteriosum (Fig 15–97). It has been suggested that the hematomas that form at this site can be contained by the surrounding structures, whereas more posterior lacerations tend to bleed extensively and do not develop false aneurysms.[133] A hoarse voice may develop because of pressure on the recurrent laryngeal nerve, and dysphagia may be present if the aneurysm presses on the esophagus. Other symptoms include chest pain, dyspnea, and shortness of breath. When small, these aneurysms often project into the aortopulmonary window and may, therefore, be invisible on plain chest radio-

graph. As they enlarge, they form a bulge projecting from the aortopulmonary window (see Fig 15–97). Chronic post-traumatic false aneurysms are saccular in shape and in time will develop calcification in the wall or in lining thrombus.[133, 143] At this stage, they are identical in appearance to degenerative saccular aneurysms on both plain chest radiographs and CT, except that the patient is often younger and there is no other evidence of atherosclerotic disease in the remainder of the aorta.

Mycotic Aneurysms

Mycotic aneurysms of the aorta are confined to patients with predisposing causes; these include intravenous drug abusers, patients with valvular disease or congenital disorders of the heart or aorta, patients who have undergone previous cardiac or aortic surgery, and immunocompromised patients. A recent review of 20 mycotic aneurysms of the aortic root serves to emphasize this point; all patients had aortic valve disease or had an infected aortic

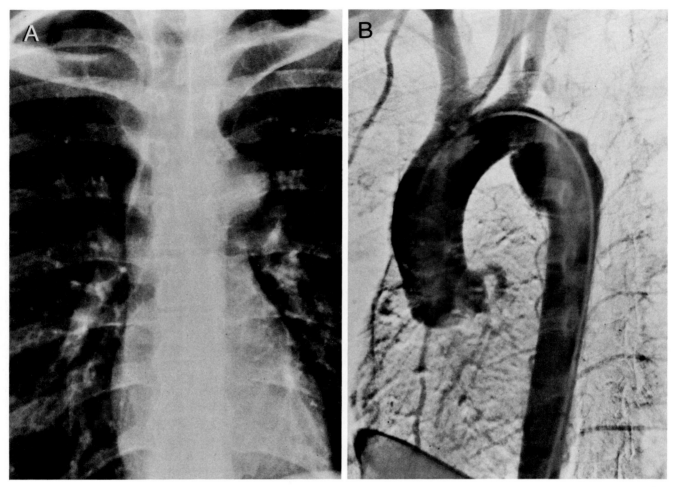

FIG 15–97.
Traumatic aortic aneurysm in a typical location in the distal aortic arch close to the level of the ligamentum arteriosum. The trauma had taken place 3 years previously. **A,** plain film. **B,** aortogram.

valve prosthesis.[92] Mycotic aneurysms may occur in any site depending on the predisposing factors. Unlike other aneurysms, the clinical presentation is usually with fever and leucocytosis. Because the process is basically a form of abscess it may be discovered first on a radionuclide scan such as an indium-111 leucocyte scintigram.[265] Mycotic aneurysms are usually saccular in shape. The major radiologic differences between mycotic aneurysms and other saccular aneurysms of the aorta are rapid enlargement and absence of calcification of the wall, because these aneurysms are rapidly fatal unless treated.

Cystic Medial Necrosis and Dissecting Hematoma

Cystic medial necrosis is characterized by deposition of acellular basophilic material within the media[77] which, when significant in amount, disrupts the structure of the aortic wall. Severe cystic medial ne-

crosis is seen in Marfan's syndrome and in an idiopathic form known as primary dilatation of the aorta. Lesser degrees of the condition are very common in older individuals, probably in response to hemodynamic stresses, such as hypertension and aortic stenosis.[77] Carlson et al.[42] examined the ascending aorta in 250 autopsies; they excluded cases of Marfan's syndrome, idiopathic dilatation of the aorta, and aortic dissection. The incidence of cystic medial necrosis increased progressively with the age of the deceased person from 10% in the first 2 decades to 60% and 64% in the 7th and 8th decades. The incidence of cystic medial necrosis was consistently higher in hypertensive patients than in normotensive subjects of comparable age. Focal aneurysms due to cystic medial necrosis usually involve the ascending aorta and are an important cause of aortic regurgitation.[162] Because much of the ascending aorta is not border-forming on the plain chest radiograph, even very large aneurysms due to cystic medial necrosis, when confined to the proximal half of the ascending aorta, may be invisible on plain chest films,[162, 291] but it may be possible to identify displaced mediastinal fat planes even if there is no visible widening of the mediastinal contour.[291] This sign is difficult to evaluate and, in general, the diagnosis is only suspected when the ascending aorta is clearly dilated. Confusion with mediastinal masses is rare, because the lesion in question is so clearly the result of dilatation of the ascending aorta.

Dissecting hematomas, sometimes inaccurately called dissecting aneurysms, are hematomas within the media of the aortic wall. They communicate with the true aortic lumen through one or more tears in the intima, the assumption being that most dissections begin within an intimal tear through which the bleeding occurs.[77] Cystic medial necrosis and hypertension are important predisposing causes.[174]

The classic de Bakey classification divided aortic dissection into types I, II, and III.[65] Type I referred to dissections which commenced in the ascending aorta and extended into the descending aorta. Type II referred to dissections confined to the ascending aorta. Type III referred to dissections which commenced just beyond the right subclavian artery and were confined to the descending aorta. The more recent classifications divide dissecting hematomas into two types depending on whether they involve the ascending aorta (type A) or are confined to the descending aorta (type B) irrespective of the site of the primary intimal tear.[4, 62, 203] The rationale for this division is that the survival of patients with ascending aortic dissections is significantly better when treated surgically, compared to those patients treated medically.[4, 62, 204] Medical treatment is based on hypotensive therapy designed to prevent propagation of the hematoma.[321] The surgical treatment entails the obliteration of the false lumen close to the entry site and, in selected cases, aortic valve replacement. Patients with acute descending aortic dissections (type B) fare equally well with medical or surgical therapy, and it is therefore recommended that such patients be treated initially with medical therapy, holding surgery in reserve.[4]

Clinically, the symptoms of acute dissection include severe chest pain—often with mid scapula radiation, circulatory shock, and pulse deficits. Ascending aortic dissections may show the signs and symptoms of left ventricular failure resulting from aortic regurgitation. Pericardial tamponade is a life-threatening complication.

In some cases, as discussed below, a dissecting hematoma can be diagnosed from plain film findings, but usually these findings cannot be relied upon either to confirm or deny the diagnosis. Although entirely normal plain chest radiographs are unusual in aortic dissection, they are occasionally encountered.

The main role of the plain chest film is to exclude other conditions. Occasionally it will provide the first clue to the diagnosis of aortic dissection.[11] A major problem in many cases is that the images are obtained with portable equipment in critically ill patients who cannot take a deep breath in and who cannot stand or sit up. All these factors make the mediastinum appear wide even in the healthy person.

Dissecting hematomas confined to the aortic root are often hidden, whereas the arch and descending aorta are border-forming structures and, therefore, dissections involving these portions of the aorta usually produce recognizable plain film signs (Fig 15–98). The widening of the aorta in dissecting hematoma tends to involve long segments, although short segmental involvement is occasionally encountered. The arch and descending aorta show uniform enlargement in many cases. Sometimes the widening is distinctly undulating in appearance; occasionally, the dissection may be manifest by a focal aneurysm of the aorta.[66] The distinction from degenerative widening and unfolding may not be possible on plain films.[154] Progressive widening over a few hours or days is an almost specific sign and is, therefore, a most important observation.

The position of calcification in the aortic wall may help one to diagnose the presence of a dissecting hematoma. The concept here is that calcification of the wall of the aorta is in atherosclerotic intimal plaques and that in aortic dissection these plaques are displaced away from the outer aortic contour.[85] In the correct clinical circumstances, atheromatous calcification more than 1.0 cm inside the aortic contour can be regarded as suggestive evidence of aortic dissection. Displacement of this degree is not a common finding, being seen in only 4% of cases in one large series.[75] The sign must be used with caution; the calcification must be unequivocally profiled against the outer aortic contour and is, therefore, of no use in the aortic arch, because the aortic knob in the frontal projection represents a foreshortened view of an obliquely curving tube. It is not a specific sign, because the wall of the aorta may be substantially thickened in degenerative disease alone, and clearly it is not applicable when the soft tissue outside the aorta is tumor or mediastinal fat.

Bleeding from a dissecting hematoma may cause recognizable mediastinal widening on plain chest ra-

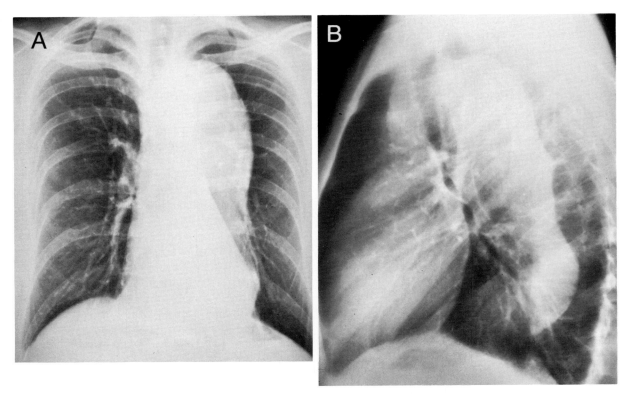

FIG 15–98.
Acute aortic dissection. Plain chest radiographs show undulating widening of the arch and descending aorta. **A,** PA radiograph. **B,** lateral radiograph.

diograph. This widening may be well-defined or ill-defined. Perihilar pulmonary consolidation may be seen due to bleeding into the lung. Pleural effusions due to seepage of blood from the mediastinum are a common accompaniment of aortic dissection; they are usually left sided or, if bilateral, are worse on the left than the right. Rupture into the pericardium is an extremely serious, often fatal complication. The presence of pericardial fluid can rarely be diagnosed using plain films.

CT provides a highly sensitive and specific technique with which to diagnose or exclude the presence of a dissecting hematoma of the aorta.* The technique used varies from center to center. A suggested protocol[322] is to perform selected pre-contrast scans at the level of the arch, the mid-ascending aorta, and the distal descending aorta (through mid-left atrium or left ventricular apex). Dynamic scans at the same three levels are then carried out; during each of three dynamic series, a 35- to 40-ml bolus injection of intravenous contrast material is rapidly administered at each level. If necessary, a slow infusion of contrast material is then continued while contiguous 1-cm sections are obtained from just above the aortic arch to the level of the diaphragm (or below, if necessary). The diagnostic features on contrast-enhanced CT scans are the exact counterparts of those seen at aortography (Fig 15–99): namely, the recognition of two lumens separated by an intimal flap (Fig 15–100). The intimal flap is seen as a curvilinear lucency within the opacified aorta. Sometimes, particularly in the aortic arch, the intimal flap may assume a serpiginous course. Plaques of calcification can frequently be seen within the displaced intima. The false lumen usually fills and empties in a delayed fashion compared with the true lumen, a finding that is best interpreted on dynamic scans at a single level. Differential opacification can be a very useful sign in cases where the intimal flap is invisible or uncertain. It should be remembered that the false lumen may be partially or, on rare occasions, totally filled by thrombus (Fig 15–101). The true lumen is usually compressed by the false lumen, sometimes to a substantial degree. The appearance of two lumina separated by an intimal flap is specific for aortic dissection, but care

*References 78, 119, 130, 138, 225, 297, and 301.

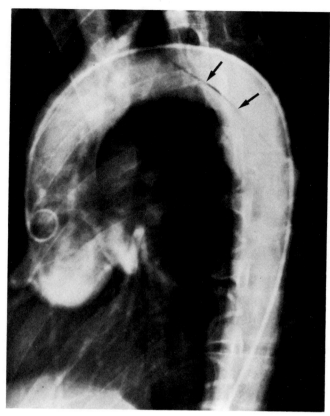

FIG 15–99.
Angiogram of a type B dissection in a patient with Marfan's syndrome showing little or no widening of the aorta but an obvious intimal flap *(arrows)* separating two lumina.

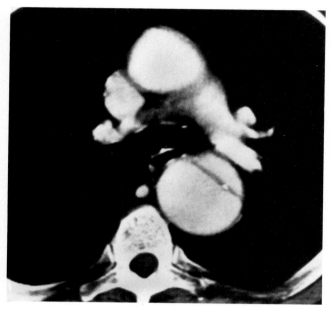

FIG 15–100.
Contrast-enhanced CT scan showing type B dissection with intimal flap, containing focal calcification, separating the two lumina. Notice the pronounced dilatation of the affected descending aorta.

must be taken not to misdiagnose an extra-aortic structure as a false lumen.[118] The innominate veins, the superior vena cava, the left superior intercostal vein, and the left pulmonary veins can all mimic a false channel, as can adjacent pleural or pericardial thickening and adjacent atelectasis of the lung (see Fig 15–96). Partial volume averaging of densities in the section above or below may closely resemble a false lumen and can give a false impression of displaced intimal calcification.

Another common but subtle sign of acute aortic dissection is a moderate increase in density of the false lumen owing to recently clotted blood.[139] This sign can only be appreciated on pre-contrast scans when it is possible to compare the density of the non-opacified true and false lumina. The shape of the opacified lumen may help. In atherosclerotic aneurysm the lumen is almost always round, whereas in aortic dissection the lumen is flattened in over half the cases.[139]

Displacement of calcified atheromatous plaques by the dissection can be demonstrated on pre-

contrast scans (Fig 15–102) and is a useful CT sign in those cases where contrast enhancement of the two lumina cannot be achieved as, for instance, when the false lumen is thrombosed. This sign is only seen in a minority of patients, however.[301] It is also possible, on occasion, to see the intimal flap even without contrast material,[301] particularly in patients who are anemic.[67] This sign should clearly not be relied upon, but could be useful if for some reason only pre-contrast CT images are available for review.

The affected portions of the aorta are often, though by no means always, enlarged. In some reports[130, 173] dilatation was always present, but in the largest series reported to date, almost 60% of patients with dissection showed no aortic dilatation.[301] Enlarged portions of the aorta should be carefully examined for the more specific signs of dissection, with dynamic scanning if necessary.[301]

Streak artifacts can mimic an intimal flap (Fig 15–103).[104, 118] Intimal flaps are gently curved structures of uniform thickness conforming to the configuration of the aorta. Streak artifacts are straight and vary in thickness. Also, their orientation may change markedly from one CT section to the next, and they often extend outside the aorta.

Distinguishing between an aortic dissection with a completely thrombosed false lumen and an atheromatous aneurysm with thrombus lining the wall of

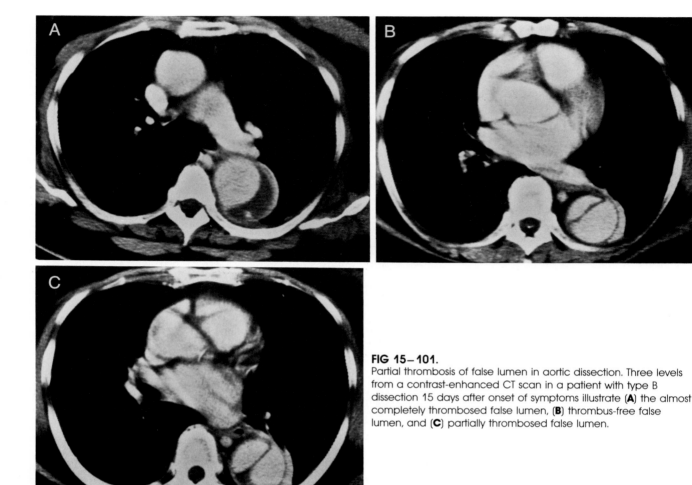

FIG 15–101.
Partial thrombosis of false lumen in aortic dissection. Three levels from a contrast-enhanced CT scan in a patient with type B dissection 15 days after onset of symptoms illustrate (**A**) the almost completely thrombosed false lumen, (**B**) thrombus-free false lumen, and (**C**) partially thrombosed false lumen.

the aorta can be difficult. The thrombosis of the false lumen means that neither the double channel nor the intimal flap can be demonstrated. In these circumstances, the displacement of intimal calcification becomes a useful sign of dissection, but it is important to realize that calcification may, on occasion, be seen lining the inner surface of the thrombus in an atherosclerotic aneurysm.[118, 139]

The choice of test for patients with possible aortic dissection is not always easy. Aortography is more invasive and subject to greater complications but has the significant advantages of being able to show aortic regurgitation and demonstrating any compromise to the arteries arising from the aorta. It can also show which arteries are perfused from which lumen and can often demonstrate with greater precision the entry point of the dissection. CT is safer and is as accurate, if not more accurate, in demonstrating the extent of the hematoma,[225] even in thrombosed

portions of the false lumen. It also allows recognition of pericardial fluid, pleural fluid, mediastinal bleeding, and any spread of hemorrhage into the lung parenchyma. MRI is not currently in routine use but no doubt will soon become so, since it provides information as good as and frequently superior to CT, but does not require contrast enhancement.

The choice of test will depend on the clinical state of the patient, the preferences of the thoracic surgeons responsible for the patient, and on the precise questions being asked. In the acute setting, especially in patients who are being considered for immediate corrective surgery, the choice probably favors angiography. If angiography will be needed in any event prior to surgery, then great care must be taken not to delay the angiogram or to compromise the examination by giving prior doses of contrast medium for a CT scan. Where it is believed that the

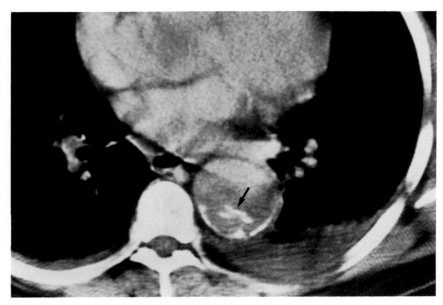

FIG 15–102.
Displaced calcification in intimal flap *(arrow)* on pre-contrast CT scan in a patient with aortic dissection.

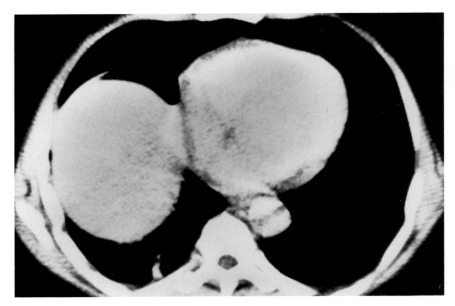

FIG 15–103.
Streak artifacts across descending aorta, mimicking an aortic dissection on a contrast-enhanced CT scan.

treatment decision can be based on the findings at CT/MRI study, then clearly CT/MRI scanning should be performed and angiography held in reserve. For example, a patient with severe chest pain, in whom the likelihood of aortic dissection is low, but whose clinical examination or plain chest films show features that require the diagnosis to be excluded, would be a good candidate for CT/MRI, as would a patient thought likely to have dissection in whom medical therapy is the treatment of choice, the prime purpose then being to confirm the diagnosis and to provide a baseline for follow-up. CT (or MRI) is clearly also the diagnostic test of choice for follow-up of a previously treated dissection.

Congenital Aneurysms

Congenital aneurysms of the aorta are rare. Almost all of those encountered in clinical practice are sinus of Valsalva aneurysms.

Normally, the media of the wall of the proximal aorta is firmly attached to the fibrous annulus of the aortic valve. In congenital aneurysm of the aortic sinus, the media avulses from its attachment to the annulus, and an aneurysm results.[77] These aneurysms most commonly arise from the posterior or right aortic sinus. An aneurysm of the posterior sinus will bulge into the right atrium, and rupture will result in an aortic to right atrial shunt. An aneurysm of the right aortic sinus will bulge into the right ventricle, and rupture will result in an aortic to right ventricular shunt. The aortic valve lies deep within the mediastinal shadow on plain chest radiograph and congenital aortic sinus aneurysms must, therefore, reach substantial size to be recognizable on plain film. Occasionally, they do reach such a size. Calcification may be visible in the wall of the aneurysm. The signs of left-to-right shunt may be visible if rupture has occurred. CT and MRI show the aneurysm to advantage.[121]

Very occasionally, aneurysms are associated with coarctation of the aorta (Fig 15–104). Whether these are truly congenital or acquired secondary to prolonged hypertension is debatable.

Aneurysms Resulting From Aortitis

Aneurysms that are the result of aortitis are rare now that syphilis is so uncommon (Fig 15–105). Takayasu's is the best known example of this group of diseases. Though more often a stenosing disease, it may, on occasion, cause saccular or fusiform aortic aneurysms (Fig 15–106).[186, 236, 335] It is a chronic inflammatory condition of unknown origin that affects the aorta, its main branches, and the pulmonary arteries. It occurs most commonly in the Orient, but has a worldwide distribution. Aneurysms in this condition may be single or multiple and may be seen anywhere in the aorta. Calcification of the wall of the aorta and of the aneurysm may be present, and aortic dissection may be a complication.

Aortic Anomalies That May Simulate a Mediastinal Mass

There are three congenital variations of the aorta that can simulate a mediastinal mass on plain chest radiographs or unenhanced CT scans: right aortic arch, double aortic arch, and pseudocoarctation of the aorta.

Right Aortic Arch

Right aortic arch is a common finding in a number of congenital heart disorders. This discussion will be confined to right aortic arch in patients without cardiac malformation, in whom the arch passes to the right of the trachea and usually descends in the right posterior mediastinum; only rarely is the descending aorta on the left. The usual branching pattern is that the left carotid artery arises first, followed by the right carotid and right subclavian arteries. The left subclavian artery arises as the fourth and most distal branch of the aortic arch. It is therefore known as an aberrant subclavian artery, to distinguish it from the so-called mirror image arrangement which is seen when right aortic arch accompanies complex congenital heart disease. (In mirror image branching, the left subclavian artery is a branch of the first vessel to arise from the aortic arch, namely the left brachiocephalic artery.) The aberrant left subclavian artery passes behind the esophagus to reach the root of the neck on the left side. The left subclavian artery may take origin from a diverticulum in the proximal descending aorta, which embryologically represents a remnant of the left arch.

The radiographic appearances (Figs 15–107 and 15–108), therefore, consist of a visible right aortic arch and a density posterior to the esophagus which varies in size from small to large. This density is sometimes due to the diverticulum and sometimes to medial displacement of the proximal descending aorta. The posterior impression on the esophagus at barium swallow and on the trachea at plain film and CT is often striking. There is also absence of a visible left aortic arch, but great caution is needed here, because either the diverticulum or the leftward displacement of the aortic arch may resemble a small

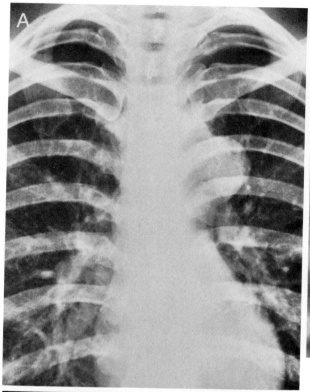

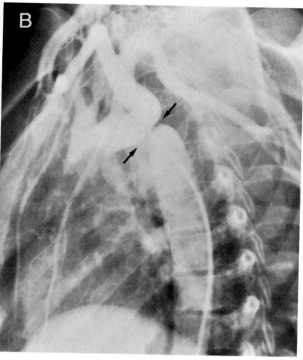

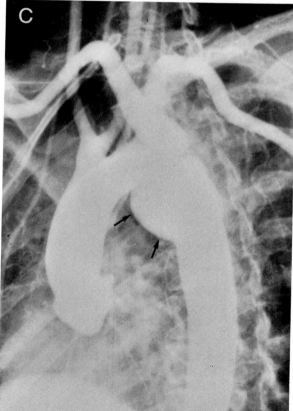

FIG 15–104.
Slowly enlarging congenital aneurysm of the aorta in a young
woman with coarctation of the aorta. **A,** plain film shows
saccular aneurysm indistinguishable from an atherosclerotic or
traumatic aneurysm (compare with Fig 15–97). **B,** early phase
of aortogram showing the coarctation *(arrows).* **C,** later phase
of the aortogram showing contrast opacification of the
aneurysm *(arrows).*

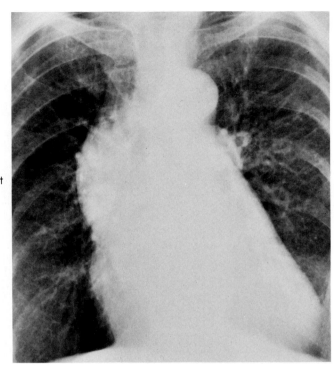

FIG 15–105.
Syphilitic aneurysm of the aorta, showing typical severe enlargement confined to the ascending aorta with calcification in the wall of the aneurysm.

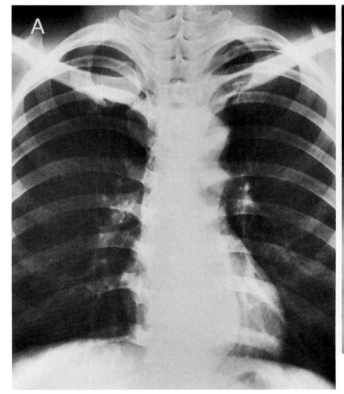

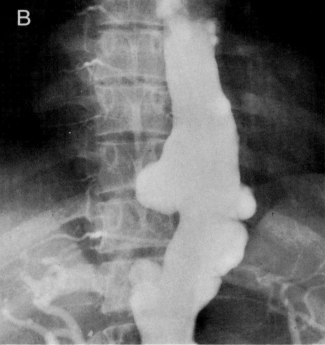

FIG 15–106.
Arteritis causing aortic aneurysms in a young Nepalese man. **A,** PA radiograph. **B,** aortogram.

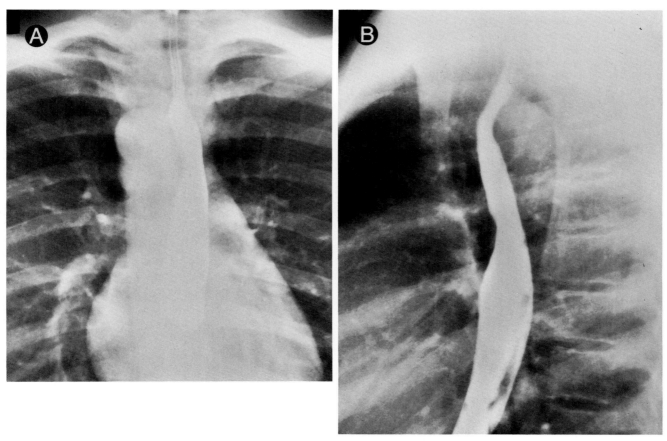

FIG 15–107.
A and **B,** right aortic arch—showing aortic arch to right of trachea but no aortic arch to left of trachea. Note the characteristic right-sided and posterior indentations on the esophagus.

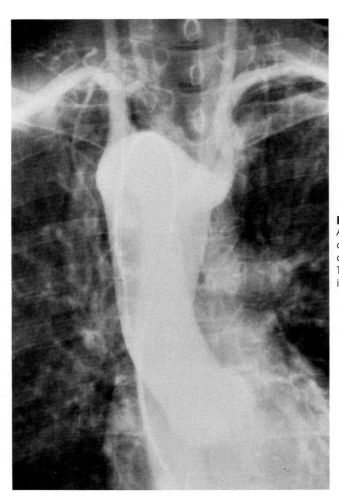

FIG 15–108.
Aortogram of right aortic arch with aberrant left subclavian artery. Note the midline position of the distal arch and the diverticulum from which the left subclavian artery takes origin. These two phenomena together give rise to the posterior impression on the esophagus shown in Figure 15–107.

left aortic knob. The descending aorta will be to the right of the midline in almost all cases.

The combination of these features makes it possible to diagnose right aortic arch with aberrant left subclavian artery on plain chest radiograph (or barium swallow study) in almost every case. CT scanning will show the same features and will also show contrast enhancement of the aorta and its branches.

Double Aortic Arch

Most patients with double aortic arch present early in life with tracheal obstruction and swallowing difficulties. Occasionally, the anomaly remains undetected until later in childhood or adult life. The two aortic arches pass to either side of the trachea and join posteriorly, at which point they often displace the trachea and esophagus forward, thus potentially causing confusion with a mass. The descending aorta is usually in the midline. The diagnostic features are:

1. The right arch is almost always larger and higher than the left arch (Fig 15–109). This observation is particularly important at barium swallow, where the arches indent the esophagus from either side.

2. At CT scanning, the branching pattern of the vessels to the head and neck is distinctive. Each arch gives rise to two vessels—a carotid and a subclavian artery—each artery of the pair lying one in front of the other (Fig 15–110).

3. The arches fuse posterior to the esophagus and trachea and may create a masslike density in the posterior mediastinum.

Pseudocoarctation of the Aorta

Pseudocoarctation of the aorta is a congenital anomaly that many authorities believe is part of the spectrum of true coarctation, but without a gradient-producing narrowing of the aorta. The aorta is kinked at the level of the ligamentum arteriosum,

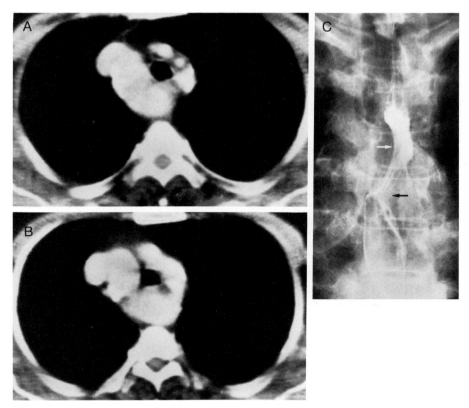

FIG 15–109.
CT scan findings in double aortic arch. **A,** contrast-enhanced CT scan at the level of the lower trachea shows right aortic arch at the same level as the two branches of the left arch. **B,** adjacent lower sections show smaller left arch at the level of the tracheal carina. **C,** barium swallow study shows two indentations corresponding to the two arches *(arrows)*. The double aortic arch was an incidental discovery in a 71-year-old man.

the same position as the usual site of coarctation (Fig 15–111). The aortic arch, therefore, rises higher than usual, the ascending aorta being more vertical and the curve of the arch tighter. The high aortic arch, or the kinking, may simulate a mass (Figs 15–112, and 15–113). Pseudocoarctation, like true coarctation, is associated with an increased tendency to aortic dissection, and then the aorta either above or below the kink may be significantly enlarged, leading to the possibility of even greater confusion with a mass (Fig 15–114).

Esophageal Tumors Presenting as Mediastinal Masses

Carcinoma of the esophagus, the most common neoplasm to affect the esophagus, only occasionally gives rise to recognizable plain film findings. The most usual sign is visible dilatation of the esophagus, which may be accompanied by recognizable thickening of the esophageal wall. Presentation as a medias-

tinal mass is almost never seen. Esophageal dilatation is usually easiest to recognize posterior to the trachea on the lateral view. The fluid-filled, dilated esophagus acts like a mass, displacing the trachea and carina forward. In healthy individuals, the lung usually invaginates posterior to the right half of the trachea, so that it is possible to see the posterior tracheal band (see Chapter 3). With esophageal dilatation, the esophagus displaces the lung, and it may be possible to recognize a thick band of tissue between air in the trachea and air in the lumen of the esophagus. This thickened band represents the combined thickness of the walls of the trachea and esophagus. In addition, in carcinoma of the esophagus, periesophageal lymphatic involvement contributes to the thickening of the posterior tracheal band.[246] As an isolated sign, increased thickness of the posterior tracheal band is of little value because the collapsed normal esophagus can interpose between the lung and the trachea and cause marked thickening of the band. However, if the sign is accompanied by for-

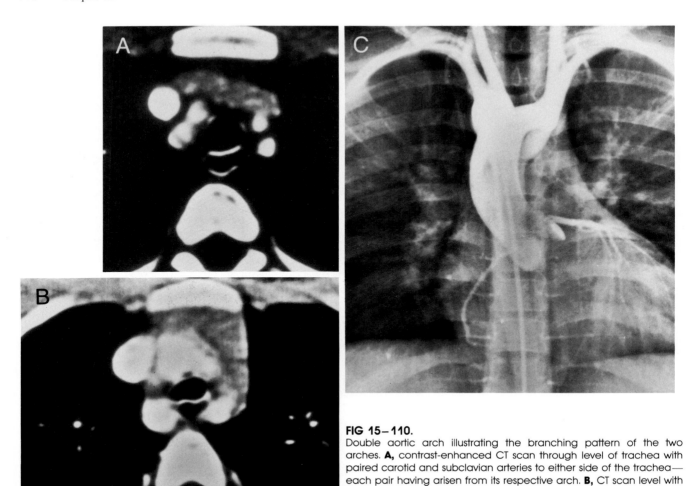

FIG 15–110.
Double aortic arch illustrating the branching pattern of the two arches. **A,** contrast-enhanced CT scan through level of trachea with paired carotid and subclavian arteries to either side of the trachea— each pair having arisen from its respective arch. **B,** CT scan level with tracheal carina showing the splitting of the ascending aorta and the two separate distal arches posterolateral to the esophagus. The patient was a 12-year-old child who presented with mild tracheal obstruction. **C,** aortogram in another child showing the anatomic features. Note the right arch is larger and higher and two main branches arise from each arch.

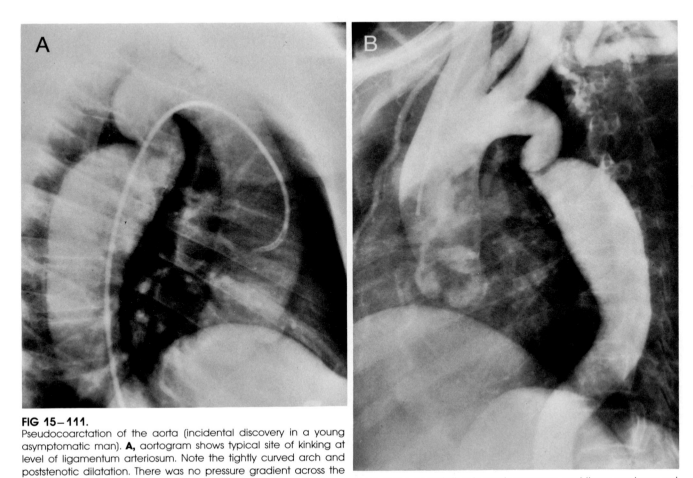

FIG 15–111.
Pseudocoarctation of the aorta (incidental discovery in a young asymptomatic man). **A,** aortogram shows typical site of kinking at level of ligamentum arteriosum. Note the tightly curved arch and poststenotic dilatation. There was no pressure gradient across the kink. **B,** true coarctation for comparison. The features are similar except that the coarctation is much narrower, and there are large collateral vessels. A pressure gradient was present.

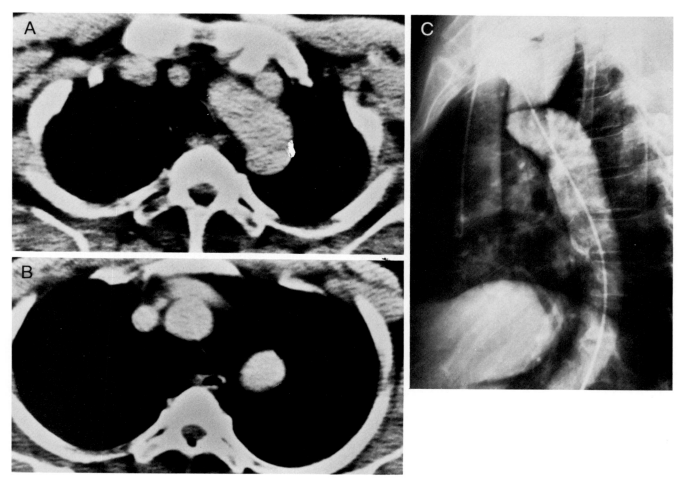

FIG 15–112.
Pseudocoarctation of the aorta simulating a mass. **A,** arch is seen in unexpectedly high position on contrast-enhanced CT scan. **B,** section 2 cm lower at the expected level of top of arch shows ascending and descending aorta. **C,** aortogram of same patient. (The plain chest radiograph in this patient is shown in Fig 15–66).

ward bowing of the trachea and anterior displacement of the carina, then esophageal dilatation can be confidently diagnosed (Fig 15–115).

Smooth muscle tumors (leiomyomas and leiomyosarcomas) may grow to a substantial size without causing dysphagia and may, therefore, present first as an asymptomatic mediastinal mass.[52] In the days when barium swallow was the automatic next test for posterior mediastinal masses, the diagnosis was readily made by observing the characteristic signs of an intramural extramucosal mass. Now, CT is often done first without preliminary barium swallow. CT shows a smooth, round, well-defined, enhancing mass in the posterior mediastinum inseparable from the esophagus (Fig 15–116). The esophagus is usually not dilated above the level of the tumor. This lack of dilatation can be an important differential di-

agnostic point in reducing the likelihood of carcinoma of the esophagus.

Hiatus Hernia

Hiatus hernias are frequent incidental findings on chest radiographs and CT examinations. They may produce pain as a result of gastroesophageal reflux and may be responsible for anemia or upper gastrointestinal bleeding. On plain chest radiograph they produce a smooth, focal widening of the posterior junction anatomy extending down to the diaphragm. Varying amounts of fat surround the hernia itself, and in most instances some air can be appreciated within the hernia on plain film; often there is a visible air-fluid level. At CT, the esophagus can be traced down into the hernia, and air (and

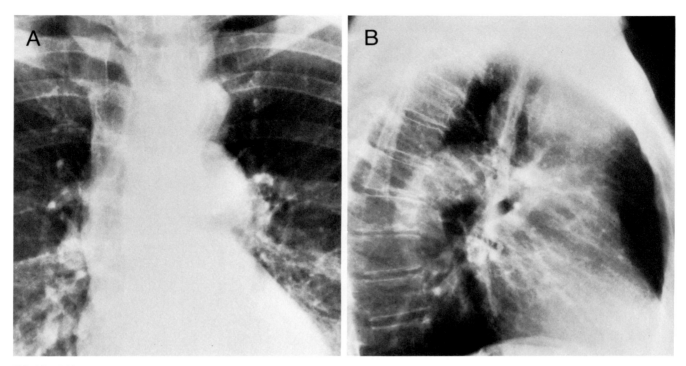

FIG 15–113.
Pseudocoarctation of the aorta. The kinked aorta is aligned such that the portion distal to the kink simulates either an enlarged pulmonary artery or a mediastinal mass. **A,** PA radiograph. **B,** lateral radiograph.

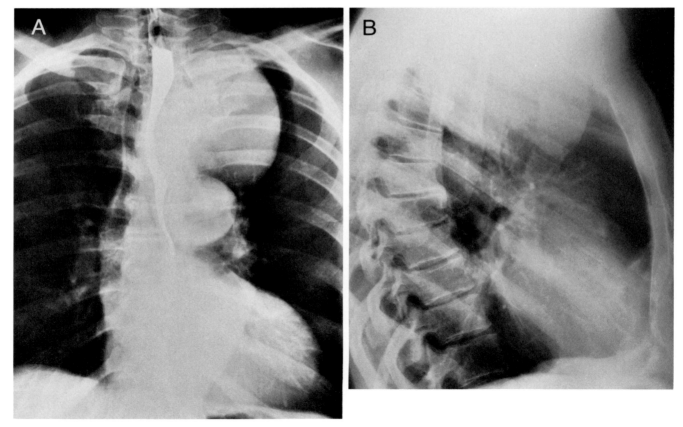

FIG 15–114.
Aneurysm formation of aortic arch proximal to pseudocoarctation. **A,** PA radiograph with barium in esophagus. **B,** lateral radiograph.

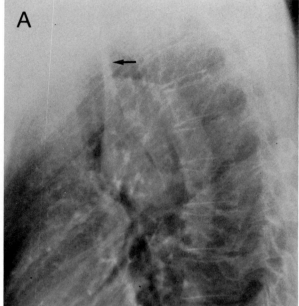

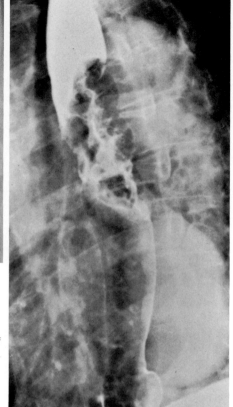

FIG 15–115.
Esophageal dilatation resulting from carcinoma of the esophagus. **A,** lateral radiograph shows forward bowing of the trachea and the thick, posterior tracheal band *(arrow).* **B,** corresponding features at barium swallow examination.

contrast material) within the lumen usually enables the diagnosis to be made without difficulty. The fat surrounding the hernia may be a striking feature. Hiatus hernias can be huge and may contain a major portion of the stomach. With large paraesophageal hernias, the stomach not infrequently undergoes organoaxial rotation and, therefore, may contain two air-fluid levels.

Hernia Through the Foramen of Bochdalek

The pleuroperitoneal hiatus in each hemidiaphragm closes during early fetal life. The major component of the developing diaphragm is the septum transversum. During the 7th week of development, the pleuroperitoneal folds fuse with the mesentery of the esophagus and migrate anteriorly to join the septum transversum, closing two large posterolateral openings. Failure of closure results in congenital diaphragmatic hernia. Small defects of closure are common and usually are not discovered until late in adult life when they appear as rounded

"humps" on one or both hemidiaphragms (Fig 15–117). They are particularly common in patients over 70 years of age. Gale found a prevalence of 6% when he reviewed the chest and abdominal CT scans of 940 individuals.[103] It is often stated that left-sided hernias are considerably more common, but Gale's review[103] revealed that left-sided hernias were approximately twice as common as those on the right, and that bilateral hernias were present in just over 15% of cases. These humps, which represent collections of herniated retroperitoneal fat and, sometimes, kidney or a portion of spleen are seen posteriorly, usually close to the spine. They are typically found on the posterior portion of the hemidiaphragm some 4 to 5 cm from the posterior attachment of the diaphragm. The herniation of the kidney may be so striking that the term intrathoracic kidney has been used.[187] The radiographic appearances of the chest in elderly individuals are sufficiently characteristic that further investigation is not warranted. When alternative causes for a diaphragmatic or paraspinal swelling are being entertained,

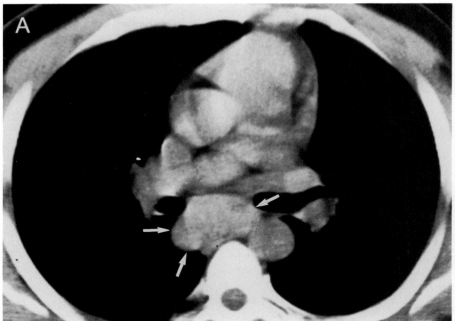

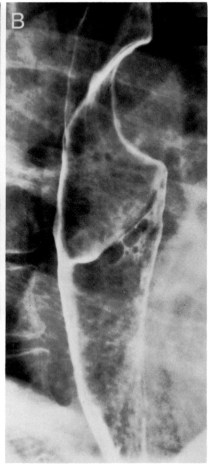

FIG 15–116.
Leiomyoma of the esophagus presenting as a mediastinal mass. **A,** contrast-enhanced CT scan shows smooth homogeneous mass centered on esophagus *(arrows)*. **B,** barium swallow study shows an intraluminal extramucosal mass.

CT scanning[103] will demonstrate the fatty nature of the hernial content and will often show the accompanying muscle defect in the diaphragm. Identifying the muscle defect may be difficult in those patients who have little retroperitoneal fat, but in most individuals there is relatively abundant subdiaphragmatic fat on the left. On the right, the liver may obscure the details of the superior portion of the right hemidiaphragm and so make it difficult to recognize a high Bochdalek defect, but typically the defects are lower and lie against retroperitoneal fat.[103] CT scanning will also reveal that the ipsilateral kidney is often in a high position. Extrapleural lipomas in contact with the diaphragm may appear similar, but they are not accompanied by a diaphragmatic defect or displacement of abdominal viscera.

Hernia Through the Foramen of Morgagni

The foramina of Morgagni are V-shaped developmental defects, also known as the space of Larrey, between the muscle origins from the sternum and adjacent ribs.[230] Hernias through the foramen of Morgagni are often confined to the right side, presumably because on the left herniation is prevented by the pericardium beneath the heart; herniation into the pericardial sac has, however, been reported in both children and adults.[278, 305] In adults, these hernias are mostly asymptomatic, although lower sternal discomfort, cough, dyspnea, and nonspecific gastrointestinal symptoms may occur.[230] On plain chest radiographs[230, 252] hernias through the foramen of Morgagni produce opacities in the right cardiophrenic angle. The shadow may be well-defined and resemble a mass, or it may be ill-defined and resemble pneumonia. The contents are mostly fat and, therefore, on plain chest radiograph the density resembles soft tissue; air-containing loops of bowel are only occasionally seen. Examination of the bowel with contrast material may show contrast medium in the hernia or may show a loop of small or large bowel hooked up toward the hernial sac. Radionuclide liver scans may show liver herniating into the chest.

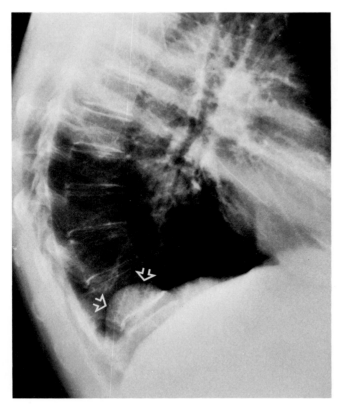

FIG 15—117.
Bochdalek hernia in a typical location on the posterior surface of the dome of the hemidiaphragm *(arrows).*

DIFFERENTIAL DIAGNOSIS OF MEDIASTINAL MASSES

The differential diagnosis of mediastinal masses is a common problem. Because the choice of likely diagnoses depends on the number of masses and their position, shape, size, and density, the radiologist must constantly construct a mental grid incorporating all these items when viewing plain radiographs and CT/MRI scans. Multiple small masses within the mediastinum are almost specific for lymphadenopathy, particularly if they are concentrated in the node-bearing areas. The nodes may be physically isolated from each other or form conglomerate masses, in which case they usually have lobular outlines. Lobulation of a single mass, though frequently seen with lymphadenopathy, is not specific, and is seen with many different types of mediastinal mass.

It has been traditional to divide mediastinal masses by their location and then to subdivide them according to their other radiographic findings. We too will use such a scheme, but some general points about density will be made first, since density is relevant whatever the site of the mass:

1. Irregular, granular, or eggshell calcification within *multiple* small mediastinal masses limits the differential diagnosis, for practical purposes, to lymphadenopathy resulting from such benign conditions as granulomatous infections (tuberculosis and histoplasmosis being the most common), coal worker's pneumoconiosis, and old sarcoidosis. Amyloidosis, treated lymphoma or metastasis may be an occasional cause. Calcification in a *solitary* mass has a wider differential diagnosis. Neural tumors may calcify, as may thymoma and teratoma, and solitary nodules in the thyroid frequently show calcification. The important practical point here is that untreated lymphoma or untreated metastatic neoplasm in lymph nodes almost never results in calcification. The exceptions are few and far between.

Aneurysms of the aorta or its major branches frequently show curvilinear calcification in their walls or in thrombus lining the aneurysm. This calcification, taken together with the observations that aneurysms always arise from and are in intimate contact with the aorta or one of its branches and that they almost always have blood swirling within them, allows a confident distinction to be made between aneurysms and other causes of mediastinal mass. Curvilinear calcification is also seen in the walls of congenital cystic lesions, notably bronchogenic and pericardial cysts, and occasionally, in cystic teratomas.

2. Uniform water density in a mass with a thin wall of uniform thickness at CT is diagnostic of a congenital cyst, the precise diagnosis depending on the location of the cyst. Variable density within a mass, even including some regions of 0 to 10 Hounsfield units, may be seen in necrotic malignant neoplasms and in benign masses that undergo cyst formation, e.g., thyroid and thymic masses. Therefore, the low density of a mass can be used to diagnose a congenital cyst only if all the above criteria are met. Irregularity of the wall and variability in the density of the remainder of the mass mean that more sinister lesions must be included in the differential diagnosis.

3. Fat density within a mass limits the possibilities to collections of normal fat (e.g., epicardial fat pads or lipomatosis resulting from high levels of circulating steroids); lipomas and liposarcomas; extramedullary hematopoiesis; and fat in cystic teratomas or thymolipoma. Fat-fluid levels within a cystic mass are pathognomonic of benign cystic teratoma. Benign lipomas and thymolipomas are composed entirely of fat containing a few thin strands of soft tissue stroma. Liposarcoma usually shows a mixture

of fat intermingled with masses of soft tissue density.

4. Intravenous contrast enhancement may show opacification of a portion of the mass at CT. The basic appearances are (a) opacification of the lumen of an aneurysm or (b) enhancement of the soft tissue component of the mass. Minor degrees of enhancement of the soft tissue component of the mass are nonspecific, but marked enhancement[282] suggests thyroid tissue; a paraganglioma, including pheochromocytoma; a neurogenic tumor; vascular malformations; or the extremely rare conditions of Castleman's disease and aggressive fibromatosis. Thyroid tissue is more intense than the other soft tissues even prior to contrast being given, and it enhances brightly after contrast material is administered.

Masses Anterior to the Ascending Aorta and the Arteries Arising From the Aortic Arch

Almost all masses in this location will be (1) thyroid masses, (2) thymic masses, (3) germ cell tumors/cysts, or (4) lymphadenopathy. Thyroid masses can usually be specifically diagnosed or excluded based on their contiguity with the thyroid gland in the neck and their high CT density on pre- and post-contrast scans. In addition, many will show cystic areas close to water density, as well as one or more areas of discrete calcification. Thymic masses and germ cell tumors can be thought of together, as most germ cell tumors arise within the thymus. Clinical and laboratory features may help distinguish between the two. For example, myasthenia gravis, red cell aplasia, and hypogammaglobulinemia are associated with thymoma, whereas high alpha fetoprotein or high human chorionic gonadotrophin levels may be seen with malignant germ cell tumors. Also, thymoma is almost unknown in patients less than 20 years old. If fat, cartilage calcification, or teeth are present in the mass, then teratoma is the diagnosis. (The only exception to this statement would be chondrosarcoma projecting from a rib or from the sternum, or the extraordinarily remote possibility of metastatic chondrosarcoma.)

The rarer causes of masses anterior to the aorta and the branches of the aortic arch are parathyroid adenoma, lymphangioma (cystic hygroma), pericardial cyst, aortic body paraganglioma, lipoma/liposarcoma or other mesenchymal tumors, or aneurysms. (Aneurysms are extremely rare in this location and, when seen, are likely to be congenital or mycotic in origin.) Many of these masses have features that permit a specific diagnosis to be made. Parathyroid ade-

nomas are usually associated with hyperparathyroidism and are only discovered because a search for an ectopic parathyroid is being made. Lymphangiomas almost always have broad contact with the root of the neck and, because they are composed largely of lymph-filled spaces, they show numerous areas of nonenhancing, water or near-water density on CT scanning. Lipomas may be indistinguishable from normal fat collections but are readily distinguished from more significant mediastinal masses. Liposarcomas show a unique mixture of fat interspersed by irregular strands or masses of soft tissue density. Aneurysms show contrast opacification of their lumina. Pericardial cysts are, in general, of uniform water density with a thin, uniform thickness wall, and they need only be considered when the mass in question is in contact with the pericardium. It should be remembered, however, that the pericardium extends to the level of the junction point between the proximal and middle thirds of the ascending aorta. Mesenchymal tumors such as fibrosarcomas or blood vessel tumors have no distinguishing features.

Paracardiac Masses

The likely diagnoses for paracardiac masses in contact with the diaphragm are pericardial cyst, diaphragmatic hernia, fat pad, or lymphadenopathy. If the mass is separated from the diaphragm, the likely differential diagnoses widen to include germ cell, mesenchymal, and pericardial tumors, and thymic masses. Approximately 20% of thymomas are found in a paracardiac location, though contact with the diaphragm is very unusual. Lack of connection with the diaphragm eliminates the possibility of a diaphragmatic hernia.

Most paracardiac masses are in the cardiophrenic angles, the right cardiophrenic angle being the site of a mass more often than the left because pericardial cysts are more often right-sided than left-sided and because foramen of Morgagni hernias can occur on the right, whereas they are usually prevented on the left by the presence of the heart. CT scanning has proved extremely helpful in the diagnosis of paracardiac masses. Most pericardial cysts are diagnosible by their uniform low density and their thin walls. Morgagni hernias are recognized by the omental fat within the hernia and sometimes by opacified bowel either within the mass or leading to it. Thus, diagnostic difficulty is confined to distinguishing thymic tumor, germ cell tumor, localized lymphadenopathy, or mesenchymal tumor. Biopsy is entirely appropriate for all these lesions.

Paratracheal, Subcarinal, and Paraesophageal Masses

These sites are considered together because the trachea, central bronchi, and esophagus are contained within a common fascial sheath. This compartment continues into the neck around the airway, the esophagus, and the pharynx. The prime considerations for nonvascular masses in these locations are lymphadenopathy, intrathoracic thyroid mass, developmental foregut cysts, esophageal tumors, hiatus hernia, and paraspinal masses encroaching on the posterior mediastinum. In terms of incidence, lymphadenopathy is by far the most frequent. Masses deep to the azygos vein in either the right paratracheal area or in the pretracheal or precarinal space are almost invariably lymphadenopathy. For masses arising in the aortopulmonary window, the only other alternative is aortic aneurysm—a diagnosis that can be readily confirmed or excluded with contrast-enhanced CT. As mentioned earlier, lymphadenopathy is frequently multifocal and, in the case of metastatic carcinoma, the primary tumor is usually already known. Bronchogenic cyst can be diagnosed with confidence if the criteria of a simple cyst are met. But many bronchogenic cysts do not show the diagnostic features of uniform low density and these are, therefore, included in the differential diagnosis of a single mass of lymph nodes. Curvilinear calcification in the wall of the cyst, though a rare sign, would enable one to distinguish between bronchogenic cyst and malignant lymphadenopathy. Thyroid masses that pass lateral to or posterior to the trachea are distinctive, partly because of the signs already described but also because thyroid masses show far greater contact, displacement, and compression of the trachea than do lymph nodes. Splitting of the trachea from the esophagus is a characteristic shared only by thyroid masses, bronchogenic cysts, esophageal tumors, and an aberrant origin of the left pulmonary artery. Aortic arch anomalies, though they deform the trachea and esophagus in various ways, do not pass between these two structures.

Esophageal tumors very rarely present as an unexpected mediastinal mass. Patients with esophageal carcinoma, the most common esophageal tumor, nearly always present with dysphagia at a time when the tumor mass is relatively small. Although the tumor can sometimes be seen as a mass on plain chest radiographs and can nearly always be recognized at CT, the diagnosis of esophageal carcinoma is made at barium swallow examination and does not form part of the differential diagnosis of a mediastinal mass. Leiomyoma or other mesenchymal tumors of the muscle layer may grow to a considerable size without causing dysphagia and may, on occasion, present as a mediastinal mass at plain chest radiography or CT scanning. The intimate relationship to the esophagus will lead to a barium swallow examination, at which time the typical features of an intramural-extramucosal esophageal mass will limit the diagnosis to leiomyoma, leiomyosarcoma or, rarely, some other tumor/cyst of the esophageal wall.

Hiatus hernia is an exceedingly common cause of enlargement of the mediastinum in the region of the lower esophagus. The plain film diagnosis is so easy and reliable that barium swallow is rarely required for diagnosis.

As discussed on p. 790, a number of vascular anomalies may mimic a mediastinal mass on plain chest radiographs and sometimes even on CT scans.

Paravertebral Masses

Strictly speaking, masses situated to either side of the vertebral column are outside the mediastinum since, according to anatomists' definitions, the mediastinum lies anterior to the spine. However, it is standard practice among radiologists and thoracic surgeons to label all masses against the spine as being posterior mediastinal masses.

Neurogenic lesions and neoplastic lymphadenopathy dominate the differential diagnosis for paraspinal masses. The neurogenic lesions consist of nerve sheath tumors (schwannoma, neurofibroma, and their malignant counterparts); ganglion cell tumors (ganglioneuroma/ganglioneuroblastoma/neuroblastoma); paragangliomas, including pheochromocytoma; lateral thoracic meningoceles; and neuroenteric cysts. Lymphadenopathy is rarely confined to the paraspinal areas; usually it is accompanied by enlarged lymph nodes in adjacent mediastinal or retroperitoneal areas. The commonest causes of posterior mediastinal lymphadenopathy are lymphoma and metastatic carcinoma from genitourinary primary tumors. The other, less common, causes of paraspinal masses include metastases from other sites; extramedullary hematopoiesis; pancreatic pseudocyst; mesenchymal tumors such as lipoma, fibroma, and hemangioma; and lesions arising from the esophagus, pharynx, spine, or aorta. The esophageal or pharyngeal lesions that may project posteriorly include leiomyoma, foregut cyst, and congenital or acquired diverticula of the esophagus. The spinal origin of lesions such as paraspinal abscess, tumors of the vertebral body that have spread into the adjacent paravertebral/mediastinal space, or hematoma from trauma to the spine are usually readily diagnosed by observing corresponding changes in the spine. Aneurysms of the descending aorta truly mimicking a mediastinal mass are uncommon. Most large aneurysms in this location are obvious dilatations of the descending aorta. Saccular aneurysms that could be confused with a mass show a broad base on the aorta and almost always have curvilinear calcification in their walls. The diagnosis is readily made at CT when opacification of the lumen can be demonstrated. Most contain thrombus within the aneurysm, but not enough to obliterate the lumen totally.

REFERENCES

1. Allen PW: The fibromatoses: A clinicopathologic classification based on 140 cases. Part 1. *Am J Surg Pathol* 1977; 1:255–270.
2. Alterman K, Shueller EF: Maturation of neuroblastoma to ganglioneuroma. *Am J Dis Child* 1970; 120:217–222.
3. Angtuaco EJC, Jimenez JF, Burrows P, et al: Lymphatic-venous malformation (lymphangiohemangioma) of mediastinum: Case report. *J Comput Assist Tomogr* 1983; 7:895–897.
4. Appelbaum A, Karp RB, Kirklin JW: Ascending vs descending aortic dissections. *Ann Surg* 1976; 183:296–300.
5. Armstrong EA, Harwood-Nash DCF, Ritz CR, et al: CT of neuroblastomas and ganglioneuromas in children. *AJR* 1982; 139:571–576.
6. Armstrong P: Tomographic evaluation of the questionably enlarged pulmonary hilum, in Armstrong P (ed): *Critical Problems in Diagnostic Radiology*. Philadelphia, JB Lippincott Co, 1983.
7. Aronberg DJ, Glazer HS, Sagel SS: MRI and CT of the mediastinum: Comparisons, controversies, and pitfalls. *Radiol Clin North Am* 1985; 23:439–448.
8. Baker HL, Berquist TH, Kispert DB, et al: Magnetic resonance imaging in a routine clinical setting. *Mayo Clin Proc* 1985; 60:75–90.
9. Bankoff MS, Daly BDT, Johnson HA, et al: Bronchogenic cyst causing superior vena cava obstruction: CT appearance. *J Comput Assist Tomogr* 1985; 9:951–952.
10. Barek L, Lautin R, Ledor S, et al: Role of CT in the assessment of superior vena caval obstruction: CT. *J Comput Tomogr* 1982; 6:121–126.
11. Baron MG: Dissecting aneurysm of the aorta. *Circulation* 1971; 63:933–943.
12. Baron RL, Lee JKT, Sagel SS, et al: Computed tomography of the abnormal thymus. *Radiology* 1982; 142:127–134.
13. Baron RL, Sagel SS, Baglan RJ: Thymic cysts following radiation therapy for Hodgkin's disease. *Radiology* 1981; 141:593–597.
14. Barrett AF, Toye DKM: Sympathicoblastoma: Radiological findings in forty-three cases. *Clin Radiol* 1963; 14:33–42.
15. Barnett SM: CT findings in tuberculous mediastinitis. *J Comput Assist Tomogr* 1986; 10:165–166.
16. Bar-Ziv J, Nogrady MB: Mediastinal neuroblastoma and ganglioneuroma. *AJR* 1975; 125:380–390.
17. Bartra P, Herrmann C, Mulder D: Mediastinal imaging in myasthemia gravis: Correlations of chest radiography, CT, MR, and surgical findings. *AJR* 1987; 148:515–519.
18. Bashist B, Ellis K, Gold RP: Computed tomography of intrathoracic goiters. *AJR* 1983; 140:455–460.
19. Bechtold RE, Wolfman NT, Karstaedt N, et al: Superior vena caval obstruction: Detection using CT. *Radiology* 1985; 157:485–487.
20. Bedros AA, Munson J, Toomey FE: Hemangioendothelioma presenting as posterior mediastinal mass in a child. *Cancer* 1980; 46:801–803.
21. Beerman PJ, Gelfand DW, Ott DJ: Pneumomediastinum after double-contrast barium enema examination: A sign of colonic perforation. *AJR* 1981; 136:197–198.
22. Bein ME, Mancuso AA, Mink JH, et al: Computed tomography in the evaluation of mediastinal lipomatosis. *J Comput Assist Tomogr* 1978; 2:379–383.
23. Benjamin SP, McCormack LJ, Effler DB, et al: Primary tumors of the mediastinum. *Chest* 1972; 62:297–303.
24. Bergstrom JF, Yost RV, Ford KT, et al: Unusual roentgen manifestations of bronchogenic cysts. *Radiology* 1973; 107:49–54.
25. Bethancourt B, Pond GD, Jones SE, et al: Mediastinal hematoma simulating recurrent Hodgkin disease during systemic chemotherapy. *AJR* 1984; 142:1119–1120.
26. Bill AH, Sumner DS: A unified concept of lymphangioma and cystic hygroma. *Surg Gynecol Obstet* 1965; 120:79–86.
27. Binder RE, Pugatch RD, Faling J, et al: Diagnosis of posterior mediastinal goiter by computer tomography. *J Comput Assist Tomogr* 1980; 4:550–552.
28. Black WC, Armstrong P, Daniel TM, et al: Computed tomography of aggressive fibromatosis in the posterior mediastinum. *J Comput Assist Tomogr* 1987; 11:153–155.
29. Black WC, Burke JW, Feldman PS, et al: CT appearance of cervical lipoblastoma. *J Comput Assist Tomogr* 1986; 10:696–698.
30. Blank N, Castellino RA: Patterns of pleural reflections of the left superior mediastinum: Normal anatomy and distributions produced by lymphadenopathy. *Radiology* 1972; 102:585–589.
31. Blewett JH, Szypulski JT: Double unilateral intrathoracic meningocele. Report of a case. *J Thorac Cardiovasc Surg* 1974; 67:481–483.

32. Boyd DP, Midell AI: Mediastinal cysts and tumors: An analysis of 96 cases. *Surg Clin North Am* 1968; 48:493–505.

33. Breatnach E, Nath PH, Delany DJ: The role of computed tomography in acute and subacute mediastinitis. *Clin Radiol* 1986; 37:139–145.

34. Brown LR, Aughenbaugh GL, Wick MR, et al: Roentgenologic diagnosis of primary corticotropin-producing carcinoid tumors of the mediastinum. *Radiology* 1982; 142:143–148.

35. Brown LR, Muhm JR, Sheedy PF, et al: The value of computed tomography in myasthenia gravis. *AJR* 1983; 140:31–35.

36. Brown LR, Reiman HM, Rosenow EC, et al: Intrathoracic lymphangioma. *Mayo Clin Proc* 1986; 61:882–892.

37. Brunner DR, Whitley NO: A pericardial cyst with high CT numbers. *AJR* 1984; 142:279–280.

38. Bryk D: Venous compression and obstruction by intrathoracic goiter. *J Can Assoc Radiol* 1974; 25:300–302.

39. Buirski G, Jordan SC, Joffe HS, et al: Superior vena caval abnormalities: Their occurrence rate, associated cardiac abnormalities and angiographic classification in a paediatric population with congenital heart disease. *Clin Radiol* 1986; 37:131–138.

40. Caffey J, Silbey R: Regrowth and overgrowth of the thymus after atrophy induced by the oral administration of adrenocorticosteroids to human infants. *Pediatrics* 1960; 26:762–770.

41. Carey LS, Ellis FH, Good CA, et al: Neurogenic tumors of the mediastinum: A clinicopathologic study. *AJR* 1960; 84:189–205.

42. Carlson RG, Lillehei CW, Edwards JE: Cystic medial necrosis of the ascending aorta in relation to age and hypertension. *Am J Cardiol* 1970; 25:411–415.

43. Carrol CL, Jeffrey RB, Federle MP, et al: CT evaluation of mediastinal infections. *J Comput Assist Tomogr* 1987; 11:449–454.

44. Carter AR, Sostman HD, Curtis AM, et al: Thoracic alterations after cardiac surgery. *AJR* 1983; 140:475–481.

45. Carter MM, Tarr RW, Mazer MJ, et al: The "aortic nipple" as a sign of impending superior vena caval syndrome. *Chest* 1985; 87:775–777.

46. Castleman B, Iverson L, Menendez VP: Localized mediastinal lymph node hyperplasia resembling thymoma. *Cancer* 1956; 9:822–830.

47. Chalmers AH, Armstrong P: Plexiform mediastinal neurofibromas: A report of two cases. *Br J Radiol* 1977; 50:215–217.

48. Chen KTK: Multicentric Castleman's disease and Kaposi's sarcoma. *Am J Surg Pathol* 1984; 8:287–293.

49. Choyke PL, Zeman RK, Gootenberg JE, et al: Thymic atrophy and regrowth in response to chemotherapy: CT evaluation. *AJR* 1987; 149:269–272.

50. Christoforidis AJ: Radiologic manifestations of histoplasmosis. *AJR* 1970; 109:478–490.

51. Cohen AJ, Sbaschnig RJ, Hochholzer L, et al: Mediastinal hemangiomas. *Ann Thorac Surg* 1987; 43:656–659.

52. Cohen AM, Cunat JS: Giant esophageal leiomyoma as a mediastinal mass. *J Can Assoc Radiol* 1981; 32:129–130.

53. Cohen AM, Creviston S, Lipuma JP, et al: NMR evaluation of hilar and mediastinal lymphadenopathy. *Radiology* 1983; 148:739–742.

54. Cohen M, Hill CA, Cangir A, et al: Thymic rebound after treatment of childhood tumors. *AJR* 1980; 135:151–156.

55. Coleman BG, Arger PH, Dalinka MK, et al: CT of sarcomatous degeneration in neurofibromatosis. *AJR* 1983; 140:383–387.

56. Coltart RS, Wraught EP: The value of radionuclide venography in superior vena caval obstruction. *Clin Radiol* 1985; 36:415–418.

57. Connell JV, Muhm JR: Radiographic manifestations of histoplasmosis: A 10 year review. *Radiology* 1976; 121:281–285.

58. Cornell SH: Calcium in the fluid of mediastinal bronchogenic cyst: A new roentgenography finding. *Radiology* 1965; 85:825–828.

59. Cox JD: Primary malignant germ cell tumors of the mediastinum. *Cancer* 1975; 36:1162–1168.

60. Cramer M, Foley WD, Palmer TE, et al: Compression of the right pulmonary artery by aortic aneurysms: CT demonstration. *J Comput Assist Tomogr* 1985; 9:310–314.

61. Crylak D, Milne ENC, Imray TJ: Pneumomediastinum: A diagnostic problem. *Crit Rev Diagn Imag* 1984; 23:75–117.

62. Daily PO, Trueblood HW, Stinson EB, et al: Management of acute aortic dissections. *Ann Thorac Surg* 1970; 10:237–247.

63. Daniel TM, Staub EW, Clark DE: Symptomatic venous compression from a mediastinal cystic lymphangioma. *Chest* 1973; 63:834–835.

64. Davis J, Mark G, Green R: Benign blood vascular tumors of the mediastinum: Report of four cases and review of the literature. *Radiology* 1978; 126:581–587.

65. DeBakey ME, Henly WS, Cooley DA, et al: Surgical management of dissecting aneurysms of the aorta. *J Thorac Cardiovasc Surg* 1965; 49:130–149.

66. Dee P, Martin R, Oudkerk M, et al: The diagnosis of aortic dissection. *Curr Probl Diagn Radiol* 1983; 12:8–55.

67. Demos TC, Posniak HV, Churchill RJ: Detection of intimal flap of aortic dissection on unenhanced CT images. *AJR* 1986; 146:601–603.

68. Dines DE, Payne WS, Bernatz PE, et al: Mediastinal granuloma and fibrosing mediastinitis. *Chest* 1979; 75:320–324.

69. Dobranowski J, Martin LFW, Bennett WF: CT evaluation of posterior mediastinal teratoma. *J Comput Assist Tomogr* 1987; 11:156–157.

70. Doppman JL, Krudy AG, Masx SJ, et al: Aspiration

of enlarged parathyroid glands for parathyroid hormone assay. *Radiology* 1983; 148:31–35.

71. Doppman JL, Oldfield EH, Chrousos CP, et al: Rebound thymic hyperplasia after treatment for Cushing's sarcoma. *AJR* 1986; 147:1145–1147.

72. Duke RA, Barrett MR, Payne SD, et al: Compression of left main bronchus and left pulmonary artery by thoracic aortic aneurysm. *AJR* 1987; 149:261–263.

73. Dyer NH: Cystic thymomas and thymic cysts: A review. *Thorax* 1967; 22:408–421.

74. Dyke PC, Mulkey DA: Maturation of ganglioneuroblastoma to ganglioneuroma. *Cancer* 1967; 20:1343–1349.

75. Earnest F, Muhm JR, Sheedy PF: Roentgenographic findings in thoracic aortic dissection. *Mayo Clin Proc* 1979; 54:43–50.

76. Edeiken J, Lee KF, Libshitz H: Intrathoracic meningocele. *AJR* 1969; 106:381–384.

77. Edwards JE: Manifestations of acquired and congenital diseases of the aorta. *Curr Probl Cardiol* 1979; 3:7–62.

78. Egan TJ, Neiman HL, Herman RJ, et al: Computed tomography in the diagnosis of aortic aneurysm dissection or traumatic injury. *Radiology* 1980; 136:141–146.

79. Eklof O, Gooding CA: Intrathoracic neuroblastoma. *AJR* 1967; 100:202–207.

80. Ellis K, Austin JHM, Jaretzki A: Radiologic detection of thymoma in patients with myasthenia gravis. *AJR* 1988; 151:873–881.

81. Ellis K, Gregg HE: Thymomas: Roentgen considerations. *AJR* 1964; 91:105–119.

82. Ellison RT, Corrao WM, Fox MJ, et al: Spontaneous mediastinal hemorrhage in patients on chronic hemodialysis. *Ann Intern Med* 1981; 95:704–706.

83. Enzi G, Biondetti PR, Fiore D, et al: Computed tomography of deep fat masses in multiple symmetrical lipomatosis. *Radiology* 1982; 144:121–124.

84. Epstein DM, Kiessel H, Gefter W, et al: MR imaging of the mediastinum: A retrospective comparison with computed tomography. *J Comput Assist Tomogr* 1984; 8:670–676.

85. Eyler WR, Clark MD: Dissecting aneurysms of the aorta: Roentgen manifestations including a comparison with other types of aneurysms. *Radiology* 1965; 85:1047–1057.

86. Faerber EN, Carter BL, Sarno RC, et al: Computed tomography of neuroblastic tumors in children. *Clin Pediatr* 1984; 23:17–21.

87. Falor WH, Kelly TR, Krabill WS: Intrathoracic goiter. *Ann Surg* 1955; 142:238–247.

88. Farmer DW, Moore E, Amparo E, et al: Calcific fibrosing mediastinitis: Demonstration of pulmonary vascular obstruction by magnetic resonance imaging. *AJR* 1984; 143:1189–1191.

89. Federle MP, Callen PW: Cystic Hodgkin's lymphoma of the thymus: Computed tomographic

appearance. *J Comput Assist Tomogr* 1979; 3:542–544.

90. Feigin DS, Eggleston JC, Siegelman SS: The multiple roentgen manifestations of sclerosing mediastinitis. *Johns Hopkins Med J* 1979; 144:8.

91. Feigin DS, Fenoglio JJ, McAllister HA, et al: Pericardial cysts: A radiologic-pathologic correlation and review. *Radiology* 1977; 125:15–20.

92. Feigl D, Feigl A, Edwards JE: Mycotic aneurysms of the aortic root: A pathologic study of 20 cases. *Chest* 1986; 90:553–557.

93. Feinstein RS, Gatewood OMB, Fishman EK, et al: Computed tomography of adult neuroblastoma. *J Comput Assist Tomogr* 1984; 8:720–726.

94. Feutz EP, Yune HY, Mandelbaum I, et al: Intrathoracic cystic hygroma. *Radiology* 1973; 108:61–66.

95. Filler RM, Traggis DG, Jaffe N, et al: Favorable outlook for children with mediastinal neuroblastoma. *J Pediatr Surg* 1972; 7:136–143.

96. Fiore D, Biondetti PR, Calabro F, et al: CT demonstration of bilateral Castleman tumors in the mediastinum. *J Comput Assist Tomogr* 1983; 7:719–720.

97. Fitch SJ, Tonkin ILD, Tonkin AK: Imaging of foregut duplication cysts. *RadioGraphics* 1986; 6:189–201.

98. Fon GT, Bein ME, Mancuso AA, et al: Computed tomography of the anterior mediastinum in myasthenia gravis. *Radiology* 1982; 142:135–141.

99. Francis IR, Glazer GM, Shapiro B, et al: Complementary roles of CT and ^{131}I-MIBG scintigraphy in diagnosing pheochromocytoma. *AJR* 1983; 141:719–725.

100. Friedman AC, Lautin E, Rothenberg L: Mach bands and pneumomediastinum. *J Can Assoc Radiol* 1981; 32:232–235.

101. Frizzera G, Banks PM, Massarelli G, et al: A systemic lymphoproliferative disorder with morphologic features of Castleman's disease. *Am J Surg Pathol* 1983; 7:211–231.

102. Gale AW, Jelihovsky T, Grant AF, et al: Neurogenic tumors of the mediastinum. *Ann Thorac Surg* 1974; 17:434–443.

103. Gale ME: Bochdalek hernia: Prevalence and CT characteristics. *Radiology* 1985; 156:449–452.

104. Gallagher S, Dixon AK: Streak artefacts of the thoracic aorta: Pseudodissection. *J Comput Assist Tomogr* 1984; 8:688–693.

105. Gamsu G, Stark DD, Webb WR, et al: Magnetic resonance imaging of benign mediastinal masses. *Radiology* 1984; 151:709–713.

106. Gelfand DW, Goldman AS, Law EJ: Thymic hyperplasia in children recovering from thermal burns. *J Trauma* 1972; 12:813–817.

107. Genereux GP, Howie JL: Normal mediastinal lymph node size and number: CT and anatomic study. *AJR* 1984; 142:1095–1100.

108. Gibbons JA, Rosencrantz H, Posey DJ, et al: Angiofollicular lymphoid hyperplasia (Castleman's tumor) resembling a pericardial cyst: Differentiation by

computerized tomography. *Ann Thorac Surg* 1981; 32:193–196.

109. Girard DE, Carlson V, Natelson EA, et al: Pneumo-mediastinum in diabetic ketoacidosis: Comments on mechanism, incidence, and management. *Chest* 1971; 60:455–459.

110. Glazer BH, Gross BH, Quint LE, et al: Normal mediastinal lymph nodes: Number and size according to American Thoracic Society mapping. *AJR* 1985; 144:261–265.

111. Glazer GM, Axel L, Moss AA: CT diagnosis of mediastinal thyroid. *AJR* 1982; 138:495–498.

112. Glazer GM, Francis IR, Gebarski K, et al: Dynamic incremental computed tomography in the evaluation of the pulmonary hili. *J Comput Assist Tomogr* 1983; 7:59–64.

113. Glazer GM, Francis IR, Shirazi KK, et al: Evaluation of the pulmonary hilum: Comparison of conventional radiography, 55° oblique tomography and dynamic computed tomography. *J Comput Assist Tomogr* 1983; 7:983–989.

114. Glazer GM, Gross BH, Francis IR, et al: Evaluation of the pulmonary hila, in Siegelman SS (ed): *Computed Tomography of the Chest*. New York, Churchill Livingstone, 1984, pp 37–58.

115. Glazer HS, Aronberg DJ, Sagel SS: Pitfalls in CT recognition of mediastinal lymphadenopathy. *AJR* 1985; 144:267–274.

116. Glickstein MF, Miller WT, Dalinka MK, et al: Paraspinal lipomatosis: A benign mass. *Radiology* 1987; 163:79–80.

117. Gobien RP, Stanley JH, Gobien BS, et al: Percutaneous catheter aspiration and drainage of suspected mediastinal abscesses. *Radiology* 1984; 151:69–71.

118. Godwin JD, Breiman RS, Speckman JM: Problems and pitfalls in the evaluation of thoracic aortic dissection by computed tomography. *J Comput Assist Tomogr* 1982; 6:750–756.

119. Godwin JD, Herfkens RL, Skioldebrand CG, et al: Evaluation of dissections and aneurysms of the thoracic aorta by conventional and dynamic CT scanning. *Radiology* 1980; 136:125–133.

120. Goldman AJ, Herrmann C, Keesey JC, et al: Myasthenia gravis and invasive thymoma: A 20 year experience. *Neurology* 1975; 25:1021–1025.

121. Gomes AS, Lois JF, George B, et al: Congenital abnormalities of the aortic arch: MR imaging. *Radiology* 1987; 165:691–695.

122. Gomori JM, Grossman RI, Goldberg HI, et al: Intracranial hematomas: Imaging by high field MR. *Radiology* 1985; 157:87–93.

123. Goodman LR, Kay HR, Teplick SK, et al: Complications of median sternotomy: Computed tomographic evaluation. *AJR* 1983; 141:225–230.

124. Goodwin RA, Loyd JE, Des Prez RM: Histoplasmosis in normal hosts. *Medicine* 1981; 60:231–266.

125. Goodwin RA, Nickell JA, Des Prez RM: Mediastinal fibrosis complicating healed primary histoplasmosis and tuberculosis. *Medicine* 1972; 51:227–246.

126. Gouliamos A, Striggaris K, Lolas C, et al: Thymic cyst. *J Comput Assist Tomogr* 1982; 6:172–174.

127. Graeber GM, Thompson LD, Ronnigen DL, et al: Cystic lesion of the thymus. *J Thorac Cardiovasc Surg* 1984; 87:295–300.

128. Gray JM, Hanson GC: Mediastinal emphysema: Aetiology, diagnosis, and treatment. *Thorax* 1966; 21:325–332.

129. Gross BH, Schneider HJ, Proto AV: Eggshell calcification of lymph nodes. *AJR* 1980; 135:1265–1268.

130. Gross SC, Barr I, Eyler WR, et al: Computed tomography in dissection of the thoracic aorta. *Radiology* 1980; 136:135–139.

131. Guit GL, Shaw PC, Ehrlich J, et al: Mediastinal lymphadenopathy and pulmonary arterial hypertension in mixed connective tissue disease. *Radiology* 1985; 154:305–306.

132. Gumbs RV, Higginbotham-Ford EA, Teal JS, et al: Thoracic extramedullary hematopoiesis in sickle-cell disease. *AJR* 1987; 149:889–893.

133. Gundry SR, Burney RE, Mackenzie JR, et al: Traumatic pseudoaneurysms of the thoracic aorta: Anatomic and radiologic correlations. *Arch Surg* 1984; 119:1055–1060.

134. Guthaner DF, Wexler L, Harell G: CT demonstration of cardiac structures. *AJR* 1979; 133:75–81.

135. Haber S: Retroperitoneal and mediastinal chemodectoma: Report of a case and review of the literature. *AJR* 1964; 92:1029–1041.

136. Halliday DR, Dahlin DC, Pugh DG, et al: Massive osteolysis and angiomatosis. *Radiology* 1964; 82:637–643.

137. Harper RAK, Guyer PB: The radiological features of thymic tumours: A review of sixty-five cases. *Clin Radiol* 1965; 16:97–100.

138. Heiberg E, Wolverson MK, Sundaram M, et al: CT findings in thoracic aortic dissection. *AJR* 1981; 136:13–17.

139. Heiberg E, Wolverson MK, Sundaram M, et al: CT characteristics of aortic atherosclerotic aneurysm versus aortic dissection. *J Comput Assist Tomogr* 1985; 9:78–83.

140. Heitzman ER: *The Mediastinum: Radiologic Correlations With Anatomy and Pathology*, ed 2. Berlin, Springer—Verlag, 1988.

141. Heitzman ER: Radiological diagnosis of mediastinal lymph node enlargement. *J Can Assoc Radiol* 1978; 29:151–157.

142. Hernandez RJ: Role of CT in evaluation of children with foregut cyst. *Pediatr Radiol* 1987; 17:265–268.

143. Heystraten FM, Rosenbusch G, Kingma LM, et al: Chronic posttraumatic aneurysm of the thoracic aorta: Surgically correctable occult threat. *AJR* 1986; 146:303–308.

144. Hirsch JH, Carter SJ, Chikos PM: Traumatic pseudoaneurysms of the thoracic aorta: Two unusual cases. *AJR* 1978; 130:157–160.

145. Hockholzer L, Theros EG, Rosen EH: Some unusual lesions of the mediastinum: Roentgenologic

and pathologic features. *Semin Roentgenol* 1979; 4:74–90.

146. Holbert BL, Libshitz HI: Superior vena caval syndrome in primary germ cell tumors. *J Can Assoc Radiol* 1986; 37:182–183.

147. Holtz S, Powers WE: Calcification in papillary carcinoma of the thyroid. *AJR* 1958; 80:997–1000.

148. Homer MJ, Wechsler RJ, Carter BL: Mediastinal lipomatosis: CT confirmation of a normal variant. *Radiology* 1978; 128:657–661.

149. Hudson TM, Vandergriend RA, Springfield DS, et al: Aggressive fibromatosis: Evaluation by computed tomography and angiography. *Radiology* 1984; 150:495–501.

150. Ikezoe J, Morimoto S, Arizawa J, et al: Ultrasonography of mediastinal teratoma. *J Clin Ultrasound* 1986; 14:513–520.

151. Irwin RS, Braman SS, Arvanitidis AN, et al: [131]I thyroid scanning in preoperative diagnosis of mediastinal goiter. *Ann Intern Med* 1978; 89:73–74.

152. Israel HL, Lenchner G, Steiner GM: Late development of mediastinal calcifications in sarcoidosis. *Am Rev Respir Dis* 1981; 124:302–305.

153. Jacobson G, Felson B, Prendergrass EP, et al: Eggshell calcifications in coal and metal miners. *Semin Roentgenol* 1967; 2:276–282.

154. Jagannath AR, Sos TA, Lockhart SH, et al: Aortic dissection: A statistical analysis of the usefulness of plain chest radiographic findings. *AJR* 1986; 147:1123–1126.

155. Jamplis RW: Infections of the mediastinum and the superior vena caval syndrome, in Shields TW (ed): *General Thoracic Surgery*, ed 2. Philadelphia, Lea & Febiger, 1983.

156. Janssen RS, Kaye AD, Lisak RP, et al: Radiologic evaluation of the mediastinum in myasthenia gravis. *Neurology* 1983; 33:534–539.

157. Kaplan JO, Morillo G, Weinfeld A, et al: Mediastinal adenopathy in myeloma. *J Can Assoc Radiol* 1980; 31:48–49.

158. Katz I, Dziadiw R: Localised mediastinal lymph node hyperplasia. *AJR* 1960; 84:206–212.

159. Kay HR, Goodman LR, Teplick SK, et al: Uses of computed tomography to assess mediastinal complications after median sternotomy. *Ann Thorac Surg* 1983; 36:706–714.

160. Kaye AD, Janssen R, Arger PH, et al: Mediastinal computed tomography in myasthenia gravis. *J Comput Tomogr* 1983; 7:273–279.

161. Keats TE, Lipscomb GE, Betts CS: Mensuration of the arch of the azygos vein and its application to the study of cardiopulmonary disease. *Radiology* 1968; 90:990–994.

162. Keene RJ, Steiner RE, Olsen EJG, et al: Aortic root aneurysm—radiographic and pathologic features. *Clin Radiol* 1971; 22:330–340.

163. Keller AR, Hochholzer L, Castleman B: Hyaline-vascular and plasma cell types of giant lymph node

hyperplasia of the mediastinum and other locations. *Cancer* 1972; 29:670–683.

164. Kim HC, Nosher J, Haas A, et al: Cystic degeneration of thymic Hodgkin's disease following radiation therapy. *Cancer* 1985; 55:354–356.

165. Kirchner SG, Heller RM, Smith CW: Pancreatic pseudocyst of the mediastinum. *Radiology* 1977; 123:37–42.

166. Kissin CM, Husband JE, Nicholas D, et al: Benign thymic enlargement in adults after chemotherapy: CT demonstration. *Radiology* 1987; 163:67–70.

167. Kittredge RD, Finby N: Pericardial cysts and diverticula. *AJR* 1967; 99:668–673.

168. Kittredge RD, Nash AD: The many facets of sclerosing fibrosis. *AJR* 1974; 122:288–298.

169. Klatte EC, Yune JY: Diagnosis and treatment of pericardial cysts. *Radiology* 1972; 104:541–544.

170. Kowolafe F: Radiological patterns and significance of thyroid calcification. *Clin Radiol* 1981; 32:571–575.

171. Krudy AG, Doppman JL, Brennan MF, et al: The detection of mediastinal parathyroid glands by computed tomography, selective arteriography, and venous sampling: An analysis of 17 cases. *Radiology* 1981; 140:739–744.

172. Kuhlman JE, Fishman EK, Wang KP, et al: Mediastinal cysts: Diagnosis by CT and needle aspiration. *AJR* 1988; 150:75–78.

173. Larde D, Belloir C, Vasile N, et al: Computed tomography of aortic dissection. *Radiology* 1980; 136:147–151.

174. Larson EW, Edwards WD: Risk factors for aortic dissection: A necropsy study of 161 cases. *Am J Cardiol* 1984; 53:849–855.

175. Levin B: The continuous diaphragm sign: A newly recognized sign of pneumomediastinum. *Clin Radiol* 1973; 24:337–338.

176. Levine GD, Rosai J: Thymic hyperplasia and neoplasia: A review of current concepts. *Hum Pathol* 1978; 9:495–515.

177. Levine TM, Wurster CF, Krespi YP: Mediastinitis occurring as a complication of odontogenic infections. *Laryngoscope* 1986; 96:747–750.

178. Levitt RG, Glazer HS, Roper CL, et al: Magnetic resonance imaging of mediastinal and hilar masses: Comparison with CT. *AJR* 1985; 145:9–14.

179. Levitt RG, Husband JE, Glazer HS: CT of primary germ-cell tumors of the mediastinum. *AJR* 1984; 142:73–78.

180. Libshitz HI, Clouser M, Zornoza J, et al: Radiographic findings of immunoblastic lymphadenopathy and related immunoblastic proliferations. *AJR* 1977; 129:875–878.

181. Light AM: Idiopathic fibrosis of mediastinum: A discussion of three cases and review of the literature. *J Clin Pathol* 1978; 31:78–88.

182. Limpert J, MacMahon H, Variakajis D: Angioimmunoblastic lympadenopathy: Clinical and radiological features. *Radiology* 1984; 152:27–30.

183. Lindfors KK, Meyer JE, Dedrick CG, et al: Thymic cysts in mediastinal Hodgkins disease. *Radiology* 1985; 156:37–41.

184. LiPuma JP, Wellman J, Stern HP: Nitrous oxide abuse: A new cause of pneumomediastinum. *Radiology* 1982; 145:602.

185. Long JA, Doppman JL, Nienhius AW: Computed tomographic studies of thoracic extramedullary hematopoiesis. *J Comput Assist Tomogr* 1980; 4:67–70.

186. Lui YQ: Radiology of aortoarteritis. *Radiol Clin North Am* 1985; 23:671–688.

187. Lundius B: Intrathoracic kidney. *AJR* 1975; 125:678–681.

188. Lyons HA, Calvy GL, Sammons BP: The diagnosis and classification of mediastinal masses: 1. A study of 782 cases. *Ann Intern Med* 1959; 51:897–932.

189. Mack JW, Heyden WH, Pauling FW, et al: Postoperative chylous pseudocyst. *J Thorac Cardiovasc Surg* 1979; 77:773–776.

190. Macklin MT, Macklin CC: Malignant interstitial emphysema of the lungs and mediastinum as an important occult complication in many respiratory diseases and other conditions. *Medicine* 1944; 23:281–358.

191. Madewell JE, Sobonya RE, Reed JC: Neurenteric cyst: RPC from the AFIP. *Radiology* 1973; 109:707–712.

192. Mahajan V, Strimlan V, van Ordstrand HS, et al: Benign superior vena cava syndrome. *Chest* 1975; 68:32–35.

193. Maier HC: Lymphatic cysts of the mediastinum. *AJR* 1955; 73:15–18.

194. Mallens WMC, Nijhius-Heddes JMA, Bakker W: Calcified lymph node metastases in bronchioloalveolar carcinoma. *Radiology* 1986; 161:103–104.

195. Margolin FR, Winfield J, Steinbach HL: Patterns of thyroid calcification: Roentgenologic-histologic study of excised specimens. *Invest Radiol* 1967; 2:208–212.

196. McLoud TC, Kalisher L, Stark P, et al: Intrathoracic lymph node metastases from extrathoracic neoplasms. *AJR* 1978; 131:403–407.

197. McMurdo KK, de Geer G, Webb WR, et al: Normal and occluded mediastinal veins: MRI imaging. *Radiology* 1986; 159:33–38.

198. McNeill AD, Groden BM, Neville AM: Intrathoracic phaeochromocytoma. *Br J Surg* 1970; 57:457–462.

199. Mendelson DS, Rose JS, Efremidis SC, et al: Bronchogenic cysts with high CT numbers. *AJR* 1983; 140:463–465.

200. Mendez G, Isikoff MB, Isikoff SK, et al: Fatty tumors of the thorax demonstrated by CT. *AJR* 1979; 133:207–212.

201. Miles J, Pennybacker J, Sheldon P: Intrathoracic meningocele: Its development and association with neurofibromatosis. *J Neurol Neurosurg Psychiatry* 1969; 32:99–110.

202. Miller DC, Walter JP, Guthaner DF, et al: Recurrent mediastinal bronchogenic cyst: Cause of bronchial obstruction and compression of superior vena cava and pulmonary artery. *Chest* 1978; 74:218–220.

203. Miller DG, Stinson EB, Oyer PE, et al: Operative treatment of aortic dissection: Experience with 125 patients over a sixteen-year period. *J Thorac Cardiovasc Surg* 1979; 78:365–382.

204. Mills SE, Teja K, Crosby IK, et al: Aortic dissection: Surgical and nonsurgical treatments compared: An analysis of seventy-four cases at the University of Virginia. *Am J Surg* 1979; 137:240–243.

205. Moncada R, Cardella R, Demos T, et al: Evaluation of superior vena cava syndrome by axial CT and CT phlebography. *AJR* 1984; 143:731–736.

206. Moncada R, Warpeha R, Pickleman J, et al: Mediastinitis from odontogenic and deep cervical infection. *Chest* 1978; 73:497–500.

207. Moore AV, Korobkin M, Powers B, et al: Thymoma detection by mediastinal CT: Patients with myasthenia gravis. *AJR* 1982; 138:217–222.

208. Moore AV, Silverman PM, Putman CE: Current concepts in computerized tomography of the mediastinum. *CRC Crit Rev Diagn Imaging* 1985; 24:1–38.

209. Morens AJ, Weismann I, Billingsley JL, et al: Angiographic and scintigraphic findings in fibrosing mediastinitis. *Clin Nucl Med* 1983; 8:167–169.

210. Morris UL, Colletti PM, Ralls PW, et al: CT demonstration of intrathoracic thyroid tissue. *J Comput Assist Tomogr* 1982; 6:821–824.

211. Müller NL, Webb WR: Imaging of the pulmonary hila. *Invest Radiol* 1985; 20:661–671.

212. Müller NL, Webb WR, Gamsu G: Subcarinal lymph node enlargement: Radiographic findings and CT correlation. *AJR* 1985; 145:15–19.

213. Müller NL, Webb WR, Gamsu G: Paratracheal lymphadenopathy: Radiographic findings and correlation with CT. *Radiology* 1985; 156:761–765.

214. Munsell WP: Pneumomediastinum: A report of 28 cases and review of the literature. *JAMA* 1967; 202:129–133.

215. Naidich DP, Khouri NF, Scott WW, et al: Computed tomography of the pulmonary hila: 1. Normal anatomy. *J Comput Assist Tomogr* 1981; 5:459–467.

216. Naidich DP, Khouri NF, Stitik FP, et al: Computed tomography of the pulmonary hila: 2. Abnormal anatomy. *J Comput Assist Tomogr* 1981; 5:468–475.

217. Nakagawa H, Huang YP, Malis LI, et al: Computed tomography of intraspinal and paraspinal neoplasms. *J Comput Assist Tomogr* 1977; 1:377–390.

218. Nakata H, Nakayama C, Kimoto T, et al: Computed tomography of mediastinal bronchogenic cysts. *J Comput Assist Tomogr* 1982; 6:733–738.

219. Nathwani BN, Rappaport H, Moran EM, et al: Malignant lymphoma arising in angioimmunoblastic lymphadenopathy. *Cancer* 1978; 41:578–606.

220. Newman A, So SK: Bilateral neurofibroma of the intrathoracic vagus nerve associated with von Recklinghausen's disease. *AJR* 1971; 112:389–392.

221. Ochsner JL, Ochsner SC: Congenital cysts of the mediastinum: 20 year experience with 42 cases. *Ann Surg* 1966; 163:909–920.

222. Olscamp G, Weisbrod G, Sanders D, et al: Castleman disease: Unusual manifestations of an unusual disorder. *Radiology* 1980; 135:43–48.

223. Olson JL, Salyer WR: Mediastinal paragangliomas (aortic body tumor): A report of four cases and a review of the literature. *Cancer* 1978; 41:2405–2412.

224. Onik G, Goodman PC: CT of Castleman's disease. *AJR* 1983; 140:691–692.

225. Oudkerk M, Overbosch E, Dee P: CT recognition of acute aortic dissection. *AJR* 1983; 141:671–676.

226. Pader E, Kirschner PA: Pericardial diverticulum. *Dis Chest* 1969; 55:344–346.

227. Panicek PM, Ewing DK, Markarian B, et al: Interstitial pulmonary hemorrhage from mediastinal hematoma secondary to aortic rupture. *Radiology* 1987; 162:165–166.

228. Papatestas AE, Alpert LI, Osserman K, et al: Studies in myasthenia gravis: Effects of thymectomy. Results on 185 patients with nonthymomatous and thymomatous myasthenia gravis, 1941–1969. *Am J Med* 1971; 50:465–474.

229. Papavasiliou C, Gouliamos A, Andreou J: The marrow heterotopia in thalassemia. *Eur J Radiol* 1986; 6:92–96.

230. Paris F, Tarazona V, Casillas M, et al: Hernia of Morgagni. *Thorax* 1973; 28:631–636.

231. Parish JM, Marschke RF, Dines DE, et al: Etiologic considerations in superior vena cava syndrome. *Mayo Clin Proc* 1981; 56:407–413.

232. Park CH, Rothermel FJ, Judge DM: Unusual calcification in mixed papillary and follicular carcinoma of the thyroid gland. *Radiology* 1976; 119:554.

233. Payne WS, Larson RH: Acute mediastinitis. *Surg Clin North Am* 1969; 49:999–1009.

234. Perez CA, Vietti T, Ackerman LV, et al: Tumors of the sympathetic nervous system in children. *Radiology* 1967; 88:750–760.

235. Perkes EA, Haller JO, Kassner EG, et al: Mediastinal cystic hygroma in infants. *Clin Pediatr* 1979; 18:168–170.

236. Peterson IM, Futhaner DF: Aortic pseudoaneurysm complicating Takayasu disease: CT appearance. *J Comput Assist Tomogr* 1986; 10:676–678.

237. Phelan MS: Castleman's giant lymph node hyperplasia. *Br J Radiol* 1982; 55:158–160.

238. Pilla TJ, Wolverson MK, Sundaram M, et al: CT evaluation of cystic lymphangiomas of the mediastinum. *Radiology* 1982; 144:841–842.

239. Polansky SM, Barwick KW, Ravin CE: Primary mediastinal seminoma. *AJR* 1979; 132:17–21.

240. Poon PY, Bronskill MJ, Henkelman M, et al: Magnetic resonance imaging of the mediastinum. *J Can Assoc Radiol* 1986; 37:173–181.

241. Price JE, Rigler LG: Widening of the mediastinum resulting from fat accumulation. *Radiology* 1970; 96:497–500.

242. Proto AV, Rost RC: CT of the thorax: Pitfalls in interpretation. *RadioGraphics* 1985; 5:693–812.

243. Pruzanski W: Lymphadenopathy associated with dysgammaglobulinaemia. *Semin Hematol* 1980; 17:44–62.

244. Pugatch RD, Braver JH, Robbins AH, et al: CT diagnosis of pericardial cysts. *AJR* 1978; 131:515–516.

245. Pugatch RD, Faling LJ, Robbins AH, et al: CT diagnosis of benign mediastinal abnormalities. *AJR* 1980; 134:685–694.

246. Putman CE, Curtis AM, Westfried M, et al: Thickening of the posterior tracheal stripe: A sign of squamous cell carcinoma of the esophagus. *Radiology* 1976; 121:533–536.

247. Quint LE, Glazer GM, Orringer MB, et al: Mediastinal lymph node detection and sizing at CT and autopsy. *Radiology* 1986; 147:469–472.

248. Reed JC, Haller KK, Feigin DS: Neural tumours of the thorax: Subject review from the AFIP. *Radiology* 1978; 126:9–17.

249. Reed JC, Sobonya RE: Morphologic analysis of foregut cysts in the thorax. *AJR* 1974; 120:851–860.

250. Rholl KS, Levitt RE, Glazer HS: Magnetic resonance imaging of fibrosing mediastinitis. *AJR* 1985; 145:255–259.

251. Rizk G, Cuteo L, Amplatz K: Rebound enlargement of the thymus after successful corrective surgery for transposition of the great vessels. *AJR* 1972; 116:528–530.

252. Robinson AE, Gooneratne NS, Blackburn WR, et al: Bilateral anteromediastinal defect of the diaphragm in children. *AJR* 1980; 135:301–306.

253. Rogers LF, Puig AW, Dooley BN, et al: Diagnostic considerations in mediastinal emphysema: A pathophysiologic-roentgenologic approach to Boerhaave's syndrome and spontaneous pneumomediastinum. *AJR* 1972; 115:495–511.

254. Rohlfing BM, Webb WR, Schlobohm RM: Ventilator-related extra-alveolar air in adults. *Radiology* 1976; 121:25–31.

255. Ross JS, O'Donovan PB, Novoa R, et al: Magnetic resonance of the chest: Initial experience with imaging and in vivo T1 and T2 calculations. *Radiology* 1984; 152:95–101.

256. Ross P, Logan W: Roentgen findings in extramedullary hematopoiesis. *AJR* 1969; 106:604–613.

257. Rubin E: Case of the winter season: Benign lipoblastoma. *Semin Roentgenol* 1979; 13:5–6.

258. Russel CF, Edis AJ, Scholz DA, et al: Mediastinal parathyroid tumors: Experience with 38 tumors requiring mediastinotomy for removal. *Ann Surg* 1981; 193:805–809.

259. Ruttley M, Mills RA: Subcutaneous emphysema and pneumomediastinum in diabetic keto-acidosis. *Br J Radiol* 1971; 44:672–674.

260. Salvatore M, Gallo A: Accessory thyroid in the anterior mediastinum: Case report. *J Nucl Med* 1975; 16:1135–1136.

261. Sandler CM, Libshitz HI, Marks G: Pneumoperitoneum, pneumomediastinum and pneumopericar-

dium following dental extraction. *Radiology* 1975; 115:539–540.

262. Schnyder PA, Gamsu G: CT of the pretracheal retrocaval space. *AJR* 1981; 136:303–308.

263. Schowengerdt CG, Suyemoto R, Main FB: Granulomatous and fibrous mediastinitis: A review and analysis of 180 cases. *J Thorac Cardiovasc Surg* 1969; 57:365–379.

264. Schulthess GK, McMurdo K, Tscholakoff D, et al: Mediastinal masses: MR imaging. *Radiology* 1986; 158:289–296.

265. Seabold JE, Binet EF, Schaefer RF: Mycotic aortic aneurysm diagnosed by In-111 leukocyte scintigraphy and computed tomography. *Clin Nucl Med* 1983; 8:486–487.

266. Seltzer RA, Mills DS, Baddock SS, et al: Mediastinal thymic cyst. *Dis Chest* 1968; 53:186–196.

267. Shapiro B, Sisson J, Kalff V, et al: The location of middle mediastinal pheochromocytomas. *J Thorac Cardiovasc Surg* 1984; 87:814–820.

268. Shenoy SS, Barua NR, Patel AR, et al: Mediastinal lymphangioma. *J Surg Oncol* 1978; 10:523–528.

269. Shin MS, Berland LL, Ho KJ: Mediastinal cystic hygromas: CT characteristics and pathogenetic consideration. *J Comput Assist Tomogr* 1985; 9:297–301.

270. Shin MS, Ho KJ: Computed tomography of primary mediastinal seminoma. *J Comput Assist Tomogr* 1983; 7:990–994.

271. Shin MS, Ho KJ: Computed tomography evaluation of bilateral bronchostenosis caused by sclerosing granulomatous mediastinitis: A complication of histoplasmosis. *J Comput Tomogr* 1984; 8:345–350.

272. Shirkhoda A, Wallace S: Computed tomography of juxtacardiac pheochromocytoma. *J Comput Tomogr* 1984; 8:207–209.

273. Shub C, Parkin TW, Lie T: An unusual mediastinal lipoma simulating cardiomegaly. *Mayo Clin Proc* 1979; 54:60–62.

274. Sickles EA, Winestock D: Bilateral intrathoracic meningoceles. *J Can Assoc Radiol* 1977; 28:79–81.

275. Siegel MJ, Nadel SN, Glazer HS, et al: Mediastinal lesions in children: Comparison of CT and MR. *Radiology* 1986; 160:241–244.

276. Siegelman SS, Scott WW, Baker RR, et al: CT of the thymus, in Siegelman SS (ed): *Computed Tomography of the Chest*. New York, Churchill Livingstone, 1984, p 260.

277. Simeone JF, Minagi H, Putman CE: Traumatic disruption of the thoracic aorta: Significance of the left apical extrapleural cap. *Radiology* 1975; 117:265–268.

278. Smith L, Lippert KM: Peritoneo-pericardial diaphragmatic hernia. *Ann Surg* 1958; 148:798–804.

279. Smith TR, Khoury PT: Aneurysm of the proximal thoracic aorta simulating neoplasm: The role of CT and angiography. *AJR* 1985; 144:909–910.

280. Snow N, Lucas AE, Grau M, et al: Purulent mediastinal abscess secondary to Ludwig's angina. *Arch Otolaryngol* 1983; 109:53–55.

281. Souadjian JV, Enriquez P, Silverstein MN, et al: The spectrum of diseases associated with thymoma. Coincidence or a syndrome? *Arch Intern Med* 1974; 134:374–379.

282. Spizarny DL, Rebner M, Gross BH: CT evaluation of enhancing mediastinal masses. *J Comput Assist Tomogr* 1987; 11:990–993.

283. Stahl JD, Goldman SM, Minkin SD, et al: Perforated duodenal ulcer and pneumomediastinum. *Radiology* 1977; 124:23–25.

284. Stebner FC, Bishop CR: Bone marrow scan and radioiron uptake of an intrathoracic mass. *Clin Nucl Med* 1982; 7:86–87.

285. Stilwell ME, Weisbrod GL, Ilves R: Spontaneous mediastinal hematoma. *J Can Assoc Radiol* 1981; 32:60–61.

286. Streiter ML, Schneider HJ, Proto AV: Steroid-induced thoracic lipomatosis: Paraspinal involvement. *AJR* 1982; 139:679–681.

287. Sullivan KL, Wechsler RJ: CT diagnosis of lymphocele. *J Comput Assist Tomogr* 1985; 9:1110–1111.

288. Sussman SK, Silverman PM, Donnal JP: CT demonstration of isolated mediastinal goiter. *J Comp Assist Tomogr* 1986; 10:863–864.

289. Suzuki M, Takashima T, Itoh H, et al: Computed tomography of mediastinal teratomas. *J Comput Assist Tomogr* 1983; 7:74–76.

290. Swenson SJ, Keller PL, Berquist TH, et al: Magnetic resonance imaging of hemorrhage. *AJR* 1985; 145:921–927.

291. Szamosi A: Radiological detection of aneurysms involving the aortic root. *Radiology* 1981; 138:551–555.

292. Tarr RW, Page DL, Glick RG, et al: Benign hemangioendothelioma involving posterior mediastinum: CT findings. *J Comput Assist Tomogr* 1986; 10:865–867.

293. Tatu WF, Pope TL Jr, Daniel TM, et al: Computed tomography of mediastinal cystic hygroma in an adult. *J Comput Tomogr* 1985; 9:233–236.

294. Teates CD: Steroid induced mediastinal lipomatosis. *Radiology* 1970; 96:501–502.

295. Teplick JG, Nedwich A, Haskin ME: Roentgenographic features of thymolipoma. *AJR* 1973; 117:873–877.

296. Theros EG: RPC of the month from the AFIP. *Radiology* 1969; 93:677–681.

297. Thorsen MK, San Dretto MA, Lawson TL, et al: Dissecting aortic aneurysms: Accuracy of computed tomographic diagnosis. *Radiology* 1983; 148:773–777.

298. Tisi GM, Friedman PJ, Peters RM, et al: Clinical staging of primary lung cancer: Official ATS statement. *Am Rev Respir Dis* 1983; 127:659–664.

299. Tomsick TA: Dental surgical subcutaneous and me-

diastinal emphysema: A case report. *J Can Assoc Radiol* 1974; 25:49–51.

300. van Heerden JA, Sheps SG, Hamberger B, et al: Pheochromocytoma: Current status and changing trends. *Surgery* 1982; 91:367–373.

301. Vasile N, Mathieu D, Keita K, et al: Computed tomography of thoracic aortic dissection: Accuracy and pitfalls. *J Comput Assist Tomogr* 1986; 10:211–215.

302. Veeze-Kuijpers B, Van Andel JG, Stiegelis WF, et al: Benign thymic cyst following mantle radiotherapy for Hodgkin's disease. *Clin Radiol* 1987; 38:289–290.

303. Victor S, Anand KV, Andappan P, et al: Malignant mediastinal chemodectoma. *Chest* 1975; 68:583–584.

304. Vyborny C, MacMahon H: Foil filters for equalized chest radiography. *Radiology* 1984; 151:524.

305. Wallace DB: Intrapericardial diaphragmatic hernia. *Radiology* 1977; 122:596.

306. Wallace S, Hill CS, Paulus DD, et al: The radiologic aspects of medullary (solid) thyroid carcinoma. *Radiol Clin North Am* 1970; 8:463–474.

307. Walter JF, Rottenberg RW, Cannon WB, et al: Giant mediastinal lymph node hyperplasia (Castleman's disease): Angiographic and clinical features. *AJR* 1978; 130:447–450.

308. Webb WR, Gamsu G: Computed tomography of the left retrobronchial stripe. *J Comput Assist Tomogr* 1983; 7:65–69.

309. Webb WR, Gamsu G, Glazer GM: Computed tomography of the abnormal pulmonary hilum. *J Comput Assist Tomogr* 1981; 5:485–490.

310. Webb WR, Gamsu G, Stark DD, et al: Evaluation of magnetic resonance sequences in imaging mediastinal tumors. *AJR* 1984; 143:723–727.

311. Webb WR, Gamsu G, Stark DD, et al: Magnetic resonance imaging of the normal and abnormal pulmonary hila. *Radiology* 1984; 152:89–94.

312. Webb WR, Hirji M, Gamsu G: Posterior wall of the bronchus intermedius: Radiographic-CT correlation. *AJR* 1984; 142:907–911.

313. Webb WR, Jensen BG, Gamsu G, et al: Coronal magnetic resonance imaging of the chest: Normal and abnormal. *Radiology* 1984; 153:729–735.

314. Webb WR, Moore EH: Differentiation of volume averaging and mass on magnetic resonance images of the mediastinum. *Radiology* 1985; 155:413–416.

315. Weinberg B, Rose JS, Efremidis SC, et al: Posterior mediastinal-teratoma (cystic dermoid): Diagnosis by computerized tomography. *Chest* 1980; 77:694–695.

316. Weinreb JC, Arger PH, Grossman R, et al: CT metrizamide myelography in multiple bilateral intrathoracic meningoceles. *J Comput Assist Tomogr* 1984; 8:324–326.

317. Weinreb JC, Mootz A, Cohen JM: MRI evaluation of mediastinal and thoracic inlet venous obstruction. *AJR* 1986; 146:679–684.

318. Weinstein JB, Aronberg DJ, Sagel SS: CT of fibrosing mediastinitis: Findings and their utility. *AJR* 1983; 141:247–251.

319. Wernecke K, Peters PE, Galanski M: Mediastinal tumors: Evaluation with suprasternal sonography. *Radiology* 1986; 159:405–409.

320. Westcott JL, Henschke CI, Berkmen Y: MR imaging of the hilum and mediastinum: Effects of cardiac gating. *J Comput Assist Tomogr* 1985; 9:1073–1078.

321. Wheat MW, Palmer RF, Bartley TD, et al: Treatment of dissecting aneurysms of the aorta without surgery. *J Thorac Cardiovasc Surg* 1965; 50:364–373.

322. White RD, Lipton MJ, Higgins CB, et al: Noninvasive evaluation of suspected thoracic aortic disease by contrast-enhanced computed tomography. *Am J Cardiol* 1986; 57:282–290.

323. Wieder S, Adams PL: Improved routine chest radiography with a trough filter. *AJR* 1981; 137:695–698.

324. Wieder S, Rabinowitz JC: Fibrous mediastinitis: A late manifestation of mediastinal histoplasmosis. *Radiology* 1977; 125:305–312.

325. Wieder S, White TJ, Salazar J, et al: Pulmonary artery occlusion due to histoplasmosis. *AJR* 1982; 138:243–251.

326. Wilson ES: Neurenteric cyst of the mediastinum. *AJR* 1969; 107:641–646.

327. Wittich GR, Karnel F, Schurawitzki H, et al: Percutaneous drainage of mediastinal pseudocysts. *Radiology* 1988; 167:51–53.

328. Woodhead PJ: Thymic enlargement following chemotherapy. *Br J Radiol* 1984; 57:932–934.

329. Woodring JH, Loh FK, Kryscio RJ: Mediastinal hemorrhage: An evaluation of radiographic manifestations. *Radiology* 1984; 151:15–21.

330. Wychulis AR, Connolly DC, McGoon DC: Pericardial cysts, tumors, and fat necrosis. *J Thorac Cardiovasc Surg* 1971; 62:294–300.

331. Wychulis AR, Payne WS, Clagett OT, et al: Surgical treatment of mediastinal tumors: A 40 year experience. *J Thorac Cardiovasc Surg* 1971; 62:379–392.

332. Wycoco D, Raval B: An unusual presentation of mediastinal Hodgkin's lymphoma on computed tomography. *J Comput Tomogr* 1983; 7:187–188.

333. Yacoub MH, Lise M: Intrathoracic cystic hygromas. *Br J Dis Chest* 1969; 63:107–111.

334. Yamato M, Fuhrman CR: Computed tomography of fatty replacement in extramedullary hematopoiesis. *J Comput Assist Tomogr* 1987; 11:541–542.

335. Yamato M, Lecky JW, Hiramatsu K, et al: Takayasu arteritis: Radiographic and angiographic findings in 59 patients. *Radiology* 1986; 161:329–334.

336. Yang WC, Zapulla R, Malis L: Neurolemmoma in lumbar intervertebral foramen. *J Comput Assist Tomogr* 1981; 5:904–906.

337. Yeh HC, Gordon A, Kirschner PA, et al: Computed tomography and sonography of thymolipoma. *AJR* 1983; 140:1131–1133.

338. Yernault JC, Kuhn G, Dumortier P, et al: "Solid" mediastinal bronchogenic cyst: Mineralogic analysis. *AJR* 1986; 146:73–74.

339. Zerhouni EA, Scott WW, Baker RR, et al: Invasive thymomas: Diagnosis and evaluation by computed tomography. *J Comput Assist Tomogr* 1982; 6:92–100.

340. Zylak CJ, Banerjee R, Galbraith PA, et al: Lung involvement in angioimmunoblastic lymphadenopathy (AIL). *Radiology* 1976; 121:513–519.

Diseases of the Airways

TRACHEAL DISORDERS

Tracheal lesions that are part of a generalized pulmonary or systemic disorder together with congenital, traumatic, and neoplastic processes are discussed in their relevant chapters elsewhere. With a few exceptions, detailed consideration in this section is given only to conditions that are essentially confined to the trachea.

The trachea may be affected by extrinsic or intrinsic processes. Extrinsic processes, particularly masses, displace and distort the trachea, while intrinsic ones cause narrowing, widening, or a mass effect.

Tracheal Narrowing

Tracheal narrowing may be long or short segment, and since the distinction is not always clearcut, both types are considered together. The important causes are listed in Table 16–1.

Tuberculosis.—Although common in the past,[305] tracheal tuberculosis is now rare. It is almost always associated with cavitary lung disease and grossly infected sputum.[62] Pathologically, there is mucosal thickening and ulceration and subsequent healing by fibrosis with stricture formation.[62] Very occasionally the trachea is involved by direct spread from adjacent nodes, and fistula formation subsequent to this is described.[2]

Scleroma.—Scleroma is a chronic progressive granulomatous infection that primarily affects the nose but may also involve the nasopharynx, larynx, trachea, and bronchi. It is caused by the gram-negative bacterium *Klebsiella rhinoscleromatis*. Scleroma is uncommon in the West, occurring mainly in Asia, North Africa, Central and South America, and Eastern Europe and affecting principally rural people from low socioeconomic groups.[62] The disease passes through three phases: catarrhal, granulomatous and proliferative, and finally scarring.[25] Patients usually present with symptoms related to the nose and paranasal sinuses, and the majority have radiographic signs of sinusitis.[25] Occasionally there will be a soft tissue mass or bone destruction suggesting a nasal carcinoma. Laryngeal involvement is usually manifest by transglottic narrowing and vocal cord thickening. There is tracheal involvement in about 5% of patients, and this is nearly always accompanied by laryngeal disease and quite often, though not necessarily, by paranasal sinus disease.[62] Either the whole or more commonly part of the trachea is involved, typically the proximal rather than the distal segment.[159] Stenoses are usually concentric and may be nodular or smooth.[94] Less commonly, there is diffuse uniform narrowing or multiple masses.[112] Bronchial involvement is described.[228]

Tracheo(broncho)pathia osteo(chondro)plastica.—This condition was first described more than 100 years ago,[358] yet it still remains a curiosity of obscure etiology. Although rare, it is more common than airway amyloidosis, a closely allied condition that some workers consider is identical.[8] In 1974, it was possible to collect 245 cases of tracheopathia from the world literature.[221]

Pathologically, the disease is characterized by the

development of cartilaginous and bony submucosal nodules[62] in the trachea and proximal airways (Fig 16–1). The nodules are typically found in the lower two thirds of the trachea and in the main, lobar, and segmental bronchi.[206] The disorder may, however, sometimes start more proximally and affect the first tracheal ring region.[368] The osteochondral nodules develop adjacent to the airway cartilages and, therefore, usually occur anterolaterally in the trachea,[206] only occasionally involving the membranous part.[345] The nodules give rise to sessile and polypoidal elevations of the mucosa, which produce airway narrowing.[368] The overlying mucosa usually remains intact but sometimes it ulcerates, causing hemoptysis.[8] The etiology of the condition is obscure, with two theories currently commanding the most support. One theory considers the nodules to be a form of ecchondrosis of the airway cartilage because of their distribution in the airways and because they have bony, cartilaginous, and fibrous connections to the cartilage rings themselves.[368] The other theory is that the

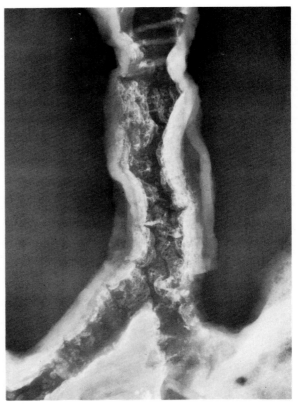

FIG 16–1.
Tracheopathia osteoplastica. Radiograph of an autopsy specimen of the trachea and main-stem bronchi opened from the back showing extensive nodular thickening of the tracheal wall. The nodules are calcified and extend down into the main-stem bronchi. Note the relative sparing of the subglottic trachea.

TABLE 16–1.
Causes of Tracheal Narrowing*

Extrinsic	
Mass lesions	Thyroid, nodes, vessels,[202] mediastinal mass
Invading lesions	Thyroid/esophageal carcinoma
Mediastinal fibrosis	Tuberculosis, histoplasmosis[357]
Intrinsic	
Congenital[29, 194]	Congenital tracheal narrowing[56]
Infective	Croup/laryngotracheobronchitis[144]
	Papillomatosis[130]
	Tuberculosis[305]
	Scleroma
	Fungal: histoplasmosis, coccidioidomycosis,[113] mucormycosis, candidiasis[62]
Granulomatous	Wegener's granulomatosis
	Sarcoidosis[43]
Neoplastic	Benign/malignant neoplasm[96]
	Lymphoma[262]
Traumatic	Tracheostomy/endotracheal intubation
	Blunt/penetrating trauma[362]
Postinflammatory[160]	Epidermolysis bullosa[332]
Depositional/dysplastic	Mucopolysaccharidoses[256]
	Chondrodysplasia punctata[186]
Immunologic	Amyloidosis[65]
	Relapsing polychondritis
Cryptogenic	Tracheopathia osteoplastica
	Saber-sheath trachea
	Idiopathic

*Modified from Berkmen YM: The trachea: The blind spot in the chest. *Radiol Clin North Am* 1984; 22:539–562.

disorder is due to amyloidosis, a condition in which cartilage and bone formation is known to occur. Several workers have in fact found evidence of amyloid in pathologic specimens from patients with tracheopathia.[8, 294, 304]

Seventy-five percent of patients are male, and presentation is usually in middle age (sixth decade), but there is a wide age range, from 11 to 78 years.[62] The common presenting symptoms are dyspnea, hoarseness, cough that is often productive, hemoptysis, and recurrent pulmonary infections.[206] The disease progresses very slowly. In one report of nine patients, seven had had symptoms for more than 10 years, and in one patient the symptoms had been present for about 20 years.[206]

The chest radiograph may be normal[206] or it may demonstrate evidence of collapse or infective consolidation. Airway calcification has diagnostic value but can be surprisingly difficult to detect.[62] Tracheal calcification (see Fig 16–1) shows as irregular or scalloped opacities lying inside the cartilage rings,[368] and though this calcification may be seen on a well-penetrated posteroanterior (PA) chest radiograph, it is better appreciated on a lateral view.[368] When the calcification extends more distally, the chest radiograph may show linear opacities radiating out from the hili, representing thickened and calcified airway walls.[8] If the tracheal air column is well seen, the irregular nodularity of the tracheal wall and the encroachment of these nodules on the lumen can be appreciated. Conventional tomography[164, 353] and particularly computed tomography (CT)[140, 253] show all these features to better advantage. The definitive diagnosis is made bronchoscopically, at which time the passage of the instrument may generate a grating sensation. It is possible, however, to miss the diagnosis even on bronchoscopy, and some patients have needed several examinations before the diagnosis was eventually made.[206]

Saber-Sheath Trachea.—This is a deformity limited to the intrathoracic part of the trachea, which is flattened from side to side such that the coronal diameter is two thirds or less of the sagittal diameter at the same level. It is virtually confined to males, who are usually more than 50 years of age, the youngest recorded patient being 37 years of age.[128] Saber-sheath trachea is strongly associated with the presence of chronic obstructive pulmonary disease (COPD); and in one series the latter was present in 93% of patients with the deformity compared with a frequency of 18% in controls.[128] The pathogenesis of the lesion is obscure, but it seems likely that it is an acquired deformity related to the abnormal pattern and magnitude of intrathoracic pressure changes in COPD.

Saber-sheath trachea can be detected on the plain chest radiograph (Fig 16–2) but is better demonstrated by plain tomography or CT (Fig 16–3). The narrowing usually affects the whole of the intrathoracic trachea with an abrupt return to normal caliber at the thoracic inlet.[129] In Greene's series[128] of 60 patients with saber-sheath trachea and 60 controls, the mean coronal diameter of the deformed tracheas was reduced to 61% and the sagittal diameter increased to 115% (see Fig 16–3), giving a mean tracheal area of 75% compared with controls. Cartilage rings are commonly calcified or ossified both pathologically and radiologically.[111, 129] The inner wall of the trachea is usually smooth (see Fig 16–3), but examples with nodular irregularity have been described.[293] The original studies described the trachea as displaying the usual changes in configuration in relation to respiration and considered the trachea

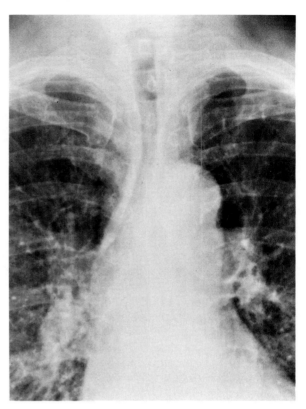

FIG 16–2.
Saber-sheath trachea. Posteroanterior radiograph in which the coronal diameter of the trachea in the cervical region is 19 mm, reducing to 9 mm in the intrathoracic portion. The transitional zone is at the level of the thoracic inlet, and the narrowing affects the whole of the intrathoracic trachea. The patient was male and had chronic bronchitis.

to be normally compliant.[128] Other workers, however, have described an abnormal degree of narrowing on forced expiration[111] and have noted that reduction in the cross-sectional area occurred mainly by apposition of the lateral walls with a little invagination of the posterior membrane.[112]

Cryptogenic Stenosis.—Intrinsic fibrotic stenoses of obscure origin have been described. These may occur at any site and can be multiple.[62]

Tracheal Widening

A number of studies* have assessed the normal tracheal dimensions in adults. In light of these data, a coronal diameter of 30 mm or more is taken as abnormal.

A limited number of disorders cause tracheal

*References 45, 95, 105, 128, 170, 184, and 342.

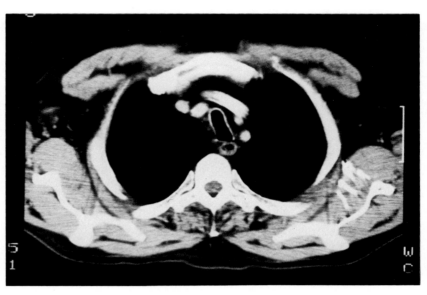

FIG 16–3.
Saber-sheath trachea. Computed tomographic scan showing the coronal diameter of the trachea at the level of the left brachiocephalic vein to be 1.0 cm vs. a sagittal diameter of 2.6 cm. This represents about a 50% coronal reduction and 15% sagittal increase in dimensions.

widening, and these are listed in Table 16–2. In some of the conditions the widening is generalized, and in others it is local, as with a tracheocele or following endotracheal tube cuff damage. In some forms of diffuse disease, widening is mild and confined to one diameter. Thus, in cystic fibrosis the sagittal diameter is increased while the coronal dimension remains normal.[137]

The most striking diffuse increase in tracheal diameter is seen in tracheobronchomegaly (Mounier-Kuhn syndrome). This is a rare abnormality of the trachea and larger airways associated with recurrent respiratory tract infection that was first described in 1932.[239] Pathologically there is atrophy of the elastic and muscular elements of both the cartilaginous and membranous parts of the trachea.[7, 184] There is evidence that points toward this being a primary process. Thus, in some patients the condition is familial with an autosomal recessive pattern of transmission.[173] There is a recognized association with ana-

TABLE 16–2.
Causes of Local and Generalized Tracheal Widening

Tracheobronchomegaly (Mounier-Kuhn syndrome)
Heritable connective tissue disorders
    Ehlers-Danlos complex[1]
    Cutis laxa[343]
Immune deficiency states/recurrent childhood infections
    Ataxia telangiectasia[193]
    Immunoglobulin deficiency[193]
    Cystic fibrosis[137]
Endotracheal cuff damage
Relapsing polychondritis[93]
Tracheocele

tomic variants of the bronchial tree,[23] and in many patients there is also a long history dating back to childhood. Some authors nevertheless consider it an acquired condition.

There are no reliable data on prevalence, but in 1,800 bronchograms there was a frequency of about 1%, and the authors considered that the condition was probably underdiagnosed.[114] It is markedly male predominant, with only about 5% of patients being female, and there is a possible racial predisposition for blacks.[23] Presentation is most commonly in the third or fourth decade, and more than three quarters of the patients have presented by the age of 40 years.[23] Symptoms, however, often date back a decade or more into childhood,[114, 184] and the disorder has even been recorded in an 18-month-old baby.[165] The typical history is of chronic cough that is characteristically loud and productive. Other clinical features include recurrent chest infections and occasionally hoarseness and dyspnea. Symptoms, therefore, closely resemble those of chronic bronchitis or bronchiectasis. Respiratory function tests show airflow obstruction and hyperinflation.[23, 114, 173] Airway compliance is increased, and dynamic collapse on expiration and cough can be demonstrated.[55, 114, 165, 184]

The diagnosis is radiological. The immediately subglottic trachea has a normal diameter but it expands as it passes to the carina (Figs 16–4 and 16–5), and this dilatation often continues into the major bronchi.[23, 114, 270] A diameter of more than 30 mm for the trachea on a PA radiograph and of more than 25 mm for main stem bronchi is required for the diagnosis. The dilatation may vary from segment

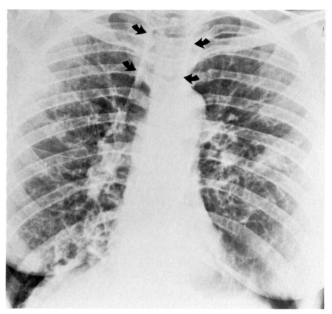

FIG 16—4.
Tracheobronchomegaly; posteroanterior radiograph. The trachea *(arrows)* is just over 3.0 cm wide. There is evidence of airflow obstruction with a low, flat right hemidiaphragm. Throughout the lungs, but particularly in the left middle and lower zones, there are line and ring opacities consistent with bronchiectasis.

to segment but overall tends to be relatively even. Atrophic mucosa prolapses between cartilage rings and gives the trachea a characteristically corrugated outline that, on a plain radiograph, is best appreciated in the lateral view.[1, 173, 325] Corrugations are particularly well shown on bronchography[23] and may become exaggerated to form sacculations or diverticula.[23, 91] Tracheal changes are well shown on CT.[79, 112, 303] The dilated proximal airways in the lung show changes of cystic or cylindrical bronchiectasis (Fig 16—6),[23, 114] and this affects particularly first- to fourth-order branches.[173] Small branches that arise from bronchiectatic segments tend to remain patent, unlike in bronchiectasis in general, where they are usually occluded by a bronchiolitis obliterans. This characteristic feature[114] is only shared by allergic bronchopulmonary aspergillosis.[296]

Dilatation of the trachea is generalized in tracheobronchomegaly. Occasionally in other conditions the trachea is locally dilated. This may be seen with a tracheocele, which is a localized ballooning of the membranous posterior tracheal wall of obscure etiology.[139] Tracheoceles tend to arise from the right posterior tracheal wall, and their size varies with transmural tracheal pressure.[325] Tracheal diverticula

may also be seen in tracheobronchomegaly and with cystic dilatation of mucous gland ducts.[325]

Tracheomalacia

Tracheomalacia is present when tracheal compliance is increased. It is usually a localized rather than a generalized process and may be congenital or acquired. Important causes are listed in Table 16—3. The increase in compliance is due to the loss of integrity of the structural components of the wall and is particularly associated with damaged or destroyed cartilage.

Tracheomalacia is diagnosed when changes in the transmural pressure gradient produce undue tracheal wall movements. Pressure gradients can be static, when generated by the Valsalva or Müller maneuvers, or dynamic when generated by inspiration, expiration, or cough. The Valsalva and Müller ma-

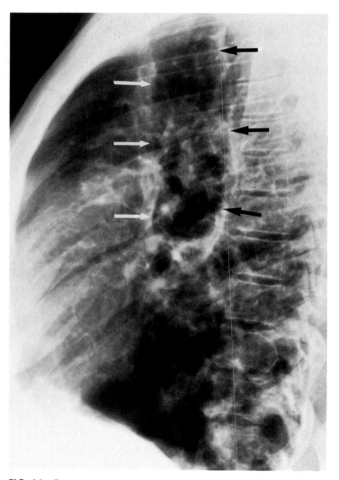

FIG 16—5.
Tracheobronchomegaly. Lateral view of trachea of the same patient as in Fig 4 showing grossly dilated trachea *(arrows)*.

TABLE 16–3.

Causes of Tracheomalacia

Congenital
  Cartilage deficiency[359]
  Generalized tracheomalacia[328]

Acquired
  Associated with endotracheal tubes and tracheostomy[275, 347]
  After closed chest trauma[93]
  After lung resection[93, 301]
  After radical neck dissection[84]
  After radiotherapy[84]
  COPD[172]
  Relapsing polychondritis[84]

neuvers are suitable for investigating the *cervical* trachea since the external pressure is always zero (atmospheric) and these procedures can produce transmural gradients that may reach 100 cm H$_2$O. Static procedures, however, fail to alter the gradient across the *thoracic* trachea[138] since, for example, with a Valsalva maneuver all thoracic contents will be subject to an identical increase in pressure. Dynamic maneuvers do not have this limitation and are therefore used to assess the compliance of intrathoracic airways.

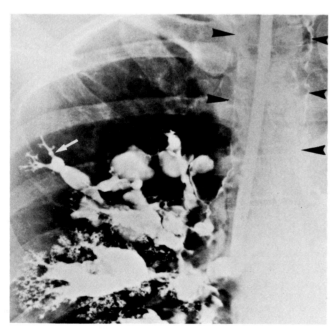

FIG 16–6.
Tracheobronchomegaly in a 53-year-old woman with recurrent lower respiratory tract infections. A bronchogram with contrast outlining the dilated trachea (3.3-cm coronal diameter; *black arrow heads*). There is varicose/cystic bronchiectasis with characteristic filling of distal bronchi *(white arrow)*, a feature otherwise seen only in allergic aspergillosis.

Until recently, the commonest cause of tracheomalacia in adults has been damage following placement of tracheostomy and endotracheal tubes. However, since the introduction of wide, low-pressure cuffs the problem has largely disappeared. Tracheostomy-related compliant segments may develop at the site of the stoma, at the level of the cuff, or in between; in this last instance, the pathogenesis is thought to be damage due to infection associated with stagnant secretions.[347] A compliant tracheal segment may or may not be accompanied by a stenosis.[108] An endotracheal tube cuff lying in a hypercompliant segment appears overinflated, and this may provide an early clue to the presence of tracheomalacia.[275]

A suspected diagnosis in the appropriate clinical setting can be confirmed with a flow-volume loop,[108] but tracheomalacic segments are best identified and characterized using fluoroscopy with video or cine recording.[93] Contrast enhancement is not necessary for these studies, but it usefully improves the image.[93] Most authors have employed conventional contrast agents, but some have used tantalum powder, which gives a dense, robust coating.[108] The trachea is studied in anteroposterior and oblique views during forced inspiration and expiration, cough, and the Valsalva and Müller maneuvers. Under these conditions a normal trachea will show narrowing both coronally and also sagittally due to invagination of the membranous posterior wall. Reliable data on the degree of narrowing to be expected is not available, and most studies have been performed in ignorance of the transmural pressure gradient generated. Several authors consider that caliber changes of more than 50% indicate increased wall compliance.[55, 172] In patients with COPD with high downstream resistance, particularly high dynamic pressure gradients can be generated across the tracheal wall, and it is likely that caliber changes of more than 50% can occur with normal tracheal compliance.[158]

Tracheal Filling Defects

In adults, tracheal filling defects are most commonly due to neoplasms, but there are a number of other causes (Table 16–4).

Ectopic Thyroid.—This is a rare cause of an intratracheal filling defect,[76, 274] with about 150 cases in the literature,[348] mostly from endemic goitrous areas.[96] Females outnumber males by about 3:1.[76] The ectopic thyroid may be histologically normal,

TABLE 16—4.

Tracheal Filling Defects*

Neoplasm[348]
  Benign (epithelial/mesenchymal)
  Malignant
    Carcinoma (squamous, adenoid cystic,
      adenocarcinoma)
    Sarcoma
    Plasmacytoma[24]
    Lymphoma
  Malignant invasion from without
Infection/granuloma
  Viral papilloma[121]
  Membranous croup
  Fungal infection
  Tuberculosis
  Rhinoscleroma
  Wegener's granulomatosis
Trauma
  Hematoma
Miscellaneous
  Ectopic thyroid
  Amyloidosis
  Tracheopathia osteoplastica
  Foreign body
  Mucoid pseudotumor[179]
  Cyst/mucocele

*Modified from Rost RC: Causes of a tracheal mass. *Semin Roentgenol* 1983; 18:4.

though it is usually goitrous. Occasionally it is malignant.[76, 96] Three quarters of intratracheal thyroid nodules are associated with extratracheal goiter. Sometimes they declare themselves years after the removal of an extratracheal goiter because of compensatory hypertrophy. Tumors may occur anywhere between subglottis and main carina,[348] but typically they are a few centimeters below the vocal cords, arising as smooth, sessile nodules from the posterolateral trachea wall.[76]

Tracheal Papilloma.—Squamous papillomas of the trachea in children are usually multiple and a manifestation of laryngeal papillomatosis with tracheobronchial dissemination.* Similar cases are rarely reported in adults.[121, 130] Solitary squamous cell papillomas of the trachea are also recognized in adults (Fig 16—7) and may undergo malignant transformation.[71, 96]

Tracheoesophageal Fistula

In the pediatric age group, tracheoesophageal fistula (TEF) is commonly congenital.[194] Occasionally

*References 54, 96, 130, 290, and 313.

such congenital fistulas may present in adults.[38, 321] Recognized causes of TEF are listed (Table 16—5), with malignant neoplasia, particularly esophageal, being the commonest in adults. Infection and trauma are the most frequent nonmalignant causes.[367]

BRONCHIECTASIS

Bronchiectasis is a chronic condition characterized by local, irreversible dilatation of bronchi, usually associated with inflammation.[106, 149] The qualification "irreversible" is included in the definition to exclude the transient airway dilatation that has been observed in pneumonia and atelectasis.* Dilatation of the airway in these circumstances is probably partly related to inflammatory changes in the wall altering compliance and to exaggerated lung stresses subsequent to collapse. Bronchiectasis may be regional or widespread. The generalized mild bronchial dilatation seen in chronic bronchitis is not considered to be a form of bronchiectasis.

Pathologically, bronchiectasis may be divided into obstructive and nonobstructive forms. The latter shows a basilar predilection and is commonly bilateral.[64] When unilateral it shows a preference for the left side.[355] The lingula and the middle lobe are also commonly affected. Grossly, bronchiectatic lungs are small in volume, gray-blue, and rubbery. Macroscopically, the airways are dilated in a variety of patterns that may be classified into two[149] or three subtypes.[285] The three-part Reid classification is

*References 17, 39, 99, 246, 261, and 315.

TABLE 16—5.

Causes of TEF in the Adult

Congenital[38, 321]
Neoplasm[222]
  Carcinoma esophagus[203]/trachea
  Lymphoma[34, 222]
Trauma
  Closed chest[143, 320]
  Penetrating[367]
  Postendoscopy/postoperative
  Endotracheal intubation[136]
  Corrosive esophagitis[11, 314]
  Esophageal foreign body[223]
  Postradiation
Infection
  Histoplasmosis[177]
  Actinomycosis[367]
  Tuberculosis
  Other bacteria

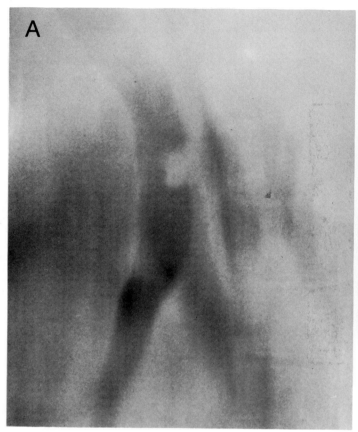

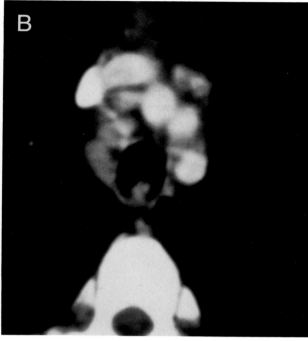

FIG 16—7.
Tracheal papilloma in an adult who presented with hemoptysis. The lesion is demonstrated **(A)** on a conventional lateral tomogram and **(B)** on computed tomography. Such lesions may become malignant.

widely used and is equally applicable to gross pathologic or bronchographic appearances. It uses the following divisions.

1. Cylindrical bronchiectasis.—This is the least severe form. Dilatation is mild, and the bronchi retain their regular and relatively straight outline (Fig 16–8). The bronchiectatic airways terminate abruptly with squared-off ends, and smaller bronchi and bronchioles are plugged with secretions. Pathologically, the number of bronchial subdivisions from the hilum to the periphery is normal.

2. Varicose bronchiectasis.—In this form, bronchial dilatation is greater and is accompanied by local constrictions that give the airway an irregular outline with a typically bulbous termination (Fig 16–9). Obstruction of small airways is more pronounced, and some are irreversibly obliterated by scarring. The number of generations of patent airways from hilum to periphery, which is normally in the order of 17 to 20, is reduced macroscopically to six or seven.

3. Cystic (saccular) bronchiectasis.—This is the most severe form of bronchiectasis (Fig 16–10), with

the airway taking on a ballooned appearance and dilating progressively as it passes distally. There is a great reduction in the number of bronchial divisions, and although the terminal sacs are subpleural they represent only fourth- or fifth-generation airways, indicating that there has been considerable parenchymal loss. Small airway branches are occluded and obliterated by a bronchiolitis obliterans. Histologically, airway walls are thickened and chronically inflamed with chronic granulation tissue, and bronchial arteries are hypertrophied. Ciliated epithelium is largely replaced by squamous epithelium or areas of squamous metaplasia that may be ulcerated. The mucosa is sometimes ulcerated or thrown into transverse ridges by circular muscle hypertrophy. Airways are surrounded by fibrosis with acute and organizing pneumonia in the adjacent parenchyma.[185]

The pathogenesis of bronchiectasis is complex, and this is borne out by the large number of recognized etiologies.[19] The two important and most commonly implicated pathogenic factors are bronchial wall weakness, often brought about by infective inflammatory damage, and an increased transmural

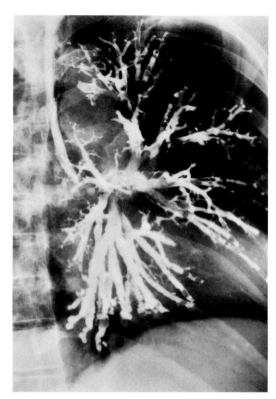

FIG 16–8.
Cylindrical bronchiectasis. Left posterior oblique projection of a left bronchogram showing cylindrical bronchiectasis affecting the whole of the lower lobe except for the superior segment. Few side branches fill. Basal airways are crowded together, indicating volume loss of the lower lobe, a common finding in bronchiectasis.

distending pressure. Recognized etiologic conditions are listed in Table 16–6.

Clinically, gross bronchiectasis is characterized by persistent cough, with copious purulent sputum and recurrent pulmonary infections. Symptoms frequently date from childhood when there may have been a history of a precipitating pneumonic event. With widespread disease there may be dyspnea and, ultimately, cor pulmonale. Such gross bronchiectasis is becoming unusual and is largely limited to patients with impaired defense mechanisms. A recognized presentation of mild bronchiectasis is recurrent hemoptysis,[101, 174] but quite often mild bronchiectasis is entirely without symptoms. This is particularly true of some forms such as that which occurs following granulomatous disease of the upper zones.

A classic description of the plain radiologic changes in bronchiectasis is that of Gudbjerg.[141] In this series only 7% of radiographs were normal, although this is a low figure judged by current clinical experience.[66, 69] Some varieties of bronchiectasis

such as occur in cystic fibrosis and the ciliary dyskinesia syndrome[244] will almost invariably show plain film changes. The following radiologic findings are described: (1) increased size and loss of definition of vascular opacities ascribed to peribronchial fibrosis; (2) visible bronchial walls, either as single thin lines or as parallel line opacities (Fig 16–11). With the latter finding the lines representing bronchial walls are more widely separated than would be expected with airways of normal diameter; (3) ring and curvilinear opacities generated by thickened airway walls seen end-on (Fig 16–12). Ring opacities tend to range in size from 5 to 20 mm and to have thin (hairline) walls. They may contain air-fluid levels (Fig 16–13); (4) dilated airways filled with secretions giving rise to broad-band shadows some 5 to 10 mm wide and several centimeters long (Figs 16–14 and 16–15). Band shadows may branch, giving V, Y, or more complex shaped opacities. They point toward the hilum. Seen end-on, such dilated fluid-filled airways generate rounded or oval nodular opacities; (5) variable vol-

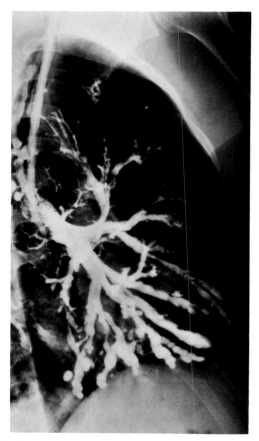

FIG 16–9.
Varicose bronchiectasis. Left posterior oblique projection of left bronchogram in a patient with the ciliary dyskinesia syndrome. All basal bronchi are affected by varicose bronchiectasis.

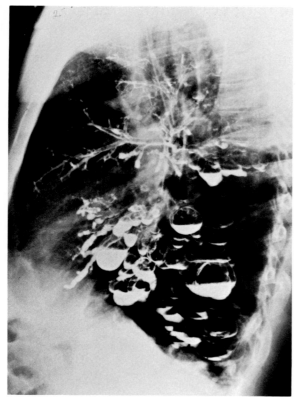

FIG 16—10.
Cystic bronchiectasis. Right lateral bronchogram showing cystic bronchiectasis affecting mainly the lower lobe and posterior segment of the upper lobe.

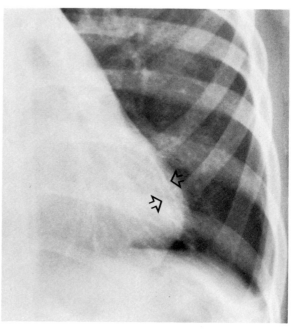

FIG 16—11.
Bronchiectasis. Posteroanterior radiograph on which thickened bronchial walls are seen as line opacities through the heart. Some lines appear paired *(arrows)* and probably represent opposite walls of a single airway. The separation of these lines is such that the airway must be dilated.

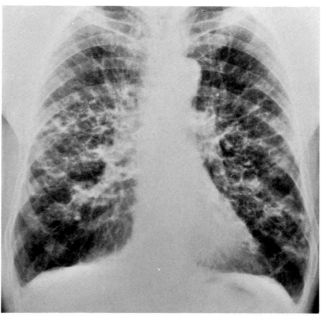

FIG 16—12.
Gross cystic bronchiectasis. Posteroanterior chest radiograph showing overinflated lungs. There is diffuse lung shadowing with nodular and linear elements. In addition, there are multiple ring opacities ranging from 3 to 15 mm.

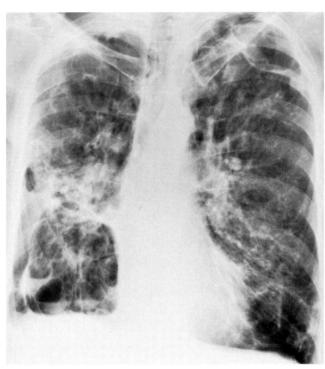

FIG 16–13.
Bronchiectasis. A patient with the ciliary dyskinesia syndrome. Overall lung volume is increased. At the left base there are multiple linear opacities due to bronchial wall thickening. On the right there is a small hydropneumothorax. Multiple ring shadows at the right base are due to bronchiectatic airways, which contain air-fluid levels.

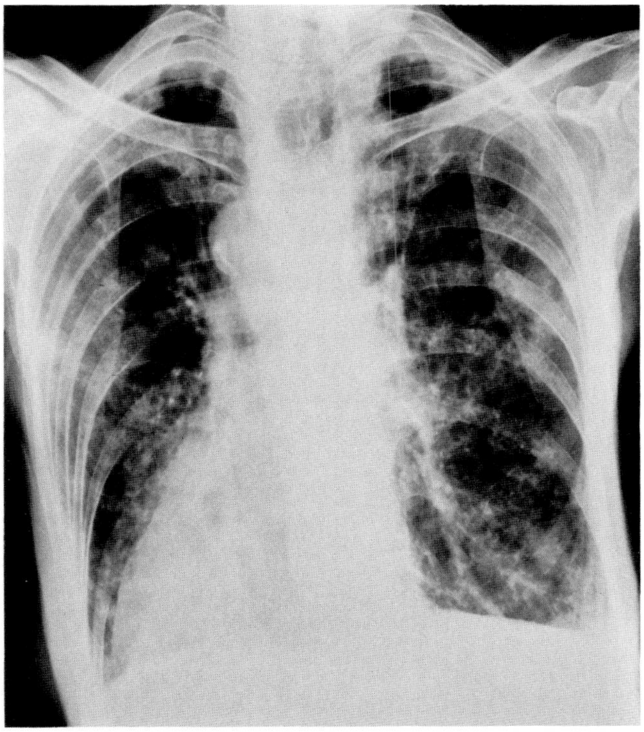

FIG 16–14.
Ciliary dyskinesia syndrome, Kartagener's syndrome. This 62-year-old woman gave a 40-year history consistent with bronchiectasis. The aortic arch, descending aorta, heart, and gastric air bubble are all on the right. There is diffuse complex pulmonary shadowing with many ring opacities. A broad branching band shadow can just be seen through the heart, representing dilated fluid-filled airways.

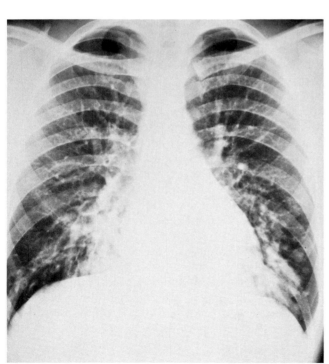

FIG 16–15.
Ciliary dyskinesia syndrome. A 20-year-old man with recurrent pneumonia, otitis, and sinusitis. In the paracardiac region, there are bilateral broad linear shadows due to dilated, fluid-filled bronchi. Like 50% of patients with ciliary dyskinesia, this patient does not have dextrocardia.

TABLE 16−6.
Causes of Bronchiectasis

Congenital	Cartilage deficiency[232, 344, 346, 359]
	Cystic bronchiectasis[6]
Postinfection	Childhood pneumonia, measles, pertussis, *Mycoplasma* pneumonia,[356] tuberculosis[247]
	Swyer-James syndrome[335]
Obstruction	Neoplasm
	Nodes (including "middle lobe syndrome")[36]
	Broncholith
	Foreign body[192]
	Bronchostenosis
Inhalation/ aspiration	Ammonia[156, 182]
	Riley-Day syndrome
	Gastric aspiration
	Heroin overdose[18]
Impaired host defense	Primary ciliary dyskinesia
	Cystic fibrosis
	Primary impaired humoral and/or cell immunity[360]
	Infantile X-linked agammaglobulinemia (Bruton's disease)
	Variable immunodeficiency[77]
	Selective immunoglobulin deficiency
	Wiskott-Aldrich syndrome
	Ataxia telangiectasia (Louis-Bar syndrome)
	Chédiak-Higashi syndrome
	Inflammatory bowel disease[53, 117]
Allergy	Allergic bronchopulmonary aspergillosis
Pulmonary fibrosis	End-stage lung[351]
	Radiation[67, 200]
Miscellaneous	Tracheobronchomegaly (Mounier-Kuhn syndrome)
	Alpha$_1$-antitrypsin deficiency[175, 178, 204]
	Obstructive azoospermia (Young's syndrome)[145, 248]
	Anhydrotic ectodermal dysplasia[277]
	Rheumatoid disease
	Ehlers-Danlos syndromes
	Marfan's syndrome
	Yellow nail syndrome
	Cryptogenic

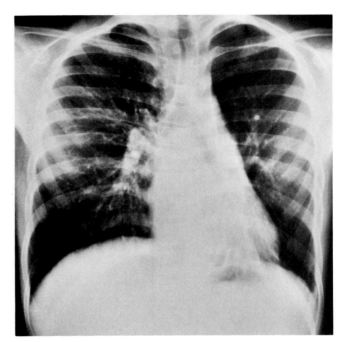

FIG 16−16.
Left lower lobe bronchiectasis. There is marked volume loss of the left lower lobe indicated by the depressed hilum, vertical left main-stem bronchus, mediastinal shift, and left-sided transradiancy. Just visible through the heart are parallel line opacities ("tubular shadows").

ume changes. In generalized forms like that associated with cystic fibrosis and the immotile cilia syndrome there is often generalized overinflation (see Figs 16−12 and 16−13).[244] Localized forms, however, are frequently accompanied by atelectasis (Fig 16−16), which may be mild and detected only by vascular crowding or fissural displacement. It may, on the other hand, be marked with a grossly collapsed airless lobe (Fig 16−17). Occasionally collateral air drift allows continued aeration of the distal lung, in which case there may be a localized increase in volume; (6) other radiologic signs include infective consolidation, evidence of scarring, bulla formation, and pleural thickening.

The definitive diagnosis of bronchiectasis is made by bronchography, though even this suffers from interpretive difficulties.[69] The types of change observed are those discussed previously under pathologic manifestations. Bronchography is an invasive and relatively unpleasant procedure, and alternative ways of diagnosing bronchiectasis have been investigated, including radionuclide scintigraphy and CT. With ventilation-perfusion (V/Q) scintiscans, there is both impaired perfusion and ventilation, with ventilation being most affected.[124] Several workers using either xenon 133 or krypton 81m have concluded that a normal V/Q scintiscan coupled with a normal chest radiograph virtually excludes bronchiectasis.[124, 326, 340] Aerosol ventilation scintigraphy, as might be expected, is less sensitive than gas ventilation scintigraphy.[15] Indium 111−labeled autologous neutrophils migrate to bronchiectatic areas of the lung, but this has not been adopted as a useful clinical technique.[70]

The CT changes in bronchiectasis have been well described[245] and include many signs that are similar to the plain radiographic findings: thick bronchial walls, either tramline or beaded; bronchial dilatation; ring opacities arranged in lines or clusters (Fig 16−18); and air-fluid levels. Bronchiectatic air-

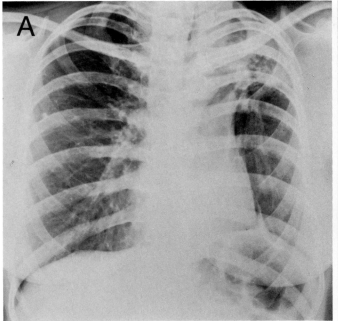

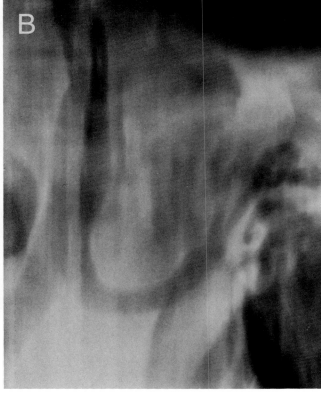

FIG 16–17.
Left upper lobe bronchiectasis. **A,** posteroanterior chest radiograph
showing a grossly collapsed left upper lobe due to previous tuber-
culosis. **B,** midlung tomogram of the left upper lobe shows bronchiectatic airways as air bronchograms in the collapsed lobe. Such airways drain well and are rarely associated with infective complications.

ways are detectable more peripherally than normal
because of their thickened walls. In judging the diameter of airways, comparison with adjacent vessels
is helpful as both should be approximately the same
size. A characteristic appearance in bronchiectasis is
the "signet ring" opacity produced by the ring
shadow of a dilated airway with its accompanying artery. Airways filled with secretions produce rounded
or flame-shaped opacities that can be identified by
following them through adjacent sections to unfilled
airways. Bullae and cystic bronchiectasis are sometimes difficult to distinguish on CT. Helpful identifying features of cystic bronchiectasis include (1) a
linear array of cysts ("string of beads"); (2) continuity of cysts with the airways proximally; (3) generally
thicker cyst walls; (4) identification of an accompanying vessel, particularly as a "signet ring" opacity.[245]
In addition to these "specific" CT findings of bronchiectasis, there may well be the nonspecific signs of
atelectasis, hyperinflation, consolidation, or pleural
thickening. False-negative CTs are produced when
airways are lost in areas of collapse and consolidation, when slice thickness and intervals are too
coarse,[260] and when bronchiectasis is cylindrical and

mild.[241, 306] Bronchiectatic changes are generally
more difficult to identify on CT in airways that are
oriented axially rather than transversely,[241] with the
middle and lingular lobes being the easiest to assess.
Overall, false-positive changes are less common than
false-negative ones.[66]

A number of studies have looked at the accuracy
of CT in detecting bronchiectasis.* Differing techniques, methods of assessment, and study populations make for difficulties in comparing these series.
In general, specificity has been high: between 90%
and 100%, with sensitivities in assessing segmental
disease ranging between 46% and 100%. Currently,
a reasonable figure to take for sensitivity is probably
about 80%. Thus, CT is useful in clinical situations
in which high specificity and moderate sensitivity are
acceptable and allows bronchography to be avoided
in most clinical situations. A good technique appears
to be the one used by Grenier et al.,[135] namely, thin
sections at 10-mm intervals throughout the lungs, allowing the advantages of high-resolution thin-
section CT without the disadvantages of needing too

*References 66, 135, 171, 234, 241, 245, and 306.

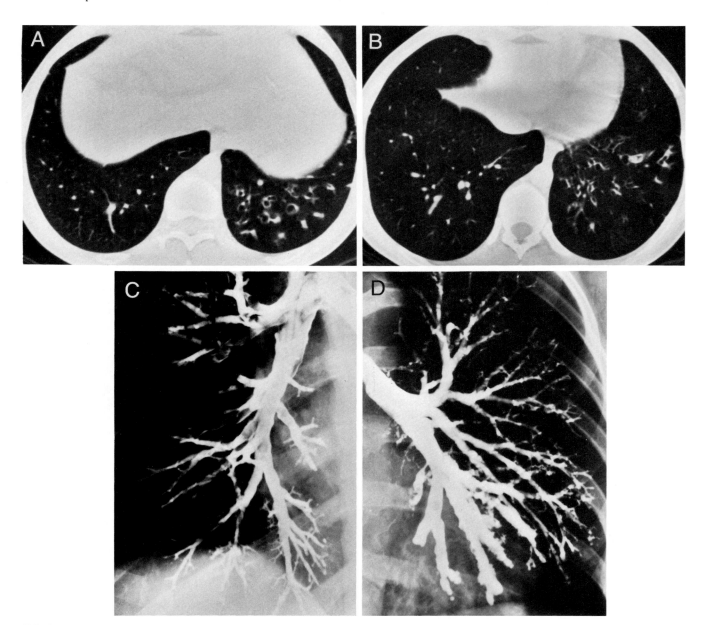

FIG 16–18.
Bronchiectasis. **A** and **B,** high-resolution thin-section (1.5-mm) computed tomographic scan showing multiple oval and rounded ring opacities in the left lower lobe. The right lung appears normal. The fact that the airways tend to be arranged in a linear fashion and to have walls of more than hairline thickness helps to distinguish these bronchiectatic airways from cysts or bullae. **C** and **D,** bronchograms on the same patient done because the patient, a 25-year-old woman, was being considered for surgery. The normality of the right bronchial tree and the bronchiectasis in the left lower lobe were confirmed.

many sections. If high sensitivity is required, such as before surgery for bronchiectasis, then bronchography may still be indicated.[260]

Ciliary Dyskinesia Syndrome (Immotile Cilia Syndrome)

The ciliary dyskinesia syndrome is one of the specific causes of bronchiectasis and, with changing patterns of etiology, it is becoming relatively more important. In this condition, first identified in 1976,[3] a variety of genetically determined defects in ciliary structure and function interfere with mucociliary clearance. This impaired clearance is associated with recurrent upper and lower respiratory tract infections.[4, 83] It has many shared features with cystic fibrosis but it is less disabling and carries a better prognosis.[244] Kartagener's syndrome (Figs 16–14 and 16–19)[181]—situs inversus, paranasal sinusitis, and bronchiectasis—is a subset of the ciliary dyskinesia syndrome (CDS), and about 50% of patients with CDS have Kartagener's syndrome.[4, 132, 244] Looked at from the point of view of dextrocardia, about one fifth of subjects with dextrocardia have Kartagener's syndrome.[229] Ciliary dyskinesia syndrome has an autosomal recessive type of transmission[291] with an equal sex incidence. Ciliary function is abnormal throughout the body, and sperm are immotile. Thus, males are infertile. Fertility in females is generally unaffected, though there are exceptions.[132] Respiratory symptoms may be delayed in onset but can generally be traced back to childhood, and CDS is even described as causing neonatal respiratory distress.[354] Symptoms are those of bronchitis, rhinitis, and sinusitis, which are universal, and otitis, which is less common. Bronchiectasis develops in childhood and adolescence (see Fig 16–15)[244] and is associated with recurrent pneumonia. Prognosis is generally good,[4] and the diagnosis is compatible with a full life span.[229] The diagnosis is regarded as established in the following circumstances: (1) complete Kartagener's syndrome; (2) men with normal situs but a classic history and immotile sperm; (3) women and children with normal situs but typical history and an affected sibling; (4) subjects with normal situs but with a classic history and ultrastructural defects of nasal or bronchial cilia on biopsy.[4] The incidental occurrence of bronchiectasis and dextrocardia in the same patient with normal cilia is described.[133]

Young's syndrome[145, 248] clinically resembles CDS. However, in Young's syndrome ciliary function is normal, and infertility is due to obstructive azoospermia. Obstruction occurs at the level of the epididymis, which is palpably enlarged. The pathogenesis of increased sinopulmonary infection in these patients is obscure.

BRONCHOLITHIASIS

The term *broncholithiasis* is generally interpreted more widely than meaning just the condition resulting from calcified material in the airway.[341] Most authors include, in addition, the effects of airway distortion or inflammation caused by calcified peribronchial nodes.[14] Nearly all cases are due to infected nodes, particularly following histoplasmosis.[73, 349] Other causal infections include tuberculosis, actinomycosis, coccidioidomycosis, and cryptococcosis. A few cases have been reported with silicosis.[57] Calcified material in an airway or luminal distortion due to peribronchial disease results in airway obstruction. This in turn leads to collapse, obstructive pneumonitis, mucoid impaction, or bronchiectasis. Fistulas can form from the airway to the esophagus,[72] pleural space, or aorta.[73] Symptoms commonly include cough, hemoptysis, and recurrent episodes of fever and purulent sputum.[73] Sometimes patients complain of a localized rhonchus. The classic symptom of lithoptysis is not common, with a frequency of just 16% in one series.[73]

In a review of the plain radiologic findings, three major types of change were distinguished:[341] (1) disappearance of a previously identified calcified nidus; (2) change in position of a calcified nidus; (3) evidence of airway obstruction including segmental or lobar atelectasis, mucoid impaction, obstructive pneumonitis, and obstructive overinflation with air trapping. There may be signs of bronchiectasis.[73] Calcified hilar or mediastinal nodes are an important feature of the radiograph, and in the presence of cough, hemoptysis, or collapse/consolidation it is important to inspect all calcifications, assessing their position and looking for evidence of movement on serial films. Movement can be difficult to detect and may just be a relatively subtle rotation.[341] Bron-

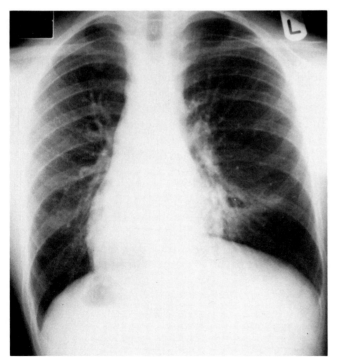

FIG 16–19.
Ciliary dyskinesia syndrome, Kartagener's syndrome. A 14-year-old boy with recurrent pneumonic episodes. There is dextrocardia and situs inversus. The left heart border is obscured by confluent nodular and linear opacities due to a bronchiectatic and shrunken left middle lobe.

choliths tend to be about twice as common on the right as on the left side, and obstructive changes particularly affect the right middle lobe.

Once the diagnosis is suspected on plain radiographs, confirmation may be sought with tomograms. Both conventional tomography[73] and CT[190, 302] have the ability to demonstrate calcification, its relationship to the airways, and any complications. In interpreting tomograms it is important to avoid misreading calcification as being within the airway when really it is adjacent. In CT, such an artifact can arise from volume averaging.[190] In conventional tomography, the mistake can be avoided by taking sections at right angles to each other. Further confirmation can be obtained by fiberoptic bronchoscopy. In some patients, this may be used therapeutically, but in others, technical difficulties and excess bleeding obviate this approach.

BRONCHIOLITIS OBLITERANS

Bronchiolitis obliterans (BO) is a descriptive term for an inflammatory process that plugs the lumen of small airways with granulation tissue and causes their ultimate destruction with obliterative scarring.[85, 215] It is not a specific disease entity but rather a nonspecific response that occurs in a variety of identified and obscure conditions.[185] It may be a generalized or local process within the lungs, but even when generalized it is usually patchy.[86] Precipitating causes are often obvious and include inhalation of toxic fumes, respiratory infections—particularly those due to viruses—systemic disorders such as rheumatoid disease, and drugs. However, a significant number of cases are cryptogenic, and in one series nearly 40% were of obscure origin.[125] Important causes are given in Table 16–7.

Bronchiolitis obliterans is well recognized following inhalation of irritant fumes. It has been most frequently described following nitrogen dioxide inhalation (silo-filler's disease),[26, 205, 231, 238] when it follows the acute symptoms after a 2- to 6-week latency.[68, 176, 273] Other fumes described include sulfur dioxide,[60, 106] ammonia,[182, 318] and hot gases.[255] Viruses are the most commonly implicated infectious agents,[5, 16, 363] particularly respiratory syncytial virus and adenovirus in children.[27] As with inhalations, there is often a latency of several weeks following infection before progressive dyspnea and radiologic opacities signal the development of BO. Nonviral infections are much less common, with some specific reports, e.g., with *Legionella pneumo-*

TABLE 16–7.
Causes of Bronchiolitis Obliterans*†

Inhalation/aspiration	Nitrogen oxides (silo-filler's disease)
	Other irritant fumes (ammonia, sulfur dioxide)
	Hot gases
	Gastric acid
After pulmonary infection	Viral (RSV, adenovirus, influenza virus)
	Bacterial (*Legionella, Bordetella*)
	Mycoplasma
	Obscure
Connective tissue disorders	Rheumatoid disease
	Polymyositis, SLE, progressive systemic sclerosis
	Sjögren's syndrome
Graft-vs.-host disease	Bone marrow transplant
	Heart-lung transplant
Drug related	Penicillamine
Cryptogenic	. . .
Local	Airway obstruction (foreign body/tumor)
	Adjacent to granuloma
	Bronchiectasis

*Modified from Epler GR, Colby TV, McLoud TC, et al: Bronciolitis obliterans organizing pneumonia. *N Engl J Med* 1985; 312:152–158.
†RSV = respiratory syncytial virus; SLE = systemic lupus erythematosus.

phila,[295] with *Mycoplasma pneumoniae,*[86] and with unidentified agents.[125] Of the connective tissue disorders[87] the association is strongest with rheumatoid disease[115, 151, 210] but has been described in polymyositis/dermatomyositis,[298] systemic lupus erythematosus,[188] progressive systemic sclerosis,[87, 125] and mixed connective tissue disease.[59] About half of the patients with rheumatoid disease and BO have been taking penicillamine,[115] and a cause-and-effect relationship has been proposed.[87, 243] Other drugs, e.g., sulfasalazine, have been implicated rarely.[361]

In the last few years an association with marrow transplants[254, 272, 288, 366] and heart-lung transplants[49] has become apparent and is probably due to acute or chronic graft-vs.-host disease.[272, 288, 366] In these patients, BO has developed 2 to 9 months after transplant and about a third of those affected have died, with many of the others having persistent disability.

Many reported cases of BO are cryptogenic, and several large series have been reported,[59, 86, 125, 339] totaling about 100 patients.

The pathologic changes of BO are described in detail in three series[86, 125, 142] and have been reviewed by Katzenstein and Askin.[185] There are two main histologic types, and the changes in both are patchy. In the commoner, there is *intraluminal* obstruction, and the terminal and respiratory bronchioles become occluded by granulomatous plugs that often extend distally into alveolar ducts. These granulomatous masses go on to fibrose. Septal inflammatory changes may occur but are relatively mild and local. Air spaces distal to occluded airways may become overinflated if they remain ventilated by collateral air drift, or they may become filled with macrophages that are often lipid-laden, giving rise to an endogenous (organizing) lipid pneumonitis. Bronchiolitis obliterans and organizing pneumonitis commonly occur together. In the less common type of BO there is *extraluminal* compression by inflammatory cell collections, particularly lymphocytes and plasma cells, that progresses to fibrosis. Airway obliteration by such scars can be easily missed.[125] If there is a significant interstitial (septal) infiltrate, then confusion with usual interstitial pneumonitis can arise. Also, if the obstructive pneumonitis element is dominant, it may be classified as a (cryptogenic) organizing pneumonia.

Clinically it is useful to separate BO into three groups: (1) BO secondary to recognized precipitating factors; (2) cryptogenic BO with organizing pneumonia (BOOP); and (3) cryptogenic BO per se. In secondary forms of the disease, progressive dyspnea and nonproductive cough develop weeks or months after the precipitating event. The cryptogenic form with organizing pneumonia (BOOP) has a distinct and relatively homogeneous pattern.[86] There is an equal sex incidence, and presentation is typically in the 40- to 60-year age group, with an age range of 21 to 75 years.[86] Dominant symptoms are dyspnea, nonproductive cough, and systemic symptoms such as malaise, fever, and weight loss. Presentation is usually delayed 2 to 6 months after the onset of initial symptoms.[59, 86, 142] The main sign in the chest is crackles on auscultation; wheezing is an unusual finding, and finger clubbing is not a feature. Respiratory function tests show a restrictive pattern and impaired gas exchange (reduced single-breath diffusing capacity), but, curiously, an obstructive pattern is uncommon.[86] The lack of an obstructive defect is possibly due to the fact that airways are occluded rather than narrowed, and the subtended lung units are subtracted.[242] Other patients are described with cryptogenic BO in whom there is no element of organizing pneumonia,[339] and these patients differ from those with BOOP in that symptoms are much more chronic and lack systemic features, and there is an obstructive ventilatory defect and often a characteristic midinspiratory squeak on auscultation.

There is a wide range of radiologic findings in

BO,[215] reflecting the variety of possible changes in the air space units beyond the obstructed airways. These units may be normal, or hyperinflated, or consolidated because of an organizing pneumonia. The main patterns are as follows.

Normal Chest Radiograph.—This is seen with inhalation, following infection, and with connective tissue disorders and transplants. It is also seen in the chronic idiopathic variety.[339]

Hyperinflation.—This is described following toxic fume inhalation[60]; in connective tissue disorders, particularly rheumatoid disease[115]; following marrow transplantation[254]; and in subacute or chronic cryptogenic disease.[46]

BOOP Pattern.—This has been described in three series.[59, 86, 142] The dominant pattern in about 75% of patients (Fig 16–20) is of consolidations, typically multifocal and bilateral and showing no zonal predilection. They can range in size from subsegmental to lobar. A variable but somewhat lower percentage of patients have "interstitial" opacities, which may be small rounded, small irregular, or coarsely linear. In addition, in one series 20% of patients showed pleural effusion or thickening and 25% had reduced lung volume,[59] while in another series two of 42 patients showed cavitation. This BOOP pattern is also seen in patients with connective tissue disorders, e.g. polydermatomyositis.[298]

Reticulonodular Patterns.—A variety of nodular patterns are seen, ranging from diffusely distributed small nodules (c 2 mm) to multiple larger nodules up to a centimeter or more, which are sometimes ill defined and can become confluent.[68, 125, 205] Nodules may be regionally distributed and show basal predominance.[146] An additional reticular element is sometimes present.

Consolidative Patterns.—These are common and in one series were found in 75% of patients.[125] They may be unifocal or multifocal,[227] and, although a bibasal distribution is common, consolidation may occur anywhere, including a pattern in the upper zones that resembles tuberculosis.[207, 361] Consolidations range in size from patchy subsegmental lesions to lobar and they may be diffuse, resembling pulmonary edema. Mixed patterns of alveolar and interstitial opacities may occur.[125]

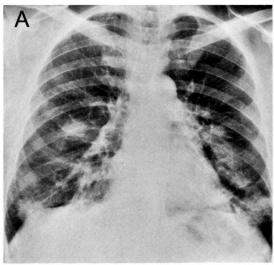

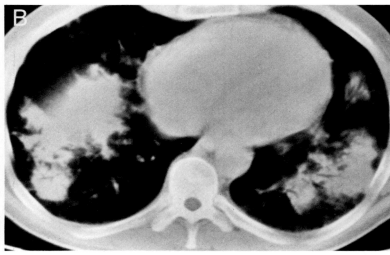

FIG 16–20.
Bronchiolitis obliterans with organizing pneumonia. The patient was a 55-year-old man who had had a viral-like syndrome during the previous 3 months and complained of increasing tiredness and dyspnea. **A,** posteroanterior radiograph. **B,** computed tomographic (CT) scan through lung bases (performed at a time when diagnosis was not known) showing multiple, nonspecific areas of consolidation, some of which have a nodular configuration. Air bronchograms are striking on CT. The diagnosis was established at open lung biopsy.

Linear Patterns.—Apart from the fine linear opacities in reticulonodular shadowing, a coarse bibasal linear pattern is described.[125]

Bronchial Wall Thickening.—This is virtually unrecorded.[142, 243]

Hypovascularity.—In a series selected on clinical grounds rather than on primarily pathologic grounds,[46, 339] seven of 13 patients showed reduction in size and number of midlung and peripheral vessels in the middle and lower zones without enlargement of main pulmonary arteries. This was accompanied by matched V/Q defects on scintiscanning.[339]

There is limited information regarding bronchography. Bronchography performed in seven of 13 patients showed principally nonfilling of side branches of fifth- and sixth-generation bronchi and lack of distal filling. Bronchiectasis was not a feature, though there was usually some loss of tapering. Airways ended abruptly with convex or squared ends.[46]

The prognosis in BOOP is good. Most patients often respond quickly to steroids, but up to a third of patients may relapse clinically and radiologically when steroid therapy is discontinued.[86] Prognosis in other forms of BO varies greatly and ranges from acute fulminant respiratory failure leading rapidly to death[166] to an indolent, chronic disorder with a time scale of many years.[339]

SWYER-JAMES' (MACLEOD'S) SYNDROME

This condition was first described in the early 1950s, and a variety of noneponymous terms have been used to identify it, in particular unilateral or lobar emphysema.[106] However, these terms may lead to confusion with, for example, congenital lobar emphysema, and the current practice of using eponymous titles seems likely to continue and is probably to be recommended. On several grounds, Swyer-James' syndrome would seem to be the most acceptable.

The first accounts were of a 6-year-old boy who had the abnormal lung removed and studied pathologically[329] and, in the following year, of nine adults aged 18 to 41 years without pathology.[214] The condition is characterized pathologically by bronchitis, bronchiolitis, bronchiolitis obliterans, and emphysema. Typically, the condition is unilateral and a whole lung is affected, but changes may be confined to a lobe or segment.[28, 283] Other recognized patterns are of segmental sparing with the rest of the lung involved[283] and of bilateral lobar or segmental disease. Bronchi and bronchioles from the fourth generation to terminal bronchioles have submucosal fibrosis causing luminal irregularity and occlusion.[283, 329] Pulmonary tissue is hypoplastic, including the pulmonary artery and its branches, which are reduced in both size and number. Lung distal to diseased airways is emphysematous and supplied by collateral air drift.

The Swyer-James syndrome is acquired and due to injury of the immature lung. It most commonly follows an acute viral infection occurring in infancy or childhood up to the age of 8 years, before the lung has completed its development.[163] Viruses implicated include adenovirus[216, 257] and measles virus.[219] Nonviral etiologies include infections such as *Mycoplasma* pneumonia,[322] tuberculosis,[271, 283] and pertussis[219] and noninfectious causes such as aspirated foreign bodies,[219, 350] irradiation,[30] and hydrocarbon ingestion.[189]

Patients are typically asymptomatic and present in adulthood with an unexpected radiologic finding. Less commonly, patients have exertional dyspnea,[219] which may be progressive, and exceptionally, quite marked[214] or repeated respiratory infections.[219, 329] Respiratory function tests show a reduced vital capacity, some airflow obstruction, and a reduced steady-state diffusing capacity.[106] Lung scintigraphy shows decreased or absent perfusion in the affected lung[352] and impaired ventilation with delayed xenon washout.[252] Although a matched perfusion/ventilation defect might raise the possibility of pulmonary artery obstruction, e.g., by a pulmonary embolus, this is rarely a diagnostic problem in the clinical setting. In addition, evidence of air trapping provided by delayed washout is not a feature of pulmonary embolism.

Findings on the plain chest radiograph are characteristic and consist of (1) unilateral transradiancy due to reduced lung perfusion (Fig 16–21, A). Should the condition be confined to a lobe, then transradiancy will be lobar. Lesser degrees of involvement are probably not detectable on the plain radiograph; (2) ipsilateral reduction in size and number of midlung and peripheral vessels (Fig 16–21, C); (3) an ipsilateral hilum that is present but small (Fig 16–21, A); (4) a normal or slightly decreased ipsilateral lung volume. The mediastinum may show some shift to the affected side at total lung capacity (TLC).[214] The fact that the ipsilateral lung volume does not increase is a helpful finding in distinguishing Swyer-James' syndrome from emphysema per se[214]; and (5) ipsilateral air trapping. This is a key finding and a sine qua non of the condition.

It can be demonstrated with an expiratory and inspiratory pair of plain PA chest roentgenograms (Fig 16–21, A and B) or by fluoroscopy. Air trapping is better shown by a forced expiratory volume (FEV_1) radiograph rather than by conventional expiratory radiography[131] as the shorter expiratory time exaggerates the differences in volume change in each lung. Alternatively, trapping can be demonstrated by xenon ventilation scintigraphy.[252]

Pulmonary angiography is usually not warranted in this condition but, when performed, has confirmed the presence of small hilar and peripheral lung vessels (Fig 16–21, C).[163, 329] Similarly, bronchograms are seldom performed now in this condition, but in the past, they have provided important information. Typically on bronchography, segmental airways are irregular in outline and end abruptly at the fifth or sixth generation in square or tapered ends,[219, 271, 283, 329] with absent filling of peripheral airways despite maneuvers designed to correct this (Fig 16–22).

The described combination of findings usually allows exclusion of other conditions that may resemble the Swyer-James syndrome. These conditions include congenital hypoplastic lung, pulmonary artery hypoplasia, and proximal interruption of the pulmonary artery. The greatest worry is that signs are being produced by a large airway obstruction causing lung hypoventilation and a compensatory reduction in perfusion. This is a problem that may only be resolved by bronchoscopy.

CHRONIC OBSTRUCTIVE AIRWAY DISEASE

Chronic obstructive airway disease (COPD, chronic airflow obstruction) is a term that encompasses a group of disorders characterized by chronic or recurrent obstruction to airflow. Four principal disorders fall under this heading: asthma, chronic bronchitis, emphysema, and bronchiectasis.[100, 333] Though some purists object to the use of all-embracing, generic terms like *chronic obstructive airway disease* or *COPD*, it becomes necessary in clinical practice, because not only are the various forms sometimes difficult to identify, but they often coexist in the same patient.

Asthma

Asthma is a recurrent disorder that is defined functionally as "a disease characterized by wide vari-

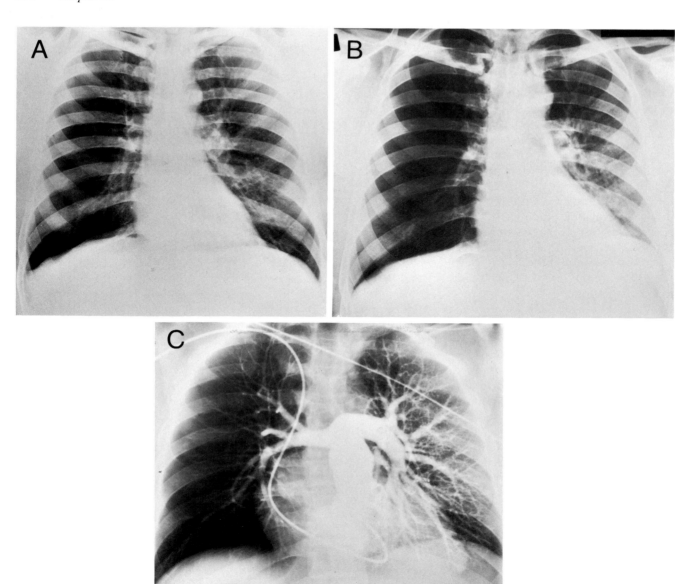

FIG 16–21.
Swyer-James (Macleod's) syndrome. **A,** posteroanterior chest radiograph on inspiration shows a transradiant right lung with a reduced number and size of vessels and a small right hilum. Lung volume on the right is probably slightly increased, and there is a blunt costophrenic angle. **B,** same patient. An expiratory radiograph demonstrates air trapping with relative elevation of the left hemidiaphragm, vascular crowding on the left, and mild mediastinal shift. **C,** same patient. Pulmonary angiogram shows a reduction in size and number of all vessels to the right lung. Compare the size of the right and left pulmonary arteries.

ations over short periods of time in resistance to air flow in intrapulmonary airways."[297] This definition does not specify the degree of variation, but it is usually taken as being 15% to 20%.

Radiologic findings in uncomplicated asthma are due to both pathologic and pathophysiologic changes. Pathologic changes have been studied largely,[58, 80] but not exclusively,[122] by examination of postmortem lungs in patients dying of asthma. Such findings represent the severe end of a spectrum of change. Grossly, the lungs are overinflated, failing to deflate because of tenacious mucus plugs in medium-sized airways. Bronchial mucosa is damaged or shed, and there are submucosal edema and inflammatory cell infiltrates of eosinophils, sometimes with lymphocytes and plasma cells causing

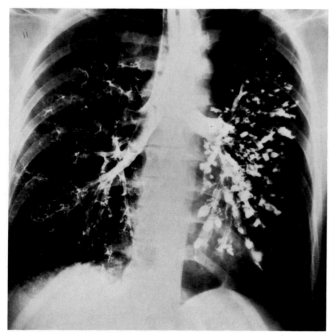

FIG 16–22.
Swyer-James' (Macleod's) syndrome. Bronchography shows diffuse bronchiectatic changes more marked in the lower zones (same patient as Fig 5–111).

bronchial wall thickening. Other changes contributing to a general thickening of the bronchial walls include mucous gland hypertrophy, basement membrane thickening, and smooth muscle hyperplasia.[162] The lung parenchyma, in addition to being generally hyperinflated, may show patchy collapse and consolidation.

Routine respiratory function tests demonstrate pathophysiologic changes in attacks but are often normal in remission. However, even in remission, results of sophisticated tests, particularly of small airway function, may be abnormal.[153, 208] In acute asthma, the findings are of increased airway resistance, increased TLC, and an increase in residual volume and functional residual capacity (FRC) with a decrease in vital capacity (VC) indicating air trapping.[226, 364] Changes in TLC and FRC may be at least 20% in an acute attack.[365] With recovery, falls in the TLC and FRC may anticipate increases in the FEV$_1$, and changes in lung volumes assessed by planimetric measurement of the chest radiograph have been used to follow the course of the disease.[220] Nonuniform ventilation and perfusion lead to mismatch and hypoxemia in attacks. Steady-state diffusing capacity for carbon monoxide is normal.

Radiographic findings in simple asthma are due to pathologic and functional changes, and in compli-

cated asthma they are due to the complications. The main radiographic findings in simple asthma in decreasing order of frequency are hyperinflation, bronchial wall thickening, and hilar prominence.

The prevalence of hyperinflation depends on many factors and is generally higher in children and in patients needing hospital admission. It is also more frequent in patients with an onset of asthma in the first or second decade than in those with a later onset.[155] Criteria for overinflation include a lung height equal to or greater than lung width,[312] a right hemidiaphragm at or below the seventh rib anteriorly, a cardiac diameter less than 11.5 cm,[311] and a retrosternal transradiancy measured 3 cm below the sternal angle of 3.5 cm or more.[155] With depression, the diaphragm tends to become less curved, but it rarely becomes flat or inverted in asthma per se.[106] The frequency of hyperinflation in adults with acute asthma has varied between approximately 20% and 70% in various series, reflecting different patient populations and hyperinflation criteria.[97, 258, 276, 369] In one series of 117 patients with a mean age of 41 years (range 13 to 75) admitted to hospital with acute asthma and in whom strict criteria for hyperinflation were applied, there was a 39% prevalence.[258] While hyperinflation is often short-lived, lasting perhaps just 24 hours,[276] it may be a permanent change, and in the study of 117 patients quoted above, 19% showed hyperinflation when in remission.[258]

In asthmatics, the walls of end-on segmental airways become thickened (more than 1 mm) and the normally invisible airways parallel to the radiograph appear as parallel- or single-line opacities (Fig 16–23). The most comprehensive study of bronchial wall thickening in asthma was that of Hodson and Trickey in 1960[154] in which they assessed the finding on plain radiographs in 190 asthmatics ranging in age from 3 to 74 years. Bronchial wall thickening was found to be more common in children, and in the small number of children analyzed it was a universal finding. Its frequency in adults was less but still surprisingly high, for example, 50% in the third and fourth decades. Bronchial wall thickening was ten times more common in patients with an infective element to their asthma (asthma-bronchitis) compared with those cases that were thought to be purely allergic. Its frequency correlated also with severity of asthma, and, in adults, bronchial wall thickening, once developed, became a permanent feature.

About 10% of asthmatic patients show slight prominence of hilar shadows. This is ascribed vari-

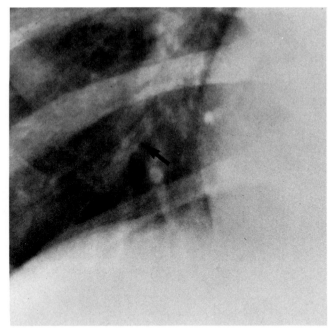

FIG 16–23.
Asthma. Localized view of the right lower zone showing bronchial wall thickening *(arrow).*

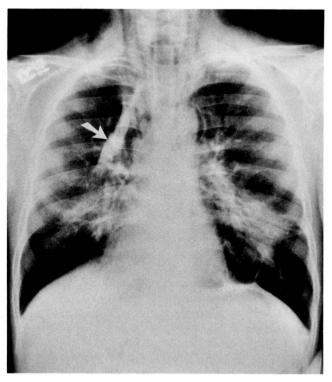

FIG 16–24.
Acute asthma. This radiograph of a 10-year-old boy shows three complications of acute asthma. In the right upper zone an oblique band shadow is due to segmental collapse *(arrow),* and in the left lower zone there is infective consolidation. The third complication is pneumomediastinum with air tracking into the neck.

ously to nodal enlargement[292] and vascular enlargement.[116, 258] Peripheral lung vessels are generally considered to be normal,[106] but some authors describe diffuse narrowing or subpleural oligemia.[116]

A number of complications associated with asthma may be detected on the chest radiograph and include (1) consolidation, (2) atelectasis/mucoid impaction, (3) pneumothorax, and (4) pneumomediastinum. Such complications are commoner in children than adults, and in one series of 479 hospital patients with a median age of nearly 4 years, 22% had abnormal radiographs, excluding signs of bronchial wall thickening and hyperinflation.[82] Other pediatric series bear these figures out.[48, 119] In adults the prevalence of similar abnormalities is generally less than 10% even in admissions for acute asthma, and only about 1% to 2% in series drawn from emergency room patients.[97, 258, 292, 369]

Consolidation in asthmatics is most commonly infective (Fig 16–24), but in some cases it will be due to eosinophilic consolidation associated with allergic aspergillosis. Collapse (Fig 16-24) ranges from subsegmental to lobar but occasionally involves a whole lung.[44] Such episodes of collapse are not necessarily associated with an acute illness, a respiratory tract infection, or a deterioration in the asthma.[161, 292] When segmental/lobar collapse occurs, the middle lobe is commonly affected both in children[82] and in

adults.[292] Collapse is due to mucoid impaction in large airways or mucus plugging in many small airways, the latter probably being the commoner mechanism.[106] It is difficult to give a frequency of occurrence of collapse per se, as in many series consolidation and collapse are considered together.[258] In adults it is probably in the order of a few percent only.[97, 292]

Pneumothorax is, unexpectedly, an unusual complication of acute asthma in adults, and in combined series consisting largely of adults with acute disease,* only three pneumothoraces in 566 patients were recorded. In a retrospective survey based on a region in the United Kingdom with over 6 million inhabitants, a frequency of pneumothorax in asthma of between 1:300 and 1:1,000 was recorded,[50] which was almost identical to figures from a large retrospective Mayo Clinic (Rochester, Minn.) study.[198] In the series reported by Burke[50] it was noted that pneumothorax did not lead to death or morbidity

*References 97, 116, 155, 258, 276, and 369.

and was usually not suspected clinically. Other workers agree that normally pneumothorax is not an important factor in mortality except when patients are being treated by positive pressure ventilation.[180] A condition that may simulate tension pneumothorax in asthmatic patients on mechanical ventilation is described. This is due to a ball valve mucus plug causing localized or unilateral obstructive hyperinflation. Close inspection of the apparent pneumothorax space will, in this situation, disclose the presence of pulmonary vessels.[250]

Pneumomediastinum in adults is as uncommon as pneumothorax, and in the combined series of 566 patients discussed above, only two had a pneumomediastinum. Pneumomediastinum is considerably commoner in children (see Fig 16–24), with a prevalence of 5.4% in 515 acute asthma admissions.[82] In children it is much commoner than pneumothorax, by a factor of 10:1 in one series.[37] Pneumopericardium has been recorded rarely.[337]

The indications for a chest radiograph in adults with asthma are not clearly established. Most authors would recommend chest radiography in all patients who are ill enough to justify admission to hospital.[97, 369] Petheram and coworkers[258] also recommend chest radiography in these circumstances, pointing out that in their series of 117 admissions, the chest radiograph showed abnormalities that altered management in 9%. Most would consider radiography essential before mechanical ventilation,[81, 276] and failure to respond to therapy is also considered an indication by some.[97, 369]

Chronic Bronchitis

Chronic bronchitis is defined, using clinical criteria, as chronic or recurrent increase in the volume of mucoid bronchial secretions sufficient to cause expectoration and occurring on most days for 3 months in 2 or more successive years, other causes for expectoration having been excluded.*

At one time chronic bronchitis was thought to be an important cause of chronic airflow obstruction, but this is no longer considered to be so.[100, 251, 259] Evidence for this view comes from clinical studies that show that chronic expectoration and airflow obstruction behave largely as independent variables.[100, 168] This is perhaps not surprising, as bronchial gland hypertrophy, the major pathologic change in chronic bronchitis, occurs in large airways,[280] whereas the dominant site of irreversible airflow ob-

*References 9, 10, 63, 100, 149, and 324.

struction is in peripheral airways less than 3.0 mm in diameter.[157, 307]

Chronic bronchitis is a common disease affecting up to 10% to 20% of the adult population in some studies.[240] It is much more common in males than females,[240] but when smoking habits are taken into account this difference is only twofold.[333] Most studies show an increasing prevalence with age. Cigarette smoking is the most important factor associated with the development of chronic bronchitis.[240] In eight combined series in England, there was a sixfold rise in prevalence of chronic bronchitis from 6.3% in nonsmokers to 40% in heavy smokers.[333] In epidemiologic studies there is a linear relationship between the amount smoked and the frequency of chronic bronchitis.[330] The quantitative contribution made by other factors to the development of chronic bronchitis is small by comparison. Such factors include occupation, environment, age, and gender. It seems that some of these factors have a stronger association with acute infective exacerbations than with chronic bronchitis itself.

The major pathologic changes are in the mucous glands, which show hypertrophy and hyperplasia and develop enlarged ducts. The enlargement of mucous glands can be quantified histologically using either the proportional mucous gland area or the Reid index—the ratio of gland thickness to bronchial wall thickness measured from epithelial basement membrane to perichondrium.[280] These indexes unfortunately do not clearly distinguish normal subjects from those with chronic bronchitis, as there is considerable overlap.[147, 334] A correlation has been demonstrated in chronic bronchitis between gland mass and sputum production.[168] Study of these indexes has shown that mucous glands also enlarge with age and in cigarette smokers.[251] There is in addition a positive association between increased mucous gland mass and emphysema,[233] probably reflecting the common etiology of smoking.

Other pathologic changes in chronic bronchitis include goblet cell hyperplasia, squamous metaplasia of the epithelium, and a variable and often mild[280] chronic inflammatory cell infiltrate.[149] Mucous plugs occur in the smaller airways, which themselves may be stenotic.[90, 224, 333] Cartilage atrophy probably occurs, but the evidence is conflicting,[126, 286, 331] and atrophy seems to be more a feature of emphysema than of chronic bronchitis.[104] Muscle hypertrophy is seen in chronic bronchitics who have episodes of wheezing.[333]

Chronic bronchitis typically presents as a persistent productive cough following an acute chest infection. Such symptoms may persist for years with normal respiratory function tests and chest radiographs. Indeed, the majority of such patients do not develop chronic airway obstruction,[106] though they are at risk from developing recurrent episodes of purulent bronchitis. Such infections cause short-term illnesses with time off work, but they have no significant long-term effect on the rate of deterioration, disability, or prognosis.[21] In addition, in these patients the annual fall in FEV_1 is within the normal range.[21, 47] In some chronic bronchitics, however, particularly those who smoke heavily, there is detectable airflow obstruction with a greater than predicted annual fall in FEV_1. These patients become dyspneic, with copious sputum, and tend to become hypoxemic.[52] Such patients may go on to develop pulmonary arterial hypertension and cor pulmonale and are at risk of respiratory failure should they have an acute infective exacerbation.

Radiologic signs in pure chronic bronchitis are poorly documented, as nearly all the available information is derived from three series of patients in whom coexistent emphysema was not excluded.[22, 308, 310] Overinflation of the lung described in these reports is in conflict with the normal TLC usually found in chronic bronchitis.[211] Overinflation and oligemia described in these studies are now generally ascribed to coexistent emphysema.

The majority of patients with chronic bronchitis have a normal chest radiograph.[110] Radiographic signs that are ascribed to chronic bronchitis include bronchial wall thickening and "increased lung markings." Bronchial wall thickening might be expected in chronic bronchitis by virtue of the known pathologic changes: mucous gland hypertrophy, cellular infiltration, and muscle hypertrophy. However, some histological studies suggest that the magnitude of these changes is small, with, in one report, an absolute increase in gland thickness of only 0.1 mm.[334] Admittedly in Reid's report,[280] the mean increase in gland thickness was 0.47 mm, but this has to be set against probable cartilage atrophy.[104] Bates and coworkers[22] described parallel line shadows on radiographs representing large airways seen side-on (tramline opacities) in 42% of patients with chronic bronchitis. However, this sign was not described by Simon and Galbraith,[308, 310] who do not consider radiologic bronchial wall thickening a part of chronic bronchitis. Airways may also be seen end-on as small ring shadows in the perihilar region. Ring shadows vary between 4 and 7 mm in diameter and most commonly represent the end-on upper lobe anterior or posterior segmental airways. This is a normal

finding, whereas side-on airways (tramline opacities) are always considered abnormal. Fraser and coworkers[104] assessed the frequency of detection of end-on airways and their wall thickness in approximately 150 controls and 150 subjects with chronic bronchitis. They found end-on airways visible in about 80% of both groups and a slight increase in wall thickness in chronic bronchitis, which was of some value in distinguishing patients with chronic bronchitis from normal subjects, though the sign was subject to significant interobserver variation. The ratio of wall thickness to external diameter in end-on airways does not correlate with the degree of airflow obstruction.[51] Another sign described in the Bates and coworkers[22] series was increased lung markings, detected in 18%. This feature again was rare in the British patients.[308, 310] The sign consists of small, ill-defined linear opacities with or without accentuation of small vascular opacities.[110] It is a very subjective sign with an obscure pathophysiologic basis. It is considered by some to be a "useful sign in support of the diagnosis of chronic bronchitis."[106]

Bronchographic findings in chronic bronchitis are largely of historic interest. They do, however, illustrate some pathophysiologic features of the disease. Dilated mucous gland ducts in the proximal airways fill with contrast in over 50% of patients (Fig 16–25).[134, 310] Gamsu et al.[109] recorded this finding in a similar percentage of normal adults, however, and it cannot be regarded as specific for chronic bronchitis. It may be significant that these latter workers used powdered tantalum rather than a liquid contrast agent. Other bronchographic findings in chronic bronchitis include incomplete peripheral airway filling,[134] squared or truncated airway ends,[279, 284, 308] lack of proximal tapering,[310] and mild irregularity of outline.[134, 310] Wall irregularity was also noted in some normal subjects.[109]

Some patients with chronic bronchitis go on to develop pulmonary arterial hypertension, and a number of studies have looked at the plain film manifestations of pulmonary arterial hypertension in mixed populations of patients with chronic airflow obstruction.[61, 152, 187, 225] In these studies the most useful signs have been the width of the right interlobar pulmonary artery and the hilar width, with or without normalization for chest size. Hilar width is the horizontal distance between right and left hilar points. In one series a hilar width of 9.5 cm or more correctly identified 72% of patients with pulmonary arterial hypertension, with an 8% false-positive rate.[152] In another series a right interlobar pulmonary artery width of 16 mm or more was true-posi-

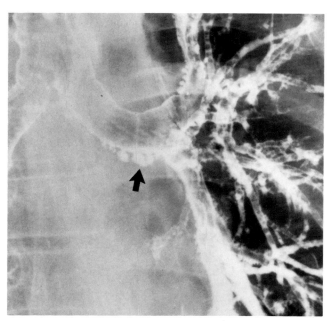

FIG 16—25.
Chronic bronchitis. Bronchogram with localized view of left hilum. Rounded collections of contrast lie adjacent to bronchial walls and are particularly well seen below the left main-stem bronchus *(arrow)*. They are caused by contrast in dilated mucous gland ducts.

tive for the identification of pulmonary arterial hypertension in 93% and false-positive in only 13%.[225]

Emphysema

Emphysema is one of the major causes of chronic airflow obstruction. It is a diagnosis that can only be made using pathologic criteria. Thus, emphysema is defined as "a condition of the lung characterized by abnormal, permanent enlargement of air-spaces distal to the terminal bronchiole accompanied by the destruction of their (air-space) walls and without obvious fibrosis. The orderly appearance of the acinus and its contents are disturbed and may be lost."[317] This definition, unlike earlier ones,[63] makes destruction of air-space walls a necessary condition, thereby excluding, for example, compensatory emphysema and other forms in which there is only air-space dilatation.

Pulmonary emphysema is worldwide in its distribution, though more frequent in polluted and industrialized societies. It is a very common condition, particularly in its milder forms, and some degree of emphysema is recorded in 50% to 70% of autopsies from various centers around the world.[319] It has a peak prevalence at about 70 years of age and is two to three times more common in males.[319]

The pathogenesis is complex, but two mechanisms stand out as being particularly important. First is structural weakness due to elastolysis, which itself may be secondary either to a constitutional disorder or to enhanced proteolysis. Second is airway obstruction caused either by loss of airway support or by inflammatory changes in the airway walls.

The most important etiologic factor by far is cigarette smoking, which exerts its effect in a variety of ways. Other inhaled pollutants have also been implicated, particularly cadmium chloride, nitrogen oxides, and phosgene. Various genetic disorders associated with emphysema are described, including alpha$_1$-antitrypsin (A_1-AT) deficiency, heritable diseases of connective tissue such as cutis laxa,[338] osteogenesis imperfecta, and Marfan's syndrome,[40] and familial emphysema. A childhood onset with hemolytic anemia is described.[13]

The pathologic classification of emphysema is based on the microscopic localization of disease within the acinus. Using such a system, it is not surprising that severe emphysema is often difficult to categorize. The principal types are (1) panacinar (panlobular), (2) centriacinar (centrilobular), (3) periacinar (paraseptal), (4) cicatricial (scar), and (5) unclassified.

1. Panacinar emphysema.—In this form the whole of the acinus is affected by dilatation and destruction. The differentiating features between alveoli and alveolar ducts are lost, pores of Kohn enlarge, and fenestrations develop between alveoli. With progressive destruction, all that eventually remains are thin strands of tissue surrounding blood vessels ("cotton candy" lung). It is the most important type of emphysema, as it is the one that is most often widespread and of severe grade and most likely, therefore, to give rise to clinically significant disease. Pathologic changes are distributed throughout the lungs but they are often basally predominant. It is the type of emphysema that occurs in A_1-AT deficiency, in Swyer-James' (Macleod's) syndrome,[317] and in familial cases. Although generally considered as the emphysema of nonsmokers, it also occurs in association with smoking-induced centrilobular emphysema.

2. Centriacinar emphysema.—In this variety of emphysema, more commonly called centrilobular, there is selective dilatation and confluence of central elements in the acinus, particularly of the respiratory bronchioles and their alveoli. The process tends to be most developed in the upper zones of the upper and lower lobes. It is strongly associated with

smoking and chronic bronchitis and it is much commoner in males. Inflammatory changes in the small airways are a common association, with plugging, mural infiltration, and fibrosis leading to stenosis, blockage, distortion, and destruction. Focal dust emphysema seen in coal workers may be considered a variety of centriacinar emphysema in which there is little airway inflammation and a more uniform distribution of disease throughout the lung.[317]

3. Periacinar emphysema.—This variety of emphysema is commonly called paraseptal, emphasizing its main feature—selective expansion of alveoli adjacent to connective tissue septa and bundles, particularly at the margins of the acinus but also subpleurally and adjacent to bronchovascular bundles. It has a tendency to develop where lung margins are sharp. Air-spaces in paraseptal emphysema often become confluent and develop into bullae, which may be sizeable. Paraseptal emphysema is the basic lesion in bullous lung disease.[316] Airway obstruction and physiologic disturbance are often minor in paraseptal emphysema despite gross bulla formation.

4. Cicatricial emphysema.—Scar emphysema is usually localized and of little clinical significance[316] except in the context of widespread scarring processes such as sarcoidosis or histiocytosis.

5. Unclassified emphysema.[149]

The classification of emphysema depends on microscopic localization of the lesions. At a macroscopic level lesions may be focal, multifocal, or widespread and may show regional predilection, e.g., upper or lower zone.

Patients with small amounts of emphysema are frequently asymptomatic.[317] Widespread emphysema, however, causes nonproductive cough and progressive exertional dyspnea. With the exception of paraseptal emphysema, the degree of disability is related to the severity of the emphysema rather than to the type.[317] There is a tendency for emphysema to be associated with the "pink puffer" type of clinical picture,[74] characterized by early dyspnea, little in the way of productive cough, and relatively normal blood gases achieved at the expense of marked dyspnea.[287] There is, however, considerable overlap with the chronic bronchitis–associated "blue bloater" end of the spectrum. Patients with this latter syndrome have productive cough, episodes of deterioration associated with infection and bronchospasm, deranged blood gases (hypoxia and hypercapnia), and a tendency to develop pulmonary arterial hypertension and cor pulmonale.[287]

Respiratory function tests in emphysema reflect three major pathologic changes: (1) small airway obstruction due to loss of mural support and inflammatory wall change, (2) loss of lung recoil, and (3) loss of alveolar surface.[287] Airway obstruction decreases peak flow and FEV_1. Lung recoil is balanced by chest wall recoil, and when the former is reduced, the chest wall moves out, and thus various static lung volumes increase (residual volume, FRC, and TLC). Reduction in the alveolar gas exchange surface is reflected in a reduction in carbon monoxide diffusion. In addition, the work of breathing is increased, and eventually hypoxemia develops, initially during sleep or exercise. Hypercapnia is not found, as responsiveness to $Paco_2$ remains intact.

Airflow obstruction in emphysema is located at two sites: (1) peripherally in small airways and (2) in large central airways. This latter component of resistance is variable and present only in expiration, particularly at low lung volumes.[103, 212] The behavior of large airways can be studied by bronchoscopy or cine bronchography.[92] The collapse of lobar and segmental airways in emphysematous subjects during forced expiration has been demonstrated,[55, 103] and pressure measurements demonstrate these to be sites of high resistance.[212, 213] Collapse of large airways is principally due to the large transmural pressures generated in emphysema during forced expiration. In addition, airway walls are probably less able to withstand such pressures because of mural atrophy[218] or altered cross-sectional geometry.[201]

A number of studies have tried to correlate chest radiographic findings and lung function tests in patients with nonspecific chronic airflow obstruction, many of whom have had emphysema. Reich and co-workers[278] found that the right lung length and the height of the arc of the right hemidiaphragm correlated well with FEV_1 and the ratio FEV_1/VC.[278] In this study, a right lung length of 30 cm or more identified 70% of the patients with airflow obstruction.[278] These workers found that if the absolute height of the right hemidiaphragm measured against the ribs were corrected for body surface area, then this too correlated well with the degree of airflow obstruction. Other workers have not found such corrections to be necessary, and, in one study of 189 patients, all but 3% of those with the height of the right hemidiaphragm at or below the right seventh rib had airflow obstruction.[51] The sensitivity of this finding, however, was low, on the order of 30% to 40%. Somewhat similar conclusions have been reported by others.[12, 78]

Radiologic findings in emphysema[267] reflect two types of change in the lung. One is the pathologic change of vascular distortion and loss, and the other is the functional one of overinflation. In the early radiologic studies, case selection of patients with emphysema lacked certainty, as it was based on clinical features and respiratory function changes[311] and not on morphologic criteria. Between 1962 and 1976, however, a number of studies correlated radiologic and pathologic findings and attempted to assess the accuracy of various signs. As Thurlbeck[333] points out, however, all these studies are to some extent flawed in that they have an excess of patients with chronic airflow obstruction, so that radiologic features of airflow obstruction will be given "disproportionate value in recognizing emphysema." In addition, in many of these studies there has been a sizeable 20% to 30% interobserver and intraobserver variation in the diagnosis of emphysema. Observer variation in the use of individual radiologic signs has also been a problem, particularly in those signs that are based on vascular changes.[183, 249, 327] Furthermore, it is difficult to give an overview of these studies, as the radiologic signs assessed, the pathologic methods used for quantifying emphysematous changes, and the various conclusions differ. Some of these studies have been critically reviewed recently.[263–265]

Many of the radiologic signs ascribed to emphysema reflect hyperinflation. The most reliable criterion is probably that of a low and flat diaphragm (Fig 16–26). In general, a right hemidiaphragm that is at or below the anterior end of the seventh rib in the midclavicular line can be considered low.[199] Flattening of a hemidiaphragm can be assessed subjectively or objectively by drawing a line from costophrenic to cardiophrenic angles and measuring the largest perpendicular to the diaphragm silhouette. A value of less than 1.5 cm indicates flattening of the diaphragm. Other less reliable signs of hyperinflation that have been used include (1) a large retrosternal space (more than 3.0 cm from the anterior surface of the aorta to the back of the sternum measured 3.0 cm below the manubriosternal junction) (Fig 16–27); (2) an obtuse costophrenic angle assessed on frontal or lateral projection (see Fig 16–27); (3) a retrosternal air-space that approaches to within 3.0 cm or less of the diaphragm (see Fig 16–27); (4) a narrow cardiac diameter, less than 11.5 cm,[309] with a vertical heart and visible lung beneath the heart (see Fig 16–26). Several reports find that signs of overinflation are the best predictors of the presence and severity of emphysema.[183, 249, 327] Nicklaus and coworkers[249] found that a flat diaphragm on the PA chest radiograph was the best

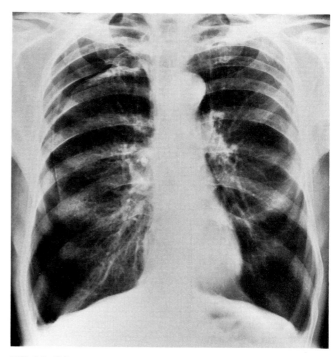

FIG 16–26.
Emphysema. A posteroanterior chest radiograph demonstrates two of the most reliable signs of emphysema: (1) depression of the right hemidiaphragm with its midpoint lying on the upper border of the seventh rib, (2) flattening of both hemidiaphragms. Other less reliable features include a narrow heart with air density below it. There is, in addition, a right pneumothorax.

predictor, detecting 94% of patients with severe emphysema, 76% with moderate, and 21% with mild, with a low false-positive rate of only 4%.

The vascular signs ascribed to emphysema include (1) areas of transradiancy (Figs 16–28 and 16–29); (2) a reduction in the number and size of pulmonary vessels and their branches, particularly in the middle or outer aspect of the lung (see Fig 16–28); (3) distortion of vessels that may be unduly straight or curved and have increased branching angles; (4) avascular areas with curvilinear hairline margins—bullae (see Fig 16–29). It is important to remember that while bullae may be a feature of generalized emphysema, they can occur as a local manifestation of paraseptal emphysema in otherwise normal lungs. Several studies have found arterial deficiency a more reliable criterion for emphysema than hyperinflation.[197, 335, 336] Using arterial deficiency alone to detect emphysema, Thurlbeck and coworkers[335] found that its accuracy was similar to that described for hyperinflation criteria by Nicklaus et al.[249] There were no false-positives, and all patients with severe, 66% with moderate, and 35% with mild emphysema were identified.

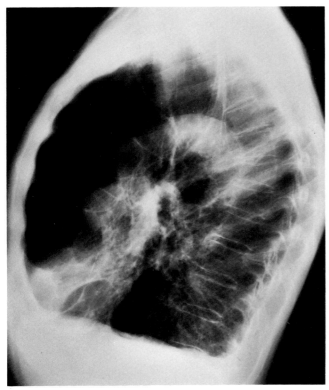

FIG 16—27.
Emphysema. Lateral chest radiograph demonstrating a characteristically large retrosternal transradiancy with increased separation of aorta and sternum measuring 4.6 cm, 3 cm below the angle of Louis and extending down to within 3 cm of the diaphragm anteriorly. Both costophrenic angles are obtuse and both hemidiaphragms flat.

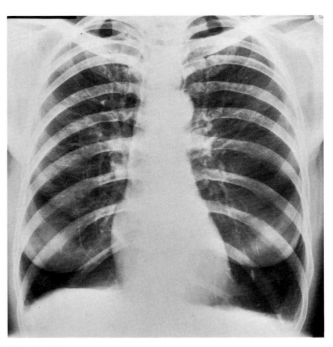

FIG 16—28.
Panacinar emphysema, alpha$_1$-antitrypsin deficiency. Large-volume lungs with low flat diaphragms. Both lower zones are hypertransradiant, and vessels within these zones are reduced in size and number and are pruned. The distribution of these changes is typical of panacinar emphysema. The patient was a 52-year-old woman. (Courtesy of Dr. P. Gishen, London.)

Thurlbeck and coworkers[335] have described another vascular pattern in emphysema in which there are increased markings peripherally on the chest radiograph (Fig 16—30). These markings are interpreted as being due to an increase in size and number of small vessels, though their exact nature has not been established. It is an appearance that is seen most commonly in the presence of pulmonary arterial hypertension, cor pulmonale, and centrilobular emphysema (see Fig 16—30). Recognition of this pattern as a manifestation of emphysema allows cases to be detected radiologically that would otherwise be missed.[335] In one series of 73 patients with chronic airflow obstruction, 63% of those with severe emphysema had this pattern.[41]

The value of the chest radiograph in assessing emphysema is by no means clear despite numerous studies. Broadly speaking, it appears that the chest radiograph detects nearly all patients with gross emphysema, about half of those with moderate emphysema, and some with mild disease. The best criteria

are not agreed on. On balance, evidence of hyperinflation is probably the most reliable, especially flattening and depression of the hemidiaphragm. Using combined data it would seem probable that both the major forms of emphysema (centriacinar and panacinar) are equally detectable,[249, 327] but not all workers agree.[183, 282] Some workers suggest that the best results are obtained using combined criteria of hyperinflation and vascular changes.[41]

When other chest conditions occur in emphysematous lungs, the radiologic appearances become modified. Thus, with consolidation and centrilobular emphysema, the emphysematous spaces produce rounded transradiancies in the air-space shadowing (Fig 16—31). With heart failure, edema may spare emphysematous lung, and the diaphragm tends to become more rounded and elevated as lung compliance falls (see Fig 16—30).[230]

Computed tomography is a more sensitive method of detecting emphysema than plain chest radiography.[31, 102, 123, 148] In addition, it can localize the changes and characterize[31] and quantitate them.[32, 102, 123, 148] The principal manifestations of emphysema on CT are (1) an overall reduction in lung density. This is quantitated by measuring atten-

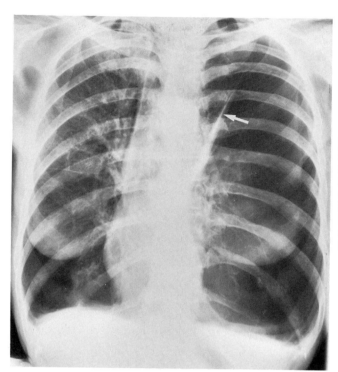

FIG 16–29.
Emphysema, alpha$_1$-antitrypsin deficiency. A female patient. Both diaphragms are low and flat. The mediastinum is displaced to the right by a large bulla, which occupies much of the left hemithorax, compressing lung tissue medially and inferiorly. Part of the wall of the bulla can be identified *(arrow)*. Vasculature is reduced in the right lower zone because of panacinar emphysema. Bulla formation is not a common feature of alpha$_1$-antitrypsin deficiency. (Courtesy of Dr. P. Gishen, London.)

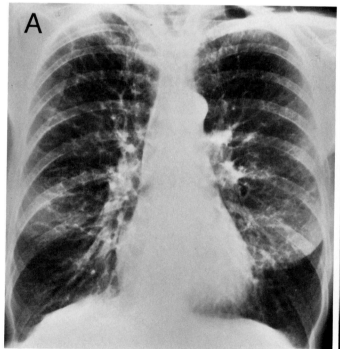

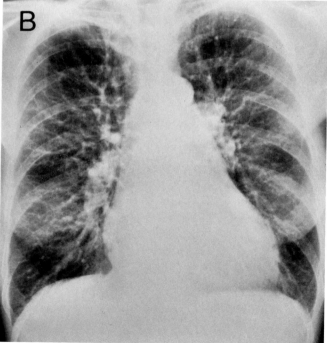

FIG 16–30.
Cor pulmonale. **A,** 50-year-old male with chronic airflow obstruction. Lungs are large in volume, the diaphragm is flat, and there is vascular attenuation at the right apex. These features suggest emphysema, and this was supported by a low carbon monoxide diffusion capacity. Lung "markings" are increased peripherally, particularly in the left midzone. **B,** the patient became chronically hypoxic and, with respiratory infections, hypercapnic. One of these episodes was associated with cor pulmonale when the patient became edematous, the heart enlarged, and hilar and lung vessels enlarged. Note that the emphysematous right upper zone shows less vascular engorgement and is relatively transradiant. Note also that the diaphragm is less depressed and more curved than before.

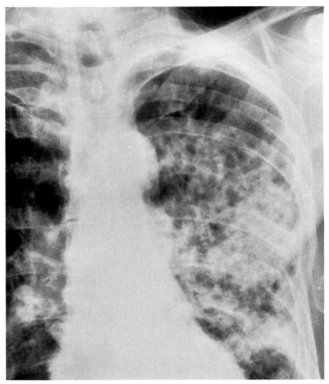

FIG 16–31.
Emphysema. A localized posteroanterior radiograph of the left upper zone shows infective consolidation superimposed on centrilobular emphysema. The emphysematous spaces create rounded transradiancies within the pneumonia.

uation values and expressing data as mean values[123] or as a histogram of attenuation values[148]; (2) localized areas of reduced attenuation that may be well or poorly defined.[123] Bullae, well-defined lesions delineated by a hairline wall, are included in these findings; (3) pruning of small vessels[31, 102, 123]; (4) vascular branching angles in excess of 80°[31]; (5) vascular distortion around low-density areas[102, 123] and vascular attenuation[31]; (6) an abnormal density gradient.[102]

A number of studies correlating CT and pathology have demonstrated the ability of CT to quantitate the amount and severity of emphysema. Foster and coworkers[102] found a positive correlation between emphysema severity and CT signs. Of the signs used, the most reliable was nonperipheral low-attenuation areas closely followed by vascular pruning and distortion. Another correlative study found that the grade of emphysema on pathologic assessment correlated with CT findings (reduced attenuation and vascular disruption) and considered CT better at detection than respiratory function tests.[32] Using 1 cm–thick scans at 1-cm intervals and windows between 800 and 1,500 Hounsfield units, Ber-

gin and coworkers[31] could distinguish between the various types of emphysema. Centriacinar emphysema is characterized by punctate holes in a homogeneous background, an upper lobe predilection, and vascular pruning if moderate or severe. In panacinar emphysema, there is a lower zone predominance of widespread low attenuation. Vessels are attenuated and their branching angles increased. The most striking feature of paraseptal emphysema is its distribution along septa, vessels, and airways and subpleurally, where it forms low-attenuation blebs and bullae. Such blebs and bullae are not pathognomonic of paraseptal emphysema and may be seen with other forms of emphysema or as isolated findings.[31]

Alpha₁-Antitrypsin Deficiency

The association between serum alpha₁-antitrypsin (A_1-AT) deficiency and COPD was first recognized in 1963,[196] and 6 years later an association with neonatal hepatitis and cirrhosis was recorded.[300]

Alpha₁-antitrypsin is a serum protein that inhibits a number of proteolytic enzymes, including trypsin, elastase, granulocyte elastase, and collagenase. It is also an acute-phase reactant. It probably has an important role in inflammatory states, preventing the damaging effects of elastases released by macrophages and particularly neutrophils. Elastase has been shown to produce emphysema in lungs when administered into the airways,[268] and the elastase of neutrophils within the lung has the same potential.[167] It is not surprising, therefore, that some patients with reduced levels of A_1-AT are at risk of developing emphysema. This effect is augmented by smoking, which appears to act by (1) causing oxidative inactivation of A_1-AT, (2) recruiting neutrophils and macrophages to the lung, and (3) reducing the resynthesis of elastin.[167] Histologically, the emphysema is of the panacinar type.[127, 299, 335]

The serum level and type of A_1-AT depends on two codominant alleles that occupy one locus. Different alleles produce different types and amounts of A_1-AT. The type of A_1-AT may be recognized by electrophoresis, and the allele producing it is designated by Pi (protease inhibitor), followed by one of a number of capital letters. By far the commonest allele is PiM, and, when homozygous (PiM/PiM), it is associated with normal A_1-AT levels. The frequency of the PiM allele in most studies from various countries has been on the order of 95% to 99%, but there are some populations in which levels below 90% have been recorded.

Some alleles are associated with low serum levels

of A_1-AT, and although there are a number of these, there are only a few that are important clinically, particularly PiZ but also PiS and Pi−, the latter having a silent allele. Homozygous PiZ individuals have about 10% to 15% of the expected serum A_1-AT level, while the heterozygotic PiZM individuals have a level of about 60%.[88] Not only are A_1-AT levels depressed, but they fail to rise in situations that stimulate a rise in acute-phase reactants. The PiZ allele has a frequency of about 1.2%, so that only one to two individuals per 10,000 of the population will be homozygotes.

A large study of 246 PiZZ patients has shown that eventually nearly every individual develops emphysema and there is a reduced life expectancy.[195] The PiZZ type of emphysema is characterized by an early onset, between 35 and 50 years of age.[89, 191, 195] Smokers present about 10 years earlier than nonsmokers,[191] and respiratory function impairment and radiologic change tend to be worse in smokers. Males outnumber females about 2:1.[120, 191] This sex difference is unexpected and possibly due to factors that operate in men other than cigarette smoking and A_1-AT deficiency.[191] Opinion is divided over the relationship of the heterozygote state (PiMZ) and respiratory disease. The consensus is that there is no definite relationship between the two, but that the heterozygote state may increase susceptibility to emphysema in the presence of other risk factors.[167]

There are radiologic changes of emphysema in about 80% of patients who are homozygous and who have COPD.[150] The striking feature of the emphysematous change is its lower zone predominance (see Fig 16−28). In a study of 165 PiZ homozygotes, 98% had lower zone involvement,[120] and in 24% this was the only zone involved. In the same series, only three of 140 patients with radiologic changes had isolated involvement of the upper or middle and upper zone.[120] Similarly, in a study of 52 PiZ patients with COPD, 67% showed isolated lower zone emphysema, whereas this pattern was seen in only 8% of PiM patients.[150] The pattern of emphysematous change in heterozygotes, such as PiMZ and PiMS phenotypes is like that in PiM individuals. Bullae are not a major feature, but they do occur (see Fig 16−29).[289]

Bullae

A bulla is an emphysematous space within the lungs that has a diameter of more than 1 cm in the distended state and that causes a local protrusion to the surface of the removed lung.[63, 281] Bullae may be single or multiple and they may represent a localized abnormality or, more commonly, be part of widespread panacinar emphysema. Occasionally they are familial.[118] Three types of bullae are recognized pathologically, types I to III.[281] Type I is usually subpleural, narrow necked, and devoid of contents and develops from a small amount of emphysematous lung that is grossly hyperinflated. In the confines of the chest it is pushed into the surrounding lung, and because it is so overinflated it is associated with redundant tongues of pleura. Type III bullae are deep in the lung with broad necks and often contain quantities of lung tissue and blood vessels. They are only mildly overinflated. Type II bullae share features of type I and III bullae. Limited data suggest that pressure in bullae is negative, like pleural surface pressure.[236]

Radiologically, a bulla produces an avascular transradiant area usually separated from the remaining lung by a thin curvilinear wall of very variable extent (Fig 16−32). Sometimes the wall is complete, but in other cases only short segments are visible, or the wall may even be completely absent, and under these circumstances bullae can be difficult to detect. It is well recognized that plain radiographs markedly underestimate the number of bullae demonstrated postmortem.[197] The wall is usually of hair-

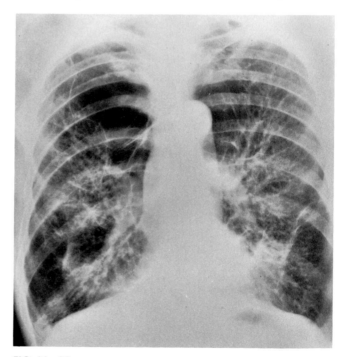

FIG 16−32.
Bullae. A patient with chronic airflow obstruction. In the right upper zone there is a large transradiant area associated with thin curvilinear opacities, representing the walls of bullae. At the right base a further transradiant zone is without curvilinear shadows.

line thickness. Sometimes segments of the wall are thicker when there are major contributions from redundant pleura or collapsed adjacent lung. Bullae due to paraseptal emphysema are much more common in the upper zones,[42] but when associated with widespread panacinar emphysema, there is a much more even distribution.[281] Bullae vary in diameter from 1 cm to ones that occupy the whole hemithorax, causing marked relaxation collapse of the adjacent lung (see Fig 16–29). They can even extend across into the opposite hemithorax, particularly by way of the anterior junctional area.[98]

Plain tomography is a more sensitive method of demonstration than plain radiography; CT is probably even more sensitive[269] and is now the investigation of choice.[98, 237] Computed tomography allows accurate assessment of the number, size, and position of bullae and is particularly useful when bullae are obscured by other lung pathology, such as diffuse interstitial fibrosis.[237] Computed tomograms taken in inspiration and expiration indicate the ex-

tent to which a bulla is ventilated, and the appearance of the rest of the lung and its modification by postural changes help in assessing the extent and degree of diffuse lung disease.[237] Computed tomography is also useful in identifying patients suitable for treatment with bullectomy.[235]

Bullae usually enlarge progressively over months or years, but the rate is variable, and a period of stability may be followed by a sudden expansion.[42] Bullae may also disappear either spontaneously[75] or following infection or hemorrhage.[42, 209, 323] The main complications of bullae are pneumothorax, infection, and hemorrhage, and an association with bronchial carcinoma has been described. When bullae become infected they usually come to contain fluid and develop an air-fluid level (Fig 16–33).[209, 217, 323] The hairline wall often becomes thickened, and indeed this may be the only sign of infection. Infected bullae differ from an abscess in that the patient is less ill, the wall of the ring shadow is less thick and has a sharp inner margin, and there is less in the way of

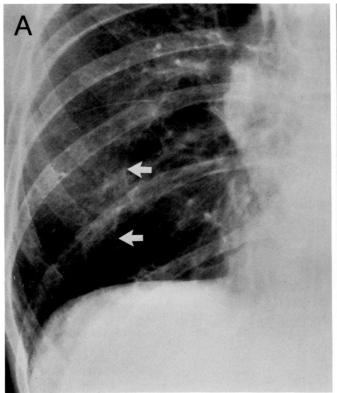

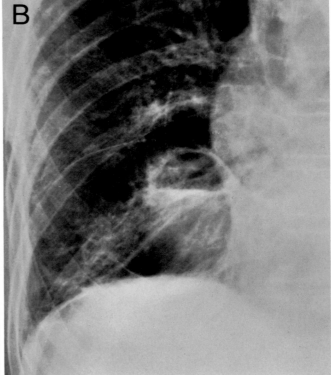

FIG 16–33.
Infected bulla. **A,** localized view of the right lower zone in a patient who does not have features of generalized emphysema. There is a subtle transradiancy inferomedially delineated by a hairline curvilinear margin *(arrows)*. **B,** 2 years later the patient presented with right-sided chest pain and cough. The bulla now contains an air-fluid level and its wall has become thickened. Gram-positive and gram-negative cocci were isolated from the sputum, and the appearances resolved with a course of antibiotics.

adjacent pneumonitis.[35, 106] Following infection, bullae often disappear.[209] Hemorrhage into the bulla is a less common complication[35, 169] that may be accompanied by hemoptysis and a drop in hemoglobin level. As with infection, the bulla may disappear after a bleed.[209] A few cases of carcinoma arising in bullae are described.[209] There is no definite evidence that this is more than a chance association, unlike the situation with a variety of lung cysts, most of which are probably congenital.[266]

Patients with isolated bullous disease are usually without signs or symptoms. Occasionally bullae produce breathlessness relieved by bullectomy.[20] The contribution of imaging to the assessment of patients before bullectomy has been reviewed.[107]

REFERENCES

1. Aaby GV, Blake HA: Tracheobronchiomegaly. *Ann Thorac Surg* 1966; 2:64–70.
2. Adenis L, Laurent JC, Charle J, et al: Tuberculose ganglionnaire mediastinale de l'adulte fistulisee dans l'oesophage. *Lille Med* 1976; 19:766–769.
3. Afzelius BA: A human syndrome caused by immotile cilia. *Science* 1976; 193:317–319.
4. Afzelius BA, Mossberg B: Editorial: Immotile cilia. *Thorax* 1980; 35:401–404.
5. Aherne W, Bird T, Court SDM, et al: Pathological changes in virus infections of the lower respiratory tract in children. *J Clin Pathol* 1970; 23:7–18.
6. Aliabadi P, Shafiepoor H: Bronchography in the recognition of congenital cystic bronchiectasis. *AJR* 1978; 131:255–257.
7. Al-Mallah Z, Quantock OP: Tracheobronchomegaly. *Thorax* 1968; 23:320–324.
8. Alroy GG, Lichtig C, Kaftori JK: Tracheobronchopathia osteoplastica: End stage of primary lung amyloidosis? *Chest* 1972; 61:465–468.
9. American College of Chest Physicians, American Thoracic Society: Pulmonary terms and symbols: A report of the ACCP-ATS Joint Committee on Pulmonary Nomenclature. *Chest* 1975; 67:583–593.
10. American Thoracic Society: Chronic bronchitis, asthma and pulmonary emphysema: A statement by the committee on diagnostic standards for nontuberculous respiratory diseases. *Am Rev Respir Dis* 1962; 85:762–768.
11. Amoury RA, Hrabovsky EE, Leoidas JC, et al: Tracheoesophageal fistula after lye ingestion. *J Pediatr Surg* 1975; 10:273–276.
12. Andersen PE, Andersen LH, Jest P: The chest radiograph in chronic obstructive lung disease compared with measurements of single-breath nitrogen washout and spirometry. *Clin Radiol* 1982; 33:51–55.
13. Anderson CE, Finklestein JZ, Nussbaum E, et al: Association of hemolytic anemia and early-onset pulmonary emphysema in three siblings. *J Pediatr* 1984; 105:247–251.
14. Arrigoni MG, Bernatz PE, Donoghue FE: Broncholithiasis. *J Thorac Cardiovasc Surg* 1971; 62:231–237.
15. Ashford NS, Buxton-Thomas MS, Flower CDR, et al: Aerosol lung scintigraphy in the detection of bronchiectasis. *Clin Radiol* 1988; 39:29–32.
16. Azizirad H, Polgar G, Borns PR, et al: Bronchiolitis obliterans. *Clin Pediatr* 1975; 14:572–584.
17. Bachman AL, Hewitt WR, Beekley HC: Bronchiectasis: A bronchographic study of 60 cases of pneumonia. *Arch Intern Med* 1953; 91:78–96.
18. Banner AS, Muthuswamy P, Shah RS, et al: Bronchiectasis following heroin-induced pulmonary edema. *Chest* 1976; 69:552–555.
19. Barker AF, Bardana EJ: Bronchiectasis: Update of an orphan disease. *Am Rev Respir Dis* 1988; 137:969–978.
20. Bateman ED, Westerman DE, Hewitson RP, et al: Pneumonectomy for massive ventilated lung cysts. *Thorax* 1981; 36:554–556.
21. Bates DV: The fate of the chronic bronchitis: A report of the 10-year follow-up in the Canadian Department of Veterans Affairs co-ordinated study of chronic bronchitis. *Am Rev Respir Dis* 1973; 108:1043–1065.
22. Bates DV, Gordon CA, Paul GI, et al: Chronic bronchitis: Report on the third and fourth stages of the co-ordinated study of chronic bronchitis in the Department of Veterans Affairs, Canada. *Med Serv J Can* 1966; 22:1–59.
23. Bateson EM, Woo-Ming M: Tracheobronchomegaly. *Clin Radiol* 1973; 24:354–358.
24. Batsakis JG, Fries GT, Goldman RT, et al: Upper respiratory tract plasmacytoma. *Arch Otolaryngol* 1964; 79:613–618.
25. Becker TS, Shum TK, Waller TS, et al: Radiological aspects of rhinoscleroma. *Radiology* 1981; 141:433–438.
26. Becklake MR, Goldman HI, Boxman AR, et al: The long-term effects of exposure to nitrous fumes. *Am Rev Tuberc* 1957; 76:398–409.
27. Becroft DMO: Bronchiolitis obliterans, bronchiectasis, and other sequelae of adenovirus type 21 infection in young children. *J Clin Pathol* 1971; 24:72–82.
28. Belcher JR, Capel L, Pattinson JN, et al: Hypoplasia of the pulmonary arteries. *Br J Dis Chest* 1959; 53:253.
29. Benjamin B, Pitkin J, Cohen D: Congenital tracheal stenosis. *Ann Otol Rhinol Laryngol* 1981; 90:364–371.
30. Berdon WE, Baker DH, Boyer J: Unusual benign and malignant sequelae to childhood radiation therapy. *AJR* 1965; 93:545–556.
31. Bergin C, Muller N, Miller RR: CT in the qualita-

tive assessment of emphysema. *J Thorac Imaging* 1986; 1:94–103.

32. Bergin C, Muller N, Nichols DM, et al: The diagnosis of emphysema: A computed tomographic–pathologic correlation. *Am Rev Respir Dis* 1986; 133:541–546.

33. Berkmen YM: The trachea: The blind spot in the chest. *Radiol Clin North Am* 1984; 22:539–562.

34. Berkmen YM, Auh YH: CT diagnosis of acquired tracheoesophageal fistula in adults. *J Comput Assist Tomogr* 1985; 9:302.

35. Bersack SR: Fluid collection in emphysematous bullae. *AJR* 1960; 83:283–292.

36. Bertelsen S, Struve-Christensen E, Aasted A, et al: Isolated middle lobe atelectasis: Aetiology, pathogenesis, and treatment of the so-called middle lobe syndrome. *Thorax* 1980; 35:449–452.

37. Bierman CW: Pneumomediastinum and pneumothorax complicating asthma in children. *AJDC* 1967; 114:42–50.

38. Black RJ: Congenital tracheo-oesophageal fistula in the adult. *Thorax* 1982; 37:61–63.

39. Blades B, Dugan DJ: Pseudobronchiectasis. *J Thorac Surg* 1944; 13:40–48.

40. Bolande RP, Tucker AS: Pulmonary emphysema and other cardiorespiratory lesions as part of the Marfan abiotrophy. *Pediatrics* 1964; 33:356–366.

41. Boushy SF, Aboumrad MH, North LP, et al: Lung recoil pressure, airway resistance, and forced flows related to morphologic emphysema. *Am Rev Respir Dis* 1971; 104:551–561.

42. Boushy SF, Kohen R, Billig DM, et al: Bullous emphysema: Clinical, roentgenologic and physiologic study of 49 patients. *Dis Chest* 1968; 54:327–334.

43. Brandstetter RD, Messina MS, Sprince NL, et al: Tracheal stenosis due to sarcoidosis. *Chest* 1981; 80:656.

44. Brashear RE, Meyer SC, Manion MW: Unilateral atelectasis in asthma. *Chest* 1973; 63:847–849.

45. Breatnach E, Abbott GC, Fraser RG: Dimensions of the normal human trachea. *AJR* 1984; 142:903–906.

46. Breatnach E, Kerr I: The radiology of cryptogenic obliterative bronchiolitis. *Clin Radiol* 1982; 33:657–661.

47. Brinkman GL, Block DL: The prognosis in chronic bronchitis. *JAMA* 1966; 197:1–7.

48. Brooks LJ, Cloutier MM, Afshani E: Significance of roentgenographic abnormalities in children hospitalized for asthma. *Chest* 1982; 82:315–318.

49. Burke CM, Theodore J, Dawkins KD, et al: Post-transplant obliterative bronchiolitis and other late lung sequelae in human heart-lung transplantation. *Chest* 1984; 86:824–829.

50. Burke GJ: Pneumothorax complicating acute asthma. *S Afr Med J* 1979; 55:508–510.

51. Burki NK, Krumpelman JL: Correlation of pulmo-nary function with the chest roentgenogram in chronic airway obstruction. *Am Rev Respir Dis* 1980; 121:217–223.

52. Burrows B, Fletcher CM, Heard BE, et al: The emphysematous and bronchial types of chronic airways obstruction. *Lancet* 1966; 1:830–835.

53. Butland RJA, Cole P, Citron KM, et al: Chronic bronchial suppuration and inflammatory bowel disease. *Q J Med* 1981; 50:63–75.

54. Caldarola VT, Harrison EG, Clagett OT, et al: Benign tumors and tumorlike conditions of the trachea and bronchi. *Ann Otol Rhinol Laryngol* 1964; 73:1042–1061.

55. Campbell AH, Young IF: Tracheobronchial collapse, a variant of obstructive respiratory disease. *Br J Dis Chest* 1963; 57:174–181.

56. Cantrell JR, Guild HG: Congenital stenosis of the trachea. *Am J Surg* 1964; 108:297–305.

57. Carasso B, Couropmitree C, Heredia R: Egg-shell silicotic calcification causing bronchoesophageal fistula. *Am Rev Respir Dis* 1973; 108:1384–1387.

58. Cardell BS: Pathological findings in deaths from asthma. *Int Arch Allergy Appl Immunol* 1956; 9:189–199.

59. Chandler PW, Shin MS, Friedman SE, et al: Radiographic manifestations of bronchiolitis obliterans with organizing pneumonia vs usual interstitial pneumonia. *AJR* 1986; 147:899–906.

60. Charan NB, Myers CG, Lakshminarayan S, et al: Pulmonary injuries associated with acute sulfur dioxide inhalation. *Am Rev Respir Dis* 1979; 119:555–560.

61. Chetty KG, Brown SE, Light RW: Identification of pulmonary hypertension in chronic obstructive pulmonary disease from routine chest radiographs. *Am Rev Respir Dis* 1982; 126:338–341.

62. Choplin RH, Wehunt WD, Theros EG: Diffuse lesions of the trachea. *Semin Roentgenol* 1983; 18:38–50.

63. Ciba Guest Symposium: Terminology, definitions, and classification of chronic pulmonary emphysema and related conditions. *Thorax* 1959; 14:286–299.

64. Clark NS: Bronchiectasis in childhood. *Br Med J* 1963; 1:80–88.

65. Cook AJ, Weinstein M, Powell RD: Diffuse amyloidosis of the tracheobronchial tree: Bronchographic manifestations. *Radiology* 1973; 107:303–304.

66. Cooke JC, Currie DC, Morgan AD, et al: Role of computed tomography in diagnosis of bronchiectasis. *Thorax* 1987; 42:272–277.

67. Cooper G, Guerrant JL, Harden AG, et al: Some consequences of pulmonary irradiation. *AJR* 1961; 85:865–874.

68. Cornelius EA, Betlach EH: Silo-filler's disease. *Radiology* 1960; 74:232–238.

69. Currie DC, Cooke JC, Morgan AD, et al: Interpretation of bronchograms and chest radiographs in pa-

tients with chronic sputum production. *Thorax* 1987; 42:278–284.

70. Currie DC, Needham S, Peters AM, et al: 111-Indium–labelled neutrophils migrate to the lungs in bronchiectasis. *Thorax* 1986; 41:256.

71. Dallimore NS: Squamous bronchial carcinoma arising in a case of multiple juvenile papillomatosis. *Thorax* 1985; 40:797–798.

72. Davis EW, Katz S, Peabody JW: Broncholithiasis, a neglected cause of bronchoesophageal fistula. *JAMA* 1956; 160:555–557.

73. Dixon GF, Donnerberg RL, Schonfeld SA, et al: Advances in the diagnosis and treatment of broncholithiasis. *Am Rev Respir Dis* 1984; 129:1028–1030.

74. Dornhorst AC: Respiratory insufficiency, Frederick W. Price Memorial Lecture. *Lancet* 1955; 1:1185–1187.

75. Douglas AC, Grant IWB: Spontaneous closure of large pulmonary bullae: A report on three cases. *Br J Tuberc* 1957; 51:335–338.

76. Dowling EA, Johnson IM, Collier FCD, et al: Intratracheal goiter: A clinicopathologic review. *Ann Surg* 1962; 156:258–267.

77. Dukes RJ, Rosenow EC, Hermans PE: Pulmonary manifestations of hypogammaglobulinaemia. *Thorax* 1978; 33:603–607.

78. Dull WL, Bohadana AB, Teculescu DB, et al: The standard chest roentgenogram for determining lung overinflation. *Lung* 1982; 160:311–314.

79. Dunne MG, Reiner B: CT features of tracheobronchomegaly. *J Comput Assist Tomogr* 1988; 12:388–391.

80. Dunnill MS: The pathology of asthma, with special reference to changes in the bronchial mucosa. *J Clin Pathol* 1960; 13:27–33.

81. Editorial: Chest radiographs in asthma. *Br Med J* 1974; 4:123–124.

82. Eggleston PA, Ward BH, Pierson WE, et al: Radiographic abnormalities in acute asthma in children. *Pediatrics* 1974; 54:442–449.

83. Eliasson R, Mossberg B, Camner P, et al: The immotile-cilia syndrome: A congenital ciliary abnormality as an etiologic factor in chronic airway infections and male sterility. *N Engl J Med* 1977; 297:1–6.

84. Ell SR, Jolles H, Galvin JR: Cine CT demonstration of nonfixed upper airway obstruction. *AJR* 1986; 146:669–677.

85. Epler GR, Colby TV: The spectrum of bronchiolitis obliterans. *Chest* 1983; 83:161–162.

86. Epler GR, Colby TV, McLoud TC, et al: Bronchiolitis obliterans organizing pneumonia. *N Engl J Med* 1985; 312:152–158.

87. Epler GR, Snider GL, Gaensler EA, et al: Bronchiolitis and bronchitis in connective tissue disease: A possible relationship to the use of penicillamine. *JAMA* 1979; 242:528–532.

88. Eriksson S: Pulmonary emphysema and alpha$_1$-antitrypsin deficiency. *Acta Med Scand* 1964; 175:197–205.

89. Eriksson S: Studies in α_1-antitrypsin deficiency. *Acta Med Scand Suppl* 1965; 432:5–85.

90. Esterley JR, Heard BE: Multiple bronchiolar stenoses in a patient with generalized airway obstruction. *Thorax* 1965; 20:309–316.

91. Ettman IK, Keel DT: Tracheal diverticulosis. *Radiology* 1962; 78:187–191.

92. Feist JH: Selective cinebronchography in obstructive and restrictive pulmonary disease. *AJR* 1967; 99:543–554.

93. Feist JH, Johnson TH, Wilson RJ: Acquired tracheomalacia: Etiology and differential diagnosis. *Chest* 1975; 68:340–345.

94. Feldman F, Seaman WB, Baker DC: The roentgen manifestations of scleroma. *AJR* 1967; 101:807–813.

95. Felson B: Letter from the editor. *Semin Roentgenol* 1983; 18:1–3.

96. Felson B: Neoplasms of the trachea and main stem bronchi. *Semin Roentgenol* 1983; 18:23–37.

97. Findley LJ, Sahn SA: The value of chest roentgenograms in acute asthma in adults. *Chest* 1981; 80:535–536.

98. Fiore D, Biondetti PR, Sartori F, et al: The role of computed tomography in the evaluation of bullous lung disease. *J Comput Assist Tomogr* 1982; 6:105–108.

99. Fleischner FG: Reversible bronchiectasis. *AJR* 1941; 46:166–172.

100. Fletcher CM, Pride NB: Definitions of emphysema, chronic bronchitis, asthma, and airflow obstruction: Twenty-five years on from the Ciba symposium. *Thorax* 1984; 39:81–85.

101. Forrest JV, Sagel SS, Omell GH: Bronchography in patients with hemoptysis. *AJR* 1976; 126:597–600.

102. Foster WL, Pratt PC, Roggli VL, et al: Centrilobular emphysema: CT-pathologic correlation. *Radiology* 1986; 159:27–32.

103. Fraser RG: The radiologist and obstructive airway disease. *AJR* 1974; 120:737–775.

104. Fraser RG, Fraser RS, Renner JW, et al: The roentgenologic diagnosis of chronic bronchitis: A reassessment with emphasis on parahilar bronchi seen end-on. *Radiology* 1976; 120:1–9.

105. Fraser RG, Pare JAP: *Diagnosis of Diseases of the Chest,* ed 2. Philadelphia, WB Saunders Co, 1977, vol 1.

106. Fraser RG, Pare JAP: *Diagnosis of Diseases of the Chest,* ed 2. Philadelphia, WB Saunders Co, 1979, vol 3.

107. Gaensler EA, Jederlinic PJ, FitzGerald MX: Patient work-up for bullectomy. *J Thorac Imaging* 1986; 1:75–93.

108. Gamsu G, Borson DB, Webb WR, et al: Structure

and function in tracheal stenosis. *Am Rev Respir Dis* 1980; 121:519–531.

109. Gamsu G, Forbes AR, Ovenfors C-O: Bronchographic features of chronic bronchitis in normal men. *AJR* 1981; 136:317–322.

110. Gamsu G, Nadel JA: The roentgenologic manifestations of emphysema and chronic bronchitis. *Med Clin North Am* 1973; 57:719–733.

111. Gamsu G, Webb WR: Computed tomography of the trachea: Normal and abnormal. *AJR* 1982; 139:321–326.

112. Gamsu G, Webb WR: Computed tomography of the trachea and mainstem bronchi. *Semin Roentgenol* 1983; 18:51–60.

113. Gardner S, Seilheimer D, Catlin F, et al: Subglottic coccidiodiomycosis presenting with persistent stridor. *Pediatrics* 1980; 66:623–625.

114. Gay S, Dee P: Tracheobronchomegaly: The Mounier-Kuhn syndrome. *Br J Radiol* 1984; 57:640–644.

115. Geddes DM, Corrin B, Brewerton DA, et al: Progressive airway obliteration in adults and its association with rheumatoid disease. *Q J Med* 1977; 46:427–444.

116. Genereux GP: Radiology and pulmonary immunopathological disease, in Steiner RE (ed): *Recent Advances in Radiology and Medical Imaging.* New York, Churchill Livingstone, Inc, 1983, vol 7, pp 213–240.

117. Gibb WRG, Dhillon DP, Zilkha KJ, et al: Bronchiectasis with ulcerative colitis and myelopathy. *Thorax* 1987; 42:155–156.

118. Gibson GJ: Familial pneumothoraces and bullae. *Thorax* 1977; 32:88–90.

119. Gilles JD, Reed MH, Simons FER: Radiologic findings in acute childhood asthma. *J Can Assoc Radiol* 1978; 29:28–33.

120. Gishen P, Saunders AJS, Tobin MJ, et al: Alpha$_1$-antitrypsin deficiency: The radiological features of pulmonary emphysema in subjects of Pi type Z and Pi type SZ: A survey by the British Thoracic Association. *Clin Radiol* 1982; 33:371–377.

121. Glazer G, Webb WR: Laryngeal papillomatosis with pulmonary spread in a 69-year-old man. *AJR* 1979; 132:820–822.

122. Glynn AA, Michaels L: Bronchial biopsy in chronic bronchitis and asthma. *Thorax* 1960; 15:142–153.

123. Goddard PR, Nicholson EM, Laszlo G, et al: Computed tomography in pulmonary emphysema. *Clin Radiol* 1982; 33:379–387.

124. Gordon I, Helms P, Fazio F: Clinical applications of radionuclide lung scanning in infants and children. *Br J Radiol* 1981; 54:576–585.

125. Gosink BB, Friedman PJ, Liebow AA: Bronchiolitis obliterans: Roentgenologic-pathologic correlation. *AJR* 1973; 117:816–832.

126. Greenberg SD, Boushy SF, Jenkins DE: Chronic bronchitis and emphysema: Correlation of pathologic findings. *Am Rev Respir Dis* 1967; 96:918–928.

127. Greenberg SD, Jenkins DE, Stevens PM, et al: The lungs in homozygous alpha$_1$-antitrypsin deficiency. *Am J Clin Pathol* 1973; 60:581–592.

128. Greene R: "Saber-sheath" trachea: Relation to chronic obstructive pulmonary disease. *AJR* 1978; 130:441–445.

129. Greene R, Lechner GL: "Saber-sheath" trachea: A clinical and functional study of marked coronal narrowing of the intrathoracic trachea. *Radiology* 1975; 115:265–268.

130. Greenfield H, Herman PG: Papillomatosis of the trachea and bronchi. *AJR* 1963; 89:45–50.

131. Greenspan RH, Sagel S, McMahon J, et al: Timed expiratory chest films in detection of air-trapping. *Invest Radiol* 1973; 8:264–265.

132. Greenstone M, Rutman A, Dewar A, et al: Primary ciliary dyskinesia: Cytological and clinical features. *Q J Med* 1988; 67:405–430.

133. Greenstone M, Rutman A, Pavia D, et al: Normal axonemal structure and function in Kartagener's syndrome: An explicable paradox. *Thorax* 1985; 40:956–957.

134. Gregg I, Trapnell DH: The bronchographic appearances of early chronic bronchitis. *Br J Radiol* 1969; 42:132–139.

135. Grenier P, Maurice F, Musset D, et al: Bronchiectasis: Assessment by thin-section CT. *Radiology* 1986; 161:95–99.

136. Grillo HC: Surgical treatment of postintubation tracheal injuries. *J Thorac Cardiovasc Surg* 1979; 78:860–875.

137. Griscom NT, Vawter GF, Stigol LC: Radiologic and pathologic abnormalities of the trachea in older patients with cystic fibrosis. *AJR* 1987; 148:691–693.

138. Griscom NT, Wohl MEB: Tracheal size and shape: Effects of change in intraluminal pressure. *Radiology* 1983; 149:27–30.

139. Gronner AT, Trevino RJ: Tracheocoele. *Br J Radiol* 1971; 44:979–981.

140. Gross BH, Felson B, Birnberg FA: The respiratory tract in amyloidosis and the plasma cell dyscrasias. *Semin Roentgenol* 1986; 21:113–127.

141. Gudbjerg CE: Roentgenologic diagnosis of bronchiectasis. *Acta Radiol* 1955; 43:209–226.

142. Guerry-Force ML, Muller NL, Wright JL, et al: A comparison of bronchiolitis obliterans with organizing pneumonia, usual interstitial pneumonia and small airways disease. *Am Rev Respir Dis* 1987; 135:705–712.

143. Guynes WA, Dickinson WE, Sutherland RD, et al: Tracheo-esophageal fistula following blunt chest trauma. *Texas Med* 1979; 75:52–53.

144. Han BK, Dunbar JS, Striker TW: Membranous laryngotracheobronchitis (membranous croup). *AJR* 1979; 133:53–58.

145. Handelsman DJ, Conway AJ, Boylan LM, et al: Young's syndrome: Obstructive azoospermia and chronic sinopulmonary infections. *N Engl J Med* 1984; 310:3–9.

146. Hawley PC, Whitcomb ME: Bronchiolitis fibrosa obliterans in adults. *Arch Intern Med* 1981; 141:1324–1327.

147. Hayes JA: Distribution of bronchial gland measurements in a Jamaican population. *Thorax* 1969; 24:619–622.

148. Hayhurst MD, MacNee W, Flenley DC, et al: Diagnosis of pulmonary emphysema by computerised tomography. *Lancet* 1984; 2:320–322.

149. Heard BE, Khatchatourov V, Otto H, et al: The morphology of emphysema, chronic bronchitis, and bronchiectasis: Definition, nomenclature, and classification. *J Clin Pathol* 1979; 32:882–892.

150. Hepper NG, Mulm JR, Sheehan WC, et al: Roentgenographic study of chronic obstructive pulmonary disease by alpha-1-antitrypsin phenotype. *Mayo Clin Proc* 1978; 53:166–172.

151. Herzog CA, Miller RR, Hoidal JR: Bronchiolitis and rheumatoid arthritis. *Am Rev Respir Dis* 1981; 124:636–639.

152. Hicken P, Green ID, Bishop JM: Relationship between transpulmonary artery distance and pulmonary artery pressure in patients with chronic bronchitis. *Thorax* 1968; 23:446–450.

153. Hill DJ, Landau LI, Phelan PD: Small airway disease in asymptomatic asthmatic adolescents. *Am Rev Respir Dis* 1972; 106:873–880.

154. Hodson CJ, Trickey SE: Bronchial wall thickening in asthma. *Clin Radiol* 1960; 11:183–191.

155. Hodson ME, Simon G, Batten JC: Radiology of uncomplicated asthma. *Thorax* 1974; 29:296–303.

156. Hoeffler HB, Schweppe I, Greenberg SD: Bronchiectasis following pulmonary ammonia burn. *Arch Pathol Lab Med* 1982; 106:686–687.

157. Hogg JC, Macklem PT, Thurlbeck WM: Site and nature of airway obstruction in chronic obstructive lung disease. *N Engl J Med* 1968; 278:1355–1360.

158. Holden WS, Ardran GM: Observations on the movements of the trachea and main bronchi in man. *J Faculty Radiol* 1957; 8:267–275.

159. Holinger PH, Gelman HK, Wolfe CK: Rhinoscleroma of the lower respiratory tract. *Laryngoscope* 1977; 87:1–9.

160. Holinger PH, Johnston KC, Basinger CE: Benign stenosis of the trachea. *Ann Otol Rhinol Laryngol* 1950; 59:837–859.

161. Hopkirk JAC, Stark JE: Unilateral pulmonary collapse in asthmatics. *Thorax* 1978; 33:207–210.

162. Hossain S: Quantitative measurement of bronchial muscle in men with asthma. *Am Rev Respir Dis* 1973; 107:99–109.

163. Houk VN, Kent DC, Fosburg RG: Unilateral hyperlucent lung: A study in pathophysiology and etiology. *Am J Med Sci* 1967; 253:406–416.

164. Howland WJ, Good CA: The radiographic features of tracheopathia osteoplastica. *Radiology* 1958; 71:847–850.

165. Hunter TB, Kuhns LR, Roloff MA, et al: Tracheo-bronchiomegaly in an 18 month old child. *AJR* 1975; 123:687–690.

166. Iannuzzi MC, Farhi DC, Bostrom PD, et al: Fulminant respiratory failure and death in a patient with idiopathic bronchiolitis obliterans. *Arch Intern Med* 1985; 145:733–734.

167. Idell S, Cohen AB: Alpha-1-antitrypsin deficiency. *Clin Chest Med* 1983; 4:359–375.

168. Jamal K, Cooney TP, Fleetham JA, et al: Chronic bronchitis: Correlation of morphological findings to sputum production and flow rates. *Am Rev Respir Dis* 1984; 129:719–722.

169. Jay SJ, Johanson WG: Massive intrapulmonary hemorrhage: An uncommon complication of bullous emphysema. *Am Rev Respir Dis* 1974; 110:497–501.

170. Jesseph JE, Merendino KA: The dimensional interrelationships of the major components of the human tracheobronchial tree. *Surg Gynecol Obstet* 1957; 105:210–214.

171. Joharjy IA, Bashi SA, Adbullah AK: Value of medium-thickness CT in the diagnosis of bronchiectasis. *AJR* 1987; 149:1133–1137.

172. Johnson TH, Mikita JJ, Wilson RJ, et al: Acquired tracheomalacia. *Radiology* 1973; 109:577–580.

173. Johnston RF, Green RA: Tracheobronchiomegaly: Report of five cases and demonstration of familial occurrence. *Am Rev Respir Dis* 1965; 91:35–50.

174. Jones DK, Cavanagh P, Shneerson JM, et al: Does bronchography have a role in the assessment of patients with haemoptysis? *Thorax* 1985; 40:668–670.

175. Jones DK, Godden D, Cavanagh P: Alpha-1-antitrypsin deficiency presenting as bronchiectasis. *Br J Dis Chest* 1985; 79:301–304.

176. Jones GR, Proudfoot AT, Hall JI: Pulmonary effects of acute exposure to nitrous fumes. *Thorax* 1973; 28:61–65.

177. Judd DR, Dubuque T: Acquired benign esophagotracheobronchial fistula. *Dis Chest* 1968; 54:237–240.

178. Kagan E, Soskolne CL, Zwi S, et al: Immunologic studies in patients with recurrent bronchopulmonary infections. *Am Rev Respir Dis* 1975; 111:441–451.

179. Karasick D, Karasick S, Lally JF: Mucoid pseudotumors of the tracheobronchial tree in two cases. *AJR* 1979; 132:459–460.

180. Karetzky MS: Asthma mortality: An analysis of 1 year's experience, review of the literature and assessment of current modes of therapy. *Medicine* 1975; 54:471–484.

181. Kartagener M: Zur pathogenese der Bronchiektasien: Bronchiektasien bei Situs viscerum inversus. *Beitr Klin Tuberk* 1933; 83:489–501.

182. Kass I, Zamel N, Dobry CA, et al: Bronchiectasis following ammonia burns of the respiratory tract: A review of two cases. *Chest* 1972; 62:282–285.

183. Katsura S, Martin CJ: The roentgenologic diagnosis of anatomic emphysema. *Am Rev Respir Dis* 1967; 96:700–706.

184. Katz I, LeVine M, Herman P: Tracheobronchiomegaly: The Mounier-Kuhn syndrome. *AJR* 1962; 88:1084–1094.

185. Katzenstein A-LA, Askin FB: *Surgical Pathology of Non-neoplastic Lung Disease.* Philadelphia, WB Saunders Co, 1982.

186. Kaufmann HJ, Mahboubi S, Spackman TJ, et al: Tracheal stenosis as a complication of chondrodysplasia punctata. *Ann Radiol* 1976; 191:203–209.

187. Keller CA, Shepard JW, Chun DS, et al: Pulmonary hypertension in chronic obstructive pulmonary disease. *Chest* 1986; 90:185–192.

188. Kinney WW, Angelillo VA: Bronchiolitis in systemic lupus erythematosus. *Chest* 1982; 82:646–649.

189. Kogutt MS, Swischuk LE, Goldblum R: Swyer-James syndrome (unilateral hyperlucent lung) in children. *AJDC* 1973; 125:614–618.

190. Kowal LE, Goodman LR, Zarro VJ, et al: CT diagnosis of broncholithiasis. *J Comput Assist Tomogr* 1983; 7:321–323.

191. Kueppers F, Black LF: α_1-Antitrypsin and its deficiency. *Am Rev Respir Dis* 1974; 110:176–194.

192. Kurklu EU, Williams MA, le Roux BT: Bronchiectasis consequent upon foreign body retention. *Thorax* 1973; 28:601–602.

193. Lallemand D, Chagnon S, Buriot D, et al: Tracheomegaly and immune deficiency syndromes in childhood. *Ann Radiol* 1981; 24:67–72.

194. Landing BH, Dixon LG: Congenital malformations and genetic disorders of the respiratory tract (larynx, trachea, bronchi, and lungs). *Am Rev Respir Dis* 1979; 120:151–185.

195. Larsson C: Natural history and life expectancy in severe alpha$_1$-antitrypsin deficiency, PiZ. *Acta Med Scand* 1978; 204:345–351.

196. Laurell CB, Ericksson S: The electrophoretic α_1 globulin pattern of serum in α_1-antitrypsin deficiency. *Scand J Clin Invest* 1963; 15:132–140.

197. Laws JW, Heard BE: Emphysema and the chest film: A retrospective radiological and pathological study. *Br J Radiol* 1962; 35:750–761.

198. Legge DA, Tiede JJ, Peters GA, et al: Death from tension pneumothorax and chlorpromazine cardiorespiratory collapse as separate complications of asthma. *Ann Allergy* 1969; 27:23–29.

199. Lennon EA, Simon G: The height of the diaphragm in the chest radiograph of normal adults. *Br J Radiol* 1965; 38:937–943.

200. Libshitz HI, Shuman LS: Radiation-induced pulmonary change: CT finding. *J Comput Assist Tomogr* 1984; 8:15–19.

201. Liddelow AG, Campbell AH: Widening of the membranous wall and flattening of the trachea and main bronchi. *Br J Dis Chest* 1964; 58:56–60.

202. Lincoln JCR, Deverall PB, Stark J, et al: Vascular anomalies compressing the oesophagus and trachea. *Thorax* 1969; 24:295–306.

203. Little AG, Ferguson MK, Demeester TR, et al: Esophageal carcinoma with respiratory tract fistula. *Cancer* 1984; 53:1322–1328.

204. Longstreth GF, Weitzman SA, Browning RJ, et al: Bronchiectasis and homozygous alpha-1-antitrypsin deficiency. *Chest* 1975; 67:233–235.

205. Lowry T, Schuman LM: "Silo-filler's disease": A syndrome caused by nitrogen dioxide. *JAMA* 1956; 162:153–160.

206. Lundgren R, Stjernberg NL: Tracheobronchopathia osteochondroplastica: A clinical bronchoscopic and spirometric study. *Chest* 1981; 80:706–709.

207. McCann BG, Hart GJ, Stokes TC, et al: Obliterative bronchiolitis and upper-zone pulmonary consolidation in rheumatoid arthritis. *Thorax* 1983; 38:73–74.

208. McCarthy D, Milic-Emili J: Closing volume in asymptomatic asthma. *Am Rev Respir Dis* 1973; 107:559–570.

209. McCluskie RA: Unusual fate of emphysematous bullae. *Thorax* 1981; 36:77.

210. MacFarlane JD, Dieppe PA, Rigden BG, et al: Pulmonary and pleural lesions in rheumatoid disease. *Br J Dis Chest* 1978; 72:288–300.

211. Macklem PT: The pathophysiology of chronic bronchitis and emphysema. *Med Clin North Am* 1973; 57:669–679.

212. Macklem PT, Fraser RG, Brown WG: Bronchial pressure measurements in emphysema and bronchitis. *J Clin Invest* 1965; 44:897–905.

213. Macklem PT, Wilson NJ: Measurement of intrabronchial pressure in man. *J Appl Physiol* 1965; 20:653–663.

214. MacLeod WM: Abnormal transradiancy of one lung. *Thorax* 1954; 9:147–153.

215. McLoud TC, Epler GR, Colby TV, et al: Bronchiolitis obliterans. *Radiology* 1986; 159:1–8.

216. Macpherson RI, Cumming GR, Chernick V: Unilateral hyperlucent lung: A complication of viral pneumonia. *J Can Assoc Radiol* 1969; 20:225–231.

217. Mahler D, D'Esopo NO: Peri-emphysematous lung infection. *Clin Chest Med* 1981; 2:51–57.

218. Maisel JC, Silvers GW, George MS, et al: The significance of bronchial atrophy. *Am J Pathol* 1972; 67:371–383.

219. Margolin HN, Rosenberg LS, Felson B, et al: Idiopathic unilateral hyperlucent lung: A roentgenologic syndrome. *AJR* 1959; 82:63–75.

220. Marmorstein BL, Cianciulli FD: Planimetric measurement of total lung capacity in asthma. *Chest* 1974; 66:378–381.

221. Martin CJ: Tracheobronchopathia osteochondroplastica. *Arch Otolaryngol Head Neck Surg* 1974; 100:290–293.

222. Martini N, Goodner JT, D'Angio GJ, et al: Tracheoesophageal fistula due to cancer. *J Thorac Cardiovasc Surg* 1970; 59:319–324.

223. Maruyama Y, Pettet JR, Green CR: Acquired esophagotracheal fistula secondary to a foreign body in the esophagus. *N Engl J Med* 1959; 260:126–127.

224. Matsuba K, Thurlbeck WM: Disease of the small airways in chronic bronchitis. *Am Rev Respir Dis* 1973; 107:552–558.

225. Matthay RA, Schwartz MI, Ellis JH, et al: Pulmonary artery hypertension in chronic obstructive pulmonary disease: Determination by chest radiography. *Invest Radiol* 1981; 16:95–100.

226. Meisner P, Hugh-Jones P: Pulmonary function in bronchial asthma. *Br Med J* 1968; 1:470–475.

227. Miki Y, Hatabu H, Takahashi M, et al: Computed tomography of bronchiolitis obliterans. *J Comput Assist Tomogr* 1988; 12:512–514.

228. Miller AH: Scleroma of larynx, trachea and bronchi. *Laryngoscope* 1949; 59:506–514.

229. Miller RD, Divertie MB: Kartagener's syndrome. *Chest* 1972; 62:130–135.

230. Milne EN, Bass H: Roentgenologic and functional analysis of combined chronic obstructive pulmonary disease and congestive cardiac failure. *Invest Radiol* 1969; 4:129–147.

231. Milne JE: Nitrogen dioxide inhalation and bronchiolitis obliterans: A review of the literature and report of case. *J Occup Med* 1969; 11:538–547.

232. Mitchell RE, Bury RG: Congenital bronchiectasis due to deficiency of bronchial cartilage (Williams-Campbell syndrome). *J Pediatr* 1975; 87:230–234.

233. Mitchell RS, Ryan SF, Petty TL, et al: The significance of morphologic chronic hyperplastic bronchitis. *Am Rev Respir Dis* 1966; 93:720–729.

234. Mootoosamy IM, Reznek RH, Osman J, et al: Assessment of bronchiectasis by computed tomography. *Thorax* 1985; 40:920–924.

235. Morgan MDL, Denison DM, Strickland B: Value of computed tomography for selecting patients with bullous lung disease for surgery. *Thorax* 1986; 41:855–862.

236. Morgan MDL, Morris J, Matthews HR: Direct measurement of pressure and gas concentrations within emphysematous bullae. *Thorax* 1987; 42:714.

237. Morgan MDL, Strickland B: Computed tomography in the assessment of bullous lung disease. *Br J Dis Chest* 1984; 78:10–25.

238. Morrissey WL, Gould IA, Carrington CB, et al: Silo-filler's disease. *Respiration* 1975; 32:81–92.

239. Mounier-Kuhn P: Dilatation de la trachee: Constatations radiographiques et bronchoscopiques. *Lyon Med* 1932; 150:106–109.

240. Mueller RE, Keble DL, Plummer J, et al: The prevalence of chronic bronchitis, chronic airway obstruction and respiratory symptoms in a Colorado City. *Am Rev Respir Dis* 1971; 103:209–228.

241. Muller NL, Bergin CJ, Ostrow DN, et al: Role of computed tomography in the recognition of bronchiectasis. *AJR* 1984; 143:971–976.

242. Muller NL, Guerry-Force ML, Staples CA, et al: Differential diagnosis of bronchiolitis obliterans with organizing pneumonia and usual interstitial pneumonia: Clinical, functional and radiologic findings. *Radiology* 1987; 162:151–156.

243. Murphy EC, Atkins CJ, Offer RC, et al: Obliterative bronchiolitis in two rheumatoid arthritis patients treated with penicillamine. *Arthritis Rheum* 1981; 24:557–560.

244. Nadel HR, Stringer DA, Levison H, et al: The immotile cilia syndrome: Radiological manifestations. *Radiology* 1985; 154:651–655.

245. Naidich DP, McCauley DI, Khouri NF, et al: Computed tomography of bronchiectasis. *J Comput Assist Tomogr* 1982; 6:437–444.

246. Nelson SW, Christoforidis A: Reversible bronchiectasis. *Radiology* 1958; 71:375–382.

247. Nelson SW, Christoforidis AJ: Bronchography in diseases of the adult chest. *Radiol Clin North Am* 1973; 11:125–152.

248. Neville E, Brewis RAL, Yeates WK, et al: Respiratory tract disease and obstructive azoospermia. *Thorax* 1983; 38:929–933.

249. Nicklaus TM, Stowell DW, Christiansen WR, et al: The accuracy of the roentgenologic diagnosis of chronic pulmonary emphysema. *Am Rev Respir Dis* 1966; 93:889–899.

250. Niederman MS, Gambino A, Lichter J: Tension ball valve mucus plug in asthma. *Am J Med* 1985; 79:131–134.

251. Niewoehner DE: New messages from morphometric studies of chronic obstructive pulmonary disease. *Semin Respir Med* 1986; 8:140–146.

252. O'Dell CW, Taylor A, Higgins CB, et al: Ventilation-perfusion lung images in the Swyer-James syndrome. *Radiology* 1976; 121:423–426.

253. Onitsuka H, Hirose N, Watanabe K, et al: Computed tomography of tracheopathia osteoplastica. *AJR* 1983; 140:268–270.

254. Ostrow D, Buskard N, Hill RS, et al: Bronchiolitis obliterans complicating bone marrow transplantation. *Chest* 1985; 87:828–830.

255. Perez-Guerra F, Walsh RE, Sagel SS: Bronchiolitis obliterans and tracheal stenosis: Late complications of inhalation burn. *JAMA* 1971; 218:1568–1570.

256. Peters ME, Arya S, Langer LO, et al: Narrow trachea in mucopolysaccharidoses. *Pediatr Radiol* 1985; 15:225–228.

257. Peters ME, Dickie HA, Crummy AB, et al: Swyer-James-MacLeod syndrome: A case with a baseline normal chest radiograph. *Pediatr Radiol* 1982; 12:211–213.

258. Petheram IS, Kerr IH, Collins JV: Value of chest radiographs in severe acute asthma. *Clin Radiol* 1981; 32:281–282.

259. Peto R, Speizer FE, Cochrane AL, et al: The relevance in adults of air-flow obstruction, but not of mucus hypersecretion, to mortality from chronic lung disease. *Am Rev Respir Dis* 1983; 128:491–500.

260. Phillips MS, Williams MP, Flower CDR: How useful is computed tomography in the diagnosis and assess-

ment of bronchiectasis? *Clin Radiol* 1986; 37:321–325.

261. Pontius JR, Jacobs LG: The reversal of advanced bronchiectasis. *Radiology* 1957; 68:204–208.

262. Pradham DJ, Rabuzzi D, Meyer JA: Primary solitary lymphoma of the trachea. *J Thorac Cardiovasc Surg* 1975; 70:938–940.

263. Pratt PC: Conventional chest films can reveal emphysema, but not COPD. *Chest* 1987; 92:8.

264. Pratt PC: Radiographic appearance of the chest in emphysema. *Invest Radiol* 1987; 22:927–929.

265. Pratt PC: Role of conventional chest radiography in diagnosis and exclusion of emphysema. *Am J Med* 1987; 82:998–1006.

266. Prichard MG, Brown PJE, Sterrett GF: Bronchiolo-alveolar carcinoma arising in longstanding lung cysts. *Thorax* 1984; 39:545–549.

267. Pugatch RD: The radiology of emphysema. *Clin Chest Med* 1983; 4:433–442.

268. Pushpakom R, Hogg JC, Woolcock AJ, et al: Experimental papain-induced emphysema in dogs. *Am Rev Respir Dis* 1970; 102:778–789.

269. Putman CE, Godwin JD, Silverman PM, et al: CT of localized lucent lung lesions. *Semin Roentgenol* 1984; 19:173–188.

270. Rahbar M, Tabatabai D: Tracheobronchiomegaly. *Br J Dis Chest* 1971; 65:65–68.

271. Rakower J, Moran E: Unilateral hyperlucent lung (Swyer-James syndrome). *Am J Med* 1962; 33:864–872.

272. Ralph DD, Springmeyer SC, Sullivan KM: Rapidly progressive air-flow obstruction in marrow transplant recipients: Possible association between obliterative bronchiolitis and chronic graft-versus-host disease. *Am Rev Respir Dis* 1984; 129:641–644.

273. Ramirez-R J, Dowell AR: Silo-filler's disease: Nitrogen dioxide–induced lung injury: Long-term follow-up and review of the literature. *Ann Intern Med* 1971; 74:569–576.

274. Randolph J, Grunt JA, Vawter GF: The medical and surgical aspects of intratracheal goiter. *N Engl J Med* 1963; 268:457–461.

275. Ravin CE, Handel DB, Kariman K: Persistent endotracheal tube cuff overdistension: A sign of tracheomalacia. *AJR* 1981; 137:408–409.

276. Rebuck AS: Radiological aspects of severe asthma. *Aust Radiol* 1970; 14:264–268.

277. Reed WB, Lopez DA, Landing B: Clinical spectrum of anhidrotic ectodermal dysplasia. *Arch Dermatol* 1970; 102:134–143.

278. Reich SB, Weinshelbaum A, Yee J: Correlation of radiographic measurements and pulmonary function tests in chronic obstructive pulmonary disease. *AJR* 1985; 144:695–699.

279. Reid L: Chronic bronchitis and emphysema: A symposium: III. Pathological findings and radiological changes in chronic bronchitis and emphysema: A. Pathological finding in chronic bronchitis. *Br J Radiol* 1959; 32:291–292.

280. Reid L: Measurement of the bronchial mucous gland layer: A diagnostic yardstick in chronic bronchitis. *Thorax* 1960; 15:132–141.

281. Reid L: *The Pathology of Emphysema*. London, Lloyd-Luke Ltd, 1967.

282. Reid L, Millard FJC: Correlation between radiological diagnosis and structural lung changes in emphysema. *Clin Radiol* 1964; 15:307–311.

283. Reid L, Simon G: Unilateral lung transradiancy. *Thorax* 1962; 17:230–239.

284. Reid LM: Correlation of certain bronchographic abnormalities seen in chronic bronchitis with the pathological changes. *Thorax* 1955; 10:199–204.

285. Reid LM: Reduction in bronchial subdivision in bronchiectasis. *Thorax* 1950; 5:233–247.

286. Restrepo GL, Heard BE: Air trapping in chronic bronchitis and emphysema: Measurements of the bronchial cartilage. *Am Rev Respir Dis* 1964; 90:395–400.

287. Robins AG: Pathophysiology of emphysema. *Clin Chest Med* 1983; 4:413–420.

288. Roca J, Granena A, Rodriguez-Roisin R, et al: Fatal airway disease in an adult with chronic graft-versus-host disease. *Thorax* 1982; 37:77–78.

289. Rosen RA, Dalinka MK, Gralino BJ, et al: The roentgenographic findings in alpha-1-antitrypsin deficiency (AAD). *Radiology* 1970; 95:25–28.

290. Rosenbaum HD, Alavi SM, Bryant LR: Pulmonary parenchymal spread of juvenile laryngeal papillomatosis. *Radiology* 1968; 90:654–660.

291. Rott HD: Kartagener's syndrome and the syndrome of immotile cilia. *Hum Genet* 1979; 46:249–261.

292. Royle H: X-ray appearances in asthma: A study of 200 cases. *Br Med J* 1952; 1:577–580.

293. Rubenstein J, Weisbrod G, Steinhardt MI: Atypical appearances of "Saber sheath" trachea. *Radiology* 1978; 127:41–42.

294. Sakula A: Tracheobronchopathia osteoplastica: Its relationship to primary tracheobronchial amyloidosis. *Thorax* 1968; 23:105–110.

295. Sato P, Madtes DK, Thorning D, et al: Bronchiolitis obliterans caused by *Legionella pneumophila*. *Chest* 1985; 87:840–842.

296. Scadding JG: The bronchi in allergic aspergillosis. *Scand J Respir Dis* 1967; 48:372–377.

297. Scadding JG: Definition of clinical categories of asthma, in Clark TJH, Godfrey S (eds): *Asthma*. London, Chapman & Hall, 1977, p 5.

298. Schwartz MI, Matthay RA, Sahn SA, et al: Interstitial lung disease in polymyositis and dermatomyositis: Analysis of six cases and review of the literature. *Medicine* 1976; 55:89–104.

299. Semple PDA, Reid CB, Thompson WD: Widespread panacinar emphysema with alpha-1-antitrypsin deficiency. *Br J Dis Chest* 1980; 74:289–295.

300. Sharp HL, Bridges RA, Krivit W, et al: Cirrhosis associated with alpha-1-antitrypsin deficiency: A previously unrecognized inherited disorder. *J Lab Clin Med* 1969; 73:934–939.

301. Shepard JO, Grillo HC, McLoud TC, et al: Right-pneumonectomy syndrome: Radiological findings and CT correlation. *Radiology* 1986; 161:661–664.

302. Shin MS, Ho KJ: Broncholithiasis: Its detection by computed tomography in patients with recurrent hemoptysis of unknown etiology. *Comput Radiol* 1983; 7:189–193.

303. Shin MS, Jackson RM, Ho KJ: Tracheobronchomegaly (Mounier-Kuhn syndrome): CT diagnosis. *AJR* 1988; 150:777–779.

304. Shuttleworth JS, Self CL, Pershing HS: Tracheopathia osteoplastica. *Ann Intern Med* 1960; 52:234–242.

305. Silverman G: Tuberculosis of the trachea and major bronchi. *Dis Chest* 1945; 11:3–17.

306. Silverman PM, Godwin JD: CT/bronchographic correlations in bronchiectasis. *J Comput Assist Tomogr* 1987; 11:52–56.

307. Silvers GW, Maisel JC, Petty TL, et al: Flow limitation during forced expiration in excised human lungs. *J Appl Physiol* 1974; 36:737–744.

308. Simon G: Chronic bronchitis and emphysema: A symposium: III. Pathological findings and radiological changes in chronic bronchitis and emphysema: B. Radiological changes in chronic bronchitis. *Br J Radiol* 1959; 32:292–294.

309. Simon G: Radiology and emphysema. *Clin Radiol* 1964; 15:293–306.

310. Simon G, Galbraith HJB: Radiology of chronic bronchitis. *Lancet* 1953; 2:850–852.

311. Simon G, Pride NB, Jones NL, et al: Relation between abnormalities in the chest radiograph and changes in pulmonary function in chronic bronchitis and emphysema. *Thorax* 1973; 28:15–23.

312. Simon G, Reid L, Tanner JM, et al: Growth of radiologically determined heart diameter, lung width, and lung length from 5–19 years, with standards for clinical use. *Arch Dis Child* 1972; 47:373–381.

313. Singer DB, Greenberg SD, Harrison GM: Papillomatosis of the lung. *Am Rev Respir Dis* 1966; 94:777–781.

314. Singh AK, Kothawla LK, Karlson KE: Tracheoesophageal and aortoesophageal fistulae complicating corrosive esophagitis. *Chest* 1976; 70:549–551.

315. Smith KR, Morris JF: Reversible bronchial dilatation: A report of a case. *Dis Chest* 1962; 42:652–656.

316. Snider GL: A perspective on emphysema. *Clin Chest Med* 1983; 4:329–336.

317. Snider GL, Kleinerman J, Thurlbeck WM, et al: The definition of emphysema: Report of a National Heart, Lung, and Blood Institute, Division of Lung Diseases workshop. *Am Rev Respir Dis* 1985; 132:182–185.

318. Sobonya R: Fatal anhydrous ammonia inhalation. *Hum Pathol* 1977; 8:293–299.

319. Sobonya RE, Burrows B: The epidemiology of emphysema. *Clin Chest Med* 1983; 4:351–358.

320. Stanbridge RD: Tracheo-esophageal fistula and bilateral recurrent laryngeal nerve palsies after blunt chest trauma. *Thorax* 1982; 37:548–549.

321. Stephens RW, Lingeman RE, Lawson LJ: Congenital tracheoesophageal fistulas in adults. *Ann Otol Rhinol Laryngol* 1976; 85:613–617.

322. Stokes D, Sigler A, Khouri NF, et al: Unilateral hyperlucent lung (Swyer-James syndrome) after severe *Mycoplasma pneumoniae* infection. *Am Rev Respir Dis* 1978; 117:145–152.

323. Stone DJ, Schwartz A, Feltman JA: Bullous emphysema: A long-term study of the natural history and the effects of therapy. *Am Rev Respir Dis* 1960; 82:493–507.

324. Stuart-Harris CH, Crofton J, Gibon JC, et al: Definition and classification of chronic bronchitis for clinical and epidemiological purposes: A report to the Medical Research Council by their committee on the aetiology of chronic bronchitis. *Lancet* 1965; 1:775–779.

325. Suprenant EL, O'Loughlin BJ: Tracheal diverticula and tracheobronchomegaly. *Dis Chest* 1966; 49:345–351.

326. Sutherland JB, Palser RF, Pagtakhan RD, et al: Xenon-133 ventilation and perfusion studies in bronchiectasis. *J Can Assoc Radiol* 1980; 31:242–245.

327. Sutinen S, Christoforidis AJ, Klugh GA, et al: Roentgenologic criteria for the recognition of non-symptomatic pulmonary emphysema. *Am Rev Respir Dis* 1965; 91:69–76.

328. Swischuk LE, Hayden CK: The trachea in children. *Semin Roentgenol* 1983; 18:7–14.

329. Swyer PR, James GCW: A case of unilateral pulmonary emphysema. *Thorax* 1953; 8:133–136.

330. Tager IB, Speizer FE: Risk estimates for chronic bronchitis in smokers: A study of male-female differences. *Am Rev Respir Dis* 1976; 113:619–625.

331. Tandon MK, Campbell AH: Bronchial cartilage in chronic bronchitis. *Thorax* 1969; 24:607–612.

332. Thompson JW, Ahmed AR, Dudley JP: Epidermolysis bullosa dystrophica of the larynx and trachea: Acute airway obstruction. *Ann Otol Rhinol Laryngol* 1980; 89:428–429.

333. Thurlbeck WM: Chronic airflow obstruction in lung disease, in Bennington JL (ed): *Major Problems in Pathology.* Philadelphia, WB Saunders Co, 1976, vol 5.

334. Thurlbeck WM, Angus GE: A distribution curve for chronic bronchitis. *Thorax* 1964; 19:436–442.

335. Thurlbeck WM, Henderson JA, Fraser RG, et al: Chronic obstructive lung disease: A comparison between clinical, roentgenologic, functional and morphologic criteria in chronic bronchitis, emphysema, asthma and bronchiectasis. *Medicine* 1970; 49:82–145.

336. Thurlbeck WM, Simon G: Radiographic appearance of the chest in emphysema. *AJR* 1978; 130:429–440.

337. Toledo TM, Moore WL, Nash DA, et al: Spontaneous pneumopericardium in acute asthma: Case re-

port and review of the literature. *Chest* 1972; 62:118–120.

338. Turner-Stokes L, Turton C, Pope FM, et al: Emphysema and cutis laxa. *Thorax* 1983; 38:790–792.

339. Turton CW, Williams G, Green M: Cryptogenic obliterative bronchiolitis in adults. *Thorax* 1981; 36:805–810.

340. Vandevivere J, Spehl M, Dab I, et al: Bronchiectasis in childhood. *Pediatr Radiol* 1980; 9:193–198.

341. Vix VA: Radiographic manifestations of broncholithiasis. *Radiology* 1978; 128:295–299.

342. Vock P, Spiegel T, Fram EK, et al: CT assessment of the adult intrathoracic cross section of the trachea. *J Comput Assist Tomogr* 1984; 8:1076–1082.

343. Wanderer AA, Ellis EF, Goltz RW, et al: Tracheobronchiomegaly and acquired cutis laxa in a child: Physiologic and immunologic studies. *Pediatrics* 1969; 44:709–715.

344. Watanabe Y, Nishiyama Y, Kanayama H, et al: Congenital bronchiectasis due to cartilage deficiency: CT demonstration. *J Comput Assist Tomogr* 1987; 11:701–703.

345. Way SPB: Tracheopathia osteoplastica. *J Clin Pathol* 1967; 20:814–820.

346. Wayne KS, Taussig LM: Probable familial congenital bronchiectasis due to cartilage deficiency (Williams-Campbell syndrome). *Am Rev Respir Dis* 1976; 114:15–22.

347. Weber AL, Grillo HC: Tracheal stenosis: An analysis of 151 cases. *Radiol Clin North Am* 1978; 16:291–308.

348. Weber AL, Grillo HC: Tracheal tumors: A radiological, clinical, and pathological evaluation of 84 cases. *Radiol Clin North Am* 1978; 16:227–246.

349. Weed LA, Andersen HA: Etiology of broncholithiasis. *Dis Chest* 1960; 37:270–277.

350. Weg JG, Krumholz RA, Hackelroad LE: Unilateral hyperlucent lung: A physiologic syndrome. *Ann Intern Med* 1965; 62:675–684.

351. Westcott JL, Cole SR: Traction bronchiectasis in end-stage pulmonary fibrosis. *Radiology* 1986; 161:665–669.

352. White RI, James AE, Wagner HN: The significance of unilateral absence of pulmonary artery perfusion by lung scanning. *AJR* 1971; 111:501–509.

353. Whitehouse G: Tracheopathia osteoplastica. *Br J Radiol* 1968; 41:701–703.

354. Whitelaw A, Evans A, Corrin B: Immotile cilia syndrome: A new cause of neonatal respiratory distress. *Arch Dis Child* 1981; 56:432–435.

355. Whitwell F: A study of pathology and pathogenesis of bronchiectasis. *Thorax* 1952; 7:213–239.

356. Whyte KF, Williams GR: Bronchiectasis after *Mycoplasma* pneumonia. *Thorax* 1984; 39:390–391.

357. Wieder S, Rabinowitz JG: Fibrous mediastinitis: A late manifestation of mediastinal histoplasmosis. *Radiology* 1977; 125:305–312.

358. Wilks S: Ossific deposits on the larynx, trachea and bronchi. *Trans Pathol Soc Lond* 1857; 8:88.

359. Williams H, Campbell P: Generalized bronchiectasis associated with deficiency of cartilage in the bronchial tree. *Arch Dis Child* 1960; 35:182–191.

360. Williams JL, Markowitz RI, Capitanio MA, et al: Immune deficiency syndromes. *Semin Roentgenol* 1975; 10:83–89.

361. Williams T, Eidus L, Thomas P: Fibrosing alveolitis, bronchiolitis obliterans, and sulphasalazine therapy. *Chest* 1982; 81:766–768.

362. Wiot JF: Tracheobronchial trauma. *Semin Roentgenol* 1983; 18:15–22.

363. Wohl MEB, Chernick V: Bronchiolitis. *Am Rev Respir Dis* 1978; 118:759–781.

364. Woolcock AJ, Read J: Lung volumes in exacerbations of asthma. *Am J Med* 1966; 41:259–273.

365. Woolcock AJ, Rebuck AS, Cade JF, et al: Lung volume changes in asthma measured concurrently by two methods. *Am Rev Respir Dis* 1971; 104:703–709.

366. Wyatt SE, Nunn P, Hows JM, et al: Airways obstruction associated with graft versus host disease after bone marrow transplantation. *Thorax* 1984; 39:887–894.

367. Wychulis AR, Ellis FH, Anderson HA: Acquired nonmalignant esophagotracheo-bronchial fistula: Report of 36 cases. *JAMA* 1966; 196:117–122.

368. Young RH, Sandstrom RE, Mark GJ: Tracheopathia osteoplastica: Clinical, radiologic and pathological correlations. *J Thorac Cardiovasc Surg* 1980; 79:537–541.

369. Zieverink SE, Harper AP, Holden RW, et al: Emergency room radiography of asthma: An efficacy study. *Radiology* 1982; 145:27–29.

Chest Trauma

SKELETAL TRAUMA

Rib fractures are commonly encountered in clinical practice, and the majority are of limited clinical significance. Certain fractures assume a greater significance by virtue of specific features.

1. The presence of fractures of certain ribs indicates a severe trauma or, alternatively, an increased likelihood of damage to certain organs. For example, the first, second, and third ribs are well protected by the shoulder girdles and the associated musculature, with the result that a considerable force is required to fracture these ribs. The possibility of damage to important structures such as the aorta and the great vessels is therefore greater.[4] However, patients with significant damage to intrathoracic vascular structures will have additional clinical and radiographic evidence of vascular damage. Thus, the finding of fractures of the first three ribs in the absence of such additional findings is no longer felt to be an indication for angiography.[12, 48] The presence of fractures of the 10th, 11th, or 12th ribs should alert one to the possibility of rupture of the liver, kidneys, or spleen.

2. The fractured rib ends may lacerate the pleura or lung with resultant bleeding or pneumothorax. This possibility constitutes perhaps the main reason for radiography in the average patient.

3. The fracturing of a large number of ribs on one side may result in a "flail" chest with inspiratory chest retraction on that side and potentially serious clinical consequences.

4. Rib fractures may be pathologic, for example in myeloma or a metastatic malignant process. These fractures are clearly of the utmost clinical significance. The diagnosis hinges on the presence of a destructive process with secondary fracturing, and it may be necessary to obtain detailed views or tomographic images in order to confirm one's suspicions. The majority of such fractures relate to metastatic neoplasm or myeloma, but on occasion the cause may be a benign process such as eosinophilic granuloma.

5. Rib fractures are commonly seen in children subjected to physical abuse.[22] Indeed the finding of occult rib fractures may be a critical clue to the fact that the child has been abused. Ordinarily rib fractures are extremely uncommon in infants and young children and, when present, can be readily attributed to a known episode of significant trauma. It is important to exclude underlying conditions that may predispose to rib fractures, such as rickets or osteogenesis imperfecta. Rib fractures in abused children are often bilateral and at varying stages of healing. Callus formation may be prominent, a feature making the fractures more readily visible.

As previously indicated, rib fractures are often clinically inconsequential. It has also to be realized that a major degree of internal thoracic trauma can occur in the absence of rib fractures. This applies particularly to the more resilient chest wall of younger individuals. The thoroughness with which one strives to determine the presence or absence of rib fractures must be determined by the particular circumstances of the case and by medicolegal considerations. Inevitably, significant amounts of time, money, and resources are expended under these circumstances—with little practical result in most cases. A thorough examination of the chest with supplementary rib detail films probably requires a minimum of five images and at least 5 to 10 minutes of room time.

There are certain fractures which have distinct or noteworthy features.

1. Stress fractures. Fractures of the first or second ribs may be stress fractures as a result, for example, of backpacking. The bony reaction and callus formation may give a spurious appearance of an apical pulmonary parenchymal process. Apical lordotic and rib detail views plus the clinical circumstances should resolve the diagnosis.

2. Cough fractures. In effect these may also be stress fractures, but they occur in older individuals in the posterolateral aspects of the lower ribs. The patient may experience localized rib pain. The condition is usually of some standing, and callus formation around the fractures may be conspicuous.

3. Excessive callus formation in cushingoid patients. Patients with Cushing's syndrome or on intensive steroid therapy are frequently osteoporotic and have an increased tendency to fractures. A very interesting and characteristic feature in these patients is the exuberant callus formation that occurs in relation to the fractures.[35] This exuberant callus may simulate a pulmonary parenchymal process.

4. Multiple rib fractures in alcoholics. Hard-core alcoholic patients frequently have multiple bilateral rib fractures in varying stages of healing. I am personally impressed with the reliability of this social indicator, which has served to alert me to other medical consequences of this condition. It surely indicates previous states of inebriation scarcely comprehensible even to the most hardened fraternity brother.

5. Pseudarthroses of ribs. On occasion rib fractures may evolve into pseudarthroses, ribs being difficult to immobilize. As with stress fractures or excessive callus formation, an unwary or unobservant physician may diagnose a parenchymal lesion.

Other skeletal injuries or their secondary effects may be encountered. The presence of a sternal fracture usually indicates a significant chest trauma, and one should be alert to the possibility of a deceleration injury to the aorta. These fractures cannot be visualized on frontal chest radiographs and may be relatively inconspicuous on lateral chest radiographs.

In the appropriate circumstances, careful attention should be paid to the sternal contours on the lateral view. Sternal fractures as such do not generally cause problems either in healing or in direct damage to adjacent structures. Costochondral separation may occur in younger individuals, and this usually indicates significant trauma. The diagnosis of costochondral separation is essentially based on the clinical findings.

Fractures of the shoulder girdle may be observed but are usually outside the concern of the pulmonologist. However, dislocation of the sternoclavicular joint with posterior displacement of the inner end of the clavicle may cause compression of the trachea and the adjacent great vessels with significant clinical consequences.[13] Dislocation of a sternoclavicular joint may be difficult or impossible to detect, particularly in a patient with major trauma in whom the radiographic examination is restricted. However, tracheal deviation may be noted and paratracheal soft tissue thickening may be apparent. Certainly clinical awareness of the possibility of such an injury is the key factor in its recognition, with the radiographs often helping to confirm the diagnosis.

Major trauma to the root of the neck may on occasion damage the phrenic nerve with resultant diaphragmatic paresis or paralysis. In a severely traumatized patient the development of lower zone or lower lobe atelectasis might not occasion much surprise. The atelectasis might be held to account for the diaphragmatic elevation rather than the reverse. Once suspected the diagnosis can be confirmed, if one chooses, by fluoroscopic or ultrasound examination.

Cervical spine trauma with spinal cord damage has obvious clinical implications for the pulmonologist. Indeed, poor clearance of secretions, with mucus plugging and secondary bacterial infection, is frequently a major problem in these individuals. However, fractures of the thoracic spine are not usually of much direct consequence to the respiratory system. The paravertebral soft tissue thickening adjacent to these fractures may, however, be conspicuous on the chest radiographs, and due allowance should be made for this, for example, in diagnosing lower lobe collapse.

PULMONARY PARENCHYMAL TRAUMA

Contusion of the lung parenchyma is frequent in major trauma and may be seen underlying the point of injury or as a contracoup lesion. The radiographic appearances are those of a diffuse ill-defined alveolar process with patchy, often confluent, shadowing in the lungs (Fig 17–1). Presumably the bleeding into the lung parenchyma must continue for a period of time following the injury; therefore, the changes should wax during that time. One should recognize, however, that it is unusual to be able to radiograph a severely injured patient within 1 hour of the trauma with all the inevitable problems of transport, resuscitation, and so on. In the majority of cases the findings are manifest at the time of the initial examination and show little tendency to increase in severity with subsequent examinations. On the contrary radiographic clearing of pulmonary contusion may be relatively rapid, and the signs of contusion have often resolved within 48 hours.

Pulmonary contusion is distributed according to the spread of a shock wave and does not localize in any anatomically recognizable pattern (i.e., strictly lobar or segmental). The interlobar fissures do not dampen the spread of the shock wave, and contusion may be seen on either side of these structures. Computed tomographic (CT) examinations are now performed with greater frequency in patients with trauma and will frequently demonstrate lung contusion with great clarity (Fig 17–2). It should be emphasized, however, that lung contusion in itself is not an indication for CT examination.

Pneumatoceles may be encountered in association with pulmonary contusion. It is postulated that the shock wave causes shearing of a portion of the lung parenchyma with escape of air into the resultant fissure. This localized internal leak of air plus the retraction of lung caused by its inherent elasticity results in a localized rounded air space in the lung parenchyma (Fig 17–3). The resultant pneumatocele may contain a variable quantity of fluid, presumably blood. Indeed if the entire space fills with blood, the result is a pulmonary *hematoma*. Pneumatoceles and hematomas may be multiple but are more commonly isolated lesions. On occasion they may be extremely large, up to 10 to 14 cm in diameter, but 2 to 5 cm is the dimension most usually encountered. It is not usual for pneumatoceles or hematomas to be apparent radiographically within a few hours of the injury. There may be two major reasons for this: (1) the initial lung contusion may be of such severity that the lesions, although present, are obscured; (2) the air leak or oozing of blood into the parenchymal space may continue for some time, thereby enlarging it. A pneumatocele does not usually have a well-defined wall, at least in the early stages following injury. The visibility of a pneumatocele is ordinarily dependent on its size, the fluid it contains, and the surrounding pulmonary contusion. It may, however, be difficult to distinguish between a pneumatocele and a hematoma that has communicated with the bronchial tree (Fig 17–4). A hematoma will become more readily visible as a circumscribed density as the surrounding pulmonary parenchymal contusion clears (Fig 17–5).

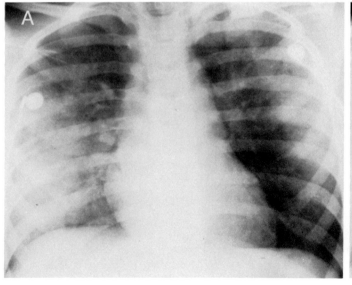 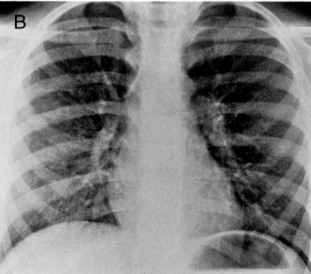

FIG 17–1.
A, radiograph of young male patient obtained within 2 hours of a motor vehicle accident. **B,** same patient 72 hours later. All evidence of pulmonary contusion has disappeared.

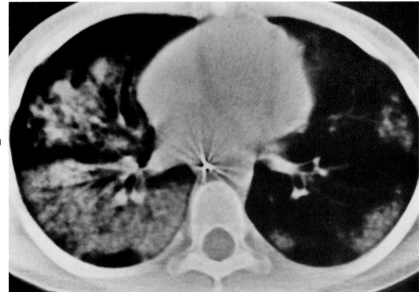

FIG 17–2.
CT scan of the patient in Figure 17–1 showing widespread patchy alveolar densities representing contused lung.

Both pneumatoceles and hematomas resolve, pneumatoceles faster than hematomas. Hematomas may take some months to resolve and may, for a considerable period, be the only visible sequela of the previous trauma. Since by this stage a hematoma will be a circumscribed lung mass, the lesion may be mistaken for a neoplasm (Fig 17–6). During the phase of resolution, a hematoma may communicate with the bronchial tree and appear as a cavitary process (Fig 17–7). Awareness of these features is important in order to avoid confusion with more serious pulmonary processes. Cavitating hematomas will resolve without treatment.

GUNSHOT, BLAST, AND STAB WOUNDS

Most gunshot wounds to the lungs seen in civilian practice are the result of low-velocity missiles. Although the missiles may fragment, there is not the devastating fragmentation of the high-velocity missile. In addition, the shock waves of low-velocity missiles are not nearly so severe or extensive in their effects. A low-velocity missile traversing the lung forms a distinct track, which may be air filled or occupied by hematoma (Fig 17–8). Surrounding this track is a variable zone of lung contusion. On occasion one may even visualize the track and be able to gauge the thickness and extent of the surrounding contusion. This observation applies particularly to cases with an air-filled track radiographed in the axis of the track. Shotgun injuries are generally severe because of the intermediate muzzle velocity of these weapons and the large mass of the shot (Fig 17–9). Shotgun injuries to the chest are stated to be nearly ten times more lethal than wounds from other weapons.[41] The pleura is inevitably involved in pulmonary damage from gunshots, and hemothorax or pneumothorax is very common. The chest radiograph is a critical factor in determining whether the pleural space should be drained. In damage confined to the lungs and pleura, drainage may be the only direct intervention that is required.

Stab wounds do not generate shock waves, and the resulting contusion of lung parenchyma is less. As with gunshot wounds, the significance of these wounds relates to the extent and severity of damage to major vascular structures and the pleura or pericardium. The actual trauma to pulmonary parenchyma is less significant.

Blast injuries are relatively uncommon. In described cases, the changes are typically bilateral and centered on the major airways, with perihilar edema and contusion.[27, 46]

TORSION OF THE LUNG

Torsion of a lung or a lobe of lung is an extremely rare but serious condition that may result from compressive trauma to the chest.[10] The victim is almost invariably a child and has usually been run over by a car. In adults, lung torsion may occur spontaneously, although usually an inciting lesion,

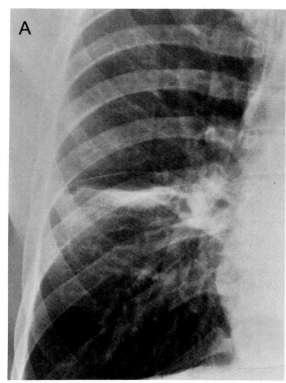

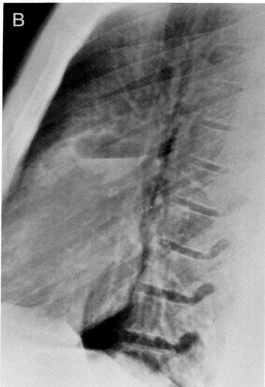

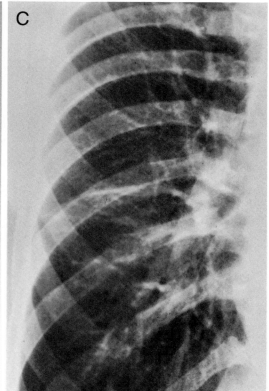

FIG 17–3.
Traumatic pneumatocele (**A** and **B**) containing a small quantity of fluid. Note that the margins of the pneumatocele are barely perceptible beyond the fluid. Six weeks later **(C)** the pneumatocele has disappeared leaving a small linear scar.

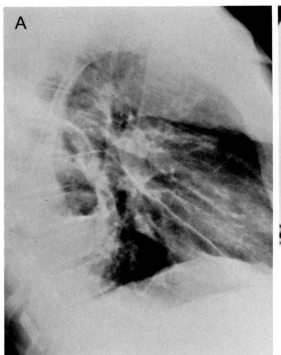

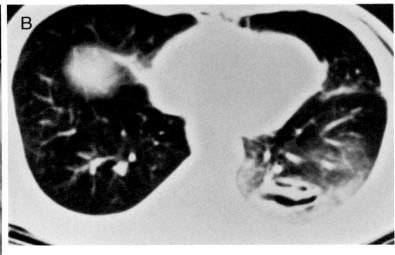

FIG 17–4.
Lateral chest radiograph **(A)** and a CT scan **(B)** show a left lower lobe air space containing fluid 1 week following a major thoracic trauma. The air space appears to have a thickened wall, but there was no clinical evidence to suggest evacuation of a hematoma. The air space had been present from the initial examination immediately after the accident and was, therefore, regarded as a pneumatocele.

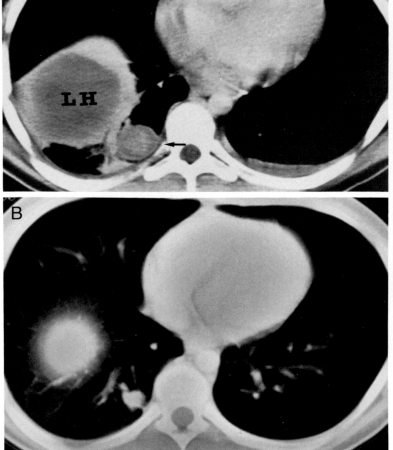

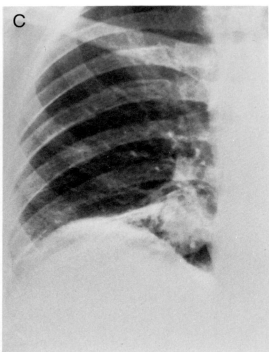

FIG 17–5.
A, CT scan of a young man involved in a motor vehicle accident. There is a large hematoma *(LH)* in the liver. A pulmonary hematoma *(arrow)* is partially obscured by right lower lobe consolidation and atelectasis. **B,** the hematoma becomes visible on a chest radiograph 1 week later. **C,** follow-up scan 6 weeks later shows a smaller well-circumscribed resolving hematoma.

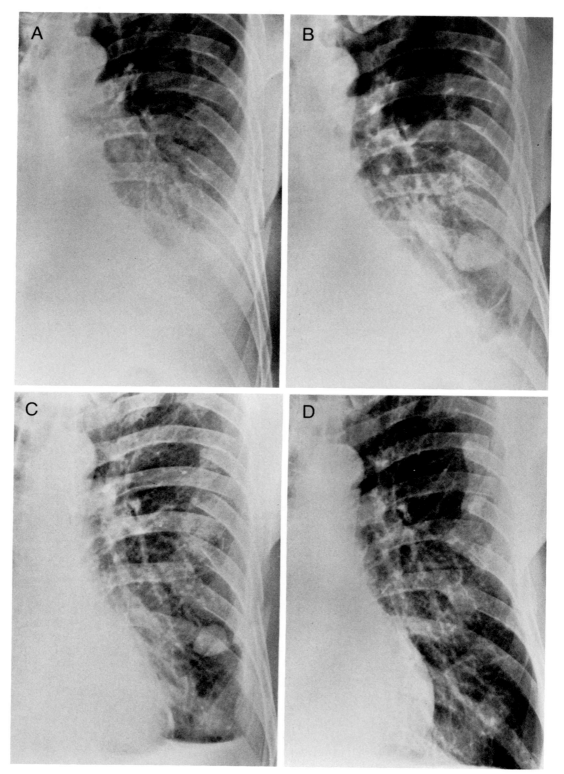

FIG 17–6.
A, admission film following major trauma to patient's left chest. There are multiple rib fractures, a left pleural effusion and left basal pulmonary parenchymal opacification. **B,** 2 days later, a pulmonary hematoma is visible. **C,** 2 weeks later the hematoma is the only residual parenchymal lesion. **D,** 6 months later the hematoma has resolved.

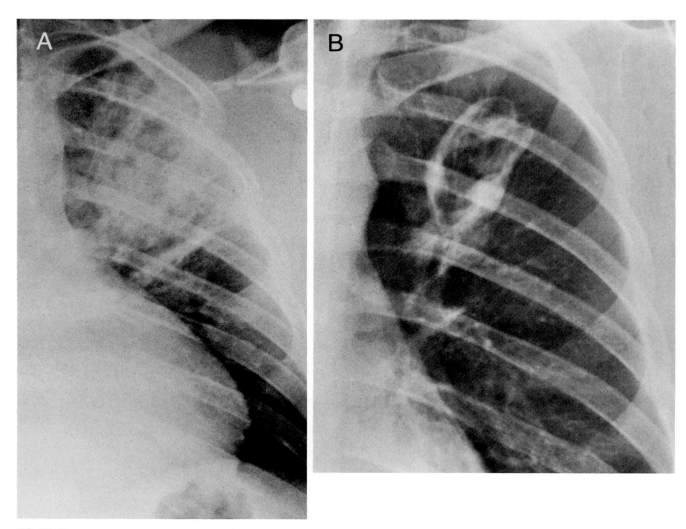

FIG 17−7.
A, left upper lobe pulmonary contusion following a motor vehicle accident. **B,** 4 weeks later, a well-circumscribed cavitary lesion represents a hematoma that has communicated with the bronchial tree and evacuated. Resolution was eventually complete.

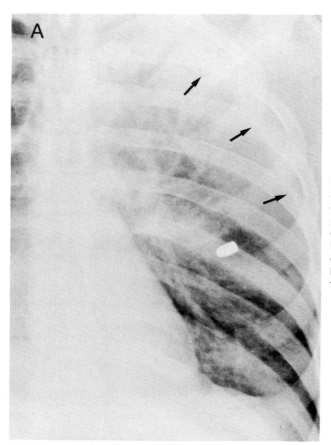

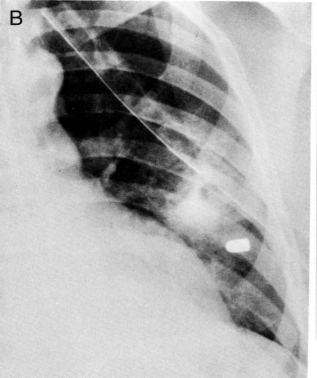

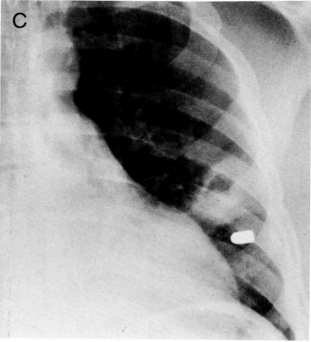

FIG 17–8.
Supine chest radiograph on admission after patient suffered gunshot wound from a handgun. **A,** hemothorax is layering posteriorly and extending round the lung laterally and over the apex *(arrows).* **B,** day 2 following chest tube drainage of the hemothorax. There is a rounded, ill-defined zone of contusion around the bullet track. **C,** day 4. The zone of contusion has become more defined, and there is a distinct air-filled bullet track.

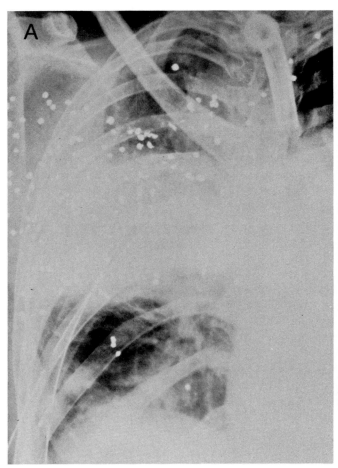

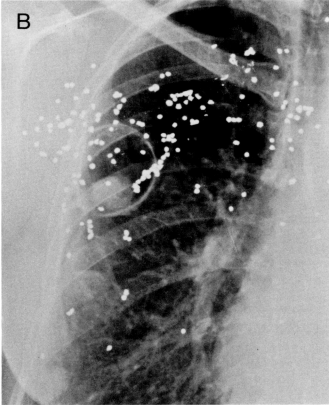

FIG 17–9.
A, massive pulmonary contusion following a shotgun wound to the chest. A hemothorax had been drained by the chest tube. **B,** ra-diograph 5 years later shows that a cavity has persisted following the shotgun wound and now contains a mycetoma.

such as a lung tumor, is present. Torsion of lung may also occur in the immediate postoperative period following thoracic surgery, usually after lobar resection.

Diagnosis of lung torsion is extraordinarily difficult. A key factor is awareness of the existence of this condition and the circumstances under which it occurs. The radiographic findings may be subdivided into:

1. The results of the torquing of the airways and the lung vessels. Airway torquing may result in an abrupt cut-off in the airway at the hilus, with the development of atelectasis. On the other hand, torquing of the hilar vessels may result in hemorrhagic infarction of lung. Thus, there is a range of findings in the lung parenchyma—from normal aeration, through varying degrees of lobar or whole lung atelectasis, to expansile consolidation of lung.

2. Anatomic malpositioning. It is only by actual identification of anatomic malpositioning that a definitive diagnosis of lung torsion can be made prior to exploration. The hilar vessels or the interlobar fissures may be observed to be rotated away from their normal position. Alternatively, if previous films are available, it might be observed that an identifiable structure such as a lung nodule has shifted position in an inexplicable fashion.

TRACHEAL OR BRONCHIAL RUPTURE

Tracheal or bronchial rupture may result from penetrating injuries. Blunt trauma must be severe to cause airway rupture, and there is likely to be significant damage to other structures such as the thoracic cage, the lungs, and the aorta. Indeed tracheobronchial rupture is associated with a 30% overall mortality, chiefly from associated injuries.[15] High-speed traffic accidents are the usual cause of tracheal or bronchial rupture. Diagnosis is by no means easy, and a significant proportion of cases go undiagnosed until complications develop either at the site of rupture (e.g., bronchial stenosis) or in the lung distal to the rupture (e.g., septic complications or persistent atelectasis) (Fig 17–10).[17, 23, 24] The findings of airway rupture are sometimes subtle and may be completely overshadowed by the other injuries. Alternatively, more obvious signs of rupture may be wrongly attributed to damage to other structures.

Basically there are two main radiographic manifestations of tracheal or bronchial rupture. The first is evidence of leakage of air at the site of rupture; the second relates to disturbed ventilation of the lung distal to the rupture. Evidence of air leakage is the most critical, and absence of air leakage makes the diagnosis of a breach in a major airway extraordinarily difficult, if not impossible. A pneumothorax is the most common finding, seen in some 60% of cases.[20] The other indication of an airway leak is the presence of a pneumomediastinum (Fig 17–11). The coexistence of a pneumothorax and a pneumomediastinum is perhaps the strongest indication of a bronchial rupture. On the other hand if the outer adventitial sleeve of the bronchus remains intact there may be no air leak, a situation that occurs in approximately 10% of cases of tracheobronchial fracture.[7] Pneumomediastinum may be the only visible sign of an air leak in ruptures of the trachea or the intramediastinal portions of the bronchi.

The pneumothorax is frequently large and under tension. Furthermore the air leak may be found to be large and persistent after insertion of pleural tubes. Radiographically the lung in these circumstances fails to reexpand. There is one unusual, but characteristic, feature that may be encountered in cases with bronchial disruption and a large pneumothorax. Normally with a pneumothorax the lung recoils inward towards the hilus. A bronchial fracture may allow the lung to sag away from the hilus inferiorly and laterally: the "fallen lung" sign (Fig

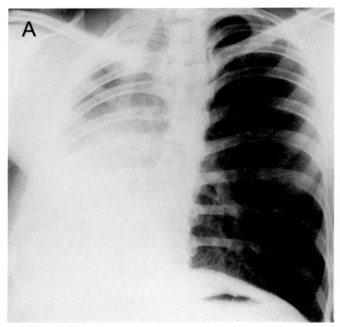

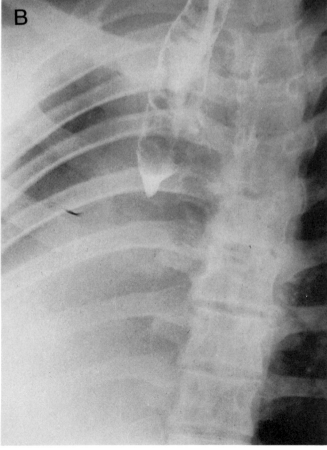

FIG 17–10.
A, chest radiograph of 18-year-old man shows total collapse of right lung. **B,** bronchogram shows total occlusion of the right bronchus, thought to result from a major accident when the patient was 9 years of age.

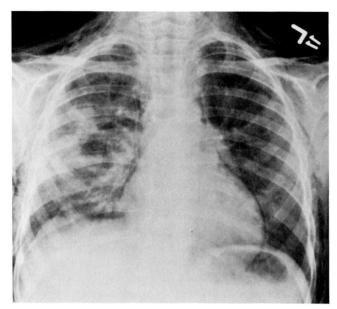

FIG 17–11.
Radiograph of young man involved in a motor vehicle accident. There is a right lung contusion with pneumatocele formation. A pneumomediastinum tracking into the neck indicated a tracheobronchial rupture.

17–12). The vascular pedicle remains intact, and the lung remains perfused, although underventilated.[31] The consequent ventilation-perfusion mismatch may result in hypoxia and cyanosis.

The presence of a pneumomediastinum is a critical finding in patients with chest trauma. A pneu-mothorax is not an infrequent accompaniment of rib fractures, and its potential significance may be overlooked. A pneumomediastinum following trauma is a more specific sign of a breach of airway integrity. Air in the mediastinum is seen as streaky lucencies in the carinal region extending superiorly as the air dissects in the tissue planes around the trachea and the aorta and the great vessels. On the margins of the mediastinum, the air dissects and elevates the mediastinal parietal pleura from the aorta and the heart. On lateral films, a pneumomediastinum is best appreciated in the retrosternal space.

The second major effect of a major airway rupture is to disturb the ventilation of the related lung. Loss of bronchial continuity, combined with hemorrhage and edema, results in atelectasis. The diagnostic problems in these cases are numerous. Collapse of a lung is usual and expected in the presence of a pneumothorax, particularly if the pneumothorax is large and under tension. Severely traumatized patients may develop atelectasis for other reasons or may have significant associated pulmonary abnormalities such as lung contusion or aspiration changes. It may be difficult to diagnose developing lung collapse: the critical finding is reduced volume of the lung relative to the other lung. Alterations in lung density may be patchy and nondescript. Atelectasis in bronchial rupture is usually persistent and unresponsive to normal therapeutic endeavors. Bronchial stenosis or occlusion at the site of rupture is a frequent consequence in the untreated case. Sep-

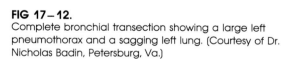

FIG 17–12.
Complete bronchial transection showing a large left pneumothorax and a sagging left lung. (Courtesy of Dr. Nicholas Badin, Petersburg, Va.)

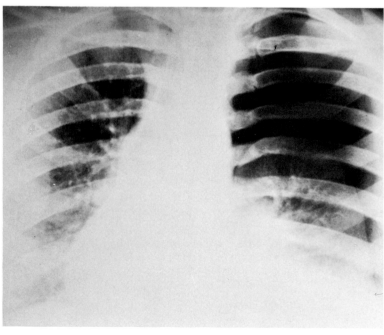

tic complications may be encountered in the affected lung.

The diagnosis of bronchial rupture is dependent on awareness of this possibility in cases of severe thoracic trauma. In a significant number of instances the diagnosis may be missed in the acute phase and may be detected only when the patient presents later with persisting lung or lobar atelectasis. It is important to perform bronchoscopy in any case in which the features described provide at least some suspicion of an airway rupture.

INJURY TO THE AORTA AND THE GREAT VESSELS

Deceleration forces can cause marked shearing stresses, particularly in zones where a structure changes from being relatively fixed to being relatively unsupported. Such a zone occurs in the aortic isthmus in the region of attachment of the ligamentum arteriosum. Below this point the descending aorta is tethered by the intercostal arteries, whereas the aortic arch is capable of movement in rapid deceleration. Transection of the aorta at this point is a major cause of death in motor vehicle or aircraft crashes. Ninety-five percent of all aortic ruptures occur in the region of the isthmus, the other 5% occur in the aortic root, presumably from posterior shearing of the aortic arch. In some cases, the degree of damage falls just short of complete transection and immediate exsanguination. In these cases the adventitial layer may just maintain the continuity of the aorta, at least for a time. However, the risk of ultimate rupture is very high, and only rarely does one encounter an old calcified post-traumatic aneurysm of the aortic isthmus. Immediate diagnosis is therefore vital, and the chest radiograph is crucial in this regard.

In the great majority of medical centers, angiography is used to make the definitive diagnosis of damage to the aorta and the great vessels. CT can enable one to diagnose the presence of aortic damage,[19] but it seems unlikely that CT will be used as a primary method of investigation in these circumstances. However, if any patient is examined by CT to investigate head trauma or possible abdominal visceral trauma, it may be reasonable to screen the aortic arch region with a few selected images. Hematoma formation is readily detected, and CT may even detect false aneurysm formation and irregularities of the aortic wall at the site of rupture.[19]

The diagnosis of damage to the aorta and the great vessels depends largely on the nature and severity of the trauma and the findings on the chest radiograph. In most cases there are no findings on clinical examination to indicate such damage.[36] The plain film findings have been comprehensively reviewed by Woodring and Dillon and are as follows[47]:

1. Diffuse widening of the mediastinum with obscuring of the aortic contours and obliteration of the aortopulmonary window (Fig 17–13). These changes result from perivascular hematoma formation. Unfortunately in many instances the chest radiographs must be obtained with the patient in the supine position and with use of a short focus-film distance. Moreover the patient may be incapable of full inspiration. The problems are compounded if the patient is short, thickset, and obese. In these circumstances a normal mediastinum can easily appear unusually wide. If it is at all possible, an upright chest film with a 6-ft focus-film distance should be obtained (Fig 17–14). It is difficult to establish reliable measurement criteria for mediastinal widening given the variations in patient positioning, body build, and age. Proposed criteria include a mediastinal width exceeding 8 cm just above the aortic knob[26] or a ratio of the width of the mediastinum to the width of the chest exceeding 0.25 at the level of the aortic knob.[40] However, although Gundry et al.[16] found mediastinal widening to be the single most reliable sign of traumatic rupture of the aorta, these authors found it impractical to base the evaluation of the mediastinum on absolute figures. Furthermore, rupture of the aorta or the great vessels may be observed with mediastinal measurements less than those quoted here.[11]

2. Evidence of hematoma displacing normal structures. Hematoma formation around the isthmus of the aorta commonly displaces the left main bronchus downward and the trachea and esophagus to the right. Depression of the left bronchus to below 40 degrees from the horizontal has been stated to be a significant indication of aortic rupture.[25] Tracheal deviation may be more difficult to assess because the trachea normally deviates to the right at the level of the aortic knob, and small degrees of patient rotation can be critical. Deviation of the esophagus—as indicated by the position of a nasogastric tube—is a good indication of hematoma formation, the esophagus normally being closely related anatomically to the isthmus and the descending aorta (Fig 17–15).[14, 43]

3. Evidence of extension of bleeding into anatomically continuous regions. Extension of bleeding in a posterior direction may cause widening of the

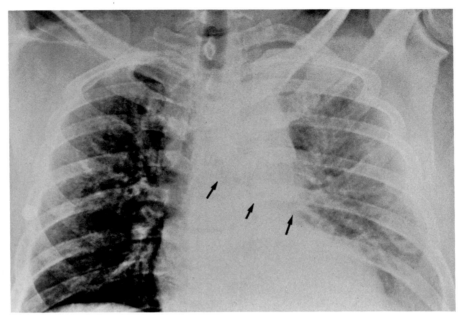

FIG 17–13.
Traumatic aortic rupture resulting from an automobile accident. Note diffuse mediastinal widening with loss of the aortic contours. A left hemothorax is present; and the left main bronchus is depressed and elongated *(arrows).*

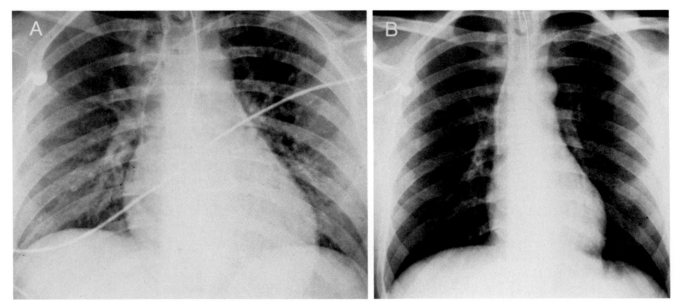

FIG 17–14.
A, chest radiograph obtained with a focus-film distance of 40 in. and the patient supine. **B,** same patient radiographed upright with a focus-film distance of 72 inches.

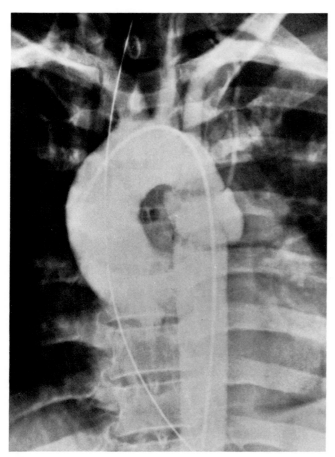

FIG 17-15.
Aortogram showing traumatic false aneurysm at the aortic isthmus. Note the wide deviation of the nasogastric tube from the aorta. Contrast this with the position of the nasogastric tube in Figure 17–14.

paravertebral lines.[34] Leakage of blood into a pleural cavity, most often the left pleural cavity, may result in the development of a hemothorax (Fig 17–16). The finding of a hemothorax in an injured patient should immediately raise the possibility of an aortic injury. Hematomas may also track out of the mediastinum over the lung apices forming apical "caps."[42] Such apical caps are particularly significant when there are no fractures of the upper ribs to account for extrapleural thickening.

There is no doubt that the diagnosis of aortic rupture is so critical that one must accept a large number of negative angiographic examinations. Mediastinal hematoma formation may indeed be present even in the absence of angiographic evidence of damage to the aorta or great vessels. In these cases the bleeding is presumably the result of small artery or venous hemorrhage.

INJURY TO THE ESOPHAGUS AND THORACIC DUCT

Rupture of the esophagus by blunt external trauma is exceedingly rare. Traumatic rupture of the esophagus usually results from a penetrating injury, including instrumentation, or as a complication of dilatation of an esophageal stricture. The radiographic features include (1) pneumomediastinum; (2) pneumothorax and/or pleural effusion, most commonly on the left side; (3) evidence of mediastinitis, including abscess formation.

Penetrating injury or surgical damage during thoracic exploration are the usual causes of injury to the thoracic duct (Fig 17–17). Damage from blunt external trauma is rare. Fluid accumulation is characteristically slow, and it may take several days for significant quantities of fluid to accumulate. The anatomic course of the thoracic duct may determine the side on which the fluid accumulates. The duct enters the thorax through the aortic opening in the diaphragm and ascends on the right anterolateral aspect of the spine. In the midthoracic region it trends to the left, to ascend on the left anterolateral aspect of the spine. Finally it arches forward to enter the venous system in the region of the junction of the left jugular and subclavian veins. The definitive diagnosis rests on determining that an effusion is chylous in appropriate clinical circumstances.

INJURY TO THE HEART AND PERICARDIUM

The heart and pericardium appear to be well protected from nonpenetrating injury, and clearly documented traumatic lesions are uncommon. Penetrating trauma, on the other hand, is ordinarily the result of a felonious assault, and patient mortality is high. The following abnormalities may be encountered following chest trauma:

1. Myocardial contusion/infarction.
2. Myocardial laceration leading to hemopericardium and tamponade.
3. Septal defects and true and false myocardial aneurysms.
4. Coronary artery damage with hemopericardium, false aneurysm formation, and infarction.
5. Chordal rupture with valve insufficiency.
6. Pneumopericardium.
7. Postpericardiectomy syndrome and constrictive pericarditis—late sequelae.

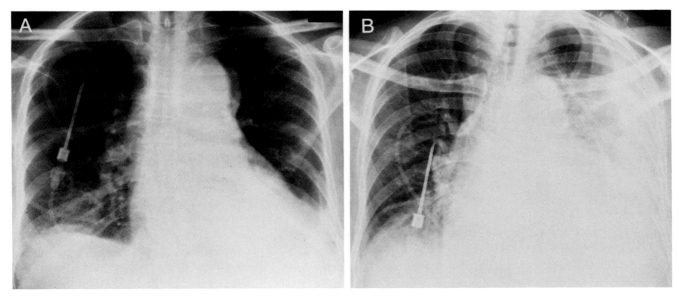

FIG 17–16.
A, mediastinal hematoma following thoracic trauma. **B,** 3 hours later a large left hemothorax has developed.

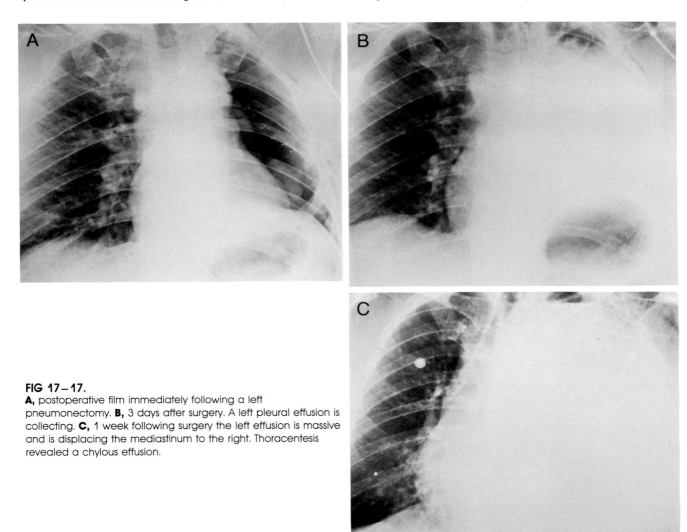

FIG 17–17.
A, postoperative film immediately following a left pneumonectomy. **B,** 3 days after surgery. A left pleural effusion is collecting. **C,** 1 week following surgery the left effusion is massive and is displacing the mediastinum to the right. Thoracentesis revealed a chylous effusion.

8. Dislocation of the heart through a pericardial tear (exceedingly rare).[21]

9. Bullet embolization.

The majority of these conditions have radiologic features that do not differ substantially from their nontraumatic equivalents. A graphic example of cardiac injury following nonpenetrating trauma is illustrated in Figures 17–18 and 17–19.

THE DIAPHRAGM

Acute rupture of the diaphragm results from either a penetrating injury or major abdominal trauma. Major abdominal trauma is usually the result of a high-speed motor vehicle accident or a fall from a considerable height. There is a high incidence of associated injury, and this is reflected in reported mortality rates of up to 20% to 25%.[30, 38] Diaphragmatic rupture resulting from abdominal trauma is more common on the left side, presumably because the liver acts as a buffer on the right. Rodriguez-Morales et al., in an analysis of 60 cases, found that 70% of diaphragmatic ruptures occurred on the left.[38] Despite the presence of a rupture in the diaphragm, herniation of abdominal contents is by no means invariable, particularly if positive pressure ventilation is used.[2] Thus, a significant number of diaphragmatic ruptures are discovered incidentally during abdominal exploration in the acute phase.[30] A number of cases remain undiagnosed during the patient's initial hospital stay only to be diagnosed later by follow-up chest radiography or when complications of visceral herniation ensue, sometimes months or years later. Delayed diagnosis of diaphragmatic rupture and herniation is particularly likely to occur in rupture of the right hemidiaphragm.[3] In those series in which all cases of diaphragmatic rupture (with or without visceral herniation) were analyzed, only some 40% to 50% of cases were identified radiographically prior to surgical intervention.[2, 30, 38] Clearly, radiographic examination must have been limited in some of these cases because of the need for urgent surgical intervention. In other cases the absence of visceral herniation rendered a radiographic diagnosis impossible. Nevertheless, there are many pitfalls in the diagnosis of diaphragmatic rupture, particularly in those cases in which additional major injury makes the radiographic examination more difficult and extended.

The diagnosis of diaphragmatic rupture can only be made or suspected if (1) there is demonstrable herniation of visceral contents through the rent in the diaphragm or (2) there is evidence of transit of fluid or air between the abdominal and pleural cavities. Herniation of hollow viscera may be readily appreciated by the characteristic gas pattern of the herniated stomach and bowel (Fig 17–20). Continuity of these loops of bowel with infradiaphragmatic bowel may be apparent, and there may be some constriction or gathering of loops at the site of the rupture. The normal diaphragmatic contours are obscured, although problems may arise if the herni-

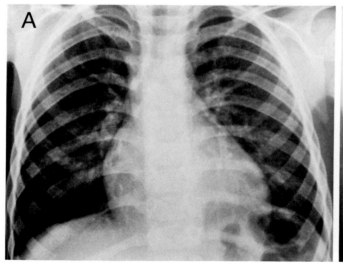 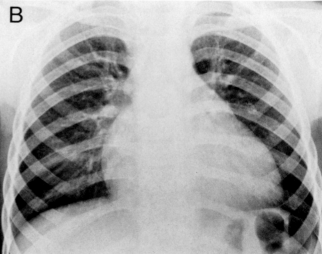

FIG 17–18.
Chest radiographs of a 3-year-old boy who was run over by a reversing car. **A,** on admission, the child's chest radiograph was normal in appearance. **B,** 2 weeks later the heart has enlarged and there is pulmonary venous congestion.

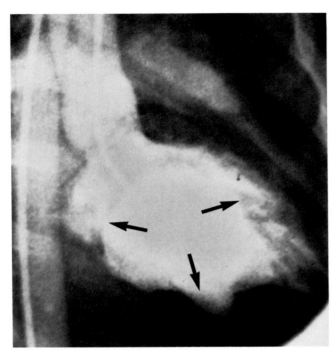

FIG 17–19.
Frame from left ventricular cineangiogram obtained in patient in Figure 17–18. There is a left ventricular aneurysm *(arrows)*.

ated stomach forms an arc-like contour simulating a paralyzed or eventrated diaphragm (Fig 17–21). The passage of a nasogastric tube may be helpful with herniations of the stomach into the left chest. The nasogastric tube will either be held up at the

esophageal hiatus or turn upward beyond the hiatus into the left chest. Studies of the gastrointestinal tract with contrast material are rarely necessary or even appropriate in the acute phase following the trauma. On the other hand, when patients present in a delayed fashion, barium studies of the stomach or the colon may, in practice, be the route to the diagnosis (Fig 17–22). Herniation of solid viscera or the omentum results in diagnostic problems and certainly accounts in large part for the difficulties in diagnosing rupture of the right hemidiaphragm. If the rupture is small and only a small knuckle of bowel herniates, this herniation may be obscured by pleural fluid and contused or collapsed lung (Fig 17–23). Diaphragmatic herniation may be simulated by post-traumatic diaphragmatic paralysis or by post-traumatic pneumatoceles. Abnormal communication between the abdominal or pleural cavities can only be inferred by the seemingly inappropriate passage of air or fluid across this barrier. For example, low-density peritoneal lavage fluid may be detected in the pleural cavity at a subsequent CT examination, or there may be an inexplicable association of a pneumothorax with a pneumoperitoneum.

Quite apart from contrast studies of the gastrointestinal tract, there are further radiologic procedures which may help one diagnose diaphragmatic rupture. CT scanning is the most likely procedure in the acute phase, and it may strongly suggest a localized herniation of bowel or omentum through the diaphragm.[18, 44] It should be emphasized that CT

FIG 17–20.
Supine chest radiograph of a young man injured in a climbing accident. The distended stomach is herniated into the left chest. There is some pleural fluid present as well as left lung contusion.

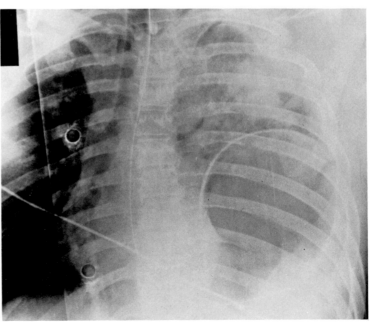

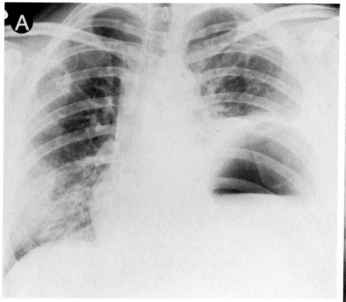

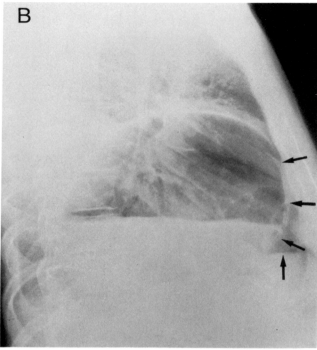

FIG 17–21.
PA **(A)** and lateral **(B)** radiographs of post-traumatic diaphragmatic hernia. The margin of the stomach wall simulates the curve of the diaphragm. However, the anterior margin of the stomach curves down to the actual level of the diaphragm (arrows).

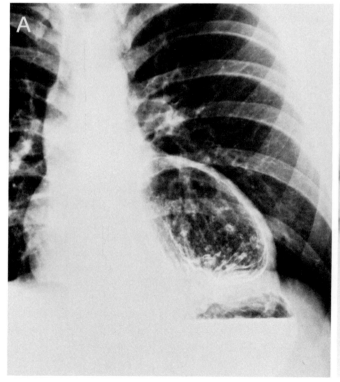

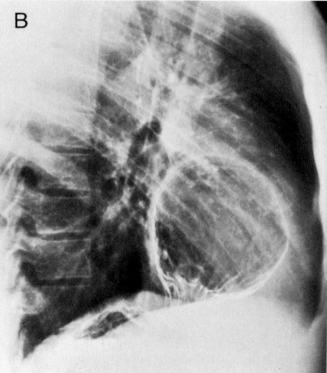

FIG 17–22.
A and **B,** chest radiographs taken after a barium study had demonstrated a diaphragmatic hernia. The herniation was believed to result from an episode of trauma that occurred some months previously.

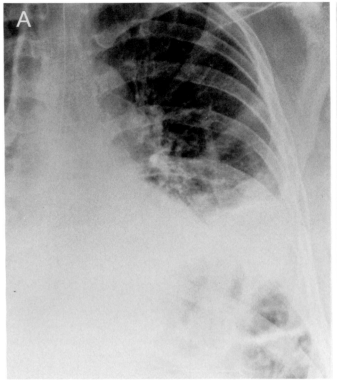

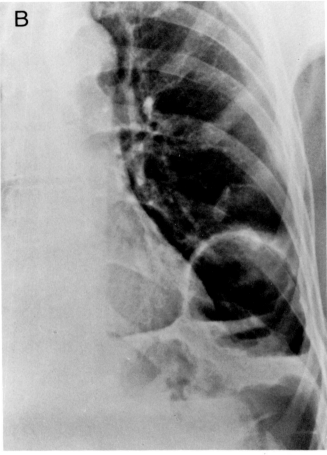

FIG 17–23.
A, young male patient radiographed soon after a stab wound to the left chest. The diaphragm was obscured by pleural fluid and consolidated or collapsed lung. The gas-filled bowel loops were thought to be under an elevated diaphragm. **B,** at a follow-up examination 2 months later, a knuckle of colon is seen to be herniating through a lateral diaphragmatic defect.

scans simply indicate focal visceral herniation and cannot demonstrate the actual defect in the diaphragm in the absence of herniation. Real-time ultrasound may also succeed in identifying visceral herniation. The diaphragm is a readily identifiable structure on real-time ultrasound studies, and bowel is also identifiable by its peristaltic movement. The difficulty with ultrasound is, however, obtaining an adequate window into the chest. Isotope liver/spleen scanning is capable of demonstrating herniation of the liver into the right chest.[3] Herniation is distinguished from upward displacement of the liver under an elevated right hemidiaphragm by a variable degree of constriction of the liver at the site of the rent in the diaphragm. It might be added parenthetically that liver/spleen scanning can also be used to diagnose the rare but interesting condition of intrathoracic splenosis.[39] This condition results from simultaneous diaphragmatic rupture and fracturing of the spleen. Splenic implants develop on the pleura and may become visible as single or multiple nodules on chest radiographs. Liver/spleen scanning will elegantly demonstrate the true nature of such nodules (Fig 17–24).

INDIRECT EFFECTS OF TRAUMA ON THE LUNGS

Severe trauma can have indirect effects on the lungs which can severely complicate the clinical and radiographic features. Basically there are three main processes that require consideration: fat embolism, adult respiratory distress syndrome, and neurogenic pulmonary edema. Only fat embolism will be described here. The other two conditions are discussed in Chapter 8.

Fat Embolism

Skeletal trauma, particularly trauma involving the pelvis and the major long bones, may cause neutral fat droplets to enter the bloodstream. These fat

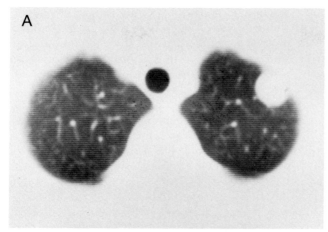

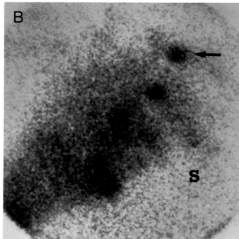

FIG 17–24.
A, CT scan of lung apices in young man showing an apical nodule. **B,** indium-111 labeled platelet stain shows uptake in the nodule *(arrow)*, indicating that the nodule is a pleural deposit of splenic tissue. There is no uptake in the splenic bed *(S)* as a result of a splenectomy 15 years earlier. (Courtesy of Dr. Marie Lee, Seattle, Washington.)

droplets are 20 to 40 μm in diameter and cause occlusions in the vascular bed of the lungs and other organs. Autopsy and special clinical studies indicate that subclinical fat embolization is much more common than is generally realized.[6, 29, 32] The term "fat embolism syndrome" is often reserved for cases in which overt clinical findings are attributable to the effects of fat embolization on the lungs and other organs such as the brain, kidneys, and skin. Fat embolization may be detected by examination of the blood and urine in as many as 90% of cases following major trauma, whereas the incidence of the fat embolism syndrome in this patient group is approximately 3%.[9]

The mechanical theory of fat embolization envis-

ages disruption of fat in the soft tissues and the bone marrow. The liberated fat enters the lacerated ends of veins in the traumatized area, possibly aided by a rise in the intramedullary pressure in bone or by movement of bony fragments. Fat embolization is stated to be less common in compound or open fractures in which a rise in intramedullary pressure is less likely. Rapid immobilization of fractures, particularly early operative fixation, decreases the incidence of fat embolization.[37]

Trauma is the major cause of fat embolism syndrome. However, fat embolization may occur in the absence of trauma in a diverse series of conditions including diabetes mellitus, acute decompression sickness, chronic pancreatitis, alcoholism, burns, severe infections, sickle cell disease, inhalational anesthesia, and renal infarction.[5] A biochemical theory of fat embolization has been proposed to account for these nontraumatic cases. According to the theory, the embolic fat is derived from circulating blood lipids and from fat mobilized from fat depots. Neutral fat in the blood is normally emulsified in the form of chylomicrons, which are less than 1 μm in diameter. During the metabolic response to stress, chylomicrons may coalesce to form fat globules up to 40 μm in diameter, and these globules are capable of causing capillary occlusion.

It seems likely, however, that the deleterious effects of fat embolization are not simply a result of vascular occlusion by neutral fat.[1, 5] Hydrolysis of neutral fat by tissue lipase forms free fatty acids that have a toxic effect on the vascular endothelium and the lung parenchyma. The result is endothelial damage leading to increased capillary permeability, and damage to the alveolar lining cells leading to loss of surfactant activity and the formation of hyaline membranes. Furthermore, platelets adhere to neutral fat, and intravascular coagulation may supervene. Excessive breakdown of platelets releases vasoactive amines such as serotonin and 5-hydroxytryptamine which, together with histamine released from damaged lung parenchyma and vasoactive amines released from the injury site, cause vasospasm and pulmonary capillary congestion. The biochemical and hematologic interactions are, therefore, complex but are almost certainly crucial to the development of the fat embolism syndrome. In rare cases, acute cor pulmonale may occur within hours of the injury and is attributable to a major degree of occlusion of the pulmonary vascular bed by neutral fat.[28] A latent period of 12 to 48 hours before the fat embolism syndrome supervenes is almost invariable, and this latent period can be readily explained by the time required to hydrolize neutral fat and for the secondary vasculitis and pneumonitis to develop.

The chief clinical manifestations of the fat embolism syndrome involve the lungs, the central nervous system, and the skin. The pulmonary manifestations are generally the first to appear: within 12 to 72 hours after the trauma the patient develops dyspnea, tachypnea, and cyanosis. The arterial oxygen tension decreases to 50 mm Hg or less. At the same time the patient may develop generalized cerebral symptoms ranging from headache and irritability through delirium and stupor to seizures and coma. Focal neurologic signs are generally absent. Fundoscopic examination may reveal petechial hemorrhages. A petechial rash appears in many, but not all cases, after 2 to 3 days. This rash is distributed over the neck and trunk.

The chest radiograph broadly reflects the severity of the syndrome. The chest radiograph may remain normal in mild cases of the fat embolization syndrome; otherwise, radiographic abnormalities develop after a 12- to 72-hour latent period. The classic response is either the development of multiple focal alveolar densities or the development of a diffuse interstitial or alveolar pulmonary edema pattern. Pleural effusions are not a feature of the fat embolization syndrome. On occasion, the degree of shadowing can become remarkably severe, yet clearing generally occurs in 7 to 14 days (Fig 17–25). On the other hand, patients may develop the adult respiratory distress syndrome with prolongation of the clinical course and a significantly increased mortality. Curtis et al.,[8] in a study of 30 patients with the fat embolization syndrome, identified 10 patients

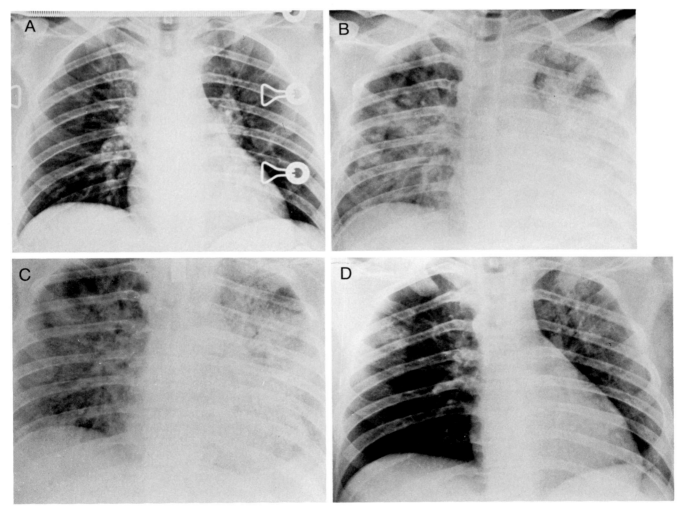

FIG 17–25.
A, admission radiograph of a young man with severe pelvic and lower extremity fractures. **B,** 72 hours later. There is severe respiratory distress with clinical evidence of the fat embolism syndrome. **C,** At 96 hours. **D,** 11 days after admission the pulmonary changes have largely regressed.

with complicating adult respiratory distress syndrome. Six of these patients died, as compared with 2 out of 18 patients with the fat embolization syndrome in an uncomplicated form. Two other patients in the series died from the effects of acute paradoxical fat embolization. All 10 patients with complicating adult respiratory distress syndrome had evidence of intravascular coagulopathy, a feature not detected in the other patients. The radiographic features of the adult respiratory distress syndrome are discussed in Chapter 8.

The development of hypoxia, particularly in a patient with a normal appearing chest radiograph, may prompt the performance of ventilation-perfusion scintigraphy. Ventilation may be expected to be normal in the fat embolism syndrome, but the perfusion scan may show multiple peripheral subsegmental defects that give the scan a diffusely mottled appearance.[33, 45] This is quite unlike the larger and more focal defects commonly associated with multiple thromboembolism.

The diagnosis of the fat embolism syndrome is based on the correlation of the clinical features, the chest radiographic appearances, and the laboratory findings, especially the results of blood gas analysis. The radiographic findings are not specific and may be found in other conditions in which trauma plays a part including pulmonary contusion, massive aspiration of gastric contents, thermal damage, toxic gas inhalation, transfusion reactions, neurogenic and other causes of pulmonary edema, and gram-negative sepsis. The latent period before the radiographic and clinical findings of the fat embolism syndrome develop is of extreme diagnostic importance. In many of the conditions mentioned, the chest radiograph is abnormal from the outset. The adult respiratory distress syndrome may supervene in any severely traumatized individual, and fat embolization as a precipitating cause may go unrecognized.

REFERENCES

1. Alho A: Fat embolism syndrome: Etiology, pathogenesis and treatment. *Acta Chir Scand* [Suppl]1980; 499:75–85.
2. Arendrup HC, Skov Jensen B: Traumatic rupture of the diaphragm. *Surg Gynecol Obstet* 1982; 154:526–530.
3. Ball T, McGory R, Smith JO, et al: Traumatic diaphragmatic hernia: Errors in diagnosis. *AJR* 1982; 138:633–637.
4. Barcia TC, Livoni JP: Indications for angiography in blunt thoracic trauma. *Radiology* 1983; 147:15–19.
5. Batra P: The fat embolism syndrome. *J Thorac Imag* 1987; 2:12–17.
6. Chan KM, Tham KT, Chiu HS, et al: Post traumatic fat embolism—its clinical and subclinical presentations. *J Trauma* 1984; 24:45–49.
7. Chesterman JT, Satsangi PN: Rupture of the trachea and bronchi by closed injury. *Thorax* 1966; 21:21–27.
8. Curtis AMcB, Knowles GD, Putman CE, et al: The three syndromes of fat embolism: Pulmonary manifestations. *Yale J Biol Med* 1979; 52:149–157.
9. Feldman F, Ellis K, Gren WM: The fat embolism syndrome. *Radiology* 1975; 114:535–542.
10. Felson B: Lung torsion: Radiographic findings in nine cases. *Radiology* 1987; 162:631–638.
11. Fisher RG, Hadlock F, Ben-Menachem Y: Laceration of the thoracic aorta and brachiocephalic arteries by blunt trauma: Report of 54 cases and review of the literature. *Radiol Clin North Am* 1981; 19:91–110.
12. Fisher RG, Ward RE, Ben-Menachem Y, et al: Arteriography and the fractured first rib: Too much for too little? *AJR* 1982; 138:1059–1062.
13. Gazak S, Davidson SJ: Posterior sternoclavicular dislocations: Two case reports. *J Trauma* 1984; 24:80–82.
14. Gerlock AJ, Muhletaler CA, Coulam CM, et al: Traumatic aortic aneurysm: Validity of esophageal tube displacement sign. *AJR* 1980; 135:713–718.
15. Guest JL, Anderson JN: Major airway injury in closed chest trauma. *Chest* 1977; 72:63–66.
16. Gundry SR, Williams S, Burney RE, et al: Indications for aortography. Radiography after blunt chest trauma: A reassessment of the radiographic findings associated with traumatic rupture of the aorta. *Invest Radiol* 1983; 18:230–237.
17. Harvey-Smith W, Bush W, Northrop C: Traumatic bronchial rupture. *AJR* 1980; 134:1189–1193.
18. Heiberg E, Wolverson MK, Hard RN, et al: CT recognition of traumatic rupture of the diaphragm. *AJR* 1980; 135:369–372.
19. Heiberg E, Wolverson MK. Sundaram M, et al: CT in aortic trauma. *AJR* 1983; 140:1119–1124.
20. Hood RM, Sloan HE: Injuries of the trachea and major bronchi. *J Thorac Cardiovasc Surg* 1959; 38:458–480.
21. Kermond AJ: The dislocated heart. An unusual complication of major chest injury. *Radiology* 1976; 119:59–60.
22. Kleinman PK: Bony thoracic trauma, in Kleinman PK (ed): *Diagnostic Imaging of Child Abuse*. Baltimore, Williams & Wilkins Co, 1987, pp 67–90.
23. Lotz PR, Martel W, Rohwedder JL, et al: Significance of pneumomediastinum in blunt trauma to the thorax. *AJR* 1979; 132:817–819.
24. Mahboubi S, O'Hara AE: Bronchial rupture in children following blunt chest trauma. *Pediatr Radiol* 1981; 10:133–138.
25. Marnocha KE, Maglinte DDT: Plain-film criteria for excluding aortic rupture in blunt chest trauma. *AJR* 1985; 144:19–21.

26. Marsh DG, Sturm JT: Traumatic aortic rupture: Roentgenographic indications for angiography. *Ann Thorac Surg* 1976; 21:337–340.

27. Martin N, Bollaert PE, Bauer P, et al: Two case reports of pulmonary blast injury. *Cah Anesthesiol* 1987; 35:133–137.

28. Mayron R, Ruiz E, Meslitz ST, et al: Tissue-fat pulmonary embolism occurring in a patient with a severe pelvic fracture. *J Emerg Med* 1985; 2:251–256.

29. McCarthy B, Mammen E, Leblanc LP, et al: Subclinical fat embolism: A prospective study of 50 patients with extremity fractures. *J Trauma* 1973; 13:9–16.

30. Morgan AS, Flanchbaum L, Esposito T, et al: Blunt trauma to the diaphragm: An analysis of 44 patients. *J Trauma* 1986; 26:565–567.

31. Oh KS, Fleischner FG, Wyman SM: Characteristic pulmonary finding in traumatic complete transection of a main stem bronchus. *Radiology* 1969; 92:371–372.

32. Palmovic V, McCarroll JR: Fat embolism in trauma. *Arch Pathol* 1965; 80:630–635.

33. Park HM, Ducret RP, Brindley DC: Pulmonary imaging in fat embolism syndrome. *Clin Nucl Med* 1986; 11:521–522.

34. Peters DR, Gamsu G: Displacement of the right paraspinous interface: A radiographic sign of acute traumatic rupture of the thoracic aorta. *Radiology* 1980; 134:599–603.

35. Resnick D: Disorders of other endocrine glands and of pregnancy, in Resnick D, Niwayama G (eds): *Diagnosis of Bone and Joint Disorders*, ed 2. Philadelphia, WB Saunders Co, 1988, pp 2287–2317.

36. Rich NM, Spencer FC: *Vascular Trauma*. Philadelphia, WB Saunders Co, 1978, pp 425–440.

37. Riska EB, Myllynen P: Fat embolism in patients with multiple injuries. *J Trauma* 1982; 22:891–894.

38. Rodriguez-Morales G, Rodriguez A, Shatney CH: Acute rupture of the diaphragm in blunt trauma: Analysis of 60 patients. *J Trauma* 1986; 26:438–444.

39. Scales FE, Lee ME: Non-operative diagnosis of intrathoracic splenosis. *AJR* 1983, 141:1273–1274.

40. Seltzer SE, D'Orsi C, Kirshner R, et al: Traumatic aortic rupture: Plain radiographic findings. *AJR* 1981; 137:1011–1014.

41. Shafer N, Wilkenfeld M, Shafer R: Gunshot wounds, in Wecht C (ed): *Legal Medicine*. Philadelphia, WB Saunders Co, 1982, pp 1–19.

42. Simeone JF, Deren MM, Cagle F: The value of the left apical cap in the diagnosis of aortic rupture. *Radiology* 1981; 139:35–37.

43. Tisnado J, Tsai FY, Alo A, et al: A new radiographic sign of acute traumatic rupture of the thoracic aorta: Displacement of the nasogastric tube to the right. *Radiology* 1977; 125:603–608.

44. Toombs BD, Sandler CM, Lester RG: Computed tomography of chest trauma. *Radiology* 1981; 140:733–738.

45. Williams AG, Mettler FA, Christie JH, et al: Fat embolism syndrome. *Clin Nucl Med* 1986; 11:495–497.

46. Williams JR, Stembridge VA: Pulmonary contusion secondary to non-penetrating chest trauma. *AJR* 1964; 91:284–290.

47. Woodring JH, Dillon ML: Radiographic manifestations of mediastinal hemorrhage from blunt chest trauma. *Ann Thorac Surg* 1984; 37:171–178.

48. Woodring JH, Fried AM, Hatfield DR, et al: Fractures of first and second ribs: Predictive value for arterial and bronchial injury. *AJR* 1982; 138:211–215.

Percutaneous Needle Biopsy and Percutaneous Empyema Drainage

Although percutaneous needle biopsy (PNB) is the procedure of choice for assessing a wide range of focal pulmonary processes, the procedure itself is not a recent development. Leyden diagnosed pneumonia by this method in 1883,[56] and Ménétier used it to diagnose lung cancer in 1886.[24] Martin and Ellis perfected the aspiration technique in 1934,[57] and several large series were reported subsequently.[20, 32] The major difficulty these early investigators encountered was imprecise placement of large needles, which caused unacceptably high rates of hemorrhage and pneumothorax.[40] The development of image intensification helped overcome the problem of accurate placement.[53] Subsequent refinements in cytopathologic diagnosis, together with the pioneering work of the Scandinavians in developing smallbore fine aspirating needles, have modernized the technique and allowed its widespread use today.[21, 23, 69, 70]

In this chapter the present state of percutaneous transthoracic biopsy of the lung, mediastinum, and hilus will be briefly reviewed. The discussion also includes a brief overview of percutaneous catheter drainage of fluid collections in the chest.

NEEDLES

There is an extensive choice of needles for PNB. The needles range in size from 16- or 17-gauge core-cutting needles[31, 55] to 22- to 23-gauge "fine"

needles for aspiration.[15, 106] The screw-type[72] or coaxial types[36, 92] are also commonly used. Recently a dual cutting edge 20-gauge needle has shown promising results.[97] The general rule is to use the smallest diameter needle possible because higher complication rates have resulted from use of the larger bore needles.[39, 77]

At the University of Virginia we generally use the 22- or 23-gauge Chiba aspiration needles for most lung biopsies because of their high yield and low complication rate.[83] To ensure the best results one must, however, have appropriate case selection, good cooperation between the radiologist and the referring pulmonologists or thoracic surgeons, and excellent cytopathologic facilities.

EQUIPMENT AND GUIDANCE

There are three major guidance techniques for PNB: fluoroscopy, computed tomography, and ultrasound. Fluoroscopy is by far the most commonly employed method. It is quicker and cheaper than the other techniques and, with high-quality image intensification, permits biopsy of almost any mediastinal or thoracic lesion, including parenchymal masses of 1 cm or larger (Fig 18–1).[49, 50] A biplane fluoroscopic system or some form of C-arm fluoroscope with good resolution is best. The major requirement is that the system have sufficient resolution to verify the position of small-caliber needles.

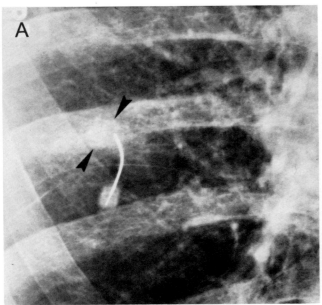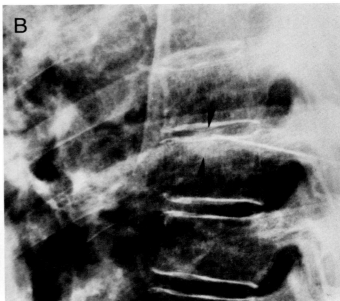

FIG 18–1.
A, anteroposterior (AP) fluoroscopic film of 22-gauge needle in the lateral aspect of a 1-cm nodule *(arrowheads).* **B,** lateral fluoroscopic film confirms position of the needle tip within the lesion *(ar-* *rowheads).* Cytologic study showed well-differentiated adenocarcinoma. We routinely document needle position with films.

Some investigators prefer computed tomographic (CT) scanning as an alternative means of guiding biopsy. CT-guided biopsy is indicated in the evaluation of small perihilar lesions, para-aortic and paramediastinal masses, aortopulmonary lesions, and lesions too small to be seen at fluoroscopy.[19, 33] CT can also be used to ensure placement of the tip of a needle within the wall of a necrotic cavity.[34] Drawbacks to the use of CT are that it is more expensive and time-consuming than fluoroscopy. Also, there is a slightly higher incidence of pneumothorax, presumably because the needle remains in the lung longer.[28] We reserve CT guidance for central lesions near vessels and small parenchymal masses that cannot be adequately seen fluoroscopically.

Real-time sonography is almost exclusively used to guide biopsies of peripheral chest wall or pleural lesions.[16, 45, 46]

TECHNIQUE

Prior to the use of PNB, the plain chest radiograph, CT scan, and any other available diagnostic information should be carefully reviewed to document the necessity of the examination and to decide which guidance technique is most appropriate. In dealing with a solitary noncalcified pulmonary nodule, it is imperative to obtain old images to check for growth and stability of the lesion. Stability of size over a 2-year period is usually a sign of benignity.[67]

We use minimal prebiopsy preparation, stipulating only that the patient not eat or drink after midnight the day before the study. We prefer, but do not routinely require, recent coagulation studies.

A radiologist explains the inherent risks of the procedure to the patient. The major risks discussed are pneumothorax, hemoptysis, and the possible need for chest tube insertion. We rarely premedicate our patients but have, on occasion, used mild sedatives for nervous individuals.

In the fluoroscopy suite, the lesion must be localized in both the AP and lateral projections. If it is a parenchymal nodule, it must be large enough to see (generally >1 cm in diameter) (see Fig 18–1). Once the lesion is identified, the most appropriate approach is determined, and the entrance site is marked before standard preparation with iodine and alcohol. Prior to needle insertion we always make sure that chest tube drainage systems are readily available in case a tension pneumothorax develops.

We then anesthetize the entrance site down to the pleura with 1% Xylocaine. A narrowly coned fluoroscopic beam is used to position the needle. The entry site should be far enough below the inferior border of the rib to avoid the neurovascular bundle. We first use the standard 22-gauge aspiration needle, selecting the needle length according to the depth of the lesion. The gloved hand or sterile forceps can be used to guide the puncture, although a commercially available needle holder is an acceptable, more expensive, alternative.[72]

The patient is warned of the impending pleural puncture and asked to try to suspend breathing without coughing. Breath holding is very important to the success of the procedure and is one of the reasons we do not premedicate our patients. Under fluoroscopic control, the needle is advanced directly toward the lesion. Once the needle is through the pleural layers, the patient is told to take quiet, shallow breaths.

The pulmonary parenchyma has a characteristic "spider web" consistency. Needle contact with the nodule can often be recognized by a smoother, more "solid" feel. Once the needle enters the lesion, placement is confirmed by fluoroscopy and can be documented by spot films if desired (see Fig 18–1). The stylet is removed while the patient suspends respiration, the needle opening being covered by the finger at all times to avoid possible air embolism. The plunger of the syringe is pulled back to aspirate material into the lumen of the needle. The aspirate is obtained by a gentle 1- to 2-cm up-and-down movement of the needle while suction is maintained. Negative pressure is released before the needle is withdrawn, and the aspirate is immediately fixed with 95% alcohol (ETOH). (The slides are prepared for us by a cytotechnologist who comes into the procedure room.) Air-dried specimens are also prepared in selected cases. The aspirate is fixed and stained in a standard manner in the pathology department and, if no malignant cells are seen, a filter of the washings of material trapped in the needle is prepared for viewing the next day.[26]

We routinely make as many as three passes into the lesion at each biopsy session, checking for pneumothorax after each pass. If no complications develop in the patient, a follow-up chest film is obtained in 4 hours. If no complications have developed by this time, outpatients are discharged, since further problems are unlikely (see "Complications of Percutaneous Needle Biopsy" later in this chapter).[73] We do not routinely instill a coagulant after the final pass, although this procedure has been suggested as a means of decreasing the rate of pneumothorax.[82]

If the aspirate does not show disease we occasionally repeat the PNB procedure the following day. This procedure has been recommended for optimum results.[100]

INDICATIONS FOR PERCUTANEOUS NEEDLE BIOPSY

The indications for PNB fall into three basic categories: diagnosing primary or metastatic cancer, diagnosing infection, and proving benignity. The need to evaluate a solitary noncalcified pulmonary nodule is probably the most frequent reason for PNB. In our experience, parenchymal lesions less than 1 cm in diameter are generally too small for successful biopsy. If the lesion is not clearly seen in both projections, we may use CT, either as the method of guidance or to define the depth of a nodule prior to performing a fluoroscopically guided biopsy. A nodule adjacent to the pleural surface is technically the easiest to investigate because of its close proximity to the chest wall.

In some instances, even if the lesion is large, its anatomic location may prevent successful biopsy. Nodules located in the lower lobes may move considerably because of diaphragmatic excursion, making the procedure more difficult. If the nodule is located posteriorly beneath the scapula, access to it may be limited, especially in older patients with limited mobility. And, of course, the uncooperative patient unable to listen to and comply with instructions may make PNB difficult regardless of the lesion's size or location.

The presence of multiple pulmonary nodules is another common reason for performing PNB. Generally the patient has a history of a primary malignancy, and biopsy is intended to confirm the clinical suspicion of metastatic disease. Although the yield of PNB in this clinical circumstance has been reported to be as low as 37.5%,[18, 105] other authors have reported 90% to 95% true positive samples in assessing metastases.[37, 40] The most accessible nodule is chosen for biopsy, either the largest one or the one nearest the pleural surface. The procedure is then identical to that for the solitary nodule. Extrapleural masses secondary to metastatic disease or myeloma are also easily sampled by PNB. The procedure in these cases does not carry the same risk of pneumothorax because the parenchyma does not have to be violated (see Fig 18–3).

The presence of hilar or mediastinal masses is another common indication for PNB.* All patients in whom such masses are suspected should have a CT examination prior to biopsy in order to delineate the exact anatomic location and characteristics of the mass. The choice of guidance technique can then be

---

*References 1, 66, 70, 71, 74, 98, 101, and 103.

made. We prefer to use fluoroscopy, when practicable, to guide the biopsy procedure because of its ease and quickness (Fig 18–2). CT guidance is preferred in evaluating hilar lesions near vessels, very small masses, or lesions for which a previous fluoroscopically guided biopsy has shown no disease.[33]

The biopsy technique is similar to that for investigating pulmonary nodules. Film documentation of the position of the needle tip within the lesion is imperative for best results (Fig 18–3). Large mediastinal masses may allow the use of larger cutting needles where necessary.[66]

In cases of suspected lymphoma, however, it may be preferable to bypass PNB and perform mediastinoscopy. The reason is that, although PNB may enable one to diagnose malignancy, the material it provides for cytologic evaluation may be insufficient to permit adequate subclassification for planning therapy (see "Results of Percutaneous Needle Biopsy" later in this chapter).[27, 99, 103]

Solitary or multiple pulmonary abnormalities suspicious for infection are also indications for PNB. These may be cavitary lesions, chronic infiltrates unresponsive to antibiotic therapy, or new focal pulmonary shadowing in the immunocompromised host.[6, 7, 10, 13, 14, 65, 76] Cavitating lesions are more challenging because the best results are obtained when the needle tip is within the wall of the lesion and not within the necrotic center. In such cases, CT guidance or bronchoscopy with endobronchial washings have been reported to be highly successful.[34]

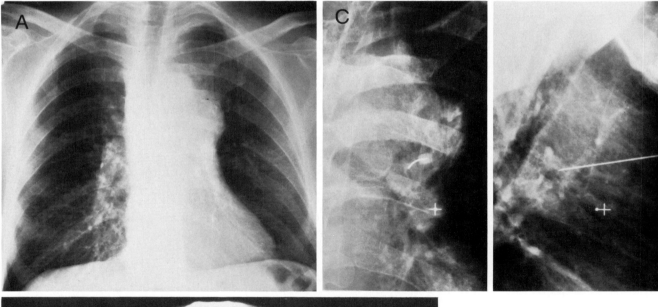

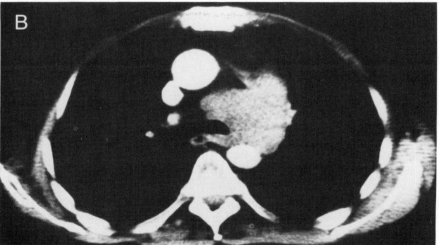

FIG 18–2.
A, posteroanterior (PA) radiograph of a 55-year-old smoker showing large mass in the region of the aortopulmonary window. **B,** CT scan confirms the presence of a large noncalcified mass. **C,** AP *(left)* and lateral *(right)* fluoroscopic spot films show the tip of the needle to be within the mass, which proved to be undifferentiated adenocarcinoma on cytologic examination. We routinely use fluoroscopy if possible because of its quickness, ease, and lower complication rate.

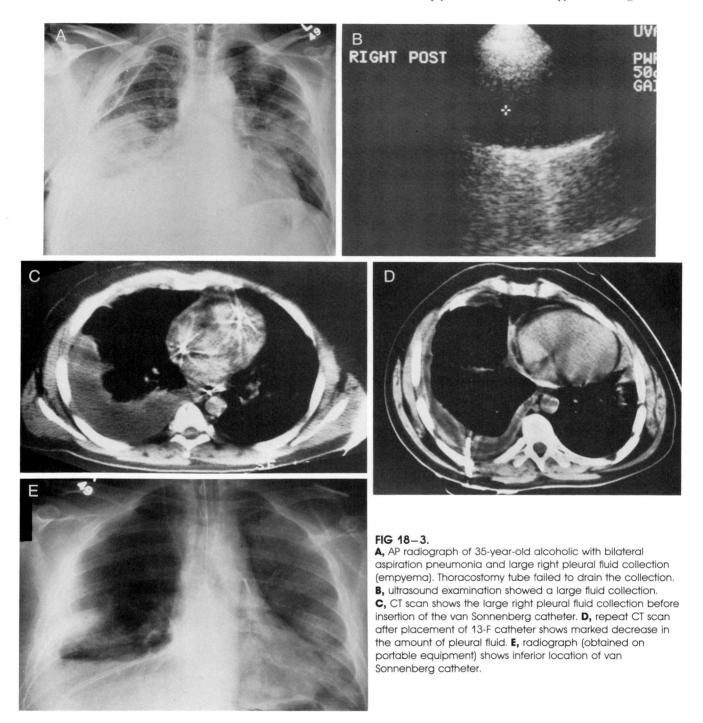

FIG 18–3.
A, AP radiograph of 35-year-old alcoholic with bilateral aspiration pneumonia and large right pleural fluid collection (empyema). Thoracostomy tube failed to drain the collection. **B,** ultrasound examination showed a large fluid collection. **C,** CT scan shows the large right pleural fluid collection before insertion of the van Sonnenberg catheter. **D,** repeat CT scan after placement of 13-F catheter shows marked decrease in the amount of pleural fluid. **E,** radiograph (obtained on portable equipment) shows inferior location of van Sonnenberg catheter.

CONTRAINDICATIONS TO LUNG BIOPSY

The only absolute contraindication to PNB is inability of the patient to cooperate well enough for the examination to be performed.

Other risk factors are only relative contraindications that should be weighed against the potential benefits of PNB (Table 18–1). The person with advanced chronic obstructive pulmonary disease is at a higher risk and needs to be appropriately informed. Coagulopathy is a relative contraindication to biopsy. If there is only a vague history of bruising or bleeding in an otherwise healthy patient, we do not require coagulation studies if we plan to employ the

TABLE 18–1.

Contraindications to Percutaneous Needle Biopsy

Absolute
 Uncooperative patient
Relative
 Advanced chronic obstructive pulmonary disease
 Coagulopathy
 Pulmonary arterial hypertension
 History of pneumonectomy

TABLE 18–2.

Reported Complications of Percutaneous Needle Biopsy

Pneumothorax
Pneumomediastinum
Heimlich valve placement
Thoracostomy tube placement
Air embolism
Hemorrhage around lesion
Minor/major hemoptysis
Hemothorax
Cardiac tamponade
Mediastinal widening
 (hematoma)
Tumor embolism
Tumor implantation of biopsy
 tract
Bronchopleural fistula
Empyema

22-gauge needle. If the patient is thrombocytopenic or on anticoagulants, we usually require coagulation studies, but unless these are markedly abnormal we will still attempt biopsy because of the low risk of serious bleeding with the small aspirating needles. If we plan to use the larger cutting needles, we routinely require appropriate coagulation studies before biopsy because of the higher risk of bleeding.

Pulmonary arterial hypertension has been viewed as a contraindication to PNB. It is a significant risk in patients with hilar lesions in whom the chance of hitting a vascular structure is greatest. However, inadvertent placement of a needle into vascular structures has not proved dangerous in some documented cases, especially when small needles are used.[52]

Finally, a prior history of pneumonectomy is a relative contraindication to PNB. But the procedure can still be undertaken in these patients if one is adequately prepared for the complications with appropriate chest tubes, valves, and water seals.

Regardless of the contraindication, both the referring physician and the radiologist must evaluate each patient in order to achieve the best clinical result. Cooperation and communication are of the utmost importance in ensuring the best diagnostic route and optimum patient care.[17]

COMPLICATIONS OF PERCUTANEOUS NEEDLE BIOPSY

Table 18–2 provides a comprehensive list of complications reported in the literature.[2, 52, 58, 61] Complication rates from pulmonary biopsy are much lower now than they were when the technique was first described, primarily because the development of new cytopathologic techniques has allowed the use of smaller caliber aspirating needles. The exact risk of complication in the individual patient varies with the clinical situation. For instance, a young nonsmoker would not run the same risk as the elderly smoker with advanced emphysema.

Pneumothorax is the most common complication of PNB and occurs in about 20% of cases.[8] However, the rate of pneumothorax has been reported to be as high as 49% in some series of elderly and high-risk patients.[9] A higher pneumothorax rate also accompanies use of the larger caliber needles.[39] Instilling a coagulant at the termination of the procedure has been reported to decrease the pneumothorax rate when the larger core coaxial needles are used.[60, 95] Approximately one in ten patients will require chest tube insertion for pneumothorax. Some authors have suggested that the risk of pneumothorax markedly increases when there is evidence of chronic obstructive pulmonary disease on the chest radiograph and obstructive airway disease on pulmonary function tests.[29]

Whenever PNB is performed, the radiologist must be prepared to place a chest tube. We always have appropriate catheters and a Heimlich valve* or water seal readily available in case a complication develops.[87] Immediate chest tube placement is necessary in patients with pneumothorax who become hypoxic or in the rare case of tension pneumothorax.

Even if no complications occur immediately, subsequent development of a pneumothorax remains a major risk. For inpatients we require close monitoring of symptoms and vital signs for 2 to 4 hours after the patient returns to bed. A follow-up radiograph of the chest is also taken 4 hours after the procedure regardless of the clinical picture. Outpatients are required to remain in the department for

*Heimlich Valve Chest Drain, Bard Parker Division of Becton-Dickinson Co., Rutherford, N.J.; TPT-1 Set. Cook, Inc., Bloomington, Ind.; Sacks Catheter, Electro-Catheter Corporation, Rahway, NJ.

4 hours following the procedure to permit close monitoring of vital signs. If a chest x-ray 4 hours after the biopsy shows no pneumothorax, the patient is discharged provided he or she is accompanied by an adult.[73, 87]

Bleeding is the other important complication of PNB. Hemoptysis, often preceded by cough, is usually minor and occurs in about 10% of cases. If hemoptysis does occur, the patient is placed in the lateral decubitus position with the biopsy side down to try to prevent blood from being aspirated into the unaffected lung. Massive hemoptysis is extremely rare.[39, 64, 100] Hemorrhage around the lesion occurs in approximately one in 20 patients. It is a significant problem in the examination of solitary pulmonary lesions because the exact site of the nodule may be obscured for subsequent passes. However, there is no association between this phenomenon and subsequent hemoptysis. Cardiac tamponade from bleeding into the pericardium has also been reported after PNB but is very rare.[51]

Other reported complications of PNB include air embolism, aspiration, infection, pneumomediastinum or mediastinal widening—especially with mediastinal and hilar lesions—and seeding of malignant cells along the needle tract.[2, 3, 54, 61] In early series in which large-bore needles were used, death was reported in up to 1% of patients.[39] Only one death has been reported when needles of 20 gauge or smaller were used.[64]

RESULTS OF PERCUTANEOUS NEEDLE BIOPSY

The overall reported yield of percutaneous mediastinal and pulmonary parenchymal biopsy for suspected carcinoma is difficult to determine because the results depend on patient selection, needle size, and the guidance system used. The size and location of the lesion, the experience of the radiologist, and the expertise of the cytotechnologist and cytopathologist are also factors. The results of the larger series will be reviewed here.*

Biopsy yields adequate cytologic material for diagnosis in approximately 90% of patients with parenchymal nodules. Some authors advocate repeating the biopsy the following day to further increase this yield.[100] The yield—that is, a true positive diagnosis of lung carcinoma in patients with lung carcinoma—ranges from 78%[90] to 99%.[75] In most centers the yield will be between 85% and 95%. Berquist

*References 9, 30, 47, 75, 80, 88, 90, 100, 101, and 103.

et al. reported a significantly diminished yield in central pulmonary parenchymal lesions and in those less than 2 cm in diameter.[9] Most of their patients were elderly, and biopsy was performed primarily for suspected metastatic disease. On the other hand, Sinner reported a yield of 97% in lesions less than 2 cm in diameter.[81] The false positive rate for malignancy is low, ranging from zero to 2%.

Those lesions that cytologists interpret as "negative for malignant disease" can be divided into two groups: (1) nodules in which a specific benign diagnosis is offered (e.g., hamartoma, infarct, and granulomatous infection); and (2) nodules in which no malignant cells are seen, but for which no specific diagnosis can be offered. In one large series, a specific benign diagnosis was made in only 16 of the 132 patients in whom the initial interpretation was "no malignant cells seen." One of these nodules was ultimately found to be a lung cancer. Furthermore, in 38 (29%) of the 132 patients, the nodule that was aspirated ultimately proved to be a malignant tumor.[11]

Therefore, if a specific benign diagnosis is established and the clinical suspicion of cancer is low, the patient may be followed with periodic chest films at 1-, 3-, 6-, and 12-month intervals for 5 years.[103] If a nonspecific benign cytologic diagnosis is made, the biopsy can be repeated.[35, 40, 80, 100] In a series of 422 patients reviewed by Westcott, 105 patients had "negative" cytologic evidence at the initial reading but, after repeat biopsy, 37 (35%) of the lesions were interpreted as malignant, which decreased the overall false negative rate from 14.3% to 1.7%.[100] The important message here is that a nonspecific benign result of PNB does not exclude carcinoma and that in any group of patients at high risk for cancer, a significant proportion of patients will, in fact, have lung cancer.[11]

With mediastinal and hilar masses, the reported rates of true positive diagnosis for suspected carcinoma or thymoma range from 85% to 95%.[1, 33, 66, 98, 101, 103] The specific benign diagnostic rate is about 30%.[86] The principal difficulty in dealing with mediastinal lesions is in the diagnosis of lymphoma, the positive diagnostic yield by PNB being only 65% to 75%.[101, 103] The most difficult lesions for the cytologist to classify are well-differentiated lymphoma and nodular sclerosing Hodgkin's disease. Larger bore needles, mediastinoscopy, and even open biopsy may be required for definitive diagnosis.[66]

PNB has been used by some investigators to obtain material for the diagnosis of pulmonary inflammatory disease.[6, 10, 13, 14, 65, 76] The best results have been obtained by Castellino and Blank, who reported a 73% diagnostic yield for focal infections in the immunocompromised host.[13]

PERCUTANEOUS DRAINAGE OF PLEURAL FLUID COLLECTIONS

Historically, fluid collections in the chest have been treated with a combination of medical and surgical methods. Lung abscesses were first treated with a course of antibiotics; if medical therapy failed they were then removed by thoracotomy and resection.[38, 104] Chronic sterile pleural fluid collections were generally drained by blind insertion of a thoracostomy tube. Without guidance other than anatomic landmarks, catheter malpositioning and inadequate drainage[63, 84] posed significant problems. Empyemas were even more difficult management problems, being usually treated with antibiotics, thoracentesis, drainage by thoracostomy tube, or operative removal.[59, 62] Blind placement of the thoracostomy tube, however, often results in incorrect placement with inadequate drainage.[58, 96] Surgery involves either rib resection with drainage or open removal of the fluid collection, and the potential morbidity of this procedure and general anesthesia, especially in the relatively unstable patient, carries significant risks.[42, 44, 78]

Radiographically directed percutaneous drainage for thoracic fluid collections emerged as a rational alternative to these standard surgical and medical therapies as a result of the refinement in angiographic interventional techniques. These procedures are now routinely performed in the pleural space, and several recent papers have reported excellent results with this technique in the management of lung abscesses and empyemas.[4, 43, 48, 79, 91, 94, 102]

Technique

Before deciding how to treat a collection in the chest, the first responsibility of the radiologist is to determine whether the fluid is within the pleural cavity or in the lung.[12, 22, 68, 93] Once the fluid has been determined to lie in the chest, the radiologist can use fluoroscopy, ultrasound, or CT scanning to guide the procedure. Because CT scanning is the most common technique reported in the literature, it will be stressed here. However, the other two methods may be used just as satisfactorily for most purposes.

The first step is to insert a small (20- to 21-gauge) needle into the fluid and aspirate some of the contents for microscopic evaluation and culture. The needle can be exchanged for a catheter or needle of sufficient bore to accept a standard J-tipped guidewire. This J guidewire is inserted and positioned so that it is in the most dependent portion of the collection. The guidewire is then used to position the appropriate catheter, which should preferably be a non-sump catheter, after progressive expansion of the site using dilators (see Fig 18–3).

The specific catheter used depends on the size and nature of the fluid collection. Small, nonviscous collections can generally be drained with the smaller catheters (8 to 12 F) which are better tolerated by the patient. Larger or more viscous collections will require catheters as large as 16 F to drain the space adequately. Catheter clotting by proteinacious fluid can be a significant problem if too small a catheter is chosen (Fig 18–4).

It is best to coil some of the catheter within the cavity, ensuring that the sideholes are in appropriate position before suturing the catheter to the skin surface. In the supine position, the catheter should be in the most dependent position within the cavity. The catheter is sutured to the skin with a Molnar disc, and the end of the catheter is then attached to a Pleur-evac Waterseal System* to allow continuous suction. A CT scan is then obtained to confirm the exact position of the catheter tip and the amount and location of any residual fluid.

In experienced hands the success rate of image-guided drainage is successful in 70% to 90% of patients. Approximately 10% of patients may require a thoracostomy tube as a supplemental procedure for adequate drainage. Complications are rare; pain, catheter clotting, and bleeding have been reported most frequently.[4, 43, 48, 79, 91, 94, 102] However, more serious sequelae such as fatal hemorrhage and hepatopleural fistulae have been reported when the pleural space is inadvertently entered during intra-abdominal drainage procedures.[12, 22, 68, 93]

In summary, percutaneous catheter drainage of pleural fluid collections is a simple, safe procedure. Its excellent overall success rate has made it an acceptable and reliable alternative to surgical intervention for treating pleural and pulmonary collections, especially in the unstable or high-risk population.

*Cook, Inc. Bloomington, Ind.; Howmedica, Queens Village, N.Y.

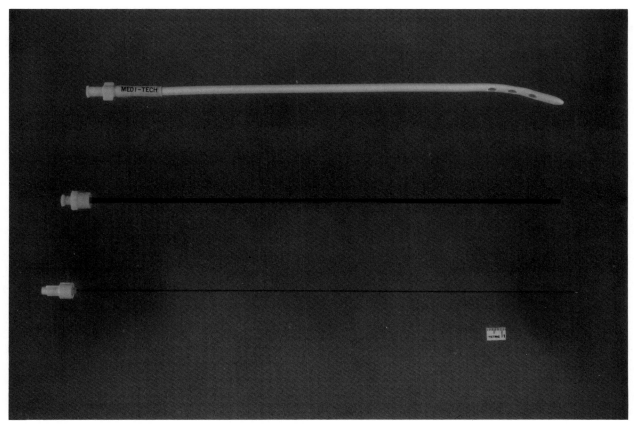

FIG 18–4.
van Sonnenberg chest catheter *(top)* , trocar *(middle)*, and introducing needle *(bottom)*.

REFERENCES

1. Adler OB, Rosenberg A, Peleg H: Fine-needle aspiration of mediastinal masses: Evaluation of 136 experiences. *AJR* 1983; 140:893–896.

2. Allison DJ: Needle biopsy of the lung. *Br J Radiol* 1978; 51:70.

3. Allison DJ, Hemingway AP: Percutaneous needle biopsy of the lung. *Br Med J* 1981; 282:875–878.

4. Aronberg DJ, Sagel SS, Jost RG, et al: Percutaneous drainage of lung abscess. *AJR* 1979; 132:282–283.

5. Baber CE, Hedlund LW, Oddson TA, et al: Differentiating empyemas and abscesses. *Radiology* 1980; 135:755–758.

6. Bandt PH, Blank N, Castellino RA: Needle diagnosis of pneumonitis: Value in high risk patients. *JAMA* 1972; 220:1578–1580.

7. Batra P, Wallace JM, Ovenfors CO: Efficacy and complications of transthoracic needle biopsy of lung in patients with pneumocystis carinii pneumonia and AIDS. *J Thorac Imag* 1987; 2:79–80.

8. Bernardino M: Percutaneous biopsy. *AJR* 1984; 142:41–45.

9. Berquist TH, Bailey PB, Cortese DA, et al: Transthoracic needle biopsy. Accuracy and complications in relation to location and type of lesion. *Mayo Clin Proc* 1980; 55:475–481.

10. Burt ME, Flye MW, Webber BL, et al: Prospective evaluation of aspiration needle, cutting needle, transbronchial, and open lung biopsy in patients with pulmonary infiltrates. *Ann Thorac Surg* 1981; 32:146–153.

11. Calhoun P, Feldman PS, Armstrong P, et al: The clinical outcome of needle aspirations of the lung when cancer is not diagnosed. *J Thorac Surg* 1986; 41:592.

12. Carrasco CH, Zornoza J, Bechtel WJ: Malignant biliary obstruction: Complications of percutaneous biliary drainage. *Radiology* 1984; 152:343–346.

13. Castellino R, Blank N: Etiologic diagnosis of focal pulmonary infection in immunocompromised patients by fluoroscopically guided percutaneous needle aspiration. *Radiology* 1979; 132:563–567.

14. Chaudhary S, Hughes WT, Feldman S, et al: Percutaneous transthoracic needle aspiration of the lung. *Am J Dis Child* 1974; 131:902–907.

15. Chin WS, Yee IS: Percutaneous aspiration biopsy of

malignant lung lesions using the Chiba needle. An initial experience. *Clin Radiol* 1978; 29:617.

16. Cinti D, Hawkins HB: Aspiration biopsy of peripheral pulmonary masses using real-time sonographic guidance. *AJR* 1984; 142:1115–1116.

17. Conces DJ Jr, Schwenk GR Jr, Doering PR, et al: Thoracic needle biopsy: Improved results utilizing the team approach. *Chest* 1987; 91:813.

18. Cortese DA, McDougall JC: Biopsy and brushing of peripheral lung cancer with fluoroscopic guidance. *Chest* 1979; 75:141–145.

19. Costello P, Duszlak EJ, Clouse ME: CT-guided biopsy: A simplified approach. *J Comput Tomogr* 1982; 6:40–42.

20. Craver LF, Binkley S: Aspiration biopsy of tumours of the lung. *J Thorac Surg* 1939; 8:439.

21. Dahlgren S, Nordenstrom B: *Transthoracic Needle Biopsy.* Chicago, Year Book Medical Publishers, 1966.

22. Dawson SL, Neff CC, Mueller PR, et al: Fatal hemorrhage after inadvertent transpleural biliary drainage. *AJR* 1983; 141:33–34.

23. Deeley TJ: *Needle Biopsy.* Glasgow, Scotland, Butterworth and Co, 1974.

24. Dick R, Heard BE, Hinson KFW, et al: Aspiration needle biopsy of thoracic lesions: An assessment of 227 biopsies. *Br J Dis Chest* 1974; 68:86.

25. Dwyer A: The displaced crus: A sign for distinguishing pleural fluid and ascites on computed tomography. *J Comput Assist Tomogr* 1978; 2:598–599.

26. Dziura BR: Fine needle aspiration of the lung: A pathologist's perspective. *J Thorac Imag* 1987; 2:49–51.

27. Erwin BC, Brynes RK, Chan WC, et al: Percutaneous needle biopsy in the diagnosis and classification of lymphoma. *Cancer* 1986; 57:1974–1078.

28. Fink I, Gamsu G, Harter LP: CT-guided aspiration biopsy of the thorax. *J Comput Assist Tomogr* 1982; 6:958–962.

29. Fish GD, Stanley JH, Miller KS, et al: Postbiopsy pneumothorax: Estimating the risk by chest radiography and pulmonary function tests. *AJR* 1988; 150:71–74.

30. Flower CDR, Verney GI: Percutaneous needle biopsy of thoracic lesions—an evaluation of 300 biopsies. *Clin Radiol* 1979; 30:215–218.

31. Frauseen CC: Aspiration biopsy with a description of a new type of needle. *N Engl J Med* 1941; 224:1054.

32. Gledhill E, Spriggs JB, Binford CH: Needle aspiration in the diagnosis of lung carcinoma. Report of experience with 75 aspirations. *Am J Clin Pathol* 1949; 19:235.

33. Gobien RP, Skucas J, Paris BS: CT-assisted fluoroscopically guided aspiration biopsy of central hilar and mediastinal masses. *Radiology* 1981; 141:443–447.

34. Gobien RP, Stanley JH, Vujic I, et al: Thoracic biopsy: CT guidance of thin-needle aspiration. *AJR* 1984; 142:827–830.

35. Gobien RP, Valicenti JF, Paris BS, et al: Thin-needle aspiration biopsy: Methods of increasing the accuracy of a negative prediction. *Radiology* 1982; 145:603–605.

36. Greene R: Transthoracic needle aspiration biopsy, in Athanasoulis CA (ed): *Interventional Radiology.* Philadelphia, WB Saunders Co, 1982, pp 587–634.

37. Haaga JR, LiPuma JP, Bryan PH, et al: Clinical comparison of small- and large-caliber cutting needles for biopsy. *Radiology* 1983; 146:665–667.

38. Hagan JL, Hardy JD: Lung abscess revisited. *Ann Surg* 1983; 197:755–762.

39. Herman PG, Hessel SJ: The diagnostic accuracy and complications of closed lung biopsies. *Radiology* 1977; 125:11.

40. House AJS: Biopsy techniques in the investigation of diseases of the lung, mediastinum, and chest wall. *Radiol Clin North Am* 1979; 17:393–412.

41. House AJ, Thomson KR: Evaluation of a new transthoracic needle for biopsy of benign and malignant lung lesions. *AJR* 1977; 129:215–220.

42. Humphrey EW: Therapy of acute empyema. *Surgery* 1966; 59:661–662.

43. Hunnam GR, Flower CDR: Radiologically-guided percutaneous catheter drainage of empyemas. *Clin Radiol* 1988; 39:121–126.

44. Ibarra-Pérez C, Selman-Lama M: Diagnosis and treatment of amebic "empyema." Report of eighty-eight cases. *Am J Surg* 1977; 134:283–287.

45. Ikezoe J, Sone S, Higashihara T, et al: Sonographically guided needle biopsy for diagnosis of thoracic lesions. *AJR* 1984; 143:229–234.

46. Izumi S, Tamaki S, Natori H, et al: Ultrasonically guided aspiration needle biopsy in disease of the chest. *Am Rev Respir Dis* 1982; 125:460–464.

47. Jereb M, Us-Krasovec M: Thin needle biopsy of chest lesions: Time-saving potential. *Chest* 1980; 78:288–290.

48. Keller FS, Rösch J, Barker AF, et al: Percutaneous interventional catheter therapy for lesions of the chest and lungs. *Chest* 1982; 81:407–412.

49. Khouri NF, Meziane MA: Transthoracic needle aspiration biopsy—optimizing the yield. *J Thorac Imag* 1987; 2:18–26.

50. Khouri NF, Stitik FP, Erozan YS, et al: Transthoracic needle aspiration biopsy of benign and malignant lung lesions. *AJR* 1985; 144:281–288.

51. Kucharczyk W, Weisbrod GL, Cooper JD, et al: Cardiac tamponade as a complication of thin needle aspiration lung biopsy. *Chest* 1982; 82:120.

52. Lalli AF, McCormack LJ, Zelch M, et al: Aspiration biopsies of chest lesions. *Radiology* 1978; 127:35–40.

53. Lalli AF, Naylor B, Whitehouse WM: Aspiration biopsy of thoracic lesions. *Thorax* 1967; 22:404.

54. Lauby VW, Burnett WE, Rosemund GP, et al: Value

and risk of biopsy of pulmonary lesions by needle aspiration. Twenty-one years experience. *J Thorac Cardiovasc Surg* 1965; 49:159–172.

55. Lee LH: A new biopsy needle and its clinical use. *AJR* 1974; 121:854.

56. Leyden T: Über infectiose pneumoni. *Dtsch Med Wochenschr* 1883; 9:52.

57. Martin HE, Ellis EB: Aspiration biopsy. *J Surg Gynecol Obstet* 1934; 59:578.

58. Maurer JR, Friedman PJ, Wing VW: Thoracostomy tube in an interlobar fissure: Radiologic recognition of a potential problem. *AJR* 1982; 139:1155–1161.

59. Mayo P, McElvein RB: Early thoracotomy for pyogenic empyema. *Ann Thorac Surg* 1966; 2:649–657.

60. McCartney R, Tait D, Stilson M, et al: A technique for the prevention of pneumothorax in pulmonary aspiration biopsy. *AJR* 1974; 120:872–875.

61. Meyer JE, Ferrucci JT, Janower ML: Fatal complications of percutaneous lung biopsy. *Radiology* 1970; 96:47–48.

62. Milfield DJ, Mattox KL, Beall AC Jr: Early evacuation of clotted hemothorax. *Ann Surg* 1978; 136:686–692.

63. Milliken JS, Moore EE, Steiner E, et al: Complications of tube thoracostomy for acute trauma. *Am J Surg* 1980; 140:738–741.

64. Milner LB, Ryan K, Gullo J: Fatal intrathoracic hemorrhage after percutaneous lung biopsy. *AJR* 1979; 132:280–281.

65. Mimica I, Donoso E, Howard JE, et al: Lung puncture in the etiological diagnosis of pneumonia. *Am J Dis Child* 1971; 122:278–282.

66. Moinuddin SM, Lee LH, Montgomery JH: Mediastinal needle biopsy. *AJR* 1984; 143:531–532.

67. Nathan MH, Collins VP, Adams RA: Differentiation of benign and malignant pulmonary nodules by growth rate. *Radiology* 1962; 79:221.

68. Neff CC, Mueller PR, Ferrucci JT, et al: Serious complications following transgression of the pleural space in drainage procedures. *Radiology* 1984; 152:335–341.

69. Nordenstrom B: A new technique for transthoracic biopsy of lung changes. *Br J Radiol* 1965; 38:550.

70. Nordenstrom B: Paraxyphoid approach to the mediastinum for mediastinography and mediastinal needle biopsy. *Invest Radiol* 1967; 2:141.

71. Nordenstrom B: Paravertebral approach to the posterior mediastinum for mediastinography and needle biopsy. *Acta Radiol* [Diagn] (Stockh) 1972; 13:298–304.

72. Nordenstrom B: New instruments for biopsy. *Radiology* 1975; 117:474.

73. Perlmutt LM, Braun SD, Newman GE, et al: Timing of chest film follow-up after transthoracic needle aspiration. *AJR* 1986; 146:1049–1050.

74. Rosenberger A, Adler O: Fine needle aspiration biopsy in the diagnosis of mediastinal lesions. *AJR* 1978; 131:239–242.

75. Sagel SS, Ferguson TB, Forrest JV, et al: Percutaneous transthoracic aspiration needle biopsy. *Ann Thorac Surg* 1978; 26:399–405.

76. Sappington SW, Favorite GO: Lung puncture in lobar pneumonia. *Am J Med Sci* 1936; 191:225–234.

77. Sargent EN, Turner AF, Gordonson J, et al: Percutaneous pulmonary needle biopsy. Report on 350 patients. *AJR* 1974; 122:758.

78. Sherman MM, Subramanian V, Berger RL: Management of thoracic empyema. *Am J Surg* 1977; 133:474–478.

79. Silverman SG, Mueller PR, Saini S, et al: Thoracic empyema: Management with image-guided catheter drainage. *Radiology* 1988; 169:5–9.

80. Sinner WN: Transthoracic needle biopsy of small peripheral malignant lung lesions. *Invest Radiol* 1973; 8:305–314.

81. Sinner WN: Complications of percutaneous transthoracic needle aspiration biopsy. *Acta Radiol* [Diagn](Stockh) 1976; 17:813.

82. Skupin A, Gomez F, Husain M, et al: Complications of transthoracic needle biopsy decreased with isobutyl 2-cyanoacrylate: A pilot study. *Ann Thorac Surg* 1987; 43:406–408.

83. Stanley JH, Fish GD, Andriole JG, et al: Lung lesions: Cytologic diagnosis by fine-needle biopsy. *Radiology* 1987; 162:389–391.

84. Stark DD, Federle MP, Goodman PC: CT and radiographic assessment of tube thoracotomy. *Radiology* 1981; 141:253–258.

85. Stark DD, Federle MP, Goodman PC: Differentiating lung abscess and empyema: Radiography and computed tomography. *AJR* 1983; 141:163–167.

86. Sterrett G, Whitaker D, Shilkin KB, et al: The fine needle aspiration cytology of mediastinal lesions. *Cancer* 1983; 51:127–135.

87. Stevens GM, Jackman RJ: Outpatient needle biopsy of the lung: Its safety and utility. *Radiology* 1984; 151:301–304.

88. Tao L-C, Pearson FG, Delarue NC, et al: Percutaneous fine-needle aspiration biopsy. *Cancer* 1980; 45:1480–1485.

89. Tepplick JG, Tepplick SK, Goodman L, et al: The interface sign: A computed tomographic sign for distinguishing pleural and intraabdominal fluid. *Radiology* 1982; 144:359–362.

90. Todd TRJ, Weisbrod G, Tao L-C, et al: Aspiration needle biopsy of thoracic lesions. *Ann Thorac Surg* 1981; 32:154–161.

91. Vainrub B, Musher DM, Guinn GA, et al: Percutaneous drainage of lung abscess. *Am Rev Respir Dis* 1978; 117:153–160.

92. vanSonnenberg E, Lin AS, Deutsch AL, et al: Percutaneous biopsy of difficult mediastinal, hilar, and pulmonary lesions by computed tomographic guidance and a modified coaxial technique. *Radiology* 1983; 148:300.

93. vanSonnenberg E, Mueller PR, Ferrucci JT Jr: Per-

cutaneous drainage of 250 abdominal abscesses and fluid collections: Part I: Results, failures, and complications. *Radiology* 1984; 151:337–341.

94. van Sonnenberg E, Nakamoto SK, Mueller PR, et al: CT and ultrasound-guided catheter drainage of empyemas after chest-tube failure. *Radiology* 1984; 151:349–353.

95. Vine HS, Kasdon EJ, Simon M: Percutaneous lung biopsy using the Lee needle and a track-obliterating technique. *Radiology* 1982; 144:921–922.

96. Webb WR, LaBerge J: Major fissure tube placement, letter to the editor. *AJR* 1983; 140:1039.

97. Weisbrod GL, Herman SJ, Tao L-C: Preliminary experience with a dual cutting edge needle in thoracic percutaneous fine-needle aspiration biopsy. *Radiology* 1987; 163:5.

98. Weisbrod GL, Lyon DJ, Tao L-C, et al: Percutaneous fine needle aspiration biopsy of mediastinal lesions. *AJR* 1984; 143:525–529.

99. Weisbrod GL, Stoneman HR, Tao L-C: Diagnosis of diffuse malignant infiltration of lung (lymphangitic carcinomatosis) by percutaneous fine-needle aspiration biopsy. *J Can Assoc Radiol* 1985; 36:238–243.

100. Westcott JL: Direct percutaneous needle aspiration of localized pulmonary lesions: Results in 422 patients. *Radiology* 1980; 137:31–35.

101. Westcott JL: Percutaneous needle aspiration of hilar and mediastinal masses. *Radiology* 1981; 141:323–329.

102. Westcott JL: Percutaneous catheter drainage of pleural effusion and empyema. *AJR* 1985; 144:1189–1193.

103. Westcott JL: Transthoracic needle biopsy of the hilum and mediastinum. *J Thorac Imag* 1987; 2:41–48.

104. Yellin A, Yellin EO, Lieberman Y: Percutaneous tube drainage the treatment of choice for refractory lung abscess. *Ann Thorac Surg* 1985; 39:266–270.

105. Zarala DC: Diagnostic fiberoptic bronchoscopy: Techniques and results of biopsy in 600 patients. *Chest* 1975; 68:12–19.

106. Zornoza J, Snow J, Lukeman JM, et al: Aspiration biopsy of discrete pulmonary lesions using a new thin needle. *Radiology* 1977; 123:519.

Index